Basics of
ANESTHESIA

Basics of
ANESTHESIA

Robert K. Stoelting, MD

Emeritus Professor
Department of Anesthesia
Indiana University School of Medicine
Indianapolis, Indiana

Ronald D. Miller, MD

Professor and Chair
Department of Anesthesia and Perioperative Care
Professor of Cellular and Molecular Pharmacology
University of California, San Francisco, School of Medicine
San Francisco, California

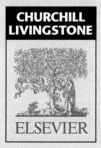

CHURCHILL
LIVINGSTONE

ELSEVIER

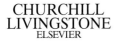

CHURCHILL
LIVINGSTONE
ELSEVIER

1600 John F. Kennedy Blvd.
Ste 1800
Philadelphia, PA 19103-2899

BASICS OF ANESTHESIA

ISBN-13: 978-0-443-06801-0
ISBN-10: 0-443-06801-1

Notice

Knowledge and best practice in this field are constantly changing. As new research and experience
broaden our knowledge, changes in practice, treatment, and drug therapy may become necessary or
appropriate. Readers are advised to check the most current information provided (i) on procedures
featured or (ii) by the manufacturer of each product to be administered, to verify the recommended
dose or formula, the method and duration of administration, and contraindications. It is the
responsibility of the practitioner, relying on his or her own experience and knowledge of the patient,
to make diagnoses, to determine dosages and the best treatment for each individual patient, and to
take all appropriate safety precautions. To the fullest extent of the law, neither the Publisher nor the
Authors assume any liability for any injury and/or damage to persons or property arising out of or
related to any use of the material contained in this book.   The Publisher

---

Library of Congress Cataloging-in-Publication Data

Stoelting, Robert K.

Basics of anesthesia/Robert K. Stoelting, Ronald D. Miller—5th ed.
        p. ; cm
     Includes bibliographical references and index.
     ISBN 0-443-06801-1
        1. Anesthesia.   I. Miller Ronald D.   II. Title.
        [DNLM: 1. Anesthesia.   WO 200 M649b 2007]
     RD81.S86 2007
     617.9′6–dc22   2006040749

Executive Publisher: Natasha Andjelkovic
Senior Developmental Editor: Heather Krehling
Publishing Services Manager: Tina K. Rebane
Senior Project Manager: Linda Lewis Grigg
Design Direction: Steven Stave

Printed in China

Last digit is the print number: 9 8 7 6 5 4 3 2 1

CONTRIBUTORS

Temitayo Ajayi, MD
Instructor of Pulmonary and Critical Care Medicine,
University of California, San Francisco, School of Medicine,
San Francisco, California

James E. Baker, MD, FRCPC
Assistant Professor of Anesthesia, University of California,
San Francisco, School of Medicine, San Francisco,
California; Assistant Professor, Department of Anesthesia,
University of Toronto Faculty of Medicine, Toronto, Ontario,
Canada

Martin S. Bogetz, MD
Professor of Anesthesia, University of California,
San Francisco, School of Medicine; Medical Director,
UCSF Surgery Center, San Francisco, California

Claire Brett, MD
Professor of Anesthesia and Pediatrics, University of
California, San Francisco, School of Medicine, San Francisco,
California

James Caldwell, MB, ChB
Professor of Anesthesia, University of California,
San Francisco, School of Medicine, San Francisco,
California

Lundy Campbell, MD
Assistant Professor of Anesthesia, University of California,
San Francisco, School of Medicine, San Francisco,
California

Lydia Cassorla, MD, MBA
Professor of Anesthesia, University of California,
San Francisco, School of Medicine, San Francisco,
California

Tina Chiu, MD
Anesthesiologist, California Pacific Medical Center,
San Francisco, California

Adam B. Collins, MD
Assistant Professor of Anesthesia, University of California,
San Francisco, School of Medicine, San Francisco,
California

Joseph F. Cotten, MD, PhD
Instructor in Anesthesia, Harvard Medical School;
Assistant in Anesthesia, Massachusetts General Hospital,
Boston, Massachusetts

Anil de Silva, MD
Professor of Anesthesia, University of California,
San Francisco, School of Medicine, San Francisco,
California

Elizabeth Donegan, MD
Associate Professor of Anesthesia, University of California,
San Francisco, School of Medicine, San Francisco, California

Rachel H. Dotson, MD
Fellow in Pulmonary and Critical Care Medicine,
Department of Medicine, University of California, San Francisco,
School of Medicine, San Francisco, California

Kenneth Drasner, MD
Professor of Anesthesia, University of California,
San Francisco, School of Medicine, San Francisco,
California

Helge Eilers, MD
Assistant Professor of Anesthesia, University of California,
San Francisco, School of Medicine, San Francisco, California

John Feiner, MD
Associate Professor of Anesthesia, University of California,
San Francisco, School of Medicine, San Francisco, California

Adrian W. Gelb, MB, ChB, DA, FRCPC
Professor of Anesthesia, University of California, San Francisco,
School of Medicine, San Francisco, California

Andrew T. Gray, MD, PhD
Associate Professor of Anesthesia, University of California,
San Francisco, School of Medicine, San Francisco, California

Michael Gropper, MD, PhD
Professor of Anesthesia and Physiology, University of California,
San Francisco, School of Medicine; Director, Critical Care
Medicine, UCSF Medical Center, San Francisco, California

Joan E. Howley, MD
Professor of Anesthesia, University of California,
San Francisco, School of Medicine, San Francisco,
California

Eric Huczko, MD, PhD
Assistant Professor of Anesthesia, University of California,
San Francisco, School of Medicine; Chief of Perioperative
Service, San Francisco Veterans Affairs Medical Center,
San Francisco, California

Samuel C. Hughes, MD
Professor of Anesthesia, University of California,
San Francisco, School of Medicine; Director, Obstetrical
Anesthesia, San Francisco General Hospital, San Francisco,
California

Andrew Infosino, MD
Associate Professor of Anesthesia and Pediatrics,
University of California, San Francisco, School of Medicine,
San Francisco, California

Anh L. Innes, MD
Fellow, Pulmonary Division, Department of Medicine,
University of California, San Francisco, School of Medicine
and UCSF Medical Center, San Francisco, California

Alicia G. Kalamas, MD
Assistant Professor of Anesthesia, University of California,
San Francisco, School of Medicine, San Francisco, California

Tin-Na Kan, MD
Instructor of Anesthesia, University of California,
San Francisco, School of Medicine, San Francisco,
California

Jeffrey A. Katz, MD
Professor of Anesthesia, University of California,
San Francisco, School of Medicine; Perioperative Medical
Director, UCSF Medical Center, San Francisco, California

Merlin D. Larson, MD
Professor of Anesthesia, University of California,
San Francisco, School of Medicine, San Francisco,
California

David J. Lee, MD
Associate Professor of Anesthesia, University of California,
San Francisco, School of Medicine; Director,
Pain Management Center, UCSF Medical Center,
San Francisco, California

Jae-Woo Lee, MD
Assistant Professor of Anesthesia, University of California,
San Francisco, School of Medicine, San Francisco,
California

Jacqueline M. Leung, MD, MPH
Professor of Anesthesia, University of California,
San Francisco, School of Medicine, San Francisco,
California

Ludwig Lin, MD
Anesthesiologist, Alta Bates/Summit Medical Center,
Berkeley, California

Lawrence Litt, PhD, MD
Professor of Anesthesia and Professor of Radiology,
University of California, San Francisco, School of Medicine,
San Francisco, California

Linda Liu, MD
Associate Professor of Anesthesia, University of California,
San Francisco, School of Medicine, San Francisco,
California

Errol Lobo, MD, PhD
Professor of Anesthesia, University of California,
San Francisco, School of Medicine, San Francisco,
California

Rachel Eshima McKay, MD
Associate Professor of Anesthesia, University of California,
San Francisco, School of Medicine, San Francisco,
California

Warren R. McKay, MD
Professor of Anesthesia, University of California,
San Francisco, School of Medicine, San Francisco,
California

Ronald D. Miller, MD
Professor and Chairman of Anesthesia, and Professor of Cellular and Molecular Pharmacology, University of California, San Francisco, School of Medicine, San Francisco, California

J. Renee Navarro, PharmD, MD
Health Science Professor of Anesthesia; Associate Dean, Academic Affairs, University of California, San Francisco, School of Medicine; Medical Director of Perioperative Services, San Francisco General Hospital, San Francisco, California

Dorre Nicholau, PhD, MD
Professor of Anesthesia, and Medical Director, Post-anesthetic Care Unit, University of California, San Francisco, School of Medicine, San Francisco, California

Claus U. Niemann, MD
Associate Professor of Anesthesia and Surgery, Division of Transplantation, University of California, San Francisco, School of Medicine, San Francisco, California

Manuel Pardo, Jr., MD
Associate Professor of Anesthesia and Sol Shnider Endowed Chair for Anesthesia Education, University of California, San Francisco, School of Medicine, San Francisco, California

Francesca Pellegrini, MD
Anesthesiologist, Department of Anesthesia, University of Ferrara, Ferrara, Italy

J. F. Pittet, MD
Professor of Anesthesia and Surgery, University of California, San Francisco, School of Medicine; Associate Investigator, Cardiovascular Research Institute, San Francisco, California

Cheng Quah, MBBS
Assistant Professor of Anesthesia, University of California, San Francisco, School of Medicine, San Francisco, California

Mark A. Rosen, MD
Professorof Anesthesia and Obstetrics, Gynecology and Reproductive Sciences, University of California, San Francisco, School of Medicine; Director, Obstetrical Anesthesia, University of California San Francisco Children's Hospital, San Francisco, California

Patricia Ann Roth, MD
Associate Professor of Anesthesia, University of California, San Francisco, School of Medicine; Medical Director, Anesthesia Support Services, UCSF Medical Center, San Francisco, California

Isobel A. Russell, MD, PhD, FACC
Professor of Anesthesia, University of California, San Francisco, School of Medicine; Chief, Cardiac Anesthesia Services, Moffitt-Long Hospitals, San Francisco, California

Muhammad Iqbal Shaikh, MD, PhD
Assistant Professor of Anesthesia, University of California, San Francisco, School of Medicine, San Francisco, California

David Shimabukuro, MDCM
Assistant Professor of Anesthesia, University of California, San Francisco, School of Medicine, San Francisco, California

Pankaj K. Sikka, MD, PhD
Assistant Professor of Anesthesia, University of California, San Francisco, School of Medicine, San Francisco, California

James Sonner, MD
Professor of Anesthesia, University of California, San Francisco, School of Medicine, San Francisco, California

Robin A. Stackhouse, MD
Professor of Anesthesia, University of California, San Francisco, School of Medicine, San Francisco, California

Robert K. Stoelting, MD
Emeritus Professor, Department of Anesthesia, Indiana University School of Medicine, Indianapolis, Indiana

Greg Stratmann, MD
Assistant Professor of Anesthesia, University of California, San Francisco, School of Medicine, San Francisco, California

Pekka Talke, MD
Professor of Anesthesia, University of California, San Francisco, School of Medicine, San Francisco, California

J. F. Tang, MD, MS
Associate Professor of Anesthesia, University of California, San Francisco, School of Medicine, San Francisco, California

Donald Taylor, MD, PhD
Assistant Professor of Anesthesia, University of California, San Francisco, School of Medicine, San Francisco, California

Art Wallace, MD, PhD
*Professor of Anesthesia, University of California,
San Francisco, School of Medicine, San Francisco,
California*

Jeanine P. Wiener-Kronish, MD
*Professor and Vice-Chair of Anesthesia and Professor of
Medicine, University of California, San Francisco, School of
Medicine; Investigator, Cardiovascular Research Institute,
San Francisco, California*

C. S. Yost, MD
*Professor of Anesthesia, University of California, San Francisco,
School of Medicine; Medical Director, Intensive Care Unit,
UCSF/Mount Zion Hospital, San Francisco, California*

William L. Young, MD
*Professor and Vice-Chair of Anesthesia and Professor of
Neurological Surgery and Neurology, University of California,
San Francisco, School of Medicine; Director, Center for
Cerebrovascular Research, UCSF Medical Center,
San Francisco, California*

PREFACE

Basics of Anesthesia was first published in 1984, with the goal of providing a concise source of information for the entire community of students of anesthesia, including medical students, physicians in training, and established practitioners. This fifth edition of *Basics of Anesthesia* continues to pursue this goal but with a significant change in authorship. In the previous editions, Drs. Stoelting and Miller were the authors of every chapter. In this fifth edition, Drs. Stoelting and Miller become the editors, as it was concluded that a current and accurate discussion of the medical specialty of anesthesiology required the use of expert contributors for each chapter. As the reader will note, this has been accomplished by utilizing, to a large extent, faculty in the Department of Anesthesia at the University of California, San Francisco, School of Medicine. However, the editors have maintained the style and format of previous editions to ensure that this edition of *Basics of Anesthesia* continues to function as an introductory textbook that succinctly presents pertinent information relevant to anesthesiology.

This fifth edition of *Basics of Anesthesia* has been expanded to include new chapters on the scope of anesthesia practice, approach to learning anesthesia, medical informatics, bioterrorism and natural disasters, and medical direction, as well as color illustrations and the liberal use of tables.

Another new feature of this edition is the addition of a teaching Web site that contains full text and illustrations. We hope it will allow for a greater usability and portability of this edition.

The editors wish to acknowledge the support of Elsevier in the preparation of this fifth edition. In particular, we are grateful to Heather Krehling and Natasha Andjelkovic for their advice and professionalism in guiding this fifth edition of *Basics of Anesthesia* to a timely publication.

Robert K. Stoelting
Ronald D. Miller

CONTENTS

Contents

Section I

INTRODUCTION

HISTORY OF ANESTHESIA

Merlin D. Larson

Although the ancient Greeks used ineffectual potions and poppy extracts to ablate surgical pain, the origins of anesthesia as we know it today began in the late 18th century. Chemists at that time were beginning to query the nature of various gases that emerged during fermentation and from heating and acidifying metallic compounds. One of these curious individuals, Joseph Priestley, a schoolmaster and congregational minister, began to ponder the nature of the gas that emerged during fermentation, and he compared the differences in the properties of this "fixed air" with a gas obtained by heating mercuric oxide. Priestley did not recognize that one gas (carbon dioxide) was produced from the other gas (oxygen) during metabolism and combustion, but his curiosity concerning the nature of gases led him to discover an anesthetic (nitrous oxide) that is still in use today.

INHALED ANESTHETICS

By exposing a solution of brass to nitric acid, Priestley obtained a gas, which he called nitrous air (nitric oxide). He then exposed this gas to a mixture of iron filings and mercury, and named this gas "dephlogisticated nitrous air," a gas known today as nitrous oxide. *Dephlogisticated* meant that it would support combustion, a fact that has meaning even today because airway fires can be supported by nitrous oxide. Priestley learned that this gas would not support life and was unable to find any practical use for it, but he speculated that it might be insufflated rectally to cure intestinal diseases.

Nitrous Oxide

The study of nitrous oxide began with the young prodigy Humphry Davy, who was destined to become one of the great scientists of the 19th century. Davy began his education in the seaport of Penzance, England, but abandoned his formal education at an early age to study the works of

Priestley and Antoine Lavoisier and to perform his own experiments on the nature of gases. He accepted the position as Superintendent of Research at the Beddoes Institute in Clifton, England, where he constructed an airtight room into which he would enter to breathe nitrous oxide. This was a bold undertaking by the young scientist because nitrous oxide at the time was thought to be a dangerous gas that could result in death if inhaled.

Davy's book on the subject stated that nitrous oxide produced feelings of exhilaration and euphoria and produced analgesia, leading him to observe, "As nitrous oxide . . . appears capable of destroying physical pain, it may probably be used with advantage during surgical operations in which no great effusion of blood takes place." Davy's work sparked an interest in nitrous oxide inhalation that spread throughout Europe and America, but the analgesic properties of the gas were ignored. Scientific exhibitions that traveled to various communities demonstrated the effects of electricity, magnetism, chemical reactions, and inhalation of nitrous oxide. For almost 50 years after the discovery of the analgesic properties of gas inhalation, physicians were inattentive to the agonizing pain and terror of surgery (Fig. 1-1).

The early 19th century witnessed a change in cultural and social beliefs that allowed the idea of painless surgery to surface. One of the first physicians to focus attention on the ablation of surgical pain was Henry Hill Hickman, who demonstrated in 1824 that inhalation of carbon dioxide could produce analgesia in animals. At the same time, Anton Mesmer and his followers claimed that they were able to induce a trancelike state that would allow surgery without the use of drugs. Although these methods were eventually proved to be unsuccessful, they initiated public awareness in the possibility of pain control and questioned the belief that only religious authorities could interpret and assuage pain (Fig. 1-2).

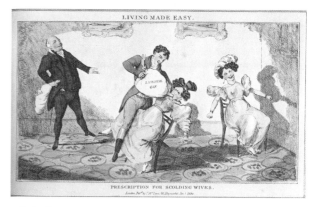

Figure 1-2 In the early 19th century, nitrous oxide provided novel entertainment for the middle class in Europe and America. Unfortunately, the analgesic properties of the gas were ignored for almost 50 years after Humphry Davy reported them. (Courtesy of the National Library of Medicine; originally published by T. McLean, 26 Haymaker, London, 1830.)

One itinerant chemist and entrepreneur, Gardner Q. Colton, is thought by some to be the dominant figure in the eventual introduction of inhalation anesthesia. Colton, who had briefly attended medical school, designed an exhibit that included a demonstration of the effects of nitrous oxide inhalation. On the night of December 10, 1844, he exhibited in the community of Hartford, Connecticut, where a young man, Samuel A. Cooley, accidentally sustained an injury to his leg while under the influence of nitrous oxide. Horace Wells, a local dentist who had an interest in painless dentistry, observed this event and asked Cooley whether any pain was felt during the injury. When he answered that he had felt no pain while under the influence of nitrous oxide, Wells arranged for Colton to administer the gas on the next morning for the extraction of one of Well's own teeth, performed painlessly by a colleague, John M. Riggs (Fig. 1-3).

Diethyl Ether

Wells was a tragic figure whose success was thwarted by an unsuccessful attempt to demonstrate the use of nitrous oxide for surgical anesthesia before an audience at the Massachusetts General Hospital. This honor instead went to his former colleague William Thomas Green Morton, who used diethyl ether vapor instead of nitrous oxide in experiments on his pets and selected dental patients. Because of the inconsistency of nitrous oxide anesthesia, Morton had shifted his attention from nitrous oxide to ether at the advice of his chemistry professor, Charles A. Jackson. On October 16, 1846, Morton used ether to produce anesthesia in Edward Gilbert Abbott for excision of a neck mass by the dean of American surgery, John C. Warren.

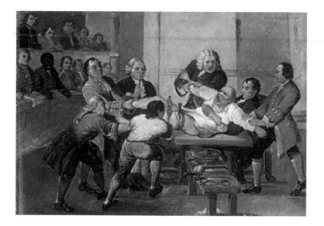

Figure 1-1 Artist unknown. Leg amputation prior to introduction of general anesthesia. (Reproduced with permission, Council of the Royal College of Surgeons of England.)

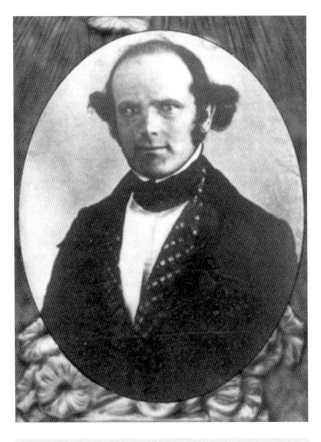

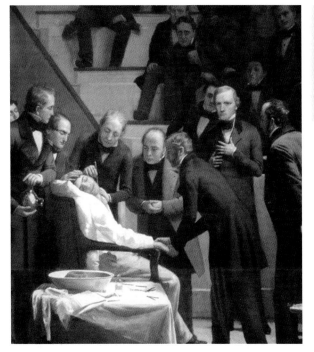

Figure 1-4 Robert Hinkley's painting from 1882 depicts the first ether anesthetic, provided on October 16, 1846, in Boston, Massachusetts. William T. G. Morton (*left*) is holding the globe inhaler, while the surgeon, John C. Warren, operates on the patient, Gilbert Abbott. (Courtesy of the Francis A. Countway Library of Medicine, Boston Medical Library, Cambridge, MA.)

Figure 1-3 Horace Wells was the first to actively promote nitrous oxide gas inhalation for pain relief during dental and surgical procedures.

Although some surgeons opposed the use of ether anesthesia, its use spread rapidly around the world after the October 16, 1846 demonstration. The Boston surgeons, who included Jacob Bigelow, George Hayworth, and John C. Warren, vigorously promoted the use of ether. Several claims were made by others to have previously used ether vapor for the same purpose. Credit for the discovery of anesthesia has therefore been given to various individuals, including Charles A. Jackson, Horace Wells, Gardner Q. Colton, William T. G. Morton, and Crawford Long, a surgeon from Athens, Georgia, who administered ether to induce surgical anesthesia in 1842 but did not publish his report until 1849 (Fig. 1-4).[1,2]

Chloroform

Ether was a relatively safe inhaled anesthetic, but it had several disadvantages, which included flammability, prolonged induction of anesthesia, delayed emergence from anesthesia, and a high incidence of nausea and vomiting. In 1847, James Y. Simpson, an obstetrician from Edinburgh, Scotland, proposed chloroform as a suitable alternative to ether. John Snow, considered by many to be the first anesthesiologist, popularized chloroform, and the drug received further endorsement from Queen Victoria of England, who inhaled the chloroform during the delivery of two of her children.

A second alternative to ether, nitrous oxide was reintroduced by Colton, who returned to Connecticut in 1863 after a brief move to California and successfully administered thousands of nitrous oxide anesthetics for dental procedures. The addition of oxygen to nitrous oxide was popularized in the late 19th century, but even with this improvement, its relative impotency limited its use for prolonged surgical interventions.

LOCAL ANESTHETICS

Paralleling the recognition of the value of inhaled gases for anesthesia, there were significant advances to establish regional anesthesia as an alternative to general anesthesia. Although the first local anesthetic, cocaine, was applied topically, the field of regional anesthesia could not have progressed without the invention of the hollow needle and syringe. The momentum for this development was the discovery of several biologically active alkaloids, such as morphine, strychnine, atropine, and brucine, which were relatively inactive when administered orally but produced dramatic effects when deposited into an open wound. In 1844, Francis Rynd developed the precursor of the syringe with a device that deposited fluids by gravity flow into tissues through a lancet wound. Alexander Wood was the first to use the hollow needle and syringe combination for treatments of patients.[3] In 1858, he reported the use of hypodermic injections of morphine for treatment of painful neuralgias. With parallel discoveries about bacterial sepsis and sterile technique, the use of injections became relatively safe. Other physicians adopted the method and used hypodermic injections of diverse drugs for various ailments.

Cocaine

Cocaine was isolated from the indigenous Andean medicinal plant *Erythroxylon coca* in 1856, and its ability to produce reliable local anesthesia of the corneal surface of the eye was demonstrated by Carl Kollar in 1884. Injections of cocaine directly into nerve trunks followed within a year. Leonard Corning performed neuraxial block in 1885, but his technique was unsafe and poorly thought out. The first true spinal anesthetic based on an understanding of injections into the cerebrospinal fluid awaited the classic experimental studies of August Bier in 1898.[4]

Procaine

The less toxic local anesthetic procaine was introduced in 1905 by Einhorn. Percutaneous blocks of the brachial plexus were first described in 1911, and the study and perfection of peripheral nerve blocks have continued to this day.

Regional Anesthetic Techniques

In addition to spinal anesthesia, other regional anesthetic techniques (i.e., neuraxial blocks) were refined in the first few decades of the 20th century with the addition of caudal and epidural neuraxial blocks. Caudal anesthesia was introduced in 1901, and it was used by Cathelin for surgical anesthesia, but the technique was found to be unreliable for operations performed on the abdomen. Identification and injection of local anesthetics into the lumbar and thoracic epidural space was first described in 1921 by Fidel Pagés, but it was not popularized until a decade later, when Achillo F. Dogliotti perfected the loss-of-resistance method to identify the epidural space.

The epidural method was introduced in the mid-20th century as an improved analgesic regimen to ablate obstetric pain. Neuraxial blocks, including spinal anesthesia, and caudal, lumbar, and thoracic epidural anesthesia, remain popular methods to provide surgical anesthesia.

METHODS FOR DELIVERY OF GENERAL ANESTHESIA

During the time of discovery of neuraxial anesthesia, the techniques for delivery of general anesthesia and the drugs used for that purpose were little changed from what was available before the 20th century. Delivery of ether or chloroform vapors or of nitrous oxide and oxygen by facemask was the standard approach, although several attempts had been made to find more suitable anesthetics. Untrained personnel were consigned the task of delivering the anesthetics, and there was only a limited interest in promoting the study of anesthesia as a scientific discipline (Fig. 1-5). However, beginning in 1930 and for the next several decades, there were significant and rapid advances in general anesthetic methods, and these improvements threatened to diminish the importance of regional anesthesia.

Tracheal Intubation

Airway devices inserted into the trachea were available before the 19th century and were used during resuscitation from drowning. The skills to perform this procedure were perfected approximately 100 years ago by otorhinolaryngology specialists, who like Chevalier Jackson, were often called to remove foreign bodies from the airway. The

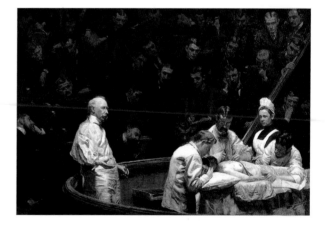

Figure 1-5 The Agnew Clinic (1889) was painted by Thomas Eakins. Young students or nurses, who had little or no prior training, usually administered anesthetics before 1900. This young anesthetist carefully observes the patient and palpates the superficial temporal artery. (Courtesy of the University of Pennsylvania, School of Medicine, Philadelphia, PA.)

Jackson laryngoscope was designed for such a purpose but was quickly modified by anesthesiologists for inserting tracheal tubes.[5] Arthur E. Guedel, Ralph M. Waters, and Ivan Macintosh were quick to point out the advantages of the tracheal tube, which included protection of the patient's airway, controlled positive-pressure ventilation of the lungs, and convenient access to the surgical field for the head and neck surgeon.

Difficult Airway

Although the sequence of intravenous or facemask induction of anesthesia followed by tracheal intubation had numerous advantages, it was hazardous if the trachea could not be intubated. Various inventions were designed to deal with this problem, including airway devices that position above the glottis, lighted stylets (i.e., flexible light wands), and fiberoptic bronchoscopes (i.e., laryngoscopes). A new concept in airway management, the laryngeal mask airway (LMA) was introduced in 1983.[6] The device surrounds the glottic opening and is often used for maintaining ventilation in selected elective surgical procedures and as an alternative to tracheal intubation in cases of difficult airway management.

NEUROMUSCULAR BLOCKING DRUGS

Arrow poisons and blowguns were an integral part of many primitive cultures. Curiosity surrounding the ingredients of the South American arrow poisons attracted the attention of the Spanish conquistadors in the early 16th century as they entered the Amazonian basin. Their accounts gained the attention of members of the medical community in Europe, who performed limited studies on animals with the small quantities that they could obtain. Sir Walter Raleigh's party reported that the native hunters were surprisingly skilled with the blowgun and preferred to use their arrow poisons instead of Western firearms, which frightened the game. The eccentric English Squire Charles Waterton took specimens of the arrow poison to England from British Guinea in 1812. In collaboration with Sir Benjamin Brodie and Francis Sibson, Waterton determined that a donkey could survive the poison if artificial respiration was provided. The active principle of the arrow poison was eventually found to derive from the bark of certain lianas (vines) that grow in the primary forests of South America. Claude Bernard accomplished localization of the effect of the drug to the neuromuscular junction in 1857.

For almost 200 years, the curare poison lacked a medical indication. During the 19th century, several physicians attempted to use unpurified extracts of the arrow poison to treat tetanus and rabies. However, the increased interest in tracheal intubation in the early 20th century and the use of controlled ventilation of the lungs stimulated interest in the use of curare during anesthesia The development of tracheal intubation and the use of curare in anesthesia were complementary innovations that combined to radically change the practice of anesthesia.[7]

The procurement of sufficient curare for clinical use resulted from the efforts of Richard Gill and his wife Ruth Gill, who had lived in Ecuador as owners of a hacienda near Banos, Ecuador, now a popular tourist attraction because of its natural hot springs. The Gills knew the native customs and were familiar with the arrow poisons of the Jivaro Indians, who live along the Paztaza and Napo rivers.

Richard Gill's interest in the drug arose after conversations with his neurologist, Walter Freeman, who suggested that Gill's obscure neurologic syndrome, characterized by intermittent spasticity, might be relieved if sufficient arrow poison could be procured for clinical testing. In 1932, Richard and Ruth Gill led an ambitious expedition into the interior jungle and returned 2 years later with 25 pounds of the curare paste. The crude preparation was delivered to associates of Squibb and Sons, who initially were unable to find clinicians to study the compound. Perplexed about what use it might have, they eventually delivered samples to Abram E. Bennett, a psychiatrist working in Omaha, Nebraska, and friend of Walter Freeman. Bennett first used the drug for spastic states with limited success, but his use of this compound to prevent the violent muscular contractions during Metrazol convulsive therapy gained acceptance as a means to prevent joint dislocations and fractures associated with these treatments.

Lewis H. Wright, an anesthesiologist and consultant to Squibb and Sons, sought out several anesthesiologists to try the drug form of curare known as Intocostrin for skeletal muscle relaxation during surgery. Initial clinical trials were unsuccessful, but in 1942, Harold R. Griffith and Enid Johnson reported their successful use of Intocostrin to relax abdominal skeletal muscles during cyclopropane anesthesia.[8] In their landmark paper, it is of interest that respiration was not assisted and the anesthetic was delivered by mask. Others quickly recognized the value of Intocostrin, and with the concomitant rise in popularity of tracheal intubation, the safe use of skeletal muscle paralysis during anesthesia was established. Subsequent years witnessed a refinement in the drugs that produce neuromuscular blockade by minimizing the autonomic side effects of the drugs and optimizing their pharmacodynamic properties (e.g., onset and duration of action, mechanism of clearance) to fit the anesthesiologist's needs.

IMPROVED INHALED AND INTRAVENOUS ANESTHETICS

A significant advance in the mid-20th century was the introduction of safe and nonflammable anesthetic vapors that gradually replaced chloroform (hepatotoxic) and ether and cyclopropane (flammable and explosive). This change occurred primarily because of advances in chemistry that allowed the halogenation of the hydrocarbon molecule. Potent nonflammable volatile liquids such as halothane, enflurane, and isoflurane were all highly successful, but the newer anesthetics represented by desflurane and sevoflurane have similar safety records with more favorable pharmacodynamic properties (Table 1-1).

Parallel advances in pharmacology and chemical research led to a progressive refinement of intravenous anesthetics from chloral hydrate to short-acting barbiturates (thiopental) and, more recently, to etomidate and propofol. With propofol, it is possible to administer anesthesia without inhaled anesthetics.

ABLATION OF THE STRESS RESPONSE

The term *anesthesia* was suggested to William Morton by Oliver Wendell Holmes in 1846 based on its Greek origin meaning "without sensation." However, some rudimentary sensations persist even during deep anesthesia, and it is therefore more appropriate to think of anesthesia as an immobile state "without perception."

The Riva Rocci method of blood pressure measurement was described in 1896, and brief anesthetic records followed soon after. These early records revealed alarming hemodynamic responses to surgical stimuli in apparently adequately anesthetized patients.

Table 1-1   Characteristics of an Ideal Inhaled Anesthetic
Absence of airway irritant effects
Absence of cerebral vasodilation
Absence of excessive myocardial depression
Absence of flammability
Absence of hepatic and renal toxicity
Bronchodilation
Compatibility with epinephrine
Easily vaporized at ambient temperature
Low blood solubility to ensure rapid induction and recovery from anesthesia
Minimal metabolism
Potency
Skeletal muscle relaxation
Suppression of excessive sympathetic nervous system activity

Surgeons soon became aware of the stresses placed on the surgical patient and devised methods to ablate the autonomic and hormonal responses to surgery. George Crile championed the concept of stress-free anesthesia in his book *Anoci-association*, published in 1911. His anesthetic method was to combine infiltration of the tissues with procaine with administration of nitrous oxide and oxygen by mask. The combination of central nervous system depression and peripheral nerve block was thought to result in significant benefits in the postoperative period. These ideas were widely disseminated at the time, but with the introduction of improved analgesics and neuromuscular blocking drugs, attention to perioperative stress reduction by combined local and general anesthesia diminished. Over the next decades, new definitions of the anesthetic state were proposed that included lack of movement, unconsciousness, and a poorly defined component of analgesia.

Balanced Anesthesia

In 1926, John S. Lundy, working at the Mayo Clinic, introduced the concept of *balanced anesthesia*. The concept emphasized the use of multiple drugs to produce unconsciousness and antinociception, provide skeletal muscle relaxation, and obliterate reflex responses. No single anesthetic drug could provide all the characteristics of an ideal general anesthesia, but a combination of intravenous analgesics, neuromuscular blocking drugs, and hypnotics given together produced the desired balanced anesthetic (see Table 1-1). Lower doses of each drug could be used because the different drugs tended to act synergistically.

Short-Acting Opioids

The introduction of short-acting opioids beginning in the 1960s had a profound influence on the practice of anesthesia. Before 1960, meperidine was commonly used during nitrous oxide–oxygen anesthesia to provide additional analgesia. Meperidine and morphine were relatively long-acting drugs and were associated with side effects that the newly developed short-acting opioids (e.g., fentanyl, sufentanil, alfentanil, remifentanil) did not produce. Today, opioids and β-adrenergic blocking drugs are widely used to control hemodynamic responses during and after surgery.

Subarachnoid Opioids

In 1979, it was reported that subarachnoid (intrathecal) and epidural opioids produced long-lasting and profound analgesia by acting on opioid receptors in the spinal cord. Combinations of local anesthetics and opioids in dilute concentrations are used commonly to provide prolonged (18 to 36 hours) postoperative pain relief with little effect on motor function or systemic blood pressure.[9] Acute pain services, often directed by anesthesiologists, were created to provide a smooth transition from intraoperative to postoperative pain control.

RECENT DEVELOPMENTS

Increased sophistication in monitoring the vital signs during anesthesia accelerated during the second half of the 20th century, a trend that coincided with an increasing complexity of surgical procedures. Anesthesia machines evolved from simple bottles and tubes to portable gas tanks and then to the large stand-alone units (i.e., workstations) prevalent today. Flowmeters, respirometers, and ventilators were eventually attached to the anesthesia machine, allowing accurate delivery of known concentrations and volumes of inspired gases.

Evaluation of gas exchange and oxygen delivery was significantly enhanced through the introduction of blood gas analysis in 1959 and the pulse oximeter in 1974.[10] End-tidal gas analysis based on infrared spectroscopy allows instantaneous evaluation of alveolar gases such as oxygen, nitrous oxide, carbon dioxide, and volatile anesthetics. Together with the studies performed in the 1960s on the end-tidal concentrations (minimum alveolar concentration [MAC]) required to prevent movement in 50% of surgical subjects, these measurements provide a useful estimate of anesthetic depth when using volatile anesthetics.[11,12]

Transesophageal echocardiography, introduced in 1979 and applied during anesthesia in 1982, allows the motions and valvular functions of the heart to be continuously monitored and is mandatory for certain surgical procedures. Brain function monitors to evaluate the effects of anesthetic drugs on the target organ are among the most recent monitors to become available.[13]

As the machines and equipment became more complex, it became apparent that universal standards and safety measures were necessary to prevent accidents from defective apparatus.[14] Professional societies arose that accredited practitioners of the art and provided standards of care for anesthesia services. The first professional society of anesthesiologists was organized in England in 1893, but associations of physician-anesthesiologists did not have significant influence until the American Society of Anesthesiologists (ASA) and the Faculty of Anesthetists of the Royal College of Surgeons were founded in the 1940s. The ASA has been a leader in organized medicine in developing standards of practice and practice guidelines for delivery of anesthesia and perioperative care of patients. Since the Anesthesia Patient Safety Foundation was founded in 1985, it has been a progressive force in prevention of anesthetic accidents and use of anesthesia simulators (i.e., mannequins) to provide education and training.[14]

Even though anesthesia is remarkably safe today, unexpected complications still occur.[15,16] Anesthesia remains a process of controlled poisoning, because all of the drugs are lethal if given improperly. Although the human brain appears to have intrinsic analgesic mechanisms, current techniques have not been able to consistently mobilize these mechanisms to combat surgical pain (Fig. 1-6).

MODERN ANESTHESIOLOGY PRACTICE

Today's anesthesiologist is expected to suppress intraoperative pain, provide preoperative counseling, maintain the *milieu interne* during surgery, and facilitate the recovery process.[17,18] For some procedures, massive transfusions and special techniques are required to sustain life. In these situations, the traditional roles of the anesthesiologist become complementary to those of maintaining fluid and electrolyte balance, preventing coagulopathy, and delivering sufficient oxygen to the vital organs. In the operating room, anesthesiologists often practice in a *care team model*, working with nurse anesthetists to provide intraoperative anesthesia care. Anesthesiologists also are experts in critical care, airway management, acute pain control, operating room management, and in the direction of ambulatory surgery centers.

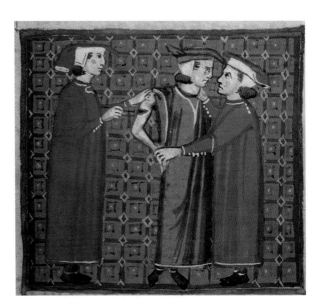

Figure 1-6 Attempts have been made over the past 500 years to control pain without drugs. In this 13th century painting, a surgeon operates while an assistant diverts the patient's attention with a fixed gaze. Mesmerism, hypnotism, and acupuncture are more recent examples of this approach to the control of surgical pain.

REFERENCES

1. Greene NM. A consideration of factors in the discovery of anesthesia and their effects on its development. Anesthesiology 1971;35:515-521.
2. Greene NM. Anesthesia and the development of surgery (1846-1896). Anesth Analg 1979;58:5-12.
3. Fink BR. Leaves and needles: The introduction of surgical local anesthesia. Anesthesiology 1985;63:77-82.
4. Larson MD. Tait and Caglieri. The first spinal anesthetic in America. Anesthesiology 1996;85:913-914.
5. Burkle CM, Zepeda FA, Bacon DR, Rose SH. A historical perspective on use of the laryngoscope as a tool in anesthesiology. Anesthesiology 2004;100:1003-1007.
6. Brain AIJ. The laryngeal mask: A new concept in airway management. Br J Anaesth 1983;55:801-805.
7. McIntyre AR. Historical background, early use and development of muscle relaxants. Anesthesiology 1959; 20:412-419.
8. Griffith HR, Johnson GE. The use of curare in general anesthesia. Anesthesiology 1942;3:418-420.
9. Sabbe MB, Yaksh TL. Pharmacology of spinal opioids. J Pain Symptom Manage 1990;5:191-203.
10. Severinghaus J, Honda Y. Pulse oximetry. Int Anesthesiol Clin 1987;25:205-216.
11. Merkle G, Eger EI. A comparative study of halothane and halopropane anesthesia: Including method for determining equipotency. Anesthesiology 1963;24:346-357.
12. Quasha AL, Eger EI, Tinker JH. Determination and application of MAC. Anesthesiology 1980;53:315-334.
13. Rampill IJ. A primer for EEG signal processing in anesthesia. Anesthesiology 1998;89:980-992.
14. Pierce EP. The 34th Rovenstine Lecture: 40 years behind the mask: Safety revisited. Anesthesiology 1996;84:965-975.
15. Lagasse RS. Anesthesia safety: Model or myth? Anesthesiology 2002;97:1609.
16. Cooper JB, Gaba DM. No myth: Anesthesia is a model for addressing patient safety. Anesthesiology 2002; 97:1335-1338.
17. Wiklund RA, Rosenbaum SH. Anesthesiology. First of two parts. N Engl J Med 1997;337:1132-1141.
18. Wiklund RA, Rosenbaum SH. Anesthesiology. Second of two parts. N Engl J Med 1997;337:1215-1219.

Chapter 2

SCOPE OF ANESTHESIA PRACTICE

Robert K. Stoelting

ANESTHESIA AS A MEDICAL SPECIALTY
   American Society of Anesthesiologists
   International Anesthesia Research Society
   American Society of Regional Anesthesia
   American Board of Anesthesiology

CERTIFIED REGISTERED NURSE ANESTHETIST
   Independent Nurse Anesthesia Practice

ANESTHESIOLOGIST ASSISTANTS

POSTGRADUATE (RESIDENCY) TRAINING IN
ANESTHESIOLOGY

ANESTHESIA PATIENT SAFETY FOUNDATION

FOUNDATION FOR ANESTHESIA EDUCATION AND
RESEARCH

ANESTHESIA SIMULATORS

HAZARDS OF WORKING IN THE OPERATING ROOM

PROFESSIONAL LIABILITY
   When an Adverse Event Occurs

RISK OF ANESTHESIA

CONTINUOUS QUALITY IMPROVEMENT

VALUE-BASED ANESTHESIA MANAGEMENT
   Office-Based Anesthesia

Since its beginning in 1842, anesthesiology has evolved into a recognized medical specialty (as affirmed by the American Medical Association and the American Board of Medical Specialties) providing continuous improvement in patient care based on the introduction of new drugs and techniques made possible in large part by research in the basic and clinical sciences. The scope of anesthesiology extends beyond the operating room to include preoperative evaluation clinics, respiratory therapy, treatment of acute postoperative pain, management of chronic pain problems, care of critically ill patients in intensive care units, and administrative responsibilities in daily management of the operating rooms. Anesthesiologists function as perioperative physicians with patient care responsibilities during the preoperative, intraoperative, and postoperative periods.

The American Society of Anesthesiologists defines anesthesiology as a discipline within the practice of medicine that specializes in the (1) medical management of patients who are rendered unconscious and/or insensible to pain and emotional stress during surgical, obstetric, and certain other medical procedures (involves preoperative, intraoperative, and postoperative evaluation and treatment of these patients); (2) protection of life functions and vital organs (brain, heart, lungs, kidneys, liver) under the stress of anesthetic, surgical, and other medical procedures; (3) management of problems in pain relief; (4) management of cardiopulmonary resuscitation; (5) management of problems in pulmonary care; and (6) management of critically ill patients in special care units.[1] The anesthesiologist's responsibilities to patients include (1) preanesthetic evaluation and treatment, (2) medical management of patients and their anesthetic procedures, (3) postanesthetic evaluation and treatment, and (4) on-site medical direction of any nonphysician who participates in the delivery of anesthesia care to the patient.[1]

As with other medical specialties, anesthesiology is represented by professional societies (American Society of Anesthesiologists, International Anesthesia Research

Society), scientific journals (*Anesthesiology*, *Anesthesia and Analgesia*), a residency review committee with delegated authority from the Accreditation Council for Graduate Medical Education to establish and ensure compliance of anesthesia residency training programs with published standards, and a medical specialty board, the American Board of Anesthesiology, that establishes criteria for becoming a certified specialist in anesthesiology.

ANESTHESIA AS A MEDICAL SPECIALTY

Anesthesia as a medical specialty evolved differently in England and the United States. Chloroform, the standard anesthetic in England, was a potent ventilatory depressant that required great skills in its administration. As a result, only physicians were considered competent to administer chloroform. In contrast, ether remained the dominant anesthetic in the United States. Unlike chloroform, ether stimulated ventilation and maintained systemic blood pressure. For these reasons, ether was thought to have a built-in protection for the patient, and its administration was often relegated to an inexperienced physician or nurse. Indeed, it was more than 60 years after the demonstration of ether anesthesia by Dr. Morton before American physicians began to devote full-time medical practice to the administration of anesthetics. For example, the first department of anesthesia was created in 1904 at the New York Medical College, with Dr. Thomas D. Buchanan as professor and chair. Dr. Arthur E. Gudel, a 1908 graduate of Indiana University School of Medicine, described the stages and planes of ether anesthesia in a monograph published in 1920. In 1923, Dr. Mary A. Ross became the first formal postgraduate trainee in anesthesiology in the United States; she received a certificate from the University of Iowa for her year of training after graduation from medical school. Dr. John S. Lundy organized a department of anesthesia at the Mayo Clinic in 1924, and Dr. Ralph M. Waters arrived at the University of Wisconsin for the same purpose in 1927. Graduates of training programs directed by Drs. Lundy and Waters continued to expand the scope of anesthesiology. Among those graduates was Dr. Emory A. Rovenstine, who in 1935 left Wisconsin to develop a department of anesthesia at Bellevue, the teaching hospital of New York University. During the next 25 years, more than 30 graduates of Dr. Rovenstine's training program became directors of departments of anesthesia.

American Society of Anesthesiologists

The first anesthesia organization in the United States was the Long Island Society of Anesthetists organized in 1905 by Dr. A. Frederick Erdmann and eight physician colleagues from the New York City area. The stated goal of this society was to "promote the art and science of anesthesia," and annual dues were $1.00. Only the London Society of Anaesthetists, founded in 1893, preceded this first society in the United States. The Long Island Society of Anesthetists grew in membership and became the New York Society of Anesthetists in 1911. The society became the American Society of Anesthetists in 1935, with 487 members and annual dues of $5.00. In 1945 the name was changed to the American Society of Anesthesiologists. This name change was intended to more accurately reflect the membership of the society, which consists of physicians with postgraduate training in anesthesia (anesthesiologists) in contrast to nonphysicians (anesthetists) who administer anesthesia (see the section "Certified Registered Nurse Anesthetist"). This semantic distinction is observed most consistently in the United States, whereas in other areas of the world (Canada, England), where only physicians administer anesthesia, the terms tend to be used interchangeably. Today, the American Society of Anesthesiologists has more than 40,000 members, which makes anesthesia the sixth largest among American medical specialties. The official seal of the American Society of Anesthesiologists depicts "vigilance" as the most important role of the anesthesiologist in the care of patients during anesthesia.

Anesthesiology, the official journal of the American Society of Anesthesiologists, was first published in July 1940, with Dr. Henry S. Ruth as the editor. This initial issue was sent to 568 members of the society and 300 additional nonmember subscribers. Today this highly respected peer-reviewed journal has a monthly worldwide circulation that exceeds 50,000.

International Anesthesia Research Society

At the same time that the New York Society of Anesthetists was evolving into the American Society of Anesthesiologists, another important organization was developing under the leadership of Dr. Francis H. McMechan, a physician practicing anesthesia in Cincinnati, Ohio. In 1919 Dr. McMechan established the National Anesthesia Research Society. This society held annual meetings, and in August 1922 the first medical journal devoted entirely to the medical specialty of anesthesiology, *Current Researches in Anesthesia and Analgesia*, appeared, with Dr. McMechan as editor. Previously, the only other source of scientific information for anesthesiology was the *American Journal of Anesthesia and Analgesia*, published since 1914 as a quarterly supplement to the *American Journal of Surgery*. In 1925, the National Anesthesia Research Society was renamed the International Anesthesia Research Society, which today continues to sponsor an annual scientific meeting and publish the journal *Anesthesia and Analgesia*.

American Society of Regional Anesthesia

The American Society of Regional Anesthesia was founded in 1923 to provide a forum for physicians interested in regional anesthesia. This society was absorbed into the American Society of Anesthetists in 1941, only to again become an independent organization in 1975. The official journal of this society, *Regional Anesthesia*, was first published in October 1976.

American Board of Anesthesiology

The American Board of Anesthesiology was incorporated as an affiliate of the American Board of Surgery in 1938. After the first voluntary examination, 87 physicians were certified as diplomates of the American Board of Anesthesiology. The American Board of Anesthesiology was recognized as an independent board by the American Board of Medical Specialties in 1941. To date, more than 30,000 anesthesiologists have been certified as diplomates of the American Board of Anesthesiology based on completing an accredited postgraduate training program, passing a written and oral examination, and meeting licensure and credentialing requirements. These diplomates are referred to as "board-certified anesthesiologists," and the certificate granted by the American Board of Anesthesiology is characterized as the primary certificate.

Starting on January 1, 2000, the American Board of Anesthesiology, similar to most other specialty boards, began to issue time-limited certificates (10-year limit). To recertify, all diplomates must participate in a program designated Maintenance of Certification in Anesthesiology (MOCA). Diplomates whose certificates are not time limited (any certificate issued before January 1, 2000) may participate voluntarily in MOCA. The MOCA program emphasizes continuous self-improvement (cornerstone of professional excellence) and evaluation of clinical skills and practice performance to ensure quality, as well as public accountability. The components include (1) a measure of professional standing (unrestricted state license), (2) a commitment to lifelong learning (formal and informal continuing medical education, (3) cognitive expertise (passing a secure written examination), and (4) evaluation of current practice.

The American Board of Anesthesiology also issues certificates in Anesthesia Pain Management and Anesthesia Critical Care Medicine to diplomates who complete 1 year of additional postgraduate training in the respective subspecialty, meet licensure and credentialing requirements, and pass a written examination. These certificates are time limited (10 years), and recertification is achieved by meeting licensure and credentialing requirements and passing a written examination.

CERTIFIED REGISTERED NURSE ANESTHETIST

It is estimated that certified registered nurse anesthetists (CRNAs) participate in more than 50% of the anesthetics administered in the United States, most often under the supervision of a physician. To become a CRNA, the candidate must earn a registered nurse degree, spend 1 year as a critical care nurse, and then complete 2 to 3 years of didactic and clinical training in the techniques of administration of anesthetics in an approved nurse anesthesia training program. The American Association of Nurse Anesthetists is responsible for the curriculum of nurse anesthesia training programs, as well as the establishment of criteria for certification as a nurse anesthetist. The activities of nurse anesthetists are typically intraoperative care of patients during anesthesia while working under the supervision (medical direction) of an anesthesiologist. This physician-nurse anesthetist team approach ("anesthesia care team") is consistent with the concept that administration of anesthesia is the practice of medicine. There may be situations when CRNAs administer anesthesia without the supervision or medical direction of an anesthesiologist.

Independent Nurse Anesthesia Practice

The traditional approaches to delivery of anesthesia care, either by the anesthesiologist alone or as part of an anesthesia care team, is under increasing pressure as CRNAs join other advance practice nurses in seeking independent privileges to practice.[2] The governors of several states have signed "opt-out" legislation that permits CRNAs in those states to administer anesthesia without physician supervision and not jeopardize Medicare reimbursement to their hospitals.

ANESTHESIOLOGIST ASSISTANTS

Anesthesiologist assistants complete a graduate-level program (about 27 months) and receive a master of medical science in anesthesia from an accredited training program (currently Case Western Reserve University, Emory University School of Medicine, South University).[3] Anesthesiologist assistants work cooperatively under the direction of the anesthesiologist as members of the anesthesia care team to implement the anesthesia care plan.

POSTGRADUATE (RESIDENCY) TRAINING IN ANESTHESIOLOGY

Postgraduate training in anesthesiology consists of 4 years of supervised experience in an approved program after the degree of doctor of medicine or doctor of osteopathy has been obtained. The first year of postgraduate training in anesthesiology consists of nonanesthesia experience (Clinical Base Year) in patient care–related specialties. The second, third, and fourth postgraduate years (Clinical Anesthesia 1 to 3) are spent learning all aspects of clinical anesthesia, including subspecialty experience in obstetric anesthesia, pediatric anesthesia, cardiothoracic anesthesia, neuroanesthesia, anesthesia for outpatient surgery, recovery room care regional anesthesia, and pain management. In addition to these subspecialty experiences, 2 months of training in critical care medicine is required.

The content of the educational experience during the clinical anesthesia years reflects the wide-ranging scope of anesthesiology as a medical specialty. Indeed, the anesthesiologist should function as the clinical pharmacologist and internist or pediatrician in the operating room. Furthermore, the scope of anesthesiology extends beyond the operating room to include acute and chronic pain management (see Chapters 39 and 43), critical care medicine (see Chapter 40), cardiopulmonary resuscitation (see Chapter 44), and research. Nonetheless, much remains to be learned, and even the mechanism of general anesthesia remains unknown.

Approximately 120 postgraduate training programs in anesthesiology are approved by the Accreditation Council for Graduate Medical Education of the American Medical Association. Approved postgraduate training programs are visited periodically (at least every 5 years) by a representative of the Anesthesia Residency Review Committee to ensure continued compliance with the published standards of quality medical education. The Anesthesia Residency Review Committee consists of members appointed by the American Medical Association, the American Society of Anesthesiologists, and the American Board of Anesthesiology.

ANESTHESIA PATIENT SAFETY FOUNDATION

The Anesthesia Patient Safety Foundation (APSF) was established under the direction of Ellison C. Pierce, Jr., MD, during his year as president of the American Society of Anesthesiologists.[4] Initial financial support for formation of the APSF was provided by the American Society of Anesthesiologists, and this financial support continues to the present. In addition, APSF receives financial support from corporations, specialty societies, and individual donors. The purpose of APSF is to "assure that no patient shall be harmed by anesthesia." To fulfill this mission, the APSF provides research grants to support investigations designed to provide a better understanding of preventable anesthetic injuries and promotes national and international communication of information and ideas about the causes and prevention of harm from anesthesia. A quarterly APSF newsletter is the most widely distributed anesthesia publication in the world and is dedicated to discussion of anesthesia patient safety issues. Anesthesiology is the only specialty in medicine with a foundation dedicated solely to issues of patient safety. The National Patient Safety Foundation, formed in 1997 by the American Medical Association, was modeled after the APSF.

FOUNDATION FOR ANESTHESIA EDUCATION AND RESEARCH

The Foundation for Anesthesia Education and Research (FAER) was established in 1986 with financial support from the American Society of Anesthesiologists. In addition, FAER receives financial support from corporations, specialty societies, and individual donors. The purpose of FAER is to encourage research, education, and scientific innovation in anesthesiology, perioperative medicine, and pain management. Over the years, FAER has funded numerous research grants and provided support for the development of academic anesthesiologists.

ANESTHESIA SIMULATORS

Anatomically correct computerized mannikins that interface with the anesthesia machine, monitors, and drugs are increasingly being used as an important educational method in training anesthesiologists and CRNAs (Fig. 2-1).[5-7] It is possible, by using the anesthesia simulator, to simulate critical incidents in anesthesia (myocardial ischemia, malignant hyperthermia, allergic reaction, pericardial tamponade, acute hemorrhage, pulmonary embolism, pneumothorax, cardiac arrest, equipment malfunction) so that the trainee or practitioner can gain or renew skills in crisis intervention without hazard to the patient. In addition to crisis management, the anesthesia simulator can be used to teach basic anesthesia skills such as airway management. Even drug pharmacokinetics may be simulated with anesthesia simulators. In addition to computerized mannikins, computer screen–based devices are available for simulation of critical incidents and the pharmacokinetics of drugs.

HAZARDS OF WORKING IN THE OPERATING ROOM

Anesthesiologists spend long hours in an environment (operating room) associated with exposure to vapors from chemicals (volatile anesthetics), ionizing radiation, and infectious agents (hepatitis viruses, human immunodeficiency virus). There is psychological stress from demands of the constant vigilance required for the care of patients during anesthesia. Furthermore, interactions with members of the operating team (surgeons, nurses) may introduce varying levels of interpersonal stress. Removal of waste anesthetic gases (scavenging) has decreased exposure to trace concentrations of these gases, although evidence that this practice has improved the health of anesthesia personnel is lacking. Universal precautions are recommended in the care of every patient in an attempt to prevent the transmission of blood-borne infections, particularly by accidental needlestick injuries.

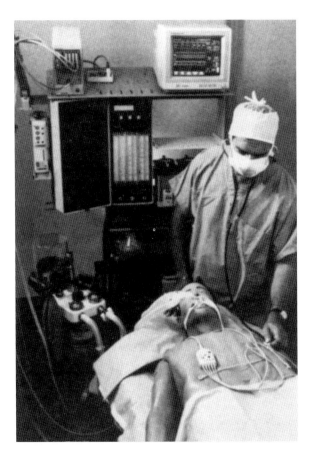

Figure 2-1 Anatomically correct computerized mannikin that interfaces with the anesthetic machine and monitors. (From Doyle DJ, Arellano R. The virtual anesthesiology training simulation system. Can J Anaesth 1995;42:267-273, with permission.)

Increased exposure to latex gloves by virtue of adherence to universal precautions has been associated with a dramatic increase in the incidence of latex sensitivity among operating room personnel, especially anesthesiologists with a preexisting history of atopy.[8] Sensitization to latex may be manifested as cutaneous sensitivity from direct contact with latex gloves or as airway changes from the inhalation of latex antigens, or both. Latex sensitivity is appropriately considered an occupational hazard of working in the operating room. Substance abuse, mental illness (depression), and suicide seem to occur with increased frequency among anesthesiologists, perhaps reflecting the impact of occupational stress.

PROFESSIONAL LIABILITY

The anesthesiologist is responsible for management and recovery from anesthesia. Physicians administering anesthetics are not expected to guarantee a favorable outcome to the patient but are required to exercise ordinary and reasonable care or skill in comparison to other anesthesiologists. That the anticipated result does not follow or that complications occur does not imply negligence (practice below the standard of care). Furthermore, an anesthesiologist is not responsible for an error in judgment unless it is viewed as inconsistent with the skill expected of every physician. As a specialist, however, an anesthesiologist is responsible for making medical judgments that are consistent with national, not local standards. Anesthesiologists maintain professional liability (malpractice) insurance that provides financial protection in the event of a court judgment against them. The best protection for the anesthesiologist against medicolegal action lies in the thorough and up-to-date practice of anesthesia, coupled with interest in the patient by virtue of preoperative and postoperative visits plus detailed records of the course of anesthesia (automated information systems provide the resource to collect and record real-time, actual data).

CRNAs can be held legally responsible for the technical aspects of the administration of anesthesia. It is likely, however, that legal responsibility for the actions of the CRNA will be shared by the physician responsible for supervising the administration of anesthesia. If an anesthesiologist employs the CRNA or advises the hospital about the qualifications or conditions of employment, the anesthesiologist may be held responsible for the CRNA's actions even though not directly involved in supervision at the time of an alleged act of negligence.

Medical students and resident physicians are not immune to court action and should be protected by professional liability insurance in the same manner as the anesthesiologist or CRNA. Insurance coverage for a medical student or resident physician is most often provided by the institution that offers the course for credit for the medical student or employs the resident physician.

When an Adverse Event Occurs

In the event of an accident or complication related to the administration of anesthesia, the anesthesiologist should promptly document the facts on the patient's medical record (see the web site for the APSF, www.apsf.org). Patient treatment should be noted and consultation with other physicians sought when appropriate. The anesthesiologist should provide the hospital and the company that writes the physician's professional liability insurance with a complete account of the incident. Should a lawsuit be threatened or legal inquiry be made concerning a patient, the anesthesiologist should promptly notify the insurance company and, when appropriate, seek legal assistance.

Most patients and families are understanding and are satisfied by frank discussion of problems (full disclosure of the facts when they are known and a physician apology) related to the administration of anesthesia. Saying "I am sorry" has not been shown to increase the risk for medicolegal action and provides the victim and family with needed understanding of the event.[9]

Malpractice is a theory arising from tort law. A tort is a civil (not criminal) wrong for which a patient can seek compensation through legal action for an alleged act of negligence by the anesthesiologist. A patient who claims injury obtains legal counsel and files a malpractice suit. Discovery depositions are taken by attorneys for both sides to elicit plaintiffs', defendants', and witnesses' opinions regarding the facts of the event; a court hearing is arranged, usually with a jury present; and witnesses for the defendant (physician) and plaintiff (patient), including experts, give testimony. The judge explains the points of law to the jury, and the jury then makes a decision, which may include a recommendation of compensation for damages. This chain of events may be interrupted at any point. For example, the plaintiff may drop the suit, or the defendant may be advised by counsel to make a settlement. A settlement can be arranged with the aid of the judge at any time during the trial before the jury verdict. Indeed, about 80% of malpractice suits are settled out of court, and of those that go to court trial, the jury finds in favor of the defendant more often than the plaintiff.

RISK OF ANESTHESIA

Approximately 28 million patients undergo anesthesia and surgery annually in the United States. Although patients may express a fear of dying during anesthesia, the fact is that anesthesia-related deaths have decreased dramatically in the last 2 decades.[10] Because fewer adverse events are being attributed to anesthesia, the professional liability insurance premiums paid by anesthesiologists have decreased.[11] The increased safety of anesthesia (especially for patients without significant coexisting diseases and undergoing elective surgery) is presumed to reflect the introduction of improved anesthesia drugs and monitoring (pulse oximetry, capnography), as well as the training of increased numbers of anesthesiologists. In one series, 244,000 patients underwent anesthesia and surgery without any mortality. This series is the basis for estimating a mortality rate from anesthesia of 1 in 250,000 anesthetics. The death rate from motor vehicle accidents is estimated to be 41 for every 250,000 accidents, and for injuries at home the death rate is estimated to be 22 for every 250,000 accidents. Despite the perceived safety of anesthesia, adverse events still occur, and not all agree that the mortality rate from anesthesia has improved as greatly as suggested by the 1 in 250,000 anesthetics.[12] It is likely that the safety of anesthesia and surgery can be improved by persuading patients to stop smoking, lose weight, avoid excess intake of alcohol, and achieve optimal

medical control of essential hypertension, diabetes mellitus, and asthma before undergoing elective operations.

When perioperative adverse events occur, it is often difficult to establish a cause-and-effect mechanism. In many instances it is impossible to separate an adverse event caused by an inappropriate action of the anesthesiologist ("lapse of vigilance," breach in the standard of care) from an unavoidable mishap (maloccurrence, coincidental event) that occurred despite optimal care.[13] Examples of adverse outcomes other than death include peripheral nerve damage, brain damage, airway trauma (most often caused by difficult tracheal intubation), intraoperative awareness, eye injury, fetal/newborn injury, and aspiration. Difficult airway management is perceived by anesthesiologists as the greatest anesthesia patient safety issue (Table 2-1).[14]

It is hoped that improved monitoring of anesthetized patients will serve to further enhance the vigilance of the anesthesiologist and decrease the role of human error in anesthetic morbidity and mortality. Indeed, human error, in part resulting from lapses in attention (vigilance), accounts for a large proportion of adverse anesthesia events.[15] A number of factors at work in the operating room environment serve to diminish the ability of the anesthesiologist to perform the task of vigilance. Prominent among these factors are sleep loss and fatigue with known detrimental effects on work efficiency and cognitive tasks (monitoring, clinical decision-making).[16] It is notable that the Anesthesia Residency Review Committee mandates that anesthesia residents not be

Table 2-1 Ten Most Important Anesthesia Patient Safety Issues as Perceived by Anesthesiologists
Difficult airway management
Production pressures (decreased time between cases in the operating room ["turnover time"], desire to avoid cancellations)
Anesthesia delivery outside the operating rooms at remote sites in the hospital
Anesthesia delivery in physicians' offices
Neurologic deficit attributed to the anesthetic technique
Presence of coronary artery disease in patients
Occupational stress for the anesthesiologist
Anesthesiologist fatigue
Medication errors
Time available for preoperative evaluation

From Stoelting RK. Results of APSF survey regarding anesthesia patient safety issues. APSF Newsletter, Spring 1999, pp 6-7. Available at http://www.apsf.org.

assigned clinical responsibilities the day after in-hospital call. The emphasis on efficiency in the operating room ("production pressures") designed to improve productivity may supersede safety and provoke the commission of errors that jeopardize patient safety. At the same time, it is important to recognize that not all adverse events during anesthesia are a result of human error and therefore preventable. For example, postoperative ulnar nerve palsy may occur despite appropriate padding and positioning during surgery, thus emphasizing that it is difficult to impossible to prevent an adverse event for which the mechanism of the injury is unknown.[17,18]

CONTINUOUS QUALITY IMPROVEMENT

Quality is a difficult concept to define in the practice of medicine. It is generally agreed, however, that attention to quality will improve patient safety and satisfaction with anesthetic care. Quality improvement programs in anesthesia are often guided by requirements of the Joint Commission on Accreditation of Healthcare Organizations (JCAHO). Quality of care is evaluated by attention to (1) structure (personnel and facilities used to provide care), (2) process (sequence and coordination of patient care activities such as performance and documentation of a preanesthetic evaluation, continuous attendance and monitoring of the patient during anesthesia), and (3) outcome. A quality improvement program focuses on measuring and improving these three basic components of care. In contrast to quality assurance programs designed to identify "outliers," continuous quality improvement (CQI) programs take a "systems" approach in recognition of the fact that random errors are inherently difficult to prevent. System errors, however, should be controllable and strategies to minimize them should be attainable. A CQI program may focus on undesirable outcomes as a way to identify opportunities for improvement in the structure and process of care.

Improvement in quality of care is often measured by a decrease in the rate of adverse outcomes. However, the relative rarity of adverse outcomes in anesthesia makes measurement of improvement difficult. To complement outcome measurement, CQI programs may focus on critical incidents and sentinel events. Critical incidents (ventilator disconnection) are events that cause or have the potential to cause injury if not noticed and corrected in a timely manner. Measurement of the occurrence rate of important critical incidents may serve as a substitute for rare outcomes in anesthesia and lead to improvement in patient safety. Sentinel events are isolated events that may indicate a systematic problem (syringe swap because of poor labeling, drug administration error related to keeping unneeded medications on the anesthesia cart).

The key factors in the prevention of patient injury related to anesthesia are vigilance, up-to-date knowledge, and adequate monitoring. Clearly, it is important to follow the standards endorsed by the American Society of Anesthesiologists. In this regard, American anesthesiology has been the unquestioned leader within organized medicine in the development and implementation of formal, published standards of practice. These standards have significantly influenced how anesthesia is practiced in the United States.

VALUE-BASED ANESTHESIA MANAGEMENT

Value-based anesthesia management defines the relationship between the cost of anesthetic management strategies and the value of this care as reflected by perioperative outcomes. Implicit in this concept of appraising costs and outcomes is identification of anesthetic management paradigms associated with the best achievable outcome at a reasonable cost in acknowledgment of the fact that economic resources are limited. Although the relationships between patient outcome and health care costs are complex, it is generally accepted that most cost-benefit relationships have a diminishing slope such that additional investment of resources generally results in only marginal increments in improvement and perhaps even declines in outcome when excessive investment of resources results in more harmful (iatrogenic complications) than beneficial effects (Fig. 2-2).[19-21] Better quality is not necessarily associated with higher cost, nor does spending less (by doing less) necessarily lead to lower quality.

It has been estimated that expenditures influenced (directly and indirectly) by anesthesiologists represent 3% to 5% of the total health care costs in the United States. Nevertheless, anesthesia drug expenses represent a small fraction of the total health care budget, and the cost of anesthetic drugs is relatively small when considered on a single-case basis; however, the large number of doses administered contributes to large aggregate costs. Although there is great emphasis on time between cases ("turnover time"), additional cases may best be accommodated on the operating room schedule by optimizing case scheduling to avoid paying overtime to salaried personnel both in the operating room and in the postanesthesia care unit.[22]

Office-Based Anesthesia

One of the most significant trends affecting health care in the last quarter of the 20th century was the development of ambulatory and office-based surgery (Fig. 2-3).[23] Increasing cost-consciousness along with better technology and short-acting anesthetic drugs has encouraged this change. To ensure patient safety, it is mandatory that policies and resources (drugs, equipment, personnel) be equivalent to that present in hospitals (single safety standard) (Table 2-2).[24,25]

Table 2-2 Evidence of a Single Safety Standard Based on Questions to Be Asked by the Patient before Agreeing to Office-Based Anesthesia

Is your office accredited for performance of surgery and administration of anesthesia?

How many of these operations have you performed and would you have this operation in an office such as yours if you were the patient?

Are you credentialed to perform this operation in a hospital or ambulatory surgery facility?

Who will administer my anesthesia and what are his/her qualifications?

Is the individual administering my anesthesia credentialed to administer anesthesia in an accredited hospital or ambulatory surgery facility?

Is the individual administering my anesthesia certified by his/her certifying organization?

When will I meet the individual responsible for administering my anesthesia?

What are the choices available to me for anesthesia?

Will the individual administering my anesthesia be in constant attendance with me during my anesthesia?

Will the anesthesia machine used for my anesthetic be modern and equivalent to the machine that would be used if I had this operation in a hospital or ambulatory surgery facility?

Will the monitors used on me during my anesthetic be the same that would be used if I had this operation in a hospital or ambulatory surgery facility?

Do you have the necessary equipment and drugs to handle any possible emergency that might occur during or after my anesthesia?

What hospital will I be admitted to should a complication occur during my anesthesia?

Is there a separate area where I will be taken to awaken from my anesthetic?

What are the qualifications of the individual who will monitor me in this recovery area?

Will the monitors used during my recovery from anesthesia be the same that would be used if I were recovering after surgery in a hospital or ambulatory surgery facility?

Is the recovery area in your office equipped in a similar manner to the recovery area in a hospital or ambulatory surgery facility?

Who is responsible for determining whether I am ready to be discharged home?

Who is ACLS certified in your office?

How is the operating room cleaned between cases?

How are the surgical instruments sterilized?

Is appropriate surgical attire worn by those in attendance during my surgery?

From Stoelting RK. APSF panel provides guidance to public, patients: Questions to ask before accepting office-based anesthesia. APSF Newsletter, Spring 2000, p 16. Available at http://www.apsf.org.

Figure 2-2 The hypothetical inputs to a productive process and the benefits derived describe a production function. As investment continues, the net benefit progressively decreases and then becomes negative (law of diminishing returns). Rationalizing rather than rationing health care technology achieves maximal benefit at the "top of the curve," a level of investment associated with the optimal investment. (From Orkin FK: Practice standards: The Midas touch or the emperor's new clothes? [editorial]. Anesthesiology 70:567-571, 1989.)

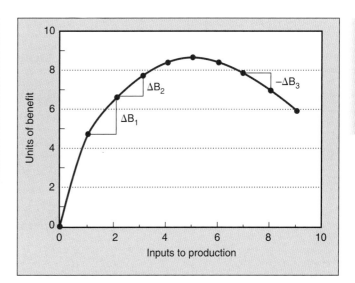

Figure 2-3 The growth of surgical procedures performed in the United States by site from 1980 to 2005. (Hospital data through 2001 from the American Hospital Association, freestanding surgery center and physician's office data through 1999, and all estimates after 1999 provided by Verispan, LLC, Chicago). (From Orkin KF, Thomas SJ. Scope of modern anesthetic practice. *In* Miller RD [ed]: Miller's Anesthesia, 6th ed. Philadelphia: Elsevier 2005, p 57.)

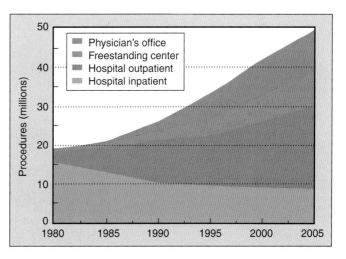

REFERENCES

1. The Scope of Practice of Nurse Anesthetists. American Society of Anesthesiologists. Available at http://www.asahq.org. Accessed January 2004.
2. Abenstein JP, Warner MA. Anesthesia providers, patient outcomes, and costs. Anesth Analg 1996;82:1273-1283.
3. American Academy of Anesthesiologist Assistants. Available at http://www.anesthetist.org.
4. Pierce EC. The 34th Rovenstine Lecture: 40 years behind the mask. Safety revisited. Anesthesiology 1996;84:965-975.
5. Doyle DJ, Arellano R. The virtual anesthesiology training simulation system. Can J Anaesth 1995;42: 267-273.

6. Gaba DM. Improving anesthesiologists' performance by simulating reality. Anesthesiology 1992;76:491-494.
7. Helmreich RL, Davies JM. Anaesthetic simulation and lessons to be learned from aviation. Can J Anaesth 1997;44:907-912.
8. Konrad C, Fieber T, Gerber H, et al. The prevalence of latex sensitivity among anesthesiology staff. Anesth Analg 1997;84:629-633.
9. Frenkel DN, Liebman CB. Words that heal. Ann Intern Med 2004;140: 482-483.
10. Cooper JB, Gaba DG. No myth: Anesthesia is a model for addressing patient safety. Anesthesiology 2002; 97:1335-1337.

11. Hallinan JT. Once seen as risky, one group of doctors changes its ways. The Wall Street Journal, June 21, 2005.
12. Lagasse RS. Anesthesia safety: Model or myth? A review of the published literature and analysis of current original data. Anesthesiology 2002;97:1609-1617.
13. Keats AS. Anesthesia mortality in perspective. Anesth Analg 1990;71: 113-119.
14. Stoelting RK. Results of APSF survey regarding anesthesia patient safety issues. APSF Newsletter, Spring 1999, pp 6-7. Available at http://www.apsf.org.
15. Cooper J, Newbower RS, Kitz RJ. An analysis of major errors and

equipment failures in anesthesia management: Considerations for prevention and detection. Anesthesiology 1984;60:34-42.

16. Weinger MB, Englund CE. Ergonomic and human factors affecting anesthetic vigilance and monitoring performance in the operating room environment. Anesthesiology 1990;73:995-1021.

17. Warner MA, Warner DO, Matsumoto JY, et al. Ulnar neuropathy in surgical patients. Anesthesiology 1999;90: 54-59.

18. Cheney FW, Domino KB, Caplan RA, et al. Nerve injury associated with anesthesia. A closed claims analysis. Anesthesiology 1999;90:1062-1069.

19. Orkin FK, Thomas SJ. Scope of modern anesthetic practice. *In* Miller RD (ed): Miller's Anesthesia, 6th ed. Philadelphia: Elsevier, 2005, pp 55-66.

20. Orkin FK. Practice standards. The Midas touch or the emperor's new clothes? [editorial] Anesthesiology 1989;70:567-571.

21. Reinhardt U. Health Care Quality Management for the 21st Century. Tampa, FL: American College of Physician Executives, 1991.

22. Dexter F, Macario A. Decrease in case duration required to complete an additional case during regularly scheduled hours in an operating room suite: A computer simulation study. Anesth Analg 1999;88:72-76.

23. Surgical Procedures 1981-2007. Chicago: SMG Marketing Group, Verispan, January 2001.

24. Stoelting RK. Office-based anesthesia growth provokes safety fears. APSF Newsletter, Spring 2000, p 1. Available at http://www.apsf.org.

25. Stoelting RK. APSF panel provides guidance to public, patients: Questions to ask before accepting office-based anesthesia. APSF Newsletter, Spring 2000, p 16. Available at http://www.apsf.org.

Chapter 3

APPROACH TO LEARNING ANESTHESIA

Manuel Pardo, Jr.

STRUCTURED APPROACH TO ANESTHESIA CARE
  Preoperative Evaluation
  Creating the Anesthesia Plan
  Preparing the Operating Room
  Managing the Intraoperative Anesthetic

For the beginning trainee, learning perioperative anesthesia care can be anxiety provoking for a number of reasons (Table 3-1). There are no proven ways to decrease the stress of starting anesthesia training. Most training programs begin with close clinical supervision by an attending anesthesiologist. More experienced trainees may offer their perspectives and practical advice. Some programs use a mannikin-based patient simulator to recreate the operating room environment.[1] Learning to practice anesthesia involves the development of flexible patient care routines, factual and theoretical knowledge, manual and procedural skills, and the mental abilities to adapt to changing situations.[2]

Table 3-1 Anxiety-Provoking Aspects of Learning Perioperative Anesthesia

Unfamiliar environment
Anesthesia machine
Electronic monitors
Anesthetic drugs
Equipment cart
Direct responsibility for patient management
Time pressure
Routine procedural aspects of anesthesia care (e.g., intravenous line placement may require more time for beginning trainees)
Fear of an unknown or unpredictable critical event (e.g., dynamic nature of the operating room environment)
Physiologic effects of surgery
Sudden problem (e.g., hypotension)

STRUCTURED APPROACH TO ANESTHESIA CARE

Anesthesiologists care for the surgical patient in the preoperative, intraoperative, and postoperative period (Table 3-2). Important patient care decisions reflect the preoperative evaluation, creating the anesthesia plan, preparing the operating room, and managing the intraoperative anesthetic.

Preoperative Evaluation

The goals of preoperative evaluation include assessing the risk of coexisting diseases, modifying risks, addressing patients' concerns, and discussing options for anesthesia care (see Chapters 13 and 14). The beginning trainee should learn the types of questions that are the most important to understanding the patient and the proposed surgery. Some specific questions and their potential importance follow.

What is the indication for the proposed surgery? Is it elective or an emergency? The indication for surgery may have particular anesthetic implications. For example, a patient requiring esophageal fundoplication will likely have severe gastroesophageal reflux disease, which may require modification of the anesthesia plan (e.g., preoperative nonparticulate antacid, intraoperative rapid-sequence induction of anesthesia). A given procedure may also have implications for anesthetic choice. Hand surgery, for example, can be accomplished with local

anesthesia, peripheral nerve blockade, or general anesthesia. The urgency of a given procedure (e.g., acute appendicitis) may preclude lengthy delay of the surgery for additional testing, without increasing the risk of complications (e.g., appendiceal rupture, peritonitis).

What are the inherent risks of this surgery? Surgical procedures have different inherent risks. For example, a patient undergoing coronary artery bypass graft has a significant risk of problems such as death, stroke, or myocardial infarction. A patient undergoing cataract extraction has a low risk of major organ damage.

Does the patient have coexisting medical problems? Does the surgery or anesthesia care plan need to be modified because of them? To anticipate the effects of a given medical problem, the anesthesiologist must understand the physiologic effects of the surgery and anesthetic and the potential interaction with the medical problem. For example, a patient with poorly controlled systemic hypertension is more likely to have an exaggerated hypertensive response to direct laryngoscopy to facilitate tracheal intubation. The anesthesiologist may change the anesthetic plan to increase the induction dose of intravenous anesthetic (e.g., propofol) and administer a short-acting β-adrenergic blocker (e.g., esmolol) before airway instrumentation. Depending on the medical problem, the anesthesia plan may require modification during any phase of the procedure.

Has the patient had anesthesia before? Were there complications such as difficult airway management? Does the patient have risk factors for difficult airway management? Anesthesia records from previous surgery can yield much useful information. The most important fact is the ease of airway management techniques such as direct laryngoscopy. If physical examination suggests some risk factors for difficult tracheal intubation, but the patient had a clearly documented uncomplicated direct laryngoscopy for recent surgery, the anesthesiologist may choose to proceed with routine laryngoscopy. Other useful historical information includes intraoperative hemodynamic and respiratory instability and occurrence of postoperative nausea.

Creating the Anesthesia Plan

After the preoperative evaluation, the anesthesia plan can be completed. The plan should list drug choices and doses in detail, as well as anticipated problems (Tables 3-3 and 3-4). Many variations on a given plan may be acceptable, but the trainee and the supervising anesthesiologist should agree in advance on the details.

Preparing the Operating Room

After determining the anesthesia plan, the trainee must prepare the operating room (Table 3-5). Routine operating room preparation includes tasks such as checking the

Table 3-2 Phases of Anesthesia Care
Preoperative Phase
Preoperative evaluation
Choice of anesthesia
Premedication
Intraoperative Phase
Physiologic monitoring and vascular access
General anesthesia (i.e., plan for induction, maintenance, and emergence)
Regional anesthesia (i.e., plan for type of block, needle, local anesthetic)
Postoperative Phase
Postoperative pain control method
Special monitoring or treatment based on surgery or anesthetic course
Disposition (e.g., home, postanesthesia care unit, ward, monitored ward, stepdown unit, intensive care unit)

Table 3-3   Sample General Anesthesia Plan

Case

A 47-year-old woman with biliary colic and well-controlled asthma requires anesthesia for laparoscopic cholecystectomy.

Preoperative Phase

Premedication

   Midazolam, 1-2 mg IV, to reduce anxiety

   Albuterol, two puffs, to prevent bronchospasm

Intraoperative Phase

Vascular access and monitoring

   Vascular access: one peripheral IV catheter

   Monitors: pulse oximetry, capnography, electrocardiogram, noninvasive blood pressure with standard adult cuff size, temperature

Induction

   Propofol, 2 mg/kg IV (may precede with lidocaine, 1.5 mg/kg IV)

   Neuromuscular blocking drug to facilitate tracheal intubation (succinylcholine, 1-2 mg/kg IV) or nondepolarizing neuromuscular-blocking drugs (rocuronium, 0.6 mg/kg)

Airway management

   Facemask: adult medium size

   Direct laryngoscopy: Macintosh 3 blade, 7.0-ID endotracheal tube

Maintenance

   Inhaled anesthetic: sevoflurane, desflurane, isoflurane

   Opioid-fentanyl: anticipate 2-4 μ/kg IV total during case

   Neuromuscular blocking drug titrated to train-of-four monitor (peripheral nerve stimulator) at the ulnar nerve*

Emergence

   Antagonize effects of nondepolarizing neuromuscular blocking drug: neostigmine, 70 μ/kg, and glycopyrrolate, 14 μ/kg IV, titrated to train-of-four monitor

   Antiemetic: dolasetron, 12.5 mg IV

   Tracheal extubation: when patient is awake, breathing, and following commands

Possible intraoperative problem and approach

   Bronchospasm: increase inspired oxygen and inhaled anesthetic concentrations, decrease surgical stimulation if possible, administer albuterol through endotracheal tube (5-10 puffs), adjust ventilator to maximize expiratory flow

Postoperative Phase

Postoperative pain control

   Patient controlled analgesia: morphine, 1 mg IV, 6-minute lock-out, no basal rate

Disposition

   Postanesthesia care unit then hospital ward

*Nondepolarizing neuromuscular blocking drug choices include rocuronium, vecuronium, pancuronium, atracurium, cisatracurium, and mivacurium.

Table 3-4   Sample Regional Anesthesia Plan

Case

A 27-year-old man requires diagnostic right shoulder arthroscopy for chronic pain. He has no known medical problems.

Preoperative Phase

Premedication: midazolam, 1-2 mg IV, to reduce anxiety

Intraoperative Phase

Type of block: interscalene

Needle: 22-gauge, nerve-stimulator needle

Local anesthetic: 1.5% mepivacaine, 25 mL

Ancillary equipment: nerve stimulator with attached cable, electrocardiographic pad for grounding

Technique: Betadine preparation, standard surface landmarks, proximity to brachial plexus identified by nerve stimulation at < 0.5 mA current

Intraoperative sedation and analgesia

   Midazolam, 0.5-1 mg IV, given every 5-10 minutes as indicated

   Fentanyl, 25-50 µg IV, given every 5-10 minutes as indicated

Postoperative Phase

Postoperative pain control: when block resolves, may treat with fentanyl, 25-50 µg IV, as needed

Disposition: postanesthesia care unit, then home

Table 3-5   Operating Room Preparation

Components	Preparation Tasks
Basic Room Setup	
Suction (S)	Check that suction is connected, working, and near the head of the bed.
Oxygen (O)	Check oxygen supply pressures (pipeline of approximately 50 psi and E-cylinder of at least 2000 psi).
	Check anesthesia machine (do positive-pressure circuit test).
Airway (A)	Two laryngoscope blades and handles
	Two endotracheal tubes of different sizes (one with and one without a stylet)
	Two laryngeal mask airways (LMA 3 and LMA 4)
	Two oral airways
	Two nasal airways
	Lidocaine or K-Y Jelly
	Bite block and tongue depressor
	Tape

Table 3-5 Operating Room Preparation—cont'd

Components	Preparation Tasks
Intravenous access (I)	Two catheter sizes
	1-mL syringe with 1% lidocaine
	Tourniquet, alcohol pads, gauze, plastic dressing, tape
Monitors (M)	Electrocardiographic pads
	Blood pressure cuff (correct size for patient)
	Pulse oximeter probe
	Capnography (breath into circuit to confirm function)
	Temperature probe
Daily Drugs to Prepare	
Premedicants	Midazolam, 2 mL at 1 mg/mL
Opioids	Fentanyl, 5 mL at 50 µg/mL
Induction drugs	Propofol, 20 mL at 10 mg/mL
	or
	Thiopental, 20 mL at 25 mg/mL
	Etomidate, 20 mL at 2 mg/mL
Neuromuscular blocking drugs	Succinylcholine, 10 mL at 20 mg/mL
	Rocuronium, 5 mL at 10 mg/mL
Vasopressors	Ephedrine, 10 mL at 5 mg/mL (dilute 50 mg/mL in 9 mL of saline)
	Phenylephrine, 10 mL at 100 µg/mL (dilute 10 mg in 100 mL of saline; label this bag and use for later cases in day)
Avoiding Drug Errors	
Tips for prevention	Look twice at the source vial being used to prepare your drug. Some vials look alike, and some drug names sound the same.
	Always label your drugs as soon as they are prepared.
	Write the drug concentration on the label.
	Discard unlabeled syringes.
Conversion of % to mg/mL	Move decimal point one place to the right (1.0% = 10 mg/mL).
	By definition, 1% = 1 g/100 mL.
	1% lidocaine is 1000 mg/100 mL, or 10 mg/mL
Conversion of 1:200,000	Memorize: 1:200,000 is 5 µg/mL (1:1000 is 1000 µg/mL or 1 mg/mL)

anesthesia machine (see Chapter 15). The specific anesthesia plan may have implications for preparing additional equipment. For example, fiberoptic tracheal intubation requires special equipment that may be kept in a cart dedicated to difficult airway management.

Managing the Intraoperative Anesthetic

Intraoperative anesthesia management generally follows the anesthesia plan, but it is always adjusted based on the patient's responses to anesthesia and surgery. The anesthesiologist must evaluate a number of different information streams and decide whether to change the patient's management. The trainee must learn to process these different information sources and attend to multiple tasks simultaneously. The general cycle of mental activity involves observation, decision-making, action, and repeat evaluation. Vigilance—being watchful and alert—is necessary for safe patient care, but vigilance alone is not enough.[3] The anesthesiologist must weigh the significance of each observation and can become overwhelmed by the amount of information or by rapidly changing information. Interpreting findings, processing information, diagnosing problems, and making management changes are often topics of discussion for the new trainee in the operating room.

REFERENCES

1. Schwid HA, Rooke GA, Carline J, et al. Evaluation of anesthesia residents using mannequin-based simulation: A multi-institutional study. Anesthesiology 2002;97:1434-1444.

2. Smith A, Goodwin D, Mort M, Pope C. Expertise in practice: An ethnographic study exploring acquisition and use of knowledge in anaesthesia. Br J Anaesth 2003;91:319-328.

3. Gaba DM. Anaesthesiology as a model for patient safety in health care. BMJ 2000;320:785-788.

MEDICAL INFORMATICS

James Caldwell

Informatics is a contraction of *information science*, which is defined as "the collection, classification, storage, retrieval, and dissemination of recorded knowledge treated both as a pure and as an applied science."[1] Medical informatics is the science of informatics as it relates to the fields within health care and biomedicine. Medical informatics is a relatively new science (term was coined in the late 1970s) that serves as an umbrella term, encompassing more specific fields, such as bioinformatics (Table 4-1). Medical informatics has two components; one is purely scientific and the other applied. The pure science of medical informatics relates to theoretical aspects of information and knowledge management. The applied component deals with how information is used in the service of patients and clinicians.

Some confusion may be caused by other terms encountered, such as *health informatics*, *medical information science*, *medical computer science*, and *computers in medicine*. These designations are being superseded by the term *medical informatics*, or they are recognized as representing only a limited area within medical informatics.

PURPOSE OF MEDICAL INFORMATICS

The purpose of medical informatics may be described as the creation and implementation of structures and processes

Table 4-1 Specialized Areas within Medical Informatics
Clinical informatics
Nursing informatics
Dental informatics
Bioinformatics
Imaging informatics
Public health informatics

that facilitate the objective of gathering data and development of knowledge and the tools to permit the application of those data and that knowledge to the clinical decision-making process at any time and place when a decision needs to be made. Clinicians use information and knowledge to make diagnoses and decide on interventions, and medical informatics is a vital tool in optimizing this process. There are many examples of information that has not been used optimally, including analysis of medical errors and the overuse and underuse of services. The judicious use of medical informatics carries the promise of decreasing medical errors.[2]

Health care professionals with knowledge of informatics improve the quality of information processing, and the quality of information processing influences the quality of health care itself. For systematic processing of information in health care, health care professionals require some level of expertise in medical informatics.

COMPUTERS IN MEDICINE

Computers are the vehicles used to realize the goals of medical informatics. Medical informatics deals with the entire domain of medicine and health care, from computer-based patient records to image processing in practice areas ranging from primary care to individual hospitals to regional health care organizations. Some areas of the field are relatively fundamental; others have an applied character. After methods and systems have been developed and made operational for one medical specialty, they can also be transferred to other specialties.

The first example of the use of computational methods relevant to medical information occurred in the U.S. census in 1890, when a punch-card system was used to process the data. In the 1960s, an early decision-support system was developed at the University of Leeds to aid in the diagnosis of acute abdominal pain. In the 1970s, the arrival of the minicomputer put the power of computing at the level of individual departments. Software tools such as UNIX allowed individuals to develop their own applications. The microcomputer or personal computer era began in the 1980s. Since then, individual physicians have had access to personal computers of increasing power at decreasing cost.

Although many individuals and departments have been enthusiastic in developing and using computer-based systems in their practice, the health care industry as a whole has been relatively slow to adopt enterprise-wide systems of managing health information. For example, less than 5% of health care institutions use electronic medical records. This situation is beginning to change, and the pace of change will accelerate. Strong external forces are driving the use of computers in health care. The Leapfrog Group is an alliance of large corporations that are major purchasers of health care, and they have strongly advocated the use of computerized physician order entry (CPOE) systems. The State of California has mandated the future use of CPOE.

The most compelling reason to incorporate computer-based information systems in medicine is that it is the only way to manage and effectively use the already vast and increasing amount of information that is available. An example is the proliferation of medications and information on their interactions. An individual physician cannot keep details of drugs and their interactions in his or her head the way an earlier generation did. More tests and services are available to and performed on patients than ever before. The result has been both overuse and underuse of tests and services. Turnover of patients in hospitals has increased, and resident work hours require multiple transfers of care in a single day. The only way to manage the array of data and to pass it on safely between the members of the care team is by electronic means. Reliance on memory and paper records will become a relic of the past.

Standards

The use of computers to manage and share information has many consequences. The first of these is that there needs to be common standards of information transfer. A simple definition of what constitutes a standard is that it is "what most people do." Standards familiar to most clinicians are the International Classification of Diseases, version 9 (ICD-9) and the Current Procedural Terminology, version 4 (CPT-4) standards for describing diseases and medical procedures, respectively. Standards may be developed in several ways. The simplest method is that the dominant vendor in an area sets the standard. An example of this is the Microsoft Windows operating system. Another approach is that a government agency such as the Health Care Finance Administration (HCFA) or National Institute for Standards and Technology (NIST) may mandate the use of an existing system. Groups of interested parties can meet and develop standards independently. If the process has been sufficiently open and rigorous, these recommendations are adopted as standards, such as the Health Level 7 (HL7) standard for clinical data interchange.

Standards have been developed and adopted in many areas of medicine, but in several crucial areas, they have not. The most complex problem is in the area of medical terminology. For example, the terms *heart attack*, *cardiac infarction*, and *myocardial infarction* mean the same thing to a clinician, but to a computer, they are three different entities. Structured systems such as the Unified Medical Language System (UMLS) and Systematized Nomenclature of Human and Veterinary Medicine (SNOMED) exist, but none has gained universal acceptance. Within the SNOMED systems, a subgroup of anesthesia-related terms is being developed. The problem of developing standardized terminology is compounded because there need to be systems of nomenclature for all areas of health care, such as nursing. Terminology needs to be standardized within a system and across systems in different areas of health care. The Data Dictionary Task Force, sponsored by the Anesthesia Patient Safety Foundation, has developed a set of common anesthesia terms that have been adopted by SNOMED and licensed by the National Library of Medicine. Common anesthesia terms are essential for optimal use of automated information systems, including anesthesia records that will reflect real-time and accurate physiologic data.[3]

Heath Insurance Portability and Accountability Act

The Health Insurance Portability and Accountability Act (HIPAA) became law on August 21, 1996. Among its many provisions are several relating to the use of electronic health care information. The requirements of HIPAA apply to all covered entities. A covered entity is one in which any patient information is transmitted electronically, no matter how small a proportion it comprises of the overall data management by the entity. Hospitals, physicians, other health care providers, health plan organizations, and their employees are covered entities. That means any clinician using any electronic means to apply or access patient information is covered by HIPAA, and the clinician must have some basic knowledge of its provisions. The two areas of most relevance are privacy and security.

Privacy

The use of computers for collecting, storing, and exchanging patient information opens up the possibility of those data falling into the wrong hands. All clinicians have an obligation to ensure that patient information is accessed only by those for whom it is appropriate in the conduct of that patient's care. An example of a breach of privacy is examination of medical information of a celebrity patient by curious health care workers.

PROTECTED HEALTH INFORMATION

If a covered entity transmits any data electronically, all protected health information (PHI), whether electronic or not, must be handled in accordance with the privacy rule. PHI is any information that can be matched to a patient, is created in the process of caring for the patient, and is kept or used in any manner—written, oral, or electronic (Table 4-2). Research records of patient care are also PHI. If all the patient identifiers are removed, the material is no longer PHI.

All patients must be provided with an official notice of privacy rights and practices, and a good faith attempt must be made to obtain a written acknowledgment of receipt of these materials. It is usually not the respon-

Table 4-2 Summary of Elements That Render Data Protected Health Information

Names
Geographic subdivisions smaller than a state
All elements of dates and the age of patients older than 89 years
Telephone and facsimile numbers and email addresses
Social security numbers, medical record numbers, health plan numbers, account numbers
Device identifiers and serial numbers
Biometric identifiers (fingerprints, voiceprints)
Photographs of the face or other identifying objects (tattoos)
Any other identifying number, characteristic, or code

sibility of an anesthesia provider to give this notice and obtain consent. Thereafter, routine use of PHI for treatment, payment, or health care operations is permitted without further consents being necessary.

Authorization

Authorization is required for release of specific elements of PHI for specific purposes outside of routine use or disclosure (e.g., application for insurance coverage, employment physical, marketing or fundraising, clinical research). The authorization document must be signed by the patient, and it must specify an expiration date or event.

Use and Disclosure

The clinician may *use* (i.e., share data within the institution) and *disclose* (i.e., share data outside the institution) PHI. An example of use of PHI is looking up results of tests in the clinical laboratory database. An example of disclosure of PHI is communicating with a patient's primary physician outside of the clinician's institution. Although many exchanges of data are covered by the *minimum necessary standard* (i.e., do not transmit more information than is absolutely necessary), this standard does not apply to treatment-related exchanges between health care providers.

PATIENTS' RIGHTS UNDER THE HEALTH INSURANCE PORTABILITY AND ACCOUNTABILITY ACT

Patients have an unlimited right to restrict or amend the use or disclosure of PHI. However, the clinician is under no obligation to treat that patient if the restrictions are considered to compromise the quality of care delivery. Patients have a right to access their records if they are part of a *designated record set*, which is defined as any data that were used to make a decision about an individual.

Security

Security is required to ensure that PHI cannot be obtained by those not authorized to have access to it. A good security system emphasizes *confidentiality*, *integrity*, and *availability*. Confidentiality means that only the appropriately authorized individuals have access to PHI. Integrity means that data can be altered only by those authorized to do so. Availability means that data are readily accessible by those who need it.

The basis of security lies in creating a culture and an infrastructure that make security possible (Table 4-3). Security starts with an appropriate culture of human behavior; this leads to an appropriate computer policy, which determines the technical mechanisms (infrastructure) to be used. Inappropriate individual behavior can defeat even the best electronic security systems. An example of human behavior that can defeat the system is a physician who carries unprotected PHI in a personal digital assistant that is left in a public place. Another example is careless discussion about patients by providers in public areas. Unless the human or organizational culture changes first, technical solutions will fail to provide security.

ELECTRONIC MEDICAL RECORD

A core function of computers in medicine is the electronic medical record, or computerized medical record. Computer databases eventually will replace paper records throughout health care. There is strong pressure from all areas of government and the private sector to implement electronic records (Tables 4-4 and 4-5). In the Veterans Administration, the medical records are almost entirely electronic; anesthesia records are a notable exception. This has resulted in decreased costs and improved outcomes. However, clinicians are wary of change, and paper records are familiar and difficult for some to relinquish.[4]

Table 4-3 Essential Practices for Maintaining Security of Electronic Protected Health Information

Do not share passwords under any circumstances.

Use a "strong" password (minimum of six characters, with at least three being a capital letter, number, or symbol).

Log off computer stations when finished with use.

Destroy all papers containing PHI in shredder or locked disposal bins (never in a trash can).

Do not leave PHI, in any form, lying around.

Do not send PHI over an unsecured email system (to your personal email account).

Do not leave PHI messages on voicemail.

Password protect all personal electronic devices with PHI.

PHI, protected health information.

An important benefit of computerization is facilitation of the adoption of evidence-based medicine (EBM).

EVIDENCE-BASED MEDICINE

EBM has been defined as "the conscientious, explicit, and judicious use of current best evidence in making decisions about the care of individual patients."[5] The practice of EBM means integrating individual clinical expertise with the best available external clinical evidence from systematic research. The optimal application of EBM requires clinical expertise in acquiring information from the patient by history, physical examination, and performance of appropriate tests, and it requires combining those results with the best available external knowledge (i.e., medical literature) and applying this knowledge to

Table 4-4 Comparison of Paper and Electronic Medical Records

Feature	Paper Records	Electronic Records
Clinician comfort	High due to familiarity	Wariness for new system
Accessibility	Only in one location	Multiple access points
Legibility	Variable, often poor	Excellent
Training required	Minimal	Extensive
Reliability	May be lost or misplaced	Must have stable infrastructure
Data entry	Almost infinite flexibility	Highly structured
Structured searching	Labor intensive	Easy
Viewing options	Limited	Almost infinite

Table 4-5 Reasons for Using Electronic Medical Records

Quality Control

Uniform data entry facilitated

Protocols and guidelines established and made accessible

Reporting of outcomes improved

Enhanced ability to benchmark performance

Patient Care

Improved accessibility of information

Computerized physician order entry

Evidence-based medicine and decision support facilitated

Errors decreased

Management and Planning

Medical records linked to other hospital systems to examine performance metrics

Revenue optimized

Forecasting improved

Research

Terminology standardized

Search capability much enhanced (identifying populations for study)

Large-scale epidemiologic studies facilitated

---

diagnosis and treatment. EBM gives less importance to intuition and more emphasis to a systematized approach to health care. This approach does not devalue individual clinical expertise, instead supplementing it.

Information Retrieval

The first step in practicing EBM is using the Internet to retrieve relevant information from the vast available repository. The days of poring over reference tomes such as the *Index Medicus* and then laboriously locating and photocopying the articles or chapters of interest are gone. Internet-based sources are usually updated frequently, in contrast to CD-based systems, which go out of date rapidly. A current scenario may be described as follows: (1) open your Web browser, (2) select a search engine, (3) type in some search terms, (4) identify the works of interest, and (5) save them directly into a citation manager or as full-text pdf files. When planning a search, the goal should be to optimize the sensitivity of the search (i.e., chance of finding what you want) and the specificity (i.e., avoid being inundated with irrelevant information).

TARGETED SEARCH STRATEGIES

A strategy for efficient searching is to start at a site that focuses on the type of information needed (Table 4-6). Alternatively, the search may be initiated at a site that deals with the specific disease entity or organ system (see Table 4-6). Another approach is to initiate the search at specific subspecialty web sites (see Table 4-6).

SEARCHING GENERAL DATABASES
Medline: The National Library of Medicine Web Site

Any person with a U.S. online account can have free access to PubMed (www.ncbi.nlm.nih.gov/PubMed). It is a comprehensive database of peer-reviewed biomedical information (see Table 4-6). To facilitate efficient searching, it has built-in search categories of therapy, diagnosis, etiology, and prognosis. Searching in PubMed is significantly enhanced by a working knowledge of its specific medical subject heading (MeSH) terms (http://www.nlm.nih.gov/mesh/MBrowser.html).

Commercial Sites

Merck Medicus (www.merckmedicus.com) is an example of a site that requires registration. It is free and provides

---

Table 4-6 Targeted Search Strategies

Evidence-Based Practices

Cochrane Library (www.cochrane.org) (database for systematic reviews and meta-analyses)

Agency for Health Care Research and Quality (www.ahrq.org)

National Guidelines Clearing House (www.guidelines.org)

Specific Disease Entity or Organ System

National Cancer Institute (www.cancer.gov)

Subspecialties

American Society of Anesthesiologists (www.asahq.org) (standards, guidelines, consensus statements)

General Databases

Medline: The National Library of Medicine (PubMed) (www.ncbi.nlm.nih.gov)

Commercial Sites

Merck Medicus (www.merckmedicus.com)

Web Search Engines

Google (www.google.com)

Scirus (www.scirus.com) (restricts searches to science-specific web pages)

access to a vast array of information, including online textbooks, Medline, medical journals, and non-Medline databases (see Table 4-6).

WEB SEARCH ENGINES

There is so much information available through search engines that it is possible to be inundated (see Table 4-6). For example, in Google, typing the query "awareness under anesthesia" generates about 120,000 hits. Putting quotation marks around the phrase limits the search to the exact phrase and reduces the number of hits to about 300. Using other modifiers, such as preceding the search phrase with "allintitle:" (Google), further limits the search to web pages with the exact title and results in only 20 hits. The hierarchy of the order in which the hits are presented may not match the quality of the content. Judging the quality of the information recovered in searches is a necessary skill in this era of easy accessibility to vast quantities of information.

Critically Evaluating the Information

There are two general source types of medical literature. The first is a primary source, and it is characterized by some amount of experimentation and generation of data. An example of this type of source is an original research article. The second type is a secondary source, which is a compilation of information from a primary source. Examples of a secondary source are systematic reviews and meta-analyses.

PRIMARY SOURCES

Title and Introduction

The title should clearly convey the hypothesis, the study population, and the basic study design. The introduction must "sell" the study to the reader. There should be a clear description of the purpose of the study or the principal hypothesis to be tested. The primary and major secondary outcomes should be objective measures and appropriate to the study question. The authors should offer persuasive justification for performing the study. The reader should be made to feel that the study is important and that it can contribute to better patient care.

Methods

The methods must be focused on and capable of addressing the primary hypothesis. In particular, the study population must be appropriate, and the numbers of subjects justified by a priori power analysis. The conduct of the study must be ethical, with proper informed consent obtained.

Results

In presenting the results, the focus must continue to be on the primary and major secondary outcome variables. Statistics are useful, but the results should pass the "eye-ball test." Significant and important differences are usually obvious to visual inspection. Beware of small "statistically significant" differences that are not obvious and of differences presented for minor variables that were not specified previously. Data should be clearly displayed, and individual data and summary statistics should be presented. All subjects should be accounted for. Significant numbers of "dropouts" that are not explained cast doubt on the validity of the results.

Discussion

The discussion should focus on the primary hypothesis or outcome. There should also be a critique of the methodology. No study is perfect, and a genuine discussion of weaknesses attests to the objectivity of the investigators. Authors are often tempted to extrapolate the results and make conclusions that are unjustified. Conclusions should relate only to the hypothesis or outcomes that were tested.

Source

Original research articles should be peer reviewed, and they are listed in databases such as Medline or EMBASE. A consequence of the growth of the World Wide Web is the proliferation of non–peer-reviewed publications. Lack of peer review does not invalidate a study, nor does peer review necessarily guarantee quality. The source of funding for the work should be stated. Studies funded by independent bodies such as the National Institutes of Health or by university or clinical departments are likely to be unbiased. Industry-sponsored studies have a predisposition to bias.

SECONDARY SOURCES

For assessing secondary material, the source is the most important predictor of quality. Reliable databases include the Cochrane Collaboration, the American College of Physicians Journal Club/Evidence-Based Medicine site, and the Database of Abstracts of Reviews of Effectiveness (DARE). These sites use experts to evaluate the primary source material and provide generally unbiased conclusions. Professional societies may sponsor reviews or publish practice guidelines. The authors are independent experts appointed by the society. Less reliable are publications by self-appointed groups of experts. Such groups sponsored by industry may not be totally unbiased in their conclusions and recommendations.

DECISION SUPPORT

Categories of Information

There are two general categories of information. *Patient-specific information* is generated from the care of an individual patient, and it includes results of a careful, thorough history and physical examination plus the results of all tests and interventions. In the computerized world, this information resides in the electronic medical record.

The other category is *knowledge-based information*, which consists of the scientific literature of health care. Computers provide the means for information retrieval and EBM. When those two information systems are combined, the result is a *decision-support system*. Decision support can also be defined as the application of information from knowledge-based systems to an individual patient. Although clinicians are initially wary of such systems, some design characteristics encourage acceptance.[4] The system should guide practice, not coerce it. The system should not block nor lock out the physician. Systems are perceived as helpful in compensating for human failure. Computer-based clinical decision–support system can enhance drug dosing, reduce errors, enhance patient safety, and improve compliance with clinical guidelines.[2,6,7]

Examples of Decision Support in Anesthesia

PERIOPERATIVE CARDIOVASCULAR EVALUATION AND TESTING

A clinician is performing a preoperative evaluation of a 59-year-old male patient, who is scheduled for unilateral total-hip arthroplasty. He has a history of essential hypertension, which was treated with a diuretic. His hip pain is managed with a nonsteroidal anti-inflammatory drug. He smoked cigarettes until 10 years ago, and he does not drink alcohol. His maternal grandfather died of a myocardial infarction when he was 63 years old; otherwise, there is no significant family medical history. He used to walk regularly and play golf twice each week. He no longer does so because of hip pain. He can climb two flights of stairs, with some slight shortness of breath. His only previous anesthetic was 20 years earlier for an appendectomy. He is obese (132 kg), and his arterial blood pressure is 146/85 mm Hg. Laboratory results show fasting glucose level of 83 mg/dL and cholesterol level of 212 mg/dL. The physician is unsure about which preoperative tests should be ordered.

The physician goes to a computer and opens PubMed. Under the search terms "preoperative," "cardiac risk assessment," and "guidelines," she finds 12 citations. On scanning the abstracts, she finds a mention of guidelines for preoperative cardiovascular evaluation published by the American College of Cardiology and the American Heart Association. She opens the search engine Google and types "American College of Cardiology." The College home page is the first hit, and she opens it. She sees a menu item called "Clinical Statements/Guidelines" and scrolls down a long list of topics until she sees "Evaluation, Cardiac." She sees "Figures and Tables" and opens Table 1, entitled "Clinical Predictors of Increased Perioperative Cardiovascular Risk (Myocardial Infarction, Heart Failure, Death)." An electrocardiogram is necessary for risk stratification in the "Minor" group listed, so she orders this test. The result is normal sinus rhythm at 82 beats/min with no abnormalities. Scanning the table shows that the only possible risk factor is uncontrolled systemic hypertension, and that is of minor grade. She next goes to Figure 1, which is an algorithm for performing the assessment. In following the algorithm, she comes on the term METs and does not know what it means. On a hunch, she opens Table 2, and there is a categorization of metabolic equivalents (METs). Returning to Figure 1 and following the algorithm takes her to step 7, which suggests that it is reasonable to proceed to surgery without further testing. As the clinician, she still has the final decision-making authority, but she is now guided by very solid information and knowledge.

DECISION SUPPORT FOR PERIOPERATIVE BETA-BLOCKADE

The clinician has the same patient as described in "Perioperative Cardiovascular Evaluation and Testing." He says that he has been talking to some friends, who tell him that he should take drugs called β-blockers before, during, and after his surgery. The clinic does not have a posted set of guidelines, so how does the physician respond?

Because Google worked well in the past, she decides to try it again. She searches on "perioperative beta blockade" (spell out Greek letters when searching), and on the list of hits is a Stanford University site designated "prophylactic perioperative beta blockade." The physician opens the page and finds exactly what she is looking for—a clear and simple set of guidelines. These guidelines suggest that the patient has two risk factors, essential hypertension and hyperlipidemia, that make him a candidate for prophylactic β-blockade. The clinician's only hesitation at this point is what drug and dose.

Another hit on the search is from the Anesthesia Patient Safety Foundation (APSF): "perioperative beta-blockade II: practical clinical application." After reading the information at this site, the physician prescribes metoprolol (25 mg) to be taken orally, twice daily until surgery. It is important that there is a mechanism to continue this therapy for at least 2 days postoperatively. Using an electronic link to the operating room schedule, the physician identifies her colleague, who will be giving anesthesia to the patient the next day. Her colleague and she discuss the search findings and agree to continue the perioperative β-adrenergic blockade as indicated in the guidelines.

PROPHYLAXIS OF POSTOPERATIVE NAUSEA AND VOMITING

An anesthesiologist is reading the preoperative clinic note for his patient for the next day. She is a 31-year-old woman scheduled for an outpatient gynecologic procedure. Written prominently on the chart is the fact that the patient's greatest concern is postoperative nausea and vomiting (PONV). According to the record, she had protracted PONV after a laparoscopic cholecystectomy 2 years earlier. She is a nonsmoker.

The physician's initial search in PubMed using the terms "postoperative nausea and vomiting" yields more than 1000 citations. Eventually, after using the additional terms "prophylaxis" and "risk factors," he narrows the number of results to fewer than 20. Two papers give him the information that he needs.[8,9] The first article suggests that this patient's risk of PONV may be as high as 79%. The second article suggests that for a patient with this level of risk, multimodal therapy with four separate interventions is warranted. He therefore decides to use ondansetron, droperidol, dexamethasone, and propofol and to avoid volatile anesthetics.

REFERENCES

1. van Bemmel JH. The structure of medical informatics. Med Inform 1984;9:175-180.
2. Bates DW, Cohen M, Leape LL, et al. Reducing the frequency of errors in medicine using information technology. J Am Med Inform Assoc 2001;8:299-308.
3. Thys DM. The role of information systems in anesthesia. APSF Newsletter 2001;summer:22-23 (www.apsf.org).
4. Beatty PCW. User attitudes to computer-based decision support in anesthesia and critical care: A preliminary survey. Internet J Anesthesiol 1999:3 (http://www.ispub.com/ostia/index.php?xmlFilePath=journals/ijeicm/vol3n1/user.xml).
5. Sackett DLW, Rosenberg WM, Muir Gray JA, et al. Evidence based medicine: What it is and what it isn't. BMJ 1996;312:71-72.
6. Hunt DL, Haynes RB, Hanna SE, et al. Effects of computer-based clinical decision support systems on physician performance and patient outcomes: A systematic review. JAMA 1998:280:1339-1346.
7. Shiffman RN, Liaw Y, Brandt CA, et al. Computer-based guideline implementation systems: A systematic review of functionality and effectiveness. J Am Med Inform Assoc 1999;6:104-114.
8. Apfel CC, Laara E, Koivuranta M, et al. A simplified risk score for predicting postoperative nausea and vomiting: Conclusions from cross-validations between two centers. Anesthesiology 1999;91:693-700.
9. Apfel CCK, Korttila K, Abdalla M, et al. A factorial trial of six interventions for the prevention of postoperative nausea and vomiting. N Engl J Med 2004;350:2441-2451.

Section II

PHARMACOLOGY

Chapter 5

BASIC PHARMACOLOGIC PRINCIPLES

Pankaj K. Sikka

Basic principles of pharmacology are derived from an understanding of pharmacokinetics and pharmacodynamics.[1] Pharmacokinetics describes the absorption, distribution, metabolism, and excretion of inhaled or injected drugs (i.e., what the body does to the drug). Pharmacodynamics describes the responsiveness of receptors to drugs and the mechanism by which these effects occur (i.e., what the drug does to the body). Receptors are the components of the cell that interact with drugs to initiate a sequence of events leading to pharmacologic effects. Selectivity of drug action also is determined by receptors that recognize specific drugs. Termination of a drug's effect occurs by metabolism, excretion, or redistribution to inactive sites. A drug may be defined as a chemical compound that produces pharmacologic effects as determined by its pharmacokinetics and pharmacodynamics.

Knowledge of the pharmacokinetics and pharmacodynamics of intravenous drugs defines the dose-response relationships of a drug and permits comparisons with other drugs.[2] The influence of altered physiologic states (e.g., aging) on drug effect can be determined. Likewise, new approaches to drug administration (e.g., computer-driven infusion pumps, patient-controlled analgesia) can be established.

PHARMACOKINETICS

The pharmacokinetic characteristics of drugs measured in healthy and ambulatory adults may be different in patients with chronic diseases (especially renal or hepatic dysfunction) and at various extremes of age, hydration, nutrition, and skeletal muscle mass.

Drug Ionization

The pharmacokinetic profile of a drug depends highly on the characteristics of the nonionized and ionized fraction of that drug (Table 5-1). The nonionized drug fraction

Table 5–1 Characteristics of Nonionized and Ionized Drug Molecules

Characteristic	Nonionized	Ionized
Pharmacologic effect	Active	Inactive
Solubility	Lipids	Water
Cross lipid barriers (renal tubules, gastrointestinal tract, placenta, blood-brain barrier)	Yes	No
Renal excretion	No	Yes
Hepatic metabolism	Yes	No

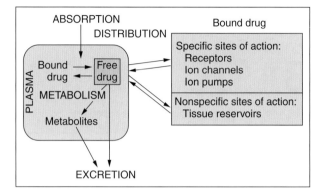

Figure 5-1 Schematic depiction of various aspects of pharmacokinetics, including absorption, distribution, metabolism, and excretion. (From Schwinn DA, Watkins WD, Leslie JB. Basic principles of pharmacology related to anesthesia. *In* Miller RD, Cucchiara RF, Miller ED, et al [eds]: Anesthesia, 4th ed. Philadelphia: Churchill Livingstone, 1994, p 44, with permission.)

tends to be pharmacologically active and lipid-soluble, whereas the ionized fraction is inactive and water soluble. The degree of ionization of a drug is a function of its pK and the pH of the surrounding fluid. When the pK and pH are identical, 50% of the drug exists in the ionized form. Small changes in pH can result in large changes in the degree of ionization, especially if the pH and pK values are similar. Acidic drugs, such as barbiturates, tend to be highly ionized at an alkaline pH, whereas basic drugs, such as opioids and local anesthetics, are highly ionized at an acid pH.

Drug Absorption

Lipid or water solubility also determines absorption and elimination characteristics of drugs. Absorption is defined as the rate at which a drug leaves its site of administration. Membrane transport occurs when drugs cross cell membranes by simple diffusion, by facilitated or carrier-mediated transport, and by active (energy-dependent) transport. Simple diffusion is a bidirectional process in which the rate of transfer of the drug is proportional to the concentration gradient. Highly lipid-soluble and small-molecular-weight drugs diffuse passively across cell membranes. Large-molecular-weight drugs are transported across cell membranes by a carrier-mediated process or an active transport system that requires energy (Fig. 5-1).[3]

FACTORS AFFECTING ABSORPTION

Absorption of a drug from its site of administration depends on several factors. Tablets with a large drug particle size may not disintegrate easily. High lipid solubility favors easy passage of drugs through membranes. A higher concentration of drug favors its absorption. Liquids or crystalloids are usually better absorbed (i.e., better solubility) than solids or colloids. A higher area of absorption and local blood supply favor absorption. Heat or vasodilatation increases drug absorption, whereas shock or vasoconstriction decreases drug absorption.

The degree of ionization of a drug affects its absorption. A nonionized drug, which is often lipid soluble, is absorbed rapidly. An ionized drug, which is often water soluble, is absorbed poorly. An acidic drug is absorbed readily from the stomach, whereas a basic drug is readily absorbed from the alkaline environment of the intestine. The amount of drug absorbed also depends on its route of administration.

Route of Administration

Intravenous administration of drugs ensures achievement of predictable plasma concentrations. Absorption of drugs after oral or intramuscular injection is often unpredictable and depends on local blood flow. Drugs absorbed from the gastrointestinal tract (principally the small intestine) enter the portal venous blood and pass through the liver before entering the systemic circulation for delivery to tissue receptors (Fig. 5-2). This is known as the *first-pass hepatic effect*, and for drugs that undergo extensive hepatic metabolism (e.g., propranolol, lidocaine), this is the reason for large differences between effective oral (i.e., drug delivered to receptors before passing through the liver) and intravenous doses. In addition to hepatic uptake, the lungs may have an important function in pharmacokinetics, as reflected by uptake of basic lipophilic amines (e.g., lidocaine, propranolol, fentanyl) into lung tissue.[4] The first-pass pulmonary effect may influence the peak arterial concentration of these drugs, and the lungs subsequently can serve as a reservoir to release drug back into the systemic circulation.

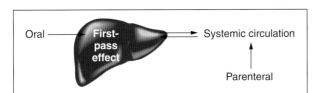

Figure 5-2 Drugs administered orally are absorbed from the gastrointestinal tract into the portal venous blood and pass through the liver (i.e., first-pass hepatic effect) before entering the systemic circulation for distribution to receptors. Conversely, intravenously administered drugs gain rapid access to the systemic circulation for delivery to receptors without an initial impact of metabolism in the liver.

Drug Distribution

The passage of a drug through cell membranes depends on the pH of the drug's environment, the degree of ionization, on the dissociation constant (pKa) of the drug, and on protein binding, molecular weight, and lipid solubility. The pKa of a drug is the pH at which the nonionized and the ionized drug concentrations are equal. Alfentanil has a more rapid onset of action than fentanyl because its pKa is close to physiologic pH, and most of the drug exists in the lipid-soluble, nonionized form at physiologic pH.

PROTEIN BINDING

The binding of a drug to proteins determines the concentration of the drug in the plasma and various other tissues. After absorption, the drug circulates in the plasma in the unbound (free) form and in the form bound to protein, which is usually albumin (acidic drugs) or α_1-acid glycoprotein (basic drugs). Protein binding acts as a temporary reservoir for a drug that prevents large fluctuations in the concentration of the unbound or free drug. However, protein binding can reduce a drug's metabolism and renal excretion by preventing its transport across renal tubular cell membranes. The binding of drugs to proteins is influenced by increasing age, hepatic and renal disease, trauma, and surgery.

ION TRAPPING

Drug distribution may be limited by the phenomenon of ion trapping, especially in the fetus. The lower pH of the fetal blood means that drugs, such as local anesthetics and opioids, that cross the placenta in the nonionized form will become ionized in the fetal circulation. Because an ionized drug cannot readily cross the placenta back to the maternal circulation, it accumulates in the fetal blood against a concentration gradient (i.e., ion trapping) (see Table 5-1).

Redistribution and Storage

After systemic absorption of drugs, the highly perfused tissues (i.e., brain, heart, kidneys, and liver) receive a proportionally larger amount of the total dose (Table 5-2). For example, approximately 75% of the cardiac output is delivered to about 10% of the total body mass. This is consistent with the rapid onset of central nervous system effects of lipid-soluble drugs (e.g., barbiturates, opioids) after their intravenous administration. As the plasma concentrations of drugs decrease below those in highly perfused tissues, drugs leave these tissues and are delivered to less well-perfused sites, such as skeletal muscles and fat. This transfer of drugs to inactive tissue sites is known as *redistribution*. Redistribution of thiopental from the brain to inactive tissue sites is principally responsible for awakening after a single dose of this drug. Repeated doses of thiopental can saturate inactive tissue sites available for redistribution, leading to delayed awakening until the metabolism can decrease plasma concentrations. Similarly, the normally short duration of action of fentanyl resulting from redistribution becomes a prolonged effect when single, large doses or continuous infusions saturate inactive tissue sites available for redistribution.

Drug Metabolism

Metabolism (principally in the liver, but to some extent also in the kidneys, lungs, and gastrointestinal tract) converts pharmacologically active, lipid-soluble drugs to water-soluble and often inactive metabolites.[5] Increased water solubility decreases the volume of distribution (Vd) of that drug and enhances its renal excretion. A lipid-soluble drug undergoes minimal renal excretion because of the ease of reabsorption from the lumens of renal tubules into pericapillary fluid. Metabolism may also result in conversion of an inactive form (prodrug) to an active drug. In some circumstances, the drug metabolite may be toxic.

Microsomal enzymes that participate in the metabolism of many drugs are located principally in hepatic smooth endoplasmic reticulum. The term *microsomal enzymes* is derived from the fact that centrifugation of homogenized hepatocytes concentrates fragments of the disrupted smooth endoplasmic reticulum in what is designated as the *microsomal fraction*. The microsomal fraction contains the cytochrome P450 system, which

Table 5–2 Body Tissue Compartments

Compartment	Body Mass (% of a 70-kg Adult)	Blood Flow (% of Cardiac Output)
Vessel-rich group	10	75
Muscle group	50	19
Fat group	20	5
Vessel-poor group	20	1

most likely constitutes a large number of protein enzymes responsible for metabolism of many foreign compounds. Enzyme induction is stimulation of microsomal enzyme activity by drugs (classically, phenobarbital) leading to accelerated metabolism of other drugs.[6] The principal determinant of microsomal enzyme activity is likely to be genetic, emphasizing the predictably large individual variations in the rate of metabolism of drugs among patients.

PHASE I AND II REACTIONS

Drugs can undergo phase I reactions (i.e., oxidation, reduction, and hydrolysis) or phase II reactions (i.e., conjugation). Oxidation (by the cytochrome P450 system), reduction (by halogenated compounds), and hydrolysis (by procaine or amides) make drugs more water soluble by introducing polar groups such as hydroxyl, amino, sulfhydryl, and carboxyl groups. Conjugation reactions involve coupling of a drug with an endogenous substrate, such as glucuronate, acetate, or an amino acid, so that they can be excreted.

Drug Excretion

Drugs are excreted unchanged or as metabolites. Sites of excretion include the kidneys (primary site), lungs, skin, bile, intestines, breast milk, saliva, and sweat. The kidneys excrete drugs by the processes of passive glomerular filtration, active tubular secretion, and passive diffusion. Nonionized drugs are easily filtered at the glomerulus, but they can diffuse back across renal tubular cell membranes, leaving only a small amount of drug in the urine. Ionized drugs are not reabsorbed after their filtration and appear unchanged in the urine. Many organic acids (e.g., penicillin) are transported across renal tubules by systems that secrete naturally occurring substances such as uric acid. Passive diffusion is a bidirectional system in which drugs diffuse across the renal tubules according to concentration, lipid solubility, and pH.

The ability of the kidneys to excrete drugs is impaired in the presence of renal damage, which may result in high plasma concentrations and prolonged durations of action. Protein binding may significantly alter the renal excretion of drugs. Hypoproteinemia may result in an increased amount of drug available for filtration. Weak acids are ionized in alkaline urine and are therefore not reabsorbed from the urine. Similarly, weak bases are ionized in acidic urine and are not reabsorbed.

Volatile anesthetics are excreted by the lungs. Drugs excreted in the bile are reabsorbed repeatedly from the intestine (enterohepatic circulation), which plays a significant role in the excretion of drugs such as vecuronium and erythromycin. Many drugs appear in breast milk, but the quantities are too small to likely affect the nursing infant.

PHARMACOKINETIC PARAMETERS

The pharmacokinetics of intravenous drugs is influenced by the Vd and the clearance of that drug from the body. The rate at which the plasma concentration of a drug decreases with time (i.e., elimination half-time) is determined by the Vd and clearance of the drug. Context-sensitive half-time and effect-site equilibration time are more useful than elimination half-time in characterizing the clinical responses to drugs.

A plot of the logarithm of the plasma concentration of drug versus time after rapid intravenous (bolus) injection depicts two distinct phases that characterize the distribution half-time of that drug (Fig. 5-3).[1] The first (alpha) phase is designated the *distribution phase*, corresponding to the initial distribution of drug from the circulation to tissues (i.e., peripheral compartments). The second (beta) phase is designated the *elimination phase*. This phase is characterized by a gradual decrease in the plasma concentration of drug and reflects its elimination from the central vascular compartment by renal and hepatic mechanisms.

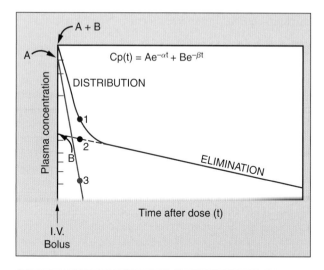

Figure 5-3 Schematic depiction of the decrease in the plasma concentration of drug with time after rapid intravenous injection into the central compartment. The initial rapid decrease in plasma concentration reflects distribution to the tissues, whereas the subsequent slow decrease in plasma concentration reflects drug elimination (i.e., clearance) by the liver and kidneys. The time necessary for the plasma concentration to decrease 50% during the distribution or elimination phase is the corresponding distribution or elimination half-time for that drug. (From Stanski DR, Watkins WD. Drug Disposition in Anesthesia. Orlando, FL: Grune & Stratton, 1982, with permission.)

Clearance

Clearance is the volume of plasma (i.e., central compartment) cleared of drug (mL/min) by renal excretion or metabolism, or both, in the liver or other organs. Clearance is one of the most important pharmacokinetic variables to be considered when defining a constant rate of intravenous drug infusion to maintain an unchanging (steady-state) plasma concentration. When the rate of drug infusion exceeds clearance, the plasma concentration increases progressively, and cumulative drug effects occur. Total clearance is additive and is a summation of clearance rates for the liver, kidneys, and other routes. Important factors determining clearance of a drug are its concentration and blood flow to the specific organ of clearance.

RENAL ELIMINATION

The kidneys are the most important organs for clearance of unchanged drugs or their metabolites. Water-soluble compounds that are not bound to proteins are excreted more efficiently than protein-bound, lipid-soluble drugs. This emphasizes the important role of metabolism in converting lipid-soluble drugs to water-soluble metabolites. Creatinine clearance or serum creatinine concentrations are useful clinical indicators of the ability of the kidneys to eliminate drugs. The magnitude of increase of these indices provides an estimate of the downward adjustment in drug dosage required to prevent accumulation of a drug in the plasma.

Volume of Distribution

Vd is a calculated number (i.e., dose of drug administered intravenously, divided by the plasma concentration) that reflects the apparent volumes of the compartments that constitute the compartmental model for that drug (Fig. 5-4).[1] Binding to plasma proteins, a high degree of ionization,

and low lipid solubility limit passage of drugs to tissues (i.e., peripheral compartments) and result in a small calculated Vd. Examples of drugs with a small Vd similar to that of extracellular fluid are neuromuscular-blocking drugs. Nonionized, lipid-soluble drugs readily pass into tissues (i.e., peripheral compartments) from the circulation (i.e., central compartment). For these drugs, plasma concentrations are low, and the calculated Vd is large. It is important to recognize that Vd does not refer to absolute anatomic volumes. Examples of such drugs are thiopental and diazepam.

Elimination Half-Time

Elimination half-time is the time necessary for the plasma concentration of drug to decrease 50% during the elimination phase (see Fig. 5-3).[1] Five elimination half-times are required for almost complete elimination of a drug. Repeated doses of drug equivalent to the initial dose at intervals more frequent than five elimination half-times will result in cumulative drug effects. Drug accumulation continues until the rate of drug elimination equals the rate of drug administered. As with drug elimination, the time necessary for a drug to achieve a steady-state plasma concentration (Cps) with intermittent doses is about five elimination half-times. A common practice is to administer a large initial intravenous dose (i.e., loading dose) of drug to achieve a therapeutic concentration rapidly and then to give continuous or intermittent intravenous injections of decreased doses of drug to match the rate of elimination and maintain an optimal and unchanging plasma concentration. In most circumstances, this is most reliably achieved by continuous intravenous infusion techniques. The maintenance dose must be adjusted downward in the presence of renal or hepatic dysfunction to prevent drug accumulation due to a prolonged elimination half-time.

Elimination half-time is the descriptor used most often to characterize a drug's pharmacokinetic behavior. However, elimination half-time is useful only in the computation of central compartment drug concentration in a one-compartment model. Elimination half-time is of little value in describing the pharmacokinetics of drugs in multicompartmental models. Of more importance to the anesthesiologist is how long it will take the plasma concentration to decrease to a level that allows the patient to awaken, rather than the slope of the plasma drug concentration curve. Elimination half-times alone provide virtually no insight into the rate of decrease in the plasma concentration after discontinuation of intravenous drug administration. Instead of focusing on elimination half-time, the anesthesiologist may wish to consider the usefulness of the context-sensitive half-time.[7]

Context-Sensitive Half-Time

Context-sensitive half-time describes the time necessary for the drug concentration to decrease to a predetermined

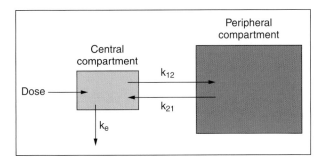

Figure 5-4 A two-compartment pharmacokinetic model. The transfer of drugs between compartments (k_{12}, k_{21}) and elimination (clearance) from the central compartment (k_e) are depicted by rate constants. (From Stanski DR, Watkins WD. Drug Disposition in Anesthesia. Orlando, FL: Grune & Stratton, 1982, with permission.)

II

percentage (e.g., 50%, 60%, 80%) after discontinuation of a continuous intravenous infusion of a specific duration; context refers to the duration of infusion. Computer simulation of multicompartmental pharmacokinetic models of drug disposition is used to calculate context-sensitive half-times for drugs administered as continuous infusions during anesthesia (Fig. 5-5).[8] Depending largely on the drug's lipid solubility and the efficiency of its clearance mechanisms, the context-sensitive half-time increases in parallel with the duration of continuous intravenous administration (see Fig. 5-5).[8] The context-sensitive half-time bears no constant relationship to the drug's elimination half-time.

For the anesthesiologist, it is important to know how long it will take for the plasma level of a drug to decrease to a level that allows the patient to awaken (Fig. 5-6). In this regard, the context-sensitive half-time may be more useful than elimination half-time, which does not consider the rate of decrease in the plasma concentration after discontinuation of intravenous drug administration.

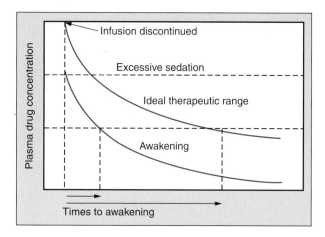

Figure 5-6 The time necessary for the plasma concentration of drug to decrease to a level associated with awakening depends on the plasma concentration present when the infusion of drug is discontinued.

Time to Recovery

The time to recovery depends on how far the plasma concentration must decrease to reach levels compatible with awakening (see Fig. 5-6). For example, if the concentration of drug administered by continuous infusion is only just above that needed for awakening, the time to recovery will be more rapid than that after a continuous infusion that maintains the plasma drug concentration at a level much higher than that associated with awakening (see Fig. 5-6). Use of brain function monitors may allow more precise titration of intravenous drug infusion rates to maintain the desired level of drug effect.

Effect-Site Equilibration

The delay between the intravenous administration of a drug and the onset of its clinical effect reflects the time necessary for the circulation to deliver the drug to its site of action (e.g., brain tissues). This delay reflects the fact that the plasma is not usually the site of drug action; the circulation is merely the route by which the drug reaches its effect site (i.e., biophase). If some parameter of drug effect can be measured (e.g., time to produce a specific effect on the electroencephalogram), the time for equilibration between drug concentration in the plasma and the drug effect can be measured. This interval is the effect-site equilibration time.

Effect-site equilibration time is a particularly relevant concept in the logical timing of intravenous drug administration. Drugs with a short effect-site equilibration time (e.g., remifentanil, alfentanil, thiopental, propofol) produce a more rapid onset of pharmacologic effect compared with drugs that have a longer effect-site equilibration time (e.g., fentanyl, sufentanil, midazolam). Knowledge of effect-site equilibration time is important in determining dosing intervals, especially when titrating intravenous drugs to a given clinical effect. Failure to appreciate the importance of effect-site equilibration time can result in unnecessary or premature administration of drug.

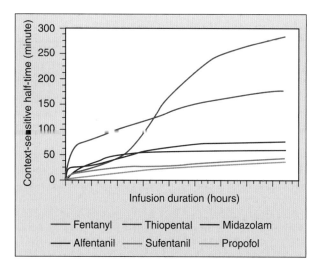

Figure 5-5 Context-sensitive half-times as a function of the duration of intravenous drug infusion for each of the computer simulated pharmacokinetic drug models.
(From Hughes MA, Glass PSA, Jacobs JR. Context-sensitive half-time in multicompartment pharmacokinetic models for intravenous anesthetic drugs. Anesthesiology 1992;76:334-341, with permission.)

Bioavailability

A drug that is absorbed from the intestine passes through the liver (i.e., first-pass effect) before it reaches the circulation. If the liver metabolizes the drug extensively, the amount of active drug reaching the circulation and its site of action will be limited. This parameter is better described as bioavailability, and it is defined as the amount of active drug that is absorbed and reaches the systemic circulation. For example, propanolol is degraded by the liver before it reaches its site of action. As a result, the dosage of a drug such as propranolol is determined by its bioavailability (see Fig. 5-2).

PHARMACODYNAMICS

The most important mechanism by which drugs exert pharmacologic effects is by the interaction of the drug with a specific protein molecule in the lipid bilayer of cell membranes (Fig. 5-7).[9] This transmembrane protein macromolecule is a receptor. A drug administered as an exogenous substance, in contrast to endogenous hormones and neurotransmitters, is an incidental "passenger" for these receptors. A drug-receptor interaction alters the function or conformation of a specific cellular component, which initiates or prevents a series of changes that characterize the pharmacologic effects of the drug.

Receptors

Receptors are excitable transmembrane proteins that are responsible for transduction of biologic signals.[10,11] Examples of receptors are voltage-sensitive ion channels, ligand-gated ion channels, and transmembrane receptors. Voltage-sensitive ion channels depend on cell membrane voltage to open and close, and they are represented by classic ion channels, such as sodium, chloride, potassium, and calcium channels. Ligand-gated ion channels, such as nicotinic cholinergic receptors and amino acid receptors (e.g., γ-aminobutyric acid [GABA]) function as receptor–ion channel complexes in which the ion channel is an integral part of a larger and more complex transmembrane protein.

GAMMA-AMINOBUTYRIC ACID RECEPTORS

Activation of GABA-chloride channels (i.e., receptors) results in cell hyperpolarization or an increase in ion conductance that prevents depolarization, thereby inhibiting neuronal activity. Such activation by benzodiazepines, barbiturates, and propofol enhances endogenous GABA-mediated inhibition in the central nervous system, providing a neurobiologic basis for the hypnotic and sedative effects of these drugs (Fig. 5-8).[12] Approximately one third of all synapses in the central nervous system are responsive to GABA.[11] Opioids and α_2-adrenergic agonists may act by inhibiting presynaptic calcium ion channels responsible for activating neurotransmitter release (see Fig. 5-8).[12]

GUANINE NUCLEOTIDE PROTEINS

Guanine (G) proteins are important intermediaries in cell communication that reflect the molecular mechanisms of actions of multiple classes of drugs, including opioids, sympathomimetics, and anticholinergics.[11] An exogenously administered drug is recognized by a specific receptor, and this receptor-ligand interaction induces conformational changes, enabling the receptor to activate a specific G protein. The activated G protein mediates the final cascade of biologic steps within the cell that ultimately lead to the pharmacologic or physiologic response characteristic of the administered drug. The effector enzyme system may

II

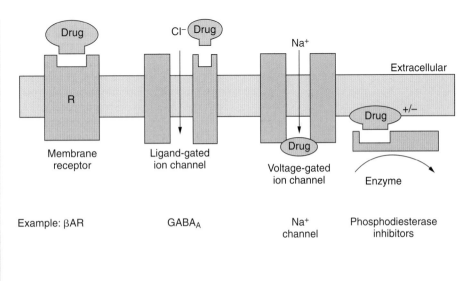

Figure 5-7 Schematic drawing of membrane-associated drug targets, including membrane (G protein–coupled) receptors, ligand-gated ion channels, voltage-sensitive ion channels, and enzymes. Potential sites of drug action are depicted. βAR, β-adrenergic receptor; GABA$_A$, γ-aminobutyric acid receptor A. (From Shafer SL, Schwinn DA. Basic principles of pharmacology related to anesthesia. *In* Miller RD, Fleisher LA, Johns RA, et al [eds]: Anesthesia, 6th ed. Philadelphia: Churchill Livingstone, 2005, p 89, with permission.)

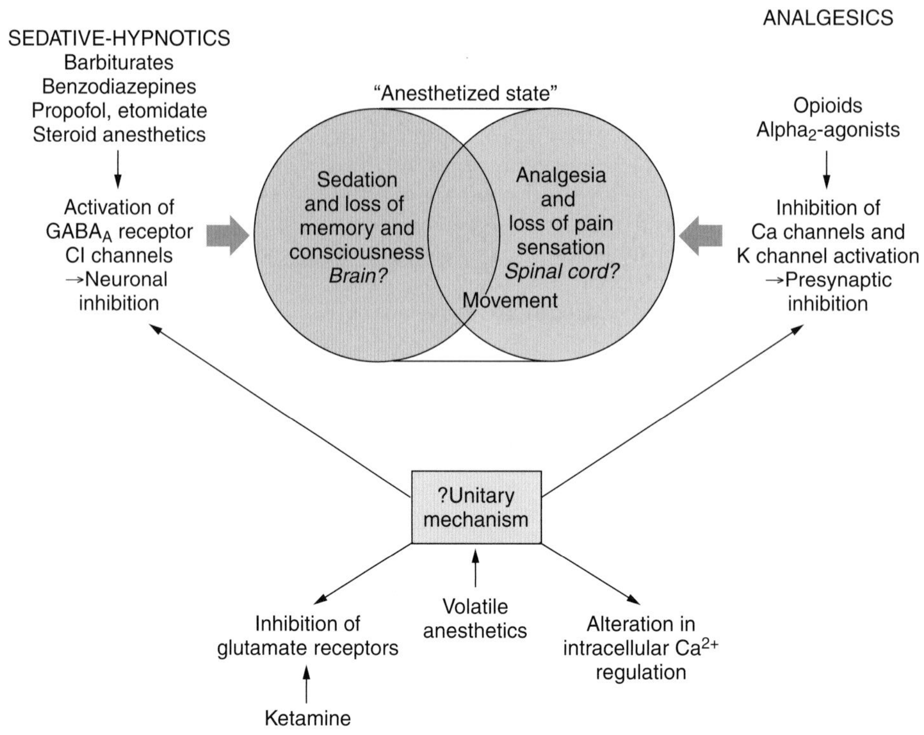

Figure 5-8 The major pathways for sedative-hypnotics and analgesics in generating the anesthetized state considered to be characteristic of volatile anesthetics. (From Lynch C, Pancrazio JJ. Snails, spiders and stereospecificity—is there a role for calcium channels in anesthetic mechanisms? Anesthesiology 1994;81:1-5, with permission.)

SEDATIVE-HYPNOTICS
Barbiturates
Benzodiazepines
Propofol, etomidate
Steroid anesthetics

Activation of $GABA_A$ receptor Cl channels →Neuronal inhibition

"Anesthetized state"

Sedation and loss of memory and consciousness *Brain?*

Analgesia and loss of pain sensation *Spinal cord?* Movement

ANALGESICS

Opioids $Alpha_2$-agonists

Inhibition of Ca channels and K channel activation →Presynaptic inhibition

?Unitary mechanism

Inhibition of glutamate receptors

Volatile anesthetics

Alteration in intracellular Ca^{2+} regulation

Ketamine

be activated or inhibited, and the ion channel may open or close in response to G protein activation.

Many different transmembrane receptors are part of the large superfamily of G protein–coupled receptors. Examples of clinically important G protein–coupled receptor systems include adrenergic, opioid, muscarinic, cholinergic, dopamine, and histamine receptors. Multiple subtypes of receptors exist, such as alpha (α_1, α_2), beta (β_1, β_2), muscarinic (μ_1, μ_2), and histamine (H_1, H_2) receptors.

ION CHANNELS

Ion channels are often characterized as voltage-sensitive or ligand-gated ion channels. Ligand-gated ion channels function as receptor–ion channel complexes in which the ion channel is an integral part of a larger and more complex transmembrane protein (e.g., glutamate activated-*N*-methyl-D-aspartate [NMDA] receptors, GABA receptors, nicotinic cholinergic receptors). The NMDA receptor may be the principal molecular target for ketamine. GABA-activated ion channels mediate the response to GABA by selectively allowing chloride ions to enter and thereby hyperpolarize neurons. Barbiturates, benzodiazepines, propofol, etomidate, and volatile anesthetics modulate GABA receptor function.

ION PUMPS

Ion pumps, as represented by Na^+/K^+-ATPase, are examples of excitable membrane proteins. Action potentials

activate sodium ion channels, allowing sodium to pass from outside to inside the cell. Na^+/K^+-ATPase then pumps sodium out of the cell in exchange for potassium, returning the cell to its original cation composition. Digitalis inhibits this energy-dependent ion pump, improving myocardial contractility.

Receptor Agonists and Antagonists

An agonist is a drug that initiates pharmacologic effects after combining with the receptor. The agonist drug therefore has a high efficacy and high affinity for the receptor. Agonist drugs, when bound to a receptor, induce stimulatory or inhibitory effects that mimic endogenous hormones and neurotransmitters. Antagonist drugs bind to receptors but are not capable of eliciting a pharmacologic response. The antagonist drug prevents receptor-mediated agonist effects by occupying agonist receptor sites. Antagonist drugs therefore have the same affinity as the agonist for the receptor, but their efficacy is poor. Antagonists can inhibit agonist effects by competitive inhibition (e.g., neuromuscular blocking drugs) or non-competitive inhibition. A drug with an affinity equal to or less than that of the agonist but with lesser efficacy is called a *partial agonist*. Some drugs produce a response below the baseline response measured in the absence of the drug. These drugs are called *inverse agonists* or *super-antagonists* (Fig. 5-9).[13]

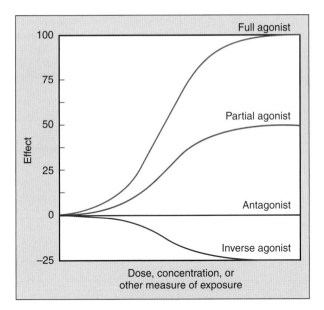

Figure 5-9 Effects of various types of ligands on receptor responses. A full agonist produces complete (100%) activation of a receptor at high concentrations, whereas partial agonist binding results in less than 100% activation, even at very high concentrations. A neutral antagonist has no inherent activity. Inverse agonists represent *superantagonists*, because binding of these ligands produces a response below the baseline response measured in the absence of drug. If the physiologic effect of the baseline levels of activated receptor is small, antagonists and inverse agonists may not be clinically distinguishable. (From Shafer SL, Schwinn DA. Basic principles of pharmacology related to anesthesia. *In* Miller RD, Fleisher LA, Johns RA, et al [eds]: Anesthesia, 6th ed. Philadelphia: Churchill Livingstone, 2005, p 86, with permission.)

Number of Receptors

The number of receptors in lipid cell membranes is dynamic, increasing (upregulation) or decreasing (downregulation) in response to specific stimuli. For example, prolonged administration of β-adrenergic agonists, as in the treatment of asthma, is associated with tachyphylaxis and a concomitant decrease in the number of β-adrenergic receptors. Conversely, chronic interference with activity of receptors, as produced by β-adrenergic antagonists, may result in increased numbers of β-adrenergic receptors such that an exaggerated response occurs if the block is abruptly reversed by discontinuation of drug therapy, as may occur in the preoperative period. Changes in the responsiveness of receptors in the absence of an increase or decrease in the number of receptors may occur with aging. More isoproterenol is necessary to increase heart

rate in the elderly compared with younger patients despite an unchanged number of receptors with aging. Variable pharmacologic responses evoked by drugs in individual patients become more predictable when dynamic changes in concentrations of receptors or alterations in responsiveness of receptors are considered.

PHARMACOLOGIC DRUG EFFECTS

Dose-Response Curves

Dose-response curves depict the relationship between the dose of drug administered (or the resulting plasma concentration) and the resulting pharmacologic effect (Fig. 5-10).[13] Logarithmic transformation of dosage is frequently used, because it permits display of a large range of doses. Dose-response curves are characterized by differences in potency, slope, efficacy, and individual responses.

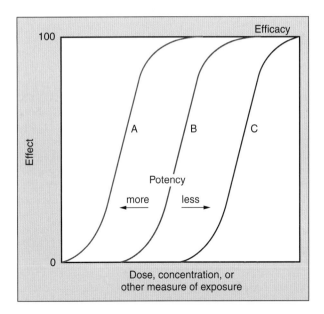

Figure 5-10 Dose or concentration versus response. A sigmoidal concentration-response curve is generated when the log drug concentration is plotted against the clinical response or effect. The concentration-response curve is shifted to the right (B to C) in the presence of a competitive antagonist or desensitization. Curve C may also represent an agonist with a lower receptor affinity or potency than curve B. Curve A represents an agonist with higher receptor affinity or potency than curve B. (From Shafer SL, Schwinn DA. Basic principles of pharmacology related to anesthesia. *In* Miller RD, Fleisher LA, Johns RA, et al [eds]: Anesthesia, 6th ed. Philadelphia: Churchill Livingstone, 2005, p. 86, with permission.)

POTENCY

The potency of a drug is depicted by its location along the dose axis of the dose-response curve. The dose required to produce a specified effect is designated as the effective dose (ED) necessary to produce that effect in a given percentage of patients (e.g., ED_{50}, ED_{90}). Increased affinity of a drug for its receptors moves the dose-response curve to the left. For clinical purposes, the potency of a drug makes little difference as long as the necessary dose of the drug can be administered conveniently.

Drug dosage is commonly calculated on the basis of body weight. When the total body weight exceeds ideal body weight, total body weight increasingly overestimates lean body mass. In adults, it is rarely necessary to scale dose to body weight of more than 80 kg for a woman or 100 kg for a man.[14]

SLOPE

The slope of the dose-response curve is influenced by the number of receptors that must be occupied before a drug effect occurs. If a drug must occupy most receptors before an effect occurs, the slope of the dose-response curve will be steep, which is characteristic of neuromuscular blocking drugs and inhaled anesthetics. This means that small increases in dose evoke large increases in drug effect. For example, a 1 minimum alveolar concentration (MAC) of a volatile anesthetic prevents skeletal muscle movement in response to a surgical skin incision in 50% (ED_{50}) of patients, whereas a further modest increase to about 1.3 MAC prevents movement in at least 95% (ED_{95}) of patients. When the dose-response curve is steep, the difference between a therapeutic and a toxic concentration may be small. This is true for volatile anesthetics that are characterized by small differences between the doses that produce desirable degrees of central nervous system depression and undesirable degrees of cardiopulmonary depression.

EFFICACY AND CEILING EFFECT

The maximal effect of a drug reflects its efficacy as depicted by a plateau in the dose-response curve. Undesirable side effects of a drug may limit dosage to below the concentration associated with its maximal effect. The degree of effect produced by increasing doses of a drug eventually reaches a steady level. This phenomenon is called the *ceiling effect*, and the dose at which it is obtained is called the *ceiling dose*. If the dose of a drug exceeds the ceiling dose, there is no further increase in the therapeutic effect, and undesirable effects may predominate. Efficacy and potency of a drug are not necessarily related.

INDIVIDUAL RESPONSES

Individual responses to a drug may vary as reflections of differences in pharmacokinetics (e.g., renal, liver or cardiac function, patient's age) or pharmacodynamics (e.g.,

enzyme activity, genetic differences). For example, benzodiazepines have a more pronounced pharmacologic effect in the elderly than in younger adults. Malignant hyperthermia, a hypermetabolic state triggered in some individuals in response to the administration of succinylcholine or volatile anesthetics, represents a genetic pharmacodynamic abnormality.

Therapeutic Index

The therapeutic index of a drug is the ratio between the lethal dose (LD_{50}) in 50% of patients and the effective dose (ED_{50}) in 50% of patients. The higher the therapeutic index of a drug, the safer it is for clinical administration because the LD is far above the ED (Fig. 5-11).[3]

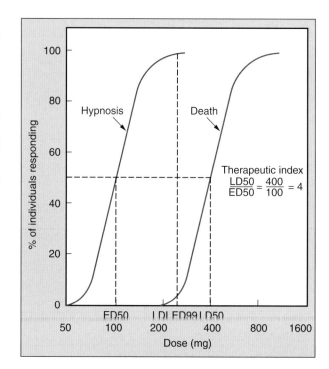

Figure 5-11 Relationships among effective dose 50 (ED_{50}), lethal dose 50 (LD_{50}), and therapeutic index. This curve was generated from experiments in which animals were injected with various doses of a sedative-hypnotic and the responses determined. ED_{50} is the dose of a drug required to produce a specific effect in 50% of patients. LD_{50} is the dose of a drug required to produce death in 50% of patients. The therapeutic index of a drug is the ratio between the LD_{50} and the ED_{50}. (From Schwinn DA, Watkins WD, Leslie JB. Basic principles of pharmacology related to anesthesia. *In* Miller RD, Cucchiara RF, Miller ED, et al [eds]: Anesthesia, 4th ed. Philadelphia: Churchill Livingstone, 1994, p 63, with permission.)

Additive and Synergistic Drug Effects

When the pharmacologic effect of two or more drugs administered together is equivalent to the summation of their individual effect, the phenomenon is called an *additive effect*. A *synergistic response* occurs when the pharmacologic effect of two or more drugs administered concomitantly is greater than the sum of the individual pharmacologic effects. *Time synergism* refers to the prolongation of action of one of the drugs (e.g., combination of lidocaine and epinephrine increases the duration of action of lidocaine).

Competitive and Noncompetitive Antagonism

Agonist and antagonist drugs compete for the same receptors. A competitive antagonist usually can be displaced from the receptor sites by administration of high doses of the agonist. A competitive antagonist shifts the dose-response curve to the right. Competitive antagonism is reversible. When bound to the receptor, a noncompetitive antagonist produces a conformational change in the receptor that results in a diminished receptor response when exposed to an agonist, even at high doses. The dose-response curve shifts to the right, the slope is reduced, and the maximum pharmacologic response diminishes. Noncompetitive antagonism may be reversible or irreversible.

Drug Stereospecificity

Molecular interactions that are the mechanistic foundation of pharmacokinetics and pharmacodynamics are stereoselective or stereospecific, emphasizing that drugs can be expected to interact with other biologic components (e.g., receptors) in a geometrically specific way.[15] When two isomers (dextro [D] and levo [L]) of opposite shape are present in equal proportions (50:50), they are referred to as a *racemic mixture*. The administration of a racemic mixture may represent pharmacologically two different drugs with distinct pharmacokinetic and pharmacodynamic properties. The two isomers of the racemic mixture may have different rates of absorption, metabolism, and excretion, as well as different affinities for receptor-binding sites. Although only one isomer is therapeutically active, it is possible that the other isomer contributes to its side effects. For example, D-bupivacaine remains in sodium ion channels for a longer period than the L-isomer, which may result in cardiotoxic effects. Ropivacaine and levobupivacaine are present only as the L-isomer and are not as likely to produce cardiotoxic effects as bupivacaine. D-Ketamine is predominantly hypnotic and analgesic, whereas L-ketamine is the likely source of this drug's unwanted side effects.

The therapeutically inactive isomer in a racemic mixture should be regarded as an impurity. A cogent theoretical argument is that studies on racemic mixtures may be scientifically flawed if the isomers exhibit different pharmacokinetics or pharmacodynamics.[15] Too often, data on drugs are presented as if only the active isomer were involved, although mixtures of stereoisomers (i.e., racemates) were studied. An estimated one third of drugs in clinical use are administered as racemic mixtures (e.g., thiopental, ketamine, bupivacaine, volatile anesthetics).

Drug Tolerance

Drug tolerance is present when a large dose of a drug is required to elicit an effect that is usually produced by the smaller (therapeutic) dose of the drug. Drug tolerance can be natural or acquired. Natural tolerance can be species or racial specific. Acquired tolerance develops in response to repeated administration of the drug and may be characterized as tissue tolerance or cross-tolerance. Tissue tolerance is confined to certain pharmacologic effects such as tolerance to the euphoric effects of morphine but not its constipating effects. Cross-tolerance occurs when an individual develops tolerance to a specific drug (e.g., alcohol) and other drugs (e.g., sedative-hypnotics, inhaled anesthetics) producing similar pharmacologic effects.

TACHYPHYLAXIS

Tachyphylaxis (i.e., acute tolerance) to the pharmacologic effects of certain drugs (e.g., ephedrine, amphetamine) may occur when they are administered at short intervals. The mechanisms responsible for tachyphylaxis are unclear but may reflect depletion of norepinephrine stores or altered dissociation of drug from its receptor sites.

Drug Dependence

Drug dependence can be defined as a psychic or physical state characterized by behavioral responses that include a compulsion to take the drug on a continuous or periodic basis to experience its psychic effects and sometimes to avoid the discomfort of its absence. Tolerance may or may not occur. A withdrawal syndrome, which can be a life-threatening situation, may develop on discontinuation of the drug.

Drug Interactions

Simultaneously administered drugs can alter each other's pharmacokinetic and pharmacodynamic behaviors. For example, ranitidine or metoclopramide can alter drug absorption by changing the pH of gastric secretions or gastrointestinal motility. Vasoconstrictors are added to local anesthetics to prolong their duration of action and decrease the risk of systemic toxicity from rapid absorption. Drugs can also displace each other from binding sites on plasma proteins, leading to complex interactions. Drug-induced stimulation or inhibition of enzyme activity can affect metabolism of concomitantly administered drugs. Alterations in hepatic blood flow or renal transport mechanisms produced by one drug may affect the clearance of other drugs. Drugs can also interact with each other at receptor sites. For example, opioids are displaced from their receptor sites by opioid antagonists. Cholinesterase inhibitors antagonize neuromuscular block by increasing the amount of acetylcholine, which displaces nondepolarizing neuromuscular blocking drugs from nicotinic receptors. Benzodiazepines and opioids act on their specific receptors to produce synergistic effects.

REFERENCES

1. Stanski DR, Watkins WD. Drug Disposition in Anesthesia. Orlando, FL: Grune & Stratton, 1982.
2. Stanski DR. The contribution of pharmacokinetics and pharmacodynamics to clinical anesthesia care. Can J Anaesth 1988;35:542-545.
3. Schwinn DA, Watkins WD, Leslie JB. Basic principles of pharmacology related to anesthesia. *In* Miller RD, Cucchiara RF, Miller ED, et al (eds): Anesthesia, 4th ed. Philadelphia: Churchill Livingstone, 1994, p 63.
4. Roerig DL, Kotrly KJ, Vucins EJ, et al. First pass uptake of fentanyl, meperidine, and morphine in the human lung. Anesthesiology 1987;67:466-472.
5. Krishna DR, Klotz U. Extrahepatic metabolism of drugs in humans. Clin Pharmacokinet 1994;26:144-150.
6. Okey AB. Enzyme induction in the cytochrome P-450 system. Pharmacol Ther 1990;45:241-245.
7. Fisher DM. (Almost) everything you learned about pharmacokinetics was (somewhat) wrong! Anesth Analg 1996;83:901-903.
8. Hughes MA, Glass PSA, Jacobs JR. Context-sensitive half-time in multicompartment pharmacokinetic models for intravenous anesthetic drugs. Anesthesiology 1992;76:334-341.
9. Schwinn DA. Adrenoceptors as models for G-protein coupled receptors: Structure, function, and regulation. Br J Anaesth 1993;71:77-85.
10. Tanelian DL, Kosek P, Mody I, MacIver MB. The role of the GABA receptor/chloride channel complex in anesthesia. Anesthesiology 1993;78:757-762.
11. Birnbaumer L, Brown AM. G proteins and the mechanisms of action of hormones, neurotransmitters, and autocrine and paracrine regulatory factors. Am Rev Respir Dis 1990;141:S106-S112.
12. Lynch C, Pancrazio JJ. Snails, spiders and stereospecificity—is there a role for calcium channels in anesthetic mechanisms? Anesthesiology 1994;81:1-5.
13. Shafer SL, Schwinn DA. Basic principles of pharmacology related to anesthesia. *In* Miller RD, Fleisher LA, Johns RA, et al (eds): Anesthesia, 6th ed. Philadelphia: Churchill Livingstone, 2005, p 89.
14. Bouillon T, Shafer SL. Does size matter? Anesthesiology 1998;89:557-560.
15. Egan TD. Stereochemistry and anesthetic pharmacology: Joining hands with the medicinal chemists. Anesth Analg 1996;83:447-450.

Chapter 6

CLINICAL CARDIAC AND PULMONARY PHYSIOLOGY

John Feiner

No specialty in medicine manages cardiac and pulmonary physiology as directly on a daily basis as anesthesiology.[1-3] An understanding of cardiorespiratory physiology prepares the anesthesiologist to manage critical and common situations in anesthesia, including hypotension, arterial hypoxemia, hypercapnia, and high peak airway pressures.

HEMODYNAMICS

Arterial Blood Pressure

Systemic blood pressure and mean arterial pressure (MAP) are commonly monitored by anesthesiologists with a blood pressure cuff or an indwelling arterial cannula. Although treatment of chronic systemic hypertension is frequently necessary, acute hypotension is a problem during many anesthetics. Hypotension varies from mild clinically insignificant reductions in MAP from general anesthesia or regional anesthesia to life-threatening emergencies. Hypotension can be severe enough to jeopardize organ perfusion, causing injury and an adverse outcome. Organs of most immediate concern are the heart and brain, followed by the kidneys, liver, and lungs. All have typical injury patterns associated with prolonged "shock." Understanding the physiology behind hypotension is critical for diagnosis and treatment.

Physiologic Approach to Hypotension

The logical treatment of acute hypotension categorizes MAP into its physiologic components:

$$MAP = SVR \times CO$$

In the equation, SVR is the systemic vascular resistance, and CO is cardiac output.

It is important to consider systolic blood pressure (SBP), diastolic blood pressure (DBP), and pulse pressure (SBP − DBP). The pulse pressure is created by the addition of stroke volume (SV) on top of a DBP within the compliant vascular tree. The aorta is responsible for most of this compliance. Increased pulse pressure can occur with an increased SV, but it most often occurs because of the poor aortic compliance that accompanies aging. Lowering DBP can have more dramatic effects on SBP if vascular compliance is poor.

SYSTEMIC VASCULAR RESISTANCE

Most drugs administered during general anesthesia and neuraxial regional anesthesia decrease SVR. Many pathologic causes can produce profound reductions in SVR, including sepsis, anaphylaxis, spinal shock, and reperfusion of ischemic organs. The calculation for SVR follows:

$$SVR = 80 \cdot \frac{MAP - CVP}{CO}$$

In the equation, MAP is the mean arterial pressure, CVP is the central venous pressure, CO is cardiac output, and the factor 80 converts units into dyne/sec/cm^5 from pressure in millimeters of mercury (mm Hg) and CO given in liters per minute (L/min).

Pulmonary artery catheterization can be used to obtain the measurements necessary for calculation of SVR, but this monitor is not usually immediately available. Signs of adequate perfusion (e.g., warm extremities, good pulse oximeter signal) may sometimes be present when hypotension is caused by low SVR. However, hypertension nearly always involves excessive vasoconstriction.

SVR is inversely proportional to the fourth power of the radius. Individually, small vessels offer a very high resistance to flow. However, total SVR is decreased when there are many vessels arranged in parallel. Capillaries, despite being the smallest blood vessels, are not responsible for most of the SVR because there are so many in parallel. Most of the resistance to blood flow in the arterial side of the circulation is in the arterioles.

CARDIAC OUTPUT

Decreased CO as a cause of hypotension may be more difficult to treat than decreased SVR. Increased CO is not usually associated with systemic hypertension, and most hyperdynamic states, such as sepsis and liver failure, are associated with decreased systemic blood pressure.

CO is defined as the amount of blood (L/min) pumped by the heart. Although the amount of blood pumped by the right heart and left heart can differ in the presence of certain congenital heart malformations, it is ordinarily assumed these amounts are the same. CO is the product of heart rate (HR) and stroke volume (SV), the net amount of blood ejected by the heart in one cycle:

$$CO = HR \times SV$$

CO can be measured clinically by thermodilution and by transesophageal echocardiography (TEE). Because CO

changes according to body size, cardiac index (CO divided by body surface area) often is used.

HEART RATE

Tachycardia and bradycardia can cause hypotension due to poor CO. The electrocardiogram (ECG), pulse oximetry, or physical examination can identify bradycardia or tachycardia. The identification of a P wave on the ECG is essential for analyzing HR. Loss of sinus rhythm and atrial contraction results in poor ventricular filling. Atrial contraction is responsible for a significant percentage of preload, even more so in patients with a poorly compliant ventricle. A slow HR may result in enhanced ventricular filling and an increased SV, but an excessively slow HR results in an inadequate CO. Tachycardia may result in insufficient time for the left ventricle to fill and result in low CO and hypotension.

EJECTION FRACTION

Ejection fraction (EF) is the percentage of ventricular blood volume that is pumped by the heart in a single contraction (SV/end-diastolic volume [EDV]). Unlike SV, the EF does not differ on the basis of body size, and an EF of 60% to 70% is considered normal. Because CO can be maintained by increasing HR, the SV should be calculated to better assess cardiac function.

PRELOAD

Preload refers to the amount the cardiac muscle is "stretched" before contraction. Preload is best defined clinically as the EDV of the heart. EDV can be measured directly with TEE. Filling pressures (e.g., left atrial pressure [LA], pulmonary capillary wedge pressure [PCWP], pulmonary artery diastolic pressure [PAD]) can also be used to assess preload. Central venous pressure (CVP) measures filling pressures on the right side of the heart, which correlates with filling pressures on the left side of the heart in the absence of pulmonary disease and when cardiac function is normal. The correlation between pressure and volume of the heart in diastole is depicted by ventricular compliance curves (Fig. 6-1). With a poorly compliant heart, normal filling pressures may not represent an adequate EDV. Likewise, trying to fill a "stiff heart" to apparently normal volumes may increase intracardiac and pulmonary capillary pressures excessively.

Frank-Starling Mechanism

The Frank-Starling mechanism is a physiologic description of the increased pumping action of the heart with increased filling. A larger preload results in increased contraction necessary to eject the added ventricular volume, resulting in a larger SV and similar EF. Reduced ventricular filling, as in hypovolemia, results in reduced SV. Small increases in preload may have dramatic effects (e.g., volume responsiveness) on SV and CO (Fig. 6-2). At higher points on the curve, little additional benefit is derived from increases in preload.

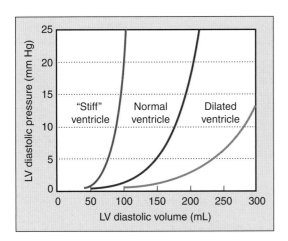

Figure 6-1 The pressure-volume relationship of the heart in diastole is shown in the compliance curves plotting left ventricular (LV) diastolic volume versus pressure. The "stiff" heart shows a steeper rise of pressure with increased volume than the normal heart. The dilated ventricle shows a much more compliant curve.

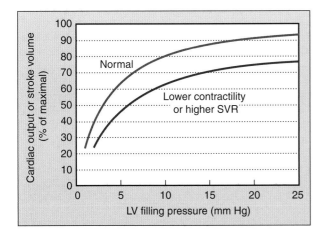

Figure 6-2 The cardiac function curve shows the typical relationship between preload, represented by left ventricular (LV) filling pressure, and cardiac function, reflected in cardiac output or stroke volume. Filling pressure can be measured as left atrial pressure or pulmonary capillary wedge pressure. At low preload, augmentation of filling results in significantly increased cardiac output. This is the steeper portion of the curve. At higher LV filling pressures, little improvement in function occurs with increased preload, and with overfilling, a decrement in function can occur because of impaired perfusion (not shown). Lower contractility or higher systemic vascular resistance (SVR) shifts the normal curve to the right and downward.

Causes of Low Preload

Causes of low preload include hypovolemia and venodilation. Hypovolemia may result from hemorrhage or fluid losses. Venodilation occurs with general anesthesia and may be even more prominent in the presence of neuraxial anesthesia. Additional causes of decreased preload include tension pneumothorax and pericardial tamponade, which prevent ventricular filling due to increased pressure around the heart, even though volume status and filling pressures are adequate. Such conditions may manifest with a systolic pressure variation (i.e., change in SBP with tidal breathing) that can be observed on an arterial blood pressure tracing. The extreme form of this is pulsus paradoxus, a pulse that changes markedly during tidal breathing. In the setting of normal or increased CVP, the presence of cardiac tamponade is likely. Systolic pressure variation is also useful in identifying hypovolemia.

Pathologic problems on the right side of the heart may prevent filling of the left ventricle. Pulmonary embolism and other causes of pulmonary hypertension prevent the right heart from pumping a sufficient volume to fill the left heart. The interventricular septum may be shifted, further constricting filling of the left heart.

AFTERLOAD

Afterload is the resistance to ejection of blood from the left ventricle with each contraction. Clinically, afterload is largely determined by SVR. When SVR is increased, the heart does not empty as completely, resulting in a lower SV, EF, and CO (Figs. 6-2 and 6-3). High SVR also causes cardiac filling pressure to increase. Low SVR improves SV and increases CO such that a low SVR is often associated with a higher CO.

Low SVR always decreases cardiac filling pressures, suggesting that preload rather than afterload is the cause of hypotension (Figs. 6-3 and 6-4). Low SVR allows greater emptying and a lower end-systolic volume (ESV), one of the hallmarks of low SVR on TEE. With the same venous return, the heart does not fill to the same EDV, resulting in lower left ventricular filling pressures (see Fig. 6-3). A similar process occurs when the SVR is increased. Such stress-induced increases in cardiac filling pressures are more pronounced in patients with poor cardiac function.

CONTRACTILITY

Contractility refers to the inotropic state of the heart, a measure of the force of contraction independent of loading conditions (preload or afterload). It can be measured for research purposes by the rate at which pressure develops in the cardiac ventricles (dP/dT) or by systolic pressure-volume relationships (see Fig. 6-4). Decreased myocardial contractility may be the explanation for hypotension. A variety of partial causes of low contractility is listed in Table 6-1.

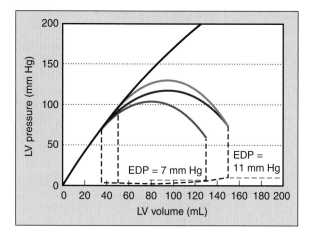

Figure 6-3 Changes in the cardiac cycle that can occur with vasodilatation are depicted. The cycle in *green* is the same cycle shown in Figure 6-4. The *red line* suggests the transition to the new cardiac cycle shown in *blue*. The systolic blood pressure has decreased to 105 mm Hg. The end-systolic volume has decreased, as has the end-diastolic volume. End-diastolic pressure (EDP) has decreased from 11 to 7 mm Hg in this example. The ejection fraction is slightly increased; however, the stroke volume may decrease, but with restoration of left ventricular (LV) filling pressures to the same level as before, the stroke volume will be higher.

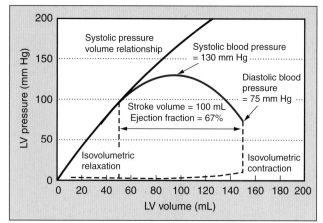

Figure 6-4 The closed drawing shows a typical cardiac cycle. Diastolic filling occurs along the typical diastolic curve from a volume of 50 mL to an end-diastolic volume (EDV) of 150 mL. Isovolumetric contraction increases the pressure in the left ventricle (LV) until it reaches the pressure in the aorta (at diastolic blood pressure) and the aortic valve opens. The LV then ejects blood, and volume decreases. Pressure in the LV and aorta reaches a peak at some point during ejection (systolic blood pressure), and the pressure then drops until the point at which the aortic valve closes (roughly the dicrotic notch). The LV relaxes, without changing volume (isovolumetric relaxation). When the pressure decreases below left atrial pressure, the mitral valve opens, and diastolic filling begins. The plot shows a normal cycle, and the stroke volume (SV) is 100 mL, ejection fraction (EF) is SV/EDV = 67%, and blood pressure is 130/75 mm Hg. The systolic pressure-volume relationship (*black*) can be constructed from a family of curves under different loading conditions (i.e., different preload) and reflects the inotropic state of the heart.

CARDIAC REFLEXES

The cardiovascular regulatory system consists of peripheral and central receptor systems that can detect various physiologic states, a central "integratory" system in the brainstem, and neurohumoral output to the heart and vascular system. A clinical understanding of cardiac reflexes is based on the concept that the cardiovascular system in the brainstem integrates the signal and provides a response through the autonomic nervous system.

Autonomic Nervous System

The heart and vascular systems are controlled by the autonomic nervous system. Sympathetic and parasympathetic efferents innervate the sinoatrial and atrioventricular nodes. Sympathetic nervous system stimulation increases HR through activation of β_1-adrenergic receptors. Parasympathetic nervous system suppression contributes to increased HR, whereas parasympathetic nervous system stimulation can profoundly slow HR through stimulation of muscarinic acetylcholine receptors in the sinoatrial and atrioventricular nodes. Conduction through the atrioventricular node is increased and decreased by sympathetic and parasympathetic nervous system inner-

Table 6-1 Decreased Myocardial Contractility as a Cause of Hypotension

Myocardial ischemia
Anesthetic drugs
Cardiomyopathy
Prior myocardial infarction
Valvular heart disease (decreased stroke volume independent of preload)

vation, respectively. Sympathetic nervous system stimulation increases myocardial contractility. Parasympathetic nervous system stimulation may decrease myocardial contractility slightly, but it has its major effect through decreasing HR.

Baroreceptors

Baroreceptors in the carotid sinus and aortic arch are activated by increased systemic blood pressure that stimulates stretch receptors to send signals through the vagus and glossopharyngeal nerves to the central nervous system. The sensitivity of baroreceptors to systemic blood pressure changes varies and is significantly altered by long-standing essential hypertension. A typical response to elevated systemic blood pressure is increased parasympathetic nervous system stimulation that decreases HR. Vagal stimulation and decreases in sympathetic nervous system activity also decrease myocardial contractility and cause reflex vasodilatation. This carotid sinus reflex can be used therapeutically to produce vagal stimulation that may be an effective treatment for supraventricular tachycardia.

The atria and ventricles are innervated by a variety of sympathetic and parasympathetic receptor systems. Atrial stretch (i.e., Bainbridge reflex) can increase HR, which may help match CO to venous return.

Stimulation of the chemoreceptors in the carotid sinus has respiratory and cardiovascular effects. Arterial hypoxemia results in sympathetic nervous system stimulation, although more profound and prolonged arterial hypoxemia can result in bradycardia, possibly through central mechanisms. A variety of other reflexes include bradycardia with ocular pressure (i.e., oculocardiac reflex) and bradycardia with stretch of abdominal viscera. The Cushing reflex is bradycardia in response to increased intracranial pressure.

Many anesthetic drugs blunt cardiac reflexes in a dose-dependent fashion, with the result that sympathetic nervous system responses to hypotension are reduced. The blunting of such reflexes represents an additional mechanism by which anesthetic drugs contribute to hypotension.

CORONARY BLOOD FLOW

The coronary circulation is unique in that a larger percentage of oxygen is extracted by the heart than in any other vascular bed, up to 60% to 70%, compared with the 25% extraction of the body as a whole. The consequence of this physiology is that the heart cannot use increased oxygen extraction as a reserve mechanism. In cases of threatened oxygen supply, vasodilatation to increase blood flow is the primary compensatory mechanism of the heart.

Coronary reserve is the ability of the coronary circulation to increase flow over the baseline state. Endogenous regulators of coronary blood flow include adenosine, nitric oxide, and adrenergic stimulation. With coronary artery stenosis, compensatory vasodilatation downstream can compensate and maintain coronary blood flow until about 90% stenosis, when coronary reserve begins to become exhausted.

Perfusion pressure of a vascular bed is usually calculated as the difference between MAP and venous pressure. Instantaneous flow through the coronary arteries varies throughout the cardiac cycle, peaking during systole. The heart is fundamentally different from other organs, because myocardial wall tension developed during systole can completely stop blood flow in the subendocardium. The left ventricle is therefore perfused predominantly during diastole. The end-diastolic pressure in the left ventricle (LVEDP) may exceed CVP and represents the effective downstream pressure. Perfusion pressure to most of the left ventricle is therefore DBP minus LVEDP. The right ventricle, with its lower intramural pressure, is perfused during diastole and systole.

PULMONARY CIRCULATION

The pulmonary circulation includes the right ventricle, pulmonary arteries, pulmonary capillary bed, and pulmonary veins, ending in the left atrium. The bronchial circulation supplies nutrients to lung tissue, and empties into the pulmonary veins and left atrium. The pulmonary circulation differs substantially form the systemic circulation in its regulation, normal pressures, and responses to drugs (Table 6-2). Use of a pulmonary artery catheter to measure pressures in the pulmonary circulation requires a fundamental understanding of their normal values and their meaning. Pulmonary hypertension may accompany several common diseases (e.g., cirrhosis of the liver, sleep apnea) and is associated with significant anesthetic-related morbidity and mortality.

Table 6-2 Normal Values for Pressures in the Venous and Pulmonary Arterial System

Value	CVP (mm Hg)	PAS (mm Hg)	PAD (mm Hg)	PAM (mm Hg)	PCWP (mm Hg)
Normal	2-8	15-30	4-12	9-16	2-12
High	>12	>30	>12	>25	>12
Pathologic	>18	>40	>20	>35	>20

CVP, central venous pressure; PAD, pulmonary artery diastolic pressure; PAM, pulmonary artery mean pressure; PAS, pulmonary artery systolic pressure, PCWP, pulmonary capillary wedge pressure.

Pulmonary Artery Pressure

PAP is much lower than systemic pressure because of low pulmonary vascular resistance (PVR). Like the systemic circulation, the pulmonary circulation accepts the entire CO and must adapt its resistance to meet different conditions.

Pulmonary Vascular Resistance

Determinants of PVR are different from SVR in the systemic circulation. During blood flow through the pulmonary circulation, resistance is thought to occur in the larger vessels, small arteries, and capillary bed. Vessels within the alveoli and the extra-alveolar vessels respond differently to forces within the lung.

The most useful physiologic model for describing changes in the pulmonary circulation is the distensibility of capillaries and the recruitment of new capillaries. This distention and recruitment of capillaries explains the changes in PVR in a variety of circumstances. Increased PAP causes distention and recruitment of capillaries, increasing the cross-sectional area and lowering PVR. Increased CO also decreases PVR through distention and recruitment. The reciprocal changes between CO and PVR maintain pulmonary pressures fairly constant over a wide range of CO.

Lung volumes have different effects on intra-alveolar and extra-alveolar vessels. At high lung volumes, intra-alveolar vessels can be compressed, whereas extra-alveolar vessels have lower resistance. The opposite is true at low lung volumes. Higher PVR occurs at high and low lung volumes. Increased PVR at low lung volumes helps to divert blood flow from collapsed alveoli, such as during one-lung ventilation.

Sympathetic nervous system stimulation can cause pulmonary vasoconstriction, but the effect is not large, in contrast to the systemic circulation, in which neurohumoral influence is the primary regulator of vascular tone. The pulmonary circulation has therefore been very difficult to treat with drugs. Nitric oxide is an important regulator of vascular tone and can be given by inhalation. Prostaglandins are vasodilators, but pharmacologic responses that can be achieved in primary pulmonary hypertension are limited.

HYPOXIC PULMONARY VASOCONSTRICTION

Hypoxic pulmonary vasoconstriction (HPV) is the pulmonary vascular response to a low P_{AO_2}. In many patients, HPV is an important adaptive response that improves gas exchange by diverting blood away from poorly ventilated areas, decreasing shunt fraction. Normal regions of the lung can easily accommodate the additional blood flow without increases in PAP. Global alveolar hypoxia, such as occurs with apnea or at high altitude, can cause significant HPV and increased PAP.

PULMONARY EMBOLI

Pulmonary emboli obstruct blood vessels, increasing the overall resistance to blood through the pulmonary vascular system. Common forms of emboli are blood clots and air, but they also include amniotic fluid, carbon dioxide, and fat emboli.

ARTERIAL THICKENING

Arteriolar thickening occurs in several clinical circumstances. It is associated with certain types of long-standing congenital heart disease. Primary pulmonary hypertension is an idiopathic disease associated with arteriolar hyperplasia. Similar changes are associated with cirrhosis of the liver (i.e., portopulmonary hypertension).

Zones of the Lung

A useful concept in pulmonary hemodynamics is West's zones of the lung. Gravity determines the way pressures change in the vascular system relative to the measurement at the level of the heart. These differences are small compared with arterial pressures, but for venous pressure and PAP, these differences are clinically significant. Every 20 cm of change in height produces a 15-mm Hg pressure difference. This can create significant positional differences in PAP that affects blood flow in the lung in various positions, such as upright and lateral positions.

In zone 1, airway pressures exceed PAP and pulmonary venous pressures. Zone 1 therefore has no blood flow despite ventilation. Normally, zone 1 does not exist, but with positive-pressure ventilation or low PAP, as may occur under anesthesia or with blood loss, zone 1 may develop. In Zone 2, airway pressure is greater than pulmonary venous pressure, but it is not greater than PAP. In Zone 2, flow is proportional to the difference between PAP and airway pressure. In Zone 3, PAP and venous pressure exceed airway pressure, and a normal blood flow pattern results (i.e., flow is proportional to the difference between PAP and venous pressure). Position can also be used therapeutically to decrease blood flow to abnormal areas of the lung and thereby improve gas exchange.

Pulmonary Edema

Fluid balance in the lung depends on hydrostatic driving forces. Excessive pulmonary capillary pressures cause fluid to leak into the interstitium and then into alveoli. The pulmonary lymphatic system is very effective in clearing fluid, but it can be overwhelmed. Hydrostatic pulmonary edema is expected with high left ventricular filling pressures, and patients become at risk of pulmonary edema as PCWP exceeds 20 mm Hg. Pulmonary edema can also occur with "capillary leak" from lung injury, such as acid aspiration.

PULMONARY GAS EXCHANGE

Oxygen

Oxygen must pass from the environment to the tissues, where it is consumed during aerobic metabolism. Arterial hypoxemia is most often defined as a low PaO_2. An arbitrary definition of arterial hypoxemia ($PaO_2 < 60$ mm Hg) is not necessary. Occasionally, arterial hypoxemia is used to describe a PaO_2 that is low relative to what might be expected based on the inspired oxygen concentration (FIO_2). *Arterial hypoxemia* (which reflects pulmonary gas exchange) is distinguished from *hypoxia*, a more general term including *tissue hypoxia*, which also reflects circulatory factors.

Mild and even moderate arterial hypoxemia (e.g., at high altitude) can be well tolerated and is not usually associated with substantial injury or adverse outcomes. Anoxia, a complete lack of oxygen, is potentially fatal and is often associated with permanent neurologic injury. Arterial hypoxemia is most significant when anoxia is threatened, and the difference between the two may be less than 1 minute.

MEASUREMENTS OF OXYGENATION

Measurements of arterial blood oxygen levels include PaO_2, arterial oxygen content (CaO_2), and oxyhemoglobin saturation (SaO_2). PaO_2 and SaO_2 are related through the oxyhemoglobin dissociation curve (Fig. 6-5). Understanding the oxyhemoglobin dissociation curve is facilitated by the ability to measure continuous oxyhemoglobin saturation with pulse oximetry (SpO_2) and measurement of PaO_2 with arterial blood gas analysis.

OXYHEMOGLOBIN DISSOCIATION CURVE

Rightward and leftward shifts of the oxyhemoglobin dissociation curve provide significant homeostatic adaptations to changing oxygen availability. P_{50}, the PO_2 at which hemoglobin is 50% saturated with oxygen, is a measurement of the position of the oxyhemoglobin dissociation curve (Table 6-3). The normal P_{50} value of adult hemoglobin is 26.8 mm Hg.

A rightward shift causes little change in loading conditions (essentially the same SaO_2 at PO_2 of 100 mm Hg), but it allows larger amounts of oxygen to dissociate from hemoglobin in the tissues. This improves tissue oxygenation. Carbon dioxide and metabolic acid shift the oxyhemoglobin dissociation curve rightward, whereas alkalosis shifts it leftward. Fetal hemoglobin is left shifted, an adaptation uniquely suited to placental physiology. Oxygen in arterial blood is bound to hemoglobin and dissolved in the plasma. The blood oxygen content is the sum of the two forms. Although amounts of dissolved oxygen are fairly trivial at normal PO_2 levels, at high FIO_2, dissolved oxygen can be physiologically and clinically important. Although under normal conditions only a fraction of the oxygen on hemoglobin (25%) can be used, all of the dissolved oxygen added while giving supplemental oxygen is used.

ARTERIAL OXYGEN CONTENT

CaO_2 is calculated based on SaO_2 and partial pressure plus the hemoglobin concentration (Fig. 6-6).

$$CaO_2 = SaO_2 (Hb \times 1.39) + 0.003 (PaO_2)$$

In the equation, Hb is the hemoglobin level, 1.39 is the capacity of hemoglobin for oxygen (1.39 mL of O_2/g of Hb fully saturated), and 0.003 mL O_2/dL/mm Hg is the solubility of oxygen. For example, if Hb = 15 g/dL and

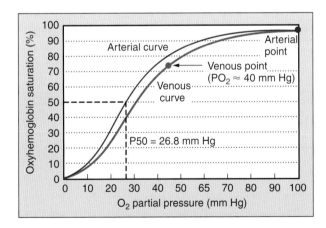

Figure 6-5 The oxyhemoglobin dissociation curve is S shaped and relates oxygen partial pressure to the oxyhemoglobin saturation. A typical arterial curve is shown in *red*. The higher PCO_2 and the lower pH of venous blood cause a rightward shift of the curve and facilitate unloading of oxygen in the tissues (*blue*). Normal adult P_{50}, the PO_2 at which hemoglobin is 50% saturated is shown (26.8 mm Hg). Normal PaO_2 of about 100 mm Hg results in a SaO_2 of about 98%. Normal PvO_2 is about 40 mm Hg, resulting in a saturation of about 75%.

Table 6-3 Events That Shift the Oxyhemoglobin Dissociation Curve

Left Shift ($P_{50} < 26.8$ mm Hg)	Right Shift ($P_{50} > 26.8$ mm Hg)
Acidosis	Alkalosis
Hypothermia	Hyperthermia
Decreased 2,3 diphosphoglycerate	Increased 2,3 diphosphoglycerate (chronic arterial hypoxemia or anemia)

P_{50}, the PO_2 at which hemoglobin is 50% saturated with oxygen.

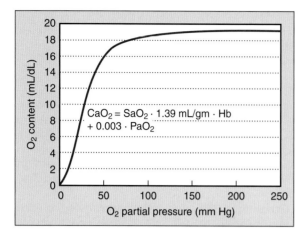

Figure 6-6 The relationship between Pa_{O_2} and oxygen content is also sigmoidal, because most of the oxygen is bound to hemoglobin. Oxygen content at the plateau of the curve ($Po_2 > 100$ mm Hg) continues to rise because dissolved oxygen still contributes a small, but not negligible, quantity.

$Pa_{O_2} = 100$ mm Hg, resulting in nearly 100% saturation, the value of Ca_{O_2} is calculated as follows:

$$Ca_{O_2} = 1.00 (15 \times 1.39) + 100 (0.003)$$
$$= 20.85 + 0.3$$
$$Ca_{O_2} = 21.15 \text{ mL/dL}$$

Dissolved oxygen can continue to provide additional Ca_{O_2}, which can be clinically significant with F_{IO_2} of 1.0

and with hyperbaric oxygen. The oxygen cascade depicts the passage of oxygen from the atmosphere to the tissues (Fig. 6-7).

DETERMINANTS OF ALVEOLAR OXYGEN PARTIAL PRESSURE

The alveolar gas equation describes transfer of oxygen from the environment into the alveoli:

$$P_{AO_2} = F_{IO_2} \bullet (P_B - P_{H_2O}) - \frac{P_{CO_2}}{RQ}$$

In the previous equation, P_B is the barometric pressure, P_{H_2O}, is the vapor pressure of water (47 mm Hg at normal body temperature of 37°C), and RQ is the respiratory quotient (the ratio of carbon dioxide production to oxygen consumption). For example, while breathing 100% oxygen ($F_{IO_2} = 1.0$) at sea level ($P_B = 760$ mm Hg, and the $P_{H_2O} = 47$ mm Hg with $Pa_{CO_2} = 40$ mm Hg, the alveolar P_{O_2} (P_{AO_2}) difference in the partial pressure of oxygen (AaD_{O_2}) is calculated as follows. RQ is usually assumed to be 0.8 on a normal diet.

$$
\begin{aligned}
P_{AO_2} &= 1.0 (760 - 47) - 40/0.8 \\
&= 713 - 50 \\
Pa_{O_2} &= 663 \text{ mm Hg}
\end{aligned}
$$

The alveolar gas equation describes the way in which inspired P_{O_2} and ventilation determine P_{AO_2}. It also describes the way in which supplemental oxygen improves oxygenation. One clinical consequence of this relationship is that supplemental oxygen can easily compensate for the adverse effects of hypoventilation (Fig. 6-8).

Figure 6-7 The oxygen cascade depicts the physiologic steps as oxygen travels from the atmosphere to the tissues. Oxygen starts at 21% in the atmosphere and is initially diluted with water vapor to about 150 mm Hg. P_{AO_2} is determined by the alveolar gas equation. Diffusion equilibrates Po_2 between the alveolus and the capillary. The A-a (alveolar to arterial) gradients occur with intrapulmonary shunt and ventilation to perfusion ($\dot{V}/\dot{Q}$) mismatch. Oxygen consumption then reduces Po_2 to tissue levels (to about 40 mm Hg).

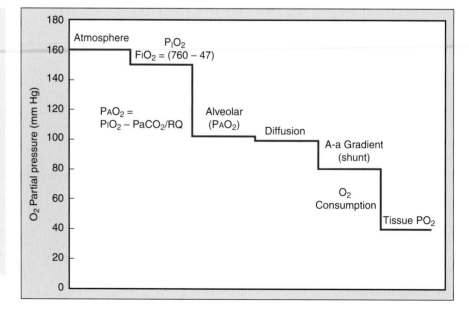

Low barometric pressure is a cause of arterial hypoxemia at high altitude. Modern anesthesia machines have safety mechanisms to prevent delivery of hypoxic gas mixtures. Nevertheless, death from delivery of gases other than oxygen is still occasionally reported because of errors in pipe connections made during construction or remodeling of operating rooms. Failure to recognize accidental disconnection of a self-inflating bag (Ambu) from its oxygen source may result in delivery of an inadequate FIO_2.

Apnea is an important cause of arterial hypoxemia, and storage of oxygen in the lung is of prime importance in delaying the appearance of arterial hypoxemia in humans. Storage of oxygen on hemoglobin is secondary, because use of this oxygen requires significant oxyhemoglobin desaturation. In contrast to voluntary breath-holding, apnea during anesthesia occurs at functional residual capacity (FRC). This substantially reduces the time to oxyhemoglobin desaturation compared with a breath-hold at total lung capacity.

The time can be estimated for SaO_2 to reach 90% when the FRC is 2.5 L and the PAO_2 is 100 mm Hg. Normal oxygen consumption is about 300 mL/min, although this is somewhat lower during anesthesia. It would take only about 30 seconds under these room air conditions to develop arterial hypoxemia. After breathing 100% oxygen, it might take 7 minutes to reach an SaO_2 of 90%. In reality, the time it takes to develop arterial hypoxemia after breathing 100% oxygen varies. Desaturation begins when sufficient numbers of alveoli have collapsed and intrapulmonary shunt develops, not simply when oxygen stores have become exhausted. In particular, obese patients develop arterial hypoxemia with apnea substantially faster than lean patients.

VENOUS ADMIXTURE

Venous admixture describes physiologic causes of arterial hypoxemia for which PAO_2 is normal. The alveolar-to-arterial oxygen (A-a) gradient reflects venous admixture. Normal A-a gradients are 5 to 10 mm Hg, but they increase with age. For example, if the arterial PO_2 on 100% oxygen were measured as 310 mm Hg, the A-a gradient can be calculated from the previous example.

$$\text{A-a gradient} = PAO_2 - PaO_2 =$$
$$663 \text{ mm Hg} - 310 \text{ mm Hg} = 353 \text{ mm Hg}$$

A picture of gas exchange can be accomplished mathematically by integrating all the effects of shunting, supplemental oxygen, and the oxyhemoglobin dissociation curve to create "isoshunt" diagrams (Fig. 6-9).

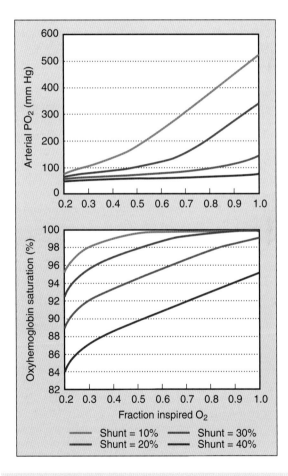

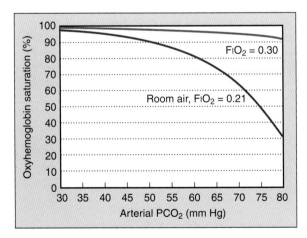

Figure 6-8 Hypoventilation decreases oxygenation, as determined by the alveolar gas equation. High $PaCO_2$ further shifts the oxyhemoglobin dissociation curve to the right. However, as little as 30% oxygen can completely negate the effects of hypoventilation.

Figure 6-9 The effect of intrapulmonary shunting and FIO_2 on PaO_2 (*top*) and SaO_2 (*bottom*) is shown graphically at shunt fractions from 10% (mild) to 40% (severe). Assumed values for these calculations are hemoglobin, 14 g/dL; $PaCO_2$, 40 mm Hg; arterial-to-venous oxygen content difference, 4 mL O_2/dL; and sea level atmospheric pressure, 760 mm Hg.

Intrapulmonary Shunt

Intrapulmonary shunt is one of the most important causes of an increased A-a gradient and the development of arterial hypoxemia. In the presence of an intrapulmonary shunt, mixed venous blood is not exposed to alveolar gas, and it continues through the lungs to mix with oxygenated blood from normal areas of the lung. This mixing lowers the PaO_2. Clinically, shunting occurs when alveoli are not ventilated, as occurs in the presence of atelectasis, or when alveoli are filled with fluid, as occurs in the presence of pneumonia or pulmonary edema. The quantitative effect of an intrapulmonary shunt is described by the shunt equation:

$$\frac{\dot{Q}s}{\dot{Q}t} = \frac{Cc'O_2 - CaO_2}{Cc'O_2 - C\bar{v}O_2}$$

In the equation, $\dot{Q}s/\dot{Q}t$ is the shunt flow relative to total flow (i.e., shunt fraction), C is the oxygen content, c' is end-capillary blood, "a" is arterial blood, and $\bar{v}$ is mixed-venous blood.

Ventilation-Perfusion Mismatch

Ventilation-perfusion ($\dot{V}/\dot{Q}$) mismatch is similar to intrapulmonary shunt ($\dot{V}/\dot{Q} = 0$), with some important distinctions. In $\dot{V}/\dot{Q}$ mismatch, disparity between the amount of ventilation and perfusion in various alveoli leads to areas of high $\dot{V}/\dot{Q}$ (i.e., well-ventilated alveoli) and areas of low $\dot{V}/\dot{Q}$ (i.e., poorly ventilated alveoli). Because of the shape of the oxyhemoglobin dissociation curve, the improved oxygenation in well-ventilated areas cannot compensate for the low PO_2 in the poorly ventilated areas, resulting in arterial hypoxemia.

Clinically, in $\dot{V}/\dot{Q}$ mismatch, administering 100% oxygen can achieve a PO_2 on the plateau of the oxyhemoglobin dissociation curve. Conversely, administering 100% oxygen in the presence of an intrapulmonary shunt only adds more dissolved oxygen by the normally perfused alveoli. Arterial hypoxemia remaining despite administration of 100% oxygen is always caused by the presence of an intrapulmonary shunt.

Diffusion Impairment

Diffusion impairment is not equivalent to low diffusing capacity. For diffusion impairment to cause an A-a gradient, equilibrium has not occurred between the PO_2 in the alveolus and the PO_2 in pulmonary capillary blood. This rarely occurs, even in patients with limited diffusing capacity. The small A-a gradient that can result from diffusion impairment is easily eliminated with supplemental oxygen, making this a clinically unimportant problem.

Venous Oxygen Saturation

Low $S\bar{v}O_2$ causes a subtle but important effect when intrapulmonary shunt is already present. Shunt is a mixture of venous blood and blood from normal regions of the lungs. If the $S\bar{v}O_2$ is lower, the resulting mixture must have a lower PaO_2. Low CO may lower $S\bar{v}O_2$ significantly.

Carbon Dioxide

Carbon dioxide is produced in the tissues and removed in the lungs by ventilation. Carbon dioxide is carried in the blood as dissolved gas, as bicarbonate, and as a small amount bound to hemoglobin as carbaminohemoglobin. Unlike the oxyhemoglobin dissociation curve, the dissociation curve for carbon dioxide is essentially linear.

HYPERCAPNIA

Hypercapnia (i.e., high $PaCO_2$) is a sign of respiratory difficulty. A $PaCO_2$ value greater than 80 mm Hg may cause carbon dioxide narcosis, possibly contributing to delayed awakening in the postanesthesia care unit. Hypercapnia may be a sign of impending respiratory failure and apnea, in which arterial hypoxemia can rapidly ensue. Although the presence of hypercapnia may be obvious if capnography is used, this monitor is not always available, and substantial hypercapnia may go unnoticed. Supplemental oxygen can prevent arterial hypoxemia despite severe hypercapnia, and an arterial blood gas analysis would not necessarily be performed if hypercapnia were not suspected (see Fig. 6-8).

DETERMINANTS OF ARTERIAL CARBON DIOXIDE PARTIAL PRESSURE

$PaCO_2$ is a balance of production and removal. If removal exceeds production, $PaCO_2$ decreases. If production exceeds removal, $PaCO_2$ increases. The resulting $PaCO_2$ is expressed by the alveolar carbon dioxide equation:

$$PaCO_2 = k \cdot \frac{\dot{V}CO_2}{\dot{V}A}$$

In the equation, k is a constant (0.863) that corrects units, $\dot{V}CO_2$ is carbon dioxide production, and $\dot{V}A$ is alveolar ventilation.

Rebreathing

Because breathing circuits with rebreathing properties are frequently used in anesthesia, elevated inspired PCO_2 is a potential cause of hypercapnia. Exhausted carbon dioxide absorbents and malfunctioning expiratory valves on the anesthesia delivery circuit are possible causes of rebreathing in the operating room that are easily detected with capnography. Use of certain transport breathing circuits may be the most common cause of clinically significant rebreathing, which may be unrecognized because capnography is not routinely used during patient transport from the operating room.

Increased Carbon Dioxide Production

Several important physiologic causes of increased carbon dioxide production may cause hypercapnia under anesthesia (Table 6-4). For example, when a tourniquet is placed on a leg, cellular carbon dioxide production does not stop, and carbon dioxide accumulates in the tissues of the leg.

Table 6-4 Causes of Increased Carbon Dioxide Production
Fever
Malignant hyperthermia
Systemic absorption during laparoscopy procedures (physiologically similar to increased production)
Thyroid storm

Increased Dead Space

Dead space includes anatomic, alveolar, and physiologic (total) dead space. Anatomic dead space represents areas of the tracheobronchial tree that are not involved in gas exchange. This includes equipment dead space, such as the endotracheal tube and tubing distal to the Y-connector of the anesthesia delivery circuit. Alveolar dead space represents alveoli that do not participate in gas exchange due to lack of blood flow. Physiologic or total dead space represents the sum of anatomic and alveolar dead space. Most pathologically significant changes in dead space represent increases in alveolar dead space.

Dead space is increased in many clinical conditions. Emphysema and other end-stage lung diseases, such as cystic fibrosis, usually involve substantial dead space. Pulmonary embolism is a potential cause of significant increases in dead space (increased Zone 1). Physiologic processes that decrease PAP, such as hemorrhagic shock, can be expected to increase dead space. Increased airway pressure and positive end-expiratory pressure (PEEP) can also increase dead space.

Quantitative estimates of dead space are described by the Bohr equation, which expresses the ratio of dead space ventilation ($\dot{V}_D$) relative to tidal ventilation ($\dot{V}_T$).

$$\frac{\dot{V}_D}{\dot{V}_T} = \frac{Pa_{CO_2} - P\bar{E}_{CO_2}}{Pa_{CO_2}}$$

In the equation, $P\bar{E}_{CO_2}$ is the mixed-expired carbon dioxide.

For example, if the Pa_{CO_2} = 40 mm Hg and the $P\bar{E}_{CO_2}$ = 20 mm Hg during controlled ventilation of the lungs, the $\dot{V}_D/\dot{V}_T$ can be calculated as follows:

$$\dot{V}_D/\dot{V}_T = (40 - 20)/40$$
$$= 20/40$$
$$\dot{V}_D/\dot{V}_T = 0.5$$

Some physiologic dead space (25% to 30%) is considered normal because some anatomic dead space is always present. The Pa_{CO_2}-PET_{CO_2} gradient is a useful indication of the presence of alveolar dead space.

Hypoventilation

Decreased minute ventilation due to decreased tidal volume or breathing frequency, or both, is the most important and common cause of hypercapnia (Fig. 6-10). Alveolar

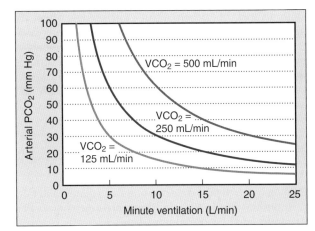

Figure 6-10 Carbon dioxide has a hyperbolic relationship with ventilation. The depicted curves are simulated with a normal resting carbon dioxide production (250 mL/min), low carbon dioxide production (125 mL/min, as during anesthesia), and increased carbon dioxide production (500 mL/min, as during moderate exercise). The value of physiologic dead space is assumed to be 30%.

ventilation ($\dot{V}_A$) combines minute ventilation and dead space ($\dot{V}_A = \dot{V}_T - \dot{V}_{DS}$). Ventilatory depressant effects of anesthetic drugs are a common cause of hypoventilation. Although increased minute ventilation can often completely compensate for elevated carbon dioxide production, rebreathing, or dead space, there is no physiologically useful compensation for inadequate minute ventilation.

If alveolar ventilation decreases by one half, Pa_{CO_2} is expected to double. This change occurs over several minutes as a new steady state develops. For example, during the first 30 to 60 seconds of apnea, Pa_{CO_2} increases significantly to mixed venous levels. Classic normal values are Pa_{CO_2} = 40 mm Hg and Pv_{CO_2} = 46 mm Hg. During apnea, Pa_{CO_2} rapidly increases about 6 mm Hg in the first minute, but this can be higher in patients with lower lung volumes or high arterial-to-venous carbon dioxide differences. After the first minute, Pa_{CO_2} increases more slowly as carbon dioxide production adds carbon dioxide to the blood, at about 3 mm Hg per minute.

DIFFERENTIAL DIAGNOSIS OF INCREASED ARTERIAL CARBON DIOXIDE PARTIAL PRESSURE

Increased Pa_{CO_2} values can be confirmed by assessing minute ventilation, capnography, and measuring an arterial blood gas value. Capnography can eliminate rebreathing. A clinical assessment of minute ventilation by physical examination and as measured by most ventilators should be adequate. Comparison of end-tidal P_{CO_2} with Pa_{CO_2} can identify abnormal alveolar dead space. Abnormal carbon dioxide production can be inferred. However, significant abnormalities of carbon dioxide physiology often are unrecognized when $PaCO_2$ is normal, because increased minute ventilation can compensate for substantial increases in dead space and carbon dioxide production. Noticing the presence of increased dead space when minute ventilation is high and $PaCO_2$ is 40 mm Hg is just as important as noticing abnormal dead space when the $PaCO_2$ is 80 mm Hg and minute ventilation is normal.

PULMONARY MECHANICS

Pulmonary mechanics concerns pressure, volume, and flow relationships in the lung and bronchial tree (Fig. 6-11). An understanding of pulmonary mechanics is essential for managing the ventilated patient. Pressures in the airway are routinely measured or sensed by the anesthesiologist providing positive-pressure ventilation.

Static Properties

The lung is made of elastic tissue that stretches under pressure (Fig. 6-12). Surface tension has a significant role in the compliance of the lung due to the air-fluid interface in the alveoli. Surfactant decreases surface tension and stabilizes small alveoli, which may otherwise tend to collapse.

The chest wall has its own compliance curve. At FRC, the chest wall tends to expand, but negative (subatmospheric) intrapleural pressure keeps the chest wall collapsed. The lungs tend to collapse, but they are held expanded due to the pressure difference from the airways to the intrapleural pressure. FRC is the natural balance point between the lungs and chest cavity.

Dynamic Properties and Airway Resistance

Airway resistance is mainly determined by the radius of the airway. For example, airway resistance is inversely proportional to the fourth power of the radius (Table 6-5). Resistance in small airways is physiologically different, because they have no cartilaginous structure or smooth muscle. Unlike capillaries, which have positive pressure inside to keep them open, small airways have zero (atmospheric) pressure during spontaneous ventilation. However, these airways are kept open by the same forces (i.e., pressure inside is greater than the pressure outside) that keep capillaries open. Negative pressure is transmitted from the intrapleural pressure, and this pressure difference keeps small airways open. When a disease process, such as emphysema, makes pleural pressure less negative, resistance in the small airways is increased, and dynamic compression occurs during exhalation.

During positive-pressure ventilation, resistance in anesthesia breathing equipment or airways manifests as

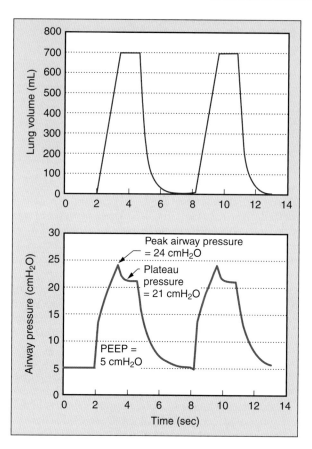

Figure 6-11 Lung volume is shown as a function of time (*top*) in a typical volume-controlled ventilator with constant flow rates. Lung volume increases at a constant rate during inspiration because of constant flow. Exhalation occurs with a passive relaxation curve. The lower panel shows the development of pressure over time. Pressure is produced from a static compliance component (see Fig. 6-12) and a resistance component. If flow is held at the plateau, a plateau pressure is reached, where there is no resistive pressure component. In this example, peak airway pressure (PAP) is 24 cm H_2O, and positive end-expiratory pressure (PEEP) is 5 cm H_2O. Dynamic compliance is tidal volume (VT)/(PAP – PEEP) = 37 mL/cm H_2O. Plateau pressure (Pplat) is 21 cm H_2O, and static compliance is VT/(Pplat – PEEP) = 44 mL/cm H_2O.

elevated airway pressures. Distinguishing airway resistance effects from static compliant components is facilitated by anesthesia machines that are equipped to provide an inspiratory pause. During ventilation, airway pressure reaches a peak inspiratory pressure, but when ventilation is paused, the pressure component from gas flow and resistance disappears, and the airway pressure decreases toward a plateau pressure (see Fig. 6-11).

Figure 6-12 A static compliance curve of a normal lung has a slight S shape. Slightly higher pressure can be required to open alveoli at low lung volumes (i.e., beginning of the curve), whereas higher distending pressures are needed as the lung is overdistended. Static compliance is measured as the change in volume divided by the change (Δ) in pressure (inspiratory pressure [PIP] – positive end-expiratory pressure [PEEP]), which is 46 mL/cm H_2O in this example.

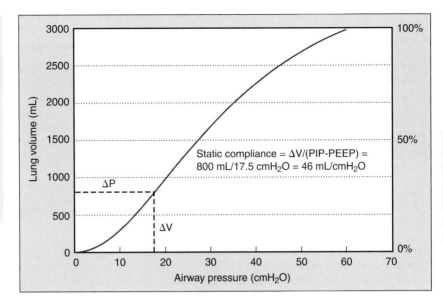

Static compliance = ΔV/(PIP-PEEP) = 800 mL/17.5 cmH_2O = 46 mL/cmH_2O

Table 6-5	Determinants of Airway Resistance
Radius of the airways	
Smooth muscle tone	
Bronchospasm	
Inflammation of the airways (asthma, chronic bronchitis)	
Foreign bodies	
Compression of airways	
Turbulent gas flow (helium a temporizing measure)	
Anesthesia equipment	

CONTROL OF BREATHING

Anesthesiologists are in a unique position to observe ventilatory control mechanisms because most drugs administered for sedation and anesthesia produce depression of breathing.

Central Integration and Rhythm Generation

Specific areas of the brainstem are involved in generating the respiratory rhythm, processing afferent signal information, and changing the efferent output to the inspiratory and expiratory muscles.

Central Chemoreceptors

Superficial areas on the ventrolateral medullary surface respond to pH and P_{CO_2}. Carbon dioxide is in rapid equilibrium with carbonic acid and therefore immediately affects the local pH surrounding the central chemoreceptors. Although the signal is transduced by protons, not carbon dioxide directly, it is acceptable to describe these chemoreceptors as carbon dioxide responsive. The central chemoreceptors are protected from rapid changes in metabolic pH by the blood-brain barrier.

Peripheral Chemoreceptors

Carotid bodies are the primary peripheral chemoreceptors in humans; aortic bodies have no significant role. Low P_{O_2}, high P_{CO_2}, and low pH stimulate the carotid bodies. Unlike the central chemoreceptors, metabolic acids immediately affect peripheral chemoreceptors. The mechanism of P_{O_2} transduction is unknown. Because of high blood flow, peripheral chemoreceptors are exposed to arterial, not venous, blood values.

Hypercapnic Ventilatory Response

Ventilation increases dramatically as Pa_{CO_2} is increased. In the presence of high P_{O_2} values, most of this ventilatory response results from the central chemoreceptors, whereas in the presence of room air, about one third of the response results from the peripheral chemoreceptors. The ventilatory response to carbon dioxide is fairly linear, although at Pa_{CO_2} levels below resting values, minute ventilation does not tend to go to zero because of an "awake" drive to breath (Fig. 6-13). At a high Pa_{CO_2} value, minute ventilation is eventually limited by maximal minute ventilation.

Lowering Pa_{CO_2} during anesthesia, as produced by assisted ventilation, results in a point at which ventilation

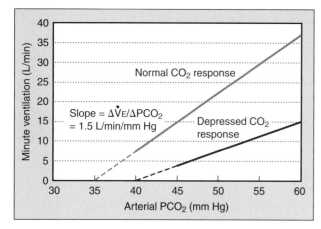

Figure 6-13 The hypercapnic ventilatory response (HCVR) is usually measured as the slope of the plot of P_{CO_2} versus minute ventilation ($\dot{V}_E$). End-tidal P_{CO_2} is usually substituted for Pa_{CO_2}. The apneic threshold, which is the carbon dioxide level at which ventilation is zero, can be extrapolated from the curve, but it is difficult to measure in awake volunteers. A depressed carbon dioxide response results from opioids, which lower the slope and raise the apneic threshold.

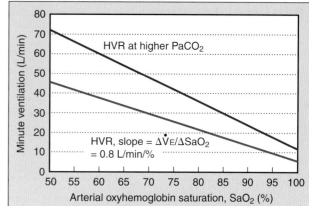

Figure 6-14 Hypoxic ventilatory response (HVR) expressed relative to Sa_{O_2} is approximately linear, which is simpler than the curvilinear response expressed as a function of Pa_{O_2}. HVR is the slope of the linear plot. HVR is higher at higher carbon dioxide concentrations. Both absolute ventilation and the slope are shifted. Low Pa_{CO_2} likewise lowers HVR.

ceases (i.e., apneic threshold). As CO_2 rises, ventilation returns at the apneic threshold, then stabilizes at a Pa_{CO_2} set-point that is about 5 mm Hg higher. Assisted ventilation is of limited value in lowering Pa_{CO_2}.

The brainstem response to carbon dioxide is slow, with 90% of steady-state ventilation being reached in about 5 minutes. When allowing the Pa_{CO_2} to rise in an apneic patient, it may take a noticeably long time to stabilize minute ventilation, which is a direct consequence of the dynamics of the central ventilatory drive.

Hypoxic Ventilatory Response

Ventilation increases as Pa_{O_2} and Sa_{O_2} decrease, reflecting stimulation of the peripheral chemoreceptors. The central response to hypoxia results in decreased minute ventilation, called *hypoxic ventilatory decline (HVD)*. The timing and combination of these effects means that in prolonged arterial hypoxemia, ventilation rises to an initial peak reflecting the rapid response of the peripheral chemoreceptors, then falls to an intermediate plateau in 15 to 20 minutes reflecting the slower addition of HVD.

Although it is P_{O_2} that affects the carotid body, it is easier to consider the hypoxic ventilatory response in terms of oxyhemoglobin desaturation because minute ventilation changes linearly with Sa_{O_2} (Fig. 6-14). The effects of hypoxia and hypercapnia on the carotid body are synergistic. At high Pa_{CO_2} levels, the response to hypoxia is much larger, whereas low Pa_{CO_2} levels can dramatically decrease responsiveness. Unlike the hypercapnic venti-

latory response, the response to hypoxia is rapid and takes only seconds to appear.

Effects of Anesthesia

Opioids, sedative-hypnotics, and volatile anesthetics have profound depressant effects on ventilation and ventilatory control. Opioid receptors are present on neurons considered responsible for respiratory rhythm generation. Sedative-hypnotics work primarily on γ-aminobutyric acid A receptors ($GABA_A$), which provide inhibitory input in multiple neurons of the respiratory system. Volatile anesthetics decrease excitatory neurotransmission. All of these drugs exert most of their depressant effects in the central integratory area and therefore clinically appear to decrease the hypoxic and hypercapnic ventilatory responses similarly. Specific effects of drugs on peripheral chemoreceptors include the inhibitory effects of dopamine and the slight excitatory effects of dopaminergic blockers such as droperidol.

Disorders of Ventilatory Control

Neonates of low postconceptual age (<60 weeks) may have episodes of apnea after anesthesia. Likewise, sudden infant death syndrome may be a result of immature ventilatory control systems. Ondine's curse, originally described after surgery near the upper cervical spinal cord, results in profound hypoventilation during sleep and anesthesia due to abnormalities in the central integratory system that seem to blunt the hypoxic and hypercapnic ventilatory responses. Idiopathic varieties of Ondine's curse have been found in children and are referred to as *primary central alveolar hypoventilation syndromes*. Morbidly obese patients and those with sleep apnea may exhibit abnormalities of ventilatory control.

Periodic breathing is commonly observed during drug-induced sedation. Mechanistically, this is most likely when peripheral chemoreceptors are activated by mild arterial hypoxemia. Continual overcorrection and undercorrection of the PaO_2 leads to oscillations of $PaCO_2$ and SaO_2.

INTEGRATION OF THE HEART AND LUNGS

The interrelationship between the heart and lungs is suggested by the Fick equation, which correlates oxygen consumption and oxygen needs at the tissue level.

$$\dot{V}O_2 = CO \bullet (CaO_2 - C\bar{v}O_2)$$

In the equation, $\dot{V}O_2$ is oxygen consumption, CO is cardiac output, CaO_2 is the arterial oxygen content, and $C\bar{v}O_2$ is the mixed venous oxygen content.

Oxygen Delivery

Oxygen delivery (DO_2) is the total amount of oxygen supplied to tissues and is a function of CO and CaO_2:

$$DO_2 = CO \bullet CaO_2$$

DO_2 can be limited by decreases in CO or CaO_2. CaO_2 can be limited by anemia or hypoxemia.

Oxygen Extraction

Different indices can be used to assess how much oxygen is removed from blood by tissues to meet their metabolic demand. Mixed venous oxygen saturation ($S\bar{v}O_2$) is normally about 75%. If tissues extract more oxygen, $S\bar{v}O_2$ may decrease. However, with high FIO_2, $S\bar{v}O_2$ may increase because of the added amount of dissolved oxygen. The most reliable figure is the calculated oxygen extraction ratio:

$$O_2 \text{ extraction} = \frac{CaO_2 - C\bar{v}O_2}{CaO_2}$$

ANEMIA

An example of threatened oxygen supply is anemia. To adapt to anemia, the body can increase CO or extract more oxygen. The normal physiologic response is to increase CO and maintain oxygen delivery. Increased HR and SV are responsible for this compensation. However, under anesthesia with a near-absent HR response, increased oxygen extraction is a more important mechanism of compensation.

METABOLIC DEMAND

Increased oxygen consumption is usually met with a combination of increased CO and increased oxygen extraction. Whereas oxygen consumption is usually constant and relatively low under anesthesia, recovery from anesthesia may be associated with significant increases in metabolic demands. Shivering and early ambulation after outpatient surgery are stresses that may affect patients still recovering from anesthesia or after significant blood loss. Increased minute ventilation is required to meet increased oxygen needs and to eliminate the extra carbon dioxide produced.

REFERENCES

1. Berne RM, Levy MN. Cardiovascular Physiology, 8th ed. St. Louis: Mosby, 2001.

2. Nunn JF. Nunn's Applied Respiratory Physiology, 4th ed. Boston: Butterworth-Heinemann, 1993.

3. West JB. Respiratory Physiology: The Essentials, 7th ed. Philadelphia: Lippincott Williams & Wilkins, 2005.

II

Chapter 7

AUTONOMIC NERVOUS SYSTEM

Muhammad Iqbal Shaikh

Involuntary regulation of cardiovascular, gastrointestinal, and thermal homeostasis of the human body occurs principally through the autonomic nervous system (ANS). Often, the success of anesthetic management depends on the maintenance of homeostasis in a variety of changing situations. In this regard, anesthesiology has been described as the practice of ANS medicine.[1]

Knowledge of the pharmacologic effects of catecholamines, sympathomimetics, antihypertensives, β-adrenergic agonists, β-adrenergic antagonists, anticholinergics, and anticholinesterases is helpful in predicting potential adverse drug reactions during the perioperative period. The most practical preoperative test for evaluation of ANS function is determination of orthostasis. ANS dysfunction is suggested by decrease in systolic blood pressure of more than 30 mm Hg and the absence of an increase in the heart rate on assuming upright posture.[2]

ANATOMY AND PHYSIOLOGY OF THE AUTONOMIC NERVOUS SYSTEM

The central ANS includes the hypothalamus, medulla, and pons. Although the cerebral cortex is the highest level of ANS integration, the hypothalamic nuclei are the principal sites for ANS organization and body responses to stress, systematic blood pressure control, and temperature regulation. The medulla and pons are vital centers for hemodynamic and ventilatory control, integrating and maintaining the automaticity of ventilation.

The peripheral ANS is divided into sympathetic nervous system (SNS, or thoracolumbar nervous system) and the parasympathetic nervous system (PNS, or craniosacral nervous system) (Fig. 7-1). Preganglionic fibers of the SNS arise from the cells in the thoracolumbar portions of the spinal cord, whereas the cell bodies of the preganglionic fibers of the PNS originate in the craniosacral region. First-order neurons of the SNS and PNS originate within the central nervous system (CNS), and preganglionic

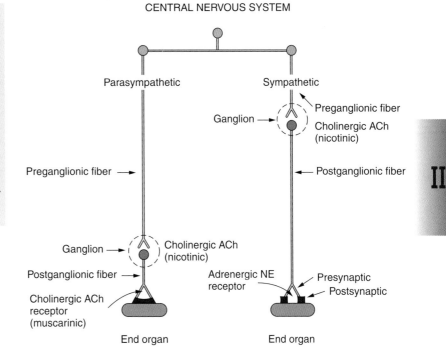

CENTRAL NERVOUS SYSTEM

Figure 7-1 Schematic diagram of the peripheral autonomic nervous system. Preganglionic fibers and postganglionic fibers of the parasympathetic nervous system release acetylcholine (ACh) as the neurotransmitter. Postganglionic fibers of the sympathetic nervous system release norepinephrine (NE) as the neurotransmitter (exceptions are fibers to sweat glands, which release ACh). (From Lawson NW, Wallfisch HK. Cardiovascular Pharmacology: A new look at the pressors. *In* Stoelting RK, Barash J (eds): Advances in Anesthesia. Chicago: Year Book Medical Publishers, 1986, pp 195-270, with permission.)

II

fibers relay impulses to second-order neurons known as the autonomic ganglia. The autonomic ganglia contain the cell bodies of the postganglionic fibers responsible for relaying the information to the effector organ. Preganglionic fibers of the SNS and PNS are myelinated (i.e., rapid-conduction fibers), and postganglionic fibers are non-myelinated. The postganglionic fibers of the SNS are distributed throughout the body and are responsible for more generalized mass reflex response. The distribution of PNS is more limited. The PNS has its terminal ganglia near the organ innervated and is more discrete in its discharge of impulses.

Sympathetic Nervous System

The preganglionic fibers of the SNS originate in the intermediolateral column of thoracic (T1 to T12) and the first three lumbar segments (L1 to L3) of the spinal cord. The myelinated motor nerves leave the spinal cord as white communicating fibers and enter one of the paired chains of 22 sympathetic ganglia. The fibers originating from these ganglia synapse within the ganglion, synapse in the ganglion at other levels and emerge as postganglionic fibers, or exit as preganglionic fibers to synapse in outlying unpaired ganglia such as celiac or mesenteric ganglia. An exception to the rule is the adrenal gland, which receives preganglionic fibers directly.

The effector organs of the SNS have adrenergic receptors, which are characterized as alpha (α) or beta (β), and dopamine (D) receptors (see Fig. 7-1). The pregan-

glionic fibers of the SNS and PNS release acetylcholine as the neurotransmitter at the preganglionic neuronal site; the postganglionic fibers release norepinephrine or dopamine as the neurotransmitter (Fig. 7-2).[3] Norepinephrine stimulates α- and β-adrenergic receptors, whereas dopamine stimulates dopamine receptors present on the effector site. Multiple classes of alpha and dopamine receptors have been identified: α_1, α_2, D_1 to D_5. The α_1-receptors are mostly localized on the postsynaptic membranes of vascular and intestinal smooth muscle and endocrine glands, and a few are present in the heart. The α_2-receptors are usually presynaptic (except in the CNS) and function in a negative-feedback loop such that their activation inhibits subsequent release of neurotransmitter. Stimulation of the α- and β-adrenergic receptors by endogenous catecholamines or synthetic agonists and antagonists produces predictable pharmacologic responses (Table 7-1).

The action of endogenously released catecholamines at the synaptic cleft is terminated by three mechanisms: uptake into the presynaptic terminals and storage into norepinephrine vesicles for reuse; extraneuronal uptake (or reuptake), in which norepinephrine is metabolized by monoamine oxidase and catecholamine-*O*-methyltransferase to form vanillylmandelic acid; and diffusion. Termination of endogenously released norepinephrine activity occurs almost entirely by uptake back into the storage vesicles. Diffusion is the predominant pathway for inactivation of effects produced by catecholamines administered exogenously.

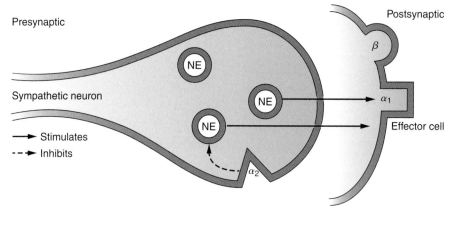

Figure 7-2 Schematic depiction of the postganglionic sympathetic nerve ending. Release of the neurotransmitter norepinephrine (NE) from the nerve ending results in stimulation of postsynaptic receptors, which are classified as α_1, β_1, and β_2. Stimulation of presynaptic α_2-receptors results in inhibition of NE release from the nerve ending. (Adapted from Ram CVS, Kaplan NM. Alpha- and beta-receptor blocking drugs in the treatment of hypertension. *In* Harvey WP (ed): Current Problems in Cardiology. Chicago: Year Book Medical Publishers, 1970, with permission.)

An important factor in the pharmacologic responses elicited by the adrenergic receptors is the dynamic state of adrenergic receptors. The density and sensitivity of α- and β-adrenergic receptors are modulated by the concentration of neurotransmitter or circulating hormone. For example, increased plasma concentrations of norepinephrine result in decreased density or sensitivity, or both, of β-adrenergic receptors in the cell membrane (i.e., downregulation).

Parasympathetic Nervous System

The PNS has its cell bodies in the brainstem and the sacral segment of the spinal cord. Cranial nerves III (oculomotor), VII (facial), IX (glossopharyngeal), and X (vagus) form the cranial outflow, whereas the sacral outflow originates from the intermediolateral gray horns of the second, third, and fourth sacral nerves. Acetylcholine is the principal neurotransmitter released at the postganglionic fibers of the PNS, but other neurotransmitters, such as vasoactive intestinal peptide, also may be released. Postganglionic fibers of the PNS that release acetylcholine as the neurotransmitter are described as cholinergic, and postsynaptic receptor sites are described as nicotinic (somatic site) and muscarinic (see Fig. 7-1). Stimulation of nicotinic or muscarinic receptors by acetylcholine or synthetic cholinergic agonists produces predictable and distinct pharmacologic responses (see Table 7-1). The action of acetylcholine at the synaptic site is terminated by acetylcholinesterase. A similar enzyme, pseudocholinesterase (i.e., plasma cholinesterase), is present in the plasma but does not appear to be physiologically important in terminating the action of acetylcholine.

CATECHOLAMINES

Catecholamines are compounds with hydroxyl groups on the 3 and 4 positions on the benzene ring of phenylethylamine (Fig. 7-3). Dopamine, norepinephrine, and epinephrine are endogenous catecholamines, which are synthesized in the nerve terminals of the SNS and adrenal medulla. They regulate most of the endogenous physiologic functions, especially during stress. Besides the endogenous catecholamines, there are a number of synthetic catecholamines; the most common are isoproterenol and dobutamine.

Pharmacologic effects produced by catecholamines reflect the ability of these substances to stimulate adrenergic receptors. All the endogenous catecholamines are ineffective after oral administration because they are conjugated and oxidized in the gastrointestinal mucosa and liver. Clinically, catecholamines are administered as continuous intravenous infusions to produce desirable pharmacologic effects, which manifest predominantly in the cardiovascular system (Table 7-2).

Dopamine

Dopamine is the immediate precursor of norepinephrine and epinephrine. This catecholamine is unique among the sympathomimetics because of its effects at multiple receptors sites depending on the dose. When administered in low doses (<3 µg/kg/min IV), dopamine stimulates D_1 receptors, which occur primarily in the renal, mesenteric, and coronary beds. Stimulation of D_1 receptors by dopamine leads to vasodilatation and associated increases in renal blood flow, glomerular filtration rate, sodium excretion (also partially due to inhibition of aldosterone), and urine

Table 7–1 Characteristics of the Autonomic Nervous System

Receptor	Effector Organ	Response to Stimulation	Synthetic Drugs	
			Agonist	*Antagonist*
Beta$_1$	Heart	Increased heart rate Increased contractility Increased conduction velocity	Dobutamine Dopamine Isoproterenol*	Metoprolol Esmolol Propranolol* Timolol* Labetalol*
	Fat cells	Lipolysis		
Beta$_2$	Blood vessels (especially skeletal and coronary arteries)	Dilation	Albuterol Ritodrine	Propranolol* Timolol* Labetalol*
	Bronchioles Uterus Kidneys Liver Pancreas	Dilation Relaxation Renin secretion Glycogenolysis Gluconeogenesis Insulin secretion		
Alpha$_1$	Blood vessels	Constriction	Phenylephrine	Prazosin Phentolamine† Labetalol
	Pancreas Intestine and bladder	Inhibition of insulin secretion Relaxation Constriction of sphincters		
Alpha$_2$	Postganglionic (presynaptic sympathetic nerve ending) Central nervous system (postsynaptic) Platelets	Inhibition of norepinephrine release Increase in potassium conductance (?) Aggregation	Clonidine Dexmedetomidine	Yohimbine Phentolamine†
Dopamine$_1$	Blood vessels	Dilation	Fenoldopam	Droperidol
Dopamine$_2$	Postganglionic (presynaptic) sympathetic nerve ending	Inhibition of norepinephrine release	Dopamine	Domperidone
Muscarinic	Heart	Decreased heart rate Decreased contractility Decreased conduction velocity	Methacholine Carbachol	Atropine Scopolamine Glycopyrrolate
	Bronchioles Salivary glands Intestine Bladder	Constriction Stimulation of secretions Contraction Relaxation of sphincters Stimulation of secretions Contraction Relaxation of sphincter		
Nicotinic	Neuromuscular junction	Skeletal muscle contraction	Succinylcholine	Nondepolarizing muscle relaxants
	Autonomic ganglia	Sympathetic nervous system stimulation		

*Produces mixed beta-1 and beta-2 effects
†Produces mixed alpha-1 and alpha-2 effects

Figure 7-3 Chemical structures of endogenous (i.e., dopamine, norepinephrine, and epinephrine) and exogenous (i.e., isoproterenol and dobutamine) catecholamines.

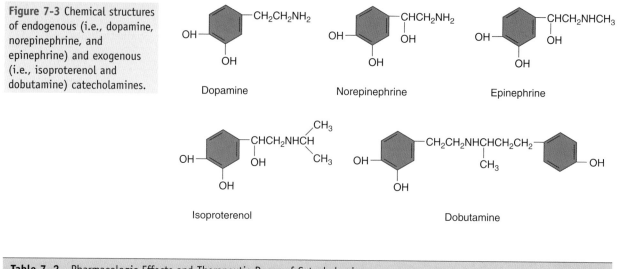

Dopamine   Norepinephrine   Epinephrine

Isoproterenol   Dobutamine

Table 7–2 Pharmacologic Effects and Therapeutic Doses of Catecholamines

Catecholamine	Mean Arterial Pressure	Heart Rate	Cardiac Output	Systemic Vascular Resistance	Renal Blood Flow	Cardiac Dysrhythmias	Preparation (mg in 250 mL)	Intravenous Dose (µg/kg/min)
Dopamine	+	+	+ + +	+	+ + +	+	200 (800 µg/mL)	2-20
Norepinephrine	+ + +	–	–	+ + +	– – –	+	4 (16 µg/mL)	0.01-0.1
Epinephrine	+	+ +	+ +	+ +	– –	+ + +	1 (4 µg/mL)	0.03-0.15
Isoproterenol	–	+ + +	+ + +	– –	–	+ + +	1 (4 µg/mL)	0.03-0.15
Dobutamine	+	+	+ + +	–	+ +	–	250 (1000 µg/mL)	2-20

+, mild increase; + +, moderate increase; + + +, marked increase; –, mild decrease; – –, moderate decrease; – – –, marked decrease.

output. Dopamine exerts a positive inotropic effect (i.e., β_1-adrenergic effect) when administered at higher doses (3 to 10 µg/kg/min IV). This inotropic effect is characterized by increased myocardial contractility without marked changes in the heart rate and systemic blood pressure. Dopamine also evokes the release of endogenous stores of norepinephrine from nerve terminals, and this predisposes the patient to cardiac dysrhythmias. At higher doses (10 to 20 µg/kg/min IV), dopamine stimulates β- and α- adrenergic receptors, whereas at doses of more than 20 µg/kg/min administered intravenously, dopamine stimulates α_1-adrenergic receptors, leading to vasoconstriction and significant increases in systemic blood pressure. Intravenous infusion of dopamine interferes with the ventilatory response to arterial hypoxemia, reflecting the role of dopamine as an inhibitory neurotransmitter at the carotid bodies. High doses of dopamine can also inhibit the release of insulin, leading to hyperglycemia.

CLINICAL USES
Dopamine is most often used in the treatment of congestive heart failure (CHF), cardiogenic shock, and septic shock.

These conditions are associated with decreased cardiac output, decreased systemic blood pressure, increased left ventricular end-diastolic pressure, and oliguria. Dopamine, because of its inotropic and chronotropic effects, increases stroke volume and cardiac output, improves systemic blood pressure, and reduces left ventricle size. Rapid metabolism of dopamine mandates its use as a continuous intravenous infusion. Extravasation of dopamine, like norepinephrine, produces intense local vasoconstriction, which may be treated by local infiltration of phentolamine. Because alkaline solutions may inactivate dopamine, it is prepared in a solution of 5% glucose in water.

Fenoldopam

Fenoldopam is a relatively selective postsynaptic D_1-agonist with no significant D_2-, α-adrenergic, or β_2-adrenergic effects (see Table 7-1). Low-dose infusion of fenoldopam (0.1 to 0.5 µg/kg/min) produces renal vasodilation and increased renal blood flow without changes in systemic blood pressure. Higher doses of fenoldopam may decrease systemic blood pressure, and the principal use of this drug is as an intravenous antihypertensive drug. A renoprotective effect of fenoldopam has not been established.

Norepinephrine

Norepinephrine is the neurotransmitter liberated by postganglionic SNS nerves. Stimulation of α_1- and β_1-receptors by norepinephrine produces vasoconstriction and increases in systolic, diastolic, and mean arterial blood pressure. Increased afterload produces baroreceptor-mediated reflex bradycardia. Cardiac output may be unchanged or decreased with an increase in coronary blood flow. Clinically, a continuous infusion of norepinephrine may be used to treat profound systemic hypotension during shock or refractory hypotension, as may occur in the early period after ligation of the vascular supply to a pheochromocytoma. The β_2-agonist effects of norepinephrine are minimal.

Epinephrine

Epinephrine stimulates α_1-, β_1-, and β_2-receptors. Low doses of epinephrine stimulate α_1-receptors in the skin, mucosa, and hepatorenal vasculature, producing vasoconstriction, whereas β_2-induced vasodilation predominates in skeletal muscles. The net effect is decreased systemic vascular resistance and a preferential distribution of cardiac output to skeletal muscles. Renal blood flow is greatly decreased during infusion of epinephrine, even with an unchanged systemic blood pressure. Stimulation of β_1-receptors increases heart rate and myocardial contractility, resulting in an increased cardiac output. Because systemic blood pressure is not greatly elevated, compensatory baroreceptor reflexes are not elicited, and cardiac output is increased. β_1-Adrenergic stimulation also increases the automaticity of the heart, which manifests as cardiac irritability, most often in the form of ventricular premature contractions.

Of all the catecholamines, epinephrine has the most significant effects on metabolism. For example, β-adrenergic stimulation from epinephrine increases adipose tissue lipolysis and liver glycogenolysis, whereas α_1-adrenergic stimulation inhibits release of insulin from the pancreas (see Table 7-1). Epinephrine release in response to surgical stimulation is a likely explanation for hyperglycemia that is often observed in the perioperative period.

CLINICAL USES

Epinephrine may be used as a continuous infusion to treat decreased myocardial contractility. Subcutaneous epinephrine is also used in combination with local anesthetics to decrease systemic absorption and to provide local hemostasis. Epinephrine is the drug of choice in the treatment of life-threatening allergic reactions or for the rapid relief of hypersensitivity reactions. It is used to restore cardiac rhythm in patients with cardiac arrest and to treat refractory bradycardia.

Isoproterenol

Isoproterenol is a synthetic catecholamine, which acts as a nonselective synthetic β-adrenergic agonist with no detectable effects on α_1-receptors. Infusion of isoproterenol increases myocardial contractility, heart rate, systolic blood pressure, and cardiac automaticity, and it decreases systemic vascular resistance in skeletal muscles and in renal and mesenteric vascular beds (i.e., β_2-adrenergic effect). The result is an increase in cardiac output, a decrease in mean arterial pressure, and a significant increase in myocardial oxygen requirements. Large doses of isoproterenol may cause tachycardia, diastolic hypotension, and a decrease in coronary blood flow leading to cardiac dysrhythmias, particularly in patients with ischemic heart disease. Although isoproterenol relieves bronchoconstriction and bronchospasm, it has largely been replaced by other highly effective, β_2-selective sympathomimetics.

CLINICAL USES

Isoproterenol may be administered as a continuous infusion to increase heart rate after heart transplantation or as a chemical pacemaker in complete heart block. Isoproterenol may be selected in patients with valvular heart disease in an attempt to decrease pulmonary vascular resistance.

Dobutamine

Dobutamine is a synthetic catecholamine obtained by substitution of a bulky aromatic group on the side chain of dopamine. Due to the center of asymmetry, the racemic mixture of dobutamine consists of positive (+) and negative (−) isomers. The (−) isomer acts on α_1-adrenergic receptors with pressor responses, and the (+) isomer is a potent β-adrenergic receptor agonist and a potent α_1-adrenergic receptor antagonist that blocks the effects of (−) dobutamine. The most prominent effect during infusion of dobutamine (2 to 20 μg/kg/min IV) is a dose-dependent increase in cardiac output with a decrease or no change in systematic vascular resistance. Dobutamine has significantly more inotropic than chronotropic effect. It enhances the automaticity of the sinus and atrioventricular node and facilitates intraventricular conduction. Dobutamine in combination with dopamine is used in treating systemic hypotension, especially in oliguric patients. Dobutamine is prepared in 5% dextrose in water, because it is inactivated in alkaline solutions.

SYMPATHOMIMETICS

Sympathomimetics are synthetic drugs obtained by dehydroxylation of hydroxyl groups at positions 3 and 4 on the benzene ring (Fig. 7-4). They are mostly used as vasopressors or inotropes (ephedrine) to reverse the downward trend in systematic blood pressure during regional

II

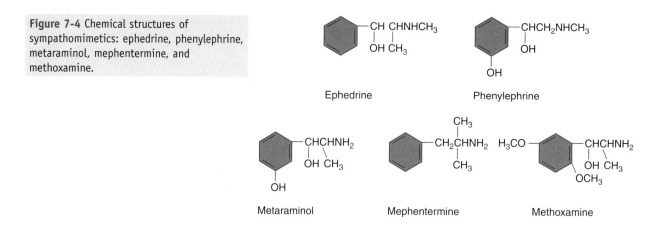

Figure 7-4 Chemical structures of sympathomimetics: ephedrine, phenylephrine, metaraminol, mephentermine, and methoxamine.

or general anesthesia. Sympathomimetics act at α- and β-adrenergic receptors by a direct effect at receptor sites or through an indirect effect by releasing endogenous norepinephrine (Table 7-3). Prolonged administration of sympathomimetics to support systematic blood pressure is not recommended.

Classification

Sympathomimetics are classified according to their selectivity for stimulating α- or β-adrenergic receptors, or both (see Table 7-3). Alternatively, sympathomimetics may be classified as direct acting (i.e., mimicking the effects of norepinephrine) or indirect acting (i.e., evoking the release of endogenous norepinephrine) (see Table 7-3). Knowing the anatomic distribution of either receptor classification and the sympathomimetic's receptor preference permits individualized selection of a drug to increase systemic blood pressure. Phenylephrine or methoxamine is used when cardiac output is adequate, as in treating hypotension after spinal or epidural anesthesia or to increase coronary perfusion in patients with coronary artery disease or aortic stenosis without chronotropic side effects.

Ephedrine is more likely to be selected when an increase in myocardial contractility is desirable.

Adverse Effects

Cardiac dysrhythmias that occur in association with administration of a sympathomimetic may reflect drug-induced β-adrenergic stimulation. Conversely, a disadvantage of using a sympathomimetic that lacks β-adrenergic effects is unopposed α-adrenergic receptor–induced peripheral vasoconstriction. Vasoconstriction results in increased diastolic blood pressure and associated baroreceptor reflex–mediated bradycardia and possible decreases in cardiac output. Antihypertensives that decrease SNS activity may decrease the pressor response elicited by an indirect-acting sympathomimetic, whereas the response to a direct-acting drug may be enhanced as receptors are sensitized (denervation hypersensitivity) by lack of tonic impulses.

Treatment of patients with tricyclic antidepressants or monoamine oxidase inhibitors (MAOIs) that increase the availability of endogenous norepinephrine introduces the potential for adverse drug interactions with sympath-

Table 7–3 Classification and Therapeutic Doses of Sympathomimetics

Sympathomimetic	Alpha$_1$	Beta$_1$	Beta$_2$	Direct (D) or Indirect (I) Action	Intravenous Dose for an Adult (mg)
Ephedrine	+ +	+ +	+	I (some D)	10-25
Phenylephrine	+ + +	–	0	D	0.05-0.2
Metaraminol	+ + +	+ +	0	I (some D)	1.5-5
Mephentermine	+	+ +	+	I	10-25
Methoxamine	+ + +	0	0	D	5-10

0, no change; +, mild stimulation; + +, moderate stimulation; + + +, marked stimulation.

omimetics. For example, administration of an indirect-acting drug such as ephedrine can elicit an exaggerated systemic blood pressure response in patients being treated with tricyclic antidepressants or MAOIs. The risk of such an adverse response seems to be greatest during the first 14 to 21 days of treatment with tricyclic antidepressants or MAOIs.[4] During this acute treatment period with antidepressants, systemic hypertension should be treated with a peripheral vasodilator, but hypotension is better managed with a decreased dose of a direct-acting drug such as phenylephrine.

Meperidine has been reported to produce hypertensive crisis, convulsions, and coma when used with MAOIs. After the period of acute treatment with antidepressants, there seems to be downregulation of receptors and a decreased likelihood of exaggerated systemic blood pressure responses. It is accepted that tricyclic antidepressants or MAOIs may be continued throughout the perioperative period without the introduction of unacceptable risk of adverse drug interaction.[5]

Ephedrine

Ephedrine is an indirect-acting sympathomimetic with α- and β-adrenergic agonist activity because it stimulates the release of norepinephrine and has some direct-acting effects. Ephedrine is also effective after oral administration. Clinically, the cardiovascular effects of ephedrine resemble those of epinephrine, but its systemic blood pressure–elevating response is less intense and lasts about 10 times longer. Intravenous administration of ephedrine results in increases in systolic and diastolic blood pressure, heart rate, and cardiac output. Systemic vascular resistance may be altered minimally because vasoconstriction (i.e., α-adrenergic stimulation) in some vascular beds is offset by vasodilation (i.e., β$_2$-adrenergic stimulation) in other areas. Patients taking β-adrenergic–blocking drugs when given ephedrine may show cardiovascular responses more typical of α-adrenergic stimulation.

Ephedrine is a commonly recommended drug for the treatment of anesthesia-induced hypotension in pregnant women. Tachyphylaxis may occur with repetitive dosing, presumably because of a persistent block of adrenergic receptors. Alternatively, tachyphylaxis may result from depletion of norepinephrine stores. β-Adrenergic stimulation produced by ephedrine may evoke cardiac dysrhythmias, especially in the presence of drugs that sensitize the heart to the effects of catecholamines.

Phenylephrine

Phenylephrine is a direct-acting sympathomimetic that increases venous constriction more than arterial constriction (i.e., α$_1$-adrenergic effect). It is less potent and longer acting than norepinephrine. Acutely, preload and afterload are increased, with a net effect of an increased

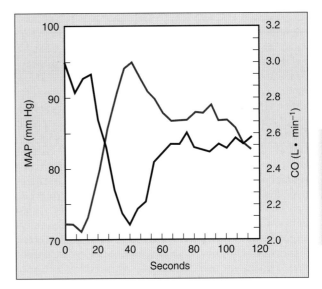

Figure 7-5 Hemodynamic responses to the rapid intravenous injection of phenylephrine. CO, cardiac output (*black line*); MAP, mean arterial pressure (*red line*). (Adapted from Schwinn DA, Reves JG. Time course and hemodynamic effects of alpha-1 adrenergic bolus administration in anesthetized patients with myocardial disease. Anesth Analg 1989;68:571-578, with permission.)

systemic blood pressure with reflex bradycardia and an associated transient decrease in cardiac output (Fig. 7-5).[6]

ANTIHYPERTENSIVES

Elevated systemic blood pressure causes pathologic changes in peripheral arterial vasculature, leading to cardiac failure, renal insufficiency, and stroke. Antihypertensives are useful in decreasing systemic blood pressure toward normal levels by selectively impairing SNS function at the heart and peripheral vasculature sites. Because these drugs are continued during the perioperative period to maintain optimal control of the systemic blood pressure, there often may be a predominance of PNS tone, and the response to sympathomimetics may be modified. During anesthesia, an exaggerated decrease in systemic blood pressure (as associated with hemorrhage, positive airway pressure, or sudden change in body position) may reflect an impaired degree of compensatory peripheral vasoconstriction. Antihypertensives that act centrally are associated with sedation and decreased anesthetic requirements (MAC).[7] An understanding of the mechanism of action of antihypertensives and the pathophysiology of associated hemodynamic changes during anesthesia helps in the optimal management of treated patients during perioperative period.

Angiotensin-Converting Enzyme Inhibitors

Angiotensin-converting enzyme (ACE) inhibitors (e.g., captopril, enalapril, lisinopril, ramipril) are uniquely valuable in the treatment of essential hypertension, postmyocardial infarction (i.e., improved survival), and diabetic nephropathy. They are also useful in treating patients with CHF and mitral regurgitation because of their cardiac-remodeling and afterload-reducing properties. ACE inhibitors have minimal CNS side effects (e.g., sedation, sexual dysfunction), resulting in improved patient compliance. Side effects associated with abrupt discontinuation of antihypertensives, such as metabolic changes (e.g., hypokalemia, hyponatremia), rebound hypertension, bronchospasm, and CHF, are not seen in patients treated with ACE inhibitors. By blocking the conversion of angiotensin I to angiotensin II, ACE inhibitors prevent angiotensin II mediated vasoconstriction. Cardiac output may remain normal or increase with filling pressure unchanged. ACE inhibitors also result in reductions in norepinephrine and plasma aldosterone levels.

SIDE EFFECTS

Captopril may cause reversible neutropenia, dermatitis, and angioedema. Enalapril produces headache, dizziness, and syncope. ACE inhibitors may cause hyperkalemia and hypotension in hypovolemic patients. ACE inhibitor therapy is continued until surgery and then reinitiated as soon as possible postoperatively.[8] There is concern, however, about potential hemodynamic instability and hypotension in patients receiving ACE inhibitors in the preoperative period. Prolonged hypotension has been observed in patients being treated with ACE inhibitors and undergoing general anesthesia for elective operations, especially if large blood or fluid shifts occur.

Clonidine

Clonidine is a centrally acting antihypertensive that stimulates α_2-adrenergic receptors in the pontomedullary region of the CNS. This stimulation inhibits SNS activity, leading to decreased outflow to the periphery. The net effect of decreased SNS activity are reductions in cardiac output, systemic vascular resistance, and systemic blood pressure.

CLINICAL USES

Acute administration of clonidine has been used to differentiate essential hypertension from suspected pheochromocytoma. Unlike patients with pheochromocytoma, the plasma concentration of norepinephrine is markedly suppressed in patients with essential hypertension. Clonidine ameliorates some of the adverse signs and symptoms of withdrawal from opioids and tobacco craving.[9] It is speculated that clonidine may replace opioid-mediated inhibition with α_2-mediated inhibition of central SNS activity.

Preoperative administration of small doses of clonidine decreases the MAC of injected and inhaled drugs, presumably reflecting the sedative and analgesic effects of this drug.[7] SNS responses evoked by direct laryngoscopy and surgical stimulation are attenuated by prior treatment with clonidine. These antihypertensive effects of clonidine may last 6 to 24 hours. Injection of clonidine into the epidural or subarachnoid space produces analgesia and, unlike opioids, does not produce depression of ventilation, pruritus, nausea, and vomiting. Bradycardia and sedation, however, may accompany this route of administration of clonidine.

SIDE EFFECTS

The major adverse effects of clonidine are dry mouth, sedation, marked bradycardia, and contact dermatitis, which occur in 15% to 20% of patients treated with a clonidine transdermal patch. Withdrawal symptoms (e.g., increased systemic blood pressure) during the preoperative and postoperative period have been described in patients who discontinued clonidine abruptly before surgery.[10] The speculated mechanism for this rebound hypertension is an acute increase in systemic vascular resistance because of the release of catecholamines. Rebound hypertension can be controlled or prevented by maintaining clonidine therapy or by substituting alternative antihypertensive drugs. Antihypertensives that act independently of central and peripheral nervous system mechanisms (e.g., peripheral vasodilators, ACE inhibitors) do not seem to be associated with rebound hypertension after sudden discontinuation of chronic therapy.[11]

Minoxidil

Minoxidil is classified as an antihypertensive used for the treatment of systemic hypertension that is refractory to other drugs. It is metabolized in the liver to an active metabolite, minoxidil sulfate, which produces arteriolar vasodilation with no effect on venous capacitance vessels. This results in decreased systemic blood pressure, reflex tachycardia, and increased cardiac output due to an increase in venous return. Minoxidil is a potent stimulator of renin secretion.

SIDE EFFECTS

Adverse effects associated with minoxidil include fluid and salt retention and reflex tachycardia with increased myocardial oxygen consumption. For these reasons, minoxidil is often administered in combination with a β-adrenergic antagonist and diuretics. Fluid retention can lead to pulmonary hypertension, reversible pericardial effusion, and cardiac tamponade, especially if renal dysfunction is present.[11] Minoxidil stimulates hair growth (i.e., hypertrichosis), and a topical preparation is available for the treatment of baldness.

Prazosin

Prazosin is a potent and selective α_1-adrenergic receptor blocker in arterioles and veins with minimal effects on α_2-adrenergic receptors. This leads to a decrease in peripheral vasomotor resistance and a decrease in venous return to the heart. Because of afterload reduction, prazosin is useful in treating patients with CHF. It is also useful in preoperative preparation of patients with pheochromocytoma. The major side effects associated with prazosin are fluid retention and orthostatic hypotension.

Hydralazine

Hydralazine causes direct relaxation of arteriolar smooth muscle without any effect on venous smooth muscle. This leads to decreased systemic blood pressure, reflex tachycardia, and increased myocardial contractility due to SNS stimulation. Hydralazine also increases plasma renin activity and causes fluid retention. Hydralazine may produce hypotension, headache, flushing, tachycardia, and angina in patients with coronary artery disease. Prolonged use can produce drug-induced lupus syndrome, serum sickness, hemolytic anemia, and rapidly progressive glomerulonephritis. Hydralazine has been used to treat hypertension during pregnancy.

Verapamil

Verapamil and diltiazem block calcium ion channels in cardiac cells, slowing heart rate, decreasing atrioventricular node conduction velocity, and increasing atrioventricular node refractoriness. These drugs are useful for treating atrioventricular node reentrant tachycardia. They are also useful in reducing ventricular rate in atrial flutter and atrial fibrillation. Because these drugs produce peripheral vasodilation, they may also be useful in patients with CHF due to chronic essential hypertension. Calcium channel blockers potentiate the effects of neuromuscular blocking agents. Combination of verapamil with a β-blocker in the treatment of hypertension may produce profound bradycardia and hypotension. Treatment with calcium entry blockers can be continued until the time of surgery without risk of significant drug interactions, especially with respect to conduction of cardiac impulses.

Labetalol

Labetalol is an antihypertensive drug that blocks α_1-receptors selectively and β-receptors nonselectively. Blockade of α_1-receptors decreases systemic vascular resistance and lowers systemic blood pressure without reflex tachycardia due to β_1-receptor block. Labetalol is eliminated through the kidneys (elimination half-time of 5.5 hours) after conjugation with hepatic glucuronide.

CLINICAL USES

Labetalol is available in intravenous and oral forms. Labetalol (0.3 to 1 mg/kg IV) is a safe and effective treatment for hypertensive emergencies in the perioperative period. Sudden increases in heart rate and systemic blood pressure that result from abrupt increases in surgical stimulation in anesthetized patients may be treated with labetalol. Although labetalol has been recommended for treatment of acute hypertension due to exogenous phenylephrine or epinephrine overdose, the β-blocking effects of this drug may be detrimental to the heart exposed to abrupt increases in afterload.[12] In this regard, administration of a peripheral vasodilating drug is preferable (see "Peripheral Vasodilators"). Labetalol may produce bronchospasm in asthmatics and CHF in patients with preexisting cardiac dysfunction. Abrupt discontinuation may precipitate withdrawal.

BETA-ADRENERGIC AGONISTS

Catecholamines stimulate β_1-, β_2-, α_1-, and α_2-adrenergic receptors. Highly selective β_2-agonists (i.e., albuterol and terbutaline) produce relaxation of bronchial, uterine, and vascular smooth muscle (see Table 7-1). Selective β_2-receptor drugs are less likely to produce adverse cardiac effects such as tachycardia or cardiac dysrhythmias as a result of direct effects on the heart. Nevertheless, reflex tachycardia, presumably caused by β_2-mediated vasodilation and subsequent hypotension, has been observed after administration of these drugs.[13] Tachyphylaxis to the effects of β_2-agonists is attributed to the decreased number and sensitivity of β-adrenergic receptors (i.e., downregulation) that occurs with chronic stimulation of these receptors.

Albuterol

Albuterol, a highly selective β_2-agonist, is used in aerosol form for the treatment of bronchospasm in asthmatics and anesthetized patients. Typically, the drug is delivered by two to three deep inhalations (each metered aerosol actuation delivers about 90 µg) 1 to 5 minutes apart. This dose may be repeated every 4 to 6 hours, and the daily dose should not exceed 16 to 20 metered aerosol actuations.

Ritodrine

Ritodrine, a selective β_2-agonist, is infused to inhibit premature uterine contractions. Several side effects, such as hypokalemia, hyperglycemia, tachycardia, and tachyphylaxis, may be associated with this infusion.[14] Hypokalemia most likely reflects sustained β-adrenergic stimulation of the sodium pump with transfer of potassium ions intracellularly. Persistent maternal hyperglycemia may evoke sufficient insulin release to cause reactive hypoglycemia in the fetus.

BETA-ADRENERGIC ANTAGONISTS

β-Adrenergic antagonists (β-blockers) are useful in the treatment of systemic hypertension, ischemic heart disease, CHF, and certain types of cardiac dysrhythmias. β-Blockers may produce a selective β_1-adrenergic block (i.e., decreased heart rate and myocardial contractility), or they may produce mixed responses: β_1- and β_2-antagonism (i.e., bronchial and vascular smooth muscle contractions) (see Table 7-1). β-Blockers such as propranolol also possess membrane-stabilizing activity. Several β-blockers (e.g., pindolol, acebutolol) activate β-receptors partially in the absence of catecholamines.

Clinical Uses

The major therapeutic effects of β-blockers are on the cardiovascular system. β-Blockers decrease systemic blood pressure by slowing the heart rate and by decreasing myocardial contractility and cardiac output. β-Blockers attenuate baroreceptor-mediated increases in heart rate associated with vasodilator therapy. This effect likely results from a decrease in the spontaneous rate of depolarization of cardiac pacemaker cells and slowing of conduction in the atrioventricular node. β-Blockers do not produce orthostatic hypotension and do not alter anesthetic requirements (i.e., MAC). It is recommended that all patients who experience acute myocardial infarction receive intravenous β-blockers (assuming no contraindications exist) as early as possible. These drugs are effective in relieving the symptom of angina pectoris and in decreasing mortality after myocardial infarction by virtue of decreasing heart rate, myocardial contractility, and myocardial oxygen requirements.

PREOPERATIVE ADMINISTRATION TO SELECTED PATIENTS

Perioperative β-blocker therapy is recommended for patients considered at risk for myocardial ischemia (e.g., patients with known coronary artery disease, positive preoperative stress tests, insulin-dependent diabetes mellitus, left ventricular hypertrophy) during high-risk surgery (e.g., vascular surgery, thoracic surgery, intra-abdominal surgery, or surgery with anticipated large blood loss).[15] The goal of preoperative therapy is a resting heart rate between 65 and 85 beats/min. All β-blockers, except those with intrinsic SNS activity, decrease mortality. Perioperative myocardial ischemia is the single most important, potentially reversible risk factor for mortality and cardiovascular complications after noncardiac surgery. Administration of atenolol for 7 days before and after noncardiac surgery in patients at risk for coronary artery disease may decrease mortality and the incidence of cardiovascular complications for as long as 2 years after surgery.[16]

Preoperatively, oral β-blocker therapy can be initiated with atenolol (50 mg), bisoprolol (5 to 10 mg daily), or metoprolol (25 to 50 mg twice daily). If the patient is seen the morning of surgery, atenolol (5 to 10 mg IV) or metoprolol (5 to 10 mg IV) can be titrated. Esmolol is an acceptable drug to achieve β-adrenergic block during surgery and postoperatively in the intensive care unit.

Side Effects

Fatigue and lethargy are commonly associated with β-blocker therapy. Hazards of β-adrenergic blockade include excessive myocardial depression and bronchoconstriction. Additive myocardial depression with volatile anesthetics can occur, but this is not a clinically significant problem. When bronchoconstriction is a possible response, as in patients with bronchial asthma or chronic obstructive pulmonary disease, it may be useful to select β-blockers with selective β_1-blocking effects. Likewise, cardioselective drugs would be logical choices for patients with peripheral vascular disease to minimize the occurrence of vasoconstriction that accompanies β_2-adrenergic block (see Table 7-1). β-Adrenergic antagonists with intrinsic sympathomimetic activity may be logical selections for treatment of patients with depressed left ventricular function or bradycardia. In patients with partial or complete atrioventricular conduction defects, β-adrenergic block may produce life-threatening bradydysrhythmias. This is particularly true in patients who are on calcium channel blockers such as verapamil.

β-Adrenergic antagonists may accentuate increases in plasma concentrations of potassium associated with infusion of potassium chloride, presumably by interfering with the mechanism necessary for movement of this ion across cell membranes.[17] Physicians must exercise caution in the use of β-blocking drugs in diabetic patients because warning signs and symptoms of hypoglycemia are blunted by β-adrenergic block. Cardioselective drugs are logical selections for patients with diabetes mellitus, because suppression of insulin secretion is produced by β_2-adrenergic block.

TREATMENT OF EXCESSIVE BETA-ADRENERGIC BLOCK

Atropine is the initial drug recommended for treatment of signs of excessive drug-induced β-block manifesting as bradycardia or atrioventricular heart block. If signs of excessive β-block persist, a specific pharmacologic treatment is administration of a β-adrenergic agonist such as isoproterenol or dobutamine. However, large doses of these drugs may be required to antagonize excessive β-block. Alternatively, calcium chloride administered intravenously (5 to 10 mg/kg IV) antagonizes excessive β-block independently of any known effect mediated by β-adrenergic receptors.

PERIOPERATIVE MANAGEMENT OF PATIENTS BEING TREATED WITH BETA-ADRENERGIC ANTAGONISTS

It must be recognized that abrupt discontinuation of treatment with β-blockers can be associated with excessive

SNS activity manifesting as systemic hypertension and myocardial ischemia. Presumably, this enhanced activity reflects an increase in the number or sensitivity of β-adrenergic receptors (i.e., upregulation) that occurs during chronic therapy. Treatment with these drugs should be maintained throughout the perioperative period. Continuous intravenous infusion of esmolol would also be effective in maintaining β-adrenergic block in patients who cannot receive oral medications during the perioperative period.

PERIPHERAL VASODILATORS

Peripheral vasodilators that are administered intravenously as a continuous infusion include sodium nitroprusside (SNP) and nitroglycerin (NTG). Conceptually, these drugs decrease systemic vascular resistance by decreasing systemic vascular resistance (SNP) or by producing venous vasodilation (thus decreasing the preload) (SNP and NTG). NTG is metabolized in the blood vessels to its active metabolite, nitric oxide, which activates guanylate cyclase to form cyclic guanine monophosphate and produce vasodilation. SNP, like NTG, increases intracellular nitric oxide that acts as an endogenous vasodilator. Cyanide toxicity and methemoglobinemia represent potential toxic effects of treatment with SNP.

Adenosine is an endogenous nucleoside present in all cells of the body. It is formed as a product of the enzymatic breakdown of adenosine triphosphate. Adenosine is a potent dilator of the coronary arteries and is capable of decreasing oxygen consumption by its antiadrenergic and negative ionotropic actions.

Clinical Uses

Peripheral vasodilators are administered to treat hypertensive crises, to produce controlled hypotension, and to facilitate left ventricular forward stroke volume in patients with acute CHF or regurgitant cardiac valve dysfunc-

tion.[18] Unlike other vasodilators, such as minoxidil and hydralazine, NTG causes only modest increases in heart rate and an overall reduction in myocardial oxygen requirements. NTG decreases venous return and cardiac output by producing venous vasodilation. Adenosine (6 mg IV) is used clinically as an alternative to verapamil to treat paroxysmal supraventricular tachycardia.

NITRIC OXIDE

Nitric oxide is a novel cellular messenger that is important in cardiovascular, immune, and nervous system functions. Inhalation of nitric oxide selectively relaxes pulmonary vasculature, with improvement in arterial oxygenation and minimal systemic cardiovascular effects.[19] Lack of systemic effects due to its binding to oxyhemoglobin makes nitric oxide a useful drug in managing patients with pulmonary hypertension. Inhaled nitric oxide also is used in diagnostic procedures such as determination of diffusion capacity across alveolar capillary membranes.

ANTICHOLINERGICS

Anticholinergics (e.g., atropine, scopolamine, glycopyrrolate) prevent the muscarinic effects of acetylcholine by competing for the same receptors as are normally occupied by the neurotransmitter. Atropine and scopolamine are tertiary amines, and they can cross lipid barriers such as the blood-brain barrier and placenta. In contrast, glycopyrrolate acts principally on peripheral cholinergic receptors, because its quaternary ammonium structure prevents it from crossing lipid barriers in significant amounts. The magnitude of anticholinergic effects may vary between drugs despite similar doses (Table 7-4). The sensitivity of peripheral cholinergic receptors differs such that low doses of an anticholinergic may be sufficient to inhibit salivation, but large doses are necessary for gastrointestinal effects.

Table 7–4 Comparative Effects of Anticholinergics Administered Intramuscularly as Pharmacologic Premedication

Effect	Atropine	Scopolamine	Glycoprrolate
Antisialagogue effect	+	+++	++
Sedative and amnesic effects	+	+++	0
Increased gastric fluid pH	0	0	±
Central nervous system toxicity	+	++	0
Relaxation of lower esophageal sphincter	++	++	++
Mydriasis and cycloplegia	+	+++	0

0, none; +, mild; ++, moderate; +++, marked.

ANTICHOLINESTERASES

Anticholinesterases are represented by quaternary ammonium (e.g., neostigmine, pyridostigmine, edrophonium) and tertiary amine (e.g., physostigmine) drugs. These drugs inhibit the enzyme acetylcholinesterase (i.e., true cholinesterase), which is normally responsible for the rapid hydrolysis of acetylcholine after its release from cholinergic nerve endings. In the presence of an anticholinesterase, acetylcholine accumulates at nicotinic and muscarinic receptor sites. Quaternary ammonium drugs cannot easily cross the blood-brain barrier such that accumulation of acetylcholine is predominantly at peripheral sites such as the nicotinic neuromuscular junction. This is the principal mechanism for drug-assisted antagonism of nondepolarizing neuromuscular blocking drugs. Conversely, physostigmine, with its tertiary amine structure, can cross the blood-brain barrier, making this an effective drug for treatment of the central anticholinergic syndrome that manifests as emergence delirium in the postanesthesia care unit (see Chapter 38).

REFERENCES

1. Lawson NW, Wallfisch HK. Cardiovascular pharmacology: A new look at the pressors. *In* Stoelting RK, Barash PG, Gallagher TJ (eds): Advances in Anesthesia. Chicago: Year Book Medical Publishers, 1986, pp 195-270.
2. Ebert TJ. Preoperative evaluation of the autonomic nervous system. *In* Stoelting RK, Barash PG, Gallagher TJ (eds): Advances in Anesthesia. St Louis: Mosby–Year Book, 1993, pp 49-68.
3. Ram CVS, Kaplan NM. Alpha- and beta-receptor blocking drugs in the treatment of hypertension. *In* Harvey WP, Leon cDe.A, Leonard JJ, et al (eds): Current Problems in Cardiology. Chicago: Year Book Medical Publishers, 1979.
4. Braverman B, McCarthy RJ, Ivankovich AD. Vasopressor challenges during chronic MAOI or TCA treatment in anesthetized dogs. Life Sci 1987;40:2587-2595.
5. Wells DG, Bjorksten AR. Monoamine oxidase inhibitors revisited. Can J Anaesth 1989;36:64-74.
6. Schwinn DA, Reves JG. Time course and hemodynamic effects of alpha-1 adrenergic bolus administration in anesthetized patients with myocardial disease. Anesth Analg 1989;68:571-578.
7. Engelman E, Lipszyc M, Gilbert E, et al. Effects of clonidine on anesthetic drug requirements and hemodynamic response during aortic surgery. Anesthesiology 1989;71:178-187.
8. Mirenda JV, Grisson TE. Anesthetic implications of the renin-angiotensin system and angiotensin-converting enzyme inhibitors. Anesth Analg 1994;72:667-683.
9. Glassman AH, Stretner F, Walsh BT, et al. Heavy smokers, smoking cessation and clonidine. Results of a double blind, randomized trial. JAMA 1988;259:2863-2866.
10. Brosky JB, Bravo JJ: Acute postoperative clonidine withdrawal syndrome. Anesthesiology 1976;44:519-523.
11. Husserl FE, Messerli FH. Adverse effects of antihypertensive drugs. Drugs 1981;22:188-210.
12. Gourdine SB, Hollinger I, Jones J, et al. New York state guidelines on the topical use of phenylephrine in the operating room. Anesthesiology 2000;92:859-864.
13. Wheeler AS, Patel KF, Spain J. Pulmonary edema during beta-2 tocolytic therapy. Anesth Analg 1981;60:695-696.
14. Moravec MA, Hurlbert BJ. Hypokalemia associated with terbutaline administration in obstetrical patients. Anesth Analg 1980;59:917-920.
15. Sjojania KG, Duncan BW, McDonald KM, et al. Safe but sound: Patient safety meets evidence-based medicine. JAMA 2002;288:508-513.
16. Mangano DT, Layug EL, Wallace A, et al. Effect of atenolol on mortality and cardiovascular morbidity after noncardiac surgery. N Engl J Med 1996;335:1713-1720.
17. Rosa RM, Silva P, Young JB, et al. Adrenergic modulation of extrarenal potassium disposal. N Engl J Med 1980;302:431-434.
18. Friederich JA, Butterworth JF. Sodium nitroprusside: Twenty years and counting. Anesth Analg 1995;81:152-162.
19. Steudel W, Hurford WE, Zapol WM. Inhaled nitric oxide: Basic biology and clinical applications. Anesthesiology 1999;91:1090-1121.

Chapter 8

INHALED ANESTHETICS

Rachel Eshima McKay, James Sonner, and Warren R. McKay

HISTORY

The discovery of inhaled anesthesia reflects the contributions of physicians and dentists in the United States and England (Fig. 8-1).[1] The most commonly used inhaled anesthetics in modern anesthesia include a single gas (i.e., nitrous oxide) and volatile liquids (i.e., halothane, enflurane, isoflurane, desflurane, and sevoflurane) (Figs. 8-2 and 8-3). None of these inhaled anesthetics meets all the criteria of an "ideal" inhaled anesthetic, and the chemical characteristics differ among the drugs (see Table 1-1 and Table 8-1).

THE FIRST INHALED ANESTHETICS

Nitrous Oxide

Nitrous oxide gas was first synthesized in 1772 by the English chemist, author, and Unitarian minister Joseph Priestley. Twenty-seven years later, Sir Humphrey Davy observed nitrous oxide's capability to produce analgesia. Davy, suffering from a toothache, administered nitrous oxide to himself and found that it relieved his pain. During Davy's tenure as research assistant to the English physician Thomas Beddoes, Davy administered nitrous oxide to numerous visitors at the Pneumatic Institute in Bristol and observed its euphoric effect. Davy eventually published a book on nitrous oxide in 1800, making the following observation: "As nitrous oxide in its extensive operation appears capable of destroying physical pain, it may probably be used with advantage during surgical operations in which no great effusion of blood takes place." It was not until 42 years later that nitrous oxide was administered prospectively to patients for relief of pain associated with surgical procedures.

Horace Wells, a 29-year-old Boston dentist, noticed the hypnotic and analgesic effects of nitrous oxide at a public exhibition in Hartford, Connecticut, in 1842. At the exhibition, Wells saw a young man painlessly sustain an

Figure 8-1 Anesthetics used in clinical practice. The history of anesthesia began with the introduction of nitrous oxide, ether, and chloroform. After 1950, all introduced drugs, with the exception of ethyl vinyl ether, have contained fluorine. All anesthetics introduced beginning with halothane have been nonflammable. (From Eger EI. Desflurane (Suprane): A Compendium and Reference. Nutley, NJ: Anaquest, 1993, pp 1-11, with permission.)

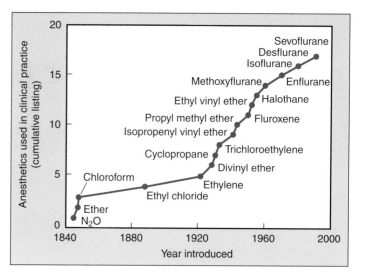

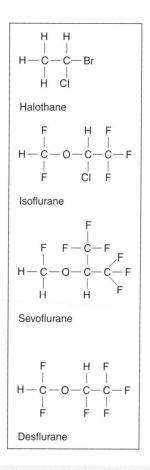

Figure 8-2 Molecular structures of potent volatile anesthetics. Halogenated volatile anesthetics are liquids at room temperature. Among the volatile anesthetics, halothane is an alkane derivative, whereas all the others are derivatives of methyl ethyl ether. Isoflurane is the chemical isomer of enflurane.

accidental cut to his shin after inhalation of nitrous oxide. The next day, Wells himself underwent a dental extraction by a fellow dentist, and he asked the exhibitionist, Gardner Quincy Coulton, to administer nitrous oxide to him during the procedure. Wells felt only minimal pain with the extraction, and he subsequently learned the method of nitrous oxide synthesis to make it available to his own patients. Soon thereafter, Wells began applying nitrous oxide to his practice to produce "painless dentistry." Two years later, he arranged to demonstrate painless surgery using nitrous oxide administration at the Massachusetts General Hospital. During administration of nitrous oxide to a young male student for a wisdom tooth extraction, the patient groaned and moved. Although the young patient stated afterward that he felt little pain during the procedure, Wells was discredited as a result of this demonstration.

Diethyl Ether

William Morton, a Boston dentist and contemporary of Wells, had observed Wells' use of nitrous oxide in his

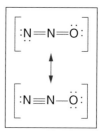

Figure 8-3 Molecular structure of nitrous oxide. Nitrous oxide is a linear molecule existing in two resonance structures. *Dots* denote nonbonding electrons.

Table 8–1 Comparative Characteristics of Inhaled Anesthetics

Characteristic	Isoflurane	Enflurane	Halothane	Desflurane	Sevoflurane	Nitrous Oxide
Blood-gas partition coefficient	1.46	1.9	2.54	0.42	0.69	0.46
Brain-blood partition coefficient	1.6	1.5	1.9	1.3	1.7	1.1
Muscle-blood partition coefficient	2.9	1.7	3.4	2.0	3.1	1.2
Fat-blood partition coefficient	45	36	51	27	48	2.3
MAC (volumes %, 30-55 years old)	1.15	1.63	0.76	6.0	1.85	104
Vapor pressure (mm Hg, 20°C)	240	172	244	669	160	
Molecular weight	184.5	184.5	197.4	168	200	44
Stable in hydrated carbon dioxide absorbent	Yes	Yes	No	Yes	No	Yes
Stable in desiccated carbon dioxide absorbent	No; carbon monoxide formation		No	No; carbon monoxide formation	No; carbon monoxide formation; exothermic reaction	
Compound A formation	No		Yes	No	Yes	
Amount metabolized (%)	0-0.2		15-40	0-0.2	5-8	

painless dentistry practice. Morton noticed parallels between nitrous oxide's effects and those obtained with diethyl ether during "ether frolics," in which ether was breathed for its inebriating effects. Like Wells, Morton applied ether in his dental practice and then asked to demonstrate its anesthetic properties at the Massachusetts General Hospital on October 16, 1846 ("ether day"). In contrast to Wells' debacle, Morton's demonstration was received with great enthusiasm. The results of successful ether anesthetics were soon published in the *Boston Medical and Surgical Journal*. Although Crawford Long administered diethyl ether to a patient in 1842, four years earlier than Morton, he did not publicize his work, and Morton therefore has traditionally been credited with the discovery of diethyl ether's capability to produce anesthesia.

Chloroform

James Simpson, an obstetrician from Edinburgh, Scotland, sought to develop an anesthetic that did not share the protracted induction, flammability, and postoperative nausea seen with diethyl ether. After considerable self-experimentation with several liquids obtained from his apothecary, he discovered the anesthetic effects of chloroform. He began to use chloroform inhalation for relief of pain during labor and delivery in 1846. Chloroform soon became popular as an inhaled anesthetic in England, although diethyl ether dominated practice in North America. Over the next few decades, chloroform was associated with several unexplained intraoperative deaths of otherwise healthy patients and with numerous cases of hepatotoxicity.

INHALED ANESTHETICS BETWEEN 1920 AND 1940

Between 1920 and 1940, ethylene, cyclopropane, and divinyl ether were introduced into use as anesthetics, gaining acceptance over the older inhalants (with the exception of nitrous oxide) by producing a faster, more pleasant induction of anesthesia and by allowing faster awakening at the conclusion of surgery. Although these agents produced anesthesia, each had serious drawbacks. Many were flammable (i.e., diethyl ether, divinyl ether, ethylene, and cyclopropane), whereas others, halogenated entirely with chlorine, were toxic (i.e., chloroform, ethyl chloride, and trichloroethylene).

FLUORINE CHEMISTRY AND MODERN INHALATIONAL ANESTHETICS

Techniques of fluorine chemistry, developed from efforts to produce the first atomic weapons, found a fortuitous, socially beneficial purpose in providing a method of synthesizing modern inhaled anesthetics.[2,3] Modern inhaled anesthetics are halogenated partly or entirely with fluorine (see Fig. 8-2). Fluorination provides greater stability and lesser toxicity.

Halothane

Halothane was introduced into clinical practice in 1956. It had several advantages compared with the older anesthetics, including nonflammability, a pleasant odor, low toxicity, and pharmacokinetic properties allowing faster induction and emergence compared with ether. After 4 years of commercial use, reports of fulminant hepatic necrosis after halothane anesthesia began to appear in cases in which other causes of liver damage were not evident. Halothane sensitizes the myocardium to the dysrhymogenic effects of catecholamines.

Methoxyflurane

Methoxyflurane was first introduced into clinical practice in 1960, and its high solubility in blood was perceived by many to be clinically advantageous. The protracted presence of anesthetic in the tissues provided ongoing sedation and analgesia to patients during the postoperative period. Within the first decade of its introduction, reports of renal failure with methoxyflurane anesthesia appeared, leading to studies confirming a dose-related nephrotoxicity because of the inorganic fluoride that resulted from the metabolism of this anesthetic.

Enflurane

Enflurane was introduced to clinical practice in 1972. Unlike halothane, it did not sensitize the heart to catecholamines, and it was not associated with hepatotoxicity. However, enflurane was metabolized to inorganic fluoride and could cause evidence of seizure activity on the electroencephalogram (EEG), especially when administered at high concentrations and in the presence of hypocapnia.

Isoflurane

Isoflurane was introduced into clinical practice in 1980. It was not associated with cardiac dysrhythmias and underwent less metabolism than halothane and enflurane. It allowed a more rapid onset of surgical anesthesia and faster awakening compared with its predecessors. Its pungency made it impractical for inhalation induction of anesthesia.

Sevoflurane and Desflurane

Sevoflurane and desflurane are halogenated exclusively with fluorine and were first synthesized during the late 1960s and 1970s, respectively.[2,3] Both were expensive and difficult to synthesize, and they were therefore not immediately considered for commercial use. In the 1980s, their development was reconsidered in light of a new appreciation that a growing proportion of anesthetic practice was taking place in the outpatient setting and that drugs halogenated exclusively with fluorine were less soluble in blood, allowing faster awakening from anesthesia (see Fig. 8-1 and Tables 8-1 and 8-2).

MECHANISM OF ACTION

Questions occur about where in the nervous system inhaled anesthetics act, what molecules they interact with to produce their effect, and the nature of the biologic interaction between anesthetic and substrate that requires an ability to measure anesthetic effects.[4] Although inhaled anesthetics have been used to provide surgical anesthesia for almost 160 years, there is no single, accepted definition of what constitutes the anesthetic state. For experimental purposes, an operational definition of immobility in response to surgical stimulation and amnesia for intraoperative events has proved useful.

Measurable Characteristics

Measurable and universal characteristics of all inhaled anesthetics include production of immobility and amnestic effects. Immobility is measured by the minimum alveolar concentration (MAC) of anesthetic required to suppress movement to a surgical incision in 50% of patients (see Table 8-2).[2,5] Unconsciousness is part of the anesthetic state, but it is impossible to measure in an immobile patient who does not remember events from surgery. Analgesia was once said to be part of the anesthetic state, but this also cannot be measured in an immobile patient who cannot remember. Surrogate measures of pain (i.e., increased heart rate or systemic blood pressure) suggest that inhaled anesthetics do not suppress the perception of painful stimuli. Some inhaled anesthetics have hyperalgesic (pain-enhancing) effects in low concentrations. Skeletal muscle relaxation is a common, but not universal, central effect of inhaled anesthetics, as evidenced by nitrous oxide, which increases skeletal muscle tone.

IMMOBILITY

Inhaled anesthetics produce immobility in large part by their actions on the spinal cord, as evidenced by determination of MAC in decerebrate animals.[6]

AMNESTIC EFFECTS

Supraspinal structures such as the amygdala, hippocampus, and cortex are considered highly probable targets for the amnestic effects of anesthetics.

CENTRAL NERVOUS SYSTEM DEPRESSION AND ION CHANNELS

There is a general agreement that inhaled anesthetics produce central nervous system depression by their actions on ion channels, which govern the electrical behavior of the nervous system.[4] The consensus is that inhaled anesthetics produce anesthesia by enhancing the function of inhibitory ion channels and by blocking the function of excitatory ion channels. Enhancing the function of inhibitory ion channels leads to hyperpolarization of the neuron. Hyperpolarization results when chloride anions enter neurons through γ-aminobutyric acid A receptors (GABA$_A$) or glycine receptors or when there is an efflux of potassium cations out of neurons through potassium ion channels. Blocking the function of excitatory ion channels prevents depolarization of the neuron by preventing the passage of positive charges into the neuron (i.e., passage of sodium ions through N-methyl-D-aspartate [NMDA] receptors or sodium channels). Anesthetics may also affect the release of neurotransmitters, and this effect may be mediated in part by ion channels that regulate the release of neurotransmitters.

BIOPHYSICAL MECHANISM OF ACTION ON ION CHANNELS

The biophysical mechanism underlying anesthetic action on ion channels, although not well understood, is crucial to our knowledge of how inhaled anesthetics work. Knowledge of how anesthetics interact with their biologic molecular targets may be sufficient to permit the design of improved new anesthetics. It is thought that inhaled anesthetics exert their effects on ion channels by binding directly to these channels, as ligands binding to a receptor. A minority view holds that inhaled anesthetics act indirectly by altering a physical property of the membrane, and in so doing, they stabilize open or closed states of ion channels.

PHYSICAL PROPERTIES

Molecular Structure

Modern inhaled anesthetics, with the exception of nitrous oxide, are halogenated hydrocarbons (see Figs. 8-2 and 8-3). Halothane lacks the ether moiety present on isoflurane, sevoflurane, and desflurane, accounting for its capability to produce ventricular cardiac dysrhythmias. Isoflurane and desflurane differ only by the substitution of one chlorine atom for fluorine. Fluorine substitution confers greater stability and resistance to metabolism.

Vapor Pressure

Nitrous oxide exists as a gas at ambient temperature, although it becomes a liquid at higher pressures. The remaining inhaled anesthetics are liquids at ambient temperatures.

VARIABLE-BYPASS VAPORIZERS

Halothane, sevoflurane, and isoflurane are delivered by variable-bypass vaporizers. The variable-bypass vaporizer contains two streams of inflowing fresh gas, one contacting a reservoir (sump) of liquid anesthetic and the other bypassing the sump. Concentration of anesthetic in the gas leaving the vaporizer is determined by the relative flow of fresh gas through the sump channel versus the bypass channel, and control of concentration occurs by adjustment of the dial on the vaporizer. Each variable-bypass vaporizer is calibrated for an individual anesthetic because vapor pressures differ (see Table 8-1).

HEATED VAPORIZER

The vapor pressure of desflurane at sea level is 700 mm Hg at 20°C (near boiling state at room temperature), and delivery by a variable-bypass vaporizer can produce unpredictable concentrations. For this reason, a specially designed vaporizer (Tec 6, Datex-Ohmeda) that heats desflurane gas to 2 atmospheres of pressure is used to accurately meter and deliver desflurane vapor corresponding to adjustments of the concentration dial by the anesthesiologist. Alternatively, there is a variable-bypass vaporizer that delivers desflurane in which gas flow is controlled through the sump and the bypass.

Stability

Anesthetic degradation by metabolism or by an interaction with carbon dioxide absorbents (especially when desiccated) produces several potentially toxic compounds.[7]

METABOLISM

Methoxyflurane produces inorganic fluoride, which is responsible for the sporadic incidence of nephrotoxicity (i.e., high-output renal failure) after prolonged anesthesia. Compound A (i.e., trifluoroethyl vinyl ether), which is produced from the breakdown of sevoflurane, and a similar compound produced from halothane have been shown to be nephrotoxic in animals after prolonged exposure. In humans, prolonged anesthesia with sevoflurane and low fresh gas flows (1 L/min) results in compound A exposure adequate to produce transient proteinuria, enzymuria, and glycosuria, but there is no evidence of increased serum creatinine concentrations or long-term deleterious

II

effects on renal function. Nevertheless, the package insert for sevoflurane recommends low fresh gas flow (<2 L/min) be restricted to less than 2 MAC hours (i.e., MAC concentration times duration of administration) of sevoflurane anesthesia.

CARBON DIOXIDE ABSORBENTS AND EXOTHERMIC REACTIONS

Variables influencing the amount of volatile anesthetic degradation on exposure to carbon dioxide absorbents and its clinical relevance include the condition (i.e., hydration and temperature) and chemical makeup of the absorbent, fresh gas flow rates, minute ventilation, and most importantly, the anesthetic itself.[8] Although desflurane and isoflurane are very stable in hydrated carbon dioxide absorbents up to temperatures of more than 60°C, full desiccation of conventional carbon dioxide absorbents containing sodium and potassium hydroxide causes degradation and carbon monoxide production from these volatile anesthetics at all temperatures (see Table 8-1). High fresh gas flow rates (especially those exceeding normal minute ventilation) accelerate the desiccation of absorbent, and the desiccation leads to accelerated degradation. Because degradation is an exothermic process, temperature of the absorbent may increase dramatically.

The exothermic reaction that results from interaction of desiccated carbon dioxide absorbent and volatile anesthetics (especially sevoflurane) can produce extremely high temperatures inside of the absorbent canister.[9,10] The temperature increase may lead to explosion and fire in the canister or anesthetic circuit. The remote risk of fire and explosion from exothermic reactions can be avoided entirely by employing measures that ensure maintenance of adequate hydration in the carbon dioxide absorbent (i.e., changing the absorbent regularly, turning fresh gas flow down or off on unattended anesthesia machines, limiting fresh gas flow rates during anesthesia, and when in doubt about the hydration of the absorbent, changing it). Commercially available carbon dioxide absorbents with decreased or absent monovalent bases (i.e., sodium hydroxide and potassium hydroxide) do not result in extensive degradation on exposure to volatile anesthetics, regardless of the state of hydration of the absorbent.

RELATIVE POTENCY OF INHALED ANESTHETICS

A comparison of relative potency between inhaled anesthetics can be described by numerous end points, but the most common parameter of comparison involves the dose required to suppress movement in 50% of patients in response to surgical incision.[5] This dose (a single point on a dose-response curve) is designated the MAC. Because

the standard deviation in the MAC is approximately 10%, 95% of patients should not move in response to incision at 1.2 MAC of the inhaled anesthetic, and 99% of patients should not move in response to incision at 1.3 MAC of the inhaled anesthetic. MAC is affected by several variables but is unaffected by gender or duration of surgery and anesthesia (Table 8-2).[5]

MAC allows potencies to be compared among anesthetics (see Table 8-1); 1.15% isoflurane is equipotent with 6% desflurane in preventing movement in response to a surgical incision in patients of a similar age and body temperature. Remarkably, MAC values for different inhaled anesthetics are additive. For example, 0.5 MAC of nitrous oxide administered with 0.5 MAC of isoflurane has the same effect as 1 MAC of any inhaled agent in preventing movement in response to incision (reflecting anesthetic-induced inhibition of reflex responses at the level of the spinal cord).[6] The concentration of anesthetic at the brain needed to prevent movement in response to a surgical incision is likely to be greater than the MAC.

PHARMACOKINETICS OF INHALED ANESTHETICS

Pharmacokinetics of inhaled anesthetics describes their uptake (absorption) from alveoli into the systemic circulation, distribution in the body, and eventual elimination by the lungs or metabolism principally in the liver (Table 8-3).[11] By controlling the inspired partial pressure (PI) (same as the concentration [%] when referring to the gas phase) of an inhaled anesthetic, a gradient is created such that the anesthetic is delivered from the anesthetic machine to its site of action, the brain. The primary objective of inhalation anesthesia is to achieve a constant and optimal brain partial pressure (Pbr) of the anesthetic.

The brain and all other tissues equilibrate with the partial pressure of the inhaled anesthetic delivered to them by the arterial blood (Pa). Likewise, the blood equilibrates with the alveolar partial pressure (PA) of the anesthetic:

$$PA \rightleftharpoons Pa \rightleftharpoons Pbr$$

Maintaining a constant and optimal PA becomes an indirect but useful method for controlling the Pbr. The PA of an inhaled anesthetic mirrors its Pbr and is the reason the PA is used as an index of anesthetic depth, a reflection of the rate of induction and recovery from anesthesia, and a measure of equal potency (see "Relative Potency of Inhaled Anesthetics"). Understanding the factors that determine the PA and the Pbr allows the anesthesiologist to skillfully control and adjust the dose of inhaled anesthetic delivered to the brain.

Table 8–2 Factors That Increase or Decrease Anesthetic Requirements

Factors Increasing MAC
Drugs
Amphetamine (acute use)
Cocaine
Ephedrine
Ethanol (chronic use)
Age
Highest at age 6 months
Electrolytes
Hypernatremia
Hyperthermia
Red hair
Factors Decreasing MAC
Drugs
Propofol
Etomidate
Barbiturates
Benzodiazepines
Ketamine
α_2-Agonists (clonidine, dexmedetomidine)
Ethanol (acute use)
Local anesthetics
Opioids
Amphetamines (chronic use)
Lithium
Verapamil
Age
Elderly patients
Electrolytes disturbance
Hyponatremia
Other factors
Anemia (hemoglobin < 5 g/dL)
Hypercarbia
Hypothermia
Hypoxia
Pregnancy

MAC, minimum alveolar concentration.

Table 8–3 Factors Determining Partial Pressure Gradients Necessary for Establishment of Anesthesia

Transfer of inhaled anesthetic from anesthetic machine to alveoli
Inspired partial pressure
Alveolar ventilation
Characteristics of anesthetic breathing system
Transfer of inhaled anesthetic from alveoli to arterial blood
Blood-gas partition coefficient
Cardiac output
Alveolar-to-venous partial pressure difference
Transfer of inhaled anesthetic from arterial blood to brain
Brain-blood partition coefficient
Cerebral blood flow
Arterial-to-venous partial pressure difference

Factors That Determine the Alveolar Partial Pressure

The PA and ultimately the Pbr of an inhaled anesthetic are determined by input (delivery) into the alveoli minus uptake (loss) of the drug from the alveoli into the pulmonary arterial blood. Input of the inhaled anesthetic depends on the PI, alveolar ventilation ($\dot{V}A$), and characteristics of the anesthetic breathing system. Uptake of the inhaled anesthetic depends on the solubility, cardiac output (CO), and alveolar-to-venous partial pressure difference (A-vD). These six factors act simultaneously to determine the PA. Metabolism and percutaneous loss of inhaled anesthetics do not significantly influence PA during induction and maintenance of anesthesia.

INSPIRED ANESTHETIC PARTIAL PRESSURE

A high PI is necessary during initial administration of an inhaled anesthetic. This initial high PI (i.e., input) offsets the impact of uptake into the blood and accelerates induction of anesthesia as reflected by the rate of increase in the PA. This effect of the PI is known as the *concentration effect*. Clinically, the range of concentrations necessary to produce a concentration effect is probably possible only with nitrous oxide (Fig. 8-4).[12]

With time, as uptake into the blood decreases, the PI should be decreased to match the decreased anesthetic uptake. Decreasing the PI to match decreasing uptake with time is critical if the anesthesiologist is to achieve the goal of maintaining a constant and optimal Pbr. For example, if the PI were maintained constant with time (input

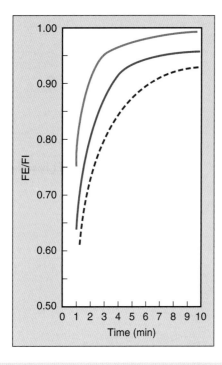

Figure 8-4 The impact of the inspired concentration (%) (FI) on the rate of increase of the alveolar (end-tidal) concentration (FE) is known as the concentration effect. The lines indicate concentrations of 85% (*green*), 50% (*blue*), and 10% (*dashed red*). (From Eger EI. Effect of inspired anesthetic concentration on the rate of rise of alveolar concentration. Anesthesiology 1963;24:153-157, with permission.)

constant), the PA (and depth of anesthesia as reflected by the Pbr) would progressively increase as uptake of the anesthetic into the blood diminished with time.

SECOND GAS EFFECT

The second gas effect is a distinct phenomenon that occurs independently of the concentration effect. The ability of the large-volume uptake of one gas (first gas) to accelerate the rate of increase of the PA of a concurrently administered companion gas (second gas) is known as the *second gas effect*. For example, the initial large volume uptake of nitrous oxide accelerates the uptake of companion gases such as volatile anesthetics and oxygen. The transient increase (about 10%) in PaO₂ that accompanies the early phase of nitrous oxide administration reflects the second gas effect of nitrous oxide on oxygen. This increase in PaO₂ has been designated *alveolar hyperoxygenation*. Increased tracheal inflow of all inhaled gases (i.e., first and second gases) and concentration of the second gases in a smaller lung volume (i.e., concentrating effect) because of the high-volume uptake of the first gas are the explanations for the second

gas effect. Although the second gas effect is based on proven pharmacokinetic principles, it is probably not a clinically significant phenomenon.

ALVEOLAR VENTILATION

Increased V̇A, like PI, promotes input of inhaled anesthetics to offset uptake into the blood. The net effect is a more rapid rate of increases in the PA and induction of anesthesia. Predictably, hypoventilation has the opposite effect, acting to slow the induction of anesthesia.

Controlled ventilation of the lungs that results in hyperventilation and decreased venous return accelerates the rate of increase of the PA by virtue of increased input (i.e., increased V̇A) and decreased uptake (i.e., decreased CO). As a result, the risk of anesthetic overdose may be increased during controlled ventilation of the lungs, and it may be appropriate to decrease the PI of volatile anesthetics when ventilation of the lungs is changed from spontaneous to controlled to maintain the PA similar to that present during spontaneous ventilation.

Another effect of hyperventilation is decreased cerebral blood flow because of any associated decrease in the PaCO₂. Conceivably, the impact of increased anesthetic input on the rate of increase of the PA would be offset by decreased delivery of anesthetic to the brain. Theoretically, coronary blood flow may remain unchanged, such that increased anesthetic input produces myocardial depression, and decreased cerebral blood flow prevents a concomitant onset of central nervous system depression.

ANESTHETIC BREATHING SYSTEM

Characteristics of the anesthetic breathing system that influence the rate of increase of the PA include the volume of the system, solubility of inhaled anesthetics in the rubber or plastic components of the system, and gas inflow from the anesthetic machine. The volume of the anesthetic breathing system acts as a buffer to slow attainment of the PA. High gas inflow from the anesthetic machine negates this buffer effect. Solubility of inhaled anesthetics in the components of the anesthetic breathing system initially slows the rate at which the PA increases. At the conclusion of an anesthetic, reversal of the partial pressure gradient in the anesthetic breathing system results in elution of the anesthetics that slows the rate at which the PA decreases.

SOLUBILITY

The solubility of inhaled anesthetics in blood and tissues is denoted by partition coefficients (see Table 8-1). A partition coefficient is a distribution ratio describing how the inhaled anesthetic distributes itself between two phases at equilibrium (when the partial pressures are identical). For example, a blood-gas partition coefficient of 10 means that the concentration of the inhaled anesthetic is 10 in the blood and 1 in the alveolar gas when the partial pressures of that anesthetic in these two phases are identical. Partition coefficients are temperature dependent. For example, the solubility of a gas in a liquid is increased when the temperature of the liquid decreases. Unless otherwise stated, partition coefficients are given for 37°C.

Blood-Gas Partition Coefficient

High blood solubility means that a large amount of inhaled anesthetic must be dissolved (i.e., undergo uptake) in the blood before equilibrium with the gas phase is reached. The blood can be considered a pharmacologically inactive reservoir, the size of which is determined by the solubility of the anesthetic in the blood. When the blood-gas partition coefficient is high, a large amount of anesthetic must be dissolved in the blood before the Pa equilibrates with the PA (Fig. 8-5).[13] Clinically, the impact of high blood solubility on the rate of increase of the PA can be offset to some extent by increasing the PI. When blood solubility is low, minimal amounts of the anesthetic have to be dissolved in the blood before equilibrium is reached such that the rate of increase of the PA and that of the Pa and Pbr are rapid (see Fig. 8-5).[13]

Tissue-Blood Partition Coefficient

Tissue-blood partition coefficients determine the time necessary for equilibration of the tissue with the Pa (see Table 8-1). This time can be predicted by calculating a time constant (i.e., amount of inhaled anesthetic that can be dissolved in the tissue divided by tissue blood flow) for each tissue. Brain-blood partition coefficients for a volatile anesthetic such as isoflurane result in time constants of about 3 to 4 minutes. Complete equilibration of any tissue, including the brain, with the Pa requires at least three time constants. This is the rationale for maintaining the PA of this volatile anesthetic constant for 10 to 15 minutes before assuming that the Pbr is similar. Time constants for less soluble anesthetics such as nitrous oxide, desflurane, and sevoflurane are about 2 minutes, and complete equilibration is achieved in approximately 6 minutes (i.e., three time constants).

Nitrous Oxide Transfer to Closed Gas Spaces

The blood-gas partition coefficient of nitrous oxide (0.46) is 34 times greater than that of nitrogen (0.014). This differential solubility means that nitrous oxide can leave the blood to enter an air-filled cavity 34 times more rapidly than nitrogen can leave the cavity to enter the blood. As a result of this preferential transfer of nitrous oxide, the volume or pressure of the air-filled cavity increases. The entrance of nitrous oxide into an air-filled cavity surrounded by a compliant wall (e.g., intestinal gas, pneumothorax, pulmonary blebs, air embolism) causes the gas space to expand. Conversely, entrance of nitrous oxide into an air-filled cavity surrounded by a noncompliant wall (e.g., middle ear, cerebral ventricles, supratentorial subdural space) causes an increase in pressure.

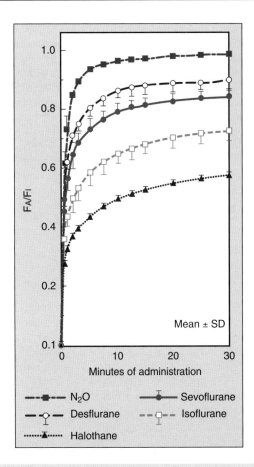

Figure 8-5 The blood-gas partition coefficient is the principal determinant of the rate at which the alveolar concentration (Fa) increases toward a constant inspired concentration (Fi). The rate of induction of anesthesia is paralleled by the rate of increase in the Fa. Despite similar blood solubility (see Table 8-1), the rate of increase of Fa is more rapid for nitrous oxide (*dashed gold line*) than for desflurane (*dashed purple line*) or sevoflurane (*solid blue line*), reflecting the impact of the concentration effect on nitrous oxide (see Fig. 8-4). Greater tissue solubility of desflurane and sevoflurane may also contribute to a slower rate of increase in the Fa of these drugs compared with nitrous oxide. (From Yasuda N, Lockhart SH, Eger EI, et al. Comparison of kinetics of sevoflurane and isoflurane in humans. Anesth Analg 1991;72:316-324, with permission.)

The magnitude of volume or pressure increase in the air-filled cavity is influenced by the PA of nitrous oxide, blood flow to the air-filled cavity, and duration of nitrous oxide administration. In an animal model, inhalation of 75% nitrous oxide doubles the volume of a pneumothorax in 10 minutes.[14] The presence of a closed pneumothorax is a contraindication to the administration of nitrous oxide. Decreasing pulmonary compliance during administration of nitrous oxide to a patient with a history of chest trauma (i.e., rib fractures) may reflect nitrous oxide–induced expansion of a previously unrecognized pneumothorax. Likewise, air bubbles associated with venous air embolism expand rapidly when exposed to nitrous oxide.

In contrast to the rapid expansion of a pneumothorax or air bubbles (i.e., venous air embolism), the increase in bowel gas volume produced by nitrous oxide is slow. The question of whether to administer nitrous oxide to patients undergoing intra-abdominal surgery is of little importance if the operation is short. Limiting the inhaled concentration of nitrous oxide to 50%, however, may be a prudent recommendation when bowel gas volume is increased (e.g., bowel obstruction) preoperatively. Following this guideline, bowel gas volume at most would double, even during prolonged operations.[14]

CARDIAC OUTPUT

The CO influences uptake into the pulmonary arterial blood and therefore PA by carrying away more or less anesthetic from the alveoli. A high CO (e.g., fear) results in more rapid uptake, such that the rate of increase in the PA and the induction of anesthesia are slowed. A low CO (e.g., shock) speeds the rate of increase of the PA because there is less uptake into the blood to oppose input. A common clinical impression is that induction of anesthesia in patients in shock is rapid.

Shunt

A right-to-left intracardiac or intrapulmonary shunt slows the rate of induction of anesthesia. This slowing reflects the dilutional effect of shunted blood containing no anesthetic on the partial pressure of anesthetic in blood coming from ventilated alveoli. A similar mechanism is responsible for the decrease in PaO_2 in the presence of a right-to-left shunt.

A left-to-right shunt (e.g., arteriovenous fistula, volatile anesthetic–induced increases in cutaneous blood flow) results in delivery to the lungs of venous blood containing a higher partial pressure of anesthetic than that present in venous blood that has passed through the tissues. As a result, a left-to-right tissue shunt offsets the dilutional effect of a right-to-left shunt on the Pa. The effect of a left-to-right shunt on the rate of increase in the Pa is detectable only if there is the concomitant presence of a right-to-left shunt. Likewise, the dilutional effect of a right-to-left shunt is greatest in the absence of a left-to-right shunt. All factors considered, it seems unlikely that the impact of a right-to-left shunt would be clinically apparent.

Wasted Ventilation

Ventilation of nonperfused alveoli does not influence the rate of induction of anesthesia because a dilutional effect on the Pa is not produced. The principal effect of wasted ventilation is the production of a difference between the PA and Pa of the inhaled anesthetic. A similar mechanism is responsible for the difference often observed between the end-tidal PCO_2 and $PaCO_2$.

ALVEOLAR-TO-VENOUS PARTIAL PRESSURE DIFFERENCES

The A-vD reflects tissue uptake of inhaled anesthetics. Highly perfused tissues (i.e., brain, heart, kidneys, and liver) account for less than 10% of body mass but receive about 75% of the CO (Table 8-4). As a result, these highly perfused tissues equilibrate rapidly with the Pa. After three time constants (6 to 12 minutes for inhaled anesthetics), about 75% of the returning venous blood is at the same partial pressure as the PA (i.e., narrow A-vD). For this reason, uptake of volatile anesthetics from the alveoli is greatly decreased after 6 to 12 minutes, as reflected by a narrowing of the PI-to-PA difference. After this time, the inhaled concentrations of volatile anesthetics should be decreased to maintain a constant PA in the presence of decreased uptake.

Skeletal muscle and fat represent about 70% of the body mass but receive less than 25% of the CO (see Table 8-5). These tissues continue to act as inactive reservoirs for anesthetic uptake for several hours. Equilibration of fat with inhaled anesthetics in the arterial blood is probably never achieved.

Recovery from Anesthesia

Recovery from anesthesia can be defined as the rate at which the PA decreases with time (Fig. 8-6).[13] In many respects, recovery is the inverse of induction of anesthesia. For example, V̇A, solubility, and CO determine the rate at which the PA decreases. Conversely, recovery from anesthesia is influenced by factors unique to this phase of the anesthetic.

DIFFERENCES FROM INDUCTION

Recovery from anesthesia differs from induction of anesthesia with respect to the absence of a concentration effect on recovery (the PI cannot be less than zero), the variable tissue concentrations of anesthetics at the start of recovery, and the potential importance of metabolism on the rate of decrease in the PA.

Table 8–4	Body Tissue Compartments	
Compartment	**Body Mass (% of a 70-kg Adult)**	**Blood Flow (% of Cardiac Output)**
Vessel-rich group	10	75
Muscle group	50	19
Fat group	20	5
Vessel-poor group	20	1

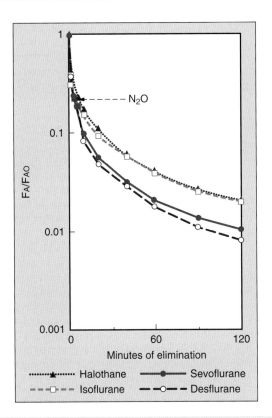

Figure 8-6 Elimination of inhaled anesthetics is reflected by the decrease in the alveolar concentration (FA) compared with the concentration present at the conclusion of anesthesia (FAO). Awakening from anesthesia is paralleled by these curves. (From Yasuda N, Lockhart SH, Eger EI, et al. Comparison of kinetics of sevoflurane and isoflurane in humans. Anesth Analg 1991;72:316-324, with permission.)

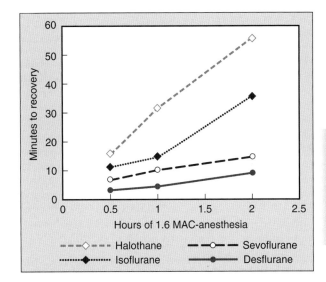

Figure 8-7 An increase in the duration of anesthesia during a constant dose of anesthetic (1.6 MAC) is associated with increases in the time to recovery (i.e., motor coordination in an animal model), with the greatest increases occurring with the most blood-soluble anesthetics. (From Eger EI. Desflurane (Suprane): A Compendium and Reference. Nutley, NJ: Anaquest, 1993, pp 1-11, with permission.)

Tissue Concentrations

Tissue concentrations of inhaled anesthetics serve as a reservoir to maintain the P_A when the partial pressure gradient is reversed by decreasing the P_I to or near zero at the conclusion of anesthesia. The impact of tissue storage depends on the duration of anesthesia and solubility of the anesthetics in various tissue compartments. For example, time to recovery is prolonged in proportion to the duration of anesthesia for a soluble anesthetic (e.g., isoflurane), whereas the impact of duration of administration on time to recovery is minimal with poorly soluble anesthetics (e.g., sevoflurane, desflurane) (Fig 8-7).[1] The variable concentrations of anesthetics in different tissues at the conclusion of anesthesia contrasts with induction of anesthesia, when all tissues initially have the same zero concentration of anesthetic.

Metabolism

An important difference between induction of anesthesia and recovery from anesthesia is the potential impact of metabolism on the rate of decrease in the P_A at the conclusion of anesthesia. In this regard, metabolism is a principal determinant of the rate of decrease in the P_A of the highly lipid-soluble methoxyflurane. Metabolism and $\dot{V}_A$ are equally important in the rate of decrease in the P_A of halothane, whereas the rate of decrease in the P_A of less lipid-soluble isoflurane, desflurane, and sevoflurane principally results from $\dot{V}_A$.[7]

CONTEXT-SENSITIVE HALF-TIME

The pharmacokinetics of the elimination of inhaled anesthetics depends on the length of administration and the blood-gas solubility of the inhaled anesthetic. As with injected anesthetics, it is possible to use computer simulations to determine context-sensitive half-times for volatile anesthetics. The time needed for a 50% decrease in anesthetic concentrations of isoflurane, desflurane, and sevoflurane is less than 5 minutes and does not increase significantly with increasing duration of anesthesia.[15] Presumably, this is a reflection of the initial phase of elimination, which is primarily a function of $\dot{V}_A$. Determination of other decrement times (80% and 90%) reveals differences between various inhaled anesthetics. For example, the

80% decrement times of desflurane and sevoflurane are less than 8 minutes and do not increase significantly with the duration of anesthesia, whereas the 80% decrement time for isoflurane increases significantly after about 60 minutes, reaching a plateau of approximately 30 to 35 minutes. The 90% decrement time of desflurane increases slightly from 5 minutes after 30 minutes of anesthesia to 14 minutes after 6 hours of anesthesia, which is significantly less than for sevoflurane (65 minutes) and isoflurane (86 minutes). Based on these simulated context-sensitive half-times, there would be little difference in recovery times among these volatile anesthetics (regardless of the duration of the drug's administration) when a pure inhalation anesthetic technique is used. The principal difference in the rates at which desflurane, sevoflurane, and isoflurane are eliminated occurs in the final 20% of the elimination process.

DIFFUSION HYPOXIA

Diffusion hypoxia may occur at the conclusion of nitrous oxide administration if patients are allowed to inhale room air. The initial high-volume outpouring of nitrous oxide from the blood into the alveoli when inhalation of this gas is discontinued can so dilute the PaO_2 that the PaO_2 decreases. The occurrence of diffusion hypoxia is prevented by filling the patient's lungs with oxygen at the conclusion of nitrous oxide administration.

EFFECTS ON ORGAN SYSTEMS

Circulatory Effects

Data collected from healthy volunteers receiving equipotent concentrations of inhaled anesthetics have demonstrated that the circulatory effects of these drugs are similar, especially during the maintenance of anesthesia (Table 8-5).[16] However, patients undergoing surgery may respond

Table 8–5 Proposed Mechanisms of Circulatory Effects
Produced by inhaled anesthetics
Direct myocardial depression
Inhibition of central nervous system and sympathetic nervous system outflow
Depression of transmission of impulses through autonomic ganglia
Attenuated carotid sinus reflex activity
Decreased formation of cyclic adenosine monophosphate
Inhibition of calcium reuptake by myocardial sarcoplasmic reticulum
Decreased influx of calcium ions through slow channels

differently from healthy volunteers. For example, factors such as coexisting disease, extremes of age, nonoptimal intravascular volume status, presence of surgical stimulation, and concurrent drugs may alter, attenuate, or exaggerate the responses expected based on data obtained from healthy volunteers.

RESPONSES DURING MAINTENANCE OF ANESTHESIA
Mean Arterial Pressure

Mean arterial pressure (MAP) decreases with increasing concentrations of desflurane, sevoflurane, isoflurane, halothane, and enflurane in a dose-dependent manner (Fig. 8-8).[16,17] With the exception of halothane, the decrease in MAP primarily reflects a decrease in systemic vascular resistance (SVR) versus a decrease in CO (Figs. 8-9 and 8-10).[16,17] In contrast, halothane lowers MAP partly or entirely by decreasing CO, whereas SVR is relatively unchanged. These findings are supported by measurements of SVR in patients receiving desflurane, sevoflurane, and isoflurane while undergoing cardiopulmonary bypass perfusion. The dose-related decrease in SVR is minimized by substitution of nitrous oxide for a portion of the volatile drug (Fig. 8-11).[18] Nitrous oxide, in contrast to the other inhaled anesthetics, causes unchanged or mildly increased MAP when administered alone to volunteers (Table 8-6).

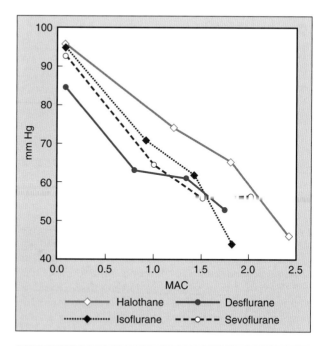

Figure 8-8 The effects of increasing concentrations (MAC) of halothane, isoflurane, desflurane, and sevoflurane on mean arterial pressure (mm Hg) when administered to healthy volunteers. (From Cahalan MK. Hemodynamic Effects of Inhaled Anesthetics. Review Courses. Cleveland: International Anesthesia Research Society, 1996, pp 14-18, with permission.)

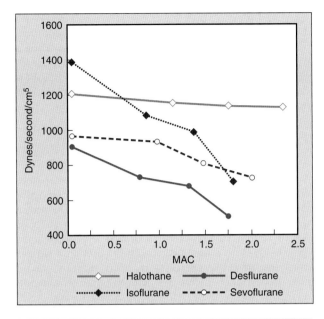

Figure 8-9 The effects of increasing concentrations (MAC) of halothane, isoflurane, desflurane, and sevoflurane on systemic vascular resistance (dynes/sec/cm⁵) when administered to healthy volunteers. (From Cahalan MK. Hemodynamic Effects of Inhaled Anesthetics. Review Courses. Cleveland: International Anesthesia Research Society, 1996, pp 14-18, with permission.)

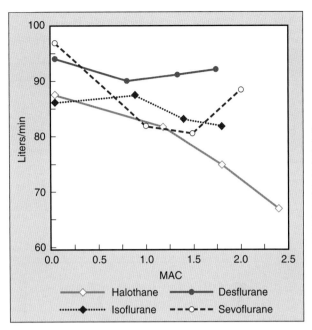

Figure 8-10 The effects of increasing concentrations (MAC) of halothane, isoflurane, desflurane, and sevoflurane on cardiac index (L/min) when administered to healthy volunteers. (From Cahalan MK. Hemodynamic Effects of Inhaled Anesthetics. Review Courses. Cleveland: International Anesthesia Research Society, 1996, pp 14-18, with permission.)

Heart Rate

Stepwise increases in the delivered concentrations of isoflurane, desflurane, and sevoflurane increase heart rates in patients and volunteers, although at different concentrations (Fig. 8-12).[16] At concentrations as low as 0.25 MAC, isoflurane causes a linear, dose-dependent heart rate increase. Heart rate increases minimally with desflurane concentrations of less than 1 MAC. When desflurane concentrations are increased, the heart rate accelerates in a linear, dose-dependent manner. In contrast to desflurane and isoflurane, heart rate in the presence of sevoflurane does not increase until the concentration exceeds 1.5 MAC.[19] However, induction with 8% sevoflurane (i.e., single-breath induction) has been associated with tachycardia in children and in adult patients undergoing controlled hyperventilation. This tachycardia may result from sympathetic nervous system stimulation associated with epileptiform brain activity.[20]

The tendency for desflurane to stimulate the circulation (i.e., increased MAP and heart rate) wanes during maintenance of anesthesia. Halothane does not increase heart rate across a wide range of concentrations (up to and exceeding 2 MAC), and this is presumed to reflect a drug-induced inhibition of baroreceptor reflex responsiveness. The dose-related increase in heart rate seen with

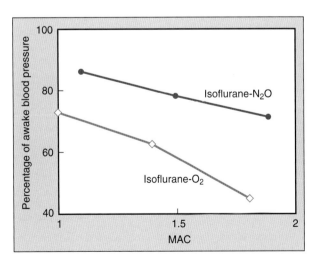

Figure 8-11 The substitution of nitrous oxide for a portion of isoflurane produces less decrease in systemic blood pressure than the same dose of volatile anesthetic alone. (From Eger EI. Isoflurane (Forane): A Compendium and Reference. Madison, WI: Ohio Medical Products, 1985, pp 1-110, with permission.)

Table 8–6 Evidence of a Sympathomimetic Effect of Nitrous Oxide Administered Alone or Added to Unchanging Concentrations of Volatile Anesthetics

Diaphoresis
Increased body temperature
Increased plasma concentrations of catecholamines
Increased right atrial pressure
Mydriasis
Vasoconstriction in the systemic and pulmonary circulations

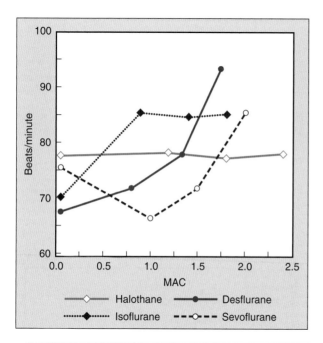

Figure 8-12 The effects of increasing concentrations (MAC) of halothane, isoflurane, desflurane, and sevoflurane on heart rate (beats/min) when administered to healthy volunteers. (From Cahalan MK. Hemodynamic Effects of Inhaled Anesthetics. Review Courses. Cleveland: International Anesthesia Research Society, 1996, pp 14-18, with permission.)

Cardiac Index

The cardiac index is minimally influenced by administration of desflurane, sevoflurane, or isoflurane over a wide range of concentrations to healthy young adults (see Fig. 8-10).[16] Transesophageal echocardiography data show that desflurane produces minor increases in the ejection fraction and left ventricular velocity of circumferential shortening compared with awake measurements.

Circulatory Effects with Rapid Concentration Increase

At concentrations of less than 1 MAC, desflurane does not increase heart rate or MAP. However, abrupt increases in inspired desflurane concentrations above 1 MAC cause transient circulatory stimulation in the absence of opioids, adrenergic blockers, or other analgesic adjuncts (Fig. 8-13).[22] To a lesser extent, isoflurane has a similar capability to evoke increases in heart rate and blood pressure. Accompanying the hemodynamic stimulation seen with abrupt increased concentrations of desflurane and isoflurane are increases in plasma epinephrine and norepinephrine concentrations and sympathetic nervous system activity. An abrupt increase in the inspired sevoflurane concentration from 1 MAC to 1.5 MAC is associated with a slight decrease in heart rate.

A stepwise increase in end-tidal desflurane concentration from 4% to 8% within 1 minute may result in a doubling of the heart rate and blood pressure above baseline. Administration of small doses of opioids, clonidine, or esmolol profoundly attenuates the heart rate and blood pressure responses to the stepwise increase in desflurane concentration. Repetition of the rapid increase in end-tidal desflurane concentration from 4% to 8% after 30 minutes results in minimal changes of the heart rate and MAP, suggesting that the receptors mediating these circulatory changes adapt to repeated stimulation. Circulatory stimulation is not seen with abrupt increases in the concentrations of sevoflurane, halothane, or enflurane up to 2 MAC (see Fig. 8-13).[22]

Sevoflurane and halothane are frequently used for inhalation induction because of their lack of pungency. Induction of anesthesia in children with halothane, but not sevoflurane, depresses myocardial contractility. In adults, maintenance of anesthesia with 1 MAC of sevoflurane or halothane in 67% nitrous oxide decreases myocardial contractility. In adults, sevoflurane can transiently increase heart rate when controlled ventilation is used.

Administration with Nitrous Oxide–Oxygen versus 100% Oxygen

Desflurane, isoflurane, and sevoflurane, administered with nitrous oxide and oxygen, decrease the MAP, SVR, cardiac index, and left ventricular stroke work index (LVSWI) in a dose-dependent manner, whereas heart rate, pulmonary artery pressure, and central venous pressure increase, consistent with the findings in which each volatile drug is

desflurane concentrations of more than 1 MAC is not significantly attenuated by partial anesthetic substitution with nitrous oxide. Isoflurane, sevoflurane, and desflurane, like halothane, diminish baroreceptor responses in a concentration-dependent manner. The transient increase in heart rate above 1 MAC seen with desflurane results from sympathetic nervous system stimulation rather than a reflex baroreceptor activity response to decreased MAP.[21]

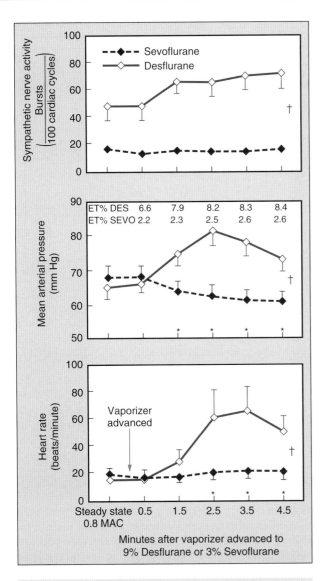

Figure 8-13 A rapid increase in the inspired concentration of sevoflurane from 0.8 MAC to 3% did not alter sympathetic nerve activity, mean arterial pressure, or heart rate. Conversely, a rapid increase in the inspired concentration of desflurane from 0.8 MAC to 9% significantly increased sympathetic nerve activity, mean arterial pressure, and heart rate (mean ± SE; *P < .05). ET, end-tidal. (From Ebert TJ, Muzi M, Lopatka CW. Neurocirculatory responses to sevoflurane in humans: A comparison to desflurane. Anesthesiology 1995;83:88-95, with permission.)

administered in oxygen alone (see Fig. 8-11).[16,17] Direct comparison reveals a more pronounced diminution of MAP, SVR, cardiac index, and LVSWI and a higher heart rate and CO when desflurane is administered in oxygen rather than in nitrous oxide at roughly equivalent MAC multiples.[17]

MYOCARDIAL CONDUCTION AND DYSRHYTHMOGENICITY

Isoflurane, sevoflurane, and desflurane do not predispose the heart to premature ventricular extrasystoles.[23] In contrast, halothane does sensitize the myocardium to premature ventricular extrasystoles, especially in the presence of catecholamines. Evidence from animal studies suggests that inhaled anesthetics suppress ventricular dysrhythmias related to myocardial ischemia, possibly as a result of prolongation of the effective refractory period.

The choice of inhaled anesthetic influences the occurrence of reflex bradydysrhythmias that may result from vagal stimulation. Children anesthetized with sevoflurane, compared with halothane, exhibit fewer episodes of decreased heart rate or sinus node arrest in response to surgical traction on the ocular muscles.

QT Interval

Inhaled anesthetics prolong the QT interval on the electrocardiogram.[24] Although each anesthetic's relative tendency to prolong the QT interval has not been compared systematically, sevoflurane should be avoided in patients with known congenital long QT syndrome (LQTS). Although sevoflurane and propofol anesthetics cause QT interval prolongation in children, neither anesthetic increases transmural dispersion of repolarization, a measure of the heterogeneous rates of repolarization of myocardial cells during phase 2 and 3 of the action potential.[25] The clinical significance of QT prolongation with sevoflurane and other inhaled anesthetics in susceptible patients is unclear. In patients with LQTS, β-adrenergic blockade is the mainstay of therapy. Patients with known long QT syndrome have been safely anesthetized with all modern inhaled anesthetics when concurrently on β-blocking drugs. Numerous malignant intraoperative arrhythmias have been reported in patients undergoing anesthesia with halothane that were subsequently attributed to undiagnosed LQTS, and none of the patients had been on β-blocking drugs.[24]

PATIENTS WITH CORONARY ARTERY DISEASE

Numerous studies in patients undergoing coronary artery bypass surgery or at risk for coronary artery disease have failed to demonstrate a difference in outcome between groups receiving inhalation (i.e., desflurane) versus intravenous (i.e., fentanyl or sufentanil) anesthetic techniques or between groups receiving one inhaled anesthetic versus another (i.e., desflurane versus isoflurane or sevoflurane versus isoflurane).[26] Concerns that isoflurane's capacity to dilate small-diameter coronary arteries might cause coronary steal, in which a patient with susceptible anatomy might develop regional myocardial ischemia as a result of coronary vasodilatation, were not valid. Volatile anesthetic drugs instead exert a protective effect on the heart, limiting the area of myocardial injury and preserving function after exposure to ischemic insult.

Anesthetic Preconditioning

The explanation for the protective benefits of volatile anesthetics against myocardial ischemia is called *anesthetic preconditioning*, and it is not explained by favorable alteration of myocardial oxygen supply-demand ratio. Evidence suggests that volatile anesthetics exert protective effects on the myocardium in the setting of compromised regional perfusion. In patients undergoing coronary artery bypass graft (CABG) surgery, maintenance with 0.2 to 1 MAC of desflurane or sevoflurane decreased the incidence of abnormally elevated troponin levels compared with patients receiving propofol.[27] Sevoflurane administered for the entire duration of CABG surgery versus prebypass or postbypass administration resulted in a lower rate of postoperative myocardial infarction compared with sevoflurane administered only in the prebypass or postbypass period, and prebypass or postbypass administration resulted in a lower risk of myocardial infarction compared with propofol anesthesia.[28]

Mechanisms of Ischemic Preconditioning

Ischemic preconditioning is a fundamental protective mechanism present in all tissues in all species. In ischemic preconditioning, exposure to single or multiple brief episodes of ischemia can confer a protective effect on the myocardium against reversible or irreversible injury with a subsequent prolonged ischemic insult. There are two distinct periods after a brief ischemic episode during which the myocardium is protected. The first period occurs for 1 to 2 hours after the conditioning episode and then dissipates. In the second period, the benefit reappears 24 hours later and can last as long as 3 days. The opening of mitochondrial ATP-sensitive potassium channels (K_{ATP}) is the crucial event that confers the protective activity, resulting from binding of various ligands to G protein–coupled receptors. Volatile anesthetics have been shown to enhance ischemic preconditioning or provide direct myocardial protection, and the K_{ATP} channels play a central role in their protective effects.[29]

Ventilation Effects

Inhaled anesthetics increase the frequency of breathing and decrease tidal volume as anesthetic concentration increases. Although minute ventilation is relatively preserved, the decreased tidal volume leads to a relatively greater proportion of dead space ventilation relative to alveolar ventilation. Gas exchange becomes progressively less efficient at deeper levels of anesthesia, and $PaCO_2$ increases proportionally with anesthetic concentration (Fig. 8-14).[1] Effects are similar among potent anesthetics at given MAC multiples. Substitution of nitrous oxide (60%) for an equivalent portion of volatile anesthetic may attenuate the increase in $PaCO_2$ at deeper levels of anesthesia.

Volunteers and patients breathing desflurane (and other volatile anesthetics) show a dose-related blunting of carbon

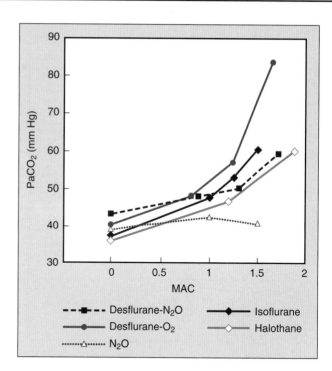

Figure 8-14 Inhaled anesthetics produce drug-specific and dose-dependent increases in $PaCO_2$. (From Eger EI. Desflurane (Suprane): A Compendium and Reference. Nutley, NJ: Anaquest, 1993, pp 1-119, with permission.)

dioxide responsiveness, which leads to apnea in subjects receiving 1.7 MAC of desflurane in oxygen (Fig 8-15).[1] Compared with volunteers, the blunting of ventilation with inhaled anesthetics may be less pronounced in patients undergoing surgery, reflecting the stimulatory effect of surgical stimulation on breathing (Fig. 8-16).[1] Volatile anesthetics all blunt the ventilatory stimulation evoked by arterial hypoxemia.[30]

CHEST WALL CHANGES

Inhaled anesthetics contribute to conformational changes in the chest wall that may influence ventilatory mechanics. Cephalad displacement of the diaphragm and inward displacement of the rib cage occur from enhanced expiratory muscle activity, and the net result contributes to reduction in functional residual capacity. Atelectasis occurs preferentially in the dependent areas of the lung and occurs to a greater extent when spontaneous ventilation is permitted.

HYPOXIC PULMONARY VASOCONSTRICTION

Inhaled anesthetics alter pulmonary blood flow, but inhibition of hypoxic pulmonary vasoconstriction is minimal. For example, arterial oxygenation is similar in patients undergoing one-lung ventilation with isoflurane

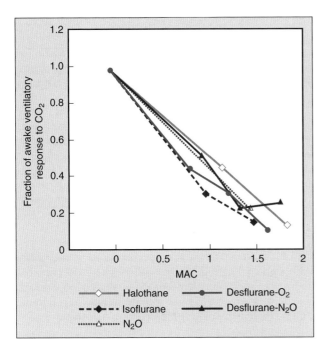

Figure 8-15 All inhaled anesthetics produce similar dose-dependent decreases in the ventilatory responses to carbon dioxide. (From Eger EI. Desflurane (Suprane): A Compendium and Reference. Nutley, NJ: Anaquest, 1993, pp 1-119, with permission.)

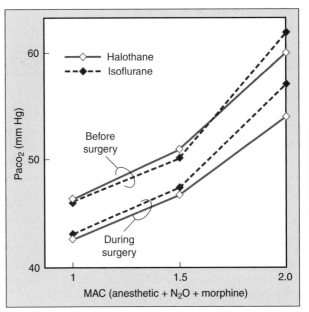

Figure 8-16 Impact of surgical stimulation on the resting Pa_{CO_2} (mm Hg) during administration of isoflurane or halothane. (From Eger EI. Desflurane (Suprane): A Compendium and Reference. Nutley, NJ: Anaquest, 1993, pp 1-119, with permission.)

versus desflurane anesthesia and sevoflurane versus propofol anesthesia.[31]

AIRWAY RESISTANCE

In the absence of bronchoconstriction, bronchodilating effects of inhaled anesthetics are small. In volunteers, isoflurane, halothane and sevoflurane, but not nitrous oxide and thiopental, decrease respiratory systemic resistance after tracheal intubation. In nonsmokers, airway resistance shows no change after tracheal intubation and desflurane anesthesia compared with a modest decrease with sevoflurane, whereas smokers show a mild, transient increase in airway resistance after tracheal intubation and desflurane anesthesia.[32]

AIRWAY IRRITANT EFFECTS

Inhaled anesthetics differ in their capacity to irritate airways (i.e., pungency). Sevoflurane, halothane, and nitrous oxide are nonpungent and cause minimal or no irritation over a broad range of concentrations. Desflurane and isoflurane are pungent, and they can irritate the airways in concentrations exceeding 1 MAC, particularly in the absence of intravenous medications (e.g., opioids, sedative-hypnotics) that decrease the perception of pungency.

Sevoflurane or halothane is selected most frequently when inhalation induction of anesthesia is desired. However, desflurane and isoflurane may be administered to surgical patients by means of a laryngeal mask airway without a greater incidence of airway irritation (e.g., coughing, breath-holding, laryngospasm, arterial oxygen desaturation) compared with sevoflurane or propofol, because maintenance usually requires concentrations of less than 1 MAC (i.e., nonirritating concentrations).[33]

Central Nervous System Effects

CEREBRAL BLOOD FLOW

Nitrous oxide administered without volatile anesthetics causes cerebral vasodilatation and increases cerebral blood flow. The cerebral metabolic rate for oxygen ($CMRO_2$) increases modestly. Coadministration of opioids, barbiturates, or propofol (but not ketamine) counteracts these effects.[34] Inhaled anesthetics do not abolish cerebral vascular responsiveness to changes in Pa_{CO_2}.[35]

Halothane, isoflurane, sevoflurane, and desflurane decrease $CMRO_2$. In normocapnic humans, these volatile anesthetics cause cerebral vasodilatation at concentrations above 0.6 MAC. There is a biphasic dose-dependent effect on cerebral blood flow. At 0.5 MAC, the decrease in $CMRO_2$ counteracts the vasodilatation such that cerebral blood flow does not change significantly. At concentrations in excess of 1 MAC, vasodilating effects predominate and cerebral blood flow increases, especially if systemic blood pressure is maintained at awake levels. The cerebral blood flow increase is relatively greater with halothane compared with isoflurane, sevoflurane, or desflurane.

INTRACRANIAL PRESSURE

Intracranial pressure increases with all of the volatile anesthetics at doses higher than 1 MAC, and autoregulation (i.e., adaptive mechanism normalizing cerebral blood flow over a wide range of systemic arterial pressures in awake patients) is impaired at concentrations of less than 1 MAC. Patients undergoing craniotomy for supratentorial tumors who receive 1 MAC of isoflurane or desflurane show decreased cerebral perfusion pressure and an arterial-venous oxygen difference for oxygen but no change in intracranial pressure.[36] However, patients undergoing pituitary tumor resection who receive 1 MAC of desflurane, isoflurane, or sevoflurane show small increases in intracranial pressure and decreased cerebral blood flow. Neurosurgical patients receiving 50% nitrous oxide plus 0.5 MAC of desflurane or isoflurane were judged to have greater brain relaxation than those receiving 1 MAC of desflurane or isoflurane without nitrous oxide. Inhaled anesthetics do not abolish cerebral vascular responsiveness to changes in $PaCO_2$.[35]

EVOKED POTENTIALS

All volatile anesthetics and nitrous oxide depress the amplitude and increase the latency of somatosensory evoked potentials in a dose-dependent manner. Evoked potentials may be abolished at 1 MAC of volatile anesthetic alone or above 0.5 MAC administered with 50% nitrous oxide. Low concentrations of volatile anesthetics (0.2 to 0.3 MAC) decrease the reliability of motor evoked potential monitoring.[37]

ELECTROENCEPHALOGRAPHIC EFFECTS

Volatile anesthetics cause characteristic, dose-dependent changes in the EEG. Increasing depth of anesthesia from the awake state is characterized by increased amplitude and synchrony. Periods of electrical silence begin to occupy a greater proportion of the time as depth increases (i.e., burst suppression). This isoelectric pattern predominates on the EEG within the range of 1.5 to 2.0 MAC.

Sevoflurane and enflurane may be associated with epileptiform activity on the EEG, especially at higher concentrations or when controlled hyperventilation is instituted. Seizure-like activity has been reported in children during sevoflurane induction, but the clinical implications of these observations are not clear.[38]

Neuromuscular Effects

Volatile anesthetics produce dose-related skeletal muscle relaxation and enhance the activity of succinylcholine and nondepolarizing neuromuscular blocking drugs. Enhancement of the relaxant effect of rocuronium is greater with desflurane than with sevoflurane or isoflurane, although all volatile anesthetics enhance skeletal muscle relaxation compared with intravenous anesthetics (e.g., propofol plus fentanyl). Elimination of volatile anesthetic enhances recovery from neuromuscular blockade. A decrease in the desflurane concentration to 0.25 MAC has a greater effect on reversal of neuromuscular block after vecuronium administration than an equipotent decrease in isoflurane concentration.

Malignant Hyperthermia

Although all potent inhaled anesthetics have the potential to trigger malignant hyperthermia, studies on humans and animals suggest less risk with desflurane, sevoflurane, and possibly isoflurane compared with halothane.

Hepatic Effects

Hepatic injury after anesthesia may be categorized as severe (immune mediated) or mild.[39]

IMMUNE-MEDIATED LIVER INJURY

Severe hepatic injury may follow anesthesia with halothane, isoflurane, sevoflurane, or desflurane. This severe form involves massive hepatic necrosis that can lead to death or necessitate liver transplantation. The mechanism for this severe injury is immunologic, requiring prior exposure to a volatile anesthetic. Halothane, isoflurane, and desflurane all undergo oxidative metabolism by cytochrome P450 enzymes to produce trifluoroacetate. The trifluoroacetate can bind covalently to hepatocyte proteins. The trifluoroacetyl-hepatocyte moieties can act as haptens, which the body recognizes as foreign and to which the immune system forms antibodies. Subsequent exposure to any anesthetic capable of producing trifluoroacetate may provoke an immune response, leading to severe hepatic necrosis.[40] Although sevoflurane is not metabolized to trifluoroacetyl products, it undergoes degradation on contact with carbon dioxide absorbent to compound A, which may act in a manner analogous to trifluoroacetate and provoke an immunologic response.

MILD LIVER INJURY

A clinically mild form of liver injury may follow administration of halothane. The main characteristic of this more common entity is modest elevation of serum transaminase levels. This mild form of liver injury is thought to be mediated by reductive metabolism of halothane and may be more likely to occur after concomitant decreases in hepatic blood flow and associated reductions in oxygen delivery to the liver.

HISTORY OF PRIOR ANESTHESIA-RELATED HEPATIC DYSFUNCTION

It is standard practice to avoid volatile anesthetics in patients who have experienced unexplained symptoms of hepatic dysfunction after inhaled anesthesia on a previous occasion. There is no evidence to suggest that volatile anesthetics are harmful to patients with preexisting hepatic disease unrelated to anesthesia.

REFERENCES

1. Eger EI. Desflurane (Suprane): A compendium and reference. Nutley, NJ: Anaquest, 1993, pp 1-11.
2. Eger EI II. History of Modern Inhaled Anesthetics: The Pharmacology of Inhaled Anesthetics, 1st ed. San Antonio, TX: Dannemiller Memorial Educational Foundation, 2000, pp 2-5.
3. Eger EI. New inhaled anesthetics. Anesthesiology 1994;80:906-922.
4. Eger EI, Koblin DD, Harris RA, et al. Hypothesis: Inhaled anesthetics produce immobility and amnesia by different mechanisms at different sites. Anesth Analg 1997;84:915-918.
5. Quasha AL, Eger EI II, Tinker JH. Determination and application of MAC. Anesthesiology 1980;53:315-334.
6. Rampill IJ. Anesthetic potency is not altered after hypothermic spinal cord transection in rats. Anesthesiology 1994;80:606-610.
7. Carpenter RL, Eger EI II, Johnson BH, et al. The extent of metabolism of inhaled anesthetics in humans. Anesthesiology 1986;65:201-205.
8. Wissing H, Kuhn I, Warnken U, Dudziak R. Carbon monoxide production from desflurane, enflurane, halothane, isoflurane, and sevoflurane with dry soda lime. Anesthesiology 2001;95:1205-1212.
9. Laster MJ, Rogh P, Eger EI. Fires from the interaction of anesthetics with desiccated absorbent. Anesth Analg 2004;99:769-774.
10. Wu J, Previte JP, Adler E, et al. Spontaneous ignition, explosion, and fire with sevoflurane and barium hydroxide lime. Anesthesiology 2004;101:534-537.
11. Eger EI II. Uptake of inhaled anesthetics: The alveolar to inspired anesthetic difference. In Eger EI II (ed): Anesthetic Uptake and Action. Baltimore: Williams & Wilkins, 1974, pp 77-96.
12. Eger EI. Effect of inspired anesthetic concentration on the rate of rise of alveolar concentration. Anesthesiology 1963;24:153-157.
13. Uasuda N, Lockard SH, Eger EI, et al. Comparison of kinetics of sevoflurane and isoflurane in humans. Anesth Analg 1992;72:316-324.

14. Eger EI II, Saidman JL. Hazards of nitrous oxide anesthesia in bowel obstruction and pneumothorax. Anesthesiology 1965;26:61-66.
15. Bailey JM. Context-sensitive half-times and other decrement times of inhaled anesthetics. Anesth Analg 1997;85:681-686.
16. Cahalan MK. Hemodynamic Effects of Inhaled Anesthetics. Review Courses. Cleveland: International Anesthesia Research Society, 1996, pp 14-18.
17. Cahalan MK, Weiskopf RB, Eger EI II, et al. Hemodynamic effects of desflurane/nitrous oxide anesthesia in volunteers. Anesth Analg 1991;73:157-164.
18. Eger EI. Isoflurane (Forane): A Compendium and Reference. Madison, WI: Ohio Medical Products, 1985, pp 1-110.
19. Malan TP, DiNardo JA, Isner RJ, et al. Cardiovascular effects of sevoflurane compared with those of isoflurane in volunteers. Anesthesiology 1995;83:918-928.
20. Yli-Hankala A, Vakkuri AP, Sarkela M, et al. Epileptiform electroencephalogram during mask induction of anesthesia with sevoflurane. Anesthesiology 1999;91:1596.
21. Ebert TJ, Perez F, Uhrich TD, Deshur MA. Desflurane-mediated sympathetic activation occurs in humans despite preventing hypotension and baroreceptor unloading. Anesthesiology 1998;85:1227-1232.
22. Ebert TJ, Muzi M, Lopatka CW. Neurocirculatory responses to sevoflurane in humans: A comparison to desflurane. Anesthesiology 1995;83:88-95.
23. Navarro R, Weiskopf RB, Moore MA, et al. Humans anesthetized with sevoflurane or isoflurane have similar arrhythmic responses to epinephrine. Anesthesiology 1994;80:545-549.
24. Booker PD, Whyte SD, Ladusans EJ. Long QT syndrome and anaesthesia. Br J Anaesth 2003;90:349-366.
25. Whyte SD, Booker PD, Buckley DG. The effects of propofol and sevoflurane on the QT interval and transmural dispersion of repolarization in children. Anesth Analg 2005;100:71-77.

26. Grundman U, Muler M, Kleinschmidt S, et al. Cardiovascular effects of desflurane and isoflurane in patients with coronary artery disease. Acta Anaesthesiol Scand 1996;40:1101-1107.
27. DeHert SG, Cromheecke S, ten Broecke PW, et al. Effects of propofol, desflurane, and sevoflurane on recovery of myocardial function after coronary surgery in elderly high-risk patients. Anesthesiology 2003;99:314-323.
28. DeHert SG, Van der Linden PJ, Cromheecke S, et al. Cardioprotective properties of sevoflurane in patients undergoing coronary surgery and cardiopulmonary bypass are related to the modalities of its administration. Anesthesiology 2004;101:299-310.
29. Zaugg M, Lucchinetti E, Spahn D, et al. Volatile anesthetics mimic cardiac preconditioning by priming the activation of the mitoK$_{ATP}$ channels via multiple signaling pathways. Anesthesiology 2002;97:4-14.
30. Sjögren D, Lindahl SGE, Sollevi A. Ventilatory responses to acute and sustained hypoxia during isoflurane anesthesia. Anesth Analg 1998;86:403-409.
31. Beck DH, Boephmer UR, Sinemus C, et al. Effects of sevoflurane and propofol on pulmonary shunt fraction during one-lung ventilation for thoracic surgery. Br J Anaesth 2001;86:38-43.
32. Goff MJ, Arain SR, Ficke DJ, et al. Absence of bronchodilation during desflurane anesthesia: A comparison to sevoflurane and thiopental. Anesthesiology 2000;93:404-408.
33. Eshima R, Maurer A, Kint T, et al. A comparison of upper airway responses during desflurane and sevoflurane administration via a laryngeal mask airway. Anesth Analg 2003;96:701-705.
34. Petersen KD, Landsfeldt U, Cold GE, et al. Intracranial pressure and cerebral hemodynamics in patients with cerebral tumors: A randomized prospective study of patients subjected to craniotomy in propofol-fentanyl, isoflurane-fentanyl, or sevoflurane-fentanyl anesthesia. Anesthesiology 2003;98:329-336.

35. Mielck F, Stephen H, Buhre W, et al. Effects of 1 MAC desflurane on cerebral metabolism, blood flow and carbon dioxide reactivity in humans. Br J Anaesth 1998;81:155-160.

36. Fraga M, Rama-Maceiras P, Rodino S, et al. The effects of isoflurane and desflurane on intracranial pressure, cerebral perfusion pressure, and cerebral arteriovenous oxygen content difference in normocapnic patients with supratentorial brain tumors. Anesthesiology 2003;98:1085-1090.

37. Lotto ML, Banoub M, Schubert A. Effects of anesthetic agents and physiologic changes on intraoperative motor evoked potentials. J Neurosurg Anesthesiol 2004;16:32-42.

38. Akeson J, Didricksson I. Convulsions on anaesthetic induction with sevoflurane in young children. Acta Anaesthesiol Scand 2004;48:405-407.

39. Martin JL. Volatile anesthetics and liver injury: A clinical update or what every anesthesiologist should know. Can J Anesth 2005;52:125-129.

40. Njoku D, Laster MJ, Gong D, et al. Biotransformation of halothane, enflurane, isoflurane and desflurane to trifluoroacetylated liver proteins: Association between protein acetylation and hepatic injury. Anesth Analg 1997;84:173-178.

Chapter 9

INTRAVENOUS ANESTHETICS

Helge Eilers

Intravenous nonopioid anesthetics have an important role in modern anesthesia practice (Table 9-1).[1-3] They are widely used to facilitate rapid induction of anesthesia or to provide sedation during monitored anesthesia care and for patients in intensive care settings. With the introduction of propofol, intravenous anesthesia also became more popular as a component of maintenance of anesthesia. However, the currently available intravenous anesthetics are not ideal anesthetic drugs in the sense of producing all and only desired effects (hypnosis, amnesia, analgesia, immobility). Therefore, "balanced anesthesia" with multiple drugs (inhaled anesthetics, sedative/hypnotics, opioids, neuromuscular blocking drugs) is generally used.

The intravenous anesthetics used for induction of general anesthesia are lipophilic and preferentially partition into highly perfused lipophilic tissues (brain, spinal cord), which accounts for their rapid onset of action. Regardless of the extent and speed of their metabolism, termination of the effect of a single bolus dose is a result of redistribution of the drug into less perfused and inactive tissues such as skeletal muscles and fat. Thus, all drugs used for induction of anesthesia have a similar duration of action for a single dose despite significant differences in their metabolism.

PROPOFOL

Propofol is the most frequently administered drug for induction of anesthesia.[1] In addition, propofol is used during maintenance of anesthesia and is a common selection for sedation in the operating room, as well as in the intensive care unit.

Physicochemical Characteristics

Propofol (2,6-diisopropylphenol) is an alkylphenol with hypnotic properties that is chemically distinct from other groups of intravenous anesthetics (Fig. 9-1). It is

Table 9–1 Drugs Classified as Intravenous Anesthetics

Isopropylphenol

   Propofol

Barbiturates

   Thiopental

   Methohexital

Benzodiazepines

   Diazepam

   Midazolam

   Lorazepam

Phencyclidine

   Ketamine

Carboxylated imidazole

   Etomidate

α_2-Adrenergic agonist

   Dexmedetomidine

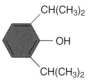

Figure 9-1 Chemical structure of 2,6-diisopropylphenol (propofol).

essentially insoluble in aqueous solutions and is therefore formulated as an emulsion containing 10% soybean oil, 2.25% glycerol, and 1.2% lecithin, the major component of the egg yolk phosphatide fraction. Because the available formulations support bacterial growth, good sterile technique is important. Although either ethylenediaminetetraacetic acid (0.05 mg/mL), metabisulfite (0.25 mg/mL), or benzyl alcohol (1 mg/mL) is added to the emulsions by the different manufacturers as retardants of bacterial growth, solutions should be used as soon as possible or at least within 6 hours after opening the propofol vial. The solutions appear milky white and slightly viscous, their pH is approximately 7, and the propofol concentration is 1% (10 mg/mL). In some countries, a 2% formulation is available. Because the emulsion contains egg yolk lecithin, susceptible patients may experience allergic reactions. The addition of metabisulfite in one of the formulations has raised concern regarding its use in patients with reactive airways (asthma) or sulfite allergies.

Pharmacokinetics

Propofol is rapidly metabolized in the liver, and the resulting water-soluble compounds are presumed to be inactive and excreted through the kidneys (Table 9-2). Plasma clearance is high and exceeds hepatic blood flow, thus indicating the importance of extrahepatic metabolism, which has been confirmed during the anhepatic phase of liver transplantation. The lungs are thought to play a major role in this extrahepatic metabolism and may account for the elimination of up to 30% of a bolus dose of propofol. The high plasma clearance of propofol explains the more complete recovery from propofol with less "hangover" than observed with thiopental. However, as with other intravenous drugs, transfer of propofol from the plasma (central) compartment and the associated termination of drug effect after a single bolus dose are mainly the result of redistribution from highly perfused (brain) to poorly perfused (skeletal muscles) compartments. Wake-up after an induction dose of propofol usually occurs within 8 to 10 minutes, as evident from the time course of the decline in plasma concentration after a single bolus dose (Fig. 9-2).[4]

CONTINUOUS INTRAVENOUS INFUSION

Rapid metabolism of propofol resulting in efficient plasma clearance in conjunction with slow redistribution from poorly perfused compartments back into the central compartment makes propofol suitable for use as a continuous intravenous infusion. The context-sensitive half-time describes the elimination half-time after a continuous infusion as a function of the duration of the infusion (Fig. 9-3).[5] The context-sensitive half-time of propofol is brief, even after a prolonged infusion, and recovery remains relatively prompt.

COMPARTMENTAL MODEL

The kinetics of propofol (and other intravenous anesthetics) after a single bolus and after continuous infusion is best described by a three-compartment model. These mathematical models have been used as the basis for the development of systems for target-controlled infusions.

Pharmacodynamics

The presumed mechanism of action of propofol is through potentiation of the chloride current mediated through the γ-aminobutyric acid type A (GABA$_A$) receptor complex.

CENTRAL NERVOUS SYSTEM

In the central nervous system (CNS), propofol primarily acts as a hypnotic and does not have any analgesic properties. It produces a decrease in cerebral blood flow (CBF) and the cerebral metabolic rate for oxygen (CMRO$_2$), which results in decreases in intracranial pressure (ICP) and intraocular pressure. The magnitude of these changes is comparable to those produced by thiopental. Although

Table 9-2 Pharmacokinetic Data for Intravenous Anesthetics

Drug	Induction Dose (mg/kg IV)	Duration of Action (min)	Vd_{ss} (min)	$T_{1/2} \alpha$ (min)	Protein Binding (%)	Clearance (mL/kg/min)	$T_{1/2} \beta$ (hr)
Propofol	1-2.5	3-8	2-10	2-4	97	20-30	4-23
Thiopental	3-5	5-10	2.5	2-4	83	3.4	11
Methohexital	1-1.5	4-7	2.2	5-6	73	11	4
Midazolam	0.1-0.3	15-20	1.1-1.7	7-15	94	6.4-11	1.7-2.6
Diazepam	0.3-0.6	15-30	0.7-1.7	10-15	98	0.2-0.5	20-50
Lorazepam	0.03-0.1	60-120	0.8-1.3	3-10	98	0.8-1.8	11-22
Ketamine	1-2	5-10	3.1	11-16	12	12-17	2-4
Etomidate	0.2-0.3	3-8	2.5-4.5	2-4	77	18-25	2.9-5.3
Dexmedetomidine	N/A	N/A	2-3	6	94	10-30	2-3

Data are for average adult patients. The duration of action reflects the duration after an average single IV dose.
N/A, not applicable; $T_{1/2} \alpha$, distribution half-time; $T_{1/2} \beta$, elimination half-time; Vd_{ss}, volume of distribution at steady state.

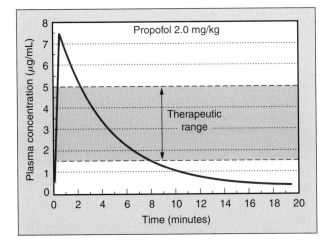

Figure 9-2 Time course of the propofol plasma concentration after a simulated single bolus injection of 2.0 mg/kg. The shape of this curve is similar for other induction drugs, although the slope and the absolute concentrations are different. (From Reves JG, Glass PSA, Lubarsky DA, McEvoy MD. Intravenous nonopioid anesthetics. In Miller RD [ed]: Miller's Anesthesia, 6th ed. Philadelphia: Churchill Livingstone, 2005.)

propofol can produce a desired decrease in ICP, the reduced CBF combined with the reduced mean arterial pressure caused by peripheral vasodilatation can critically decrease cerebral perfusion pressure.

Animal studies suggest that propofol is neuroprotective during focal ischemia to the same extent as thiopental or isoflurane. When administered in large doses, propofol produces burst suppression in the electroencephalogram (EEG), an end point that has been used for the administration of intravenous anesthetics for neuroprotection during neurosurgical procedures. Occasionally, excitatory effects such as twitching or spontaneous movement can be observed during induction of anesthesia with propofol. Although these effects may resemble seizure activity, most studies and reports support an anticonvulsant effect of propofol, and it may be safely administered to patients with seizure disorders.[1]

CARDIOVASCULAR SYSTEM

When compared with equianesthetic doses of other induction drugs, propofol produces the most pronounced decrease in systemic blood pressure. This effect can be attributed to profound vasodilatation, whereas a direct myocardial depressant effect is controversial. Vasodilation occurs in both the arterial and venous circulation and leads to reductions in preload and afterload. The effect on systemic blood pressure is more pronounced with increased age, in patients with reduced intravascular fluid volume, and with rapid injection. Propofol markedly inhibits the normal baroreflex response and produces only a small increase in heart rate, thus further exacerbating its hypotensive effect. Profound bradycardia and asystole after the administration of propofol have been described in healthy adults despite prophylactic anticholinergics.[6]

RESPIRATORY SYSTEM

Propofol is a potent respiratory depressant and generally produces apnea after an induction dose. A maintenance infusion will reduce minute ventilation through reductions in tidal volume and respiratory rate, with the effect on tidal volume being more pronounced. In addition, the

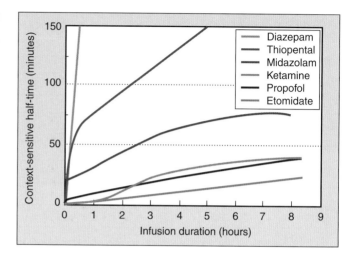

Figure 9-3 Context-sensitive half-time for the most commonly used intravenous anesthetics. Propofol, etomidate, and ketamine have the smallest increase in context-sensitive half-times, with prolonged infusions making these drugs more suitable for use as continuous infusions. (From Reves JG, Glass PSA, Lubarsky DA, McEvoy MD. Intravenous nonopioid anesthetics. In Miller RD [ed]: Miller's Anesthesia, 6th ed. Philadelphia: Churchill Livingstone, 2005.)

ventilatory response to hypoxia and hypercapnia is reduced. Propofol causes a greater reduction in upper airway reflexes than thiopental does, which makes it well suited for instrumentation of the airway, such as placement of a laryngeal mask airway. When compared with thiopental, propofol decreases the incidence of wheezing after induction of anesthesia and tracheal intubation in healthy and asthmatic patients.[7]

OTHER EFFECTS

An interesting and desired side effect of propofol is its antiemetic activity. Similar to thiopental and unlike volatile anesthetics, propofol does not potentiate neuromuscular blockade. However, studies have found good intubating conditions after propofol induction without the use of neuromuscular blocking agents. Unexpected tachycardia occurring during propofol anesthesia should prompt laboratory evaluation for possible metabolic acidosis (propofol infusion syndrome).[8]

Clinical Uses

Pain on injection is a common complaint and can be reduced by premedication with an opioid or coadministration with lidocaine. Dilution of propofol and the use of larger veins for injection can reduce the incidence and severity of injection pain.

INDUCTION AND MAINTENANCE OF ANESTHESIA

Propofol (1 to 2.5 mg/kg IV) is most commonly administered for induction of general anesthesia. Increasing age, reduced cardiovascular reserve, or premedication with benzodiazepines or opioids reduces the required induction dose, whereas children need higher doses (2.5 to 3.5 mg/kg IV). Generally, titration of the induction dose helps prevent severe hemodynamic changes. Propofol is also often used for maintenance of anesthesia either as part of a balanced anesthesia regimen in combination with volatile anesthetics, nitrous oxide, sedative-hypnotics, and

opioids or as part of a total intravenous anesthetic technique, usually in combination with opioids. Therapeutic plasma concentrations for maintenance of anesthesia normally range between 3 and 8 µg/mL (typically requiring a continuous infusion rate between 100 and 200 µg/kg/min) when combined with nitrous oxide or opioids.

SEDATION

Propofol is a popular choice for sedation of mechanically ventilated patients in the intensive care unit and for sedation during procedures in or outside the operating room. The required plasma concentration is 1 to 2 µg/mL, which will normally necessitate a continuous infusion rate between 25 and 75 µg/kg/min. Because of its pronounced respiratory depressant effect and its narrow therapeutic range, propofol should be administered only by individuals trained in airway management.

ANTIEMETIC

Subanesthetic bolus doses of propofol or a subanesthetic infusion can be used to treat postoperative nausea and vomiting (10 to 20 mg IV, 10 µg/kg/min as an infusion).

BARBITURATES

Before the introduction of propofol and its increasing use for induction of anesthesia, the intravenous anesthetics most commonly used for induction were barbiturates (thiopental, methohexital).[2]

Physicochemical Characteristics

Barbiturates are derived from barbituric acid (lacks hypnotic properties) through substitutions at the N1, C2, and C5 positions (Fig. 9-4). Based on their substitution at position 2, barbiturates used for induction of anesthesia can be grouped into thiobarbiturates, substituted with a

Table 9-3 Summary of the Pharmacodynamic Effects of Commonly Used Intravenous Anesthetics

	Propofol	Thiopental	Midazolam	Ketamine	Etomidate	Dexmedetomidine
Dose for induction of anesthesia (mg/kg IV)	1.5-2.5	3-5	0.1-0.3	1-2	0.2-0.3	
Systemic blood pressure	Decreased	Decreased	Unchanged to decreased	Increased	Decreased	Decreased
Heart rate	Unchanged to decreased	Increased	Unchanged	Increased	Unchanged to increased	Decreased
Systemic vascular resistance	Decreased	Decreased	Unchanged to decreased	Increased	Unchanged to decreased	Decreased
Ventilation	Decreased	Decreased	Unchanged	Unchanged	Unchanged to decreased	Unchanged
Respiratory rate	Decreased	Decreased	Unchanged	Unchanged	Unchanged to decreased	Unchanged
Response to carbon dioxide	Decreased	Decreased	Unchanged	Unchanged	Decreased	Unchanged
Cerebral blood flow	Decreased	Decreased	Unchanged	Increased to unchanged	Decreased	Unchanged
Cerebral metabolic requirements for oxygen	Decreased	Decreased	Unchanged	Increased to unchanged	Decreased	Unchanged to decreased
Intracranial pressure	Decreased	Decreased	Unchanged	Unchanged to increased	Decreased	Unchanged
Anticonvulsant	Unclear	Yes	Yes	Unclear	No	
Anxiolysis	No	No	Yes	No	No	Yes?
Analgesia	No	No	No	Yes	No	No?
Emergence delirium	No?	No	No	Yes	No	No
Nausea and vomiting	Decreased	Unchanged	Unchanged to decreased	Unchanged	Increased	Unchanged
Adrenocortical suppression	No	No	Yes?	No	Yes	No
Pain on injection	Yes	No	No	No	No	No

sulfur (thiopental), or oxybarbiturates, substituted with an oxygen (methohexital). Hypnotic, sedative, and anticonvulsant effects, as well as lipid solubility and onset time, are determined by the type and position of substitution.

Thiopental and methohexital are formulated as sodium salts mixed with anhydrous sodium carbonate. After reconstitution with water or normal saline, the solutions (2.5% thiopental and 1% methohexital) are alkaline with a pH higher than 10. Although this property prevents bacterial growth and helps increase the shelf life of the solution after reconstitution, it will lead to precipitation when mixed with acidic drug preparations such as neuromuscular blocking drugs. These precipitates can irreversibly block intravenous delivery lines if mixing occurs during administration. Furthermore, accidental injection into an artery or infiltration into paravenous tissue will cause extreme pain and may lead to severe tissue injury.

Several barbiturates, including thiopental and methohexital, have optical isomers with different potencies. However, the available formulations are racemic mixtures, and their potencies reflect the summation of the potencies of the individual isomers.

Figure 9-4 Structure of barbituric acid and its derivatives.

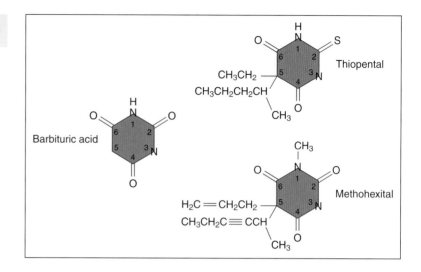

Pharmacokinetics

Barbiturates, except for phenobarbital, undergo hepatic metabolism most importantly by oxidation, but also by N-dealkylation, desulfuration, and destruction of the barbituric acid ring structure. The resulting metabolites are inactive and excreted through urine and, after conjugation, through bile. In contrast, phenobarbital is mainly eliminated unchanged through renal excretion. Chronic administration of barbiturates or the administration of other drugs that induce oxidative microsomal enzymes (enzyme induction) enhances barbiturate metabolism. Through stimulation of aminolevulinic acid synthetase, the production of porphyrins is increased. Therefore, barbiturates should not be administered to patients with acute intermittent porphyria.

Methohexital is cleared more rapidly by the liver than thiopental is and thus has a shorter elimination half-time. This accounts for faster and more complete recovery after methohexital administration. Although thiopental is metabolized slowly and has a long elimination half-time, recovery after a single bolus administration is comparable to methohexital and propofol because it depends on redistribution to inactive tissue sites rather than metabolism (Fig. 9-5).[9] However, even single-bolus induction doses of thiopental can, in some cases, lead to psychomotor impairment that lasts up to several hours. If administered as repeated boluses or as a continuous infusion, especially when using larger doses to produce burst suppression on the EEG, recovery from the effects of thiopental will be markedly prolonged because of the long context-sensitive half-time (see Fig. 9-3).

Pharmacodynamics

The mechanism of action for the effect of barbiturates in the CNS presumably involves both enhancement of inhibitory neurotransmission and inhibition of excitatory transmission. Although the effects on inhibitory transmission probably result from activation of the $GABA_A$ receptor complex, the effects on excitatory transmission are less well understood.

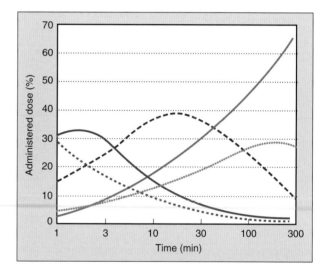

Figure 9-5 After rapid intravenous injection of thiopental, the percentage of the administered dose remaining in blood (*yellow line*) rapidly decreases as the drug moves from blood to highly perfused vessel-rich tissues (*blue line*), especially the brain. Subsequently, thiopental is redistributed to skeletal muscles (*red line*) and, to a lesser extent, to fat (*pink line*). Ultimately, most of the administered dose of thiopental undergoes metabolism (*green line*). (From Saidman LJ. Uptake, distribution, and elimination of barbiturates. *In* Eger EI [ed]: Anesthetic Uptake and Action. Baltimore: Williams & Wilkins, 1974, pp 264-284, with permission.)

CENTRAL NERVOUS SYSTEM

Barbiturates produce dose-dependent CNS depression ranging from sedation to general anesthesia when administered in induction doses.[2] They do not have analgesic properties, and in fact some evidence suggests that they may reduce the pain threshold and thus could be classified as an antianalgesic. Barbiturates are potent cerebral vasoconstrictors and produce predictable decreases in CBF, cerebral blood volume, and ICP. As a result, they decrease $CMRO_2$ in a dose-dependent manner up to a maximum dose at which the EEG becomes flat-line. The ability of barbiturates to decrease ICP and $CMRO_2$ makes these drugs useful in the management of patients with space-occupying intracranial lesions. Furthermore, they may provide neuroprotection from focal cerebral ischemia (stroke, surgical retraction, temporary clips during aneurysm surgery), but probably not from global cerebral ischemia (cardiac arrest). An exception to the generalization that barbiturates decrease electrical activity on the EEG is methohexital, which activates epileptic foci, thus facilitating their identification during surgery designed to ablate these sites. For the same reason, methohexital is also a popular choice for anesthesia to facilitate electroconvulsive therapy.

CARDIOVASCULAR SYSTEM

Administration of barbiturates for induction of anesthesia typically produces modest decreases in systemic blood pressure that are smaller than those produced by propofol. This decrease in systemic blood pressure is principally due to peripheral vasodilation and reflects barbiturate-induced depression of the medullary vasomotor center and decreased sympathetic nervous system outflow from the CNS. Although barbiturates blunt the baroreceptor reflex, compensatory increases in heart rate limit the decrease in blood pressure and make it transient. Moreover, dilation of peripheral capacitance vessels leads to pooling of blood and decreased venous return, thus resulting in the potential for reduced cardiac output and systemic blood pressure. Indeed, exaggerated decreases in systemic blood pressure are likely to follow the administration of barbiturates to patients with hypovolemia, cardiac tamponade, cardiomyopathy, coronary artery disease, or cardiac valvular disease because such patients are less able to compensate for the effects of peripheral vasodilation. Hemodynamic effects are also more pronounced with larger doses and rapid injection. The negative inotropic effects of barbiturates, which are readily demonstrated in isolated heart preparations, are usually masked in vivo by baroreceptor reflex–mediated responses.

RESPIRATORY SYSTEM

Barbiturates are respiratory depressants and lead to decreased minute ventilation through reduced tidal volumes and respiratory rate. Anesthetic induction doses of thiopental and methohexital typically induce transient apnea, which will be more pronounced if other respiratory depressants are also administered. Barbiturates also decrease the ventilatory responses to hypercapnia and hypoxia. Resumption of spontaneous breathing after an anesthetic induction dose of a barbiturate is characterized by a slow breathing rate and decreased tidal volume. Suppression of laryngeal reflexes and cough reflexes is not as profound as after propofol administration, which makes barbiturates an inferior choice for airway instrumentation in the absence of neuromuscular blocking drugs. Furthermore, stimulation of the upper airway or trachea (secretions, laryngeal mask airway, direct laryngoscopy, tracheal intubation) during inadequate depression of airway reflexes may result in laryngospasm or bronchospasm. This phenomenon is not unique to barbiturates but is true in general when the drug dose is inadequate to suppress the airway reflexes.

SIDE EFFECTS

Accidental intra-arterial injection of barbiturates results in excruciating pain and intense vasoconstriction, often leading to severe tissue injury involving gangrene.[2] Aggressive therapy is directed at reversing the vasoconstriction to maintain perfusion and reduce the drug concentration mainly by dilution. Approaches to treatment include blockade of the sympathetic nervous system (stellate ganglion block) in the involved extremity. It is likely that barbiturate crystal formation results in the occlusion of more distal and small-diameter arteries and arterioles. Barbiturate crystal formation in veins is less hazardous because of the ever-increasing diameter of veins. Accidental subcutaneous injection (extravasation) of barbiturates results in local tissue irritation, thus emphasizing the importance of using dilute concentrations of barbiturates (2.5% thiopental, 1% methohexital). If extravasation occurs, some recommend local injection of the tissues with 0.5% lidocaine (5 to 10 mL) in an attempt to dilute the barbiturate concentration.

Life-threatening allergic reactions to barbiturates are rare, with an estimated occurrence of 1 in 30,000 patients. However, barbiturate-induced histamine release can occasionally be seen.

Clinical Uses

The principal clinical uses of barbiturates are rapid intravenous induction of anesthesia and treatment of increased ICP or to provide neuroprotection from focal cerebral ischemia.[2] A continuous intravenous infusion of a barbiturate such as thiopental is seldom used to maintain anesthesia because of its long context-sensitive half-time and prolonged recovery period (see Fig. 9-3).[5]

INDUCTION OF ANESTHESIA

Administration of thiopental (3 to 5 mg/kg IV) or methohexital (1 to 1.5 mg/kg IV) produces induction of

II

anesthesia (unconsciousness) in less than 30 seconds. Patients may experience a garlic or onion taste during induction of anesthesia.

Succinylcholine or a nondepolarizing neuromuscular blocking drug is often administered shortly after the barbiturate to produce skeletal muscle relaxation and facilitate tracheal intubation. The combination of a barbiturate, usually thiopental, and succinylcholine administered intravenously in rapid succession is the classic drug regimen used for "rapid-sequence induction of anesthesia." An important advantage of rapid-sequence induction of anesthesia is avoidance of facemask ventilation and early tracheal intubation with a cuffed tube (provides protection against aspiration in at-risk patients). Although thiopental is the drug that has traditionally been used in this setting, propofol is also a frequent choice.

For patients who are not at increased risk for aspiration, an alternative approach to the rapid intravenous induction of anesthesia is the administration of small doses of barbiturates (thiopental, 0.5 to 1.0 mg/kg IV), followed by placement of the facemask on the patient's face and delivery of an inhaled anesthetic such as sevoflurane to complete the induction of anesthesia. The low dose of barbiturate improves patient acceptance of the facemask and negates any unpleasant memory of the pungency of the inhaled anesthetic. This slow induction of anesthesia helps titrate the anesthetic effect more carefully and thereby avoids exaggerated hemodynamic responses. A slower induction with careful titration can also be accomplished by using only intravenous anesthetics, but propofol would probably be a more logical choice for this application because it has a shorter context-sensitive half-time (see Fig. 9-3).[5] Rectal administration of a barbiturate such as methohexital (20 to 30 mg/kg) may be used to facilitate induction of anesthesia in mentally challenged and uncooperative pediatric patients.

NEUROPROTECTION

Traditionally, an isoelectric EEG indicating maximal reduction of $CMRO_2$ has been used as the end point for barbiturate administration with the goal of neuroprotection. More recent data demonstrating equal protection after smaller doses have challenged this practice.[2] One risk of the use of high-dose barbiturate therapy to decrease ICP or to provide protection against focal cerebral ischemia (cardiopulmonary bypass, carotid endarterectomy, thoracic aneurysm resection) is the associated hypotension, which could lead to critically reduced cerebral perfusion pressure and may require the administration of vasoconstrictors to maintain adequate perfusion pressure.

BENZODIAZEPINES

Benzodiazepines commonly used in the perioperative period include diazepam, midazolam, and lorazepam, as well as the selective benzodiazepine antagonist flumazenil.[3] Benzodiazepines are unique among the group of intravenous anesthetics in that their action can readily be terminated by administration of their selective antagonist flumazenil. Their most desired effects are anxiolysis and anterograde amnesia, which are extremely useful for premedication.

Physicochemical Characteristics

The chemical structure of the benzodiazepines contains a benzene ring fused to a seven-member diazepine ring, hence their name (Fig. 9-6). The three commonly used benzodiazepines in the perioperative setting are all highly lipophilic, with midazolam having the highest lipid solubility. All three drugs are highly protein bound, mainly to serum albumin. Although they are used as parenteral formulations, all three drugs are absorbed after oral administration. Other possible routes of administration include intramuscular, intranasal, and sublingual. Exposure of the acidic midazolam preparation to the physiologic pH of blood causes a change in the ring structure that renders the drug more lipid soluble, thus

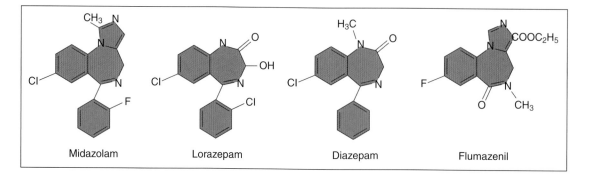

Midazolam   Lorazepam   Diazepam   Flumazenil

Figure 9-6 Chemical structure of the most commonly used benzodiazepines and their antagonist flumazenil.

speeding its passage across the blood-brain barrier and its onset of action.

Pharmacokinetics

The highly lipid-soluble benzodiazepines rapidly enter the CNS, which accounts for their rapid onset of action, followed by redistribution to inactive tissue sites and subsequent termination of the drug effect (see Table 9-2). Metabolism of benzodiazepines occurs in the liver through microsomal oxidation (*N*-dealkylation and aliphatic hydroxylation) or glucuronide conjugation. Microsomal oxidation, the primary pathway for metabolism of midazolam and diazepam, is more susceptible to external factors such as age, diseases (hepatic cirrhosis), and the administration of other drugs that modulate the efficiency of the enzyme systems.

Diazepam undergoes hepatic metabolism to active metabolites (desmethyldiazepam and oxazepam) that may contribute to the prolonged effects of this drug. By contrast, midazolam is selectively metabolized by hepatic CYP4503A4 to a single dominant and inactive metabolite, 1-hydroxymidazolam. Furthermore, the short duration of action of a single dose of midazolam is due to its lipid solubility, which leads to rapid redistribution from the brain to inactive tissue sites. Despite its prompt passage into the brain, midazolam is considered to have a slower effect-site equilibration time than propofol and thiopental. In this regard, intravenous doses of midazolam should be sufficiently spaced to permit the peak clinical effect to be recognized before a repeat dose is considered.

The elimination half-time of diazepam greatly exceeds that of midazolam, thus suggesting that the CNS effects of diazepam are probably prolonged in comparison to midazolam, especially in elderly patients. Midazolam has the shortest context-sensitive half-time, which makes it the only one of the three benzodiazepine drugs suitable for continuous infusion (see Fig. 9-5).[5]

Pharmacodynamics

Benzodiazepines work through activation of the $GABA_A$ receptor complex and enhancement of GABA-mediated chloride currents, thereby leading to hyperpolarization of neurons and reduced excitability (Fig. 9-7).[10] There are specific binding sites for benzodiazepines on the γ-subunits of $GABA_A$ receptors, which explains why they were initially termed benzodiazepine receptors. Consistent with its greater potency, midazolam has an affinity for benzodiazepine receptors that is approximately twice that of diazepam.

GABA receptors that are responsive to benzodiazepines occur almost exclusively on postsynaptic nerve endings in the CNS, with the greatest density being in the cerebral cortex. The anatomic distribution of $GABA_A$ receptors (restricted to the CNS) is consistent with the minimal

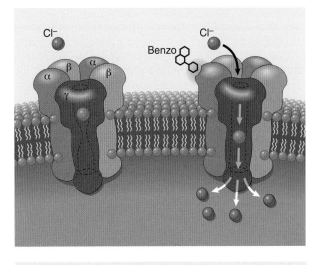

Figure 9-7 Schematic depiction of the γ-aminobutyric acid (GABA) receptor forming a chloride ion channel. Benzodiazepines (Benzo) attach selectively to α-subunits and are presumed to facilitate the action of the inhibitory neurotransmitter GABA on the α-subunits. (From Mohler H, Richards JG. The benzodiazepine receptor: A pharmacological control element of brain function. Eur J Anesthesiol 1988;2:15-24, with permission.)

effects of these drugs outside the CNS. Indeed, the magnitude of depression of ventilation and the development of hypotension after the administration of benzodiazepines are lower than that observed when barbiturates are used for induction of anesthesia (Table 9-3).

SPECTRUM OF EFFECTS

The wide spectrum of effects of benzodiazepines is similar for all drugs in this class, although potencies for individual effects may vary between drugs.[3] The most important effects of benzodiazepines are their sedative-hypnotic action and their amnestic properties (anterograde amnesia). In addition, benzodiazepines function as anticonvulsants and are used to treat seizures. These effects are mediated through the α_1-subunits of the GABA receptor, whereas anxiolysis and muscle relaxation are mediated through the γ-subunits. The site of action for muscle relaxation is in the spinal cord, and it requires much higher doses than the other effects do.

SAFETY PROFILE

Benzodiazepines have a very favorable side effect profile and, when administered alone, cause only minimal depression of ventilation and the cardiovascular system, which makes them relatively safe even in larger doses. Another advantage, as well as argument for their safety, is the ability to promptly antagonize the CNS effects of benzodiazepines with the selective benzodiazepine antagonist flumazenil.

CENTRAL NERVOUS SYSTEM

Like propofol and barbiturates, benzodiazepines decrease $CMRO_2$ and CBF, but to a smaller extent. In contrast to propofol and thiopental, midazolam is unable to produce an isoelectric EEG, thus emphasizing that there is a ceiling effect on benzodiazepine-induced decreases in $CMRO_2$. Patients with decreased intracranial compliance demonstrate little or no change in ICP after the administration of midazolam. Benzodiazepines have not been shown to possess neuroprotective properties. They are potent anticonvulsants for the treatment of status epilepticus, alcohol withdrawal, and local anesthetic–induced seizures.

CARDIOVASCULAR SYSTEM

Midazolam, as used for induction of anesthesia, produces a greater decrease in systemic blood pressure than comparable doses of diazepam do. These changes are most likely due to peripheral vasodilatation inasmuch as cardiac output is not changed. Consequently, the effect of midazolam on systemic blood pressure is exaggerated in hypovolemic patients.

RESPIRATORY SYSTEM

Benzodiazepines produce minimal depression of ventilation, although transient apnea may follow rapid intravenous administration of midazolam for induction of anesthesia, especially in the presence of opioid premedication. Benzodiazepines decrease the ventilatory response to carbon dioxide, but this effect is not usually significant if they are administered alone. More severe respiratory depression can occur when benzodiazepines are administered together with opioids.[11]

SIDE EFFECTS

Allergic reactions to benzodiazepines are extremely rare to nonexistent. Pain during intravenous injection and subsequent thrombophlebitis are most pronounced with diazepam and reflect the poor water solubility of this benzodiazepine. It is the organic solvent, propylene glycol, required to dissolve diazepam that is most likely responsible for pain during intramuscular or intravenous administration, as well as for the unpredictable absorption after intramuscular injection. Midazolam is more water soluble (but only at low pH), thus obviating the need for an organic solvent and decreasing the likelihood of exaggerated pain or erratic absorption after intramuscular injection or pain during intravenous administration.

Clinical Uses

Benzodiazepines are used for (1) preoperative medication, (2) intravenous sedation, (3) intravenous induction of anesthesia, and (4) suppression of seizure activity. The slow onset and prolonged duration of action of lorazepam limit its usefulness for preoperative medication or induction of anesthesia, especially when rapid and sustained awakening at the end of surgery is desirable. Flumazenil (8 to 15 µg/kg IV) may be useful for treating patients experiencing delayed awakening, but it must be kept in mind that the duration of action of the antagonist is brief (about 20 minutes) and resedation may occur.

PREOPERATIVE MEDICATION AND SEDATION

The amnestic, anxiolytic, and sedative effects of benzodiazepines are the basis for the use of these drugs for preoperative medication. Midazolam (1 to 2 mg IV) is effective for premedication, sedation during regional anesthesia, and brief therapeutic procedures.[3,12] When compared with diazepam, midazolam produces a more rapid onset, with greater amnesia and less postoperative sedation. Midazolam is the most commonly used oral premedication for children. For example, 0.5 mg/kg administered orally 30 minutes before induction of anesthesia provides reliable sedation and anxiolysis in children without producing delayed awakening.[13]

The synergistic effects between benzodiazepines and other drugs, especially opioids and propofol, can be used to achieve better sedation and analgesia. However, the combination of these drugs greatly enhances their respiratory depression and may lead to airway obstruction or apnea.[11] Benzodiazepine effects, as well as its synergistic effects, are more pronounced with increasing age, and therefore dose reduction and careful titration may be necessary.

INDUCTION OF ANESTHESIA

Though not generally used as the main intravenous induction drug, general anesthesia can be induced by the administration of midazolam (0.1 to 0.3 mg/kg IV). The onset of unconsciousness, however, is slower than after the administration of thiopental, propofol, or etomidate. Onset of unconsciousness is facilitated when a small dose of opioid (fentanyl, 50 to 100 µg IV) is injected 1 to 3 minutes before midazolam is administered. Despite the possible production of lesser circulatory effects, it is unlikely that the use of midazolam or diazepam for induction of anesthesia offers any advantages over barbiturates or propofol. Delayed awakening is a potential disadvantage of administering a benzodiazepine for the induction of anesthesia.

SUPPRESSION OF SEIZURE ACTIVITY

The efficacy of benzodiazepines, especially diazepam, as anticonvulsants is consistent with the ability of these drugs to enhance the inhibitory effects of GABA, particularly in the limbic system. Indeed, diazepam (0.1 mg/kg IV) is often effective in abolishing seizure activity produced by local anesthetics, alcohol withdrawal, and status epilepticus.

KETAMINE

Ketamine, a phencyclidine derivative introduced into clinical use in 1965, is different from most other intravenous anesthetics in that it produces significant analgesia.[1] The characteristic cataleptic state observed after an induction dose of ketamine is known as "dissociative anesthesia," wherein the patient's eyes remain open with a slow nystagmic gaze (cataleptic state).

Physicochemical Characteristics

Ketamine is a partially water-soluble and highly lipid-soluble derivative of phencyclidine (Fig. 9-8). It is between 5 and 10 times more lipid soluble than thiopental. Of the two stereoisomers the S-(+) form is more potent than the R-(−) isomer. Only the racemic mixture of ketamine (10, 50, 100 mg/mL) is available in the United States.

The use of ketamine has always been limited by its unpleasant psychomimetic side effects, but its unique features make it a very valuable alternative in certain settings, mostly because of the potent analgesia with minimal respiratory depression. Most recently it has become popular as an adjunct administered at subanalgesic doses to limit or reverse opioid tolerance.

Pharmacokinetics

The high lipid solubility of ketamine ensures a rapid onset of the drug's effect. Like other intravenous induction drugs, the effect of a single bolus injection is terminated by redistribution to inactive tissue sites. Metabolism occurs primarily in the liver and involves N-demethylation by the cytochrome P450 system. Norketamine, the primary active metabolite, is less potent (one third to one fifth the potency of ketamine) and is subsequently hydroxylated and conjugated into water-soluble inactive metabolites that are excreted in urine. Ketamine is the only intravenous anesthetic that has low protein binding (12%) (see Table 9-2).

Pharmacodynamics

The mechanism of action of ketamine is complex, but the major effect is probably produced through inhibition of the N-methyl-D-aspartate receptor complex.[1] If ketamine is administered as the sole anesthetic, amnesia is not as complete as with the administration of a benzodiazepine. Reflexes are often preserved, but it cannot be assumed that patients are able to protect their upper airway. The

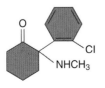

Figure 9-8 Chemical structure of ketamine.

eyes remain open and the pupils are moderately dilated with a nystagmic gaze. Frequently, lacrimation and salivation are increased, and premedication with an anticholinergic drug may be indicated to limit this effect (see Table 9-3).

EMERGENCE REACTIONS

The unpleasant emergence reactions after ketamine administration are the main factor limiting its use. Such reactions may include vivid colorful dreams, hallucinations, out-of-body experiences, and increased and distorted visual, tactile, and auditory sensitivity. These reactions can be associated with fear and confusion, but a euphoric state may also be induced, which explains the potential for abuse of the drug. Children usually have a lower incidence of and less severe emergence reactions. Combination with a benzodiazepine may be indicated to limit the unpleasant emergence reactions and also increase amnesia.

CENTRAL NERVOUS SYSTEM

In contrast to the intravenous anesthetics, ketamine is considered to be a cerebral vasodilator that increases CBF, as well as $CMRO_2$. For these reasons, ketamine has traditionally not been recommended for use in patients with intracranial pathology, especially increased ICP. Nevertheless, these perceived undesirable effects on CBF may be blunted by the maintenance of normocapnia.[14] Despite the potential to produce myoclonic activity, ketamine is considered an anticonvulsant and may be recommended as treatment of status epilepticus when more conventional drugs are ineffective.

CARDIOVASCULAR SYSTEM

Ketamine can produce significant, but transient increases in systemic blood pressure, heart rate, and cardiac output, presumably by centrally mediated sympathetic stimulation. These effects, which are associated with increased cardiac work and myocardial oxygen consumption, are not always desirable and can be blunted by coadministration of benzodiazepines, opioids, or inhaled anesthetics. Though more controversial, ketamine is considered to be a direct myocardial depressant. This property is usually masked by its stimulation of the sympathetic nervous system, but it may become apparent in critically ill patients with limited ability to increase their sympathetic nervous system activity.

RESPIRATORY SYSTEM

Ketamine is not thought to produce significant respiratory depression. When used as a single drug, the respiratory response to hypercapnia is preserved and blood gases remain stable. Transient hypoventilation and, in rare cases, a short period of apnea can follow rapid administration of large intravenous doses for induction of anesthesia. The ability to protect the upper airway in the presence of ketamine cannot be assumed despite the presence of active airway reflexes. Especially in children, the risk for laryngospasm because of increased salivation has to be considered and can be reduced by premedication with an anticholinergic. Ketamine relaxes bronchial smooth muscles and may be helpful in patients with reactive airways and in the management of patients experiencing bronchoconstriction.

Clinical Uses

The unpleasant emergence reactions after the administration of ketamine have restricted its use in the perioperative period.[15] Nevertheless, ketamine's unique properties, including profound analgesia, stimulation of the sympathetic nervous system, bronchodilation, and minimal respiratory depression, make it an important alternative to the other intravenous anesthetics and a desirable adjunct in many cases. Moreover, ketamine can be administered by multiple routes (intravenous, intramuscular, oral, rectal, epidural), thus making it a useful option for premedication in mentally challenged and uncooperative pediatric patients.

INDUCTION AND MAINTENANCE OF ANESTHESIA

Induction of anesthesia can be achieved with ketamine, 1 to 2 mg/kg intravenously or 4 to 6 mg/kg intramuscularly. Though not commonly used for maintenance of anesthesia, the short context-sensitive half-time makes ketamine a consideration for this purpose (see Fig. 9-3).[5] For example, general anesthesia can be achieved with the infusion of ketamine, 15 to 45 µg/kg/min, plus 50% to 70% nitrous oxide or by ketamine alone, 30 to 90 µg/kg/min.

ANALGESIA

Small bolus doses of ketamine (0.2 to 0.8 mg/kg IV) may be useful during regional anesthesia when additional analgesia is needed (cesarean section under neuraxial anesthesia with an insufficient regional block). Ketamine provides effective analgesia without compromise of the airway. An infusion of a subanalgesic dose of ketamine (3 to 5 µg/kg/min) during general anesthesia and in the early postoperative period may be useful to produce analgesia or reduce opioid tolerance and opioid-induced hyperalgesia.[16]

ETOMIDATE

Etomidate, first synthesized in 1964 and introduced into clinical use in 1972, is an intravenous anesthetic with hypnotic but not analgesic properties and with minimal hemodynamic effects.[1] The pharmacokinetics of etomidate makes it suitable for use as a continuous infusion, but mainly because of its endocrine side effects it is not more widely used.

Physicochemical Characteristics

Etomidate is a carboxylated imidazole derivative that has two optical isomers (Fig. 9-9). The available preparation

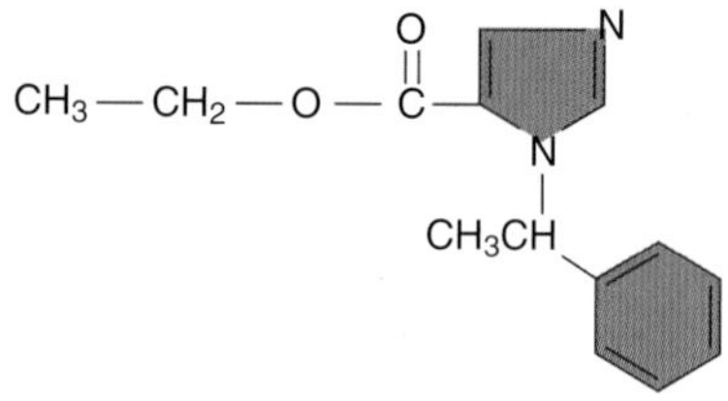

Figure 9-9 Chemical structure of etomidate.

contains only the active D-(+) isomer, which has hypnotic properties. The drug is poorly soluble in water and is therefore supplied as a 2-mg/mL solution in 35% propylene glycol. The solution has a pH of 6.9 and thus does not cause problems with precipitation like thiopental does.

Pharmacokinetics

An induction dose of etomidate produces rapid onset of anesthesia, and recovery depends on redistribution to inactive tissue sites, comparable to thiopental and propofol. Metabolism is primarily by ester hydrolysis to inactive metabolites, which are then excreted in urine (78%) and bile (22%). Less than 3% of an administered dose of etomidate is excreted as unchanged drug in urine. Clearance of etomidate is about five times that for thiopental, as reflected by a shorter elimination half-time (see Table 9-2). The duration of action is linearly related to the dose, with each 0.1 mg/kg providing about 100 seconds of unconsciousness. Because of its minimal effects on hemodynamics and short context-sensitive half-time, larger doses, repeated boluses, or continuous infusions can safely be administered (see Fig. 9-3).[5] Etomidate, like most other intravenous anesthetics, is highly protein bound (77%), primarily to albumin.

Pharmacodynamics

Etomidate appears to have GABA-like effects and seems to primarily act through potentiation of $GABA_A$-mediated chloride currents, like most other intravenous anesthetics.[1]

CENTRAL NERVOUS SYSTEM

Etomidate is a potent cerebral vasoconstrictor, as reflected by decreases in CBF and ICP. These effects of etomidate are similar to those produced by comparable doses of thiopental. Despite its reduction of $CMRO_2$, etomidate failed to show neuroprotective properties in animal studies, and human studies are lacking. The frequency of excitatory spikes on the EEG after the administration of etomidate is greater than with thiopental. Similar to methohexital, etomidate may activate seizure foci, manifested as fast activity on the EEG. In addition, spontaneous movements characterized as myoclonus occur in more than 50% of patients receiving etomidate, and this myoclonic activity may be associated with seizure-like activity on the EEG.

CARDIOVASCULAR SYSTEM

A characteristic and desired feature of induction of anesthesia with etomidate is cardiovascular stability after bolus injection.[1] In this regard, systemic blood pressure decreases are modest or absent and principally reflect decreases in systemic vascular resistance. Therefore, the systemic blood pressure–lowering effects of etomidate are probably exaggerated in the presence of hypovolemia, and optimization of the patient's intravascular fluid volume status before induction of anesthesia should be achieved. Etomidate produces minimal changes in heart rate and cardiac output. The depressive effects of etomidate on myocardial contractility are minimal at concentrations used for induction of anesthesia.

RESPIRATORY SYSTEM

The depressant effects of etomidate on ventilation are less pronounced than those of barbiturates, although apnea may occasionally follow rapid intravenous injection of the drug. Depression of ventilation may be exaggerated when etomidate is combined with inhaled anesthetics or opioids.

ENDOCRINE SYSTEM

Etomidate causes adrenocortical suppression by producing a dose-dependent inhibition of 11β-hydroxylase, an enzyme necessary for the conversion of cholesterol to cortisol (Fig. 9-10).[17] This suppression lasts 4 to 8 hours after an induction dose of etomidate. Despite concerns regarding the use of etomidate for induction of anesthesia based on its adrenocortical depression, no outcome studies have demonstrated an adverse effect on outcome.

Clinical Uses

Etomidate is an alternative to propofol and barbiturates for the rapid intravenous induction of anesthesia, especially in patients with compromised myocardial contractility. After a standard induction dose (0.2 to 0.3 mg/kg IV), the onset of unconsciousness is comparable to that achieved by thiopental and propofol. There is a high incidence of pain during intravenous injection of etomidate, and this pain may be followed by venous irritation. Involuntary myoclonic movements are common but may be masked by the concomitant administration of neuromuscular blocking drugs. Awakening after a single intravenous dose of etomidate is rapid, with little evidence of any residual depressant effects. Etomidate does not produce analgesia, and postoperative nausea and vomiting may be more common than after the administration of thiopental or propofol. The principal limiting factor in the clinical use of etomidate for induction of anesthesia is its ability to transiently depress adrenocortical function.[17] Theoretically, this suppression may be either desirable for stress-free anesthesia or undesirable if it prevents useful protective responses against stresses that accompany the perioperative period.

DEXMEDETOMIDINE

Dexmedetomidine is a highly selective α_2-adrenergic agonist.[18] Recognition of the usefulness of α_2-agonists is based on observations of decreased anesthetic requirements

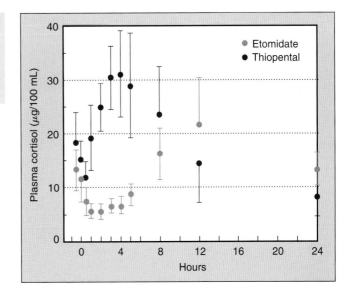

Figure 9-10 Etomidate, but not thiopental, is associated with decreases in the plasma concentrations of cortisol. *P < .05 versus thiopental, mean ± SD. (From Fragen RT, Shanks CA, Molteni A, et al. Effects of etomidate on hormonal responses to surgical stress. Anesthesiology 1984;61:652-656, with permission.)

in patients receiving chronic clonidine therapy. The effects of dexmedetomidine can be antagonized with α_2-antagonist drugs.

Physicochemical Characteristics

Dexmedetomidine is the active *S*-enantiomer of medetomidine, a highly selective α_2-adrenergic agonist and imidazole derivative that is used in veterinary medicine. Dexmedetomidine is water soluble and available as a parenteral formulation (Fig. 9-11).

Pharmacokinetics

Dexmedetomidine undergoes rapid hepatic metabolism involving conjugation, *N*-methylation, and hydroxylation, followed by conjugation. Metabolites are excreted through urine and bile. Clearance is high, and the elimination half-time is short (see Table 9-2). However, there is a significant increase in the context-sensitive half-time from 4 minutes after a 10-minute infusion to 250 minutes after an 8-hour infusion.

Pharmacodynamics

Dexmedetomidine produces its selective α_2-agonist effects through activation of CNS α_2-receptors. Hypnosis presumably results from stimulation of α_2-receptors in the locus ceruleus, and the analgesic effect originates at the level of the spinal cord. The sedative effect produced by dexmedetomidine has a different quality than that produced by other intravenous anesthetics in that it more resembles a physiologic sleep state through activation of endogenous sleep pathways. Dexmedetomidine is likely to be associated with a decrease in CBF without significant changes in ICP and $CMRO_2$ (see Table 9-3). It has the potential for the development of tolerance and dependence.

CARDIOVASCULAR SYSTEM

Dexmedetomidine infusion results in moderate decreases in heart rate and systemic vascular resistance and, consequently, decreases in systemic blood pressure. A bolus injection may produce transient increases in systemic

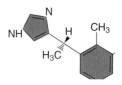

Figure 9-11 Chemical structure of dexmedetomidine.

blood pressure and pronounced decreases in heart rate, an effect that is probably mediated through activation of peripheral α_2-adrenergic receptors. Bradycardia associated with dexmedetomidine infusion may require treatment. Heart block, severe bradycardia, or asystole have been observed and may result from unopposed vagal stimulation. The response to anticholinergic drugs is unchanged.

RESPIRATORY SYSTEM

The effects of dexmedetomidine on the respiratory system are a small to moderate decrease in tidal volume and very little change in the respiratory rate. The ventilatory response to carbon dioxide is unchanged. Although the respiratory effects are mild, upper airway obstruction as a result of sedation is possible. In addition, dexmedetomidine has a synergistic sedative effect when combined with other sedative-hypnotics.

Clinical Uses

Dexmedetomidine is principally used for the short-term sedation of intubated and ventilated patients in an intensive care setting.[18] In the operating room, dexmedetomidine may be used as an adjunct to general anesthesia or to provide sedation as during awake fiberoptic tracheal intubation or during regional anesthesia. When administered during general anesthesia, dexmedetomidine (0.5- to 1-μg/kg loading dose over a period of 10 to 15 minutes, followed by an infusion of 0.2 to 0.7 μg/kg/hr) decreases the dose requirements for inhaled and injected anesthetics. Awakening and the transition to the postoperative setting may benefit from dexmedetomidine-produced sedative and analgesic effects without respiratory depression.

REFERENCES

1. Stoelting RK, Hillier SC. Nonbarbiturate intravenous anesthetic drugs. *In* Pharmacology and Physiology in Anesthetic Practice, 4th ed. Philadelphia: Lippincott Williams & Wilkins, 2006, pp 155-178.
2. Stoelting RK, Hillier SC. Barbiturates. *In* Pharmacology and Physiology in Anesthetic Practice, 4th ed. Philadelphia: Lippincott Williams & Wilkins, 2006, pp 127-139.
3. Stoelting RK, Hillier SC. Benzodiazepines. *In* Pharmacology and Physiology in Anesthetic Practice, 4th ed. Philadelphia: Lippincott Williams & Wilkins, 2006, pp 140-154.
4. Reves JG, Glass PSA, Lubarsky DA, McEvoy MD. Intravenous nonopioid anesthetics. *In* Miller RD (ed): Miller's Anesthesia, 6th ed. Philadelphia: Churchill Livingstone, 2005, pp 317-378.
5. Hughes MA, Glass PSA, Jacobs JR. Context-sensitive half-time in multicompartmental pharmacokinetic models for intravenous anesthetic drugs. Anesthesiology 1992;76:334-341.

6. Tramer MR, Moore RA, McQuay HJ. Propofol and bradycardia: Causation, frequency, and severity. Br J Anesth 1997;78:642-651.
7. Eames WO, Rooke GA, Sai-Chuen R, et al. Comparison of the effects of etomidate, propofol, and thiopental on respiratory resistance after tracheal intubation. Anesthesiology 1996;84:1307-1311.
8. Burrow BK, Johnson ME, Packer DL. Metabolic acidosis associated with propofol in the absence of other causative factors. Anesthesiology 2004;101:239-241.
9. Saidman LJ. Uptake, distribution, and elimination of barbiturates. *In* Eger EI (ed): Anesthetic Uptake and Action. Baltimore: Williams & Wilkins 1974, pp 264-284.
10. Mohler H, Richards JG. The benzodiazepine receptor: A pharmacological control element of brain function. Eur J Anesthesiol 1988;2:15-24.
11. Bailey PL, Pace NL, Ashburn MA, et al. Frequent hypoxemia and apnea after sedation with midazolam and fentanyl. Anesthesiology 1990;73:826-830.
12. Reves JG, Fragen RJ, Vinik HR, et al. Midazolam: Pharmacology and uses. Anesthesiology 1985;62:310-324.
13. Cote CJ, Cohen IT, Suresh S, et al. A comparison of three doses of a commercially prepared oral midazolam syrup in children. Anesth Analg 2002;94:37-43.
14. Albanese J, Arnaud S, Rey M, et al. Ketamine decreases intracranial pressure and electroencephalographic activity in traumatic brain injury patients during propofol sedation. Anesthesiology 1997;87:1328-1324.
15. Kohrs R, Durieux ME. Ketamine: Teaching an old drug new tricks. Anesth Analg 1998;87:1186-1193.
16. Himmelseher S, Durieux ME. Ketamine for perioperative pain management. Anesthesiology 2005;102:211-220.
17. Fragen RT, Shanks CA, Molteni A, et al. Effects of etomidate on hormonal responses to surgical stress. Anesthesiology 1984;61:652-656.
18. Kamibayashi T, Maze M. Clinical uses of alpha$_2$-adrenergic agonists. Anesthesiology 2000;93:1345-1349.

II

Chapter 10

OPIOIDS

Robert K. Stoelting

Opioid is the term used to describe all exogenous substances, natural and synthetic, that bind specifically to opioid receptors and produce some agonist (morphine-like) effects (Table 10-1).[1] Opioids are unique in producing analgesia without loss of touch, proprioception, or consciousness.

STRUCTURE-ACTIVITY RELATIONSHIPS

The potency of opioids is closely related to the stereo-chemical structure of the molecule, with levo-isomers being the most active. The naturally occurring form of morphine is the levo-isomer (L-morphine). Semisynthetic opioids result from minor modification of the morphine molecule (Fig. 10-1). Synthetic opioids contain the phenanthrene nucleus of morphine but are manufactured by synthesis rather than chemical modification of morphine. The principal pharmacodynamic difference between opioids is potency and rate of equilibration between plasma and the site of drug effect (e.g., central nervous system [CNS]).

MECHANISM OF ACTION

General Actions of Opioids

Opioids act as agonists at stereospecific opioid receptors in the CNS and outside the CNS in peripheral tissues.[2] Opioids mimic the actions of endogenous peptide opioid receptor ligands (i.e., endorphins) by binding to opioid receptors, resulting in activation of pain-modulating (antinocieptive) systems. The principal effect of opioid receptor activation is a decrease in neurotransmission, which results mostly from presynaptic inhibition of neuro-transmitter (e.g., acetylcholine, dopamine, norepinephrine, substance P) release.[3] The effect of opioid receptor activation is increased potassium conductance, leading to hyperpolarization of cellular membranes. Depression of

Table 10–1 Clinically Used Opioid Agonists and Comparative Potency

Drug	Relative Potency
Morphine	1
Meperidine	0.1
Fentanyl	75-125
Sufentanil	500-1000
Alfentanil	10-25
Remifentanil	250

cholinergic transmission in the CNS may result in opioid-induced inhibition of acetylcholine release from nerve endings, producing significant analgesic and other side effects (depression of ventilation) of opioids.

Opioid Receptors

Opioid receptors are classified as mu, delta, and kappa receptors (Table 10-2).[4] These receptors belong to a superfamily of guanine (G) protein–coupled receptors, whose activation results in inhibition of adenyl cyclase and inhibition of ion movement across calcium and potassium channels. These effects ultimately result in decreased neuronal activity.

Mu or morphine-preferring receptors are principally responsible for supraspinal and spinal analgesia. Activation of a subpopulation of mu receptors (μ_1) is speculated to produce analgesia, whereas μ_2 receptors are responsible for hypoventilation, bradycardia, and physical dependence. Nevertheless, cloning of the mu receptor does not confirm the existence of separate and distant mu receptor subtypes, and it is possible that such subtypes result from post-translational modification of a common protein.[5]

NEURAXIAL OPIOIDS

Placement of opioids in the epidural or subarachnoid space to manage acute or chronic pain is based on the knowledge that opioid receptors (principally mu receptors) are present in the substantia gelatinosa of the spinal cord. Analgesia produced by neuraxial (spinal or epidural) opioids, in contrast to intravenous administration of opioids or regional anesthesia with local anesthetics, is not associated with sympathetic nervous system denervation, skeletal muscle weakness, or loss of proprioception. Analgesia is dose related (e.g., epidural dose is 5 to 10 times the subarachnoid dose) and specific for visceral rather than somatic pain.

Analgesia that follows epidural placement of opioids reflects diffusion of the drug across the dura to gain access to mu opioid receptors on the spinal cord and the systemic absorption to produce effects similar to those that would follow intravenous administration of the opioid. Poorly

II

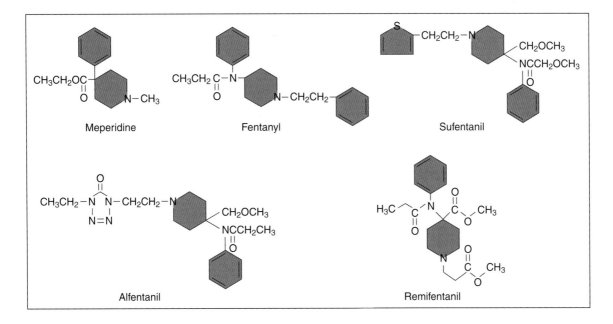

Figure 10-1 Chemical structures of opioid agonists commonly administered in the perioperative period: meperidine, fentanyl, sufentanil, alfentanil, and remifentanil.

Table 10–2   Classification of Opioid Receptors

Features	Mu$_1$	Mu$_2$	Kappa	Delta
Effects	Analgesia (supraspinal, spinal)	Analgesia (spinal)	Analgesia (supraspinal, spinal)	Analgesia (supraspinal, spinal)
	Euphoria	Depression of ventilation	Dysphoria, sedation	Depression of ventilation
	Low abuse potential	Physical dependence	Low abuse potential	Physical dependence
	Miosis		Miosis	
		Constipation (marked)		Constipation (marked)
	Bradycardia			
	Hypothermia			
	Urinary retention		Diuresis	Urinary retention
Agonists	Endorphins	Endorphins	Dynorphins	Enkephalins
	Morphine	Morphine		
	Synthetic opioids	Synthetic opioids		
Antagonists	Naloxone	Naloxone	Naloxone	Naloxone
	Naltrexone	Naltrexone	Naltrexone	Naltrexone
	Nalmefene	Nalmefene	Nalmefene	Nalmefene

Adapted from Atcheson R, Lambert DG. Update on opioid receptors. Br J Anesth 1994;73:132-134.

lipid-soluble opioids (e.g., morphine) result in a slower onset of analgesia but have a longer duration of action than lipid-soluble opioids (e.g., fentanyl, sufentanil).

Pharmacokinetics

Opioids placed in the epidural space undergo significant systemic absorption and passage into the subarachnoid space. Penetration of the dura is greatly influenced by lipid solubility, with fentanyl and sufentanil passing across the dura much more rapidly than morphine. Epidural administration of morphine, fentanyl, and sufentanil produces opioid blood concentrations that are similar to those produced by intramuscular injection of an equivalent dose.[6] Vascular absorption after intrathecal administration of opioids is insignificant.

Cephalad movement of opioids in the cerebrospinal fluid (CSF) depends on lipid solubility. For example, lipid-soluble opioids such as fentanyl and sufentanil are limited in cephalad migration by uptake into the spinal cord, whereas less lipid-soluble morphine remains in the CSF for transfer to more cephalad locations. Coughing or straining, but not body position, can affect opioid movement in the CSF.

Side Effects

The side effects of neuraxial opioids result from the presence of drug in the CSF or systemic circulation, or both (Table 10-3).[1] Typically, most side effects are dose dependent. The most common side effects after neuraxial opioids are used to treat acute postoperative pain are pruritus, nausea and vomiting, urinary retention, and depression of ventilation.

Early depression of ventilation occurs within 2 hours of neuraxial injection of the opioid. Delayed depression of ventilation typically occurs 6 to 12 hours after epidural or intrathecal administration of morphine and reflects cephalad migration of the opioid in the CSF and subsequent interaction with opioid receptors located in the ventral medulla. Factors that increase the risk of delayed depression of ventilation, especially concomitant use of any intravenous opioid or sedative, must be considered in determining the dose of a neuraxial opioid (Table 10-4).[1,6]

DETECTION OF DEPRESSION OF VENTILATION

Detection of depression of ventilation induced by neuraxial opioids may be difficult. Arterial hypoxemia and hypercarbia may develop despite a normal breathing rate.

Table 10–3   Side Effects of Neuraxial Opioids
Pruritus
Nausea and vomiting
Urinary retention
Depression of ventilation
Sedation
Central nervous system excitation
Activation of latent viral infections
Sexual dysfunction
Water retention

Table 10-4 Factors That Increase the Risk of Depression of Ventilation

High opioid dose

Low lipid solubility of opioids

Concomitant administration of parenteral opioids or other sedatives

Lack of opioid tolerance

Advanced age

Patient position (?)

Increased intrathoracic pressure

Pulse oximetry reliably detects opioid-induced arterial hypoxemia, and supplemental oxygen is an effective treatment.[7] Capnography provides early warning that opioid-induced hypoventilation is occurring. A slow breathing rate (<8 breaths/min) may accompany opioid-induced depression of ventilation. Perhaps the most reliable clinical sign of depression of ventilation is a depressed level of consciousness, possibly caused by hypercarbia. Naloxone (0.25 µg/kg/min IV) is effective in reversing the depression of ventilation produced by neuraxial opioids.

OPIOID AGONISTS

Opioid agonists include but are not limited to morphine, meperidine, fentanyl, sufentanil, alfentanil, and remifentanil. The most notable feature in the clinical use of opioids is the extraordinary variation in dose requirements for achievement of analgesia.[8] This interindividual variation emphasizes that usual doses of opioids may produce clinical responses ranging from inadequate to excessive opioid effects.

Morphine

Morphine is the prototype opioid agonist with which all other opioids are compared. In humans, morphine produces analgesia, euphoria, sedation, and a decreased ability to concentrate. The cause of pain persists, but even small doses of morphine increase the threshold to pain and modify the perception of noxious stimulation such that it is no longer experienced as pain. Continuous, dull pain is relieved by morphine more effectively than sharp, intermittent pain. In contrast to nonopioid analgesics, morphine is effective against pain arising from the viscera, as well as from skeletal muscles, joints, and integumental structures. Analgesia is most prominent when opioids are administered before the painful stimulus occurs (i.e., preemptive analgesia).[9] This is a pertinent consideration in administering an opioid to patients before the acute surgical stimulus. In the absence of pain, however, the administration of morphine may produce dysphoria rather than euphoria.

PHARMACOKINETICS

Clearance of opioids principally occurs by hepatic metabolism, but large differences in lipid solubility account for pharmacokinetic differences between opioids (Table 10-5).[1]

Morphine is well absorbed after intramuscular administration, with an onset of effect in 15 to 30 minutes and a peak effect in 45 to 90 minutes. The duration of action is about 4 hours. Absorption of morphine from the gastrointestinal tract is not reliable. Morphine is usually

Table 10-5 Pharmacokinetics of Opioid Agonists

Drug	pK	Percent Nonionized (pH 7.4)	Protein Binding (%)	Clearance (mL/min)	Volume of Distribution (L)	Elimination Half-Time (hr)	Context-Sensitive Half-Time (min)	Effect-Site (Blood/Brain) Equilibration Time (min)*
Morphine	7.9	23	35	1050	334	1.7-3.3		
Meperidine	8.5	7	70	1020	305	3-5		
Fentanyl	8.4	8.5	84	1530	335	3.1-6.6	260	6.8
Sufentanil	8.0	20	93	900	123	2.2-4.6	30	6.2
Alfentanil	6.5	89	92	238	27	1.4-1.5	60	1.4
Remifentanil	7.3	58	66-93	4000	30	0.17-0.33	4	1.1

* Rate of equilibration between plasma and the site of drug effect.
Data from Stoelting RK, Hillier SC. Opioid agonists and antagonists. *In* Pharmacology and Physiology in Anesthetic Practice. Philadelphia, Lippincott Williams & Wilkins, 2006, pp 87-124.

administered intravenously in the perioperative period, eliminating the unpredictable influence of drug absorption. The peak effect (equilibration time between the blood and brain) after intravenous administration of morphine is delayed compared with opioids such as fentanyl and alfentanil, requiring about 15 to 30 minutes.

Only a small amount of administered morphine gains access to the CNS. For example, it is estimated that less than 0.1% of morphine that is administered intravenously has entered the CNS at the time of the peak plasma concentration. Reasons for poor penetration of morphine into the CNS include relatively poor lipid solubility and rapid conjugation (metabolism) with glucuronic acid. Morphine-3-glucuronide is pharmacologically inactive, whereas morphine-6-glucuronide may produce analgesia and depression of ventilation by its actions at mu receptors.[10] Elimination of morphine glucuronides may be impaired in patients with renal failure, causing an accumulation of metabolites and unexpected ventilatory depressant effects. Gender may affect opioid-induced analgesia, as reflected by a greater analgesic potency and slower speed of onset of morphine in women than men.[11]

SIDE EFFECTS

Side effects described for morphine are also characteristic of other opioid agonists, although the incidence and magnitude may vary. Naloxone is a specific pharmacologic antagonist of opioid-induced analgesia and depression of ventilation.

Cardiovascular System

The administration of morphine, even in large doses (1 mg/kg IV), to supine and normovolemic patients is unlikely to cause direct myocardial depression or hypotension. Conversely, changing from the supine to standing position may produce orthostatic hypotension and syncope, presumably reflecting drug-induced impairment of compensatory sympathetic nervous system responses. Morphine can evoke decreases in systemic blood pressure due to drug-induced histamine release, especially with rapid intravenous administration of large doses. Morphine-induced bradycardia results from increased parasympathomimetic effects. Synthetic and short-short acting opioids do not evoke the release of histamine. Opioids do not sensitize the heart to catecholamines. The combination of an opioid agonist with nitrous oxide or a benzodiazepine results in decreases in systemic blood pressure that do not accompany administration of these drugs when administered alone.

Ventilation

All opioid agonists produce dose-dependent and gender-specific depression of ventilation, primarily through an agonist effect at μ_2 receptors, leading to a direct depressant effect on brainstem ventilation centers.[4] This depression of ventilation is characterized by decreased responsiveness of these ventilatory centers to carbon dioxide, as reflected by an increase in the resting $PaCO_2$ and displacement of the carbon dioxide response curve to the right. Depression of ventilation produced by opioid agonists persists for several hours, as demonstrated by decreased ventilatory responses to carbon dioxide. High doses of opioids may result in apnea, but the patient remains conscious and able to initiate a breath if asked to do so. Clinically, depression of ventilation produced by opioid agonists manifests as a decreased frequency of breathing that is often accompanied by a compensatory increase in tidal volume.

Central Nervous System

Opioids, even in high doses, do not reliably produce unconsciousness, especially in young patients, emphasizing that these drugs cannot be considered true anesthetics. In the absence of hypoventilation, opioids act as cerebral vasoconstrictors to decrease cerebral blood flow and possibly intracranial pressure (ICP). These drugs must be used with caution in patients with head injury because depression of ventilation and accumulation of carbon dioxide can result in undesirable increases in ICP. Opioids do not produce evidence of seizure activity on the electroencephalogram, nor do they alter the responses to neuromuscular blocking drugs. Miosis produced by opioid agonists is caused by excitatory action on the oculomotor nerve.

Skeletal muscle rigidity, especially of the thoracoabdominal muscles (i.e., stiff-chest syndrome), is common when large doses of opioid agonists (most common with fentanyl) are rapidly administered intravenously. The skeletal muscle rigidity may reflect actions at opioid receptors and involve interactions with dopaminergic and γ-aminobutyric acid (GABA)–responsive neurons. Skeletal muscle rigidity can be severe enough to interfere with adequate ventilation and oxygenation. Administration of a neuromuscular blocking drug or an opioid antagonist is effective for terminating opioid-induced skeletal muscle rigidity.

The contribution of opioids to total anesthetic requirements can be quantified by determining the decrease in the minimum alveolar concentration (MAC) of a volatile anesthetic in the presence of opioids. Opioids can be shown to decrease MAC for volatile anesthetics in a dose-related manner until a ceiling effect is reached (about 50% decrease), beyond which additional doses of opioid fail to further decrease anesthetic requirements for the volatile anesthetic.[12] This observation casts doubt on the ability of opioid agonists to provide total amnesia reliably in every patient, even with high doses.

Sedation

Postoperative titration of morphine frequently induces sedation that precedes the onset of analgesia.[13] The usual recommendation for morphine titrations includes a short interval between boluses (5 to 7 minutes) to allow evaluation of its clinical effect. The assumption that sleep occurs when pain is relieved is not necessarily accurate, and morphine-induced sedation should not be considered as an indicator of appropriate analgesia during intravenous morphine titration.

Biliary and Gastrointestinal Tract

Opioids can cause spasm of biliary smooth muscle, resulting in increases in intrabiliary pressure that may be associated with epigastric distress or biliary colic. This pain may be confused with angina pectoris. Naloxone can relieve pain caused by biliary spasm, but it does not affect myocardial ischemia. Nitroglycerin can relieve pain due to biliary spasm or myocardial ischemia. Opioids, especially morphine, decrease peristaltic activity and enhance the tone of the pyloric sphincter, contributing to delayed gastric and intestinal tract emptying. Opioid-induced enhancement of bladder sphincter tone may make spontaneous urination difficult.

Nausea and Vomiting

Opioid-induced nausea and vomiting are caused by direct stimulation of dopamine receptors in the chemoreceptor trigger zone in the floor of the fourth cerebral ventricle. Activation of these dopamine receptors as a mechanism for opioid-induced nausea and vomiting is consistent with the antiemetic efficacy of dopamine receptor antagonists such as butyrophenones. Conversely, morphine depresses the vomiting center in the medulla. As a result, intravenous administration of morphine produces less nausea and vomiting than intramuscular administration, presumably because opioid administered intravenously reaches the vomiting center as rapidly as it reaches the chemoreceptor trigger zone. Nausea and vomiting are relatively uncommon in recumbent patients given morphine, suggesting that a vestibular component may contribute to opioid-induced nausea and vomiting.

Tolerance and Physical Dependence

Tolerance (i.e., development of the need to increase the dose of opioid agonist to achieve the same analgesic effect previously achieved with a lower dose) and dependence (i.e., addiction) are major limitations to the clinical use of opioids. Tolerance usually requires about 25 days to develop with analgesic doses of morphine, but some degree of physical dependence may occur after 48 hours of continuous medication.[14] The miotic and constipating effects of opioids persist, whereas tolerance to the depression of ventilation develops. When opioid dependence occurs, discontinuation of the opioid agonist produces a typical withdrawal-abstinence syndrome (e.g., diaphoresis, insomnia, restlessness, abdominal cramps, nausea and vomiting, diarrhea) that reaches a peak in 72 hours and then declines over the next 7 to 10 days (Table 10-6).[14]

Long-term pharmacodynamic tolerance characterized by opioid insensitivity may persist for months or years in some individuals, and it most likely represents persistent

		Table 10-6 Time Course of Opioid Withdrawal	
Drug	**Onset (Hours)**	**Peak Intensity (Hours)**	**Duration (Days)**
Morphine	6-18	36-72	7-10
Heroin	6-18	36-72	7-10
Meperidine	2-6	8-12	4-5
Fentanyl	2-6	8-12	4-5
Methadone	24-48	3-21 days	6-7 weeks

Data from Mitra S, Sinatra RS. Perioperative management of acute pain in the opioid-dependent patient. Anesthesiology 2004;101:212-227.

neural adaptive changes.[14] Prolonged exposure to opioids activates N-methyl-D-aspartate receptors and is important in the development of opioid tolerance and increased pain sensitivity. Downregulation of spinal glutamate receptors also likely accompanies opioid tolerance.

Modulate Immune Function

Opioids may alter immunity through neuroendocrine effects by direct effects on the immune system.[15] Prolonged exposure to opioids appears more likely than short-term exposure to produce immunosuppression, especially in susceptible persons, and abrupt withdrawal may induce immunosuppression. This modulation of immune function is reflected by alterations in the biochemical and proliferative properties of the various cellular components of the immune system.

Meperidine

Meperidine is a synthetic opioid that is about one tenth as potent as morphine. Structurally, mepcridine is similar to atropine, and it possesses a mild atropine-like antispasmodic effect. Unlike morphine, meperidine is well absorbed from the gastrointestinal tract. The principal metabolite of meperidine, normeperidine, produces CNS stimulation in high concentrations. Meperidine is uniquely effective in suppressing postoperative shivering that may result in detrimental increases in metabolic oxygen consumption. The antishivering effects of meperidine may reflect stimulation of kappa receptors and a drug-induced decrease in the shivering threshold, which does not occur with alfentanil, clonidine, propofol, or volatile anesthetics.[16]

Orthostatic hypotension is more frequent and profound than after comparable doses of morphine. Unlike morphine, meperidine rarely causes bradycardia, but it may increase heart rate, reflecting its modest atropine-like effects. For the same reasons, mydriasis rather than miosis is likely to accompany administration of meperidine. Large doses of meperidine decrease myocardial contractility, an effect that is unique among the opioids. Administration of meperidine to patients receiving antidepressant drugs (e.g., monoamine oxidase inhibitors, fluoxetine) may evoke the serotoninic syndrome (i.e., autonomic nervous system instability with systemic hypertension, tachycardia, diaphoresis, hyperthermia, agitation, and hyperreflexia).[17]

Fentanyl

Fentanyl is a synthetic opioid agonist structurally related to meperidine. As an analgesic, fentanyl is 75 to 125 times more potent than morphine.

PHARMACOKINETICS

A single dose of fentanyl administered intravenously has a more rapid onset and shorter duration of action than morphine. Fentanyl is a substrate for hepatic cytochrome P450 enzymes (CYP3A) and is susceptible to drug interactions that reflect interference with enzyme activity (less likely than with alfentanil).[18] Despite the clinical impression that fentanyl has a rapid onset, there is a distinct time lag between the peak plasma concentration and peak slowing on the electroencephalogram. This delay reflects the effect-site equilibration time between blood and the brain for fentanyl, which is 6.4 minutes (see Table 10-5).[1] The greater potency and more rapid onset of action reflect the greater lipid solubility of fentanyl compared with that of morphine, which facilitates its passage across the blood-brain barrier. Likewise, the short duration of action of a single dose of fentanyl reflects its rapid redistribution to inactive tissue sites such as fat and skeletal muscles, with an associated decrease in the plasma concentration of the drug. When multiple intravenous doses of fentanyl are administered or there is a continuous infusion of the drug, progressive saturation of these inactive tissue sites occurs. As a result, the plasma concentration of fentanyl does not decrease rapidly, and the duration of analgesia, as well as depression of ventilation, may be prolonged. As the duration of continuous intravenous infusion of fentanyl increases beyond about 2 hours, the context-sensitive half-time of this opioid becomes greater than that of sufentanil (Fig. 10-2).[19] This reflects saturation of inactive redistribution tissue sites with fentanyl during prolonged infusion and return of the opioid from peripheral compartments to the plasma.

SIDE EFFECTS

The side effects of fentanyl resemble those of morphine, except that histamine release and hypotension do not accompany even rapid intravenous administration of large doses of this opioid. In contrast, prior administration of a benzodiazepine (and presumably other injected or inhaled anesthetics) alters the cardiovascular response to fentanyl. Bradycardia may be prominent after the administration of fentanyl. Analgesic concentrations of fentanyl greatly potentiate the effects of other depressant or sedative drugs (e.g., benzodiazepines). For example, an opioid-benzodiazepine combination displays marked synergism with respect to hypnosis and depression of ventilation. Inhibition of CYP3A4 enzyme, as produced by the protease inhibitor ritonavir, can delay the clearance of fentanyl, resulting in prolonged effects of this opioid.[20]

CLINICAL USES

Fentanyl is administered clinically in a wide range of doses. Low doses of fentanyl (1 to 2 μg/kg IV) (or equivalent doses of sufentanil or alfentanil) are injected to provide analgesia. Injection of an opioid such as fentanyl before painful surgical stimulation occurs may decrease the subsequent amount of opioid required in the postoperative period to provide analgesia (i.e., preemptive analgesia). Fentanyl (2 to 20 μg/kg IV) may be administered as an adjuvant to inhaled anesthetics in an attempt to blunt circulatory responses to direct laryngoscopy for tracheal intubation or to sudden changes in the level of surgical stimulation. Conversely, opioids are frequently not useful when administered intraoperatively after surgical stimulation has evoked systemic hypertension. Intraoperative tachycardia, however, may respond to small intravenous

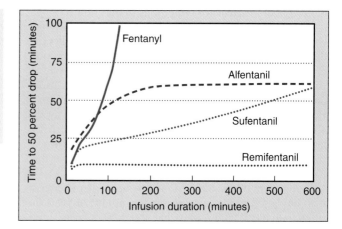

Figure 10-2 Computer simulation–derived, context-sensitive half-times (i.e., time necessary for the plasma concentration to decrease 50% after discontinuation of the opioid infusion) as a function of the duration of the intravenous infusion. (From Egan TD, Lemmens JHM, Fiset P, et al. The pharmacokinetics of the new short-acting opioid remifentanil (GI87084B) in healthy adult male volunteers. Anesthesiology 1993;79:881-892, with permission.)

doses of opioids. Timing of the intravenous injection of fentanyl to prevent or treat such responses should consider the effect-site equilibration time, which is prolonged for fentanyl compared with alfentanil and remifentanil. Large doses of fentanyl (50 to 150 μg/kg IV) have been used alone to produce surgical anesthesia. Large doses of fentanyl as the sole anesthetic have the advantage of stable hemodynamics, whereas possible patient awareness is a disadvantage because opioids are not complete anesthetics. Fentanyl may also be administered as a transmucosal preparation or transdermal preparation to produce analgesia.[1]

Sufentanil

Sufentanil is an analog of fentanyl, with an analgesic potency that is 5 to 10 times that of fentanyl. The effect-site equilibration time of sufentanil resembles that of fentanyl (see Table 10-5).[1] A rapid redistribution to inactive tissue sites terminates the effect of small doses, but a cumulative effect can accompany large or repeated doses. The context-sensitive half-time of sufentanil is less than that for alfentanil for continuous intravenous infusions of up to 8 hours (see Fig. 10-2).[19] After termination of a sufentanil infusion, the decrease in the plasma drug concentration is accelerated by metabolism and by continued redistribution of sufentanil into peripheral compartments. Depression of ventilation and bradycardia may be more profound with sufentanil than with fentanyl. Use of large doses of potent opioids such as sufentanil may produce skeletal muscle rigidity that makes ventilation of the lungs difficult.

Alfentanil

Alfentanil is an analog of fentanyl that is one fifth to one tenth as potent and has one third the duration of action.

A unique advantage of alfentanil compared with fentanyl and sufentanil is the more rapid onset of action (effect-site equilibration time of about 1.4 minutes) after intravenous administration (see Table 10-5).[1] The rapid effect-site equilibration characteristic of alfentanil is a result of the low pK of this opioid, and almost 90% of the drug exists in the lipid-soluble nonionized form at physiologic pH. The rapid peak effect of alfentanil at the brain is useful when an opioid is required to blunt the response to a single, brief stimulus such as tracheal intubation or performance of a retrobulbar block.[21] A 10-fold interindividual variation in systemic clearance of alfentanil, as reflected by widely differing plasma concentrations despite fixed-dose administration, most likely results from differences in CYP3A4 enzyme activity between individuals.[18]

Remifentanil

Remifentanil is a selective opioid agonist with analgesic potency similar to that of fentanyl. It has a blood-brain equilibration time (effect-site equilibration time of about 1.1 minutes) similar to that of alfentanil (see Table 10-5).[1]

PHARMACOKINETICS

Remifentanil is structurally unique because of its ester linkage, which renders it susceptible to hydrolysis by nonspecific plasma and tissue esterases (different from pseudocholinesterase, which hydrolyzes succinylcholine and mivacurium) to inactive metabolites (Fig. 10-3).[19] This unique pathway of metabolism imparts to remifentanil brevity of action, precise and rapidly titratable effects due to its rapid onset and offset, noncumulative effects, and rapid recovery after discontinuation of its intravenous infusion. The context-sensitive half-time for

Figure 10-3 Remifentanil undergoes hydrolysis by nonspecific plasma and tissue esterases (major pathway) to pharmacologically inactive metabolites. (From Egan TD, Lemmens JHM, Fiset P, et al. The pharmacokinetics of the new short-acting opioid remifentanil (GI87084B) in healthy adult male volunteers. Anesthesiology 1993;79:881-892, with permission.)

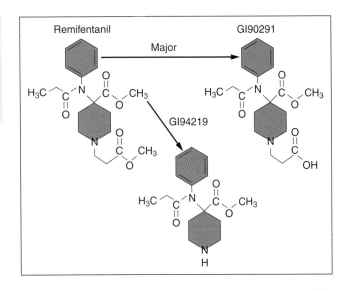

remifentanil is independent of the duration of infusion, and it is estimated to be about 4 minutes (see Fig. 10-2).[19]

CLINICAL USES

The clinical uses of remifentanil reflect the unique pharmacokinetic profile of this opioid. In cases in which a profound analgesic effect is desired transiently, remifentanil may be useful. Anesthesia can be induced with remifentanil (1 μg/kg IV) administered over 60 to 90 seconds. Remifentanil can be used as the analgesic component of a general anesthetic (0.05 to 2.0 μg/kg/min IV) or sedation technique, with the ability to rapidly recover from undesirable effects such as opioid-induced depression of ventilation or excessive sedation. Before cessation of the remifentanil infusion, a longer-acting opioid should be administered to ensure analgesia when the patient awakens. The combination of remifentanil and propofol is synergistic resulting in severe depression of ventilation.[22] Intermittent remifentanil administered as patient-controlled analgesia is an effective and reliable analgesic during labor and delivery.[23] The rapid onset and offset of action of remifentanil makes it possible to quickly adjust the required level of sedation in mechanically ventilated critically ill patients.[24]

ACUTE OPIOID TOLERANCE

Postoperative analgesic requirements in patients receiving relatively large doses of remifentanil intraoperatively are often surprisingly high, suggesting remifentanil may be associated with acute opioid tolerance.[25] Nevertheless, not all data support the development of acute opioid tolerance after remifentanil-based anesthesia.[26]

OPIOID AGONIST-ANTAGONISTS

Opioid agonist-antagonists are represented by drugs that bind to mu receptors, where they produce limited responses (i.e., partial agonists) or no effect (i.e., antagonists) (Fig. 10-4).[1] These drugs often exert partial agonist actions at other receptors, including kappa and delta receptors. Antagonist properties of these drugs can attenuate the efficacy of subsequently administered opioid agonists. However, the antagonist properties of these drugs have been used to advantage to provide postoperative analgesia, with the hope that associated depression of ventilation will be minimal.

Side effects of opioid agonist-antagonists are similar to those of opioid agonists, and these drugs may cause dysphoric reactions. Advantages of opioid agonist-antagonists are the ability to produce analgesia with limited depression of ventilation and a low potential to produce physical dependence. These drugs exhibit a ceiling effect, and increasing the dose beyond a certain point does not produce additional pharmacologic effects.

OPIOID ANTAGONISTS

General Characteristics

Minor changes in the structure of an opioid agonist can convert the drug into an opioid antagonist at one or more of the opioid receptors (Fig. 10-5).[1] The high affinity for the opioid receptors characteristic of pure opioid antagonists results in displacement of the opioid agonist from the mu receptors. After this displacement, the binding of the

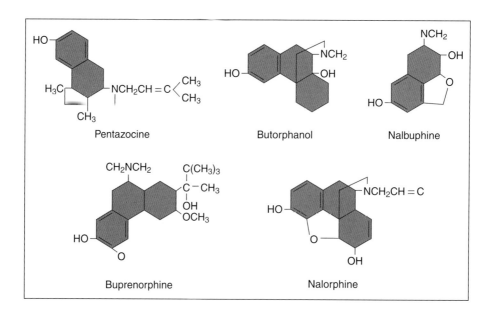

Figure 10-4 Chemical structures of opioid agonist-antagonist drugs: pentazocine, butorphanol, nalbuphine, buprenorphine, and nalorphine.

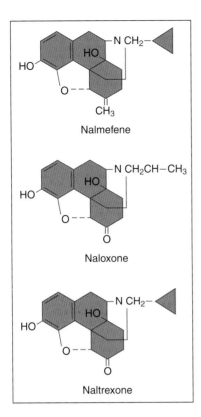

Figure 10-5 Chemical structures of opioid antagonist drugs: nalmefene, naloxone, and naltrexone.

pure antagonist does not activate the mu receptors, and antagonism occurs.

Naloxone

Naloxone (1 to 4 µg/kg IV) promptly reverses opioid-induced analgesia and depression of ventilation. The short duration of action of naloxone (30 to 45 minutes) is presumed to result from its rapid removal from the brain with the return of opioid effects unless supplemental doses of naloxone are administered. A continuous infusion of naloxone (3 to 5 µg/kg/hr IV) may be an alternative to repeated intermittent intravenous doses of naloxone. Cardiovascular stimulation after the intravenous administration of naloxone manifests as increased sympathetic nervous system activity, presumably reflecting the abrupt reversal of analgesia and the sudden perception of pain. This increased sympathetic nervous system activity may manifest as tachycardia, systemic hypertension, pulmonary edema, and cardiac dysrhythmias, including ventricular fibrillation.

REFERENCES

1. Stoelting RK, Hillier SC. Opioid agonists and antagonists. *In* Pharmacology and Physiology in Anesthetic Practice. Philadelphia: Lippincott Williams & Wilkins, 2006, pp 87-124.
2. Stein C. The control of pain in peripheral tissue by opioids. N Engl J Med 1995;332:1685-1690.
3. deLeon-Cassosla OA, Lema MJ. Postoperative epidural opioid analgesia: What are the best choices? Anesth Analg 1996;83:867-875.
4. Atcheson R, Lambert DG. Update on opioid receptors. Br J Anaesth 1994;73:132-134.
5. Lambert DG. Recent advances in opioid pharmacology. Br J Anaesth 1998;81:1-2.
6. Chaney MA. Side effects of intrathecal and epidural opioids. Can J Anaesth 1995;42:891-903.
7. Bailey PL, Rhondeau S, Schafer PG, et al. Dose-response pharmacology of intrathecal morphine in human volunteers. Anesthesiology 1993;79:49-59.
8. Auburn F, Monsel S, Langeron O, et al. Postoperative titration of intravenous morphine in the elderly patient. Anesthesiology 2002;96:17-23.
9. Woolf CJ, Wall PD. Morphine sensitive and morphine insensitive actions of C-fibers input on the rat spinal cord. Neurosci Lett 1998;64:221.
10. Vaughn CW, Connor M. In search of a role for the morphine metabolite morphine-3-glucuronide. Anesth Analg 2003;97:311-312.
11. Sarton E, Olofsen E, Romberg R, et al. Sex differences in morphine analgesia: A experimental study in healthy volunteers. Anesthesiology 2000;93:1245-1254.
12. Lang E, Kapila A, Shlugman D, et al. Reduction of isoflurane minimal alveolar concentration by remifentanil. Anesthesiology 1996;85:721-728.
13. Paqueron X, Lumbroso A, Mergoni P, et al. Is morphine-induced sedation synonymous with analgesia during intravenous morphine titration? Br J Anaesth 2002;89:697-701.
14. Mitra S, Sinatra RS. Perioperative management of acute pain in the opioid-dependent patient. Anesthesiology 2004;101:212-217.
15. Ballantyne JC, Mao J. Opioid therapy for chronic pain. N Engl J Med 2003;349:1943-1953.
16. Ikeda T, Sessler DI, Tayefeh F, et al. Meperidine and alfentanil do not reduce the gains or maximum intensity of shivering. Anesthesiology 1998;88:858-865.
17. Tissot TA. Probable meperidine-induced serotoninic syndrome in a patient with a history of fluoxetine use. Anesthesiology 2003;98:1511-1512.
18. Ibrahim AE, Feldman J, Darim A, et al. Simultaneous assessment of drug interactions with low- and high-extraction opioids: Application to parecoxib effects on the pharmacokinetics and pharmacodynamics of fentanyl and alfentanil. Anesthesiology 2003;98:853-861.
19. Egan TD, Lemmens JHM, Fiset P, et al. The pharmacokinetics of the new short-acting opioid remifentanil (GI87084B) in healthy adult male volunteers. Anesthesiology 1993;79:881-892.

20. Olkkola KT, Palkama VJ, Neuvonen PJ. Ritonavir's role in reducing fentanyl clearance and prolonging its half-life. Anesthesiology 1999;91:681-685.

21. Miller DR, Martineau RJ, O'Brien H, et al. Effects of alfentanil on the hemodynamic and catecholamine response to tracheal intubation. Anesth Analg 1993;76:1040-1046.

22. Niewenhuijs DJF, Olofsen E, Romberg RR, et al. Response surface modeling of remifentanil-propofol interaction on cardiorespiratory control and bispectral index. Anesthesiology 2003;98:312-322.

23. Evron S, Glezerman M, Sadan O, et al. Remifentanil: A novel systemic analgesic for labor pain. Anesth Analg 2005;100:233-238.

24. Dahaba AA, Grabner T, Rehak PH, et al. Remifentanil versus morphine analgesia and sedation for mechanically ventilated critically ill patients. A randomized double blind study. Anesthesiology 2004;101:640-646.

25. Guignard B, Bossard AE, Coste C, et al. Acute opioid tolerance. Intraoperative remifentanil increases postoperative pain and morphine requirement. Anesthesiology 2000;93:409-417.

26. Gustorff B, Hanlik G, Hoerauf KH, et al. The absence of acute tolerance during remifentanil infusion in volunteers. Anesth Analg 2002;94:1223-1228.

LOCAL ANESTHETICS

Kenneth Drasner

Local anesthesia can be defined as loss of sensation in a discrete region of the body caused by disruption of impulse generation or propagation. Local anesthesia can be produced by various chemical and physical means, and these effects may or may not be reversible. In routine clinical practice, local anesthesia is produced by a narrow class of compounds, and recovery is normally spontaneous, predictable, and complete.

HISTORY

Cocaine's systemic toxicity, its irritant properties when placed topically or around nerves, and its substantial potential for physical and psychological dependence generated interest in identification of an alternative local anesthetic. Since cocaine, was known to be a benzoic acid ester (Fig. 11-1), developmental strategies focused on this class of chemical compounds. Although benzocaine was identified before the turn of the century, its poor water solubility restricted its use to topical anesthesia, for which it still finds some limited application in modern clinical practice. The first useful injectable local anesthetic, procaine, can be considered the prototype on which all commonly used anesthetics are based. The procaine molecule is derived from an aromatic acid (*para*-aminobenzoic acid) and an amino alcohol, yielding a structure with three distinct regions: an aromatic head, which imparts lipophilicity; a terminal amine tail, a proton acceptor that imparts hydrophobicity; and a hydrocarbon chain attached to the aromatic acid by an ester linkage (Fig. 11-2). Several other derivatives of *para*-aminobenzoic acid were developed as local anesthetics during the first half of the past century, most notably tetracaine and chloroprocaine, both embodying modifications of the aromatic ring (Fig. 11-3).

In 1948, lidocaine was introduced, and it was the first departure from the amino-ester series. Being derived from an aromatic amine (i.e., xylidine) and an amino acid, the hydrocarbon chain and the aromatic head of the

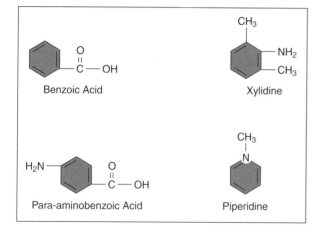

Figure 11-1 Important components of local anesthetics: benzoic acids, xylidine, *para*-aminobenzoic acid, and piperidine.

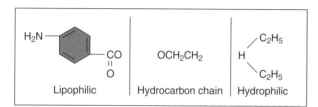

Figure 11-2 Local anesthetics consist of a lipophilic and hydrophilic portion separated by a connecting hydrocarbon chain.

lidocaine molecule are linked by an amide bond (rather than an ester), imparting greater stability. This molecular structure also averts the allergic reactions commonly associated with ester anesthetics (which result from sensitivity to the cleaved aromatic acid). Because of these favorable properties, lidocaine became the template for the development of a series of amino-amide anesthetics (see Fig. 11-3).

Most amino-amide local anesthetics (e.g., lidocaine) are derived from xylidine, including mepivacaine, bupivacaine, ropivacaine, and levobupivacaine (see Fig. 11-1). In contrast to lidocaine, the terminal amino portion of these newer compounds is contained within a piperidine ring (see Fig. 11-1), and the series is commonly referred to as pipecholyl xylidines. Ropivacaine and levobupivacaine share an additional distinctive characteristic; they are single enantiomers rather than racemic mixtures. They are products of a developmental strategy that takes advantage of the differential stereoselectivity of neuronal and cardiac sodium ion channels to reduce the

potential for cardiac toxicity (see "Adverse Effects"). Because they are amides, all of the newer local anesthetics require biotransformation in the liver rather than undergoing ester hydrolysis in plasma, as is the case for the amino-esters.

MECHANISMS OF ACTION AND FACTORS AFFECTING BLOCK

Nerve Conduction

Local anesthetics block the transmission of the action potential by inhibition of voltage-gated sodium ion channels. Under normal or resting circumstances, the neural membrane is characterized by a negative potential of roughly −90 mV (the potential inside the nerve fiber is negative relative to the extracellular fluid). This negative potential is created by active outward transport of sodium and inward transport of potassium ions, combined with a membrane that is relatively permeable to potassium and relatively impermeable to sodium ions. With excitation of the nerve, there is an increase in the membrane permeability to sodium ions, causing a decrease in the transmembrane potential. If a critical potential is reached (i.e., threshold potential), there is a rapid and self-sustaining influx of sodium ions resulting in depolarization, after which the resting membrane potential is re-established. From an electrophysiologic standpoint, local anesthetics block conduction of neural transmission by decreasing the rate of depolarization in response to excitation, preventing achievement of the threshold potential. They do not alter the resting transmembrane potential, and they have little effect on the threshold potential.

Anesthetic Effect and the Active Form of the Local Anesthetic

Local anesthetics exert their electrophysiologic effects by blocking sodium ion conductance. This effect is primarily mediated by interaction with specific receptors that are within the inner vestibule of the sodium ion channel. The commonly used injectable local anesthetics exist in two forms that are in dynamic equilibrium, an uncharged base and a protonated or charged quaternary amine. Evidence suggests that it is the charged form of the local anesthetic molecule that binds to the receptor and is responsible for the predominant action of these drugs. However, the situation is a bit more complex, as the charged structure is highly hydrophilic, and relatively incapable of penetrating the nerve membrane to reach its site of action. The neutral base plays a critical role in the local anesthetic effect by permitting the anesthetic to penetrate the nerve membrane to gain access to the receptor (Fig. 11-4).[1] After penetration, re-equilibration occurs, permitting the charged form of the local anesthetic to bind. These

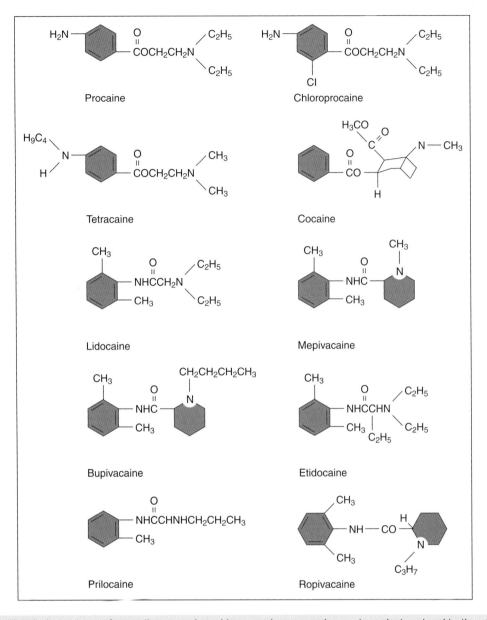

Figure 11-3 Chemical structures of ester (i.e., procaine, chloroprocaine, tetracaine, and cocaine) and amide (i.e., lidocaine, mepivacaine, bupivacaine, etidocaine, prilocaine, and ropivacaine) local anesthetics.

drugs may also reach the sodium channel laterally (i.e., hydrophobic pathway). To add further complexity, this mechanism, although attractive, cannot completely account for all of the local anesthetic effect. For example, benzocaine only exists in an uncharged form, and it is not affected by pH, but it still possesses local anesthetic activity. One unproven theory suggests that such effects are mediated by expansion of the nerve membrane resulting in constriction of the sodium ion channels.

Sodium Ion Channel State, Anesthetic Binding, and Use-Dependent Block

According to the modulated receptor model, sodium ion channels alternate between several conformational states, and local anesthetics bind to these different conformational states with different affinities. During excitation, the sodium channel moves from a resting-closed state to an activated-open state, with passage of sodium ions and consequent depolarization. After depolarization, the channel

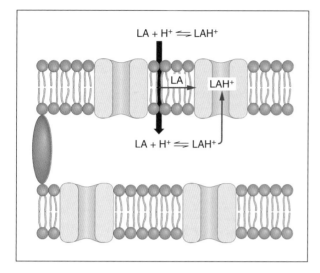

Figure 11-4 During diffusion of local anesthetic across the nerve sheath and membrane to receptor sites within the inner vestibule of the sodium channel, only the uncharged base (LA) can penetrate the lipid membrane. After reaching the axoplasm, ionization occurs, and the charged cationic form (LAH⁺) attaches to the receptor. Anesthetic may also reach the channel laterally (i.e., hydrophobic pathway). (From Covino BG, Scott DB, Lambert DH. Handbook of Spinal Anesthesia and Analgesia. Philadelphia: WB Saunders, 1994, p 7, with permission.)

assumes an inactivated-closed conformational state. Local anesthetics bind to the activated and inactivated states more readily than the resting state, attenuating conformational change. Drug dissociation from the inactivated conformational state is slower than from the resting state. Thus, repeated depolarization produces more effective anesthetic binding. The electrophysiologic consequence of this effect is progressive enhancement of conduction blockade with repetitive stimulation, an effect referred to as *use-dependent* or *frequency-dependent block*. For this reason, selective conduction blockade of nerve fibers by local anesthetics may in part be related to the characteristic frequency of activity of the nerve.

Critical Role of pH

The relative proportion of charged and uncharged local anesthetic molecules is a function of the dissociation constant of the drug and the environmental pH. Recalling the Henderson-Hasselbalch equation, the dissociation constant (Ka) can be expressed as follows:

$$pKa = pH - \log[\text{base}]/[\text{conjugate acid}]$$

If the concentration of the base and conjugate acid are equivalent, the latter component of the equation cancels (because $\log 1 = 0$). Thus, the pKa provides a useful way to describe the propensity of a local anesthetic to exist in a charged or an uncharged state. The lower the pKa, the greater is the percent of un-ionized fraction at a given pH. For example, the highly lipophilic compound benzocaine has a pKa of 3.5, and the molecule exists solely as the neutral base under normal physiologic conditions. In contrast, because the pKa values of the commonly used injectable anesthetics are between 7.6 and 8.9, less than one half of the molecules are un-ionized at physiologic pH (Table 11-1). Because local anesthetics are poorly soluble in water, they are generally marketed as water-soluble hydrochloride salts. These hydrochloride salt solutions are acidic, contributing to the stability of local anesthetics but potentially impairing the onset of a block. Bicarbonate is sometimes added to local anesthetic solutions to increase the un-ionized fraction in an effort to hasten the onset of anesthesia. Other conditions that lower pH, such as tissue acidosis produced by infection, may likewise have a negative impact on the onset and quality of local anesthesia.

Lipid Solubility

Lipid solubility of a local anesthetic affects its tissue penetration and its uptake in the nerve membrane. This physiochemical property impacts the fundamental characteristics of local anesthetics. Lipid solubility is ordinarily expressed as a partition coefficient, which is determined by comparing the solubility of the drug in a nonpolar solvent, such as *n*-heptane or octanol, with the solubility in an aqueous phase, generally water or buffered solution. Although results may vary depending on the specific methodology, lipid solubility generally correlates with local anesthetic potency and duration of action, and to a lesser extent, it varies inversely with latency or the time to onset of local anesthetic effect. Duration of the local anesthetic effect also correlates with protein binding, which likely serves to retain anesthetic within the nerve.

When considering physiochemical characteristics as they relate to the local anesthetic effect, it is important to appreciate that measures of anesthetic activity may also be impacted by the in vitro or in vivo system in which these effects are determined. For example, tetracaine is approximately 20 times more potent than bupivacaine when assessed in isolated nerve, but these drugs are generally equipotent when assessed in intact in vivo systems. Even within in vivo systems, comparisons among local anesthetics may vary based on the model or the specific site of application (spinal versus peripheral block) because of secondary effects such as the inherent vasoactive properties of the anesthetic.

Table 11-1 Comparative Pharmacology and Current Use of Local Anesthetics

Classification and Compounds	pKa	Nonionized (%) at pH 7.4	Potency*	Max. Dose (mg) for Infiltration†	Duration after Infiltration (min)	Topical	Infiltration	Intravenous Regional	Peripheral Block	Epidural	Spinal‡
Esters											
Procaine	8.9	3	1	500	45-60	No	Yes	No	Yes	No	Yes
Chloroprocaine	8.7	5	2	600	30-60	No	Yes	No	Yes	Yes	Yes (?)
Tetracaine	8.5	7	8			Yes	No	No	No	No	Yes
Amides											
Lidocaine	7.9	24	2	300	60-120	Yes	Yes	Yes	Yes	Yes	Yes (?)
Mepivacaine	7.6	39	2	300	90-180	No	Yes	No	Yes	Yes	Yes (?)
Prilocaine	7.9	24	2	400	60-120	No	Yes	Yes	Yes	Yes	Yes (?)
Bupivacaine, levobupivacaine	8.1	17	8	150	240-480	No	Yes	No	Yes	Yes	Yes
Ropivacaine	8.1	17	6	200	240-480	No	Yes	No	Yes	Yes	Yes

*Relative potencies vary based on experimental model or route of administration.
†Dosage should take into account the site of injection, use of a vasoconstrictor, and patient-related factors.
‡Use of lidocaine, mepivacaine, prilocaine, and chloroprocaine for spinal anesthesia is controversial and evolving (*see text*).

Differential Local Anesthetic Blockade

Nerve fibers can be classified according to fiber diameter, presence (type A and B) or absence (type C) of myelin, and function (Table 11-2). Nerve fiber diameter influences conduction velocity; a larger diameter correlates with more rapid nerve conduction. The presence of myelin also increases conduction velocity. This effect results from insulation of the axolemma from the surrounding media, forcing current to flow through periodic interruptions in the myelin sheath (i.e., nodes of Ranvier). With respect to local anesthetic effect, conduction blockade is predictably absent if at least three successive nodes of Ranvier are exposed to adequate concentrations of local anesthetics. However, the observation that sensitivity to local anesthetic blockade is inversely related to nerve fiber diameter probably does not reflect cause and effect. There is evidence to suggest that large, myelinated nerve fibers are more sensitive to local anesthetic blockade than smaller, unmyelinated fibers.[2] Nonetheless, in clinical practice, progressive increases in the concentrations of local anesthetics result in interruption of transmission of autonomic, sensory, and motor neural impulses and therefore production of autonomic nervous system blockade, sensory anesthesia, and skeletal muscle paralysis. The mechanisms underlying this divergence between clinical experience and experimental data are poorly understood, but they may be related to the anatomic and geographic arrangement of nerve fibers, variability in the longitudinal spread required for neural blockade, effects on other ion channels, and inherent impulse activity.

PROPENSITY TO INDUCE DIFFERENTIAL BLOCKADE

Local anesthetics are not equivalent in their propensity to induce differential blockade. For example, for equivalent analgesic or local anesthetic effect, etidocaine produces more profound motor block than bupivacaine. This characteristic makes bupivacaine a more valuable drug, particularly for use in labor or for postoperative pain management, and it accounts for etidocaine's limited use in clinical anesthesia. Attempts to identify local anesthetics with far greater sensory selectivity have been largely unsuccessful, although such effects can be achieved with alternative compounds under certain circumstances, such as that achieved with spinal administration of opioids.

Spread of Local Anesthesia after Injection

When local anesthetics are deposited around a peripheral nerve, they diffuse from the outer surface (mantle) toward the center (core) of the nerve along a concentration gradient (Fig. 11-5).[3] As a result, nerve fibers located in the mantle of the mixed nerve are blocked first. These mantle fibers are generally distributed to more proximal anatomic structures, whereas distal structures are innervated by fibers near the core. This anatomic arrangement accounts for the initial development of proximal anesthesia with subsequent distal involvement as local anesthetic diffuses to reach more central core nerve fibers. Consequently, skeletal muscle paralysis may precede the onset of sensory blockade if the motor nerve fibers are more peripheral. The sequence of onset and recovery from conduction blockade of sympathetic, sensory, and motor nerve fibers in a mixed peripheral nerve depends as much or more on the anatomic location of the nerve fibers within the mixed nerve as on their intrinsic sensitivity to local anesthetics.

PHARMACOKINETICS

Local anesthetics differ from most therapeutic agents in that drug is deposited at the target site, and systemic absorption and circulation attenuate or curtail its effect rather than deliver the drug to its intended site of action. High plasma concentrations of local anesthetics after absorption from injection sites are undesirable and are a link to their potential toxicity. Peak plasma concentrations achieved are determined by the rate of systemic uptake and, to a lesser extent, the rate of clearance of the

Type	Fiber Subtype	Diameter (μm)	Conduction Velocity (m/sec)	Function
A (myelinated)	Alpha	12-20	80-120	Proprioception, large motor
	Beta	5-15	60-80	Small motor, touch, pressure
	Gamma	3-8	30-80	Muscle tone
	Delta	2-5	10-30	Pain, temperature, touch
B (myelinated)		3	5-15	Preganglionic autonomic
C (unmyelinated)		0.3-1.5	0.5-2.5	Dull pain, temperature, touch

Table 11-2 Classification of Nerve Fibers

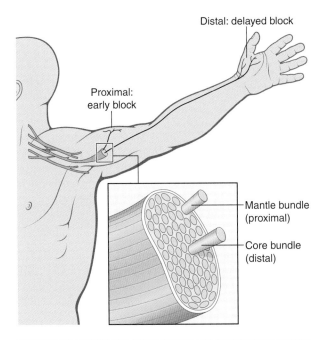

Distal: delayed block

Proximal:
early block

Mantle bundle
(proximal)

Core bundle
(distal)

Figure 11-5 Local anesthetics deposited around a peripheral nerve diffuse along a concentration gradient to block nerve fibers on the outer surface (mantle) before more centrally located (core) fibers. This accounts for early manifestations of anesthesia in more proximal areas of the extremity.

local anesthetic. Uptake is affected by several factors related to the physiochemical properties of the local anesthetic and local tissue blood flow. Uptake tends to be delayed for local anesthetics with high lipophilicity and protein binding.

Local Anesthetic Vasoactivity

Anesthetics differ somewhat in their vasoactivity, but most are vasodilators at clinically relevant concentrations, although this effect varies with site of injection. Such differences may be clinically important. For example, the lower systemic toxicity of S (–) ropivacaine compared with the R (+) enantiomer in part may result from its vasoconstrictive activity (see "Adverse Effects"). The variable effect of vasoconstrictors added to local anesthetic solutions used for spinal anesthesia is another example. In contrast to lidocaine or bupivacaine, tetracaine produces a significant increase in spinal cord blood flow. As would be predicted, prolongation of spinal anesthesia by epinephrine or other vasoconstrictors is more pronounced with tetracaine than with other commonly used spinal anesthetics.

Metabolism

The amino-ester local anesthetics undergo hydrolysis, whereas the amino-amide local anesthetics undergo metabolism by hepatic microsomal enzymes. The lungs are also capable of extracting local anesthetics such as lidocaine, bupivacaine, and prilocaine from the circulation. The rate of this metabolism and first-pass pulmonary extraction may influence toxicity (see "Systemic Toxicity"). In this regard, the relatively rapid hydrolysis of the ester local anesthetic chloroprocaine makes it less likely to produce sustained plasma concentrations than other local anesthetics, particularly the amino-amides. However, patients with atypical plasma cholinesterase levels may be at increased risk of developing excessive plasma concentrations of chloroprocaine or other ester local anesthetics due to absent or limited plasma hydrolysis. Hepatic metabolism of lidocaine is extensive, and clearance of this local anesthetic from plasma parallels hepatic blood flow. Liver disease or decreases in hepatic blood flow, as occur with congestive heart failure or general anesthesia, can decrease the rate of metabolism of lidocaine. Low water solubility of local anesthetics usually limits renal excretion of the parent compound to less than 5% of the injected dose.

Vasoconstrictors

Addition of a vasoconstrictor (usually 1,200,000 or 5 μg/mL of epinephrine) to local anesthetic solutions used for infiltration, peripheral block, and epidural or spinal anesthesia produces local vasoconstriction, which limits systemic absorption of local anesthetic and prolongs the duration of action while having little effect on the onset of anesthesia. Decreased systemic absorption of local anesthetic increases the likelihood that the rate of metabolism will match the rate of absorption, decreasing the possibility of systemic toxicity. However, systemic absorption of epinephrine may contribute to cardiac dysrhythmias or accentuate systemic hypertension in vulnerable patients. Epinephrine should also be avoided when performing peripheral nerve blocks in areas that may lack collateral flow (e.g., digital blocks). In contrast, epinephrine-induced vasoconstriction decreases local bleeding and may provide added benefit when combined with local anesthetics used for infiltration anesthesia.

ADVERSE EFFECTS

Important adverse effects of local anesthetics, although rare, may occur from systemic absorption, local tissue toxicity, allergic reactions, and drug-specific effects.

Systemic Toxicity

Systemic toxicity of local anesthetics results from excessive plasma concentrations of these drugs, most often from accidental intravascular injection during performance of nerve blocks. Less often, excessive plasma concentrations result from absorption of local anesthetics from tissue injection sites. The magnitude of local anesthetic systemic absorption depends on the dose injected, the specific site of injection, and the inclusion of a vasoconstrictor in the local anesthetic solution. Systemic absorption of local anesthetic is greatest after injection for intercostal nerve blocks and caudal anesthesia, intermediate after epidural anesthesia, and least after brachial plexus blocks (Fig. 11-6).[4]

Clinically significant systemic toxicity results from effects on the central nervous system and cardiovascular system. Establishment of maximal acceptable local anesthetic doses for performance of regional anesthesia is an attempt to limit plasma concentrations that can result from systemic absorption of these drugs (see Table 11-1). However, standard dosage recommendations are not evidence based, and they fail to take into account the specific injection site and patient-related factors.[5] Nonetheless, dosage recommendations represent guidelines for providing a starting point from which adjustments based on clinical circumstances and evolving evidence can be made.

CENTRAL NERVOUS SYSTEM TOXICITY

Increasing plasma concentrations of local anesthetics produce circumoral numbness, facial tingling, restlessness, vertigo, tinnitus, and slurred speech, culminating in tonic-clonic seizures. Local anesthetics are neuronal depressants, and onset of seizures is thought to reflect selective depression of cortical inhibitory neurons, leaving excitatory pathways unopposed. However, higher doses may affect inhibitory and excitatory pathways, resulting in central nervous system depression and even coma. These effects generally parallel anesthetic potency.

Arterial hypoxemia and metabolic acidosis can occur rapidly during seizure activity. Acidosis potentiates the central nervous system toxicity of the local anesthetics.

Early tracheal intubation to facilitate ventilation of the patient's lungs and maintenance of oxygenation may be prudent. Neuromuscular blocking drugs can stop the peripheral manifestations of seizure activity but not the underlying central nervous system activity. Treatment must include administration of drugs to stop the central nervous system manifestations of seizure activity. Diazepam (0.1 mg/kg IV) is an effective drug, as are small doses of thiopental (1 to 2 mg/kg IV), which are usually more immediately accessible. Hyperventilation should be considered, because it can reduce $PaCO_2$, and the resultant decrease in cerebral blood flow may reduce delivery of local anesthetic to the brain.

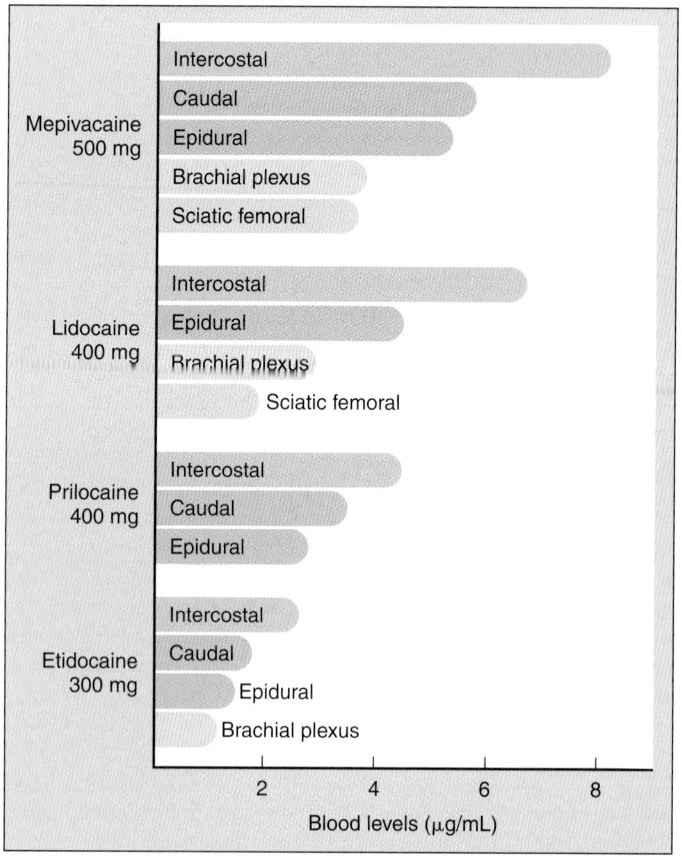

Figure 11-6 Peak plasma concentrations of local anesthetics resulting during performance of various types of regional anesthetic procedures. (From Covino BD, Vassals HG. Local Anesthetics: Mechanism of Action in Clinical Use. Orlando, FL: Grune & Stratton, 1976, with permission.)

CARDIOVASCULAR SYSTEM TOXICITY

The cardiovascular system is more resistant to the toxic effects of local anesthetics than the central nervous system. Nevertheless, high plasma concentrations of local anesthetics can produce profound hypotension due to relaxation of arteriolar vascular smooth muscle and direct myocardial depression. Part of the cardiac toxicity reflects the ability of local anesthetics to block cardiac sodium ion channels. As a result, cardiac automaticity and conduction of cardiac impulses are impaired, manifesting on the electrocardiogram as prolongation of the PR interval and widening of the QRS complex. Local anesthetics may also produce profound direct cardiac toxicity, and they are not all equivalent in this regard. For example, the ratio of the dose required to produce cardiovascular collapse compared with that producing seizures for lidocaine is about twice that for bupivacaine. Such findings support the concept that bupivacaine has greater cardiac toxicity, which has been the driving force for development of single-enantiomer anesthetics, such as ropivacaine and levobupivacaine.

Allergic Reactions

Allergic reactions to local anesthetics are rare, despite the frequent use of these drugs. It is estimated that less than 1% of all adverse reactions to local anesthetics are caused by allergic mechanisms. Most adverse responses attributed to allergic reactions are instead manifestations of systemic toxicity due to excessive plasma concentrations of the local anesthetic. Hypotension associated with syncope may be psychogenic or vagally mediated, whereas tachycardia and palpitations may occur from systemic absorption of epinephrine.

CROSS-SENSITIVITY

The amino-ester local anesthetics, which produce metabolites related to *para*-aminobenzoic acid, are more likely to evoke hypersensitivity reactions than the amino-amides. Although cross-sensitivity does not exist between classes of local anesthetics, allergic reactions may also be caused by methylparaben or similar compounds that resemble *para*-aminobenzoic acid, which are used as preservatives in commercial formulations of ester and amide local anesthetics. Although patients known to be allergic to ester local anesthetics can receive amide local anesthetics, this recommendation assumes that the local anesthetic was responsible for evoking the initial allergic reaction, rather than a common preservative.

DOCUMENTATION

Documentation of allergy to local anesthetics is based principally on clinical history (e.g., rash, laryngeal edema, hypotension, bronchospasm). However, elevations of serum tryptase, a marker of mast cell degranulation, may have some value with respect to confirmation, and intradermal testing may help establish the local anesthetic as the offending antigen if other drugs (e.g., sedative-hypnotics, opioids) have been administered concurrently.

SPECIFIC LOCAL ANESTHETICS

Amino-Esters

PROCAINE

The earliest injectable local anesthetic, procaine, enjoyed extensive use during the first half of the past century, primarily as a spinal anesthetic. Its instability and the considerable potential for hypersensitivity reactions resulted in limited use after the introduction of lidocaine. Concerns regarding *transient neurologic symptoms* (TNS) associated with spinal lidocaine (see "Lidocaine") have renewed interest in procaine as a spinal anesthetic. However, limited data suggest that procaine offers only small advantage with respect to TNS, and spinal procaine is associated with a significantly higher incidence of nausea.[6]

TETRACAINE

Tetracaine is still commonly used for spinal anesthesia. As such, it has a fairly long duration of action, particularly if used with a vasoconstrictor, although this combination results in a surprisingly high risk of TNS.[7] Tetracaine is available as a 1% solution or as niphanoid crystals; the crystal form is preferable because of the relative instability of the anesthetic in solution. Tetracaine is rarely used for epidural anesthesia or peripheral nerve blocks because of its slow onset, profound motor blockade, and potential toxicity when administered at high doses. Although it is an ester, its rate of metabolism is one fourth that of procaine and one tenth that of chloroprocaine.

CHLOROPROCAINE

Chloroprocaine initially gained popularity as an epidural anesthetic, particularly in obstetrics because its rapid hydrolysis virtually eliminated concern about systemic toxicity and fetal exposure to the local anesthetic. Neurologic injury was presumed to occur from accidental intrathecal injection of high doses of chloroprocaine intended for the epidural space. Some early experimental studies attributed this toxicity to the preservative, sodium bisulfite, contained in the commercial formulation.[8] However, other early experimental data sharply conflicted, whereas more recent studies not only fail to demonstrate neurotoxicity from intrathecal bisulfite, but instead suggest a neuroprotective effect for this compound.[9] In any event, a formulation of chloroprocaine devoid of preservatives and antioxidants is available.

Chloroprocaine has been used principally to produce epidural anesthesia of a relatively short duration. Epidural administration of chloroprocaine is sometimes avoided because it impairs the anesthetic or analgesic action of epidural bupivacaine and of opioids used concurrently or sequentially.[10] Chloroprocaine has been recently evaluated as a spinal anesthetic,[11,12] reflecting clinical concerns related to the possible toxicity of lidocaine placed in the subarachnoid space,[13] and the low doses required for spinal anesthesia would not be predicted to produce toxicity.[9] These initial reports are encouraging, but may be too limited to support off-label use as a spinal anesthetic at the time of this writing. Additionally, despite the controversy, chloroprocaine solutions used for spinal anesthesia should be bisulfite-free.

Amino-Amide Local Anesthetics

LIDOCAINE

Lidocaine has been the most commonly used and versatile local anesthetic. It is used for local topical and regional intravenous applications, peripheral nerve block, and spinal and epidural anesthesia. Although recent issues have led to restricted use of lidocaine for production of spinal anesthesia, this local anesthetic remains popular for all other applications, including epidural anesthesia.

Potential neurotoxicity (i.e., cauda equina syndrome) when lidocaine is administered for spinal anesthesia (especially continuous spinal anesthesia) has emerged.[13] Most of the initial injuries resulted from neurotoxic concentrations of anesthetic in the caudal region of the subarachnoid space achieved by the combinaion of maldistribution and relatively high doses of anesthetic administered through small-gauge spinal catheters. However, even doses of lidocaine routinely used for single-injection spinal anesthesia (75 to 100 mg) have been associated with neurotoxicity.[14]

TNS represents a syndrome of pain and/or dysesthesia that most often follows even modest intrathecal doses of lidocaine (but near zero incidence with bupivacaine).[15,16] These symptoms were initially called *transient radicular irritation*, but this term was later abandoned in favor of TNS because of the lack of certainty regarding their cause. In addition to the use of intrathecal lidocaine, cofactors that contribute to the occurrence of TNS include the lithotomy position, positioning for knee arthroscopy, and outpatient status.[17] In contrast, local anesthetic concentration, the presence of glucose, concomitant administration of epinephrine, and technique-related factors such as the size or type of needle do not alter the incidence of TNS.[17]

Symptoms of TNS generally manifest within the first 12 to 24 hours after surgery, most often resolve within 3 days, and rarely persist beyond a week. Although self-limited, the pain can be quite severe, often exceeding that induced by the surgical procedure and rarely requiring rehospitalization for pain control. Nonsteroidal anti-inflammatory drugs are often fairly effective and should be used as first-line treatment. TNS is not associated with sensory loss, motor weakness, or bowel and bladder dysfunction. The etiology and significance of these symptoms remain to be established, but discrepancies between factors afffecting TNS and experimental animal toxicity cast doubt that TNS and persistent neurologic deficits (e.g., cauda equina syndrome) are mediated by the same mechanism.

MEPIVACAINE

Mepivacaine was the first in the series of pipecholyl xylidines, combining the piperidine ring of cocaine with the xylidine ring of lidocaine (see Figs. 11-1 and 11-3). This resulted in an anesthetic with characteristics very similar to lidocaine, although with less vasodilation, and a slightly longer duration of action. The clinical use of mepivacaine parallels lidocaine, with the exception that it is relatively ineffective as a topical local anesthetic. As a spinal anesthetic, it appears to have a low, although not insignificant, incidence of TNS.

PRILOCAINE

Prilocaine was introduced into clinical practice with the anticipation that its rapid metabolism and low acute toxicity (central nervous system toxicity about 40% less than lidocaine) would make it a useful drug. Unfortunately, administration of high doses (>600 mg) may result in clinically significant accumulation of the metabolite, *ortho*-toluidine, an oxidizing compound capable of converting hemoglobin to methemoglobin. Prilocaine-induced methemoglobinemia spontaneously subsides and can be reversed by the administration of methylene blue (1 to 2 mg/kg IV over 5 minutes). Nevertheless, the capacity to induce dose-related methemoglobinemia has limited the clinical acceptance of this local anesthetic.

Similar to other anesthetics, prilocaine has recently received attention as a spinal anesthetic, owing to dissatisfaction with spinal lidocaine. Available data, albeit limited, suggest prilocaine has a duration of action similar to lidocaine with a much lower incidence of transient neurologic symptoms. However, prilocaine is not currently approved for use in the United States, nor is there any formulation available that would be appropriate for intrathecal administration.

BUPIVACAINE

Bupivacaine is a congener of mepivacaine, with a butyl rather than a methyl tail off the piperidine ring, a modification that imparts a longer duration of action. This characteristic, combined with its high-quality sensory anesthesia relative to motor blockade, has established bupivacaine as the most commonly used local anesthetic for epidural anesthesia during labor and for postoperative pain management. Bupivacaine is also commonly used for peripheral nerve block, and it has a relatively unblemished record as a spinal anesthetic.

Refractory cardiac arrest has been associated with the use of 0.75% bupivacaine when accidentally injected intravenously during attempted epidural anesthesia, and this concentration is no longer recommended for epidural anesthesia.[18] The most likely mechanism for bupivacaine's cardiotoxicity relates to the nature of its interaction with cardiac sodium ion channels.[19] When electrophysiologic differences between anesthetics are compared, lidocaine is found to enter the sodium ion channel quickly and to leave quickly. In contrast, recovery from bupivacaine blockade during diastole is relatively prolonged, making it far more potent with respect to depressing the maximum upstroke velocity of the cardiac action potential (Vmax) in ventricular cardiac muscle. As a result, bupivacaine has been labeled a "fast-in, slow-out" local anesthetic. This characteristic likely creates conditions favorable for unidirectional block and reentry. Other mechanisms may contribute to bupivacaine's cardiotoxicity, including disruption of atrioventricular nodal conduction, depression of myocardial contractility, and indirect effects mediated by the central nervous system.[20] This potential for cardiotoxicity places important limitations on the total dose of bupivacaine, and it underscores the critical role of fractional dosing during regional block. However, cardiotoxicity is not a concern when infusions of dilute solutions of bupivacaine are administered epidurally for labor or for postoperative pain or when small doses are administered for spinal anesthesia.

Single-Enantiomer Local Anesthetics

Concern for bupivacaine cardiotoxicity focused attention on the stereoisomers of bupivacaine and on its homolog, ropivacaine.

STEREOCHEMISTRY

Isomers are different compounds that have the same molecular formula. Subsets of isomers that have atoms connected by the same sequence of bonds but that have different spatial orientations are called *stereoisomers*. *Enantiomers* are a particular class of stereoisomers that exist as mirror images. The term *chiral* is derived from the Greek *cheir* for "hand," because the forms can be considered non-superimposable mirror images. Enantiomers have identical physical properties except for the direction of the rotation of the plane of polarized light. This property is used to classify the enantiomer as *dextrorotatory* (+) if the rotation is to the right or clockwise and as *levorotatory* (–) if it is to the left or counterclockwise. A *racemic* mixture is a mixture of equal parts of enantiomers and is optically inactive because the rotation caused by the molecules of one isomer is canceled by the opposite rotation of its enantiomer. Chiral compounds can also be classified on the basis of absolute configuration, generally designated as *R* (rectus) or *S* (sinister). Enantiomers may differ with respect to specific biologic activity. For example, the *S* (–) enantiomer of bupivacaine has inherently less cardiotoxicity than its *R* (+) mirror image.

ROPIVACAINE

Ropivacaine (levopropivacaine) is the *S* (–) enantiomer of the homolog of mepivacaine and bupivacaine with a propyl tail on the piperidine ring. In addition to a more favorable interaction with cardiac sodium ion channels, ropivacaine has a greater propensity to produce vasoconstriction, which may contribute to its reduced cardiotoxicity. In vitro and in vivo studies provide support for the reduced cardiotoxicity of ropivacaine compared with bupivacaine.

Motor blockade is less pronounced, and electrophysiologic studies raise the possibility that C fibers are preferentially blocked, together suggesting that ropivacaine may produce greater differential block. However, as expected from its lower lipid solubility, ropivacaine was found to be less potent than bupivacaine. The question of potency is critical to any comparison of these anesthetics; if more drug needs to be administered to achieve a desired effect, the apparent benefits with respect to cardiotoxicity (or differential block) may not exist when more appropriate equipotent comparisons are made. It appears that ropivacaine offers some advantage with respect to cardiotoxicity, but it has no clinically significant benefit over bupivacaine with respect to differential block. Consequently, the added expense of this local anesthetic compared with bupivacaine seems justified only in circumstances in which relatively high doses of local anesthetic are administered, such as those used to achieve major peripheral nerve block or surgical epidural anesthesia.

LEVOBUPIVACAINE

Levobupivacaine is the single *S* (–) enantiomer of bupivacaine. Similar to ropivacaine, cardiotoxicity is reduced, but there is no advantage over bupivacaine with respect to differential blockade. As with ropivacaine, the clinically significant advantage of this compound over the racemic mixture is restricted to situations in which relatively high doses of anesthetic are administered.

Eutectic Mixture of Local Anesthetics

The keratinized layer of the skin provides an effective barrier to diffusion of topical anesthetics, making it difficult to achieve anesthesia of intact skin by topical application. However, a combination of 2.5% lidocaine and 2.5% prilocaine cream (i.e., eutectic mixture of local anesthetics [EMLA]) is available for this purpose. This mixture has a lower melting point than either component, and it exists as an oil at room temperature that is capable of overcoming the barrier of the skin. EMLA cream is particularly useful in children for relieving pain associated with venipuncture or placement of an intravenous catheter, although it may take up to an hour before adequate topical anesthesia is produced.

II

FUTURE LOCAL ANESTHETICS

Local anesthetics play a central role in modern anesthetic practice. However, despite major advances in pharmacology and techniques for administration over the past century, this class of compounds has a relatively narrow therapeutic index with respect to their potential for neurotoxicity and for adverse cardiovascular and central nervous system effects. Toxicity has been the prominent force behind the evolution of these compounds and the manner in which they are used. Data demonstrate that the neurotoxicity of these compounds does not result from blockade of the voltage-gated sodium channel, indicating that local anesthetic effect and toxicity are not mediated by a common mechanism.[21] Compounds binding to alternative sites at the sodium ion channel may display far greater affinity for neuronal over cardiac channels. The future may see the development of anesthetics with far better therapeutic advantage.

REFERENCES

1. Covino BG, Scott DB, Lambert DH. Handbook of Spinal Anesthesia and Analgesia. Philadelphia: WB Saunders, 1994, p 7.
2. Gissen AJ, Covino BG, Gregus J. Differential sensitivities of mammalian nerve fibers to local anesthetic agents. Anesthesiology 1980;53:467-474.
3. Winnie AP, Tay CH, Patel KP, et al. Pharmacokinetics of local anesthetics during plexus blocks. Anesth Analg 1977;56:852-861.
4. Covino B, Vassallo H. Local Anesthetics: Mechanisms of Action and Clinical Use. New York: Grune & Stratton, 1976.
5. Rosenberg PH, Veering BT, Urmey WF. Maximum recommended doses of local anesthetics: A multifactorial concept. Reg Anesth Pain Med 2004;29:564-575.
6. Hodgson PS, Liu SS, Batra MS, et al. Procaine compared with lidocaine for incidence of transient neurologic symptoms. Reg Anesth Pain Med 2000;25:218-222.
7. Sakura S, Sumi M, Sakaguchi Y, et al. The addition of phenylephrine contributes to the development of transient neurologic symptoms after spinal anesthesia with 0.5% tetracaine. Anesthesiology 1997;87:771-778.

8. Gissen A, Datta S, Lambert D. The chloroprocaine controversy. II. Is chloroprocaine neurotoxic? Reg Anesth 1984;9:135-144.
9. Taniguchi M, Bollen AW, Drasner K. Sodium bisulfite: Scapegoat for chloroprocaine neurotoxicity? Anesthesiology 2004;100:85-91.
10. Eisenach JC, Schlairet TJ, Dobson CE 2nd, Hood DH. Effect of prior anesthetic solution on epidural morphine analgesia. Anesth Analg 1991;73:119-123.
11. Drasner K. Chloroprocaine spinal anesthesia: Back to the future? Anesth Analg 2005;100:549-552.
12. Kouri ME, Kopacz DJ, Spinal-2 chloroprocaine: A comparison with lidocaine in volunteers. Anesth Analg 1991;73:119-123.
13. Drasner K. Local anesthetic neurotoxicity: Clinical injury and strategies that may minimize risk. Reg Anesth Pain Med 2002;27:576-580.
14. Drasner K. Lidocaine spinal anesthesia: A vanishing therapeutic index? Anesthesiology 1997;87:469-472.
15. Schneider M, Ettlin T, Kaufmann M, et al. Transient neurologic toxicity after hyperbaric subarachnoid anesthesia with 5% lidocaine. Anesth Analg 1993;76:1154-1157.

16 Hampl KF, Schneider MC, Ummenhofer W, Drewe J. Transient neurologic symptoms after spinal anesthesia. Anesth Analg 1995;81:1148-1153.
17. Freedman JM, Li DK, Drasner K, et al. Transient neurologic symptoms after spinal anesthesia: An epidemiologic study of 1,863 patients. Anesthesiology 1998;89:633-641.
18. Albright GA. Cardiac arrest following regional anesthesia with etidocaine or bupivacaine. Anesthesiology 1979;51:285-287.
19. Clarkson CW, Hondeghem LM. Mechanism for bupivacaine depression of cardiac conduction: Fast block of sodium channels during the action potential with slow recovery from block during diastole. Anesthesiology 1985;62:396-405.
20. Bernards CM, Artu AA. Hexamethonium and midazolam terminate dysrhythmias and hypertension caused by intracerebroventricular bupivacaine in rabbits. Anesthesiology 1991;74:89-96.
21. Sakura S, Bollen AW, Ciriales R, Drasner K. Local anesthetic neurotoxicity does not result from blockade of voltage-gated sodium channels. Anesth Analg 1995;81:338-346.

Chapter 12

NEUROMUSCULAR BLOCKING DRUGS

Ronald D. Miller

Neuromuscular blocking drugs (NMBDs) interrupt transmission of nerve impulses at the neuromuscular junction (NMJ) and thereby produce paresis or paralysis of skeletal muscles. On the basis of electrophysiologic differences in their mechanisms of action and duration of action, these drugs can be classified as depolarizing NMBDs (mimic the actions of acetylcholine [ACh]) and nondepolarizing NMBDs (interfere with the actions of ACh), the latter of which are further subdivided into long-, inter-mediate-, and short-acting drugs (Table 12-1). Succinyl-choline (SCh) is the only depolarizing NMBD used clinically. It is also the only NMBD that has both a rapid onset and ultrashort duration of action. Among the non-depolarizing NMBDs, rocuronium most closely resembles the onset characteristics of SCh.

CLINICAL USES

The principal clinical uses of NMBDs are to produce skeletal muscle relaxation for facilitation of tracheal intubation and to provide optimal surgical working conditions. NMBDs may also be administered in emergency departments, cardiopulmonary resuscitation situations, and the intensive care unit setting to facilitate mechanical ventilation of the patient's lungs. Of prime importance is to recognize that NMBDs lack analgesic or anesthetic effects and must not be used to render an inadequately anesthetized patient paralyzed. Ventilation of the lungs must be mechanically provided whenever significant skeletal muscle weakness is produced by these drugs. Clinically, intraoperative evaluation of neuromuscular blockade is typically provided by visually monitoring the mechanical response (twitch response) produced by electrical stimulation of a peripheral nerve (usually a branch of the ulnar or facial nerve) delivered from a peripheral nerve stimulator (see the section "Monitoring the Effects of Nondepolarizing Neuromuscular Blocking Drugs").

Table 12–1 Classification of Neuromuscular Blocking Drugs
Depolarizing (rapid onset and ultrashort-acting)
Succinylcholine
Nondepolarizing
Long-acting
Pancuronium
Intermediate-acting
Vecuronium
Rocuronium
Atracurium
Cisatracurium
Short-acting
Mivacurium

Choice of Neuromuscular Blocking Drug

The choice of NMBD is influenced by its speed of onset, duration of action, route of elimination, and associated side effects, such as drug-induced changes in systemic arterial blood pressure or heart rate, or both. Rapid onset and brief duration of skeletal muscle paralysis, characteristic of SCh, are useful when tracheal intubation is the reason for administering an NMBD. Because of its rapid onset time, rocuronium is often used to facilitate tracheal intubation, but its duration of action is much longer than that of SCh. Although SCh can be administered as a continuous intravenous infusion, nondepolarizing NMBDs are usually selected when longer periods of neuromuscular blockade are needed. When rapid onset of skeletal muscle paralysis is not necessary, it is acceptable to induce skeletal muscle relaxation by the administration of long- or intermediate-acting nondepolarizing NMBDs to facilitate tracheal intubation.

NEUROMUSCULAR JUNCTION

The NMJ consists of a prejunctional motor nerve ending separated from the highly folded postjunctional membrane of the skeletal muscle by a synaptic cleft (Fig. 12-1).[1] Neuromuscular transmission is initiated by arrival of an impulse at the motor nerve terminal with an associated influx of calcium ions and resultant release of the ligand ACh. ACh binds to nicotinic cholinergic receptors (the ligand-gated channel) on postjunctional membranes and thereby causes a change in membrane permeability to ions, principally potassium and sodium. This change in

permeability and movement of ions causes a decrease in the transmembrane potential from about –90 mV to –45 mV (threshold potential), at which point a propagated action potential spreads over the surfaces of skeletal muscle fibers and leads to muscular contraction. ACh is rapidly hydrolyzed (within 15 msec) by the enzyme acetylcholinesterase (true cholinesterase), thus restoring membrane permeability (repolarization) and preventing sustained depolarization. Acetylcholinesterase is primarily located in the folds of the end-plate region, which places it in close proximity to the site of action of ACh.

Release of Acetylcholine

ACh is synthesized in the motor nerve terminal, and the protein synapsin anchors the ACh vesicle to the release site of the terminal. Some of the ACh is then released and the rest is held in reserve for response to a stimulus. Presynaptic receptors, aided by calcium, facilitate replenishment of the motor nerve terminal, which can be stimulated by SCh and neostigmine and depressed by small doses of nondepolarizing NMBDs.

Postjunctional Receptors

Postjunctional receptors are glycoproteins consisting of five subunits (Fig. 12-2).[2] The subunits of the receptor are arranged such that a channel is formed that allows the flow of ions along a concentration gradient across cell membranes. This flow of ions is the basis of normal neuromuscular transmission. Extrajunctional receptors retain the two α-subunits but may have an altered γ- or δ-subunit by the substitution of an ε-unit.

The two α-subunits are the binding sites for ACh and the sites occupied by NMBDs. For example, occupation of one or both α-subunits by a nondepolarizing NMBD causes the ion channel to remain closed, and ion flow to produce depolarization cannot occur. SCh attaches to α-sites and causes the ion channel to remain open (mimics ACh), thereby resulting in prolonged depolarization. Large doses of nondepolarizing NMBDs (large molecules) may also act to occlude the channel and in this way prevent the normal flow of ions. Neuromuscular blockade secondary to occlusion of the channels is resistant to drug-enhanced antagonism with anticholinesterase drugs. The lipid environment around cholinergic receptors can be altered by drugs such as volatile anesthetics, thus changing the properties of the ion channels.

Extrajunctional Receptors

Postjunctional receptors are confined to the area of the end plate precisely opposite the prejunctional receptors, whereas extrajunctional receptors (the ε-unit is replaced by γ-subunits) are present throughout skeletal muscles. Extrajunctional receptor synthesis is normally suppressed

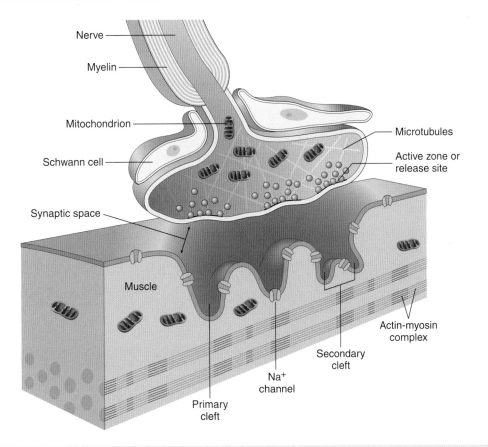

Figure 12-1 Adult neuromuscular junction with the three cells that constitute the synapse: the motor neuron (i.e., nerve terminal), muscle fiber, and Schwann cell. The motor neuron from the ventral horn of the spinal cord innervates the muscle. Each fiber receives only one synapse. The motor nerve loses its myelin and terminates on the muscle fiber. The nerve terminal, covered by a Schwann cell, has vesicles clustered about the membrane thickenings, which are the active zones, toward its synaptic side and mitochondria and microtubules toward its other side. A synaptic gutter, made up of a primary and many secondary clefts, separates the nerve from the muscle. The muscle surface is corrugated, and dense areas on the shoulders of each fold contain acetylcholine receptors. Sodium channels are present at the clefts and throughout the muscle membrane. (From Martyn JAJ. Neuromuscular physiology and pharmacology. In Miller RD [ed]: Miller's Anesthesia, 6th ed. Philadelphia: Churchill Livingstone, 2005.)

by neural activity. Prolonged inactivity, sepsis, and denervation or trauma (burn injury) to skeletal muscles may be associated with a proliferation of extrajunctional receptors. When activated, extrajunctional receptors stay open longer and permit more ions to flow, which in part explains the exaggerated hyperkalemic response when SCh is administered to patients with denervation or burn injury. Proliferation of these receptors also accounts for the resistance or tolerance to nondepolarizing NMBDs, as can occur with burns or prolonged (several days) mechanical ventilation of the lungs.

STRUCTURE-ACTIVITY RELATIONSHIPS

NMBDs are quaternary ammonium compounds that have at least one positively charged nitrogen atom that binds to the α-subunit of postsynaptic cholinergic receptors (Fig. 12-3). In addition, these drugs have structural similarities to the endogenous neurotransmitter ACh. For example, SCh is two molecules of ACh linked by methyl groups. The long, slender, flexible structure of ACh allows it to bind to and activate cholinergic receptors. The bulky rigid molecules that are characteristic of nondepolarizing

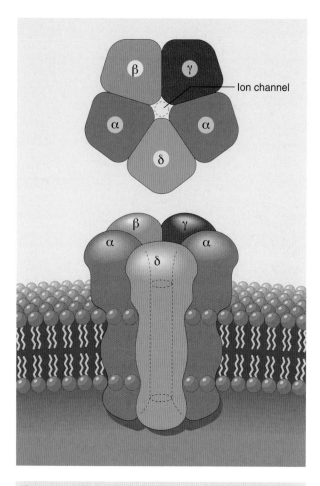

Figure 12-2 The postjunctional nicotinic cholinergic receptor consists of five subunits (α, α, β, γ, δ) arranged to form an ion channel. (From Taylor P. Are neuromuscular blocking agents more efficacious in pairs? Anesthesiology 1985;63:1-3, with permission.)

DEPOLARIZING NEUROMUSCULAR BLOCKING DRUGS

SCh is the only depolarizing NMBD used clinically. Furthermore, it is the only NMBD with both a rapid onset and ultrashort duration of action. Typically, doses of 0.5 to 1.5 mg/kg intravenously are administered and produce a rapid onset of skeletal muscle paralysis (30 to 60 seconds) that lasts 5 to 10 minutes. These characteristics make SCh ideal for providing rapid skeletal muscle paralysis to facilitate tracheal intubation. SCh has been used clinically for more than 50 years. Despite consistent industrial efforts, no drug has been developed that is better than SCh for tracheal intubation.[3] Although an intravenous dose of 0.5 mg/kg may be adequate, 1.0 to 1.5 mg/kg is commonly administered to facilitate tracheal intubation. If a subparalyzing dose of a nondepolarizing NMBD (pretreatment with 5% to 10% of its 95% effective dose [ED_{95}]) is administered 2 to 4 minutes before injection of SCh to blunt fasciculations, the dose of SCh should be increased by about 70%. Although ideal for facilitating tracheal intubation, SCh has many adverse effects. As an alternative, a longer-acting nondepolarizing NMBD, such as rocuronium, may be chosen.

Characteristics of Blockade

SCh mimics the action of ACh and produces a sustained depolarization of the postjunctional membrane. Skeletal muscle paralysis occurs because a depolarized postjunctional membrane and inactivated sodium channels cannot respond to subsequent release of ACh (hence, the designation depolarizing neuromuscular blockade). Depolarizing neuromuscular blockade is also referred to as phase I blockade. Phase II blockade is present when the postjunctional membrane has become repolarized but still does not respond normally to ACh (desensitization neuromuscular blockade). The mechanism of phase II blockade is unknown but may reflect the development of nonexcitable areas around the end plates that become repolarized but nevertheless prevent the spread of impulses initiated by the action of ACh. With the initial dose of SCh, subtle signs of a phase II blockade begin to appear (fade to tetanic stimulation).[4] Phase II blockade, which resembles the blockade produced by nondepolarizing NMBDs, predominates when the dose of SCh exceeds 3 to 5 mg/kg IV (Table 12-2).

The sustained depolarization produced by the initial administration of SCh is initially manifested as transient generalized skeletal muscle contractions known as fasciculations. Furthermore, the sustained opening of sodium channels produced by SCh is associated with leakage of potassium from the interior of cells sufficient to increase plasma concentrations of potassium by about 0.5 mEq/L. With proliferation of extrajunctional receptors and damaged muscle membranes, many more channels will leak potassium and thereby lead to acute hyperkalemia.

NMBDs, though containing portions similar to ACh, do not activate cholinergic receptors.

Nondepolarizing NMBDs are either aminosteroid compounds (pancuronium, vecuronium, rocuronium) or benzylisoquinolinium compounds (atracurium, cisatracurium, mivacurium). Pancuronium is the bisquaternary aminosteroid NMBD most closely related to ACh structurally. The ACh-like fragments of pancuronium give the steroidal molecule its high degree of neuromuscular blocking activity. Vecuronium and rocuronium are monoquaternary analogs of pancuronium. Aminosteroid NMBDs lack hormonal activity. Benzylisoquinolinium derivatives are more likely than aminosteroid derivatives to evoke the release of histamine, presumably reflecting the presence of a tertiary amine.

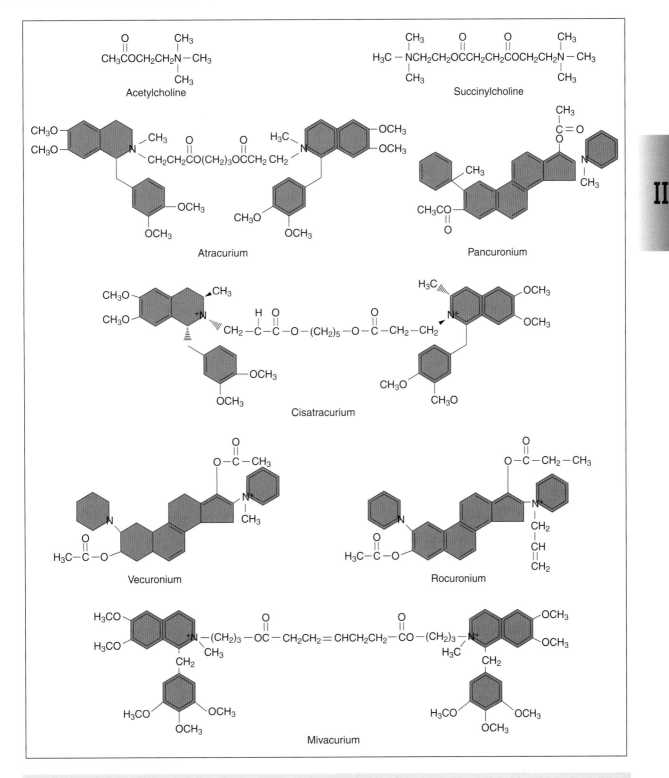

Figure 12-3 Chemical structure of acetylcholine and neuromuscular blocking drugs.

Table 12–2 Comparison of Depolarizing (Succinylcholine) and Nondepolarizing (Rocuronium) Neuromuscular Blocking Drugs

| | Succinylcholine | | Rocuronium |
	Phase I	Phase II	
Administration of rocuronium	Antagonize	Augment	Augment
Administration of succinylcholine	Augment	Augment	Antagonize
Administration of neostigmine	Augment	Antagonize	Antagonize
Fasciculations	Yes		No
Response to single electrical stimulation (single twitch)	Decreased	Decreased	Decreased
Train-of-four ratio	>0.7	<0.3	<0.3
Response to continuous (tetanus) electrical stimulation	Sustained	Unsustained	Unsustained
Post-tetanic facilitation	No	Yes	Yes

Metabolism

Hydrolysis of SCh to inactive metabolites is accomplished by plasma cholinesterase (pseudocholinesterase) produced in the liver (Fig. 12-4). Plasma cholinesterase has an enormous capacity to hydrolyze SCh at a rapid rate (ACh is metabolized even more rapidly) such that only a small fraction of the original intravenous dose reaches the NMJ. Because plasma cholinesterase is not present at the NMJ, the neuromuscular blockade produced by SCh is terminated by its diffusion away from the NMJ into extracellular fluid. Therefore, plasma cholinesterase influences the duration of action of SCh by controlling the amount of SCh that is hydrolyzed before reaching the NMJ. Liver disease must be severe before decreases in the synthesis of plasma cholinesterase are sufficient to prolong the effects of SCh. Potent anticholinesterases, as used in the treatment of myasthenia gravis, and certain chemotherapeutic drugs (nitrogen mustard, cyclophosphamide) may so decrease plasma cholinesterase activity that prolonged skeletal muscle paralysis follows the administration of SCh.

ATYPICAL PLASMA CHOLINESTERASE

Atypical plasma cholinesterase lacks the ability to hydrolyze ester bonds in drugs such as SCh and mivacurium. The presence of this atypical enzyme is often recognized only after an otherwise healthy patient experiences prolonged skeletal muscle paralysis (>1 hour) after the administration of a conventional dose of SCh or mivacurium. Subsequent determination of the dibucaine number permits diagnosis of the presence of atypical plasma cholinesterase. Dibucaine is an amide local anesthetic that inhibits normal plasma activity by about 80%, whereas the activity of atypical enzyme is inhibited by about 20% (Table 12-3). It is important to recognize that the dibucaine number reflects the quality of plasma cholinesterase (ability to metabolize SCh and mivacurium) and not the quantity of

enzyme that is circulating in plasma. For example, decreases in plasma cholinesterase activity because of liver disease or anticholinesterases are often associated with a normal dibucaine number.

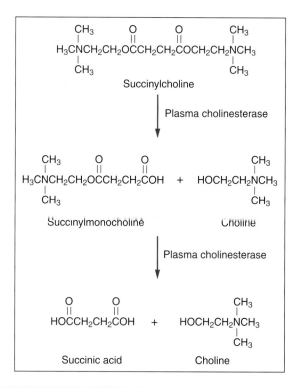

Figure 12-4 The brief duration of action of succinylcholine is due to its rapid hydrolysis in plasma by cholinesterase enzyme to inactive metabolites (succinylmonocholine has $1/20$ to $1/80$ the activity of succinylcholine at the neuromuscular junction).

Table 12-3 Variants of Plasma Cholinesterase and Duration of Action of Succinylcholine

Variants of Plasma Cholinesterase	Type of Butylcholinesterase	Incidence	Dibucaine Number (% Inhibition of Enzyme Activity)	Duration of Succinylcholine-Induced Neuromuscular Blockade (min)
Homozygous, typical	UU	Normal	70-80	5-10
Heterozygous	UA	1/480	50-60	20
Homozygous, atypical	AA	1/3200	20-30	60-180

Adverse Side Effects

Adverse side effects after the administration of SCh are numerous and may limit or even contraindicate the use of this NMBD in certain patients (Table 12-4). SCh usually should not be given to patients 24 to 72 hours after major burns, trauma, and extensive denervation of skeletal muscles because it may result in acute hyperkalemia and cardiac arrest.[5] Administration of SCh to apparently healthy boys with unrecognized muscular dystrophy has resulted in acute hyperkalemia and cardiac arrest.[6] For this reason, the Food and Drug Administration has issued a warning against the use of SCh in children, except for emergency control of the airway.

CARDIAC DYSRHYTHMIAS

Sinus bradycardia, junctional rhythm, and even sinus arrest may follow the administration of SCh. These responses reflect the action of SCh at cardiac postganglionic muscarinic receptors, where this drug mimics the normal effects of ACh (Table 12-5). Cardiac dysrhythmias are most likely to occur when a second intravenous dose of SCh is administered about 5 minutes after the first dose.

Table 12-4 Adverse Side Effects of Succinylcholine

Cardiac dysrhythmias
Sinus bradycardia
Junctional rhythm
Sinus arrest
Fasciculations
Hyperkalemia
Myalgia
Myoglobinuria
Increased intraocular pressure
Increased intragastric pressure
Trismus

Intravenous administration of atropine or subparalyzing doses of nondepolarizing NMBDs (pretreatment) 1 to 3 minutes before SCh decreases the likelihood of these cardiac responses. Atropine administered intramuscularly with the preoperative medication does not reliably protect against SCh-induced decreases in heart rate. The effects of SCh at autonomic nervous system ganglia also mimic the actions of the neurotransmitter ACh and may be manifested as ganglionic stimulation with associated increases in systemic blood pressure and heart rate (see Table 12-5).

HYPERKALEMIA

Hyperkalemia sufficient to cause cardiac arrest may follow the administration of SCh to patients with unhealed skeletal muscle injury, as produced by third-degree burns or trauma, or with denervation injury, as caused by spinal cord transection, and lead to skeletal muscle atrophy. The risk for hyperkalemia in these patients increases with time and usually peaks 7 to 10 days after the injury. There is evidence that increased release of potassium after the administration of SCh (doses as small as 20 mg IV) can begin within 2 to 4 days after denervation injury. In addition, extrajunctional receptors and hyperkalemia will develop in any patient who is immobile (critical care patients) for several days if SCh is given. For example, cardiac arrest has occurred when SCh has been used for emergency endotracheal intubation in the intensive care unit. The duration of susceptibility to the hyperkalemic effects of SCh is unknown, but the risk is probably decreased 3 to 6 months after denervation injury. All factors considered, it might be prudent to avoid administration of SCh to any patient more than 24 hours after a burn injury, extensive trauma, or spinal cord transection.

Presumably, the risk of a hyperkalemic response in burn patients diminishes with healing of the skeletal muscles damaged by the burn injury. Yet vulnerability to hyperkalemia is complicated. The common explanation of proliferation of extrajunctional receptors (not proved to occur after burn injury), thus providing more sites for potassium to leak outward across cell membranes during depolarization, is oversimplified.[7] Pretreatment with nondepolarizing NMBDs minimally influences the magnitude of potassium release evoked by SCh and cannot

Table 12–5 Autonomic Nervous System and Histamine-Releasing Effects of Neuromuscular Blocking Drugs

Drug*	Nicotinic Receptors at Autonomic Ganglia	Cardiac Postganglionic Muscarinic Receptors	Histamine Release
Succinylcholine	Modest stimulation	Modest stimulation	Minimal
Pancuronium	None	Modest blockade	None
Vecuronium	None	None	None
Rocuronium	None	None	None
Atracurium	None	None	Slight†
Cisatracurium	None	None	None
Mivacurium	None	None	Slight†

*ED_{95} equivalent doses.
†Occurs only with doses estimated to be 2 to 3 × ED_{95}.

be relied on as a safeguard. The presence of acute extensive trauma or upper motor neuron injury may also place patients at risk for SCh-induced hyperkalemia. Patients with renal failure are not susceptible to exaggerated release of potassium, and SCh can be safely administered to these patients, assuming that they do not have uremic neuropathy.

MYALGIA
Postoperative skeletal muscle myalgia, manifested particularly in the muscles of the neck, back, and abdomen, may follow the administration of SCh. Myalgia localized to neck muscles may be described as a "sore throat" by the patient and incorrectly attributed to the previous presence of a tracheal tube. Young adults undergoing minor surgical procedures that permit early ambulation seem most likely to complain of myalgia. It is speculated that unsynchronized contractions of skeletal muscle fibers (fasciculations) associated with generalized depolarization lead to myalgia. Prevention of fasciculations by prior administration of subparalyzing doses of a nondepolarizing NMBD (pretreatment) or lidocaine will decrease the incidence but not totally prevent myalgia.[8] Magnesium will prevent fasciculations, but not myalgia. Nonsteroidal anti-inflammatory drugs are effective in treating the myalgia.

INCREASED INTRAOCULAR PRESSURE
SCh causes a maximum increase in intraocular pressure 2 to 4 minutes after its administration. This increase in intraocular pressure is transient and lasts only 5 to 10 minutes. The mechanism by which SCh increases intraocular pressure is unknown, although contraction of extraocular muscles with associated compression of the globe has been presumed to contribute. The concern that contraction of extraocular muscles could cause extrusion of intraocular contents in the presence of an open eye injury has resulted in the common clinical practice of

avoiding the administration of SCh to these patients. This theory has never been substantiated and is challenged by the report of patients with an open eye injury in whom intravenous administration of SCh did not cause extrusion of global contents.[9] Furthermore, there is evidence that contraction of extraocular muscles does not contribute to the increase in intraocular pressure that accompanies the administration of SCh.[10]

INCREASED INTRACRANIAL PRESSURE
Increases in intracranial pressure after the administration of SCh do not consistently occur (Fig. 12-5).[11]

INCREASED INTRAGASTRIC PRESSURE
SCh causes unpredictable increases in intragastric pressure. When intragastric pressure does increase, it seems to be related to the intensity of fasciculations, thus emphasizing the potential value of preventing this skeletal muscle activity by prior administration of a subparalyzing dose of a nondepolarizing NMBD. An unproven hypothesis is that this increased intragastric pressure may cause passage of gastric fluid and contents into the esophagus and pharynx with a subsequent risk for pulmonary aspiration.

TRISMUS
Incomplete jaw relaxation with masseter jaw rigidity after a halothane-SCh sequence is not uncommon in children (occurs in about 4.4% of patients) and is considered a normal response. In extreme cases this response may be so severe that the ability to mechanically open the patient's mouth is limited. The difficulty lies in separating the normal response to SCh from the masseter rigidity that may be associated with malignant hyperthermia. Because SCh is not recommended for use in children, except for emergency airway control, trismus is less of an issue.

Figure 12-5 Mean intracranial pressure (ICP) did not change significantly when succinylcholine, 1 mg/kg IV, was administered to patients with neurologic injury (Glasgow Coma Scale score of 6). (From Kovarik WD, Mayberg TS, Lam AM, et al. Succinylcholine does not change intracranial pressure, cerebral blood flow velocity, or the electroencephalogram in patients with neurologic injury. Anesth Analg 1994;78:469-473, with permission).

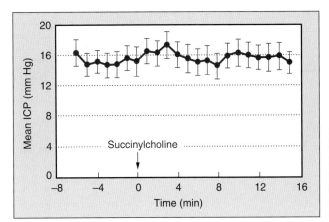

II

NONDEPOLARIZING NEUROMUSCULAR BLOCKING DRUGS

Nondepolarizing NMBDs are classified clinically as long, intermediate, and short acting (see Table 12-1). These drugs act by competing with ACh for α-subunits at the postjunctional nicotinic cholinergic receptors and preventing changes in ion permeability. As a result, depolarization cannot occur (hence, the designation nondepolarizing neuromuscular blockade), and skeletal muscle paralysis develops. Unlike depolarizing muscle relaxants, SCh skeletal muscle fasciculations do not accompany the onset of nondepolarizing neuromuscular blockade. Differences in onset, duration of action, rate of recovery, metabolism, and clearance influence the clinical decision to select one drug versus another (Table 12-6).

Pharmacokinetics

Nondepolarizing NMBDs, because of their quaternary ammonium groups, are highly ionized, water-soluble compounds at physiologic pH and possess limited lipid solubility. As a result, these drugs cannot easily cross lipid membrane barriers, such as the blood-brain barrier, renal tubular epithelium, gastrointestinal epithelium, or placenta. Therefore, nondepolarizing NMBDs do not produce central nervous system effects, renal tubular reabsorption is minimal, oral administration is ineffective, and maternal administration does not adversely affect the fetus. Redistribution of nondepolarizing NMBDs also exerts a role in the pharmacokinetics of these drugs.

Many of the variable pharmacologic responses of patients to nondepolarizing NMBDs can be explained by differences in pharmacokinetics, which can be changed by many factors, such as hypovolemia, hypothermia, and the presence of hepatic or renal disease (or both). Renal and hepatic elimination is aided by access to a large fraction of the administered drug because of the high degree of ionization, which maintains high plasma concentrations of nondepolarizing NMBDs and also prevents renal reabsorption of excreted drug.

Renal disease markedly alters the pharmacokinetics of only the long-acting nondepolarizing NMBDs, such as pancuronium. The intermediate-acting NMBDs are eliminated by the liver (rocuronium), by metabolism by plasma cholinesterase (mivacurium), by Hofmann elimination (atracurium or cisatracurium), or by a combination of these mechanisms.

Pharmacodynamic Responses

The absence of age-related changes in the responsiveness of the NMJ (changes in pharmacodynamics) is confirmed by similar dose-response curves in elderly and young adults (Figs. 12-6 and 12-7).[12,13] Enhancement of neuromuscular blockade by volatile anesthetics reflects a pharmacodynamic action as manifested by decreased plasma concentrations of nondepolarizing NMBDs required to produce a given degree of neuromuscular blockade in the presence of volatile anesthetics. In addition to volatile anesthetics, other drugs, such as aminoglycoside antibiotics, local anesthetics, cardiac antiarrhythmic drugs, dantrolene, magnesium, lithium, and tamoxifen (an antiestrogenic drug), may enhance the neuromuscular blockade produced by nondepolarizing NMBDs. A few drugs may diminish the effects of a nondepolarizing NMBD, including calcium, corticosteroids, and anticonvulsant (phenytoin) drugs.[14] Some neuromuscular diseases can be associated with altered pharmacodynamic responses (myasthenia gravis, Duchenne's muscular dystrophy). Burn injury causes resistance to the effects of nondepolarizing NMBDs, as reflected by the need to establish a higher plasma concentration of drug to achieve the same pharmacologic effect as in patients without a burn injury. There is resistance to the effects of nondepolarizing NMBDs in skeletal muscles affected by a cerebral vascular accident, perhaps reflecting proliferation of extrajunctional receptors that respond to ACh.

Table 12–6 Comparative Pharmacology of Nondepolarizing Neuromuscular Blocking Drugs

	ED$_{95}$ (mg/kg)	Onset to Maximum Twitch Depression (min)	Duration to Return to ≥25%*	Intubating Dose (mg/kg)	Continuous Infusion (mg/kg/min)	Renal Excretion (% Unchanged)	Hepatic Degradation (%)	Biliary Excretion (% Unchanged)	Hydrolysis in Plasma
Pancuronium	0.07	3-5	60-90	0.1		80	10	5-10	No
Vecuronium	0.05	3-5	20-35	0.08-0.1	1	15-25	20-30	40-75	No
Rocuronium	0.3	1-2	20-35	0.6-1.2		10-25	10-20	50-70	No
Atracurium	0.2	3-5	20-35	0.4-0.5	6-8	NS	NS	NA	Enzymatic, spontaneous
Cisatracurium	0.05	3-5	20-35	0.1	1-1.5	NS	NS	NS	Spontaneous
Mivacurium	0.08	2-3	12-20	0.25	5-6	NS	NS	NS	Enzymatic

*Control twitch height (minutes).
NS, not significant

144

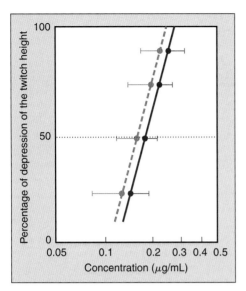

Figure 12-6 The absence of age-related changes in the responsiveness of the neuromuscular junction to long-acting nondepolarizing neuromuscular blocking drugs such as pancuronium is confirmed by the similarity of plasma concentrations necessary to produce comparable responses in young adults (*red circles*) and elderly individuals (*blue circles*). (From Duvaldestin P, Saada J, Berger JL, et al. Pharmacokinetics, pharmacodynamics, and dose-response relationship of pancuronium in control and elderly subjects. Anesthesiology 1982;56:36-40, with permission.)

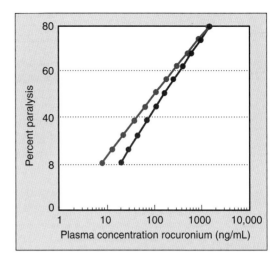

Figure 12-7 The plasma concentration of rocuronium necessary to produce a specific degree of paralysis is not different in elderly (*red circles*) and young adults (*blue circles*). (From Matteo RS, Ornstein E, Schwartz AE, et al. Pharmacokinetics and pharmacodynamics of rocuronium [ORG 9426] in elderly surgical patients. Anesth Analg 1993;77:1193-1197, with permission.)

Cardiovascular Effects

Nondepolarizing NMBDs may exert minor cardiovascular effects through drug-induced release of histamine, effects on cardiac muscarinic receptors, or effects on nicotinic receptors at autonomic ganglia (see Table 12-5). Transient hypotension can occur with atracurium and mivacurium, but usually with large doses (>0.4 and 0.15 mg/kg, respectively.) The relative magnitude of the circulatory effects varies from patient to patient and depends on factors such as underlying autonomic nervous system activity, blood volume status, preoperative medication, drugs administered for maintenance of anesthesia, and concurrent drug therapy.

Critical Care Medicine and Critical Illness Myopathy and Polyneuropathy

A small fraction of patients with asthma (receiving corticosteroids) or acutely injured patients with multiple organ system failure (including sepsis) who require mechanical ventilation of the lungs for prolonged periods (usually more than 6 days) may manifest prolonged skeletal muscle weakness on recovery that is augmented by the skeletal muscle paralysis produced by NMBDs. These patients exhibit moderate to severe quadriparesis with or without areflexia, but they usually retain normal sensory function. The time course of the weakness is unpredictable, and in some patients the weakness may progress and persist for weeks or months. The pathophysiology of this myopathy is not well understood. Therefore, NMBDs should be given for 2 days or less and only after the use of analgesics, sedatives, and adjustments to ventilator settings have been maximally used. Although myopathy occurs autonomously, administration of NMBDs can augment the severity of this condition. SCh should be used with caution to facilitate endotracheal intubation in critically ill patients because of reports of cardiac arrest, presumably caused by acute hyperkalemia.

Allergic Reactions

NMBDs are the triggering drugs for more than 50% of the anaphylactic and anaphylactoid reactions occurring during anesthesia; such reactions occur at a rate between 1 in 1000 and 1 in 25,000 anesthetics. SCh is the most common offender. Even though it does not release histamine, rocuronium was identified as producing an increased risk for allergic reactions in France and Norway, with no confirmation from other countries. More recently, a follow-up study from Norway of 83 cases of anaphylaxis during general anesthesia revealed that 77% of these reactions were mediated by immunoglobulin E and 93% were associated with NMBDs, with SCh being the most common drug.[15] There may be cross-sensitivity between all NMBDs because of the presence of a common antigenic component, the quaternary ammonium group. Anaphylactic reactions after the first exposure to an NMBD may reflect sensitization from previous contact with cosmetics or soaps that also contain antigenic quaternary ammonium groups.

LONG-ACTING NONDEPOLARIZING NEUROMUSCULAR BLOCKING DRUGS

Pancuronium

Pancuronium is a bisquaternary aminosteroid nondepolarizing NMBD with an ED_{95} of 70 μg/kg; it has an onset of action of 3 to 5 minutes and a duration of action of 60 to 90 minutes (see Table 12-6 and Fig. 12-3). An estimated 80% of a single dose of pancuronium is eliminated unchanged in urine. In the presence of renal failure, plasma clearance of pancuronium is decreased 30% to 50%, thus resulting in a prolonged duration of action. An estimated 10% to 40% of pancuronium undergoes hepatic deacetylation to inactive metabolites, with the exception of 3-desacetylpancuronium, which is approximately 50% as potent as pancuronium at the NMJ.

CARDIOVASCULAR EFFECTS

Pancuronium typically produces a modest 10% to 15% increase in heart rate, mean arterial pressure, and cardiac output. The increase in heart rate reflects pancuronium-induced selective blockade of cardiac muscarinic receptors (atropine-like effect), principally in the sinoatrial node. Indeed, the heart rate responses evoked by pancuronium still occur in patients treated with β-adrenergic antagonists. The magnitude of the heart rate increase evoked by pancuronium seems to be more dependent on the preexisting heart rate (an inverse relationship) than on the dose or rate of pancuronium administration. Marked increases in heart rate in response to pancuronium seem more likely to occur in patients with altered atrioventricular conduction of cardiac impulses, such as may occur in the presence of atrial fibrillation. The modest increase in systemic blood pressure and cardiac output after the administration of pancuronium reflects the effect of heart rate on cardiac output in the absence of changes in systemic vascular resistance. The cardiac-stimulating effects of pancuronium could contribute to increased myocardial oxygen requirements and the development of myocardial ischemia in patients with coronary artery disease. Histamine release and autonomic ganglion blockade are not produced by pancuronium.

INTERMEDIATE-ACTING NONDEPOLARIZING NEUROMUSCULAR BLOCKING DRUGS

Vecuronium, rocuronium, atracurium, and cisatracurium are classified as intermediate-acting nondepolarizing NMBDs. In contrast to the long-acting nondepolarizing NMBD pancuronium, these drugs possess efficient clearance mechanisms that minimize the likelihood of significant cumulative effects (progressively longer duration of action) with repeated injections or continuous intravenous infusions.

When compared with pancuronium, these drugs have (1) a similar onset of maximum neuromuscular blockade, with the exception of rocuronium, which is unique because of its rapid onset, which can (with large doses) parallel that of SCh; (2) approximately one third the duration of action (hence the designation *intermediate acting*); (3) a 30% to 50% more rapid rate of recovery; (4) minimal to absent cumulative effects; and (5) minimal to absent cardiovascular effects. Drug-enhanced antagonism of the neuromuscular blockade produced by intermediate-acting nondepolarizing NMBDs is facilitated by the concomitant spontaneous recovery that occurs after rapid clearance of the drug.

Vecuronium

Vecuronium is a monoquaternary aminosteroid nondepolarizing NMBD with an ED_{95} of 50 μg/kg that produces an onset of action of 3 to 5 minutes and a duration of action of 20 to 35 minutes (see Fig. 12-3 and Table 12-6). This drug undergoes both hepatic and renal excretion. Metabolites are pharmacologically inactive, with the exception of 3-desacetylvecuronium, which is approximately 50% to 70% as potent as the parent compound. The increased lipid solubility of vecuronium as compared with pancuronium also facilitates biliary excretion of vecuronium. The effect of renal failure on the duration of action of vecuronium is small, but repeated or large doses may result in prolonged neuromuscular blockade. Vecuronium is typically devoid of circulatory effects, even with rapid intravenous administration of doses that exceed $3 \times ED_{95}$, thus emphasizing its lack of vagolytic effects or associated histamine release.

Rocuronium

Rocuronium is a monoquaternary aminosteroid nondepolarizing NMBD with an ED_{95} of 0.3 mg/kg that has an onset of action of 1 to 2 minutes and a duration of action of 20 to 35 minutes (see Table 12-6 and Fig. 12-3). The lack of potency of rocuronium in comparison to vecuronium is an important factor in determining the rapid onset of neuromuscular blockade produced by this drug. Conceptually, when a large number of molecules are administered, the result is a larger number of molecules that are available to diffuse to the NMJ. Thus, a rapid onset of action is more likely to be achieved with a less potent drug such as rocuronium. The onset of maximum single twitch depression after the intravenous administration of rocuronium at 3 to 4 × ED$_{95}$ (1.2 mg/kg) resembles the onset of action of SCh after the intravenous administration of 1 mg/kg (Fig. 12-8).[16] However, the large doses of rocuronium (3 to 4 × ED$_{95}$) needed to mimic the onset time of SCh produce a duration of action resembling that of pancuronium. Furthermore, rocuronium administered at a dose of 1 to 2 × ED$_{95}$ (0.6 mg/kg) does not produce intubation conditions as good as SCh does, and larger doses (1.2 mg/kg) of rocuronium are required.[17]

Clearance of rocuronium is largely as unchanged drug in bile, with deacetylation not occurring. Renal excretion of the drug may account for as much as 30% of a dose, and administration of this drug to patients in renal failure could result in a longer duration of action, especially with repeated doses or prolonged intravenous infusion. Cardiovascular effects or the release of histamine does not follow the rapid intravenous administration of even large doses of rocuronium.[18]

Atracurium

Atracurium is a bisquaternary benzylisoquinolinium nondepolarizing NMBD (mixture of 10 stereoisomers) with an ED$_{95}$ of 0.2 mg/kg that produces an onset of action of 3 to 5 minutes and a duration of action of 20 to 35 minutes (see Table 12-6 and Fig. 12-3). Clearance of this drug is by a chemical mechanism (spontaneous nonenzymatic degradation at normal body temperature and pH known as *Hofmann elimination*) and a biologic mechanism (ester hydrolysis by nonspecific plasma esterases). Laudanosine is the major metabolite of both pathways. This metabolite is not active at the NMJ but may, in high concentrations, cause central nervous system stimulation. The two routes of metabolism occur simultaneously and are independent of hepatic and renal function, as well as plasma cholinesterase activity. As such, the duration of atracurium-induced neuromuscular blockade is similar in normal patients and those with absent or impaired renal or hepatic function or those with atypical plasma cholinesterase (emphasizes that ester hydrolysis of atracurium is unrelated to the plasma cholinesterase responsible for the hydrolysis of SCh and mivacurium). Hofmann elimination and ester hydrolysis account for the lack of cumulative drug effects and the unaltered duration of action of atracurium, even in patients with renal or hepatic failure. Ester hydrolysis accounts for an estimated two thirds of degraded atracurium.

CARDIOVASCULAR EFFECTS

Systemic blood pressure and heart rate changes do not usually accompany the rapid intravenous administration of atracurium in doses up to 2 × ED$_{95}$. Rapid intravenous administration of 3 × ED$_{95}$ may produce transient increases in heart rate and decreases in systemic blood pressure.[19] Plasma histamine concentrations increase transiently and parallel the heart rate and systemic blood pressure changes.

Cisatracurium

Cisatracurium is a benzylisoquinolinium nondepolarizing NMBD with an ED$_{95}$ of 50 μg/kg that has an onset of action of 3 to 5 minutes and a duration of action of 20 to 35 minutes (see Table 12-6 and Fig. 12-3).[20] Structurally, cisatracurium is an isolated form of 1 of the 10 stereoisomers of atracurium. This drug principally undergoes degradation by Hofmann elimination to laudanosine. Plasma concentrations of laudanosine after the administration of cisatracurium are far lower than after

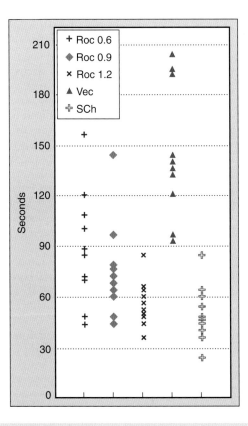

Figure 12-8 The onset to maximum twitch depression is similar after the intravenous administration of rocuronium (Roc) at doses of 0.9 mg/kg and 1.2 mg/kg and succinylcholine (SCh), 1 mg/kg. Vec, vecuronium. (From Magorian TT, Flannery KB, Miller RD. Comparison of rocuronium, succinylcholine and vecuronium for rapid sequence induction of anesthesia. Anesthesiology 1993;79:913-918, with permission.)

equivalent doses of atracurium. Presumably, the greater potency of cisatracurium than atracurium results in fewer molecules being administered and therefore lower plasma concentrations of metabolites. In contrast to atracurium, nonspecific plasma esterases do not seem to be involved in the clearance of cisatracurium. The organ-independent clearance of cisatracurium means that this nondepolarizing NMBD, like atracurium, can be administered to patients with renal or hepatic failure without a change in its duration of action. Cisatracurium, in contrast to atracurium, is devoid of histamine-releasing effects, so cardiovascular changes do not accompany the rapid intravenous administration of even large doses of cisatracurium.

SHORT-ACTING NONDEPOLARIZING NEUROMUSCULAR BLOCKING DRUGS

Mivacurium

Mivacurium is a benzylisoquinolinium nondepolarizing NMBD with an ED_{95} of 80 µg/kg that has an onset of action of 2 to 3 minutes and a duration of action of 12 to 20 minutes (see Table 12-6 and Fig. 12-3). As such, the duration of action of mivacurium is approximately twice that of SCh and 30% to 40% that of the intermediate-acting nondepolarizing NMBDs. Mivacurium consists of three stereoisomers, with the two most active isomers undergoing hydrolysis by plasma cholinesterase at a rate equivalent to 88% that of SCh. Hydrolysis of these two isomers is responsible for the short duration of action of mivacurium. As with SCh, hydrolysis of mivacurium is decreased and its duration of action increased in patients with atypical plasma cholinesterase (see Table 12-3).

Spontaneous recovery from the neuromuscular blocking effects of mivacurium is rapid, and the need for drug-enhanced antagonism may be negated if the residual neuromuscular block is shown to be clinically dissipated.[21] Furthermore, neostigmine decreases plasma cholinesterase activity and could theoretically slow the hydrolysis of mivacurium. Nevertheless, moderate levels of mivacurium-induced neuromuscular blockade are readily antagonized by neostigmine. This apparent paradox is most likely due to the fact that neostigmine is a better antagonist of true cholinesterase than plasma cholinesterase. Edrophonium has little or no effect on the activity of plasma cholinesterase.

CARDIOVASCULAR EFFECTS

Cardiovascular responses to mivacurium are usually minimal at doses up to $2 \times ED_{95}$. Rapid administration of mivacurium at $3 \times ED_{95}$ may evoke sufficient histamine release to transiently decrease systemic blood pressure and increase the heart rate.

MONITORING THE EFFECTS OF NONDEPOLARIZING NEUROMUSCULAR BLOCKING DRUGS

Evaluation of the mechanically evoked responses produced by electrical stimulation delivered from a peripheral nerve stimulator is the most reliable method to monitor the pharmacologic effects of NMBDs. Use of a peripheral nerve stimulator permits titration of the NMBD to produce the desired pharmacologic effect, and at the conclusion of surgery the responses evoked by the nerve stimulator are used to judge spontaneous recovery from an NMBD-induced neuromuscular blockade, which is facilitated by the administration of anticholinesterase drugs (e.g., neostigmine) (see the section "Drug-Assisted Antagonism of Nondepolarizing Neuromuscular Blocking Drugs").

Most often, superficial electrodes or subcutaneous needles (must have a metal hub) are placed over the ulnar nerve at the wrist or elbow or the facial nerve on the lateral aspect of the face, and a supramaximal electrical stimulus is delivered from the peripheral nerve stimulator.[22,23] The adductor pollicis muscle is innervated solely by the ulnar nerve, which accounts for the popularity of placing stimulating electrodes from the peripheral nerve stimulator over the ulnar nerve. Facial nerve stimulation and observation of the orbicularis oculi muscle, though difficult to quantitate, may be a consideration when mechanically evoked responses to stimulation of the ulnar nerve are not visible because of positioning of the upper extremities. Another consideration is the observation that monitoring the response of the orbicularis oculi muscle to facial nerve stimulation more closely reflects the onset of neuromuscular blockade at the larynx than does the response of the adductor pollicis to ulnar nerve stimulation (Fig. 12-9).[24] Moreover, the onset of neuromuscular blockade after the administration of nondepolarizing NMBDs is more rapid, but less intense at the laryngeal muscles (vocal cords) than at the peripheral muscles (adductor pollicis) (Fig. 12-10).[25] In this regard, the period of laryngeal paralysis may be dissipating before a maximum effect is reached at the adductor pollicis. In contrast, the onset of neuromuscular blockade at the laryngeal muscles and at the muscles innervated by the ulnar nerve is similar when SCh is administered (see Fig. 12-10).[25] Thus, monitoring the twitch response at the adductor pollicis is more likely to parallel the intensity of the drug-induced effect at the laryngeal adductors when SCh is administered.

Patterns of Stimulation

Mechanically evoked responses used for monitoring the effects of NMBDs include the single twitch response, train-of-four (TOF) ratio, double burst suppression, tetanus, and post-tetanic stimulation (Figs. 12-11 to 12-14).[22,23] These mechanically evoked responses are evaluated

Figure 12-9 The effects of rocuronium (in terms of maximum depression of the single twitch response) are less intense and the duration of action is less at the adductor muscles of the larynx than at the adductor pollicis. (From Meistelman C, Plaud B, Donati F. Rocuronium [ORG 9426] neuromuscular blockade at the adductor muscles of the larynx and adductor pollicis in humans. Can J Anaesth 1992;39:665-669, with permission.)

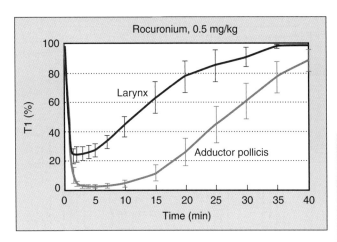

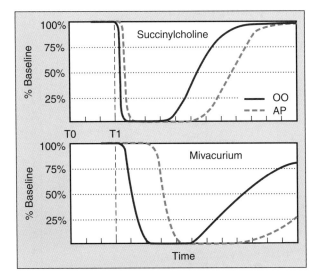

Figure 12-10 The maximum onset of twitch depression after the administration of mivacurium (also true for intermediate-acting neuromuscular blocking drugs) is more rapid when the twitch response is monitored at the orbicularis oculi (OO) muscle than at the adductor pollicis (AP). The onset of maximum twitch depression after the administration of succinylcholine is similar at both skeletal muscles. (From Sayson SC, Mongan PD. Onset of action of mivacurium chloride: A comparison of neuromuscular blockade monitoring at the adductor pollicis and the orbicularis oculi. Anesthesiology 1994;81:35-42, with permission.)

twitch response recovers to a percentage of control height (see Table 12-6).

The response to peripheral nerve stimulation can be used to answer the following questions:

1. Is the neuromuscular blockade adequate for surgery?
2. Is the neuromuscular blockade excessive?
3. Can this neuromuscular blockade be antagonized?

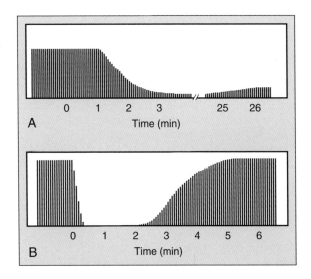

Figure 12-11 Schematic illustration of the onset and recovery from the neuromuscular blocking effects of a nondepolarizing (**A**) or a depolarizing (**B**) neuromuscular blocking drug ("0 time" indicates injection of the neuromuscular blocking drug) as depicted by the mechanically evoked single twitch response to repeated electrical stimulation of the nerve. (Modified from Viby-Mogensen J. Clinical assessment of neuromuscular transmission. Br J Anaesth 1982;54:209-223, with permission.)

visually, manually by touch (tactile), or by recording. The depth of neuromuscular blockade may be defined as the percentage of a predetermined inhibition of twitch response from control height (ED$_{95}$, dose necessary to depress the twitch response 95%) and the duration of drug effect as the time from drug administration until the

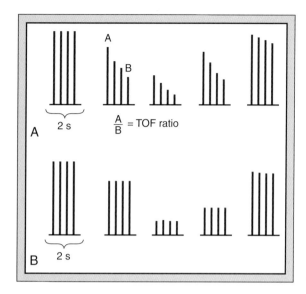

Figure 12-12 Schematic illustration of the mechanically evoked response to train-of-four (TOF) electrical stimulation of the nerve after injection of a nondepolarizing neuromuscular blocking drug (**A**) or a depolarizing (succinylcholine) neuromuscular blocking drug (**B**). The TOF ratio is less than 1 (fades) only in the presence of effects at the neuromuscular junction produced by a nondepolarizing neuromuscular blocking drug. (Modified from Viby-Mogensen J. Clinical assessment of neuromuscular transmission. Br J Anaesth 1982;54:209-223, with permission.)

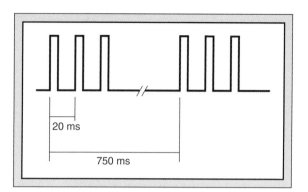

Figure 12-13 Schematic illustration of the stimulation pattern of double burst stimulation (three electrical impulses at 50 Hz separated by 750 msec). (From Bevan DR, Donati F, Kopman AF. Reversal of neuromuscular blockade. Anesthesiology 1992;77:785-792, with permission.)

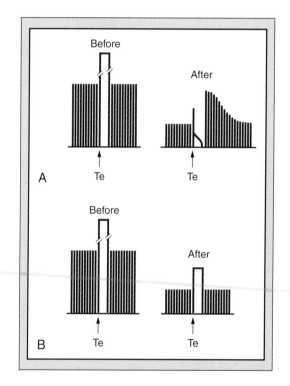

Figure 12-14 Schematic illustration of the evoked response to tetanic (Te) stimulation (50 Hz for 5 seconds) before and after the intravenous injection of a nondepolarizing neuromuscular blocking drug (**A**) or a depolarizing (succinylcholine) neuromuscular blocking drug (**B**). (Modified from Viby-Mogensen J. Clinical assessment of neuromuscular transmission. Br J Anaesth 1982;54:209-223, with permission.)

Depression of the twitch response greater than 90% or elimination of two to three twitches of the TOF correlates with acceptable skeletal muscle relaxation for performance of intra-abdominal surgery in the presence of an adequate concentration of volatile anesthetic. If all twitches from TOF stimulation are absent, more NMBD should not be given until some twitch is present. If some of the twitches from TOF stimulation are present, antagonism is likely to be successful (see the section "Drug-Assisted Antagonism of Nondepolarizing Neuromuscular Blocking Drugs").

TRAIN-OF-FOUR STIMULATION

TOF (four electrical stimulations at 2 Hz delivered every 0.5 second) is based on the concept that ACh is depleted by successive stimulations. Only four twitches are necessary because subsequent stimulation fails to further alter the release of additional ACh. In the presence of effects produced at the NMJ by nondepolarizing NMBDs, the height of the fourth twitch is lower than that of the first twitch, thereby allowing calculation of a TOF ratio (fade) (see Fig. 12-12).[22] Recovery of the TOF ratio to greater than 0.7 correlates with complete return to control height of a single twitch response. In the presence of effects produced at the NMJ by SCh, the TOF ratio remains near 1.0 because the height of all four twitch responses is decreased by a similar amount (phase I blockade) (see Fig. 12-12).[22] A TOF ratio of less than 0.3 in the presence of SCh reflects phase II blockade (see Table 12-2).

DOUBLE BURST SUPPRESSION

Accurate estimation of the TOF ratio is not reliable clinically by either visual or manual assessment. Difficulty in estimating the TOF ratio may be due to the fact that the two middle twitch responses interfere with comparison of the first and last twitch response. In this regard, double burst suppression (two bursts of three electrical stimulations separated by 750 msec) is perceived by the observer as two separate twitches (see Fig. 12-13).[23] The observer's ability to detect a TOF ratio less than 0.3 is improved with double burst suppression, but the ability to conclude that the TOF ratio is greater than 0.7 is still not ensured.[26] In contrast to the difficulty in quantifying the TOF ratio, determination of the number of electrically evoked twitch responses to TOF stimulation is more likely to be reproducible. For example, the fourth twitch can be observed when the first twitch is equivalent to 30% to 40% of control twitch height, which corresponds to a TOF ratio of about 0.35. Counting the number of visible TOF responses may be helpful in predicting the ease with which neuromuscular blockade can be antagonized with an anticholinesterase drug (Table 12-7) (see the section "Drug-Assisted Antagonism of Nondepolarizing Neuromuscular Blocking Drugs").[23]

TETANUS

Tetanus (continuous or tetanic electrical stimulation for 5 seconds at about 50 Hz) is an intense stimulus for the release of ACh at the NMJ. In the presence of effects produced at the NMJ by nondepolarizing NMBDs, the response to tetanus is not sustained (fades), whereas in the presence of SCh-induced effects at the NMJ, the response to tetanus is greatly decreased but does not fade with a phase I blockade (see Fig. 12-14).[22] A sustained response to tetanus is present when the TOF ratio is greater than 0.7. At the cessation of tetanus, there is an increase in the immediately available stores of ACh such that the subsequent twitch responses are transiently enhanced (post-tetanic facilitation) (see Fig. 12-14).[22]

DRUG-ASSISTED ANTAGONISM OF NONDEPOLARIZING NEUROMUSCULAR BLOCKING DRUGS

Drug-assisted (pharmacologic) antagonism of the effects of nondepolarizing NMBDs as achieved by the intravenous administration of an anticholinesterase drug (usually neostigmine, but possibly edrophonium or pyridostigmine) may be recommended on a routine basis. Even if all tests of the adequacy of normal neuromuscular function are normal, 50% of the receptors at the NMJ may still be occupied by an NMBD. Although it is not known how many receptors are necessary for adequate skeletal muscle strength, when in doubt, it is better to have as many receptors free of the effects of NMBDs as possible (see Table 12-7).[23] Unequivocal clinical confirmation (sustained head lift or leg lift, or both, for 5 seconds, tongue depressor test) provides assurance of adequate recovery (spontaneous and drug assisted) from the effects of NMBDs.

Anticholinesterase Drugs

Anticholinesterase drugs are typically administered during the time when spontaneous recovery from the neuromuscular blockade is occurring so that the effect of the pharmacologic antagonist adds to the rate of spontaneous recovery from the nondepolarizing NMBD. In this regard, the rapid spontaneous recovery rate characteristic of

Table 12–7	Choice of Anticholinesterase Drug		
TOF Visible Twitches	**Estimated TOF Fade**	**Anticholinesterase Drug and Dose (mg/kg IV)**	**Anticholinergic Drug and Dose (µg/kg IV)†**
None*		Not recommended	Not recommended
≤2	++++	Neostigmine 0.07	Glycopyrrolate, 7, or atropine, 15
3-4	+++	Neostigmine 0.04	Glycopyrrolate, 7, or atropine, 15
4	++	Edrophonium 0.5	Atropine 7
4	0	Edrophonium 0.25	Atropine 7

*Postpone drug-assisted antagonism until some evoked response is visible.
†Administered simultaneously with an anticholinesterase drug.
++++, marked; +++, moderate; ++, minimal; 0, none; TOF, train-of-four.
Adapted from Bevan DR, Donati F, Kopman AF. Reversal of neuromuscular blockade. Anesthesiology 1992;77:785-792, with permission.)

intermediate- and short-acting NMBDs is an advantage over a long-acting drug such as pancuronium. For example, the incidence of weakness in the postoperative period despite drug-assisted antagonism is more frequent in patients receiving pancuronium than an intermediate- or short-acting NMBD.

Anticholinesterase drugs, such as neostigmine, accelerate the already established pattern of spontaneous recovery at the NMJ by inhibiting the activity of acetyl-cholinesterase and thereby leading to the accumulation of ACh at nicotinic (NMJ) and muscarinic sites. Increased amounts of ACh in the region of the NMJ improve the chance that two ACh molecules will bind to the α-subunits of the nicotinic cholinergic receptors (see Fig. 12-2). This alters the balance of the competition between ACh and a nondepolarizing NMBD in favor of the neurotransmitter (ACh) and restores neuromuscular transmission. In addition, anticholinesterase drugs may generate antidromic action potentials and repetitive firing of motor nerve endings (presynaptic effects).

The quaternary ammonium structure of anticholinesterase drugs greatly limits their entrance into the central nervous system such that selective antagonism of the peripheral nicotinic effects of nondepolarizing NMBDs at the NMJ is possible. For example, the peripheral cardiac muscarinic effects of anticholinesterase drugs (bradycardia) are attenuated by the prior or simultaneous intravenous administration of atropine or glycopyrrolate.

Factors Influencing the Success of Antagonism of Neuromuscular Blocking Drugs

Factors influencing the success of drug-assisted antagonism of NMBDs include (1) the intensity of the neuromuscular blockade at the time that the pharmacologic antagonist is administered, (2) the choice of antagonist drug, (3) the dose of antagonist drug, (4) the rate of spontaneous recovery from the NMBD, and (5) the concentration of the inhaled anesthetic.

Neostigmine is the most commonly administered antagonist. The greater the spontaneous recovery, as judged by the response to peripheral nerve stimulation, the more rapidly that complete recovery will occur from neostigmine administration. Although large doses of neostigmine will result in more rapid antagonism, the maximum dose should be limited to 60 to 70 µg/kg. Antagonism will be more rapid in the presence of an NMBD with rapid elimination (atracurium instead of pancuronium). The rate of antagonism can also be hastened by reducing the concentration of the volatile anesthetic.

Evaluation of the Adequacy of Antagonism

Adequacy of recovery (spontaneous and drug assisted) from the neuromuscular blocking effects produced by nondepolarizing NMBDs should be determined by the result of multiple tests of skeletal muscle strength (Table 12-8).[27] Even though a TOF ratio greater than 0.7 has been recommended, visual estimation of the TOF is neither accurate nor reliable. In the absence of an accurately measured TOF ratio, a sustained response to tetanus or the ability to maintain head lift for 5 to 10 seconds usually indicates a TOF ratio greater than 0.7. Grip strength is also a useful indicator of recovery from the effects of NMBDs. Although a TOF ratio higher than 0.7 or its equivalent provides evidence of the patient's ability to sustain adequate ventilation, the pharyngeal musculature may still be weak and upper airway obstruction remains a risk.[28-30] Furthermore, diplopia, dysphagia, an increased risk of aspiration, and a decreased ventilatory response

Table 12–8 Clinical Tests of Neuromuscular Transmission

Test	Normal Function	% of Receptors Occupied*	Comment
Tidal volume	5 mL/kg	80	Insensitive
Train-of-four	No fade	70	Somewhat uncomfortable
Vital capacity	At least 20 mL/kg	70	Requires patient cooperation
Sustained tetanus (50 Hz)	No fade	60	Uncomfortable
Double burst suppression	No fade	60	Uncomfortable
Head lift	180 Degrees for 5 sec	50	Requires patient cooperation
Handgrips	Sustained for 5 sec	50	Requires patient cooperation

*Approximate percentage of receptors occupied when the response returns to its normal value.
Adapted from Naguib M, Lien CA. Pharmacology of muscle relaxants and their antagonists. *In* Miller RD (ed): Miller's Anesthesia, 6th ed. Philadelphia: Churchill Livingstone, 2005.

to hypoxia in the presence of a TOF ratio greater than 0.7 emphasize the value of more sensitive clinical methods for assessing neuromuscular function, such as sustained head lift or leg lift (or both) for 5 seconds or an evaluation of masseter muscle strength (tongue depressor test).[28-31]

Allowing spontaneous recovery from NMBDs without the aid of drug-assisted antagonism (administration of an anticholinesterase drug) is not recommended unless there is compelling clinical evidence that significant residual neuromuscular blockade does not persist. Avoidance of drug-assisted antagonism (neostigmine) for fear of increasing the incidence of postoperative nausea and vomiting is not warranted.[31]

When the initial response to an anticholinesterase drug seems inadequate, the following questions should be answered before additional antagonist drug is administered:

1. Has sufficient time elapsed for the anticholinesterase drug to antagonize the nondepolarizing NMBD (15 to 30 minutes)?
2. Is the degree of neuromuscular blockade too intense to be antagonized?
3. Is acid-base and electrolyte status normal?
4. Is body temperature normal?
5. Is the patient taking any drugs that could interfere with antagonism?
6. Has clearance of the nondepolarizing NMBD from plasma been decreased by renal or hepatic dysfunction (or by both)?

Answers to these questions will often provide the reason for failure of anticholinesterase drugs to adequately antagonize nondepolarizing neuromuscular blockade.

A New Antagonist of Neuromuscular Blocking Drugs

A γ-cyclodextrin (sugammadex) is under development that antagonizes steroidal NMBDs, especially rocuronium, by encapsulating them.[32] This mechanism of action is totally different from that of neostigmine in that no action on any cholinesterase takes place. Furthermore, no cardiovascular effects occur. If clinical studies succeed, rocuronium could be used to facilitate tracheal intubation and then be immediately reversed. This would markedly reduce the need for SCh.

FUTURE ADMINISTRATION TECHNIQUES

Currently, NMBDs are given by intermittent bolus administration. In the future, perhaps more sophisticated continuous techniques will be developed.[33]

REFERENCES

1. Martyn JAJ. Neuromuscular physiology and pharmacology. *In* Miller RD (ed): Miller's Anesthesia, 6th ed. Philadelphia: Churchill Livingstone, 2005.
2. Taylor P. Are neuromuscular blocking agents more efficacious in pairs? Anesthesiology 1985;63:1-3.
3. Miller RD: Will succinylcholine ever disappear? Anesth Analg 2004;98:1674-1675.
4. Naguib M, Lien CA, Aken J, et al. Posttetanic potentiation and fade in the response to tetanic and train-of-four stimulation during succinylcholine-induced block. Anesth Analg 2004;98:1686-1691.
5. Gronert GA, Theye RA. Pathophysiology of hyperkalemia induced by succinylcholine. Anesthesiology 1975;43:89-99.
6. Rosenberg H, Gronert GA. Intractable cardiac arrest in children given succinylcholine. Anesthesiology 1992;77:1054.
7. Martyn JAJ, Richtsfeld M. Succinylcholine-induced hyperkalemia in acquired pathologic states. Anesthesiology 2006;104:158-169.
8. Schreiber JU, Lysakowski C, Fuchs-Binder T, et al. Prevention of succinylcholine-induced fasciculation and myalgia. Anesthesiology 2005;103:877-884.
9. Libonati MM, Leahy JJ, Ellison D. The use of succinylcholine in open eye surgery. Anesthesiology 1985;62:637-640.
10. Kelly RE, Dinner M, Turner LS, et al. Succinylcholine increases intraocular pressure in the human eye with the extraocular muscles detached. Anesthesiology 1993;79:948-952.
11. Kovarik WD, Mayberg TS, Lam AM, et al. Succinylcholine does not change intracranial pressure, cerebral blood flow velocity, or the electroencephalogram in patients with neurologic injury. Anesth Analg 1994;78:469-473.
12. Duvaldestin P, Saada J, Berger JL, et al. Pharmacokinetics, pharmacodynamics, and dose-response relationship of pancuronium in control and elderly subjects. Anesthesiology 1982;56:36-40.
13. Matteo RS, Ornstein E, Schwartz AE, et al. Pharmacokinetics and pharmacodynamics of rocuronium (ORG 9426) in elderly surgical patients. Anesth Analg 1993;77:1193-1197.
14. Richard A, Girard F, Girard DC, et al. Cisatracurium-induced neuromuscular blockade is affected by chronic phenytoin or carbamazepine treatment in neurosurgical patients. Anesth Analg 2005;100:538-544.
15. Harboe T, Guttormsen AB, Irgene A, et al. Anaphylaxis during anesthesia in Norway. Anesthesiology 2005;102:897-903.
16. Magorian TT, Flannery KB, Miller RD. Comparison of rocuronium, succinylcholine and vecuronium for rapid sequence induction of anesthesia. Anesthesiology 1993;79:913-918.
17. Sluga M, Vmmenhofer W, Studer W, et al. Rocuronium versus succinylcholine for rapid sequence induction of anesthesia and endotracheal intubation. Anesth Analg 2005;101:1356-1361.
18. Levy JH, Davis GK, Duggan J, et al. Determination of the hemodynamics and histamine release of rocuronium (ORG 9426) when administered in increased doses under N_2O/O_2-sufentanil anesthesia. Anesth Analg 1994;78:318-321.
19. Basta SJ, Ali HH, Savarese JJ, et al. Clinical pharmacology of atracurium besylate (BW 33A): A new nondepolarizing muscle relaxant. Anesth Analg 1982;61:723-729.

20. Mellinghoff H, Radbruch L, Diefenbach C, et al. A comparison of cisatracurium and atracurium: Onset of neuromuscular block after bolus injection and recovery after subsequent infusion. Anesth Analg 1996;83:1072-1075.

21. Naguib M, Selim M, Bakhamees HS, et al. Enzymatic versus pharmacologic antagonism of profound mivacurium-induced neuromuscular blockade. Anesthesiology 1996;84:1051-1059.

22. Viby-Mogensen J. Clinical assessment of neuromuscular transmission. Br J Anaesth 1982;54:209-223.

23. Bevan DR, Donati F, Kopman AF. Reversal of neuromuscular blockade. Anesthesiology 1992;77:785-792.

24. Meistelman C, Plaud B, Donati F. Rocuronium (ORG 9426) neuromuscular blockade at the adductor muscles of the larynx and adductor pollicis in humans. Can J Anaesth 1992;39:665-669.

25. Sayson SC, Mongan PD. Onset of action of mivacurium chloride: A comparison of neuromuscular blockade monitoring at the adductor pollicis and the orbicularis oculi. Anesthesiology 1994;81:35-42.

26. Kopman AF, Yee PS, Neuman GG. Relationship of the train-of-four fade to the clinical signs and symptoms of residual paralysis in awake volunteers. Anesthesiology 1997;86:765-771.

27. Naguib M, Lien CA. Pharmacology of muscle relaxants and their antagonists. *In* Miller RD (ed): Miller's Anesthesia, 6th ed. Philadelphia: Churchill Livingstone, 2005.

28. Eikermann M, Blobner M, Groeben H, et al. Postoperative upper airway obstruction after recovery of the TOF-ratio of the adductor pollicis muscle from neuromuscular blockade. Anesth Analg (in press).

29. Ericksson LI. Evidence-based practice and neuromuscular monitoring: It's time for routine quantitative assessment. Anesthesiology 2003;98:1042-1048.

30. Ericksson LI. The effects of residual neuromuscular blockade and volatile anesthetics on the control of ventilation. Anesth Analg 1999;89:243-251.

31. Cheng CR, Sessler DI, Apfel C. Does neostigmine administration produce a clinically important increase in postoperative nausea and vomiting? Anesth Analg 2005;101:1349-1355.

32. Kopman AF. Suggammadex: A revolutionary approach to neuromuscular antagonism. Anesthesiology 2006;104:718-723.

33. Eleveld DJ, Proost JH, Wierda JMKH. Evaluation of a closed-loop muscle relaxant control system. Anesth Analg 2005;101:758-764.

Chapter 13

PREOPERATIVE EVALUATION AND MEDICATION

Rachel Dotson, Jeanine P. Wiener-Kronish, and Temitayo Ajayi

PREOPERATIVE EVALUATION

The Joint Commission for the Accreditation of Healthcare Organizations has mandated that anesthesiologists perform a preoperative evaluation of patients undergoing anesthesia. The American Society of Anesthesiologists (ASA) has adopted standards for preoperative evaluation of patients that include the requirements that an anesthesiologist shall be responsible for (1) determining the medical status of the patient, (2) developing a plan of anesthesia care, and (3) reviewing with the patient or a responsible adult the proposed care plan (see Appendix).[1] An important aspect of the preoperative visit is to inform the patient and other interested adults about events to expect on the day of surgery and to discuss the risks associated with anesthesia (Table 13-1).

History

The preoperative evaluation should establish the state of health of patients, especially their exercise tolerance, their present illness, and the interactions that they have had with their physicians (Table 13-2). An assessment of mental status should also be made. Documentation of the medications that a patient is taking is needed, as well as any use of drugs, including alcohol and tobacco (Table 13-3). It is important to document previous anesthetics and whether there were any complications, which surgeries have been performed, and any previous medical illnesses. An assessment of all drug allergies and family history of malignant hyperthermia needs to be documented. Documentation of significant patient wishes, including prohibition of the administration of blood or suspension of do-not-resuscitate orders, needs to be made.

Goals of the preoperative evaluation are to (1) inform the patient of the risk so that an informed consent can be made, (2) educate the patient regarding the anesthesia and events to take place in the perioperative period, (3)

Table 13-1 Perioperative Events That May Be Discussed with the Patient Preoperatively

Risks associated with anesthesia (depends on the patient's desire to know)

Nausea and vomiting

Myalgia

Dental injury

Peripheral neuropathy

Cardiac dysrhythmias

Myocardial infarction

Atelectasis

Aspiration

Stroke

Allergic drug reactions

Death (very unlikely)

Preoperative insomnia and medication available for its treatment

Time, route of administration, and expected effects from the preoperative medication

Time of anticipated transport to the operating room

Anticipated duration of surgery

Awakening after surgery in the postanesthesia care unit

Probable presence of catheters on awakening (tracheal, gastric, bladder, venous, arterial)

Time of expected discharge to the hospital room or to home with an escort after surgery

Magnitude of postoperative discomfort and methods available for its treatment

Table 13-2 Specific Areas That May Be Investigated in the Preoperative History

Previous Adverse Responses Related to Anesthesia

Allergic reactions

Sleep apnea

Prolonged skeletal muscle paralysis

Delayed awakening

Nausea and vomiting

Hoarseness

Myalgia

Hemorrhage

Jaundice

Post–dural puncture headache

Adverse response in relatives

Central Nervous System

Cerebrovascular insufficiency

Seizures

Cardiovascular System

Exercise tolerance

Angina pectoris

Previous myocardial infarction

Hypertension

Rheumatic fever

Claudication

Tachydysrhythmias

Lungs

Exercise tolerance

Dyspnea and orthopnea

Cough and sputum production

Bronchial asthma

Cigarette consumption

Pneumonia

Recent upper respiratory tract infection

Liver

Alcohol consumption

Hepatitis

answer questions and reassure the patient and family, (4) notify the patient about the prohibition of ingesting food, and (5) instruct the patient about which medications to take on the day of surgery or which medications to stop taking. A final goal is to use the operative experience to motivate the patient to more optimal health and improved health outcomes. Examples of this last goal are to encourage patients to stop smoking before and after their procedures and to administer β-adrenergic receptor blocking agents to patients at risk for cardiac complications (Fig. 13-1).[2-5]

Questions that should be addressed include the following:

Table 13-2 Specific Areas That May Be Investigated in the Preoperative History—cont'd

Kidneys

Dialysis dependency

Chronic renal insufficiency

Skeletal and Muscular Systems

Arthritis

Osteoporosis

Weakness

Endocrine System

Diabetes mellitus

Thyroid gland dysfunction

Adrenal gland dysfunction

Coagulation—History of DVT, PE

Bleeding tendency

Easy bruising

Hereditary coagulopathies

Reproductive System

Menstrual history

Pregnancy

Dentition

Dentures

Caps

Table 13-3 Current Drug Use and Potential Interactions with Drugs Administered in the Perioperative Period

Drug	Adverse Effects
Alcohol abuse	Tolerance to anesthetic drugs
β-Antagonists	Bradycardia Bronchospasm Impaired sympathetic nervous system responses Myocardial depression
Antibiotics	Prolongation of the effects of neuromuscular blocking drugs
Antihypertensives	Impaired sympathetic nervous system responses
Aspirin	Bleeding tendency
Benzodiazepines	Tolerance to anesthetic drugs
Calcium channel blockers	Hypotension
Digitalis	Cardiac dysrhythmias or conduction disturbances
Diuretics	Hypokalemia Hypovolemia
Monoamine oxidase inhibitors	Exaggerated responses to sympathomimetic drugs if previous treatment was acute
Tricyclic antidepressants	Exaggerated responses to sympathomimetic drugs if previous treatment was acute

III

Is the patient in optimal health?

Can or should the patient's physical or mental condition be improved before surgery?

Does the patient have any health problems or use any medication that could unexpectedly influence perioperative events?

Preoperative Physical Examination

The preoperative physical examination needs to include an evaluation of the airway; the cardiovascular status of the patient, including an assessment of body mass index, systemic blood pressure, and hemoglobin saturation with oxygen; and an examination of the heart and lungs (Table 13-4). Routine preoperative laboratory tests need not be ordered if a patient is in optimal medical condition for daily living and the procedure is minimally invasive (Table 13-5).[6] Preoperative labora-

tory testing frequently fails to uncover pathologic conditions and is inefficient in screening for abnormalities in asymptomatic patients. Therefore, routine laboratory tests in patients at low risk are rarely beneficial and should be ordered only when a patient is symptomatic or has a specific disease (Tables 13-6 and 13-7). Optimal preoperative assessment requires a complete history and physical examination to determine whether the patient has an abnormality that warrants laboratory tests.

Information obtained during the preoperative evaluation needs to be available to the surgeon and to the anesthesiologist who ultimately delivers the anesthetic. This is often accomplished through electronic information systems. Perioperative interventions, including the administration of β-blockers, will need to be continued, and this information needs to be available in the patient's record.

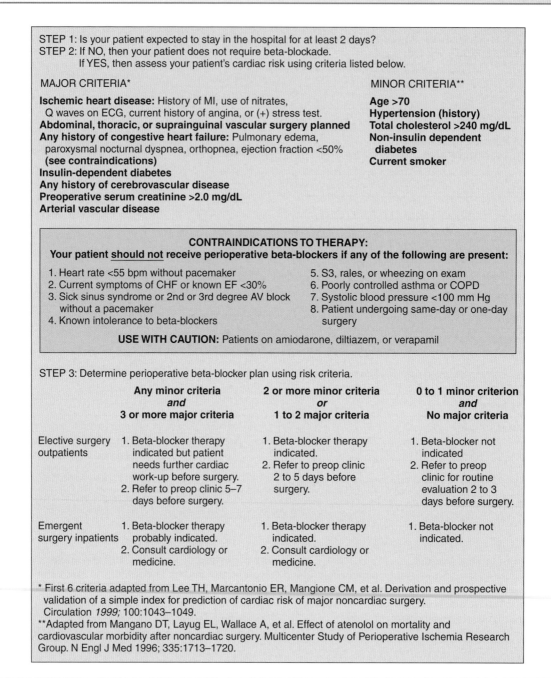

STEP 1: Is your patient expected to stay in the hospital for at least 2 days?
STEP 2: If NO, then your patient does not require beta-blockade.
          If YES, then assess your patient's cardiac risk using criteria listed below.

MAJOR CRITERIA*

Ischemic heart disease: History of MI, use of nitrates,
   Q waves on ECG, current history of angina, or (+) stress test.
Abdominal, thoracic, or suprainguinal vascular surgery planned
Any history of congestive heart failure: Pulmonary edema,
   paroxysmal nocturnal dyspnea, orthopnea, ejection fraction <50%
   (see contraindications)
Insulin-dependent diabetes
Any history of cerebrovascular disease
Preoperative serum creatinine >2.0 mg/dL
Arterial vascular disease

MINOR CRITERIA**

Age >70
Hypertension (history)
Total cholesterol >240 mg/dL
**Non-insulin dependent
   diabetes**
Current smoker

CONTRAINDICATIONS TO THERAPY:
Your patient should not receive perioperative beta-blockers if any of the following are present:

1. Heart rate <55 bpm without pacemaker
2. Current symptoms of CHF or known EF <30%
3. Sick sinus syndrome or 2nd or 3rd degree AV block
   without a pacemaker
4. Known intolerance to beta-blockers

5. S3, rales, or wheezing on exam
6. Poorly controlled asthma or COPD
7. Systolic blood pressure <100 mm Hg
8. Patient undergoing same-day or one-day
   surgery

USE WITH CAUTION: Patients on amiodarone, diltiazem, or verapamil

---

STEP 3: Determine perioperative beta-blocker plan using risk criteria.

| | **Any minor criteria
and
3 or more major criteria** | **2 or more minor criteria
or
1 to 2 major criteria** | **0 to 1 minor criterion
and
No major criteria** |
|---|---|---|---|
| Elective surgery outpatients | 1. Beta-blocker therapy indicated but patient needs further cardiac work-up before surgery.
2. Refer to preop clinic 5–7 days before surgery. | 1. Beta-blocker therapy indicated.
2. Refer to preop clinic 2 to 5 days before surgery. | 1. Beta-blocker not indicated
2. Refer to preop clinic for routine evaluation 2 to 3 days before surgery. |
| Emergent surgery inpatients | 1. Beta-blocker therapy probably indicated.
2. Consult cardiology or medicine. | 1. Beta-blocker therapy indicated.
2. Consult cardiology or medicine. | 1. Beta-blocker not indicated. |

* First 6 criteria adapted from Lee TH, Marcantonio ER, Mangione CM, et al. Derivation and prospective
  validation of a simple index for prediction of cardiac risk of major noncardiac surgery.
  Circulation *1999;* 100:1043–1049.
**Adapted from Mangano DT, Layug EL, Wallace A, et al. Effect of atenolol on mortality and
cardiovascular morbidity after noncardiac surgery. Multicenter Study of Perioperative Ischemia Research
Group. N Engl J Med 1996; 335:1713–1720.

Figure 13-1 Perioperative β-blocker protocol. AV, atrioventricular; CHF, congestive heart failure; COPD, chronic obstructive pulmonary disease; ECG, electrocardiogram; EF, ejection fraction; MI, myocardial infarction. (UCSF β-Blocker form.)

Overall Assessment of Perioperative Risk

Perioperative risk encompasses the risks that the patient brings to the procedure because of health problems; the risk associated with the planned surgery, including its impact on the function of organs; and the interaction of the anesthesia, patient, and surgery (Table 13-8). The greater the number of patients with whom anesthesiologists and surgeons have interacted for specific procedures, the less the perioperative risk for the patient. This may be due to not only the increased skill of the anesthesiologists and surgeons but also the knowledge and availability of the staff involved in the perioperative care of the patients.

Table 13-4 Specific Areas That May Be Investigated in the Preoperative Physical Examination

Central Nervous System

Level of consciousness

Evidence of peripheral sensory or skeletal muscle dysfunction

Cardiovascular System

Auscultation of the heart (heart rate, rhythm, murmur)

Systemic blood pressure (supine and standing)

Peripheral pulses (arterial cannulation site)

Veins (access sites)

Peripheral edema

Lungs

Auscultation of the lungs (rales, wheezes)

Pattern of breathing

Anatomy of the thorax (emphysema)

Upper Airway

Cervical spine mobility

Temporomandibular mobility

Prominent central incisors

Diseased or artificial teeth

Ability to visualize the uvula

Thyromental distance

Coagulation

Bruising

Petechiae

An investigation from Britain in 1987 documented a 30-day crude mortality rate after surgery and anesthesia of about 0.8%.[7] Anesthesia was considered to be the sole cause of death in only 1 in 185,000 cases and a major contributor to death in 7 of 10,000 cases. More recently, between 1992 and 1994, perioperative deaths within 48 hours of an operation occurred in 347 of 184,472 patients, or about 0.2%.[7] Mortality was attributed to anesthesia-related events in about 1 in 13,322 procedures (a rate of 0.01%) in an urban hospital setting and more often in patients with underlying illnesses.[7] Thus, anesthesia-related mortality is very low. Investigations have suggested that equipment failure is a very minor cause of anesthesia mishaps and that human error is the major cause of anesthesia-related problems.[7]

Emergency surgery is associated with increased risk, as is vascular surgery.[8] Procedures involving large blood loss or fluid shifts are considered high-risk surgeries and often have an incidence of cardiac death and nonfatal myocardial infarction of greater than 5%. In contrast, ophthalmologic surgery and surgeries that are superficial or involve endoscopy are extremely safe and have an incidence of cardiac death and nonfatal myocardial infarction of less than 1%. Intermediate-risk surgeries include carotid surgery, head and neck surgery, intraperitoneal and intrathoracic surgery, orthopedic surgery, and prostate surgery.[8]

American Society of Anesthesiologists Classification

The ASA Physical Status classification allows an overall description of the status of the patient and correlates well with patient outcomes (Table 13-9).[8]

CLINICAL EVALUATION OF PATIENTS FOR CARDIAC RISK

The preoperative history should characterize the duration, severity, and stability of any cardiopulmonary symptoms. The patient's baseline functional status can be informative, and one should decipher whether functional limitations are cardiac in etiology or due to other conditions, such as claudication, pulmonary disease, arthritis, or deconditioning.[9,10] Cardiac risk factors must be identified, including age, male gender, cigarette smoking, diabetes mellitus, hypercholesterolemia, systemic hypertension, obesity, sedentary lifestyle, and family history of coronary artery disease.[4] A baseline electrocardiogram should be reviewed for evidence of previous myocardial infarction, ischemic changes, conduction abnormalities, or left ventricular hypertrophy. Additional testing should be considered if indicated by the history or physical examination, but only if the test results will alter the patient's management. The surgery itself is also important to consider because prolonged procedures (>5 hours), urgent surgeries, and major thoracic, abdominal, and vascular surgeries are considered higher risk.[4]

Clinical Predictors of Cardiac Risk

Several investigations have identified major risk factors for perioperative cardiac complications.[3] Perioperative cardiac events have been associated with six independent variables (Table 13-10). The presence of zero, one, two, or more than three variables is associated with cardiac complication rates of 0.4%, 0.9%, 7%, and 11%, respectively.[3] Based on the Revised Cardiac Index, patients with more than two variables are at moderate (7%) to high risk (11%) for perioperative cardiac events.[3]

III

Table 13-5 Preoperative Test Recommendations in Asymptomatic Patients Scheduled for Elective Operations

| Age (yr) | General Anesthesia | | Sedation for MAC and Regional Technique (Men and Women) | Nerve Block (Local) (Men and Women) |
	Men	Women		
<40	None	Hb or Hct?* Pregnancy test?	None	None
40-50	ECG	Hb or Hct?* Pregnancy test?	None	None
50-64	Hb or Hct?* ECG	Hb or Hct?* ECG	Hb or Hct*	None
65-74	Hb or Hct ECG Creatinine/BUN* Glucose*	Hb or Hct* ECG Creatinine/BUN* Glucose*	Hb or Hct* ECG†	Hb or Hct*
>74	Hb and Hct* ECG Creatinine/BUN* Glucose* Chest x-ray?	Hb and Hct* ECG Creatinine/BUN* Glucose* Chest x-ray?	Hb and Hct* ECG† Creatinine/BUN* Glucose*	Hb and Hct* ECG†

*Should be based on history or physical examination.
†Within 12 months.
BUN, blood urea nitrogen; ECG, electrocardiogram; Hb, hemoglobin; Hct, hematocrit; MAC, monitored anesthesia care.
Modified from Roizen MF, Cohn S. Preoperative evaluation for elective surgery: What laboratory tests are needed? *In* Stoelting RK, Barash PG, Gallagher TJ (eds): Advances in Anesthesia, vol 10. Chicago: Mosby–Year Book, 1993, pp 25-43.

Pharmacologic Preoperative Prophylaxis

β-BLOCKERS
Evidence supports the perioperative administration of β-blockers to decrease cardiac events and mortality.[2,11,12] A randomized controlled trial of 200 patients with coronary artery disease or cardiac risk factors who were under-going noncardiac surgery documented a significant decrease in cardiovascular mortality and higher event-free survival rates in patients treated perioperatively with atenolol versus placebo.[2] Although the principal effect was attributed to the decrease in cardiovascular

Table 13-6 Unexpected Abnormalities Detected on a Preoperative Electrocardiogram

Atrial fibrillation
Atrioventricular heart block
ST changes suggestive of myocardial ischemia
Atrial premature contractions
Ventricular premature contractions
Left or right ventricular hypertrophy
Prolonged QT interval
Tall peaked T waves
Evidence of pre-excitation syndrome
Evidence of a previous myocardial infarction

Table 13-7 Unexpected Abnormalities Detected on a Preoperative Chest Radiograph

Tracheal deviation
Mediastinal masses
Pulmonary masses
Pulmonary blebs
Aortic aneurysm
Pulmonary edema
Pneumonia
Atelectasis
Fractures of the ribs or vertebrae
Cardiomegaly
Dextrocardia

Table 13-8 Considerations That Influence the Choice of Anesthetic Technique

Coexisting diseases that may or may not be related to the reason for surgery
Site of the surgery
Body position of the patient during elective or emergency surgery
Likelihood of increased amounts of gastric contents
Age of the patient
Preference of the patient

Table 13-10 Independent Risk Factors Associated with Perioperative Cardiac Events

High-risk surgery
History of ischemic heart disease
Congestive heart failure
Cerebrovascular disease
Diabetes mellitus requiring insulin therapy
Preoperative serum creatinine >2.0 mg/dL

mortality observed in the first 6 to 8 months, the survival benefit persisted over the 2-year follow-up period. To determine the effects of perioperative β-blockade on vascular surgery patients, a randomized multicenter trial examined the effect of bisoprolol on cardiac-related mortality and nonfatal myocardial infarction within 30 days of major vascular surgery in high-risk patients.[13] High risk was defined as the presence of at least one cardiac risk factor (age >70 years, angina, previous myocardial infarction by history or Q waves on the electrocardiogram, compensated congestive heart failure or a history of congestive heart failure, current treatment of ventricular dysrhythmias, current treatment of diabetes mellitus, limited exercise capacity, and dobutamine echocardiography consistent with inducible ischemia). Significantly decreased rates of cardiac-related mortality and nonfatal myocardial infarction in the bisoprolol group resulted in premature termination of the trial by the study's safety committee.[13]

The dose of β-blocker should be titrated to a target resting heart rate of less than 65 beats/min.[12,14] β-Blockers should be avoided in patients with asthma and used

III

Table 13-9 Physical Status Classification of the American Society of Anesthesiologists

Physical Status Classification	Description
PS-1	A normal healthy patient
PS-2	A patient with mild systemic disease that results in no functional limitations Examples: Hypertension, diabetes mellitus, chronic bronchitis, morbid obesity, extremes of age
PS-3	A patient with severe systemic disease that results in functional limitations Examples: Poorly controlled hypertension, diabetes mellitus with vascular complications, angina pectoris, previous myocardial infarction, pulmonary disease that limits activity
PS-4	A patient with severe systemic disease that is a constant threat to life Examples: Congestive heart failure, unstable angina pectoris, advanced pulmonary, renal, or hepatic dysfunction
PS-5	A moribund patient who is not expected to survive without the operation Examples: Ruptured abdominal aneurysm, pulmonary embolus, head injury with increased intracranial pressure
PS-6	A declared brain-dead patient whose organs are being removed for donor purposes
Emergency operation (E)	Any patient in whom an emergency operation is required Example: An otherwise healthy 39-year-old woman who requires dilatation and curettage for moderate but persistent vaginal bleeding (PS-1E)

From information in American Society of Anesthesiologists. New classification of physical status. Anesthesiology 1963;24:111.

judiciously in those with chronic obstructive pulmonary disease (COPD) when spirometry demonstrates a significant bronchodilator response.

α₂-AGONISTS

If β-blockers are contraindicated in patients at risk for perioperative cardiac complications, α_2-agonists (clonidine, dexmedetomidine, or mivazerol) should be considered as an alternative for cardioprotection.[15] α_2-Agonists have also been shown to reduce perioperative cardiac events (myocardial ischemia) after cardiac and noncardiac surgery (vascular surgery). α_2-Agonists may provide these benefits by dilation of poststenotic coronary arteries and mitigation of perioperative hemodynamic disturbances.[15,16] Additionally, α_2-agonists provide pain relief, thus decreasing the need for analgesics. It is not known whether combination therapy with an α_2-agonist and β-blocker produces an additive or synergistic effect.

Coronary Revascularization

Data fail to show any benefit from coronary artery revascularization by coronary artery bypass grafting (CABG) or percutaneous coronary artery intervention for the sole purpose of reducing perioperative cardiac events.[17] Therefore, coronary artery revascularization should be reserved for patients who have indications for the procedure (patients with advanced coronary artery disease in whom CABG may provide a survival benefit or cardiac symptoms that are unstable or refractory to medical therapy) independent of the planned surgery. For patients who have undergone percutaneous coronary artery stenting preoperatively for independent indications, elective noncardiac surgery should be deferred for a minimum of 6 weeks to allow endothelialization of the stents and completion of antiplatelet therapy.[18]

Guidelines

Practice guidelines for perioperative cardiovascular risk assessment have been published. The American College of Cardiology/American Heart Association Task Force published guidelines in which it was emphasized that preoperative intervention is seldom necessary unless clinically indicated independent of surgery and should be limited to patients who are likely to benefit from such testing, intervention, or therapy.[5] Another algorithm is based on clinical predictors (major, intermediate, and minor), including previous cardiovascular evaluation and treatment, functional capacity (defined in metabolic equivalents), risks specific for the intended surgery, and if indicated, results of noninvasive cardiac testing. Alternatively, a proposed strategy aimed at reducing the risk for cardiac events with pharmacologic therapy, rather than simply categorizing a patient as low, intermediate, or high risk, has been advocated.[19]

PREOPERATIVE EVALUATION OF PATIENTS WITH PULMONARY DISEASE

It is estimated that 5% to 10% of all surgical patients and 9% to 40% of those undergoing abdominal surgery will experience postoperative pulmonary complications.[20] Postoperative pulmonary complications in nonthoracic surgery are associated with significant morbidity and have been shown to increase the length of hospitalization. The first step in reducing postoperative pulmonary complications is to identify patients at increased risk.

Risk Factors for Postoperative Pulmonary Complications

Although the clinical significance varies, atelectasis, postoperative pneumonia, acute respiratory distress syndrome, and postoperative respiratory failure are often grouped together in studies of risk factors for postoperative pulmonary complications. Mild to moderate obesity as a risk factor for postoperative pulmonary complications remains controversial.[21] However, obese patients often have a higher incidence of comorbid conditions, which may contribute to the risk for pulmonary complications.[22] Pulmonary complications after nonthoracic surgery are more frequent than cardiac complications and are associated with greater increases in hospital length of stay.[23]

Although most studies have reported a lower risk for pulmonary complications with epidural or spinal anesthesia than with general anesthesia, the results are mixed. Nonetheless, it may be reasonable to consider spinal or epidural anesthesia, or even regional block if possible, for surgery in patients at high risk for pulmonary complications.

POSTOPERATIVE RESPIRATORY FAILURE

Postoperative respiratory failure is commonly defined as an inability to extubate the patient's trachea 48 hours after surgery. Risk factors for postoperative respiratory failure may be divided into those that are patient specific and those that are surgery specific (Table 13-11). The 30-day death rate in patients with postoperative respiratory failure is much higher than that in patients not experiencing this complication (27% versus 1%).[23,24] Renal and fluid status and preoperative respiratory status are the principal patient-specific risk factors for postoperative respiratory failure (Table 13-12).[23,24]

Respiratory Risk Index Score

A respiratory risk index score can be used to predict the probability of postoperative respiratory failure (Tables 13-12, 13-13 and 13-14).[23,24] Although this risk index score permits general estimates of risk in patients undergoing a variety of surgical procedures, it does not include data from the physical examination or pulmonary function tests, which are commonly used to assist in risk prediction before surgery. The ability of the risk score index to

Table 13-11 Risk Factors for Postoperative Respiratory Failure

Patient Specific

General health status

  Age

  Functional status

  Cancer

  Alcohol use

Pulmonary status

  Smoking

  Chronic obstructive pulmonary disease

  Increased body mass index

Neurologic status

  Impaired sensorium

Cardiac status

  Myocardial infarction

Renal and fluid status

  Renal failure

  Blood transfusions

Surgery Specific

Location of the incision relative to the diaphragm

Emergency operation

Type of anesthesia (regional, general)

Table 13-12 Preoperative Predictors of Postoperative Respiratory Failure

Variable	Odds Ratio (95% Confidence Interval)
Type of surgery	
Abdominal aortic aneurysm	14.3 (12.0-16.9)
Thoracic	8.14 (7.17-9.25)
Neurosurgery, upper abdominal, or peripheral vascular	4.21 (3.80-4.67)
Neck	3.10 (2.40-4.01)
Other surgery*	1.00 (reference)
Emergency surgery	3.12 (2.83-3.43)
Albumin <30 g/L	2.53 (2.28-2.80)
Blood urea nitrogen >30 mg/dL	2.29 (2.04-2.56)
Partially or fully dependent status	1.92 (1.74-2.11)
History of chronic obstructive pulmonary disease	1.81 (1.66-1.98)
Age (yr)	
≥70	1.91 (1.71-2.13)
60-69	1.51 (1.36-1.69)
<60	1.00 (reference)

*Other surgeries include ophthalmologic, ear, nose, mouth, lower abdominal, extremity, dermatologic, spine, and back surgery.
Adapted from Arozullah AM, Daley J, Henderson WG, Khuri SF. National Veterans Administration Surgical Quality Improvement Program. Ann Surg 2000;232:242-253.

predict postoperative respiratory failure in predominantly healthy patients undergoing elective nonthoracic surgery is uncertain because the data used to develop this index were from patients who were all males with a high burden of comorbid conditions and almost a third of the surgeries were intrathoracic or performed on an emergency basis.[23,24]

SITE OF SURGERY

The risk for postoperative respiratory complications is most strongly related to the surgical site, and the risk increases as the incision approaches the diaphragm. Upper abdominal and thoracic surgery carries the greatest risk for postoperative pulmonary complications, ranging from 10% to 40%.[25] The risk is much lower for laparoscopic cholecystectomy (0.3% to 0.4%) than for open cholecystectomy (13% to 33%).[26]

CHRONIC OBSTRUCTIVE PULMONARY DISEASE

Patients with COPD have an increased risk for postoperative pulmonary complications.[27] Such patients should

be treated aggressively before surgery if they do not have optimal reduction of symptoms and airflow obstruction on physical examination or if they do not have optimal exercise capacity. Although there are few data on the preoperative benefit of individual drugs, a combination of bronchodilators, physical therapy, antibiotics, smoking cessation, and corticosteroids may reduce the risk for postoperative pulmonary complications in this patient population. The incidence of perioperative bronchospasm is increased in patients with asthma.[28] Before surgery, patients should be free of wheezing.

Chest Radiograph

Routine preoperative chest radiographs are still widely used, although the preponderance of the evidence does not support their broad utilization. For example, a retrospective study conducted to evaluate a protocol for selec-

III

Table 13-13 Respiratory Failure Risk Index

Preoperative Predictor	Point Value
Type of surgery	
Abdominal aortic aneurysm	27
Thoracic	21
Neurosurgery, upper abdominal, or peripheral vascular	14
Neck	11
Emergency surgery	11
Albumin <30 g/L	9
Blood urea nitrogen >30 mg/dL	8
Partially or fully dependent status	7
History of chronic obstructive pulmonary disease	6
Age (yr)	
≥70	6
60-69	4

Adapted from Arozullah AM, Daley J, Henderson WG, Khuri SF. National Veterans Administration Surgical Quality Improvement Program. Ann Surg 2000;232:242-253.

operative chest radiographs, 15% of the radiographs were considered useful by the anesthesiologist and only 5% had an impact on the surgical plan or anesthetic management.[29] The ASA has stated that chest radiographs are not indicated on the basis of age or preexisting respiratory condition unless there is a surgical indication or a clear clinical change or need to establish the presence or absence of a defined pulmonary condition.[1]

Pulmonary Function Testing

Although there is consensus that all candidates for lung resection should undergo preoperative pulmonary function testing, such testing should be performed selectively in patients undergoing other surgical procedures.[1,20,30] Furthermore, clinical findings are generally more predictive of pulmonary complications than are the results obtained from pulmonary function studies. Even patients at high risk as defined by pulmonary function studies can undergo surgery with an acceptable risk for pulmonary complications.[31] Pulmonary function studies may be helpful in patients with COPD or asthma if it remains uncertain whether the degree of airflow obstruction has been optimally reduced. However, the results of preoperative pulmonary function testing alone should not be used to cancel nonthoracic surgery.

Arterial Blood Gases

A $Paco_2$ higher than 45 mm Hg has been reported to be a strong risk factor for pulmonary complications.[32] However, in another report, an elevated $Paco_2$ was not associated with increased mortality or morbidity in surgical patients undergoing lung resection.[31] Therefore, arterial blood gas analysis alone should not be used to exclude patients from surgery.

tive ordering of preoperative chest radiographs according to the patient's clinical status, medical history, and scheduled surgery showed that abandonment of routine ordering of preoperative chest radiographs did not produce adverse effects on patient care.[29] Of patients who received pre-

Table 13-14 Respiratory Failure Risk Index Scores for Phase I and Phase II Patients*

Class	Point Total	N (%)[†]	Predicted Probability of PRF	% RF (Phase I)	% RF (Phase II)
1	≤10	39,567 (48%)	0.5%	0.5%	0.5%
2	11-19	18,809 (23%)	2.2%	2.1%	1.8%
3	20-27	13,865 (17%)	5.0%	5.3%	4.2%
4	28-40	7,976 (10%)	11.6%	11.9%	10.1%
5	>40	1,502 (2%)	30.5%	30.9%	26.6%

*Phase I included patients enrolled between October 1, 1991, and December 31, 1993, at 44 Veterans Affairs Medical Centers (VAMC). Phase II included patients enrolled between January 1, 1994, through August 31, 1995, at all 132 VAMCs that perform surgery.
†Number of phase I subjects in each risk class.
PRF, postoperative respiratory failure; RF, respiratory failure.
Adapted from Arozullah AM, Daley J, Henderson WG, Khuri SF. National Veterans Administration Surgical Quality Improvement Program. Ann Surg 2000;232:242-253.

Preventive Strategies

Despite some variability in the risk factors for postoperative pulmonary complications, there are several risk reduction strategies intended to provide optimal lung mechanics that can be used throughout the perioperative period, including lung expansion maneuvers and pain control. Deep-breathing exercises, which are a component of chest physical therapy, and incentive spirometry have been studied most extensively,[33] Preoperative education in lung expansion maneuvers appears to reduce postoperative pulmonary complications to a greater degree than does instruction that begins after surgery.[33] Intermittent positive-pressure breathing and continuous positive airway pressure, though effective, are not recommended routinely because of their relatively high cost and the risk for treatment-associated complications.

Smoking Cessation

The risk for postoperative pulmonary complications among smokers as opposed to nonsmokers is greatly increased.[34] The length of preoperative smoking cessation necessary to decrease this risk is not clear.[35] It is generally accepted that the increased incidence of postoperative pulmonary complications in smokers can be reduced significantly by persuading the patient to stop smoking before surgery, although there is no consensus on the minimal or optimal duration of preoperative abstinence. Carbon monoxide and nicotine elimination occurs after 12 to 24 hours. Indeed, the major benefit from discontinuing smoking in the immediate preoperative period appears to be a decrease in carboxyhemoglobin content and better oxygen availability to tissues.[34] There is also evidence that the sensitive upper airway reflexes of smokers are reduced by abstinence. A few days may greatly improve ciliary beating, and 1 to 2 weeks provides a significant reduction in sputum volume.[34]

Prevention of Venous Thromboembolism

In patients undergoing general surgery without thromboprophylaxis, rates of deep vein thrombosis and fatal pulmonary embolism range from 15% to 30% and from 0.2% to 0.9%, respectively (Tables 13-15 and 13-16).[22,36]

III

Table 13-15 Risk Factors for Venous Thromboembolism

Risk Factors (1 Point Each)	Risk Factors (2 Points Each)	Risk Factors (3 Points Each)
Age 41-60 yr	Age 61-70 yr	Age >70 yr
Bed confinement/immobilization >12 hours	Major surgery	Acquired thrombophilia
Central line	Malignancy	Inherited thrombophilia*
Estrogen therapy	Multiple trauma	Previous history of PE
Family history of DVT or PE	Previous history of idiopathic DVT	
General anesthesia time >2 hours	Spinal cord injury with paralysis	
Hyperviscosity syndromes		
Inflammatory bowel disease		
Laparoscopic surgery		
Leg swelling, ulcers, stasis, varicose veins		
MI/CHF		
Obesity (>20% over IBW or BMI >30)		
Pregnancy or <1 month postpartum		
Previous history of operative DVT		
Stroke with paralysis		
Total risk factor score: Low = 0, Moderate = 1-2, High = 3-4, Very high = >4.		

*Thrombophilia includes factor V Leiden, prothrombin variant mutations, anticardiolipin antibody syndrome, antithrombin, protein C or protein S deficiency, hyperhomocysteinemia, and myeloproliferative disorders.
BMI, body mass index; CHF, congestive heart failure; DVT, deep vein thrombosis; IBW, ideal body weight; MI, myocardial infarction; PE, pulmonary embolism.
Adapted from the UCSF Medical Center Adult Venous Thromboembolism Risk Assessment and Prophylaxis Order Form.

Table 13-16 Thromboembolic Risk Stratification for Surgery Patients

Low risk	Uncomplicated surgery in patients <40 years of age with minimal immobility postoperatively and no risk factors
Moderate risk	Any surgery in patients aged 40-60 years Major surgery in patients >40 years of age and no other risk factors Minor surgery in patients with 1 or more risk factors
High risk	Surgery in patients aged >60 years Major surgery in patients aged 40-60 years with one or more risk factors
Very high risk	Major surgery in patients >40 years of age with previous venous thromboembolism, cancer, or known hypercoagulable state, major orthopedic surgery, elective neurosurgery, multiple trauma, or acute spinal cord injury

Adapted from Gutt CN, Oniu T, Wolkener F, et al. Prophylaxis and treatment of deep vein thrombosis in general surgery. Am J Surg 2005;189:14-22.

Prevention strategies include the use of low-dose unfractionated heparin, low-molecular-weight heparin, and intermittent pneumatic compression stockings.[36,37] The use of graded compression elastic stockings alone is associated with a 44% reduction in risk.[37] However, low-dose unfractionated heparin and low-molecular-weight heparin are the most effective therapies in reducing the incidence of deep vein thrombosis, with a 68% to 76% reduction in risk. The two heparin preparations appear to be equally effective in preventing deep vein thrombosis in general surgery patients.[36] Nonetheless, there are discrepant findings in regard to the bleeding complications associated with each therapy. Some studies have reported significantly fewer wound hematomas and bleeding complications with low-molecular-weight heparin, whereas other trials have shown that low-molecular-weight heparin causes more bleeding than low-dose unfractionated heparin does.[36]

Routine use of thromboprophylaxis is recommended in surgical patients who are older than 40 years or undergoing major surgical procedures. The type and duration of surgery clearly influence the risk for deep vein thrombosis. Most individuals undergoing outpatient surgery appear to have a low frequency of deep vein thrombosis.

When compared with no thromboprophylaxis, both subcutaneous low-dose unfractionated heparin and low-molecular-weight heparin have been shown to reduce the risk for pulmonary embolism by at least 60%. In moderate-risk patients, fixed low-dose unfractionated heparin (5000 units every 12 hours) or low-molecular-weight heparin (3400 anti–factor Xa units or equivalent) once daily is sufficient.[22] Compression elastic stockings are effective when used alone in moderate-risk patients in whom anticoagulants are contraindicated.[22]

PREOPERATIVE MEDICATION

Management of anesthesia begins with preoperative psychological preparation of the patient and administration of a drug or drugs selected to elicit specific pharmacologic responses. This initial psychological and pharmacologic component of anesthetic management is referred to as preoperative medication.[38] Ideally, all patients should enter the preoperative period free of anxiety, sedated but easily arousable, and fully cooperative.

Psychological Preparation

Psychological preparation is provided by the anesthesiologist's preoperative visit and interview with the patient and family members. The incidence of anxiety is lower in patients visited by the anesthesiologist preoperatively than in those receiving only pharmacologic premedication and no visit. Nevertheless, a shortage of time and the fact that some patients' problems do not lend themselves to reassurance may limit the anxiolytic value of the preoperative interview.

Pharmacologic Premedication

Pharmacologic premedication is typically administered orally or intramuscularly 1 to 2 hours before the anticipated induction of anesthesia.[38] For outpatient surgery, premedication may be administered intravenously in the immediate preoperative period. The goals of pharmacologic premedication are multiple and must be individualized to meet each patient's unique requirements. Furthermore, multiple different drugs or combinations of drugs may be selected to achieve the same goals (Tables 13-17 and 13-18).

The appropriate drug or drugs and doses to be used for pharmacologic premedication can be selected only after the psychological and physiologic condition of the patient has been evaluated (Tables 13-19 and 13-20). The choice of drug and dose must take into account multiple factors. Certain types of patients should not receive depressant pharmacologic drugs in an attempt to decrease preoperative anxiety and produce sedation (Table 13-21). A patient who requests to be "asleep" before being transported to the operating room must be assured that this is neither a desired nor a safe goal of pharmacologic premedication.

Table 13-17 Primary Goals of Pharmacologic Premedication

Relief of anxiety (anxiolysis)

Sedation

Analgesia

Amnesia

Antisialagogue effect

Increase in gastric fluid pH

Decrease in gastric fluid volume

Attenuation of sympathetic nervous system reflex responses

Decrease in anesthetic requirements

Prophylaxis against allergic reactions

Table 13-18 Secondary Goals of Pharmacologic Premedication

Decrease in cardiac vagal activity—better achieved with the intravenous injection of an anticholinergic (atropine) just before the time of anticipated need

Facilitation of induction of anesthesia—not necessary in view of the availability of potent intravenous induction drugs

Postoperative analgesia—better achieved with neuraxial opioids or the intravenous injection of an opioid just before the painful surgical stimulus (preemptive analgesia) and/or just before awakening

Prevention of postoperative nausea and vomiting—better achieved with the intravenous injection of an antiemetic just before awakening versus withholding treatment and treating the symptoms if necessary

III

Table 13-19 Drugs and Doses Used for Pharmacologic Premedication before Induction of Anesthesia*

Classification	Drug	Typical Adult Dose (mg)	Route of Administration
Benzodiazepines	Midazolam	1-2.5	IV
	Diazepam	5-10	Orally, IV
	Lorazepam	0.5-2	Orally, IV
Opioids	Morphine	5-15	IV
	Fentanyl	25-100 µg	IV
Antihistamines	Diphenhydramine	12.5-25	Orally, IV
α_2-Agonists	Clonidine	0.1-0.3	Orally, transdermal**
Antiemetics	Droperidol[†]	1.25	IV
	Dolasetron	12.5	IV
	Ondansetron	4	IV
Anticholinergics	Atropine	0.3-0.6	IV
	Glycopyrrolate	0.1	IV
H_2 antagonists	Cimetidine	200-300	Orally
	Ranitidine	150	Orally
	Famotidine	20-40	Orally
Antacids	Nonparticulate	15-30 mL	Orally
Proton pump inhibitors	Omeprazole	20	Orally
	Pantoprazole	40	IV
Gastrointestinal stimulants	Metoclopramide	10	Orally, IV

*Doses are to be titrated to patient's condition and age.
**24 hours for full effect.
[†]Rare incidence of prolonged QT interval on the electrocardiogram.
IM, intramuscular; IV, intravenous.

Table 13-20	Determinants of Drug Choice and Dose
Patient age and weight	
Physical status	
Level of anxiety	
Tolerance of depressant drugs	
Previous adverse experience with drugs used for preoperative medication	
Allergies	
Elective or emergency surgery	
Inpatient or outpatient surgery	

Table 13-21	Is Depressant Pharmacologic Premedication Indicated?	
No	**Yes**	
Newborn (<1 year of age)	Cardiac surgery	
Elderly	Cancer surgery	
Decreased level of consciousness	Coexisting pain	
Intracranial pathology	Regional anesthesia	
Severe pulmonary disease		
Hypovolemia		

Drugs Administered for Pharmacologic Premedication

Several classes of drugs are available to facilitate achievement of the desired goals for pharmacologic premedication in each individual patient (see Table 13-19). These drugs are administered orally if possible as opposed to intramuscularly to improve patient comfort. The small volume of water (up to 150 mL) used to facilitate oral administration of drugs introduces no hazards related to gastric fluid volume. Ultimately, selection of specific drugs is based on a consideration of the desirable goals to be achieved balanced against any potential undesirable effects of these drugs.

BENZODIAZEPINES

Benzodiazepines are the most commonly administered drugs for production of sedation and relief of anxiety before elective surgery. These drugs act on specific brain receptors to produce selective anxiolytic effects at doses that do not produce excessive sedation or cardiopulmonary depression. In addition, these drugs, particularly midazolam and lorazepam, produce suppression of recall of events that occur after their administration (anterograde amnesia).

Disadvantages of benzodiazepines as used for pharmacologic premedication include excessive and prolonged sedation in occasional patients. Flumazenil, a specific benzodiazepine antagonist, is effective in reversing undesirable or unacceptably persistent effects of these drugs. Though not widely appreciated, benzodiazepines administered for preoperative medication may interfere with the release of cortisol in response to stress.[39]

OPIOIDS

Advantages of the use of opioids for pharmacologic premedication include the absence of direct myocardial depression and the production of analgesia in patients who are experiencing pain preoperatively or who will require insertion of invasive monitors before induction of anesthesia. Discomfort associated with the institution of a regional anesthetic is another possible indication for use of an opioid as pharmacologic premedication. Administration of an opioid in the preoperative medication (preemptive analgesia) may decrease the need for parenteral analgesics in the early postoperative period.[40]

Morphine and meperidine are the most commonly used opioids for pharmacologic premedication. Morphine is well absorbed after intramuscular injection, with a peak effect in 45 to 90 minutes. After intravenous administration the peak effect of morphine usually occurs within 20 minutes. Inclusion of morphine in the preoperative medication decreases the likelihood that undesirable increases in heart rate will accompany surgical stimulation during the administration of volatile anesthetics.[41] Pharmacologic premedication with intramuscular administration of opioids may seem reasonable when a nitrous oxide–opioid anesthetic is planned. The opioid, however, may be just as logically given intravenously immediately before the induction of anesthesia. In this regard, fentanyl is often administered intravenously immediately before the induction of anesthesia.

Adverse effects of opioids used for pharmacologic premedication include depression of the medullary ventilatory center, as evidenced by decreased responsiveness to carbon dioxide, and orthostatic hypotension secondary to relaxation of peripheral vascular smooth muscle. Orthostatic hypotension will be further exaggerated if opioids are administered to patients with decreased intravascular fluid volume. Nausea and vomiting most likely reflect opioid-induced stimulation of the chemoreceptor trigger zone in the medulla. The delayed gastric emptying produced by morphine may alter the rate of absorption of orally administered drugs, increase the risk for pulmonary aspiration, and result in nausea and vomiting. Recumbency seems to minimize nausea and vomiting after the administration of opioids, thus suggesting that stimulation of the vestibular apparatus may also be important in production of this undesirable effect. Nevertheless, opioids may be avoided for this reason in patients undergoing outpatient surgery or those having operations (gynecologic and ophthalmologic operations) known to be associated with a high incidence of nausea and vomiting. Opioid-induced smooth muscle constriction may be manifested as choledochoduodenal sphincter spasm, which has caused some anesthesiologists to question the use of opioids in patients with biliary tract disease. The pain associated with opioid-induced biliary tract spasm may be difficult to differentiate from angina pectoris. In this regard, nitroglycerin will relieve any pain associated with both conditions, whereas administration of an opioid antagonist, naloxone, relieves only the pain that is due to opioid-induced biliary tract spasm. An annoying side effect of opioids used as pharmacologic premedication is pruritus, which may be particularly prominent around the nose.

ANTIHISTAMINES

Antihistamines are occasionally used for pharmacologic premedication because of their sedative and antiemetic properties. Promethazine has a new warning from the FDA—associated with apnea in children and deaths.

Prophylaxis against Allergic Reactions

Diphenhydramine (25 to 50 mg orally) has been recommended as pharmacologic premedication to provide prophylaxis against intraoperative allergic reactions in patients who have a history of chronic atopy or are undergoing procedures (radiographic dye studies) known to be associated with allergic reactions. An H_2 antagonist such as cimetidine (300 mg orally) should be administered with diphenhydramine. This combination of an H_1 antagonist (diphenhydramine) and an H_2 antagonist (cimetidine) acts by occupying peripheral receptor sites normally responsive to histamine, thus decreasing manifestations of any subsequent drug-induced release of histamine. Prednisone (50 mg orally or other doses) may also be added to this prophylactic regimen. Even with this prophylactic regimen, however, drug-induced allergic reactions may still occur in highly sensitive patients.

α_2-AGONISTS

Clonidine is a centrally acting α_2-agonist that acts as an antihypertensive drug. Administered as preoperative medication (0.1 mg bid or 0.1 mg patch), this drug produces sedation and attenuation of the autonomic nervous system reflex responses (hypertension, tachycardia, catecholamine release) associated with preoperative anxiety and surgical stimulation. Administration of clonidine (titrate to effect) in the preoperative medication may decrease the incidence of preoperative myocardial ischemia in patients with suspected or documented coronary artery disease.[42] Dose requirements for inhaled and injected anesthetics are also decreased in patients receiving clonidine as preoperative medication. Bradycardia and dry mouth are possible side effects when α_2-agonists are administered as part of the pharmacologic premedication.

ANTIEMETICS

Nausea and vomiting are unpleasant symptoms that rarely harm patients. Nevertheless, prophylactic administration of an antiemetic in the preoperative medication may be recommended with the goal of decreasing the incidence of postoperative nausea and vomiting. In this regard, females undergoing gynecologic operations and patients undergoing ophthalmologic operations are at high risk for this unpleasant symptom.

Drugs used in the preoperative medication for prophylaxis against postoperative nausea and vomiting include serotonin antagonists (ondansetron, tropisetron, granisetron, dolasetron), gastrointestinal prokinetics (metoclopramide), and phenothiazines (perphenazine). The butyrophenone droperidol is a proven effective antiemetic, but its clinical use is tempered by concern this drug may increase the QT interval on the electrocardiogram. Antiemetics are often administered intravenously before the end of surgery. Disadvantages of routine prophylactic administration of antiemetics include (1) increased cost, especially if serotonin antagonists are administered; (2) orthostatic hypotension; and (3) the fact that some patients vomit with or without prophylaxis.

ANTICHOLINERGICS

Routine inclusion of anticholinergics as part of the pharmacologic premedication is not necessary. The most frequent reasons for administering anticholinergics are (1) production of an antisialagogue effect, (2) production of sedative and amnesic effects, and (3) prevention of reflex bradycardia (Table 13-22). Anticholinergics have inherent side effects that need to be considered when selecting these drugs as preoperative medication (Table 13-23). Furthermore, anticholinergics are not predictably effective in increasing gastric fluid pH or decreasing gastric fluid volume.

Antisialagogue Effect

The need for including an anticholinergic in the preoperative medication to produce an antisialagogue effect has been questioned inasmuch as the currently used inhaled and injected anesthetics (ketamine being an exception) do not stimulate excessive upper airway secretions. Nevertheless, a decrease in secretions during general anesthesia, particularly when a tracheal tube is in place, is a desirable effect of an anticholinergic administered preoperatively. An antisialagogue effect is particularly important for intraoral operations, for bronchoscopy, or when topical anesthesia is necessary because excessive secretions may interfere with the surgery or impair production of topical anesthesia by diluting the local anesthetic. Administration of an anticholinergic for an antisialagogue effect is not necessary when regional anesthesia is planned.

Scopolamine is about three times more potent as an antisialagogue than atropine is. For this reason, scopolamine is often selected when both an antisialagogue effect and

III

Table 13-22 Comparative Effects of Anticholinergics Administered Intramuscularly as Pharmacologic Premedication

	Atropine	Scopolamine	Glycopyrrolate
Antisialagogue effect	+	+++	++
Sedative and amnesic effects	+	+++	0
Central nervous system toxicity	+	++	0
Relaxation of lower esophageal sphincter	++	++	++
Mydriasis and cycloplegia	+	+++	0

0, none; +, mild; ++, moderate; +++, marked.

Table 13-23 Undesirable Side Effects of Anticholinergics

Central nervous system toxicity
Tachycardia
Relaxation of the lower esophageal sphincter
Mydriasis and cycloplegia
Increase in body temperature
Drying of airway secretions
Increased physiologic dead space

sedation are desired results of preoperative medication. Glycopyrrolate may be preferentially selected when an antisialagogue effect, in the absence of sedation, is desired. As an antisialagogue, glycopyrrolate is about twice as potent as atropine and has a longer duration of action. To decrease the period of discomfort from a dry mouth and throat, an anticholinergic can be administered intramuscularly just before the patient is transported to the operating room or intravenously just before the induction of anesthesia. Nevertheless, anxiety, fluid deprivation before elective surgery, and other drugs used for pharmacologic premedication may produce a dry mouth and throat, even in the absence of an anticholinergic.

Sedative and Amnesic Effects

Atropine and scopolamine are tertiary amines that can cross lipid barriers, including the blood-brain barrier. The resulting sedative and amnesic effects reflect penetrance of these drugs into the central nervous system. Scopolamine, more than atropine, produces useful sedative effects, particularly in combination with benzodiazepines or opioids as used for pharmacologic premedication. It is estimated that the sedative and amnesic effects of scopolamine are 8 to 10 times greater than those of atropine. Glycopyrrolate, as a quaternary ammonium

compound, cannot easily cross the blood-brain barrier and thus does not produce significant sedative or amnesic effects.

Prevention of Reflex Bradycardia

Use of anticholinergics in the pharmacologic premedication for prevention of reflex bradycardia is a secondary objective because the dose and timing of intramuscular administration are not appropriate for the period when bradycardia is most likely to occur. The logical approach, particularly in children with increased vagal activity, is to administer atropine or glycopyrrolate intravenously shortly before the anticipated need. Bradycardia has been observed after induction of anesthesia with propofol, thus causing some to recommend prior intravenous injection of atropine when vagal stimulation is likely to occur in association with the use of this intravenous anesthetic.

Undesirable Side Effects

Undesirable side effects of anticholinergics are multiple and must be considered in the decision to use these drugs for pharmacologic premedication (see Table 13-23).

Central Nervous System Toxicity

The central nervous system toxicity (central anticholinergic syndrome) produced by anticholinergics is manifested as delirium or prolonged somnolence after anesthesia. This undesirable response is more likely to follow the administration of scopolamine than atropine, but the incidence should be low with the doses used for pharmacologic premedication. Nevertheless, elderly patients may be uniquely susceptible to central nervous system toxicity secondary to atropine or scopolamine. Central nervous system toxicity is unlikely after the administration of glycopyrrolate because this drug cannot easily cross the blood-brain barrier. It must be recognized that the toxicity attributed to the anticholinergic may also represent an uninhibited response to pain as the depressant effects of the anesthetic dissipate.

Central anticholinergic syndrome presumably reflects blockade of muscarinic cholinergic receptors in the central nervous system. Physostigmine (up to 2 mg IV; for life-threatening anticholinergic toxicity administer 1 mg/min) is a specific treatment of the central nervous system toxicity caused by scopolamine or atropine in view of the ability of this tertiary amine anticholinesterase to cross the blood-brain barrier. Neostigmine and pyridostigmine are not effective anticholinesterase antidotes because their quaternary ammonium structure prevents these drugs from easily entering the central nervous system.

Tachycardia

Scopolamine and glycopyrrolate, which have minimal cardioaccelerator effects, may be more logical selections than atropine for pharmacologic premedication when an increased heart rate would be undesirable, as in patients with mitral stenosis and atrial fibrillation. Nevertheless, the most likely cardiac response after the intramuscular administration of atropine, glycopyrrolate, or scopolamine for pharmacologic premedication is slowing of the heart rate, presumably reflecting a weak cholinergic agonist effect of these drugs.

H_2 ANTAGONISTS

H_2 antagonists counter the ability of histamine to induce secretion of gastric fluid with a high concentration of hydrogen ions. Therefore, these drugs offer a pharmacologic approach for increasing gastric fluid pH before the induction of anesthesia. Routine prophylactic use of an H_2 antagonist in the pharmacologic premedication, though advocated by some, is not recommended (Table 13-24).[43] However, inclusion of an H_2 antagonist in the pharmacologic premedication may be a consideration in patients thought to be at increased risk for pulmonary aspiration (parturients, morbid obesity, symptoms of esophageal reflux, anticipated difficult airway management). An objection to the routine inclusion of H_2 antagonists in the preoperative medication is the concept that all therapies should be individualized and tailored to fit specific patients, their diseases, and the particular preoperative circumstances. More important, the incidence of pulmonary aspiration and serious morbidity is sufficiently low in patients undergoing elective surgery that the cost of preventing one serious complication of pulmonary aspiration by the routine use of prophylactic medications such as H_2 antagonists would be very high.[44] Furthermore, these drugs are not 100% effective (an inherent failure rate).[38] H_2 antagonists will not alter the pH of gastric fluid that is present before administration of the drug, nor will they facilitate gastric emptying. Under no circumstances can preoperative medication with H_2 antagonists be substituted for an anesthetic technique that includes placement of a cuffed tracheal tube or maintenance of consciousness to protect the lungs from inhalation of gastric fluid.

Table 13-24 Summary of Pharmacologic Recommendations to Reduce the Risk for Pulmonary Aspiration

Medication Type and Examples	Recommendation
Antiemetics	No routine use
Antacids	No routine use
Anticholinergics	No use
Gastric acid secretion blockers	No routine use
Gastrointestinal stimulants	No routine use
Combinations of the above medications	No routine use

Modified from Warner MA, Caplan RA, Epstein BS, et al. Practice guidelines for preoperative fasting and the use of pharmacologic agents to reduce the risk of pulmonary aspiration: Application to healthy patients undergoing elective procedures. Anesthesiology 1999;90:896-905.

ACID SUPPRESSION

Antacids administered 15 to 30 minutes before induction of anesthesia are nearly 100% effective in increasing gastric fluid pH to greater than 2.5. The efficacy of antacids may be dependent to some extent on patient movement to facilitate complete mixing with gastric fluid. Nonparticulate antacids, such as sodium citrate, effectively increase gastric fluid pH to greater than 2.5 and do not produce significant pulmonary dysfunction should inhalation of fluid containing antacids occur.

In contrast to H_2 antagonists, administration of antacids is effective in increasing the pH of gastric fluid that is present in the stomach at the time of administration (no lag time). This desirable effect, however, is predictably associated with an increased gastric fluid volume that does not occur with H_2 antagonists. Nevertheless, withholding antacids because of concern for increasing gastric fluid volume is not warranted. As with H_2 antagonists, routine inclusion of antacids in the pharmacologic premedication is not recommended (see Table 13-24).[43] Rather, antacids are more appropriately administered to selected patients who are judged by the anesthesiologist to be at increased risk for pulmonary aspiration. Intravenous administration of a proton pump inhibitor will achieve acid suppression within hours. Intravenous formulations in the United States include esomeprazole, lansoprazole, and pantoprazole.

GASTROINTESTINAL PROKINETICS

Gastrointestinal prokinetics (metoclopramide, cisapride) may be considered as part of the pharmacologic premedication in selected patients because of the ability of these drugs to stimulate gastric emptying (see Table 13-24).[43] An antiemetic effect of these drugs is not a consistent observation. Of interest, the antibiotic erythromycin promotes gastric emptying and has been advocated as a pharmacologic method to decrease the risk for aspiration before emergency anesthesia and surgery.[45]

Metoclopramide

Metoclopramide speeds gastric emptying by selectively increasing the motility of the upper gastrointestinal tract and relaxing the pyloric sphincter. The onset of metoclopramide's effect is 30 to 60 minutes after oral administration and 1 to 3 minutes after intravenous injection. The drug may be useful in pharmacologic preoperative medication intended to decrease gastric fluid volume in at-risk patients (diabetics with gastroparesis, parturients, patients who have recently ingested solids and require emergency surgery for disease unrelated to the gastrointestinal tract, anticipated difficult airway management). Nonetheless, metoclopramide does not guarantee gastric emptying, and its beneficial effects may be offset by the concomitant or prior administration of anticholinergics, opioids, or antacids.[38] The ability of metoclopramide to increase lower esophageal sphincter tone may also be negated by inclusion of atropine in the preoperative medication. Metoclopramide does not predictably alter gastric fluid pH. Side effects of metoclopramide include abdominal cramping if rapidly administered intravenously and occasional neurologic dysfunction reflecting passage into the central nervous system and production of dopamine receptor blockade. Administration of metoclopramide in the presence of known or suspected gastrointestinal obstruction is not recommended.

Premedication for Outpatients

When administering pharmacologic preoperative medication to outpatients, the introduction of persistent drug effects that delay emergence from anesthesia or prevent early discharge (nausea and vomiting) after elective and usually minor surgery must be avoided.

Fasting before Elective Surgery

Fasting before elective surgery ("NPO after midnight") is based on the historical presumption that absence of intake of solids and fluids will minimize gastric fluid volume at the time of induction of anesthesia and thus decrease the risk for pulmonary aspiration of gastric contents, especially in vulnerable patients (Table 13-25).[46] Nevertheless, complete gastric emptying can never be guaranteed, regardless of the duration of fasting. Furthermore, solid food passes through the stomach at variable and unpredictable rates, sometimes taking up to 12 hours, especially if a high fat content is present. Conversely, clear liquids have a 50% emptying time of just 12 to 20 minutes. Therefore, it seems illogical to have a single guideline for

Table 13-25 Patient Characteristics Associated with an Increased Risk for Aspiration

Elderly
Decreased consciousness
Increased intragastric pressure
Increased acid production (gastric ulcers, gastritis, esophagitis)
Gastric and intestinal hypomotility (bowel obstruction, pregnancy, obesity, diabetes mellitus, renal failure, electrolyte disorders)
Recent food intake
Impaired esophageal sphincter control (hiatal hernia, gastroesophageal reflux disease)
Neuromuscular incoordination
Presence of a nasogastric tube (definitive data lacking except for ventilator-associated pneumonia)

solid food and clear liquid ingestion before induction of anesthesia for elective operations. Indeed, fears that ingestion of clear fluids in the 2 hours preceding induction of anesthesia would increase gastric fluid volume at the time of induction of anesthesia are unfounded.[43] When more than 2 hours has elapsed after the ingestion of clear liquids, endogenous gastric fluid secretion is the principal determinant of the volume and pH of gastric fluid, and a longer fluid fast does not improve the gastric environment. Preoperative anxiety has not been documented to slow gastric emptying.[47] Although opioids may slow gastric emptying, it has not been verified that this drug-induced effect influences the rate of emptying of clear liquids.

The recommendations for fasting before elective surgery have been modified from the previously strict adherence to prohibition against the intake of solids and liquids for several hours before induction of anesthesia for elective surgery. Specifically, clear liquids (water, fruit juices without pulp, carbonated beverages, clear tea, black coffee) are permitted up to 2 hours before the induction of anesthesia for elective operations (Table 13-26).[43] A longer fasting interval is required for milk and solid foods (see Table 13-26).[43] It is acceptable to administer drugs (pharmacologic premedication, medications being taken by the patient preoperatively) with up to 150 mL of water in the hour preceding induction of anesthesia. Preoperative oral nutrition with a special carbohydrate-rich beverage does not appear to increase gastric fluid volume or acidity.[48] Existing guidelines do not clarify the management of patients who have known gastric emptying problems.[49]

Table 13-26 Summary of Fasting Recommendations to Reduce the Risk for Pulmonary Aspiration*

Ingested Material	Minimum Fasting Period (Applies to All Ages)
Clear liquids (water, pulp-free juices, carbonated beverages, clear tea, black coffee)	2 hours
Breast milk	4 hours
Infant formula	6 hours
Nonhuman milk	6 hours
Light meal (typically consists of toast and clear liquids; meals that include fried or fatty foods or meat may prolong the gastric emptying time)	6 hours

These recommendations apply to healthy patients undergoing elective operations exclusive of parturients. Following these recommendations does not guarantee that gastric emptying has occurred.
Adapted from Warner MA, Caplan RA, Epstein BS, et al. Practice guidelines for preoperative fasting and the use of pharmacologic agents to reduce the risk of pulmonary aspiration: Application to healthy patients undergoing elective procedures. Anesthesiology 1999;90:896-905.

Table 13-27 Suggestions for Preoperative Medication for Adults Undergoing Elective Surgery*

Patient visit and interview by the anesthesiologist
Benzodiazepine (orally) to treat insomnia the night before surgery
Benzodiazepine (orally) 1 to 2 hours before induction of anesthesia (administer with up to 150 mL of water)
Opioid (intramuscularly or intravenously) instead of benzodiazepines if analgesia is desired before induction of anesthesia
Possible use of an H_2 antagonist (orally) or a proton pump inhibitor (orally) 1 to 2 hours before induction of anesthesia, especially in patients considered to be at increased risk for pulmonary aspiration

*See Table 13-19 for doses.

PROPHYLAXIS FOR ASPIRATION

Aspiration is estimated to occur in 1 in 3200 operations and is a relatively uncommon event.[50] However, when anesthesia-related aspiration occurs and leads to acute lung injury, this complication is associated with 10% to 30% of anesthesia-related deaths.[50] The administration of proton pump inhibitors suppresses acid secretion in response to all primary stimulants, including histamine, gastrin, and acetylcholine, and these inhibitors are not associated with tolerance. Omeprazole, 20 mg administered orally the evening before or 2 hours before surgery, is the equivalent to sodium citrate.[50] Suppression of acid within 20 minutes can also be achieved by administering pantoprazole, 40 mg intravenously.

Suggestions for Preoperative Medication

The best drug or drug combination to achieve the desired goals of pharmacologic premedication is not known and is often influenced by the individual anesthesiologist's previous experience (Table 13-27).

REFERENCES

1. Pasternak LR. ASA practice guidelines for preanesthetic assessment. Int Anesthesiol Clin 2002;40:31-46.
2. Mangano DT, Layug EL, Wallace A, et al. Effect of atenolol on mortality and cardiovascular morbidity after noncardiac surgery. Multicenter Study of Perioperative Ischemia Research Group. N Engl J Med 1996; 335:1713-1720.
3. Lee TH, Marcantonio ER, Mangione CM, et al. Derivation and prospective validation of a simple index for prediction of cardiac risk of major noncardiac surgery. Circulation 1999;100:1043-1049.
4. Fleisher LA, Eagle KA. Guidelines on perioperative cardiovascular evaluation: What have we learned over the past 6 years to warrant an update? Anesth Analg 2002; 94:1378-1389.
5. Eagle KA, Berger PB, Calkins H, et al. ACC/AHA Guideline Update for Perioperative Cardiovascular Evaluation for Noncardiac Surgery— Executive Summary. A report of the American College of Cardiology/ American Heart Association Task Force on Practice Guidelines (Committee to Update the 1996 Guidelines on Perioperative Cardiovascular Evaluation for Noncardiac Surgery). Anesth Analg 2002;94:1052-1064.
6. Roizen MF, Cohn S. Preoperative evaluation for elective surgery: What laboratory tests are needed? *In* Stoelting RK, Barash PG, Gallagher TJ (eds): Advances in Anesthesia, vol 10. Chicago: Mosby–Year Book, 1993, pp 25-43.
7. Fleisher L. Risk of anesthesia. *In* Miller RD (ed): Miller's Anesthesia, 6th ed. Philadelphia: Elsevier, 2005, pp 893-927.
8. American Society of Anesthesiologists. New classification of physical status. Anesthesiology 1963;24:111.

9. Fleisher LA, Eagle KA. Screening for cardiac disease in patients having noncardiac surgery. Ann Intern Med 1996;124:767-772.

10. Hollenberg SM. Preoperative cardiac risk assessment. Chest 1999;115:51S-57S.

11. Auerbach AD, Goldman L. Beta-blockers and reduction of cardiac events in noncardiac surgery: Clinical applications. JAMA 2002;287:1445-1447.

12. Auerbach AD, Goldman L. Beta-blockers and reduction of cardiac events in noncardiac surgery: Scientific review. JAMA 2002;287:1435-1444.

13. Poldermans D, Boersma E, Bax JJ, et al. The effect of bisoprolol on perioperative mortality and myocardial infarction in high-risk patients undergoing vascular surgery. Dutch Echocardiographic Cardiac Risk Evaluation Applying Stress Echocardiography Study Group. N Engl J Med 1999;341:1789-1794.

14. Cohn SL, Goldman L. Preoperative risk evaluation and perioperative management of patients with coronary artery disease. Med Clin North Am 2003;87:111-136.

15. Wijeysundera DN, Naik JS, Beattie WS. Alpha-2 adrenergic agonists to prevent perioperative cardiovascular complications: A meta-analysis. Am J Med 2003;114:742-752.

16. Wallace AW, Galindez D, Salahieh A, et al. Effect of clonidine on cardiovascular morbidity and mortality after noncardiac surgery. Anesthesiology 2004;101:284-293.

17. McFalls EO, Ward HB, Moritz ET, et al. Coronary-artery revascularization before elective major vascular surgery. N Engl J Med 2004;351:2795-2804.

18. Wilson SH, Fasseas P, Orford JL, et al. Clinical outcome of patients undergoing non-cardiac surgery in the two months following coronary stenting. J Am Coll Cardiol 2003; 42:234-240.

19. Grayburn PA, Hillis LD. Cardiac events in patients undergoing noncardiac surgery: Shifting the paradigm from noninvasive risk stratification to therapy. Ann Intern Med 2003;138:506-511.

20. Mitchell CK, Smoger SH, Pfeifer MP, et al. Multivariate analysis of factors associated with postoperative pulmonary complications following general elective surgery. Arch Surg 1998;133:194-198.

21. Flum DR, Salem L, Elrod JA, et al. Early mortality among medicare beneficiaries undergoing bariatric surgical procedures. JAMA 2005;294:1903-1908

22. Gutt CN, Oniu T, Wolkener F, et al. Prophylaxis and treatment of deep vein thrombosis in general surgery. Am J Surg 2005;189:14-22.

23. Arozullah AM, Daley J, Henderson WG, et al. Multifactorial risk index for predicting postoperative respiratory failure in men after major noncardiac surgery. The National Veterans Administration Surgical Quality Improvement Program. Ann Surg 2000;232:242-253.

24. Arozullah AM, Khuri SF, Henderson WG, et al. Development and validation of a multifactorial risk index for predicting postoperative pneumonia after major noncardiac surgery. Ann Intern Med 2001; 135:847-857.

25. Kroenke K, Lawrence VA, Theroux JF, et al. Postoperative complications after thoracic and major abdominal surgery in patients with and without obstructive lung disease. Chest 1993; 104:1445-1451.

26. McAlister FA, Bertsch K, Man J, et al. Incidence of and risk factors for pulmonary complications after nonthoracic surgery. Am J Respir Crit Care Med 2005;171:514-517.

27. Smetana GW. Preoperative pulmonary evaluation. N Engl J Med 1999;340:937-944.

28. Warner DO, Warner MA, Barnes RD, et al. Perioperative respiratory complications in patients with asthma. Anesthesiology 1996;85:460-467.

29. Rucker L, Frye EB, Staten MA. Usefulness of screening chest roentgenograms in preoperative patients. JAMA 1983;250:3209-3211.

30. Fisher BW, Majumar SR, McAlister FA. Predicting pulmonary complications after nonthoracic surgery: A systematic review of blinded studies. Am J Med 2002;112:219-225.

31. Fishman A, Martinez F, Naunheim K, et al. A randomized trial comparing lung-volume-reduction surgery with medical therapy for severe emphysema. N Engl J Med 2003;348:2059-2073.

32. Jayr C, Matthay MA, Goldstone J, et al. Preoperative and intraoperative factors associated with prolonged mechanical ventilation. A study in patients following major abdominal vascular surgery. Chest 1993; 103:1231-1236.

33. Celli BR, Rodriquez KS, Snider GL. A controlled trial of intermittent positive pressure breathing, incentive spirometry, and deep breathing exercises in preventing pulmonary complications after abdominal surgery. Am Rev Respir Dis 1984; 130:12-15.

34. Moores LK. Smoking and postoperative pulmonary complications. An evidence-based review of the recent literature. Clin Chest Med 2000;21:139-146.

35. Warner DO. Preoperative smoking cessation: How long is long enough? Anesthesiology 2005;102:883-884.

36. Geerts WH, Pineo GF, Heit JA, et al. Prevention of venous thromboembolism: The Seventh ACCP Conference on Antithrombotic and Thrombolytic Therapy. Chest 2004;126:338S-400S.

37. Agu OG, Hamilton G, Baker D. Graduated compression stockings in the prevention of venous thromboembolism. Br J Surg 1999;86:992-1004.

38. White PF. Pharmacologic and clinical aspects of preoperative medication. Anesth Analg 1986;65:963-974.

39. Kay J, Fingling JW, Raff H. Epidural triamcinolone suppresses the pituitary-adrenal axis in human subjects. Anesth Analg 1994;79:501-505.

40. Katz J, Kavanagh BP, Sandler AN, et al. Preemptive analgesia. Clinical evidence of neuroplasticity contributing to postoperative pain. Anesthesiology 1992;77:439-446.

41. Cahalan MK, Lutz FW, Eger EI II, et al. Narcotics decrease heart rate during inhalational anesthesia. Anesth Analg 1987;66:166-170.

42. Quintin L, Bouilloc Z, Butin E, et al. Clonidine for major vascular surgery in hypertensive patients: A double-blind, controlled, randomized study. Anesth Analg 1996;83:687-695.

43. Warner MA, Caplan RA, Epstein BS, et al. Practice guidelines for preoperative fasting and the use of pharmacologic agents to reduce the risk of pulmonary aspiration: Application to healthy patients undergoing elective procedures. Anesthesiology 1999;90:896-905.

44. Warner MA, Warner ME, Weber JG. Clinical significance of pulmonary aspiration during the perioperative period. Anesthesiology 1993;78:56-62.

45. Kopp VJ, Mayer DC, Shaheen NJ. Intravenous erythromycin promotes gastric emptying prior to emergency anesthesia. Anesthesiology 1997; 87:703-705.

46. McIntyre JWR. Evolution of 20th century attitudes to prophylaxis of pulmonary aspiration during anaesthesia. Can J Anaesth 1998;45:1024-1030.

47. Lydon A, McGinley J, Cooke T, et al. Effect of anxiety on the rate of gastric emptying of liquids. Br J Anaesth 1998;81:522-525.

48. Hausel J, Nygren J, Thorell A, et al. Randomized clinical trial of the effects of oral preoperative carbohydrates on postoperative nausea and vomiting after laparoscopic cholecystectomy. Br J Surg 2005;92:415-421.

49. Jellish WS, Kartha V, Fluder E, et al. Effect of metoclopramide on gastric fluid volumes in diabetic patients who have fasted before elective surgery. Anesthesiology 2005;102:904-909.

50. Pisegna JR, Martindale RG. Acid suppression in the perioperative period. J Clin Gastroenterol 2005; 39:10-16.

III

Chapter 14

CHOICE OF ANESTHETIC TECHNIQUE

Donald Taylor

ANESTHETIC TECHNIQUE
   General Anesthetic
   Regional Anesthetic
   Peripheral Nerve Block
   Monitored Anesthesia Care

PREPARATION FOR ANESTHESIA

PHARMACOECONOMICS

The preoperative anesthetic evaluation (see Chapter 13) provides a database with which to make decisions regarding risk assessment and perioperative management. Regardless of the site (dedicated preanesthesia clinic, inpatient hospital visit, or primary care clinic) and health care provider performing the preoperative evaluation, final assessment of its adequacy is the responsibility of the anesthesiologist providing the anesthetic care for the patient.[1] The anesthesiologist is ultimately responsible for (1) determining the medical status of the patient, (2) developing a plan of anesthesia care, and (3) reviewing with the patient or a responsible adult the proposed care plan. After review of the patient's medical history and laboratory and other test results from the patient's medical record, confirmation by a focused physical examination, and review of the patient's fasting status, the anesthesiologist chooses the anesthetic technique.

ANESTHETIC TECHNIQUE

The anesthesiologist selects as the anesthetic technique a (1) general anesthetic, (2) regional anesthetic (see Chapter 17), (3) peripheral nerve block (see Chapter 18), or (4) monitored anesthetic care (MAC). The choice of anesthetic technique (or combination of techniques) is determined by surgical and patient considerations; frequently, more than one anesthetic technique is appropriate (Table 14-1). Patient safety, the ability of the surgeon to perform the procedure, and patient comfort during and after the procedure are important issues. Intraoperative and postoperative monitoring considerations may influence the choice of anesthetic technique. For example, if rapid neurologic evaluation is needed, a general anesthetic with short-acting drugs or a regional anesthetic may be selected. Conversely, if intraoperative transesophageal echocardiography is required, a general endotracheal anesthetic will probably be preferred. There are few circumstances in which a specific anesthetic technique

Table 14-1 Considerations That Influence the Choice of Anesthetic Technique

Preference of the patient, anesthesiologist, and surgeon

Coexisting diseases that may or may not be related to the reason for surgery (gastroesophageal reflux, diabetes mellitus, asthma)

Site of surgery

Body position of the patient during surgery

Elective or emergency surgery

Likelihood of increased amounts of gastric contents at the time of induction of anesthesia

Suspected difficult airway management and tracheal intubation

Duration of surgery or procedure

Patient age

Anticipated recovery time

Postanesthesia care unit discharge criteria

has been demonstrated to be safer or more efficacious than another technique,[2,3] but anesthesiologists may perform better with techniques with which they are more experienced. During residency training, it is preferable to gain exposure to as many anesthetic techniques as possible.

Unpleasant side effects associated with anesthesia may influence the choice of anesthetic technique. Because the relative safety of different anesthetic techniques is often viewed as similar, patient satisfaction may become the principal determinant of the anesthetic technique selected. Assuming equivalent safety, both the anesthesiologist and patient are likely to place the greatest importance on avoidance of pain, followed by vomiting, nausea, and to a lesser extent, urinary retention, myalgia, and pruritus. For some patients, avoiding an awake technique is the predominant concern, perhaps because of anxiety. For these patients, even in the absence of pain, the sights, sounds, and smells of the operating or procedure room are an experience to be avoided.[4,5]

An ideal anesthetic technique would incorporate optimal patient safety and satisfaction, provide excellent operating conditions for the surgeon, allow rapid recovery, and avoid postoperative side effects. In addition, it would be low in cost, allow early transfer or discharge from the postanesthesia care unit (see Chapter 38), optimize postoperative pain control (see Chapter 39), and permit optimal operating room efficiency, including turnover times. It is the responsibility of the anesthesiologist to evaluate the medical condition and unique needs of each patient, select

an acceptable anesthetic technique, and make this recommendation to the patient.

An informed patient who has an understanding of the anesthetic techniques available and the needs for accomplishing the surgery is likely to be comfortable with the anesthetic technique recommended by the anesthesiologist. Consent for anesthesia requires an informed patient, and "coercion" by the anesthesiologist should not be used to obtain consent for an anesthetic technique that the patient does not desire. On reaching this decision, the anesthesiologist should document the relevant findings, American Society of Anesthesiologists (ASA) classification, anesthetic technique, and a statement noting that the patient understands and accepts the plan and accompanying risks (see Table 13-9).

General Anesthetic

General anesthesia may be initiated by the administration of intravenous drugs or inhalation of a volatile anesthetic with or without nitrous oxide.

INTRAVENOUS INDUCTION OF ANESTHESIA

Induction of general anesthesia (loss of consciousness) in adult patients is most often accomplished by the intravenous administration of drugs (propofol, thiopental, or etomidate) that produce rapid onset of unconsciousness (see Chapter 9). After loss of consciousness, the anesthesiologist may place a laryngeal mask airway (LMA) and/or administer a neuromuscular blocking drug intravenously to produce skeletal muscle relaxation for facilitation of direct laryngoscopy before tracheal intubation (see Chapter 16). The intravenous injection of a drug to produce unconsciousness followed immediately by a neuromuscular blocking drug that produces a rapid onset of skeletal muscle paralysis (succinylcholine, rocuronium, mivacurium) is referred to as "rapid-sequence" induction of anesthesia. Frequently, the patient is breathing oxygen (3 to 5 L/min) via a facemask (preoxygenation) before rapid-sequence induction of anesthesia. Preoxygenation is intended to replace nitrogen (denitrogenation) in the patient's functional residual capacity (about 2500 mL of 21% oxygen) with oxygen. This practice should increase the margin of safety during periods of upper airway obstruction or apnea (drug induced during direct laryngoscopy for tracheal intubation) that may accompany induction of anesthesia. In healthy awake patients, the increase in arterial hemoglobin oxygen saturation achieved with eight vital capacity breaths of 100% oxygen over a period of 60 seconds is similar to that achieved by breathing 100% oxygen for 3 minutes at normal tidal volumes.[6] Four vital capacity breaths over a 30-second period also increases arterial oxygenation, but the time until hemoglobin desaturation is shorter than in patients breathing oxygen for 3 minutes or taking eight deep breaths.

III

Rapid-Sequence Induction of Anesthesia

A typical rapid-sequence induction of anesthesia includes preoxygenation followed by the administration of a nonparalyzing (defasciculating) dose of a nondepolarizing neuromuscular blocking drug (pancuronium, 1 to 2 mg IV or its equivalent) and succinylcholine (1 to 2 mg/kg IV). Cricoid pressure may be applied by an assistant just before the onset of drug-induced unconsciousness and loss of protective upper airway reflexes. Rocuronium, though not as rapid in onset as succinylcholine, is used as an alternative when a depolarizing muscle relaxant is contraindicated. It is common practice to administer an opioid (fentanyl, 1 to 2 μg/kg IV or its equivalent) 1 to 3 minutes before administration of the induction drug. The opioid is intended to blunt the subsequent pressor and heart rate responses to direct laryngoscopy and tracheal intubation and also to initiate preemptive analgesia. Remifentanil and alfentanil undergo more rapid blood-brain equilibration than fentanyl does and thus may be more reliable in blunting the sympathetic nervous system responses evoked by direct laryngoscopy and tracheal intubation.[7]

With the onset of unconsciousness, the patient's head is positioned to optimize patency of the upper airway, and positive-pressure inflation of the patient's lungs with oxygen is instituted. Direct laryngoscopy for tracheal intubation is initiated only after the onset of skeletal muscle paralysis (often verified by a peripheral nerve stimulator), which is typically 45 to 90 seconds after the administration of succinylcholine. Rocuronium, 2 to 3 × the 95% effective dose (ED_{95}), may be the nondepolarizing neuromuscular blocking drug alternative to succinylcholine for facilitation of tracheal intubation. Facilitation of tracheal intubation by skeletal muscle paralysis with pancuronium, vecuronium, atracurium, cisatracurium, or mivacurium is possible if it is acceptable to wait 3 to 5 minutes for their peak pharmacologic effect.

Monitoring of arterial hemoglobin oxygen saturation with a pulse oximeter provides early warning should arterial oxygen desaturation occur during the period of apnea required for tracheal intubation. It is mandatory that proper placement of the tube in the trachea be confirmed after direct laryngoscopy (Table 14-2). After tracheal intubation, it may be prudent to insert a gastric tube through the mouth to decompress the stomach and remove any easily accessible fluid. This orogastric tube should be removed at the conclusion of anesthesia. When gastric suction is needed postoperatively, normally the tube should be inserted through the nares rather than the mouth.

INHALATION INDUCTION OF ANESTHESIA

An alternative to rapid-sequence induction of anesthesia is the inhalation of sevoflurane (nonpungent) with or without nitrous oxide.[8] Prior intravenous administration of a "sleep dose" of an induction drug may be used if an intravenous catheter is in place. Desflurane produces a rapid onset of effect but is not selected for inhalation

Table 14-2 Evidence of a Patent Upper Airway after Induction of Anesthesia

The upper part of the chest expands and the reservoir bag partially empties during inspiration
The reservoir bag refills during exhalation
Capnography reveals cyclic waveforms decreasing to zero during inhalation and a plateau peak (>20 mm Hg) during exhalation
The pulse oximeter continues to read >95%
Bilateral breath sounds are present

induction because of its airway irritant effects. Inhalation or "mask induction" of anesthesia is most often selected for pediatric patients when prior insertion of a venous catheter is not practical. The resurgence of interest in inhalation induction of anesthesia in adults is based on its potential safety inasmuch as spontaneous ventilation is maintained and patients regulate their own depth of anesthesia, thereby avoiding excessive concentrations of sevoflurane, which will suppress ventilation.[9,10] Sevoflurane may also be useful when difficult airway management is anticipated because of the absence of salivation and preservation of spontaneous breathing. The traditional "awake look" in a patient with a suspected difficult airway, which included titration of intravenous drugs until the patient tolerated direct laryngoscopy, has been modified to include spontaneous ventilation of high concentrations of sevoflurane until laryngoscopic evaluation is possible.

Characteristics of Inhalation Induction with Sevoflurane

Loss of consciousness typically occurs within about 1 minute when breathing 8% sevoflurane. LMA placement can usually be achieved within 2 minutes after administering 7% sevoflurane by facemask.[9] The addition of nitrous oxide to the inspired gas mixture does not add significantly to the induction sequence. Prior administration of benzodiazepines may facilitate inhalation induction, whereas opioids may complicate this technique by increasing the likelihood of apnea.[10]

A technique for induction of anesthesia with sevoflurane includes priming the circuit (emptying the reservoir bag and opening the adjustable pressure-limiting ["pop-off"] valve), dialing the vaporizer setting to 8% while using a fresh gas flow of 8 L/min, and maintaining this flow for 60 seconds before applying the facemask to the patient. At this point a single breath from end-expiratory volume to maximum inspiration followed by deep breathing typically produces loss of consciousness in 1 minute.

After inhalation induction of anesthesia, a depolarizing or nondepolarizing neuromuscular blocking drug is administered intravenously to provide the skeletal muscle relaxation needed to facilitate direct laryngoscopy for tracheal intubation. If the anesthesiologist decides to not place a tube in the trachea, anesthesia is maintained by inhalation through a facemask or LMA.

MAINTENANCE OF ANESTHESIA

The objectives during maintenance of general anesthesia are amnesia, analgesia, skeletal muscle relaxation, and control of the sympathetic nervous system responses evoked by noxious stimulation. These objectives are achieved most often by the use of a combination of drugs that may include inhaled or injected drugs (or both), with or without neuromuscular blocking drugs. Each drug selected should be administered on the basis of a specific goal that is relevant to that drug's known pharmacologic effects at therapeutic doses. For example, it is not logical to administer high concentrations of volatile anesthetics to produce skeletal muscle relaxation when neuromuscular blocking drugs are specific for achieving this goal. Likewise, it is not acceptable to obscure skeletal muscle movement by administering excessive amounts of neuromuscular blocking drugs because of insufficient doses of anesthetics. The selective use of drugs for their specific pharmacologic effects permits the anesthesiologist to tailor the anesthetic to the patient's medical condition and any unique needs introduced by the surgery.

Despite its lack of potency, nitrous oxide is the most frequently administered inhaled anesthetic. Typically, nitrous oxide (50% to 70% inhaled concentration) is administered in combination with a volatile anesthetic or opioid, or both. It is important to remember that it is the partial pressure of an inhaled anesthetic that produces its pharmacologic effect. For example, 60% inhaled nitrous oxide administered at sea level exerts a partial pressure of 456 mm Hg (60% of the total barometric pressure of 760 mm Hg). The same inhaled concentration of nitrous oxide (or a volatile anesthetic) administered at an altitude where the barometric pressure is less than 760 mm Hg exerts a decreased pharmacologic effect because the partial pressure of the anesthetic that can be achieved in the brain is lower.

Volatile anesthetics have the advantage of high potency, and they can be readily controlled in terms of the concentration delivered from the anesthetic machine so that the dose can be titrated to produce a desired response, including skeletal muscle relaxation and prompt awakening. The excessive sympathetic nervous system responses evoked by noxious stimulation are predictably attenuated by volatile anesthetics. Dose-dependent cardiac depression is a major disadvantage of volatile anesthetics (see Chapter 8). Indeed, a volatile drug is seldom administered as the sole anesthetic but is more often administered in combination with nitrous oxide. Substitution of nitrous oxide for a portion of the dose of the volatile anesthetic allows a decrease in the delivered concentration of the volatile drug, resulting in less cardiac depression despite the same total dose of anesthetic drugs. Volatile anesthetics

may provide inadequat analgesic effects, may be associated with postoperative hepatic dysfunction, and introduce the possibility of carbon monoxide production should they be exposed to desiccated carbon dioxide absorbents that contain strong bases.

In certain instances it is acceptable to administer neuromuscular blocking drugs to ensure lack of patient movement and permit a decrease in the delivered concentration of volatile anesthetics. This use of neuromuscular blocking drugs, however, must not be interpreted as an endorsement for the administration of an inadequate dose of anesthetic that is obscured by skeletal muscle paralysis. In this regard, intraoperative awareness is a recognized risk of minimal concentrations of anesthetic drugs ("light anesthesia"), especially when patient movements are obscured by drug-induced skeletal muscle paralysis.

Opioids that generally do not depress the cardiovascular system are combined most often with nitrous oxide (see Chapter 10). In patients with normal left ventricular function, however, the lack of opioid-induced cardiovascular depression and the absence of attenuation of sympathetic nervous system reflexes may be manifested as systemic hypertension. When this occurs, the addition of low concentrations of a volatile anesthetic to the delivered gases is often effective in returning the increased systemic blood pressure to an acceptable level. Neuromuscular blocking drugs are often necessary, even in the absence of the need for skeletal muscle relaxation, because adequate doses of opioids administered in the presence of nitrous oxide are unlikely to prevent patient movement in response to painful stimulation. Another disadvantage of injected drugs versus inhaled anesthetics is an inability to accurately titrate and maintain a therapeutic concentration of the injected drug. This disadvantage can be offset to some extent by continuous intravenous infusion of the injected anesthetic at a rate previously determined in other patients to be associated with therapeutic concentrations in blood. Brain function monitoring (bispectral index, entropy, auditory evoked potentials) may be helpful in titrating the dose of inhaled or injected anesthetic drugs to produce the desired degree of central nervous system depression (see Chapter 20).[11]

Regional Anesthetic

A neuraxial regional anesthetic (spinal, epidural, caudal) is selected when maintenance of consciousness during surgery is desirable (see Chapter 17). Spinal anesthesia and epidural anesthesia each have advantages and disadvantages that may make one or the other technique better suited to a specific patient or surgical procedure. Spinal anesthesia (1) takes less time to perform, (2) produces a more rapid onset of better-quality sensory and motor anesthesia, and (3) is associated with less pain during surgery. The principal advantages of epidural anesthesia are (1) a lower risk for post–dural puncture

III

headache, (2) less systemic hypotension if epinephrine is not added to the local anesthetic solution, (3) the ability to prolong or extend the anesthesia through an indwelling epidural catheter, and (4) the option of using the epidural catheter to provide postoperative analgesia. Skeletal muscle relaxation and contraction of the gastrointestinal tract are also produced by a regional anesthetic.

Patients may have preconceived and erroneous conceptions about regional anesthesia that will require the anesthesiologist to reassure them regarding the safety of this technique. The only absolute contraindication to spinal or epidural anesthesia is patient refusal. Certain preexisting conditions increase the relative risk of these techniques, and the anesthesiologist must balance the perceived benefits of this technique before proceeding (Table 14-3). Disadvantages of this anesthetic technique include the occasional failure to produce sensory levels of anesthesia that are adequate for the surgical stimulus and the decrease in systemic blood pressure that may accompany the peripheral sympathetic nervous system blockade produced by the regional anesthetic, particularly in the presence of hypovolemia.

A regional anesthetic technique is most often selected for surgery that involves the lower part of the abdomen or the lower extremities in which the level of sensory anesthesia required is associated with minimal sympathetic nervous system blockade.[12,13] This should not, however, imply that a general anesthetic is an unacceptable technique for similar types of surgery.

For procedures lasting between 20 and 90 minutes, intravenous regional anesthesia (IVRA, or Bier block) may be used.[2] IVRA provides reliable anesthesia for both the upper and lower extremities, although the latter may be more problematic because of the size of the lower extremities in adults. After the application of a tourniquet and exsanguination of the extremity, lidocaine (0.5%) is commonly administered into a catheter previously placed in the involved extremity. Double tourniquets (distal cuff inflated over the area where local anesthetic has infiltrated with time) help ameliorate tourniquet pain. Intravenous analgesics such as ketorolac may be useful for treatment of patient discomfort during IVRA. IVRA is more cost-effective than general anesthesia or brachial plexus block for outpatient hand surgery.

Peripheral Nerve Block

A peripheral nerve block is most appropriate as a technique of anesthesia for superficial operations on the extremities (see Chapter 18). Advantages of peripheral nerve blocks include maintenance of consciousness and the continued presence of protective upper airway reflexes. The isolated anesthetic effect produced by a peripheral nerve block is particularly attractive in patients with chronic pulmonary disease, severe cardiac impairment, or inadequate renal function. For example, insertion of a vascular shunt in the upper extremity for hemodialysis in a patient who may have associated pulmonary and cardiac disease is often accomplished with anesthesia provided by a peripheral nerve block of the brachial plexus. Likewise, avoidance of the need for neuromuscular blocking drugs in this type of patient circumvents the possible prolonged effect produced by these drugs in the absence of renal function.

A disadvantage of peripheral nerve block as an anesthetic technique is the unpredictable attainment of adequate sensory and motor anesthesia for performance of the surgery. The success rate of a peripheral nerve block is often related to the frequency with which the anesthesiologist uses this anesthetic technique. Patients must be cooperative for a peripheral nerve block to be effective. For example, acutely intoxicated and agitated patients are not ideal candidates for a peripheral nerve block.

Monitored Anesthesia Care

MAC is defined by the ASA as a procedure in which an anesthesiologist is requested or required to provide anesthetic services; the anesthesiologist is responsible for preoperative evaluation, care during the procedure, and management after the procedure.[14,15] This responsibility includes (1) diagnosis and treatment of clinical problems during the procedure; (2) support of vital functions; (3) administration of sedatives, analgesics, hypnotics, anesthetic drugs, or other medications as necessary for patient safety; (4) psychological support and physical comfort; and (5) provision of other services as needed to complete the procedure safely. The care of a patient undergoing MAC is held to the same standard as any other anesthetic technique, given that the level of sedation may progress rapidly, go beyond consciousness, and lead to an "unplanned" general anesthetic (specifically defined by the ASA as any instance in which the patient loses consciousness as defined by the ability to respond purposefully). When this occurs, extra care may be needed in monitoring to prevent airway mishaps such as upper airway obstruction and arterial hypoxemia, as reflected by the pulse oximeter reading.

Table 14-3 Conditions That May Increase the Risk Associated with Spinal or Epidural Anesthesia
Hypovolemia
Increased intracranial pressure
Coagulopathy (thrombocytopenia) (see Table 39-6)
Sepsis
Infection at the cutaneous puncture site
Preexisting neurologic disease (multiple sclerosis?)

While caring for a patient under MAC, it is important to consider the total dose of local anesthetic administered by the surgeon and the risk for local anesthetic toxicity, with an eye to potentially toxic doses (see Chapter 11). In addition to monitoring the patient, the anesthesiologist makes the decision to administer supplemental oxygen (may not be necessary if pulse oximeter readings are acceptable while breathing room air), typically by nasal cannula. In addition to oxygen, the anesthesiologist may administer drugs intravenously to provide anxiolysis (midazolam), sedation (propofol), and analgesia (remifentanil, ketorolac, ketamine). Depending on the patient and the procedure, fulfilling one or all of these goals (anxiolysis, sedation, and analgesia for arthroscopic surgery) may be needed. Opioid administration during MAC may be useful but also requires careful monitoring of oxygenation and ventilation. Inhaled anesthetics (nitrous oxide, sevoflurane) administered in concentrations below the threshold of loss of consciousness may be useful during infiltration of local anesthetic solutions, especially for brief periods while patients are not tolerating the procedure because of agitation or inadequate analgesia. MAC may facilitate avoidance of side effects (sympatholysis, respiratory depression, delayed emergence) and can be particularly cost-effective in comparison to general or regional anesthetics in the ambulatory care setting.

PREPARATION FOR ANESTHESIA

Preparation for anesthesia after the preoperative medication has been administered and the patient is transported to the operating room is similar regardless of the anesthetic technique that has been selected (Table 14-4). On arrival in the operating room, the patient is identified and the planned surgery reconfirmed. The patient's medical record, including the nurse's notes, is consulted by the anesthesiologist to learn of any unexpected changes in the patient's medical condition, vital signs, or body temperature and to determine that the preoperative medication and, if indicated, prophylactic antibiotics have been administered. Likewise, any laboratory data that have become available since the anesthesiologist's previous visit should be reviewed.

Initial preparation for anesthesia, regardless of the technique of anesthesia selected, usually begins with insertion of a catheter in a peripheral vein and application of a blood pressure cuff. This initial preparation may be accomplished in a holding area or in the operating room. The use of separate rooms (induction rooms) distinct from the operating room for induction of anesthesia is not recommended by some because of the questionable safety of routinely moving anesthetized patients with the necessary attached equipment from one area to another. An exception to this recommendation may be the performance of peripheral nerve blocks or institution

Table 14-4 Routine Preparation before Induction of Anesthesia Independent of the Anesthetic Technique Selected

Anesthesia machine (see Table 15-9)

   Attach an anesthetic breathing system with a properly sized facemask

   Occlude the patient end of the anesthetic breathing system and fill with oxygen from the anesthesia machine ("flush valve") (applying manual pressure to the distended reservoir bag checks for leaks in the anesthetic breathing system and confirms the ability to provide positive-pressure ventilation of the patient's lungs with oxygen)

Check the anesthetic breathing system valves

Calibrate the oxygen analyzer with air and oxygen and set alarm limits

Check the carbon dioxide absorbent for color change

Check the liquid level of vaporizers

Confirm proper function of the mechanical ventilator

Confirm the availability and function of wall suction

Check the final position of all flowmeter, vaporizer, and monitor (visual and audible alarm) settings

Monitors

   Blood pressure

   Pulse oximetry

   Electrocardiography

   Capnography

Drugs

   Local anesthetic (lidocaine)

   Induction drug (propofol, thiopental, etomidate)

   Opioid (fentanyl, sufentanil, alfentanil, remifentanil)

   Benzodiazepine (midazolam, diazepam)

   Anticholinergic (atropine, glycopyrrolate)

   Sympathomimetic (ephedrine, phenylephrine)

   Succinylcholine

   Nondepolarizing neuromuscular blocking drug (mivacurium, rocuronium, atracurium, vecuronium, cisatracurium, pancuronium)

   Anticholinesterase (neostigmine, edrophonium)

   Opioid antagonist

   Benzodiazepine antagonist

Continued

III

Table 14-4 Routine Preparation before Induction of Anesthesia Independent of the Anesthetic Technique Selected—cont'd

Catecholamine to treat an allergic reaction (epinephrine)
Equipment
Intravenous solution and connecting tubing
Catheter for vascular cannulation
Suction catheter
Oral and/or nasal airway
Laryngeal mask airway
Tracheal tube
Nasogastric tube
Temperature probe

of epidural anesthesia in a holding area so that the block is in place when the operating room becomes available. Likewise, an epidural catheter for postoperative pain management may be placed in the holding area before transport of the patient to the operating room and induction of general anesthesia. Monitors such as the pulse oximeter, electrocardiogram, and peripheral nerve stimulator are also applied while the patient is still awake. Immediately before induction of anesthesia, baseline vital signs (systemic blood pressure, heart rate, cardiac rhythm, arterial hemoglobin oxygen saturation, breathing rate) and the corresponding time are recorded.

Regardless of the anesthetic technique selected, the provider should verify that the anesthesia machine is present and functional (in certain circumstances such as anesthesia for cardioversion, a breathing circuit may suffice) and that specific drugs and equipment are always immediately available (see Table 14-4), including suctioning capability, adequate monitoring (systemic blood pressure, electrocardiography, pulse oximetry, capnography, body temperature), airway equipment (appropriately sized facemask, oral airway, nasal airway, LMA, laryngoscope with appropriate functional blades), materials for venous access, and drugs appropriate for emergency intravenous induction and resuscitation (induction drugs, neuromuscular blocking drugs, vasopressors, including ephedrine and phenylephrine).

PHARMACOECONOMICS

The desire for cost containment often leads to recommendations that low-cost drugs (antiemetics, intravenous induction drugs, volatile anesthetics, neuromuscular blocking drugs) be used in preference to newer, but more expensive drugs with desirable pharmacologic profiles.[16] The ultimate goal must be to obtain the best results (low toxicity, rapid awakening, absence of nausea and vomiting) at the most practical cost. A useful method to decrease the cost of volatile anesthetics is the use of low fresh gas flow (2 L/min) during maintenance of anesthesia.[17]

REFERENCES

1. Practice Advisory for Preoperative Evaluation. A report by the American Society of Anesthesiologists Task Force on Preanesthetic Evaluation. Anesthesiology 2000;96:485.
2. Chan V, Peng P, Kaszas Z, et al. A comparative study of general anesthesia, intravenous regional anesthesia, and axillary block for outpatient hand surgery: Clinical outcome and cost analysis. Anesth Analg 2001;93:1181-1184.
3. Arbous M, Grobbee D, van Kleef J, et al. Mortality associated with anaesthesia: A qualitative analysis to identify risk factors. Anaesthesia 2001;56:1141-1153.
4. Rashiq S, Bray P. Relative value to surgical patients and anesthesia providers of selected anesthesia related outcomes. BMC Med Inform Decis Mak 2003;3:3.
5. Macario A, Weinger M, Carney S, et al. Which clinical anesthesia outcomes are important to avoid? The perspective of patients. Anesth Analg 1999;89:652-658.
6. Brake AS, Tara SK, Aouadad MT, et al. Preoxygenation: Comparison of maximal breathing and tidal volume breathing techniques. Anesthesiology 1999;91:612-616.
7. Jhaveri R, Joshi P, Batenhorst R, et al. Dose comparison of remifentanil and alfentanil for loss of consciousness. Anesthesiology 1997;87:253-259.
8. Doi M, Ikeda K. Airway irritation produced by volatile anaesthetics during brief inhalation: Comparison of halothane, enflurane, isoflurane and sevoflurane. Can J Anaesth 1993;40:122-128.
9. Muzi M, Robinson BJ, Ebert TJ, et al. Induction of anesthesia and tracheal intubation with sevoflurane in adults. Anesthesiology 1996;85:536-541.
10. Muzi M, Colinco MD, Robinson BJ, et al. The effects of premedication on inhaled induction of anesthesia with sevoflurane. Anesth Analg 1997;85:1143-1148.
11. Hall D, Weaver J, Ginsberg S, et al. Bispectral EEG index monitoring of high-dose nitrous oxide and low-dose sevoflurane sedation. Anesth Prog 2002;49:56-62.
12. Rodgers A, Walker N, Schug S, et al. Reduction of postoperative morbidity and mortality with epidural or spinal anesthesia: Results from overview of randomized trials. BMJ 2000;321:1493-1497.
13. Horlocker TT, Wedel DJ, Benzon H, et al. Regional anesthesia in the anticoagulated patient: Defining the risks. Reg Anesth Pain Med 2003;28:172-197.
14. Position on Monitored Anesthesia Care. ASA House of Delegates, amended October 2005 (www.ashq.org).
15. Ghisi D, Aanelli A, Tosi M, et al. Monitored anesthesia care. Minerva Anestesiol 2005;71:533-538.
16. Eger EI, White PF, Bogetz MS. Clinical and economic factors important to anaesthetic choice for day-case surgery. Pharmacoeconomics 2000;17:245-262.
17. Dion P. The cost of anesthetic vapors. Can J Anaesth 1992;39:633-638.

Chapter 15

ANESTHESIA DELIVERY SYSTEMS

Patricia Ann Roth and Joan E. Howley

An anesthesia delivery system consists of the anesthesia workstation (anesthesia machine) and anesthetic breathing system (circuit), which permit delivery of known concentrations of inhaled anesthetics and oxygen to the patient, as well as removal of the patient's carbon dioxide. Carbon dioxide can be removed either by washout (delivered gas flow >5 L/min from the anesthesia machine) or by chemical neutralization.

ANESTHESIA WORKSTATION

The anesthesia machine has evolved from a simple pneumatic device to a complex integrated computer-controlled multicomponent workstation (Figs. 15-1 and 15-2).[1] The components within the anesthesia workstation function in harmony to deliver known concentrations of inhaled anesthetics to the patient. The multiple components of the anesthesia workstation include what was previously recognized as the anesthesia machine (the pressure-regulating and gas-mixing components), vaporizers, anesthesia breathing circuit, ventilator, scavenging system, and respiratory and physiologic monitoring systems (electrocardiogram, systemic blood pressure, body temperature, arterial hemoglobin saturation with oxygen, and inhaled and exhaled concentrations of oxygen, carbon dioxide, and anesthetic gases and vapors) (Table 15-1).[1] Alarm systems to signal apnea or disconnection of the anesthetic breathing system from the patient are included. The alarms present on the pulse oximeter and capnograph must be audible to the anesthesiologist. Most anesthesia machines are powered by both electric and pneumatic power.

The anesthesia workstation ultimately provides delivery of medical gases and the vapors of volatile anesthetics at known concentrations to the common gas outlet. These gases enter the anesthetic breathing system to be delivered to the patient by spontaneous or mechanical ventilation. Exhaled gases are passed through a carbon dioxide absorbent and are either returned to the patient after carbon

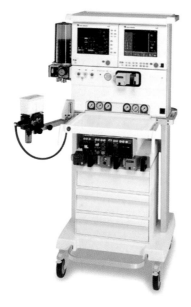

Figure 15-1 GE/Datex-Ohmeda S/5 Anesthesia Delivery Unit (ADU) workstation.

dioxide is removed or scavenged from the breathing system to the waste gas removal limb.

Fail-Safe

Anesthesia machines are equipped with a fail-safe valve designed to prevent the delivery of hypoxic gas mixtures from the machine in the event of failure of the oxygen supply. This valve shuts off or proportionally decreases the flow of all gases when the pressure in the oxygen delivery line decreases to less than 30 psi. This safety measure will protect against unrecognized exhaustion of oxygen delivery from a cylinder attached to the anesthesia machine or from a central source. This valve, however, does not prevent the delivery of 100% nitrous oxide when the oxygen flow is zero but gas pressure in the circuit of the anesthesia machine is maintained. In this situation, an oxygen analyzer is necessary to detect the delivery of a hypoxic gas mixture. Far superior to the fail-safe valve or an oxygen analyzer is the continuous presence of a vigilant anesthesiologist.

Ohmeda machines have a chain connecting the oxygen and nitrous oxide flowmeter knobs. This connection prevents oxygen flow from being terminated while nitrous oxide flow continues and prevents delivery of nitrous oxide without the flow of oxygen. Dräger machines prevent the flow of nitrous oxide without the presence of oxygen flow with a pressure control piston. Until the oxygen flowmeter is turned on, nitrous oxide will not flow.

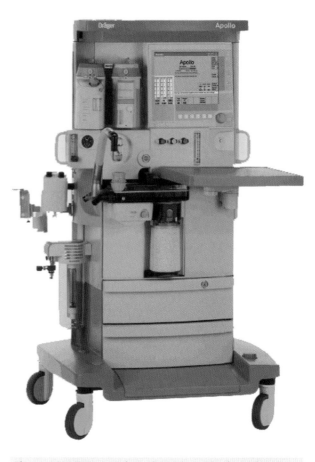

Figure 15-2 Dräger Narkomed 6000 anesthesia workstation.

Table 15–1 Common Features of Anesthesia Machines
Inlet of hospital pipeline for compressed gases (oxygen, nitrous oxide, and air)
Inlet of compressed gas cylinders
Pressure regulators to reduce pipeline and tank pressure to safe and consistent levels
Fail-safe device
Flowmeters to control the amount of gases delivered to the breathing limb
Vaporizers for adding volatile anesthetic gas to the carrier gas
Common gas line through which compressed gases mixed with a volatile agent enter the breathing limb
Breathing limb, including an oxygen analyzer, inspiratory one-way valve, circle system, expiratory gas sampling line, spirometer to measure the respiratory rate and volume, expiratory one-way valve, adjustable pressure-limiting valve, carbon dioxide absorbent, reservoir bag, mechanical ventilator, and scavenger system

Compressed Gases

Gases used in the administration of anesthesia (oxygen, nitrous oxide, air) are most often delivered to the anesthesia machine from a central supply source located in the hospital (Fig. 15-3).[2] Hospital-supplied gases enter the operating room from a central source through pipelines to color-coded wall outlets (yellow for air, blue for nitrous oxide, and green for oxygen). Color-coded pressure hoses are connected to the wall outlet by gas-specific diameter fittings that are not interchangeable (diameter index safety system, which is designed to prevent misconnections of pipeline gases). Oxygen or air from a central supply source may also be used to power (pneumatic driven) the ventilator on the anesthesia machine.

Gas enters the anesthesia machine through pipeline inlet connections that are gas specific (threaded noninter-

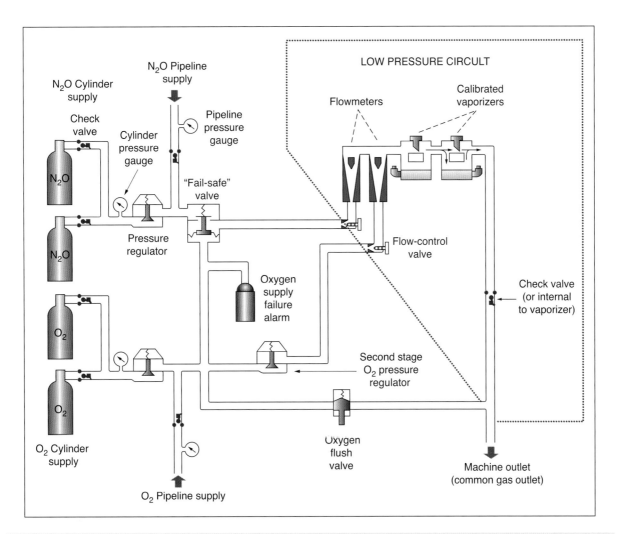

Figure 15-3 Schematic diagram of the internal circuitry of an anesthesia machine. Oxygen and nitrous oxide enter the anesthesia machine through a central supply line (most common); alternatively (infrequently), they are provided from gas cylinders attached to pin-indexed yokes on the machine. Check valves prevent transfilling of gas cylinders or flow of gas from cylinders into the central supply line. Pressure regulators decrease pressure in the tubing from the gas cylinders to about 50 psi. The fail-safe valve prevents flow of nitrous oxide if the pressure in the oxygen supply circuit decreases to less than 30 psi. Needle valves control gas flow to rotameters (flowmeters). Agent-specific vaporizers provide a reliable means to deliver preselected concentrations of a volatile anesthetic. An interlock system allows only one vaporizer to be in the "on" (delivery) setting at a time. After mixing in the manifold of the anesthesia machine, the total fresh gas flow enters the common outlet for delivery to the patient through the anesthetic breathing system (circuit). (Adapted from Check-Out. A Guide for Preoperative Inspection of an Anesthetic Machine. Park Ridge, IL: American Society of Anesthesiologists, 1987, pp 1-14, with permission.)

changeable connections) to minimize the possibility of a misconnection. The gas must be delivered from the central supply source at an appropriate pressure (about 50 psi) for the flowmeters on the anesthesia machine to function properly.

Anesthesia machines are also equipped with cylinders of oxygen and nitrous oxide for use should the central gas supply fail (see Fig. 15-3).[2] Color-coded cylinders are attached to the anesthesia machine by a hanger yoke assembly, which consists of two metal pins that correspond to holes in the valve casing of the gas cylinder (pin indexed) (Table 15-2). This design makes it impossible to attach an oxygen cylinder to any yoke on the anesthesia machine other than that designed for oxygen. Otherwise, a cylinder containing nitrous oxide could be attached to the oxygen yoke, which would result in the delivery of nitrous oxide when the oxygen flowmeter was activated. Color-coded pressure gauges (green for oxygen, blue for nitrous oxide) on the anesthesia machine indicate the pressure of the gas in the corresponding gas cylinder (see Table 15-2).

CALCULATION OF CYLINDER CONTENTS

The pressure in an oxygen cylinder is directly proportional to the volume of oxygen in the cylinder. For example, a full oxygen cylinder (E size) contains about 625 L of oxygen at a pressure of 2000 psi and half this volume when the pressure is 1000 psi. Therefore, it is possible to accurately calculate how long a given flow rate of oxygen can be maintained before the cylinder is empty. In contrast to oxygen, the pressure gauge for nitrous oxide does not indicate the amount of gas remaining in the cylinder because the pressure in the gas cylinder remains at 750 psi as long as any liquid nitrous oxide is present. When nitrous oxide leaves the cylinder as a vapor, additional liquid is vaporized to maintain an unchanging pressure in the cylinder. After all the liquid nitrous oxide is vaporized, the pressure begins to decrease, and it can be assumed that about 75% of the contents of the gas cylinder have been exhausted. Because

a full nitrous oxide cylinder (E size) contains about 1590 L, approximately 400 L of nitrous oxide remains when the pressure gauge begins to decrease from its previously constant value of 750 psi. Vaporization of a liquefied gas (nitrous oxide), as well as expansion of a compressed gas (oxygen), absorbs heat, which is extracted from the metal cylinder and the surrounding atmosphere. For this reason, atmospheric water vapor often accumulates as frost on gas cylinders and in valves, particularly during high gas flow from these tanks. Internal icing does not occur because compressed gases are free of water vapor.

Flowmeters

Flowmeters on the anesthesia machine precisely control and measure gas flow to the common gas inlet (see Fig. 15-3).[2] Measurement of the flow of gases is based on the principle that flow past a resistance is proportional to pressure. Typically, gas flow enters the bottom of a vertically positioned and tapered (the cross-sectional area increases upward from site of gas entry) glass flow tube. Gas flow into the flowmeter tube raises a bobbin- or ball-shaped float. The float comes to rest when gravity is balanced by the fall in pressure caused by the float. The upper end of the bobbin or the equator of the ball indicates the gas flow in milliliters or liters per minute. Proportionality between pressure and flow is determined by the shape of the tube (resistance) and the physical properties (density and viscosity) of the gas. The flowmeters are initially calibrated for the indicated gas at the factory. Because few gases have the same density and viscosity, flowmeters are not interchangeable with other gases. The scale accompanying an oxygen flowmeter is green, whereas the scale for the nitrous oxide flowmeter is blue.

Gas flow exits the flowmeters and passes into a manifold (mixing chamber) located at the top of the flowmeters (see Fig. 15-3).[2] The oxygen flowmeter should be the last in the sequence of flowmeters, and thus oxygen should be the last gas added to the manifold. This arrangement

Table 15-2	Characteristics of Compressed Gases Stored in E Size Cylinders That May Be Attached to the Anesthesia Machine			
Characteristic	**Oxygen**	**Nitrous Oxide**	**Carbon Dioxide**	**Air**
Cylinder color	Green*	Blue	Gray	Yellow*
Physical state in cylinder	Gas	Liquid and gas	Liquid and gas	Gas
Cylinder contents (L)	625	1590	1590	625
Cylinder weight empty (kg)	5.90	5.90	5.90	5.90
Cylinder weight full (kg)	6.76	8.80	8.90	
Cylinder pressure full (psi)	2000	750	838	1800

*The World Health Organization specifies that cylinders containing oxygen for medical use be painted white, but manufacturers in the United States use green. Likewise, the international color for air is white and black, whereas cylinders in the United States are color-coded yellow.

reduces the possibility that leaks in the apparatus proximal to oxygen inflow can diminish the delivered oxygen concentration, whereas leaks distal to that point result in loss of volume without a qualitative change in the mixture. Nevertheless, an oxygen flowmeter tube leak can produce a hypoxic mixture regardless of the flowmeter tube arrangement (Fig. 15-4).[3] Indeed, flowmeter tube leaks are a hazard reflecting the fragile construction of this component of the anesthesia machine. Subtle cracks may be overlooked and result in errors in delivered flow.

Gases mix in the manifold and flow to an outlet port on the anesthesia machine, where they are directed into either a vaporizer or an anesthetic breathing system (see Fig. 15-3).[2] For emergency purposes, provision is made for delivery of a large volume of oxygen (35 to 75 L/min) to the outlet port through an oxygen flush valve that bypasses the flowmeters and manifold. The oxygen flush valve allows direct communication between the oxygen high-pressure circuit and the low-pressure circuit (see Fig. 15-3).[2] Activation of the oxygen flush valve during a mechanically delivered inspiration from the anesthesia machine ventilator permits the transmission of high airway pressure to the patient's lungs, with the possibility of barotrauma.

VAPORIZERS

Volatile anesthetics are liquids at room temperature and atmospheric pressure. Vaporization, which is the conversion of a liquid to a vapor, takes place in a closed container, referred to as a vaporizer. The vapor concentration resulting from vaporization of a volatile liquid anesthetic must be delivered to the patient with the same accuracy and predictability as other gases (nitrous oxide, oxygen).

Physics of Vaporization

The molecules that make up a liquid are in constant random motion. In a vaporizer containing a volatile liquid anesthetic, there is an asymmetric arrangement of intermolecular

forces applied to the molecules at the liquid-oxygen interface. The result of this asymmetric arrangement is a net attractive force pulling the surface molecules into the liquid phase. This force must be overcome if surface molecules are to enter the gas phase, where their relatively sparse density constitutes a vapor. The energy necessary for molecules to escape from the liquid is supplied as heat. The heat of vaporization of a liquid is the number of calories required at a specific temperature to convert 1 g of a liquid into a vapor. The heat of vaporization necessary for molecules to leave the liquid phase is greater when the temperature of the liquid decreases.

Vaporization in the closed confines of a vaporizer ceases when equilibrium is reached between the liquid and vapor phases such that the number of molecules leaving the liquid phase is the same as the number re-entering. The molecules in the vapor phase collide with each other and the walls of the container, thereby creating pressure. This pressure is termed vapor pressure and is unique for each volatile anesthetic. Furthermore, vapor pressure is temperature dependent such that a decrease in the temperature of the liquid is associated with a lower vapor pressure and fewer molecules in the vapor phase. Cooling of the liquid anesthetic reflects a loss of heat (heat of vaporization) necessary to provide energy for vaporization. This cooling is undesirable because it lowers the vapor pressure and limits the attainable vapor concentration.

Vaporizer Classification and Design

Vaporizers are classified as agent-specific, variable-bypass, flow-over, temperature-compensated (equipped with an automatic temperature-compensating device that helps maintain a constant vaporizer output over a wide range of temperatures), and out-of-circuit vaporizers (Fig. 15-5).[1] These contemporary vaporizers are unsuitable for the controlled vaporization of desflurane, which has a vapor pressure near 1 atm (664 mm Hg) at 20°C. For this reason, a desflurane vaporizer is electrically heated to 23°C to 25°C and pressurized with a backpressure regulator to 1500 mm Hg to create an environment in which the anesthetic has relatively lower, but predictable volatility.

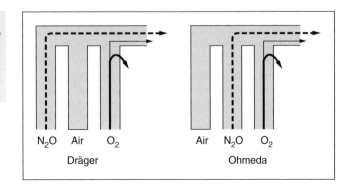

Figure 15-4 Oxygen flow tube leak. An oxygen flow tube leak can produce a hypoxic mixture regardless of the flow tube arrangement (From Brockwell RC. Inhaled anesthetic delivery systems. *In* Miller RD [ed]: Miller's Anesthesia, 6th ed. Philadelphia: Churchill Livingstone, 2005, with permission.)

III

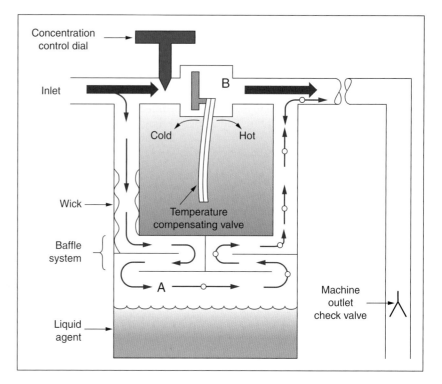

Figure 15-5 Schematic diagram of the agent-specific Ohmeda Tec vaporizer. Counterclockwise rotation of the concentration control dial diverts a portion of the total fresh gas flow through the vaporizing chamber (A), where wicks saturated with liquid anesthetic ensure a large gas-liquid interface for efficient vaporization. A temperature-compensating valve diverts more or less fresh gas flow through the vaporizing chamber to offset the effects of changes in temperature on the vapor pressure of the liquid anesthetic (temperature-compensated vaporizer). Gases saturated with the vapor of the liquid anesthetic join gases that have passed through the bypass chamber (B) for delivery to the machine outlet check valve. When the concentration control dial is in the off position, no fresh gas inflow enters the vaporizing chamber. (From Brockwell RC, Andrews JJ. Delivery systems for inhaled anesthetics. *In* Barash PG, Cullen BF, Stoelting RK [eds]: Clinical Anesthesia. Philadelphia: Lippincott Williams & Wilkins, 2006, pp 557-594, with permission.)

Variable bypass describes dividing (splitting) the total fresh gas flow through the vaporizer into two portions. The first portion of the fresh gas flow (20% or less) passes into the vaporizing chamber of the vaporizer, where it becomes saturated (flow-over) with the vapor of the liquid anesthetic. The second portion of the fresh gas flow passes through the bypass chamber of the vaporizer. Both portions of the fresh gas flow mix at the patient outlet side of the anesthesia machine. The proportion of fresh gas flow diverted through the vaporizing chamber, and thus the concentration of volatile anesthetic delivered to the patient, is determined by the concentration control dial. The scale on the concentration control dial is in volume percent for the specific anesthetic drug. A temperature-sensitive bimetallic strip or an expansion element influences proportioning of total gas flow between the vaporizing and bypass chambers as the vaporizer temperature changes (temperature compensated) (see Fig. 15-5).[1] For example, as the temperature of the liquid anesthetic in the vaporizer chamber decreases, the temperature-sensing elements allow increased gas inflow into this chamber to offset the effect of decreased anesthetic liquid vapor pressure.

Vaporizers are often constructed of metals with high thermal conductivity (copper, bronze) to further minimize heat loss. As a result, vaporizer output is nearly linear between 20°C and 35°C.[3] Designation of vaporizers as agent specific and out of circuit emphasizes that these devices are calibrated to accommodate a single volatile anesthetic and are isolated from the anesthetic breathing system.

Tipping of vaporizers can cause liquid anesthetic to spill from the vaporizing chamber into the bypass chamber with a resultant increased vapor concentration exiting from the vaporizer. Nevertheless, the likelihood of tipping is minimized because vaporizers are secured to the anesthesia machine and there is little need to move them. Leaks associated with vaporizers are most often due to a loose filler cap.

Commonly, two to three agent-specific vaporizers are present on the anesthesia machine. A safety interlock mechanism ensures that only one vaporizer at a time can be turned on. Turning on a vaporizer requires depression of a release button on the concentration dial, followed by counterclockwise rotation of the dial. This prevents accidental movement of the dial from the off to the on position. The location of the filler port on the lower portion of the vaporizer minimizes the likelihood of overfilling of the vaporizing chamber (>125 mL) with liquid anesthetic. A window near the filler port permits visual verification of the level of liquid anesthetic in the vaporizing chamber. Use of an agent-specific keyed filler device prevents placement of a liquid anesthetic into the vaporizing chamber that is different from the drug for which the vaporizer was calibrated. This is uniquely important for desflurane because its vapor pressure is near 1 atm and accidental placement of desflurane in a contemporary vaporizer could result in an anesthetic overdose.[4] As with anesthesia machines, periodic maintenance (usually every 12 months) is recommended by the manufacturers of vaporizers.

ANESTHETIC BREATHING SYSTEMS

The function of anesthetic breathing systems is to deliver oxygen and anesthetic gases to the patient and to eliminate carbon dioxide. Conceptually, the anesthetic breathing system is a tubular extension of the patient's upper airway. Anesthetic breathing systems can add considerable resistance to inhalation because peak flows as high as 60 L/min are reached during spontaneous inspiration. This resistance is influenced by unidirectional valves and connectors. The components of the breathing system, particularly the tracheal tube connector, should have the largest possible lumen to minimize this resistance to breathing. Right-angle connectors should be replaced with curved connectors to minimize resistance. Substituting controlled ventilation of the patient's lungs for spontaneous breathing can offset the increased resistance to inhalation imparted by anesthetic breathing systems.

Anesthetic breathing systems are classified as open, semiopen, semiclosed, and closed according to the presence or absence of (1) a gas reservoir bag in the circuit, (2) rebreathing of exhaled gases, (3) means to chemically neutralize exhaled carbon dioxide, and (4) unidirectional valves (Table 15-3). The most commonly used anesthetic breathing systems are the (1) Mapleson F (Jackson-Rees) system, (2) Bain circuit, and (3) circle system.

Mapleson Breathing Systems

In 1954, Mapleson analyzed and described five different arrangements of fresh gas inflow tubing, reservoir tubing, facemask, reservoir bag, and an expiratory valve to administer anesthetic gases (Fig. 15-6).[5] These five different semiopen anesthetic breathing systems are designated Mapleson A to E. The Mapleson F system, which is a Jackson-Rees modification of the Mapleson D system, was added later. The Bain circuit is a modification of the Mapleson D system (Fig. 15-7).[6]

FLOW CHARACTERISTICS
The Mapleson systems are characterized by the absence of valves to direct gases to or from the patient and the absence of chemical carbon dioxide neutralization. Because there is no clear separation of inspired and expired gases, rebreathing occurs when inspiratory flow exceeds the fresh gas flow. The composition of the inspired mixture depends on how much rebreathing takes place. The amount of rebreathing associated with each system is highly dependent

Table 15–3 Classification of Anesthetic Breathing Systems

System	Gas Reservoir Bag	Rebreathing of Exhaled Gases	Chemical Neutralization of Carbon Dioxide	Unidirectional Valves	Fresh Gas Inflow Rate*
Open					
Insufflation	No	No	No	None	Unknown
Open drop	No	No	No	None	Unknown
Semiopen					
Mapleson A, B, C, D	Yes	No†	No	One	High
Bain	Yes	No†	No	One	High
Mapleson E	No	No†	No	None	High
Mapleson F (Jackson-Rees)	Yes	No†	No	One	High
Semiclosed					
Circle	Yes	Partial	Yes	Three	Moderate
Closed					
Circle	Yes	Total	Yes	Three	Low

*High, greater than 6 L/min; moderate, 3 to 6 L/min; low, 0.3 to 0.5 L/min.
†No rebreathing of exhaled gases only when fresh gas inflow is adequate.

Figure 15-6 Anesthetic breathing systems classified as semiopen Mapleson **A** through **F**. FGF, fresh gas flow. (Modified from Willis BA, Pender JW, Mapleson WW. Rebreathing in a T-piece: Volunteer and theoretical studies of Jackson-Rees modification of Ayre's T-piece during spontaneous respiration. Br J Anaesth 1975;47:1239-1246, with permission.)

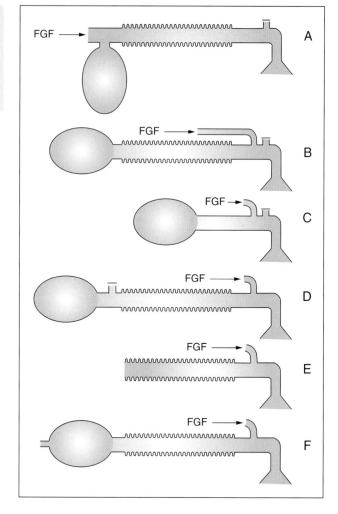

Figure 15-7 Schematic diagram of the Bain system showing fresh gas flow (FGF) entering a narrow tube within the larger corrugated expiratory limb (A). The only valve in the system (B) is an adjustable pressure-limiting (overflow) valve located near the FGF inlet and reservoir bag (C). (Modified from Bain JA, Spoerel WE. A streamlined anaesthetic system. Can Anaesth Soc J 1972;19:426-435, with permission.)

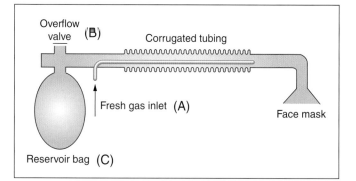

on the fresh gas flow rate. The optimal fresh gas flow may be difficult to determine. It is necessary to adjust the fresh gas flow when changing from spontaneous and controlled ventilation. Monitoring end-tidal CO_2 is the best method to determine the optimal fresh gas flow. The performance of these circuits is best understood by studying the gas disposition at end exhalation during spontaneous and controlled ventilation (Fig. 15-8).[7]

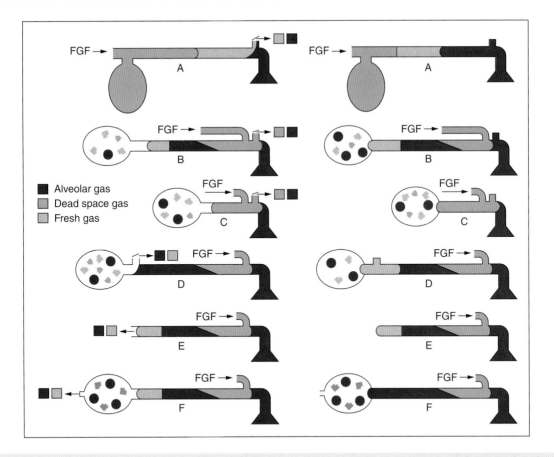

Figure 15-8 Gas disposition at end exhalation during spontaneous ventilation (*left*) or controlled ventilation (*right*) of the lungs in semiopen Mapleson **A** through **F** anesthetic breathing systems. The relative efficiency of different Mapleson systems for preventing rebreathing during spontaneous ventilation is **A > DF > C > B**. The relative efficiency of different Mapleson systems for preventing rebreathing during controlled ventilation is **DF > B > C > A**. FGF, fresh gas flow. (Modified from Sykes MK. Rebreathing circuits. A review. Br J Anaesth 1968;40:666-674, with permission.)

Mapleson F (Jackson-Rees) System

The Mapleson F (Jackson-Rees) system is a T-piece arrangement with a reservoir bag and an adjustable pressure-limiting overflow valve on the distal end of the gas reservoir bag (see Fig. 15-6).[5] The degree of rebreathing when using this anesthetic breathing system is influenced by the method of ventilation (spontaneous versus controlled) and adjustment of the pressure-limiting overflow valve (venting). Fresh gas flow equal to two to three times the patient's minute ventilation is recommended to prevent rebreathing of exhaled gases.

FLOW CHARACTERISTICS

During spontaneous ventilation, exhaled gases pass down the expiratory limb and mix with fresh gases (see Fig. 15-8).[7] The expiratory pause allows the fresh gas to push the exhaled gases down the expiratory limb. With the next inspiration, the inhaled gas mixture comes from the fresh gas flow and from the expiratory limb, including the reservoir bag.

CLINICAL USES

The Mapleson F system is commonly used for controlled ventilation during transport of intubated patients. It is also popular for pediatric anesthesia because it has minimal dead space and offers minimal resistance because there are no moving parts except the pressure-limiting overflow valve. The Mapleson F system may be used for both spontaneous and controlled ventilation. It is inexpensive, can be used with a facemask or endotracheal tube, is lightweight, and can be repositioned easily. Pollution of the atmosphere with anesthetic gases when using this system can be decreased by adapting it to scavenging systems.

DISADVANTAGES

Disadvantages of the Mapleson F system include (1) the need for high fresh gas inflow to prevent rebreathing, (2) the possibility of high airway pressure and barotrauma should the overflow valve become occluded, and (3) the lack of humidification. Lack of humidification can be offset by allowing the fresh gas to pass through an in-line heated humidifier.

Bain System

The Bain circuit is a coaxial version of the Mapleson D system in which the fresh gas supply tube runs coaxially inside the corrugated expiratory tubing (see Fig. 15-7).[6] The fresh gas tube enters the circuit near the reservoir bag, but the fresh gas is actually delivered at the patient end of the circuit. The exhaled gases are vented through the overflow valve near the reservoir bag. The Bain circuit may be used for both spontaneous and controlled ventilation. Prevention of rebreathing during spontaneous ventilation requires a fresh gas flow of 200 to 300 mL/kg/min and a flow of only 70 mL/kg/min during controlled ventilation.

ADVANTAGES

Advantages of the Bain circuit include (1) warming of the fresh gas inflow by the surrounding exhaled gases in the corrugated expiratory tube, (2) conservation of moisture as a result of partial rebreathing, and (3) ease of scavenging waste anesthetic gases from the overflow valve. It is lightweight, easily sterilized, and reusable. It is useful when access to the patient is limited, such as during head and neck surgery.

DISADVANTAGES

Hazards of the Bain circuit include unrecognized disconnection or kinking of the inner fresh gas tube. The outer expiratory tube should be transparent to allow inspection of the inner tube.

Circle System

The circle system is the most popular anesthetic breathing system in the United States. It is so named because its essential components are arranged in a circular manner (Fig. 15-9).[3] The circle system prevents rebreathing of carbon dioxide by chemical neutralization of carbon dioxide with carbon dioxide absorbents.

CLASSIFICATION

A circle system can be classified as semiopen, semiclosed, or closed, depending on the amount of fresh gas inflow (see Table 15-3). In a semiopen system, very high fresh gas flow is used to eliminate rebreathing of gases. A semiclosed system is associated with rebreathing of gases and is the most commonly used breathing system in the United States. In a closed system, the inflow gas exactly matches that being consumed by the patient. As a result of rebreathing of exhaled gases in the semiclosed and closed circle systems, there is (1) some conservation of airway moisture and body heat and (2) decreased pollution of the surrounding atmosphere with anesthetic gases when the fresh gas inflow rate is set at less than the patient's minute ventilation.

DISADVANTAGES

Disadvantages of the circle system include (1) increased resistance to breathing because of the presence of unidirec-

Figure 15-9 Schematic diagram of the components of a circle absorption anesthetic breathing system. Rotation of the bag/vent selector switch permits substitution of an anesthesia machine ventilator (V) for the reservoir bag (B). The volume of the reservoir bag is determined by the fresh gas inflow and adjustment of the adjustable pressure-limiting (APL) valve. (From Brockwell RC, Andrews JJ. Delivery systems for inhaled anesthetics. *In* Barash PG, Cullen BF, Stoelting RK [eds]: Clinical Anesthesia. Philadelphia: Lippincott Williams & Wilkins, 2006, pp 557-594, with permission.)

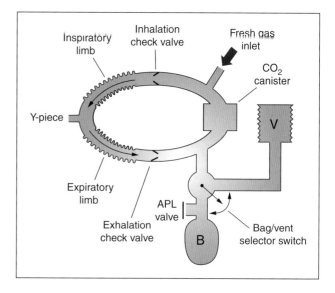

tional valves and carbon dioxide absorbent, (2) bulkiness with loss of portability, and (3) enhanced opportunity for malfunction because of the complexity of the apparatus.

IMPACT OF REBREATHING

Rebreathing of exhaled gases in a semiclosed circle system influences the inhaled anesthetic concentrations of these gases. For example, when uptake of the anesthetic gas is high, as during induction of anesthesia, rebreathing of exhaled gases depleted of anesthetic greatly dilutes the concentration of anesthetic in the fresh gas inflow. This dilutional effect of uptake is offset clinically by increasing the delivered concentration of anesthetic. As uptake of anesthetic diminishes, the impact of dilution on the inspired concentration produced by rebreathing of exhaled gases is lessened.

COMPONENTS

The circle system consists of (1) a fresh gas inlet, (2) inspiratory and expiratory unidirectional valves, (3) inspiratory and expiratory corrugated tubing, (4) a Y-piece connector, (5) an adjustable pressure-limiting (APL) valve, also referred to as an overflow or "pop-off" valve, (6) a reservoir bag, (7) a canister containing carbon dioxide absorbent, (8) a bag/vent selector switch, and (9) a mechanical anesthesia ventilator (see Fig. 15-9).[3]

Fresh Gas Inlet and Unidirectional Valves

Fresh gas enters the circle system through a connection from the common gas outlet of the anesthesia machine. Two unidirectional valves are situated in different limbs of the corrugated tubing such that one functions for inhalation and the other for exhalation. These valves (1) permit positive-pressure breathing and (2) prevent the rebreathing of exhaled gases until they have passed through the carbon dioxide absorbent canister and have had their oxygen content replenished. Rebreathing and hypercapnia can occur if the unidirectional valves stick in the open position, and total occlusion of the circuit can occur if they are stuck in the closed position. If the expiratory valve is stuck in the closed position, breath stacking and barotrauma can occur. If the unidirectional valves are functioning properly, the only dead space in the circle system is between the Y-piece and the patient.

Corrugated Tubing

The inspiratory and expiratory corrugated tubes serve as conduits for delivery of gases to and from the patient. Their large bore provides minimal resistance, and the corrugations provide flexibility, resist kinking, and promote turbulent instead of laminar flow. During positive-pressure ventilation, some of the delivered gas distends the corrugated tubing and some is compressed within the circuit, which leads to a smaller delivered tidal volume.

Y-Piece Connector

A Y-piece connector at the patient end of the circuit has (1) a curved elbow, (2) an outer diameter of 22 mm to fit inside a facemask, and (3) an inner diameter of 15 mm to fit onto an endotracheal tube connector.

Adjustable Pressure-Limiting Valve

When the "bag/vent" selector switch is set to "bag," the APL (overflow or "pop-off") valve (1) allows venting of excess gas from the breathing system into the waste gas scavenging system and (2) can be adjusted to allow the anesthesiologist to provide assisted or controlled ventilation of the patient's lungs by manual compression of the gas reservoir bag. The APL valve should be fully open during spontaneous ventilation so that circuit pressure remains negligible throughout inspiration and expiration.

Reservoir Bag

When the "bag/vent" selector switch is set to "bag," the gas reservoir bag maintains an available reserve volume of gas to satisfy the patient's spontaneous inspiratory flow rate (up to 60 L/min), which greatly exceeds conventional fresh gas flows (commonly 3 to 5 L/min) from the anesthesia machine. The bag also serves as a safety device because its distensibility limits pressure in the breathing circuit to less than 60 cm H_2O, even when the APL valve is closed.

Closed Anesthetic Breathing System

In a closed anesthetic breathing system, there is total rebreathing of exhaled gases after absorption of carbon dioxide, and the APL valve or relief valve of the ventilator is closed. A closed system is present when the fresh gas inflow into the circle system (150 to 500 mL/min) satisfies the patient's metabolic oxygen requirements (150 to 250 mL/min during anesthesia) and replaces anesthetic gases lost by virtue of tissue uptake. If sidestream gas analyzers are used, the analyzed gas exiting the analyzer must be returned to the breathing system to maintain a closed system.

ADVANTAGES

Advantages of a closed circle anesthetic breathing system over a semiclosed circle anesthetic breathing system include (1) maximal humidification and warming of inhaled gases, (2) less pollution of the surrounding atmosphere with anesthetic gases, and (3) economy in the use of anesthetics.

DISADVANTAGES

A disadvantage of a closed circle anesthetic breathing system is an inability to rapidly change the delivered concentration of anesthetic gases and oxygen because of the low fresh gas inflow.

III

DANGERS OF CLOSED ANESTHETIC BREATHING SYSTEM

The principal dangers of a closed anesthetic breathing system are delivery of (1) unpredictable and possibly insufficient concentrations of oxygen and (2) unknown and possibly excessive concentrations of potent anesthetic gases.

Unpredictable Concentrations of Oxygen

Unpredictable and possibly insufficient delivered concentrations of oxygen when using a closed anesthetic breathing system are more likely if nitrous oxide is included in the fresh gas inflow. For example, decreased tissue uptake of nitrous oxide with time in the presence of unchanged uptake of oxygen can result in a decreased concentration of oxygen in the alveoli (Table 15-4). Therefore, the use of an oxygen analyzer placed on the inspiratory or expiratory limb of the circle system is mandatory when nitrous oxide is delivered through a closed anesthetic breathing system.

Unknown Concentrations of Potent Anesthetic Gases

Exhaled gases, devoid of carbon dioxide, form a major part of the inhaled gases when a closed anesthetic breathing system is used. This means that the composition of the inhaled gases is influenced by the concentration present in the exhaled gases. The concentration of anesthetic in exhaled gases reflects tissue uptake of anesthetic. Initially, tissue uptake is maximal, and the concentration of anesthetic

---

Table 15–4 Alveolar Gas Concentration with a Closed Circle Anesthetic Breathing System

Example 1

Gas inflow is nitrous oxide, 300 mL/min, and oxygen, 300 mL/min, for 15 minutes. Nitrous oxide uptake by tissues at the time is 200 mL/min, and oxygen consumption is 250 mL/min. Alveolar gas after tissue uptake consists of 100 mL nitrous oxide and 50 mL oxygen. The alveolar concentration of oxygen (F_{AO_2}) is

$$F_{AO_2} = 50 \text{ mL oxygen}/(100 \text{ mL nitrous oxide} + 50 \text{ mL oxygen}) \times 100 = 33\%$$

Example 2

Gas inflow as in Example 1, but the duration of administration is 1 hour. At this time, tissue uptake of nitrous oxide has decreased to 100 mL/min, but oxygen consumption remains unchanged at 250 mL/min. Alveolar gas after tissue uptake consists of 200 mL nitrous oxide and 50 mL oxygen. The alveolar concentration of oxygen (F_{AO_2}) is

$$F_{AO_2} = 50 \text{ mL oxygen}/(200 \text{ mL nitrous oxide} + 50 \text{ mL oxygen}) \times 100 = 20\%$$

---

in the exhaled gases is minimal. Subsequent rebreathing of these exhaled gases dilutes the inhaled concentration of anesthetic delivered to the patient. Therefore, high inflow concentrations of anesthetic are necessary to offset maximal tissue uptake. Conversely, only small amounts of anesthetic need to be added to the inflow gases when tissue uptake has decreased. The unknown impact of tissue uptake on the concentration of anesthetic in exhaled gases makes it difficult to estimate the inhaled concentration delivered to the patient through a closed anesthetic breathing system. This disadvantage can be partially offset by administering higher fresh gas inflow (3 L/min) for about 15 minutes before instituting the use of a closed anesthetic breathing system. This approach permits elimination of nitrogen from the lungs and corresponds to the time of greatest tissue uptake of anesthetic.

ANESTHESIA MACHINE VENTILATORS

When the "bag/vent" selector switch is set to "vent," the gas reservoir bag and APL valve are eliminated from the circle anesthetic system and the patient's ventilation is delivered from the mechanical anesthesia ventilator. Anesthesia ventilators are powered by compressed gas, electricity, or both. Most conventional anesthesia machine ventilators are pneumatically driven by oxygen or air that is pressurized and, during the inspiratory phase, routed to the space inside the ventilator casing between the compressible bellows and the rigid casing. Pressurized air or oxygen entering this space forces the bellows to empty its contents into the patient's lungs through the inspiratory limb of the breathing circuit. This pressurized air or oxygen also causes the ventilator relief valve to close, thereby preventing inspiratory anesthetic gas from escaping into the scavenging system.

Oxygen is preferable to air as the ventilator driving gas because if there is a leak in the bellows, the fraction of inspired oxygen will be increased. If there is a leak in the bellows in a ventilator driven by 50 psi oxygen or air, peak inspiratory pressures will rise. During exhalation, the driving gas is either vented into the room or directed to the scavenging system, and the bellows refills as the patient exhales. Some newer anesthesia machines have mechanically driven piston-type ventilators. The piston operates much like the plunger of a syringe to deliver the desired tidal volume or airway pressure to the patient.

Bellows

Ventilators with bellows that rise during exhalation (standing or ascending bellows) are preferred because the bellows will not rise (fill) if there is a leak in the anesthesia breathing system or the system becomes accidentally disconnected (Fig. 15-10).[8] Ventilators with bellows that descend during exhalation (hanging or descending

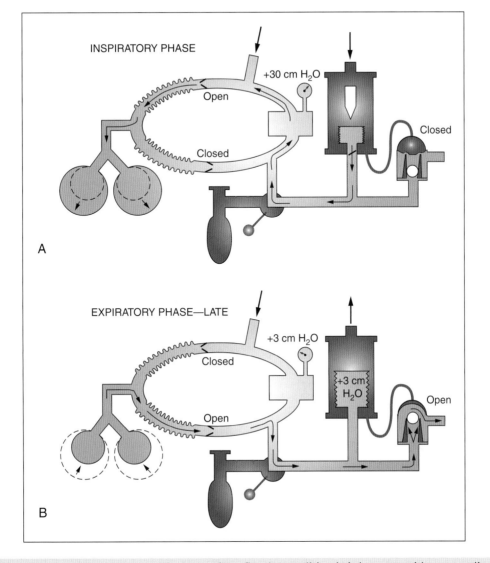

Figure 15-10 Inspiratory (**A**) and expiratory (**B**) phases of gas flow in a traditional circle system with an ascending bellows anesthesia ventilator. The bellows physically separates the driving gas circuit from the patient's gas circuit. The driving gas circuit is located outside the bellows, and the patient's gas circuit is inside the bellows. During the inspiratory phase (A), the driving gas enters the bellows chamber and causes the pressure within it to increase. This increased pressure causes the ventilator's relief valve to close, thus preventing anesthetic gas from escaping into the scavenging system, and the bellows to compress, thereby delivering the anesthetic gas within the bellows to the patient's lungs. During the expiratory phase (B), the driving gas exits the bellows chamber. The pressure within the bellows chamber and the pilot line decline to zero, which causes the mushroom portion of the ventilator's relief valve to open. Gas exhaled by the patient fills the bellows before any scavenging occurs because a weighted ball is incorporated into the base of the ventilator's relief valve. Scavenging occurs solely during the expiratory phase because the ventilator's relief valve is open only during expiration. (From Andrews JJ. The Circle System. A Collection of 30 Color Illustrations. Washington, DC: Library of Congress, 1998, with permission.)

bellows) are potentially dangerous because the bellows will continue to rise and fall during a disconnection. Whenever a ventilator is used, a disconnect alarm must be activated and audible.

Humidity and Heat Exchange in the Breathing Circuit

The upper respiratory tract (especially the nose) functions as the principal heat and moisture exchanger (HME) to bring inspired gas to body temperature and 100% relative humidity in its passage to the alveoli. Water is removed from medical gases (cylinders or piped) to prevent corrosion and condensation. Tracheal intubation or the use of a laryngeal mask airway bypasses the upper airway and thus leaves the tracheobronchial mucosa the burden of heating and humidifying inspired gases. Humidification of inspired gases by the lower respiratory tract in intubated patients can lead to dehydration of the mucosa, impaired ciliary function, impaired surfactant function, inspissation of secretions, atelectasis, and a rise in the alveolar-to-arterial gradient. Breathing of dry and room-temperature gases in intubated patients is associated with water and heat loss from the patient. Heat loss is more important than water loss, and the most important reason to provide heated humidification in intubated patients is to decrease heat loss and associated decreases in body temperature, especially in infants and children, who are rendered poikilothermic by general anesthesia.

Humidification

Humidification is a form of vaporization in which water vapor (moisture) is added to the gases delivered by the anesthetic breathing system to minimize water and heat loss. The water formed and the heat generated by chemical neutralization of carbon dioxide help humidify and heat the gases in the breathing circuit. Humidifiers used for anesthesia and in the intensive care unit include (1) HME humidifiers, (2) heated water vaporizers, and (3) nebulizers.

HEAT AND MOISTURE EXCHANGER HUMIDIFIERS
HME humidifiers are devices that when placed between the endotracheal tube and Y-piece of the circle system, conserve some of the exhaled water and heat and return it to the inspired gases. They contain a porous hydrophobic or hygroscopic membrane that traps exhaled humidified gases and returns them to the patient on inspiration. Bacterial and viral filters can be incorporated in HME humidifiers to convert them into heat- and moisture-exchanging filters (HMEFs).

Advantages
The advantages of HME humidifiers over other types of humidifiers are that they are (1) simple and easy to use, (2) lightweight, (3) not dependent on an external power source, (4) disposable, and (5) low cost.

Disadvantages
The disadvantages of HME humidifiers are that they (1) are not as effective as heated water vaporizers and humidifiers in maintaining patient temperature, (2) add resistance and increase the work of breathing and therefore should be used with caution in spontaneously ventilating patients, (3) can become clogged with patient secretions or blood, and (4) can increase dead space, which can cause significant rebreathing in pediatric patients. Special low-volume HMEs are available for pediatric patients.

HEATED WATER VAPORIZERS AND HUMIDIFIERS
Heated water vaporizers and humidifiers are used to deliver a relative humidity higher than that delivered by HME humidifiers. Heated water vaporizers are more frequently used in pediatric anesthesia and intensive care unit patients. Risks associated with the use of heated water vaporizers and humidifiers include (1) thermal injury, (2) nosocomial infection, (3) increased work of breathing, and (4) increased risk of malfunction because of the complexity of these systems.

NEBULIZERS
Nebulizers produce a mist of microdroplets of water suspended in a gaseous medium. The quantity of water droplets delivered is not limited by the temperature of the carrier gas. In addition to water, nebulizers are used to deliver medications to peripheral airways.

POLLUTION OF THE ATMOSPHERE WITH ANESTHETIC GASES

There is unproven concern that chronic exposure to low concentrations of inhaled anesthetics could pose a health hazard to operating room personnel. The Occupational Safety and Health Administration (OSHA) presently has no required exposure limits regulating nitrous oxide and halogenated anesthetics. In the operating room, OSHA recommends that the concentration of nitrous oxide not exceed 25 ppm and exposure concentrations of volatile anesthetics not exceed 2 ppm. Recommendations regarding waste anesthetic gases have been made by the American Society of Anesthesiologists (Table 15-5).[9]

Control of pollution of the atmosphere with anesthetic gases requires (1) scavenging of waste anesthetic gases, (2) periodic preventive maintenance of anesthesia equipment, (3) attention to the anesthetic technique, and (4) adequate ventilation of the operating rooms.

Scavenging Systems

Scavenging is the collection and subsequent removal of vented gases from the operating room. The excess gas comes from either the APL valve if the bag/vent selector switch is set to "bag" or from the ventilator relief valve if the bag/vent selector switch is set to "vent." All excess gas from the patient exits the breathing system through these valves. In addition, when the bag/vent selector switch is set to vent, some anesthetic breathing systems direct the drive gas inside the bellows canister to the scavenging system. The amount of delivered gas used to anesthetize a patient commonly far exceeds the patient's needs. The anesthesiologist must be certain that the scavenging system

Table 15–5 Recommendations of the American Society of Anesthesiologists Task Force on Waste Anesthetic Gases

Waste anesthetic gases should be scavenged.

Appropriate work practices should be used to minimize exposure to waste anesthetic gases.

Personnel working in areas where waste anesthetic gases may be present should be educated regarding (1) current studies on the health effects of exposure to waste anesthetic gases, (2) appropriate work practices to minimize exposure, and (3) machine checkout and maintenance procedures.

There is insufficient evidence to recommend routine monitoring of trace concentrations of waste anesthetic gases in the operating room and postanesthesia care unit.

There is insufficient evidence to recommend routine medical surveillance of personnel exposed to trace concentrations of waste anesthetic gases, although each institution should have a mechanism for employees to report suspected work-related health problems.

From McGregor DG, Baden JM, Bannister C, et al. Waste anesthetic gases: Information for the management in anesthetizing areas and the postanesthesia care unit (PACU). Park Ridge, IL: American Society of Anesthesiologists, 1999.

is operational and adjusted properly to ensure adequate scavenging. If sidestream gas analyzers are used, the analyzed gas exiting the analyzer must be directed to the scavenging system or returned to the breathing system.

Scavenging systems may be characterized as active or passive. An active system is connected to the hospital's vacuum system and gases are drawn from the machine by a vacuum. A passive system is connected to the hospital's ventilation duct and waste gases flow out of the machine on their own.

Many anesthesia machines provide scavenging with a waste gas receiver mounted on the side of the anesthesia machine. Advantages of this system include (1) a needle valve that allows the clinician to manually adjust the amount of vacuum flow through the scavenging system, (2) a needle valve that can be adjusted such that the 3-L reservoir bag will be slightly inflated and appear to "breathe" with the patient, and (3) unlike other active scavenging systems, a waste gas receiver that does not require a strong vacuum to operate.

HAZARDS
Hazards of scavenging systems include (1) obstruction of the scavenging pathways, which can result in excessive positive pressure in the breathing circuit and possible

barotrauma, and (2) excessive vacuum applied to the scavenging system, which can cause negative pressures in the breathing system. Scavenging systems contain two relief valves to minimize these hazards. If gas accumulates in the scavenging system and cannot leave the anesthesia machine properly, the positive-pressure relief valve opens when the pressure reaches 10 cm H_2O to allow the gas to escape into the room. If negative pressure is applied to the scavenging system, the negative-pressure relief valve opens and allows room air to be drawn in (instead of drawing gas from the patient). Additionally, if the amount of fresh gas flow exceeds the capacity of the scavenging system, the excess waste anesthetic gas exits the scavenging system through the positive-pressure relief valve and pollutes the operating room.

Periodic Preventive Maintenance of Anesthesia Equipment

High-pressure leakage of nitrous oxide can occur as a result of faulty yolks attaching the nitrous oxide tank to the anesthesia machine or faulty connections from the central nitrous oxide gas supply to the anesthesia machine. Low-pressure leakage of anesthetic gases can occur because of leaks inside the anesthesia machine and leaks between the machine and patient. Periodic preventive maintenance of the anesthesia machine by qualified service representatives is recommended.

Anesthetic Technique

Anesthetic techniques that can lead to operating room pollution include (1) poorly fitting facemasks (2) flushing the anesthetic delivery circuit, (3) filling anesthetic vaporizers, (4) the use of uncuffed endotracheal tubes, (5) failure to turn off the nitrous oxide flow or vaporizers at the end of the anesthesia, and (6) the use of semiopen breathing circuits such as the Jackson-Rees, which are difficult to scavenge.

Adequate Room Ventilation

The air in the operating room should be exchanged at least 15 times per hour by the operating room ventilation system. This rate should be checked periodically by the hospital's clinical engineering department.

ELIMINATION OF CARBON DIOXIDE

Open and semiopen breathing systems eliminate carbon dioxide by venting all exhaled gases to the atmosphere. Semiclosed and closed breathing systems eliminate carbon dioxide by chemical neutralization. Chemical neutralization is accomplished by directing the exhaled gases through a carbon dioxide absorber, which consists of a canister (usually transparent) containing carbon dioxide absorbent

III

granules. Gas flow through the absorber during exhalation is usually from top to bottom. A space at the base of the absorber allows the collection of dust and water.

Carbon Dioxide Absorbents

SODA LIME

Soda lime granules consist of water, calcium hydroxide, and small amounts of sodium and potassium hydroxide that serve as activators (Table 15-6). Soda lime granules fragment easily and produce alkaline dust, which can lead to bronchospasm if inhaled. Silica is added to the granules to provide hardness and minimize alkaline dust formation.

Neutralization of carbon dioxide with soda lime begins with reaction of carbon dioxide with water present in the soda lime granules and the subsequent formation of carbonic acid (Table 15-7). Carbonic acid then reacts with the hydroxides present in the soda lime granules to form carbonates (with bicarbonates as intermediates), water, and heat.

The water formed from the neutralization of carbon dioxide, the water present in the soda lime granules, and the water condensed from the patient's exhaled gases leach the alkaline bases from the soda lime granules and produce a slurry containing NaOH and KOH in the bottom of the canister. These monovalent bases can be corrosive to the skin.

AMSORB PLUS®

Amsorb® was introduced in the year 2000, and an improved version, Amsorb Plus®, has replaced Amsorb® in the United States.[10] Amsorb Plus® granules consist of water, calcium hydroxide, and calcium chloride (see Table 15-6).

Table 15-7 Chemical Neutralization of Carbon Dioxide

Soda Lime

$$CO_2 + H_2O \rightarrow H_2CO_3$$

$$H_2CO_3 + 2NaOH \text{ (or KOH)} \rightarrow Na_2CO_3 \text{ (or } K_2CO_3) + 2H_2O + \text{Heat}$$

$$Na_2CO3 \text{ (or } K_2CO_3) + Ca(OH)_2 \rightarrow CaCO_3 + 2NaOH \text{ (or KOH)}$$

$$H_2CO_3 + Ca(OH)_2 \rightarrow CaCO_3 + 2H_2O + \text{Heat}$$

Amsorb Plus

$$CO_2 + H_2O \rightarrow H_2CO_3$$

$$H_2CO_3 + Ca(OH)_2 \rightarrow CaCO_3 + 2H_2O + \text{Heat}$$

Neutralization of carbon dioxide with Amsorb Plus® begins with reaction of carbon dioxide with water present in the Amsorb Plus® granules and the subsequent formation of carbonic acid (see Table 15-7). Carbonic acid then reacts with the calcium hydroxide present in the Amsorb Plus® granules to form calcium bicarbonate, carbonate, water, and heat.

Unlike soda lime, Amsorb Plus® does not contain the strong monovalent bases NaOH or KOH (see Table 15-6). Amsorb Plus® contains $CaOH_2$, and this ingredient alone minimizes the risks associated with the degradation of inhaled anesthetics. The $CaCl_2$ contained in Amsorb Plus® further minimizes these risks by acting as a humectant and thereby allowing for greater availability of water. Calcium sulfate and polyvinylpyrrolidine are added to increase hardness.

Table 15-6 Comparison of Carbon Dioxide Absorbents

	Soda Lime	Amsorb Plus®
Contents		
Ca(OH)$_2$ (%)	76-81	>80
NaOH (%)	4	0
KOH (%)	1	0
Water (%)	14-19	13-18
Remaining balance	—	CaCl$_2$
Method of hardness	Silica	Calcium sulfate and polyvinylpyrrolidine
Mesh size	4-8	4-8
Generation of compound A with sevoflurane	Yes	No
Generation of carbon monoxide with inhaled anesthetics	Yes	No
Risk of exothermic reactions and fire in the presence of sevoflurane	No	No

HEAT OF NEUTRALIZATION

The water formed by the neutralization of carbon dioxide with soda lime and Amsorb Plus® is useful for humidifying the gases and for dissipating some of the heat generated in these exothermic reactions. The heat generated during the neutralization of carbon dioxide can be detected by warmness of the canister. Failure of the canister to become warm should alert the anesthesia provider to the possibility that chemical neutralization of carbon dioxide is not taking place.

Efficiency of Carbon Dioxide Neutralization

The efficiency of carbon dioxide neutralization is influenced by the size of the carbon dioxide granules and the presence or absence of channeling in the carbon dioxide canister.

ABSORBENT GRANULE SIZE

The optimal absorbent granule size represents a compromise between absorptive efficiency and resistance to airflow through the carbon dioxide absorbent canister. Absorbent efficiency increases as absorbent granule size decreases because the total surface area coming in contact with carbon dioxide increases. The smaller the absorbent granules, however, the smaller the interstices through which gas must flow and the greater the resistance to flow.

Absorbent granule size is designated as mesh size, which refers to the number of openings per linear inch in a sieve through which the granular particles can pass. The granular size of carbon dioxide absorbents in anesthesia practice is between 4 and 8 mesh, a size at which absorbent efficiency is maximal with minimal resistance. A 4-mesh screen means that there are four quarter-inch openings per linear inch. An 8-mesh screen has eight eighth-inch openings per linear inch.

CHANNELING

Channeling is the preferential passage of exhaled gases through the carbon dioxide absorber canister via pathways of low resistance such that the bulk of the carbon dioxide absorbent granules are bypassed. Channeling resulting from loose packing of absorbent granules can be minimized by gently shaking the canister before use to ensure firm packing of the absorbent granules. Carbon dioxide absorbent canisters are designed to facilitate uniform dispersion of exhaled gas flow through the absorbent granules.

ABSORPTIVE CAPACITY

Absorptive capacity is determined by the maximum amount of carbon dioxide that can be absorbed by 100 g of carbon dioxide absorbent. Channeling of exhaled gases through the absorbent granules can substantially decrease their efficiency. Carbon dioxide absorber canister design also influences the absorptive capacity of the carbon dioxide absorbent.

INDICATORS

Carbon dioxide absorbents contain a pH-sensitive indicator dye that changes color when the carbon dioxide absorbent granules are exhausted. When the absorptive components of the granules are exhausted, carbonic acid accumulates and produces a change in the pH and thus in the indicator dye color.

Soda lime contains the indicator dye ethyl violet, which changes granule color from white to purple when exhausted. Over time, exhausted granules may revert to their original white color even though absorptive capacity does not recover with time. On reuse, the dye quickly produces the purple color change again. Amsorb Plus® contains an indicator dye that changes granule color from white to purple when exhausted and, once changed, does not revert to its original color.

Degradation of Inhaled Anesthetics

Desiccated soda lime may degrade sevoflurane, isoflurane, enflurane, and desflurane to carbon monoxide. Soda lime, either moist and containing a normal water complement or dry, degrades sevoflurane and halothane to unsaturated nephrotoxic compounds (compound A). In contrast, Amsorb Plus®, either desiccated or moist, does not degrade inhaled anesthetics.

GENERATION OF CARBON MONOXIDE

Degradation of inhaled anesthetics by desiccated soda lime can lead to significant concentrations of carbon monoxide that can produce carboxyhemoglobin concentrations reaching 30% or higher.[11] Production of carbon monoxide and carboxyhemoglobin increases with (1) the inhaled anesthetic used (desflurane = enflurane > isoflurane >> halothane = sevoflurane), (2) low fresh gas flows, (3) higher concentrations of inhaled anesthetics, (4) higher absorbent temperatures, and (5) dry absorbent.

GENERATION OF COMPOUND A

Degradation of sevoflurane by soda lime can result in the production of compound A, which is a dose-dependent nephrotoxin in rats.[12] Compound A is toxic to humans exposed to the greatest concentrations clinically achievable if these concentrations are applied in excess of more than 4 to 6 hours. Production of compound A with soda lime increases with (1) low fresh gas flows, (2) higher concentrations of sevoflurane, (3) higher absorbent temperatures, and (4) absorbent desiccation.

DESICCATION

Desiccation of soda lime increases the degradation of inhaled anesthetics. The retrograde flow (from bottom to top) of fresh gas through the carbon dioxide absorber can desiccate the absorbent. This may be affected by a number of factors, including (1) the design of the anesthesia breathing system, (2) the presence or absence of a breathing reservoir bag, (3) whether the APL valve is open or closed, (4) the relative resistance through the components of the breathing circuit, (5) the fresh gas flow rate, (6) the inspiratory-to-expiratory ratio, (7) the use of HMEs, and (8) scavenger suction. With conventional breathing system design, removing the breathing bag, opening the APL valve, and occluding the Y-piece all enhance retrograde flow and desiccation of the carbon dioxide absorbent. For example, without a patient attached to the conventional circle system, a fresh gas flow rate of 5 L/min or higher through the carbon dioxide absorbent can cause desiccation of the absorbent, particularly if a breathing bag is absent from the breathing circuit. Absence of the breathing bag facilitates retrograde flow through the circle system because the inspiratory valve produces some resistance to flow and thus causes fresh gas flow to take the retrograde path of least resistance (bottom to top) through the carbon dioxide absorbent and out the breathing bag terminal, which does not have a breathing bag attached. Desiccation requires a prolonged period (usually 48 hours) of retrograde gas flow. Accordingly, most instances of increased blood concentrations of carboxyhemoglobin occur in patients anesthetized on a Monday after continuous flow of oxygen (flowmeter accidentally left on) through the carbon dioxide absorbent over the weekend.

FIRE AND EXTREME HEAT IN THE BREATHING SYSTEM

Desiccation of the carbon dioxide absorbent Baralyme (no longer clinically available) can lead to fire within the circle system with sevoflurane use.[13] A poorly characterized chemical reaction between sevoflurane and Baralyme can produce sufficient heat and combustible degradation products to lead to the spontaneous generation of fires within the carbon dioxide absorber canister and breathing circuit. Cases of extreme heat without fire associated with desiccated soda lime have been reported in Europe. To avoid this problem, anesthesiologists should make every effort to not use desiccated carbon dioxide absorbents.

RECOMMENDATIONS REGARDING SAFE USE OF CARBON DIOXIDE ABSORBENTS

The Anesthesia Patient Safety Foundation has published suggested steps regarding the selection of carbon dioxide absorbents and steps to take should desiccation of the carbon dioxide absorbent be a potential risk (Table 15-8).[14]

CHECKING ANESTHESIA MACHINE AND CIRCLE SYSTEM FUNCTION

The Food and Drug Administration checkout procedures apply only to conventional anesthesia machines (Table 15-9).[15] Because checkout procedures for newer anesthesia machines vary, the user must refer to the operator's manual for special checkout procedures and precautions. An understanding of the anesthesia machine used is mandatory for the anesthesiologist to practice safe anesthesia.

Table 15–8 Consensus Statement and Recommendations of the Anesthesia Patient Safety Foundation (APSF) Task Force on Carbon Dioxide Absorbent Desiccation

The APSF recommends the use of carbon dioxide absorbents whose composition is such that exposure to volatile anesthetics does not result in significant degradation of the volatile anesthetic.

The APSF further recommends that there should be institutional, hospital, and/or departmental policies regarding steps to prevent desiccation of carbon dioxide absorbent should they choose conventional carbon dioxide absorbents that may degrade volatile anesthetics when absorbent desiccation occurs.

When absorbents are used that may degrade volatile anesthetics, conference attendees generally agreed that users could take the following steps, consistent with ECRI recommendations:

   1. Turn off all gas flow when the machine is not in use.

   2. Change the absorbent regularly, on Monday morning for instance.

   3. Change absorbent whenever the color change indicates exhaustion.

   4. Change all absorbent, not just one canister in a two-canister system.

   5. Change the absorbent when uncertain of the state of hydration, such as if fresh gas flow has been left on for an extensive or indeterminate period.

   6. If compact canisters are used, consider changing them more frequently.

From Olympio MA. Carbon dioxide absorbent desiccation safety conference convened by APSF. Anesthesia Patient Safety Foundation Newsletter. Summer 2005, pp 25-29 (www.apsf.org).

Table 15-9 Anesthesia Apparatus Checkout Recommendations, 1993

This checkout, or a reasonable equivalent, should be conducted before the administration of anesthesia. These recommendations are valid only for an anesthesia system that conforms to current and relevant standards and includes an ascending bellows ventilator and at least the following monitors: capnograph, pulse oximeter, oxygen analyzer, respiratory volume monitor (spirometer), and breathing system pressure monitor with high- and low-pressure alarms. This is a guideline that users are encouraged to modify to accommodate differences in equipment design and variations in local clinical practice. Such local modifications should undergo appropriate peer review. Users should refer to the operator's manual for the manufacturer's specific procedures and precautions, especially the manufacturer's low-pressure leak test (step 5).

Emergency Ventilation Equipment

*1. **Verify that backup ventilation equipment is available and functioning.**

High-Pressure System

*2. **Check the oxygen cylinder supply.**
   a. Open the O_2 cylinder and verify that it is at least half full (about 1000 psi).
   b. Close the cylinder.

*3. **Check the central pipeline supplies.**
   a. Check that hoses are connected and pipeline gauges read about 50 psi.

Low-Pressure System

*4. **Check the initial status of the low-pressure system.**
   a. Close the flow control valves and turn the vaporizers off.
   b. Check the fill level and tighten the vaporizers' filler caps.

*5. **Perform a leak check of the machine's low-pressure system.**
   a. Verify that the machine master switch and flow control valves are turned off.
   b. Attach a "suction bulb" to the common fresh gas outlet.
   c. Squeeze the bulb repeatedly until fully collapsed.
   d. Verify that the bulb stays fully collapsed for at least 10 seconds.
   e. Open one vaporizer at a time and repeat steps c and d as above.
   f. Remove the suction bulb and reconnect the fresh gas hose.

*6. **Turn on the machine master switch and all other necessary electrical equipment.**

*7. **Test the flowmeters.**
   a. Adjust the flow of all gases through their full range and check for smooth operation of floats and undamaged flow tubes.
   b. Attempt to create a hypoxic O_2/N_2O mixture and verify correct changes in flow and/or alarm.

Scavenging System

*8. **Adjust and check the scavenging system.**
   a. Ensure proper connections between the scavenging system and both the APL (pop-off) valve and the ventilator relief valve.
   b. Adjust the waste gas vacuum (if possible).
   c. Fully open the APL valve and occlude the Y-piece.
   d. With minimum O_2 flow, allow the scavenger reservoir bag to collapse completely and verify that the absorber pressure gauge reads about zero.
   e. With the O_2 flush activated, allow the scavenger reservoir bag to distend fully, and then verify that the absorber pressure gauge reads <10 cm H_2O.

Breathing System

*9. **Calibrate the O_2 monitor.**
   a. Ensure that the monitor reads 21% in room air.
   b. Verify that the low-O_2 alarm is enabled and functioning.
   c. Reinstall the sensor in the circuit and flush the breathing system with O_2.
   d. Verify that the monitor now reads greater than 90%.

Continued

Table 15–9   Anesthesia Apparatus Checkout Recommendations, 1993—cont'd

10. **Check the initial status of the breathing system.**
    a. Set the selector switch to "bag" mode.
    b. Check that the breathing circuit is complete, undamaged, and unobstructed.
    c. Verify that adequate CO_2 absorbent is present.
    d. Install the breathing circuit accessory equipment (e.g., humidifier, PEEP valve) to be used during the procedure.

11. **Perform a leak check of the breathing system.**
    a. Set all gas flows to zero (or minimum).
    b. Close the APL (pop-off) valve and occlude the Y-piece.
    c. Pressurize the breathing system to about 30 cm H_2O with an O_2 flush.
    d. Ensure that the pressure remains fixed for at least 10 seconds.
    e. Open the APL (pop-off) valve and ensure that the pressure decreases.

Manual and Automatic Ventilation Systems

12. **Test the ventilation systems and unidirectional valves.**
    a. Place a second breathing bag on the Y-piece.
    b. Set the appropriate ventilator parameters for the next patient.
    c. Switch to the automatic ventilation (ventilator) mode.
    d. Fill the bellows and breathing bag with an O_2 flush and then turn the ventilator ON.
    e. Set the O_2 flow to minimum and other gas flows to zero.
    f. Verify that during inspiration the bellows delivers the appropriate tidal volume and that during expiration the bellows fills completely.
    g. Set the fresh gas flow to about 5 L/min.
    h. Verify that the ventilator bellows and simulated lungs fill and empty appropriately without sustained pressure at end expiration.
    i. Check for proper action of the unidirectional valves.
    j. Exercise the breathing circuit accessories to ensure proper function.
    k. Turn the ventilator OFF and switch to the manual ventilation (bag/APL) mode.
    l. Ventilate manually and ensure inflation and deflation of the artificial lungs and appropriate feel of system resistance and compliance.
    m. Remove the second breathing bag from the Y-piece.

Monitors

13. **Check, calibrate, and/or set the alarm limits of all monitors.**
    Capnometer   Pulse oximeter
    Oxygen analyzer   Respiratory volume monitor (spirometer)
    Pressure monitor with high and low airway alarms

Final Position

14. **Check the final status of the machine.**
    a. Vaporizers off
    b. APL valve open
    c. Selector switch to "bag"
    d. All flowmeters to zero
    e. Patient suction level adequate
    f. Breathing system ready to use

*If an anesthesia provider uses the same machine in successive cases, these steps need not be repeated or may be abbreviated after the initial checkout.
APL, adjustable pressure limiting; PEEP, positive end-expiratory pressure.
From Food and Drug Administration. Anesthesia Apparatus Checkout Recommendations, Rockville, MD, 1993.

A complete anesthesia machine and circle system function checkout procedure should be performed each day before the first case (see Table 15-9, steps 1 through 14).[15] An abbreviated checkout should be performed before each subsequent use that day (see Table 15-9, steps 10 through 14).[15] The most important preoperative checks are (1) calibration of the oxygen monitor, (2) a leak check of the machine's low-pressure system, and (3) a leak check of the breathing system. It is also essential to verify backup ventilation equipment, including whether a self-inflating bag is available and functioning before rendering a patient apneic.

Calibration of the Oxygen Monitor

The oxygen monitor is the only machine safety device that detects problems downstream from the flowmeters (see Table 15-9, step 9).[15] The other machine safety devices (the fail-safe valve, the oxygen supply failure alarm, and the proportioning system) are all upstream from the flowmeters.

Leak Check of the Machine's Low-Pressure System

A leak check of the machine's low-pressure system is performed to confirm the integrity of the anesthesia machine from the flowmeters to the common gas outlet (see Table 15-9, step 5) (Fig 15-11).[15,16] It evaluates the portion of the anesthesia machine that is downstream from all safety devices, except the oxygen monitor. The low-pressure circuit is the most vulnerable part of the anesthesia machine because the components located within this area are the ones most subject to breakage and leaks. It is mandatory that the machine's low-pressure system be checked because leaks in this circuit can lead to hypoxia or patient awareness, or both.

The leak test of the low-pressure system for some anesthesia machine designs varies, and the anesthesiologist must refer to the operator's manual for instructions. Newer anesthesia machines use self-checks of the machine's low-pressure system, but internal vaporizer leaks will not be detected unless each vaporizer is turned on individually during the low-pressure system self-test.

III

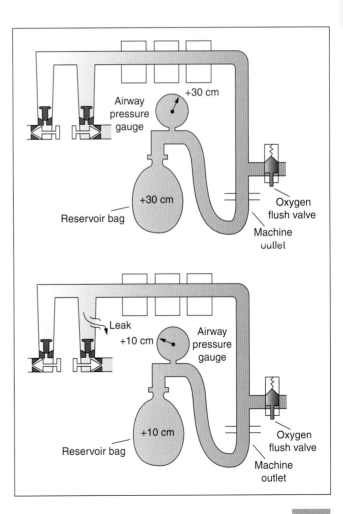

Figure 15-11 A positive-pressure leak test is performed before each case by occluding the outlet of the circle anesthesia system to create a pressure of 30 cm H_2O within the anesthetic breathing system as depicted on the airway pressure gauge. The absence of a low-pressure leak in the anesthesia machine and circle system is verified by a sustained positive pressure reading on the airway pressure gauge. Should the airway pressure gauge show decreasing pressure over 10 seconds, the anesthesiologist must perform a further machine check to determine the cause of the leak. Failure to discover the cause of the leak could jeopardize the ability to provide positive-pressure ventilation of the patient's lungs during the anesthesia. (From Andrews JJ. Understanding Anesthesia Machines. Cleveland, OH: International Anesthesia Research Society Review Course Lectures, 1988, p 78, with permission.)

Leak Check of the Breathing System

A leak check of the breathing system must be performed before every procedure (see Table 15-9, step 11).[15] This test does not check the integrity of the unidirectional valves inasmuch as the breathing system will pass the leak check even if the unidirectional valves are incompetent or stuck shut (see Table 15-9, step 12).[15]

REFERENCES

1. Brockwell RC, Andrews JJ. Delivery systems for inhaled anesthetics. *In* Barash PG, Cullen BF, Stoelting RK (eds): Clinical Anesthesia. Philadelphia: Lippincott Williams & Wilkins, 2006, pp 557-594.
2. Check-Out. A Guide for Preoperative Inspection of an Anesthetic Machine. Park Ridge, IL: American Society of Anesthesiologists, 1987, pp 1-14.
3. Brockwell RC. Inhaled anesthetic delivery systems. *In* Miller RD (ed): Miller's Anesthesia, 6th ed. Philadelphia: Churchill Livingstone, 2005.
4. Andrews JJ, Johnston RV, Kramer GC. Consequences of misfilling contemporary vaporizers with desflurane. Can J Anaesth 1993;40:71-74.
5. Willis BA, Pender JW, Mapleson WW. Rebreathing in a T-piece: Volunteer and theoretical studies of Jackson-Rees modification of Ayre's T-piece during spontaneous respiration. Br J Anaesth 1975;47:1239-1246.
6. Bain JA, Spoerel WE. A streamlined anaesthetic system. Can Anaesth Soc J 1972;19:426-435.
7. Sykes MK. Rebreathing circuits: A review. Br J Anaesth 1968;40:666-674.
8. Andrews JJ. The Circle System. A Collection of 30 Color Illustrations. Washington, DC: Library of Congress, 1998.
9. McGregor DG, Baden JM, Bannister C, et al. Waste Anesthetic Gases: Information for the Management in Anesthetizing Areas and the Postanesthesia Care Unit (PACU). Park Ridge, IL: American Society of Anesthesiologists, 1999.
10. Murray JM, Renfrew CW, Bedi A, et al. Amsorb. A new carbon dioxide absorbent for use in anesthetic breathing systems. Anesthesiology 1999;91:1342-1348.
11. Baxter PJ, Garton K, Kaharasch ED. Mechanistic aspects of carbon monoxide formation from volatile anesthetics. Anesthesiology 1998;89:929-941.
12. Kharasch ED, Frink EJ, Artru A, et al. Long-duration low-flow sevoflurane and isoflurane effects on postoperative renal and hepatic function. Anesth Analg 2001;93:1511-1520.
13. Lester M, Roth P, Eger EI. Fires from the interaction of anesthetics with desiccated absorbent. Anesth Analg 2004;99:769-774.
14. Olympio MA. Carbon dioxide absorbent desiccation safety conference convened by APSF. Anesthesia Patient Safety Foundation Newsletter. Summer 2005, pp 25-29 (www.apsf.org).
15. Anesthesia Apparatus Checkout Recommendations. Rockville, MD: Food and Drug Administration, 1993.
16. Andrews JJ. Understanding Anesthesia Machines. Cleveland, OH: International Anesthesia Research Society Review Course Lectures, 1988, p 78.

Chapter 16

AIRWAY MANAGEMENT

Robin A. Stackhouse and Andrew Infosino

Competence in airway management is a critical skill for safely administering anesthesia. Difficult or failed airway management is the major factor in anesthesia-related morbidity (dental damage, pulmonary aspiration, airway trauma, unanticipated tracheostomy, anoxic brain injury, cardiopulmonary arrest) and mortality.[1] The incidence of difficult mask ventilation (defined as an inability to maintain SpO_2 at greater than 90% or an inability to prevent/reverse the signs of inadequate ventilation) ranges from 0.09% to 5%.[2] Difficult tracheal intubation (defined as successful intubation requiring more than three attempts or taking longer than 10 minutes) occurs in 1.1% to 3.8% of patients. Failed tracheal intubation occurs at an incidence of 0.0001% to 0.02%.[3]

Competence in airway management requires (1) knowledge of the anatomy and physiology of the airway, (2) ability to assess the patient's airway for the anatomic features that correlate with difficult airway management, (3) skill with the many devices for airway management, and (4) appropriate application of the American Society of Anesthesiologists (ASA) algorithm for difficult airway management (Fig. 16-1).[1]

ANATOMY AND PHYSIOLOGY OF THE UPPER AIRWAY

Nose and Mouth

Air is warmed and humidified as it passes through the nares during normal breathing. Resistance to airflow through the nasal passages is twice that through the mouth and accounts for approximately two thirds of total airway resistance. The ophthalmic and maxillary divisions of the trigeminal nerve (cranial nerve V) provide innervation to the nasal mucosa as the anterior ethmoidal, nasopalatine, and sphenopalatine nerves (Fig. 16-2).[4]

The palatine nerves branch from the sphenopalatine ganglion to innervate the hard and soft palate. The

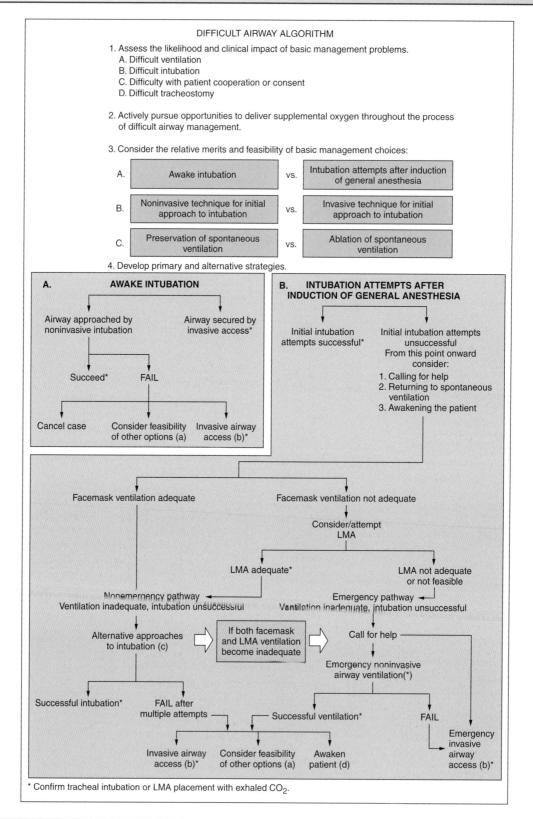

Figure 16-1 Guidelines for management of a difficult airway. LMA, laryngeal mask airway. (From Caplan RA, Benumof JL, Berry FA, et al. Practice guidelines for management of the difficult airway. Anesthesiology 2003;98:1269-1277, with permission.)

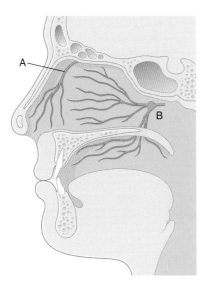

Figure 16-2 Innervation of the nasal cavity. A diagram of the lateral wall of the nasal cavity illustrates its sensory nerve supply. The anterior ethmoidal nerve, a branch of the ophthalmic division of the trigeminal nerve, supplies the anterior third of the septum and lateral wall (A). The maxillary division of the trigeminal nerve via the sphenopalatine ganglion supplies the posterior two thirds of the septum and the lateral wall (B). (From Ovassapian A. Fiberoptic Endoscopy in Anesthesia and Critical Care. New York: Raven Press, 1990, pp 57-79, with permission.)

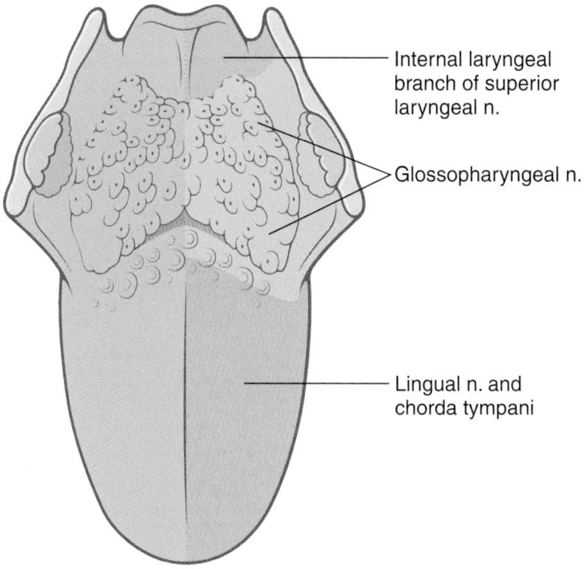

Figure 16-3 Sensory innervation of the tongue. (From Stackhouse RA. Fiberoptic airway management. Anesthesiol Clin North Am 2002;20:933-951.)

III

mandibular division of the trigeminal nerve forms the lingual nerve, which provides sensation to the anterior two thirds of the tongue. The posterior third of the tongue, the soft palate, and the oropharynx are innervated by the glossopharyngeal nerve (cranial nerve IX) (Fig. 16-3).[5]

Pharynx

The nasal and oral cavities are connected to the larynx and esophagus by the pharynx. The pharynx is a musculo-fascial tube that can be divided into the nasopharynx, the oropharynx, and the hypopharynx. The nasopharynx is separated from the oropharynx by the soft palate. The epiglottis demarcates the border between the oropharynx and the hypopharynx. Innervation is by way of cranial nerves IX (glossopharyngeal) and X (vagus) (Figs. 16-4 and 16-5).[6] The vagus nerve provides sensation to the hypopharynx through the internal branches of the superior laryngeal nerves (see Fig. 16-5).[6]

Airway resistance may be increased by prominent lymphoid tissue in the nasopharynx. The tongue is the predominant cause of resistance in the oropharynx. Obstruc-

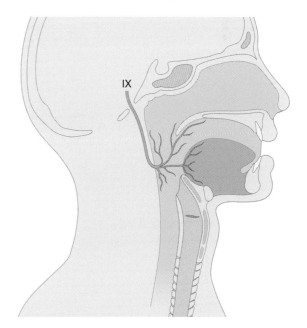

Figure 16-4 Sensory distribution of the glossopharyngeal nerve. (From Patil VU, Stehling LC, Zauder HL. Fiberoptic Endoscopy in Anesthesia. St Louis: CV Mosby, 1983.)

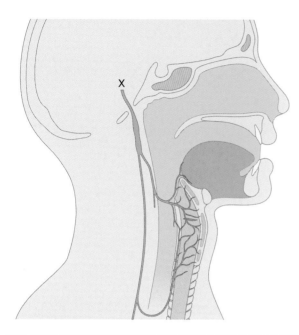

Figure 16-5 Sensory distribution of the vagus nerve. (From Patil VU, Stehling LC, Zauder HL. Fiberoptic Endoscopy in Anesthesia. St Louis: CV Mosby, 1983.)

tion by the tongue is increased by relaxation of the genioglossus muscle during anesthesia.

Larynx

The adult larynx is between the third and the sixth cervical vertebrae.[7] It functions in the modulation of sound and separates the trachea from the esophagus during swallowing. This protective mechanism, when exaggerated, becomes laryngospasm. The larynx is composed of muscles, ligaments, and cartilages (thyroid, cricoid, arytenoids, corniculates, and epiglottis). The vocal cords are formed

by the thyroarytenoid ligaments and are the narrowest portion of the adult airway. The anterior-posterior dimension of the vocal cords is approximately 23 mm in males and 17 mm in females. The vocal cords are 6 to 9 mm in the transverse plane but can expand to 12 mm. This calculates to a glottic aperture of 60 to 100 mm. An understanding of the motor and sensory innervation of the laryngeal structures is important for performing anesthesia of the upper airway (Table 16-1).

Trachea

The trachea begins at the sixth cervical vertebra and extends to the carina, which overlies the fifth thoracic vertebra. It is 10 to 15 cm long and supported by 16 to 20 horseshoe-shaped cartilages. The most cephalad cartilage, the cricoid, is the only one that has a full ring structure. It is shaped like a signet ring, wider in the cephalocaudal dimension posteriorly.

AIRWAY ASSESSMENT

History and Anatomic Examination

The patient's airway history should be evaluated to determine whether there are any medical, surgical, or anesthetic factors that have implications for airway management. Patients who have had a previous problem with airway management should have been informed of the problem, the apparent reasons for the difficulty, how tracheal intubation was accomplished, and the implication for future anesthetics. The previous anesthetic record should contain a description of the airway difficulties, what airway management techniques were used, and whether they were successful.[1] Patients with a history of difficult airway management can be registered with the Medic Alert system, which allows 24-hour-a-day access to the pertinent information.

Studies of anatomic variables and their implications for difficult airway management have shown that there is

Table 16–1	Motor and Sensory Innervation of Larynx	
Nerve	**Sensory**	**Motor**
Superior laryngeal (internal division)	Epiglottis Base of tongue Supraglottic mucosa Thyroepiglottic joint Cricothyroid joint	None
Superior laryngeal (external division)	Anterior subglottic mucosa	Cricothyroid (adductor tensor)
Recurrent laryngeal	Subglottic mucosa Muscle spindles	Thyroarytenoid Lateral cricoarytenoid Interarytenoid (adductors) Posterior cricoarytenoid (adductor)

low sensitivity, specificity, and positive predictive value for any single test (Table 16-2).[8] Correlation is better with a combination of tests. These tests are based on examination of the oropharyngeal space, neck mobility, submandibular space, and submandibular compliance. Various congenital and acquired disease states have a correlation with difficult airway management (Tables 16-3 and 16-4).

OROPHARYNGEAL SPACE

Mallampati proposed a classification system (Mallampati score) to correlate the oropharyngeal space with the ease of direct laryngoscopy and tracheal intubation.[9] With the observer at eye level, the patient holds the head in a neutral position, opens the mouth maximally, and protrudes the tongue without phonating. The airway is classified according to the visible structures (Fig. 16-6).[10]

Class I: The soft palate, fauces, uvula, and tonsillar pillars are visible.
Class II: The soft palate, fauces, and uvula are visible.
Class III: The soft palate and base of the uvula are visible.
Class IV: The soft palate is not visible.

Table 16–2 Components of the Preoperative Airway Physical Examination

Airway Examination Component	Nonreassuring Findings
Length of upper incisors	Relatively long
Relationship of the maxillary and mandibular incisors during normal jaw closure	Prominent overbite (maxillary incisors anterior to the mandibular incisors)
Relationship of the maxillary and mandibular incisors during voluntary protrusion of the mandible	Patient cannot bring the mandibular incisors anterior to (in front of) the maxillary incisors
Interincisor distance	Less than 3 cm
Visibility of the uvula	Not visible when the tongue is protruded with the patient in a sitting position (Mallampati class greater than II)
Shape of the palate	Highly arched or very narrow
Compliance of the mandibular space	Stiff, indurated, occupied by a mass, or nonresilient
Thyromental distance	Less than three fingerbreadths
Length of the neck	Short
Thickness of the neck	Thick
Range of motion of the head and neck	Patient cannot touch the tip of the chin to the chest or cannot extend the neck

Table 16–3 Congenital Syndromes Associated with Difficult Endotracheal Intubation

Syndrome	Description
Trisomy 21	Large tongue, small mouth make laryngoscopy difficult Small subglottic diameter possible Laryngospasm is common
Goldenhar (oculoauriculovertebral anomalies)	Mandibular hypoplasia and cervical spine abnormality make laryngoscopy difficult
Klippel-Feil	Neck rigidity because of cervical vertebral fusion
Pierre Robin	Small mouth, large tongue, mandibular anomaly
Treacher Collins (mandibular dysostosis)	Laryngoscopy is difficult
Turner	High likelihood of difficult tracheal intubation

Table 16–4 Pathologic States That Influence Airway Management

Pathologic State	Difficulty
Epiglottitis (infectious)	Laryngoscopy may worsen obstruction
Abscess (submandibular retropharyngeal, Ludwig's angina)	Distortion of the airway renders facemask ventilation or tracheal intubation extremely difficult
Croup, bronchitis, pneumonia	Airway irritability with a tendency for cough, laryngospasm, bronchospasm
Papillomatosis	Airway obstruction
Tetanus	Trismus renders oral tracheal intubation impossible
Traumatic foreign body	Airway obstruction
Cervical spine injury	Neck manipulation may traumatize the spinal cord
Basilar skull fracture	Nasotracheal intubation attempts may result in intracranial tube placement
Maxillary or mandibular injury	Airway obstruction, difficult facemask ventilation and tracheal intubation Cricothyroidotomy may be necessary with combined injuries
Laryngeal fracture	Airway obstruction may worsen during instrumentation Endotracheal tube may be misplaced outside the larynx and worsen the injury
Laryngeal edema (after intubation)	Irritable airway Narrowed laryngeal inlet
Soft tissue neck injury (edema, bleeding, subcutaneous emphysema)	Anatomic distortion of the upper airway Airway obstruction
Neoplastic upper airway tumors (pharynx, larynx)	Inspiratory obstruction with spontaneous ventilation
Lower airway tumors (trachea, bronchi, mediastinum)	Airway obstruction may not be relieved by tracheal intubation Lower airway is distorted
Radiation therapy	Fibrosis may distort the airway or make manipulation difficult
Inflammatory rheumatoid arthritis	Mandibular hypoplasia, temporomandibular joint arthritis, immobile cervical vertebrae, laryngeal rotation, and cricoarytenoid arthritis make tracheal intubation difficult
Ankylosing spondylitis	Fusion of the cervical spine may render direct laryngoscopy impossible
Temporomandibular joint syndrome	Severe impairment of mouth opening
Scleroderma	Tight skin and temporomandibular joint involvement make mouth opening difficult
Sarcoidosis	Airway obstruction (lymphoid tissue)
Angioedema	Obstructive swelling renders ventilation and tracheal intubation difficult
Endocrine or metabolic acromegaly	Large tongue Bony overgrowths
Diabetes mellitus	May have decreased mobility of the atlanto-occipital joint
Hypothyroidism	Large tongue and abnormal soft tissue (myxedema) make ventilation and tracheal intubation difficult
Thyromegaly	Goiter may produce extrinsic airway compression or deviation
Obesity	Upper airway obstruction with loss of consciousness Tissue mass makes successful facemask ventilation difficult

There is a correlation between the Mallampati score, what can be seen on direct laryngoscopy, and the ease of intubation. The laryngoscopic view is classified according to the Cormack and Lehane score (Fig. 16-7).[11],[12]

Grade 1: Most of the glottis is visible.
Grade 2: Only the posterior portion of the glottis is visible.
Grade 3: The epiglottis, but no part of the glottis can be seen.
Grade 4: No airway structures are visualized.

In conjunction with the Mallampati classification, the interincisor gap, the size and position of the maxillary and mandibular teeth, and the conformation of the palate should be assessed.[1] An interincisor gap of less than 3 cm correlates with difficulty achieving a line of view on direct laryngoscopy.[13] Mandibular prominence or a receding mandible also correlates with a poor laryngoscopic view. Overbite results in a reduction in the effective interincisor gap when the patient's head and neck are optimally positioned for direct laryngoscopy. Micrognathia limits the pharyngeal space (tongue positioned more posterior) and the space in which the soft tissues are going to be displaced during direct laryngoscopy. This causes the glottic structures to be anterior to the line of vision during direct laryngoscopy. Various genetic syndromes and acquired disease states limit the pharyngeal space and are difficult to assess on physical examination.

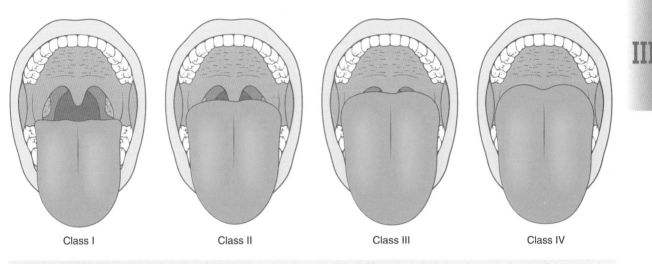

| Class I | Class II | Class III | Class IV |

Figure 16-6 Mallampati classification. (From Samsoon GLT, Young JRB. Difficult tracheal intubation: A retrospective study. Anaesthesia 1987;42:487-490, with permission.)

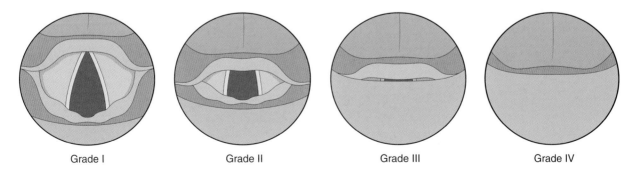

| Grade I | Grade II | Grade III | Grade IV |

Figure 16-7 Four grades of laryngoscopic view. Grade I is visualization of the entire laryngeal aperture, grade II is visualization of just the posterior portion of the laryngeal aperture, grade III is visualization of only the epiglottis, and grade IV is visualization of just the soft palate. (From Cormack RS, Lehane J. Difficult tracheal intubation in obstetrics. Anaesthesia 1984;39:1105-1111; and Williams KN, Carli F, Cormack RS. Unexpected, difficult laryngoscopy: A prospective survey in routine general surgery. Br J Anaesth 1991;66:38-44, with permission.)

III

ATLANTO-OCCIPITAL EXTENSION/NECK MOBILITY

Flexion of the neck, by elevating the head approximately 10 cm, aligns the laryngeal and pharyngeal axes. Extension of the head on the atlanto-occipital joint is important for aligning the oral and pharyngeal axes to obtain a line of vision during direct laryngoscopy (Fig. 16-8). These maneuvers place the head in the "sniffing" position and bring the three axes into optimal alignment. Atlanto-

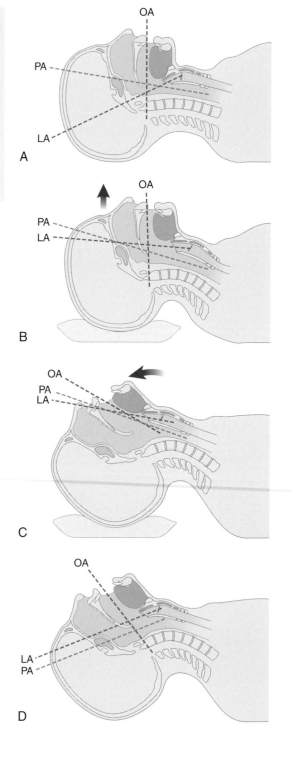

Figure 16-8 Schematic diagram showing alignment of the oral axis (OA), pharyngeal axis (PA), and laryngeal axis (LA) in four different head positions. Each head position is accompanied by an *inset* that magnifies the upper airway (the oral cavity, pharynx, and larynx) and superimposes, as a variously bent *bold dotted line*, the continuity of these three axes with the upper airway. **A,** The head is in a neutral position with a marked degree of nonalignment of the OA, PA, and LA. **B,** The head is resting on a large pad that flexes the neck on the chest and the LA with the PA. **C,** The head is resting on a pad (which flexes the neck on the chest) with concomitant extension of the head on the neck, which brings all three axes into alignment (sniffing position). **D,** Extension of the head on the neck without concomitant elevation of the head.

occipital extension is quantified by the angle traversed by the occlusal surface of the maxillary teeth when the head is fully extended from the neutral position. More than 30% limitation of atlanto-occipital joint extension from a norm of 35 degrees is associated with an increased incidence of difficult tracheal intubation.

THYROMENTAL/STERNOMENTAL DISTANCE

A thyromental distance (mentum to thyroid cartilage) less than 6 to 7 cm correlates with a poor laryngoscopic view. This is typically seen in patients with a receding mandible or a short neck. It creates a more acute angle between the oral and pharyngeal axes and limits the ability to bring them into alignment. This distance is often estimated in fingerbreadths. Three ordinary fingerbreadths approximates this distance. If the sternomental distance is used, it should measure more than 12.5 to 13.5 cm.

SUBMANDIBULAR COMPLIANCE

The submandibular space is the area into which the soft tissues of the pharynx must be displaced to obtain a line of vision during direct laryngoscopy. Anything that limits the size of this space or compliance of the tissue will decrease the amount of anterior displacement that can be achieved. Ludwig's angina, tumors, radiation scarring, burns, and previous neck surgery are conditions that can decrease submandibular compliance.

BODY HABITUS

Obesity has been associated with an increased incidence of difficult airway management. Proper positioning, with a wedge-shaped bolster behind the patient's back, results in a more optimal sniffing position. However, the problems of decreased functional residual capacity (FRC) with subsequent decreased time to arterial oxygen desaturation and more difficult mask ventilation secondary to decreased compliance still persist.

Cricothyroid Membrane and Cricothyrotomy

When routine airway management techniques have failed, the end point of the ASA difficult airway algorithm is to attain airway control by emergency invasive access (see Fig. 16-1).[1] The devices that are available for these emergency techniques are designed for accessing the airway through the cricothyroid membrane (cricothyrotomy). The cricothyroid membrane can be identified by first locating the thyroid cartilage and then sliding the fingers down the neck to the membrane, which lies just below. Alternatively, in patients who do not have a prominent thyroid cartilage, identification of the cricoid cartilage can be achieved by beginning palpation of the neck at the sternal notch and sliding the fingers up the neck until a cartilage that is wider and higher (cricoid cartilage) than those below is felt.

AIRWAY MANAGEMENT TECHNIQUES

Ventilation with a Facemask

Much attention has focused on devices to obviate the problem of difficult tracheal intubation. Failure to place an endotracheal tube is not the actual cause of the severe adverse outcomes related to difficult airway management. The primary problem is an inability to oxygenate, ventilate, prevent aspiration, or a combination of these factors. Prospectively identifying patients at risk for difficult facemask ventilation, ensuring the ability to ventilate the patient's lungs before administering longer-acting anesthetics and neuromuscular blocking drugs, and developing proficient facemask ventilation skills are critical to the practice of anesthesia.

PREDICTORS OF DIFFICULT FACEMASK VENTILATION

Independent variables associated with difficult facemask ventilation are (1) age older than 55 years, (2) a body mass index greater than 26 kg/m^2, (3) a beard, (4) lack of teeth, and (5) a history of snoring.[2] Advancing age, obesity, and snoring are indicators that there will be decreased compliance and increased resistance during facemask ventilation. An appropriately sized facemask and oral and nasal airways may help mitigate these factors. A beard or lack of teeth may result in an inability to develop adequate positive pressure from the anesthesia breathing circuit. With the caveat that the patient's dentures are well adhered, allowing the teeth to be left in during induction of anesthesia may be advantageous. An oral airway will often give enough structure to the oral tissues to allow facemask ventilation in edentulous patients.

FACEMASK CHARACTERISTICS

Facemasks are available in a variety of sizes. Clear masks have the benefit of allowing visualization of fogging, skin color, and signs of regurgitation. The facemask should fit over the bridge of the nose with the upper border aligned with the pupils. The sides should seal just lateral to the nasolabial folds, and the bottom of the facemask should seat between the lower lip and the chin. Most facemasks come with a hooked rim around the 22-mm orifice that attaches to the anesthesia breathing circuit. This rim allows straps to be used to hold the facemask in place when a patient is breathing spontaneously.

TECHNIQUE

The facemask is held to the patient's face with the fingers of the anesthesiologist's left hand lifting the mandible (chin lift, jaw thrust) to the facemask. Pressure on the submandibular soft tissue should be avoided because it can cause airway obstruction. The anesthesiologist's left thumb and index figure apply counterpressure on the facemask. Displacement of the mandible, atlanto-occipital joint extension, chin lift, and jaw thrust combine to maximize the pharyngeal space. Differential application of pressure with individual fingers can improve the seal attained of the facemask. The anesthesiologist's right hand is used to generate positive pressure by compressing the reservoir bag of the anesthesia breathing circuit. Ventilating pressure should be less than 20 cm H_2O to avoid insufflation of the stomach.

In instances in which the airway cannot be maintained with only one hand on the facemask, a two- or three-handed facemask technique can be used (Fig. 16-9). If not trained in airway management, the assistant can help by squeezing the reservoir bag while the anesthesiologist uses the right hand to mirror the hand position of the left and improve the facemask seal. When the second person is skilled in

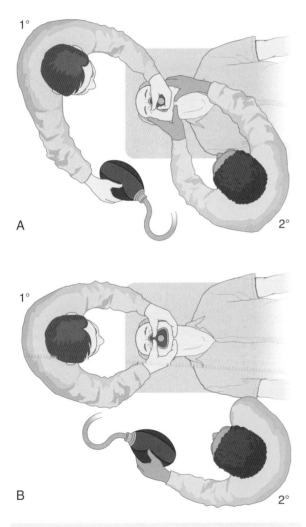

Figure 16-9 Optimal facemask ventilation. **A,** Two-person effort when the second person knows how to perform a jaw thrust. **B,** Two-person effort when the second person can only squeeze the reservoir bag. (From Benumof J. Airway Management Principles and Practice. St. Louis: Mosby-Year Book, 1996, pp 143-156.)

airway management, the anesthesiologist maintains the standard hand position and the assistant uses both hands to generate an optimal seal.

AIRWAY ADJUNCTS

Airway adjuncts should be used if it is difficult to generate sufficient positive pressure for adequate ventilation with the anesthesia breathing circuit. Oral and nasal airways are designed to create an air passage by displacing the tongue from the posterior pharyngeal wall. Aligning the airway with the patient's profile and approximating the anatomic path that it will take can be used to estimate the appropriate size. The distal tip of the airway should be at the angle of the mandible when the proximal end is just anterior to the mouth (oral airway) or the nose (nasal airway). An oral airway may generate a gag reflex or cause laryngospasm in an awake or lightly anesthetized patient. Nasal airways are better tolerated at lighter planes of anesthesia. However, nasal airways are relatively contraindicated in patients with coagulation or platelet abnormalities and those with basilar skull fractures.

Endotracheal Intubation

Endotracheal intubation may be considered in every patient receiving general anesthesia (Table 16-5). Orotracheal intubation by direct laryngoscopy in anesthetized patients is routinely chosen unless specific circumstances dictate a different approach. Equipment and drugs used for tracheal intubation include a properly sized endotracheal tube, laryngoscope, functioning suction catheter, appropriate anesthetic drugs, and equipment for providing positive-pressure ventilation of the lungs with oxygen.

Elevation of the patient's head 8 to 10 cm with pads under the occiput (shoulders remaining on the table) and extension of the head at the atlanto-occipital joint serve to align the oral, pharyngeal, and laryngeal axes such that the passage and line of vision from the lips to the glottic opening are most nearly a straight line. The height of the operating table should be adjusted so that the patient's face is near the level of the standing anesthesiologist's xiphoid

Table 16–5 Indications for Endotracheal Intubation
Provide a patent airway
Prevent inhalation (aspiration) of gastric contents
Need for frequent suctioning
Facilitate positive-pressure ventilation of the lungs
Operative position other than supine
Operative site near or involving the upper airway
Airway maintenance by mask difficult

cartilage. If not opened by extension of the head, the patient's mouth may be manually opened by counter pressure of the right thumb on the mandibular teeth and right index finger on the maxillary teeth. Simultaneously, the patient's lower lip can be rolled away with the anesthesiologist's left index finger to prevent bruising by the laryngoscope blade.

CRICOID PRESSURE

Cricoid pressure (Sellick's maneuver) is applied by an assistant exerting downward external pressure with the thumb and index finger on the cricoid cartilage to displace the cartilaginous cricothyroid ring posteriorly and thus compress the underlying esophagus against the cervical vertebrae (Fig. 16-10). Conceptually, this maneuver should prevent spillage of gastric contents into the pharynx during the period from induction of anesthesia (unconsciousness) to successful placement of a cuffed tracheal tube. It is difficult to precisely judge the magnitude of downward external pressure (about 5 kg is recommended) that needs to be exerted on the cricoid cartilage to reliably occlude the esophagus. Furthermore, stimulation of the pharynx, as by external pressure on the cricoid cartilage, may evoke an upper airway reflex characterized by a decrease in lower esophageal sphincter pressure, which could favor the passage of gastric contents into the esophagus.[14] For this reason, it may be recommended that cricoid pressure be applied before the induction of anesthesia in selected patients. Although the application of cricoid pressure is often performed, it is important to recognize that aspiration has occurred during such application and data supporting the efficacy of cricoid pressure are not available.[15] Furthermore, downward external pressure on the cricoid cartilage may displace the esophagus laterally rather than resulting in compression of it by the esophagus.

USE OF THE LARYNGOSCOPE

The laryngoscope consists of a battery-containing handle to which blades with a light (bulb or fiberoptic) may be attached and removed interchangeably (Fig. 16-11). The laryngoscope is held in the anesthesiologist's left hand near the junction between the handle and blade of the laryngoscope. The blade is then inserted in the right side of the patient's mouth so that the incisor teeth are avoided and the tongue is deflected to the left, away from the lumen of the blade. Pressure on the teeth or gums must be avoided as the blade is advanced forward and centrally toward the epiglottis. The anesthesiologist's wrist is held rigid as the laryngoscope is lifted along the axis of the handle to cause anterior displacement of the soft tissues and bring the laryngeal structures into view. The handle should not be rotated as it is lifted to prevent using the patient's upper teeth or gums as a fulcrum with the blade of the laryngoscope as a lever.

Curved (Macintosh) Blade

The tip of the curved blade is advanced into the space between the base of the tongue and the pharyngeal surface of the epiglottis (Fig. 16-12A). Forward and upward movement of the blade exerted along the axis of the laryngoscope handle stretches the hyoepiglottic ligament, elevates the epiglottis, and exposes the glottic opening.

Straight (Miller) Blade

The tip of the straight blade is passed beneath the laryngeal surface of the epiglottis (see Fig. 6-12B). Forward and upward movement of the blade exerted along

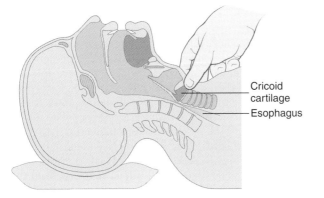

Figure 16-10 Cricoid pressure is provided by an assistant exerting downward pressure with the thumb and index finger on the cricoid cartilage (approximately 5-kg pressure) so that the cartilaginous cricothyroid ring is displaced posteriorly and the esophagus is thus compressed (occluded) against the underlying cervical vertebrae.

Cricoid cartilage
Esophagus

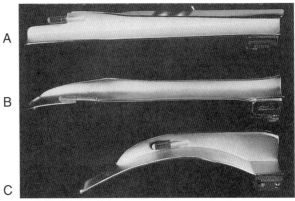

Figure 16-11 Examples of detachable laryngoscope blades that can be used interchangeably on the same handle, including a straight blade (**A**), a straight blade with a curved distal tip (**B**), and a curved blade (**C**).

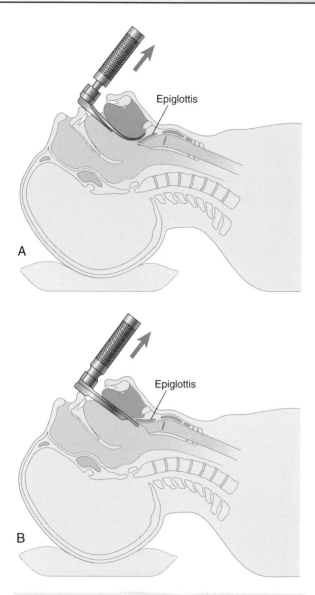

Figure 16-12 Schematic diagram depicting the proper position of the laryngoscope blade for exposure of the glottic opening. **A,** The distal end of the curved blade is advanced into the space between the base of the tongue and the pharyngeal surface of the epiglottis. **B,** The distal end of the straight blade is advanced beneath the laryngeal surface of the epiglottis. Regardless of blade design, forward and upward movement exerted along the axis of the laryngoscope handle, as denoted by the *arrows*, serves to elevate the epiglottis and expose the glottic opening.

the axis of the laryngoscope handle directly elevates the epiglottis to expose the glottic opening. Depression or lateral movement of the patient's thyroid cartilage externally on the neck with the anesthesiologist's right hand may facilitate exposure of the glottic opening.

Flex Tip (Heine, CLM) Blade
This blade is similar to a Macintosh blade, but it has a hinged tip that is controlled by a lever that is triggered with the thumb of the anesthesiologist's left hand during direct laryngoscopy. The laryngoscope is inserted into the vallecula, and then the lever is deployed to increase the lift on the hyoepiglottic ligament.

CHOICE OF LARYNGOSCOPE BLADE
The choice of laryngoscope blade is often based on the personal preference of the anesthesiologist. Advantages cited for the curved blade include less trauma to teeth with more room for passage of the tracheal tube and less bruising of the epiglottis because the tip of the blade should not touch this structure. The advantage cited for the straight blade is better exposure of the glottic opening. Laryngoscope blades are numbered according to their length. A Macintosh 3 or 4 blade or a Miller 2 or 3 blade is the standard intubating blade for adult patients.

ENDOTRACHEAL TUBE SIZES
Endotracheal tube sizes are specified according to their internal diameter (ID), which is marked on each tube (Table 16-6). Tracheal tubes are available in 0.5-mm ID increments. The endotracheal tube also has lengthwise centimeter markings starting at the distal tracheal end to permit accurate determination of the length inserted past the patient's lips. Tracheal tubes are most often made of clear, inert polyvinyl chloride plastic that molds to the contour of the airway after softening on exposure to body temperature. Tracheal tube material should also be radiopaque to ascertain the position of the distal tip relative to the carina and be transparent to permit visualization of secretions or airflow as evidenced by condensation of water vapor in the lumen of the tube ("breath fogging") during exhalation.

TECHNIQUE
The endotracheal tube is held in the anesthesiologist's right hand like a pencil and introduced into the right side of the patient's mouth with the natural curve directed anteriorly. It should be advanced toward the glottis from the right side of the mouth as midline insertion usually obscures visualization of the glottic opening. The tube is advanced until the proximal end of the cuff is 1 to 2 cm past the vocal cords, which should place the distal end of the tube midway between the vocal cords and carina. At this point, the laryngoscope blade is removed from the patient's mouth. The cuff of the endotracheal tube is inflated with air to create a seal against the tracheal mucosa. This seal facilitates positive-pressure ventilation of the lungs and decreases the likelihood of aspiration of pharyngeal or gastric contents. Use of the minimum volume of air in a low-pressure high-volume cuff that prevents leaks during positive ventilation pressure (20 to 30 cm H_2O) minimizes the likelihood of mucosal ischemia

Table 16–6 Endotracheal Tube, Suction Catheter, and Stylet Size Based on Age and Weight

Age (yr)	Weight (kg)	Endotracheal Tube ID (mm)	Suction Catheter (French)	Stylet (French)
Premature	<1.5	2.5	6	6
Premature	1.5-2.5	3.0	6	6
Newborn	3.5	3.5	8	6
1	10	4.0	8	6
2-3	15	4.5	10	6
4-6	20	5.0	10	10
7-9	30	5.5	12	10
10-12	40	6.0	14	10
13-15	50	6.5	14	14
>16	>60	7.0	18	14

ID, internal diameter.

resulting from prolonged pressure on the tracheal wall. Nevertheless, there is probably no period of tracheal intubation that does not produce some laryngotracheal damage. For example, ciliary denudation has been found to occur predominantly over the tracheal rings and underlying the cuff site after only 2 hours of intubation and with tracheal wall pressure below 25 mm Hg. Distention of the small pilot balloon attached to the inflation tube leading to the cuff confirms cuff inflation. After confirmation of correct placement, the tracheal tube is secured in position with tape.

Noting the depth of insertion as determined by the centimeter markings on the tracheal tube at the upper incisor teeth or gums helps predict a midtrachea position of the distal end of the tube. Securing the orotracheal tube at the upper incisor teeth or gums at the 23-cm mark in men and the 21-cm mark in women should reliably place the distal end of the tube in the midtrachea and thus minimize the likelihood of accidental endobronchial intubation.[16] Furthermore, if a cuffed tube is properly placed in the midtrachea, the anesthesiologist can easily detect, by external palpation, cuff distention in the suprasternal notch during rapid inflation of the cuff.

ENDOTRACHEAL TUBE STYLETS

A variety of endotracheal tube stylets may be used in selected patients to facilitate endotracheal intubation.

Gum Elastic Bougie

A gum elastic bougie is a 60-cm-long, 15-French stylet with a 40-degree curve approximately 3.5 cm from the distal tip. It has been used successfully in patients with a poor laryngoscopic view. It is passed under the epiglottis and into the airway. A characteristic bumping may be felt as the bougie moves down the trachea over the tracheal cartilages.

Schroeder Stylet

The Schroeder stylet is a disposable, plastic articulating stylet that allows the angle of the endotracheal tube to be adjusted to the correct angle while performing direct laryngoscopy and tracheal intubation. It can be used for both oral and nasal intubation.

Frova Intubating Introducer

The Frova Intubating Introducer is a 65-cm stylet with a distal angulated tip and an internal channel to accommodate a stiffening stylet or allow jet ventilation. It is available in an adult and pediatric size (Fig. 16-13).[17]

Lighted Stylets

Lighted stylets (lightwands) consist of a malleable stylet with a light at the distal tip. The endotracheal tube is mounted on the stylet, and a "hockey stick" curve is placed in the distal third of the tube (Table 16-7) (Fig. 16-14).[17] The assembled device is advanced in the midline of the airway until a well-circumscribed glow is seen through the anterior surface of the neck. As the device is advanced further, the light should remain distinct as it is seen to travel down the neck and disappear under the sternal notch. A diffuse glow indicates that there is more soft tissue being transilluminated and the device is in the esophagus rather than the trachea.

Lighted stylets do not require movement of the head or neck and can be used in patients with limited mouth opening. These devices have been useful in patients with cervical spine instability, limited interincisor gap, poor

Figure 16-13 A, The Schroeder directional stylet (courtesy of Parker Medical, Englewood, CO) and **B,** the Frova Intubating Introducer (courtesy of Cook Critical Care, Bloomington, IN). (From Hagberg CA. Special devices and techniques. Anesthesiol Clin North Am 2002;20:907-932.)

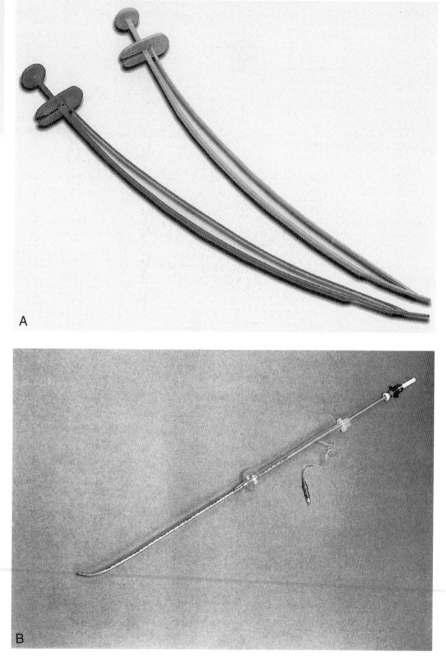

dentition, severe overbite, and facial trauma. Lighted stylets are relatively contraindicated in patients with oropharyngeal pathology (laryngeal fractures, pharyngeal masses or abscesses, foreign body) because they are passed blindly and may cause damage. There is a higher failure rate when lighted stylets are used in patients with thick necks and dark skin.[17]

Seeing Optical Stylet

The Seeing Optical Stylet (SOS) is a semimalleable, stainless steel high-resolution fiberoptic endoscope that is available in adult and pediatric sizes (Fig. 16-15).[17] The endotracheal tube is mounted on the SOS, and it is advanced through the upper airway just as a lighted stylet. The SOS offers the advantage of visualization of the airway

Table 16–7 Lighted Stylets (Lightwands) Appropriate for Each Endotracheal Tube Size

Tracheal Tube Size (ID)	Trachlight, Laerdal	Intubating Fiber Optic Stylette, Sun Medical	Fiber Optic Malleable Lighted Stylet, Anesthesia Associates
2.5	—	—	—
3.0	Infant	—	Pediatric
3.5	Infant	—	Pediatric
4.0	Infant	Pediatric	Pediatric
4.5	Child	Pediatric	Pediatric
5.0	Child	Pediatric	Adult
5.5	Child	Adult	Adult
6.0	Adult	Adult	Adult
6.5	Adult	Adult	Adult
7.0	Adult	Adult	Adult
7.5	Adult	Adult	Adult

ID, internal diameter.

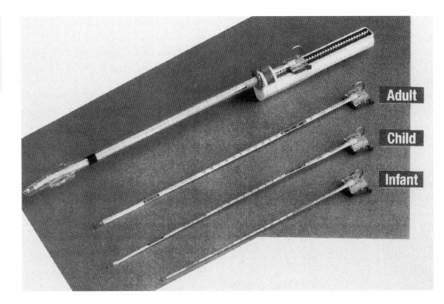

Figure 16-14 Trachlight (courtesy of Laerdal Medical Corp., Long Beach, CA). (From Hagberg CA. Special devices and techniques. Anesthesiol Clin North Am 2002;20:907-932.)

structures as it is advanced. As with any fiberoptic scope, the view is dependent on the amount of space that is present. Maneuvers that increase the pharyngeal space (chin lift, jaw thrust, tongue traction) improve the field of view when using the SOS. The adult-size SOS requires a 5.5 mm ID endotracheal tube or larger. The pediatric-size SOS can be used with endotracheal tubes 3.0 to 5.0 mm ID. The SOS does not require head or neck movement or a large interincisor gap.

CONFIRMATION OF ENDOTRACHEAL INTUBATION

Confirmation of placement of the tube in the trachea rather than the esophagus is verified by clinical assessment and identification of carbon dioxide in the patient's exhaled tidal volume. The immediate and sustained presence of carbon dioxide in the exhaled gases from the tracheal tube as detected by capnography (end-tidal P_{CO_2} >30 mm Hg for three to five consecutive breaths) is the most reliable confirmatory sign of tracheal placement of the tube.

Figure 16-15 Seeing Optical Stylet system (courtesy of Clarus Medical, Minneapolis, MN).

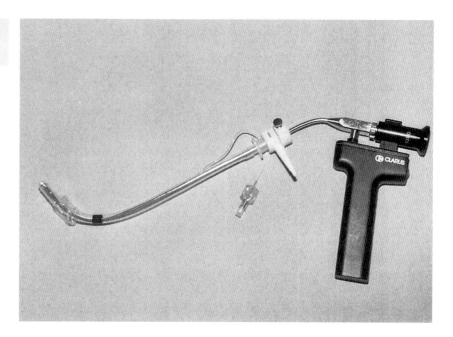

Carbon dioxide will not be persistently present in exhaled gases from a tube accidentally placed in the esophagus.

Symmetric bilateral movement of the chest with manual compression of the reservoir bag on the anesthesia breathing circuit combined with the presence of bilateral breath sounds on apical or midaxillary auscultation of the lungs (or both) is commonly confirmed after tracheal intubation. A characteristic feel of the reservoir bag, associated with normal lung compliance during manual inflation of the lungs and the presence of expiratory refilling of the bag, is evaluated. Condensation of water in the tube lumen (breath fogging) during exhalation is evidence of tracheal placement of the tube. Progressive decreases in arterial hemoglobin oxygen saturation as evident on the pulse oximeter may alert the anesthesiologist to a previously unrecognized esophageal intubation.

Fiberoptic Endotracheal Intubation

INDICATIONS
Fiberoptic endotracheal intubation is most frequently chosen when it is anticipated or known that a patient's trachea will be difficult to intubate by direct laryngoscopy. It is ideally suited to these situations because the technique can be performed before inducing general anesthesia, thus eliminating the risk of failed tracheal intubation and failed ventilation in anesthetized patients.

Fiberoptic endotracheal intubation is recommended for patients with unstable cervical spines. The technique does not require movement of the patient's neck, and it can be performed before induction of general anesthesia, thereby allowing for evaluation of the patient's neurologic function after tracheal intubation and surgical positioning.

Patients who have sustained an injury to the upper airway from either blunt or penetrating trauma are at risk for the endotracheal tube creating a false passage by exiting the airway through the disrupted tissue during direct laryngoscopy. By performing a fiberoptic intubation, not only can the injury be assessed, but the tracheal tube can also be placed beyond the level of the injury and thus eliminate the risk of causing subcutaneous emphysema, which could compress and further compromise the airway.

CONTRAINDICATIONS
An absolute contraindication to fiberoptic endotracheal intubation is a lack of time. The technique requires time to set up the equipment and prepare the patient's airway for tracheal intubation. Therefore, if immediate airway management is required, another technique should be used.

A number of circumstances make fiberoptic endotracheal intubation relatively contraindicated because the chance of success is diminished or it poses certain risks for the patient. Because the field of vision through a fiberoptic bronchoscope (laryngoscope) depends on the presence of space around the scope, anything that impinges on upper airway size (edema of the pharynx or tongue, infection, hematoma, infiltrating masses) will make tracheal intubation more difficult. Inflating the cuff of the endotracheal tube to hold the pharyngeal walls open may be helpful. Blood and secretions easily soil the optics of a fiberoptic bronchoscope. An inability to keep the tip clean will result in failure. Administering an antisialagogue to the patient before initiating fiberoptic intubation, suctioning, and maintaining the pharyngeal space can minimize soiling. Another relative contraindication to fiberoptic intubation is the presence of a pharyngeal abscess, which could be disrupted as the endotracheal tube is advanced and result in aspiration of purulent material.

TECHNIQUE

Fiberoptic tracheal intubation may be performed through an oral or nasal approach, with the patient awake or anesthetized. In general, the nasal route is easier because the angle of curvature of the endotracheal tube naturally approximates that of the patient's upper airway. When performing an oral fiberoptic tracheal intubation, a more anterior curvature is required, which may be accomplished by using one of the commercially available intubating oral airways. Nasal fiberoptic tracheal intubation tends to be less of a stimulus for the gag reflex. The gag reflex can be overcome with adequate topical anesthesia and local anesthetic blocks. The risk of inducing bleeding is higher when the nasal route is used, however, and therefore relatively contraindicated in patients with platelet abnormalities or coagulation disorders. Oral fiberoptic tracheal intubation is preferable in patients who have a contraindication to the vasoconstrictors required for nasal intubation (pregnant women, some patients with heart disease).

The decision to perform fiberoptic tracheal intubation in an awake versus an anesthetized patient is dependent on the risk of losing airway control. It is always safest to maintain spontaneous breathing if there is a question about the ability to manage the patient's airway.

PATIENT PREPARATION

The procedure should be explained to the patient along with assurance that the patient will be made as comfortable as possible. An antisialagogue (glycopyrrolate, 0.2 mg IV) should be administered to inhibit the formation of secretions that can obscure fiberoptic visualization. Sedation choices are numerous, but the depth of sedation should be titrated to reflect individual patient needs. Topical anesthesia and local anesthetic blocks are then administered.

Nose and Nasopharynx

The nasal mucosa must be anesthetized and vasoconstricted, which is typically done with either a 4% cocaine solution or a combination of 3% lidocaine/0.25% phenylephrine. Local anesthetic solutions can be applied on soaked cotton-tipped swabs or pledgets.

Tongue and Oropharynx

Topicalization may be achieved by aerosolized local anesthetic or by bilateral block of the glossopharyngeal nerve at the base of each anterior tonsillar pillar. Approximately 2 mL of 2% lidocaine injected at a depth of 0.5 cm is sufficient to block the glossopharyngeal nerves. Aspiration with the syringe before injecting the local anesthetic solution is necessary to ensure that the needle is not intravascular or through the tonsillar pillar.

Larynx and Trachea

Topicalization or nerve blocks may be used for the larynx and trachea. Local anesthetic may be sprayed, aerosolized, or nebulized into the airway. It should be noted that the larger particle size of a spray tends to cause it to be deposited in the pharynx, with only a small proportion reaching the trachea. Conversely, the small particle size of a nebulized spray is carried more effectively into the trachea, but also into the smaller airways, where the anesthetic is not needed and undergoes more rapid systemic absorption. Lidocaine is the preferred topical local anesthetic because of its broad therapeutic window. Benzocaine can cause methemoglobinemia even in therapeutic doses. Tetracaine has a very narrow therapeutic window, and the maximum allowable dose (1.2 mg/kg) can easily be exceeded. Cetacaine is a mixture of benzocaine and tetracaine and has the disadvantages of each local anesthetic.

Superior Laryngeal Nerve Block

Injecting local anesthetic solution bilaterally, in the vicinity of the superior laryngeal nerves where they lie between the greater cornu of the hyoid bone and the superior cornu of the thyroid cartilage as they traverse the thyrohyoid membrane to the submucosa of the piriform sinus, blocks the internal branch of the superior laryngeal nerve. The overlying skin is cleaned with alcohol or povidone-iodine (Betadine). The cornua of the hyoid bone or the thyroid cartilage may be used as a landmark. A 22- to 25-gauge needle is "walked" off the cephalad edge of the thyroid cartilage or the caudal edge of the hyoid bone, and approximately 2 mL of local anesthetic solution is injected.

Transtracheal Block

For a transtracheal block, the skin is prepared and a 20-gauge IV catheter is advanced through the cricothyroid membrane while simultaneously aspirating with an attached syringe filled with 4 mL of local anesthetic solution. When air is aspirated, the catheter is advanced into the trachea and the needle is withdrawn. The syringe is reattached to the catheter, aspiration of air is reconfirmed, and the local anesthetic solution is rapidly injected.

FIBEROPTIC LARYNGOSCOPY

Fiberoptic laryngoscopy has revolutionized the anesthesiologist's ability to safely care for patients at risk for difficult airway management and associated adverse side effects (arterial hypoxemia, hypoventilation, aspiration of gastric contents). Endotracheal tubes may be placed in the trachea with the aid of fiberoptic laryngoscopy through a nasal or oral approach in awake or sedated patients.

Nasal Fiberoptic Intubation

Nasal fiberoptic intubation involves the use of a lubricated endotracheal tube that is at least 1.5 mm larger than the diameter of the fiberoptic bronchoscope. Softening the endotracheal tube in warm water before use makes it less likely to cause mucosal trauma or submucosal tunneling. The endotracheal tube is advanced through the nose into the pharynx by aiming perpendicular to the plane of the patient's face just above the inferior border of the nasal alar rim. If resistance is met at the back of the nasopharynx, 90 degrees of counterclockwise rotation allows the endotracheal tube to pass less traumatically because the bevel then faces the posterior pharyngeal wall.

Secretions should be suctioned before inserting the fiberoptic bronchoscope through the endotracheal tube. It is essential that the fiberoptic bronchoscope exit the tip of the endotracheal tube and not the Murphy eye. The fiberoptic bronchoscope and the endotracheal tube are manipulated to bring the larynx into view, and the bronchoscope is advanced into the trachea.

Inflation of the endotracheal tube cuff during advancement of the fiberoptic bronchoscope in the pharynx serves to create an enlarged pharyngeal space. Because secretions tend to adhere to the pharyngeal walls, endotracheal tube cuff inflation also helps keep the optics of the fiberoptic bronchoscope from being obscured. The inflated cuff further aims the tip of the endotracheal tube anteriorly.

The target should always be kept in the center of the anesthesiologist's field of vision by flexion and rotation as the fiberoptic bronchoscope is slowly advanced. As the fiberoptic bronchoscope passes through the vocal cords, the tracheal rings will become visible. The scope is advanced to just above the carina, and then the endotracheal tube is threaded over the scope. Force should not be exerted if resistance is encountered when advancing the endotracheal tube because the fiberoptic bronchoscope can become kinked and result in diversion of the endotracheal tube into the esophagus and a damaged fiberoptic bronchoscope. Resistance to advancement often means that the endotracheal tube is caught on a vocal cord, which can be relieved by rotating the tracheal tube as it is gently advanced. The appropriate depth of endotracheal tube placement can be verified by observing the distance between the carina and the tip of the endotracheal tube as the fiberoptic bronchoscope is withdrawn. If there is any resistance when removing the fiberoptic bronchoscope, it is either through the Murphy eye or kinked in the pharynx. In both instances, the endotracheal tube and the scope must be withdrawn together to avoid damaging the fiberoptic bronchoscope.

Awake Oral Fiberoptic Intubation

When performing awake oral fiberoptic intubation, the patient's upper airway is anesthetized (local anesthetic topicalization and/or superior laryngeal nerve block, and transtracheal block), with nasal topicalization omitted.

Asleep Oral/Nasal Fiberoptic Intubation

Fiberoptic intubation under general anesthesia should be considered only if adequate oxygenation and ventilation can be maintained. Both nasal intubation and oral tracheal intubation are possible, and the technique can be performed with the patient breathing spontaneously or under controlled ventilation. A nasal airway can be placed and connected to the anesthesia breathing circuit with a 15-mm connector. When providing an airway in this manner, it is preferable to use an intravenous anesthetic technique because those in the room will be exposed to the anesthetic vapors if volatile anesthetics are insufflated to maintain anesthesia.

An important difference in performing fiberoptic laryngoscopy in an anesthetized patient is that the soft tissues of the pharynx, in contrast to the awake state, tend to relax and limit space for visualization with the fiberoptic bronchoscope. Using jaw thrust or a tonsil retractor, expanding the endotracheal tube cuff in the pharynx, or applying traction on the tongue may overcome this problem. It is advisable to have a second person trained in anesthesia delivery assisting when a fiberoptic intubation is performed under general anesthesia because it is difficult to maintain the patient's airway, be attentive to the monitors, and perform the fiberoptic intubation alone.

When using the nasal approach, topical anesthesia for the nasal mucosa is not required, but vasoconstriction is necessary to increase the diameter of the passage and to decrease the risk of bleeding. For the nasal or the oral approach, topical anesthesia or blocks to inhibit the reflexes of the pharynx, vocal cords, and trachea are useful because the airway reflexes are still intact and the patient may cough, develop laryngospasm, or reflux gastric contents.

The curvature of the endotracheal tube is not optimal for oral tracheal intubation, and an appropriately sized oral intubating airway serves as a more effective channel. Care must be taken to maintain the intubating airway in a midline position. Alternatively, a laryngeal mask airway (LMA) provides an excellent channel for awake oral fiberoptic intubation.

PATIL-SYRACUSE MASK

The Patil-Syracuse mask is designed with a port that will accommodate an endotracheal tube and a fiberoptic bronchoscope through a diaphragm. This device allows for spontaneous or controlled ventilation while fiberoptic nasal or oral intubation is being performed.

AINTREE AIRWAY EXCHANGE CATHETER

The Aintree catheter is an airway exchange catheter with connectors that allow ventilation with an anesthesia breathing circuit or jet ventilator. It differs from other exchange catheters by having a lumen of adequate size to accommodate a fiberoptic bronchoscope.

Rigid Fiberoptic Laryngoscopes

Rigid fiberoptic laryngoscopes include the Bullard laryngoscope, the UpsherScope, the WuScope system, and the GlideScope (Fig. 16-16A to C). These devices are all anatomically shaped, rigid fiberoptic laryngoscopes with a light source for use in patients who have conditions (limited mouth opening, inability to flex the neck) that can make traditional laryngoscopy and tracheal intubation difficult or impossible. All fiberoptic techniques are hindered if upper airway secretions obscure the optics, thus emphasizing the value of prior administration of an antisialagogue.

WUSCOPE SYSTEM

The WuScope is available in two adult sizes and consists of a three-part bivalve scope that can be disassembled for removal after tracheal intubation (see Fig. 16-16A). The laryngoscope blade is tubular, which helps generate space in the pharynx for a greater field of vision while minimizing contact of the fiberoptic system with pharyngeal secretions. It has a channel that allows instillation of medications or oxygen insufflation.

An endotracheal tube is loaded into the channel of the scope. Tracheal intubation is accomplished as with the other rigid laryngoscopes, followed by release and removal of the anterior portion of the bivalve and then removal of the posterior portion and handle by following the curvature of the airway.[17]

BULLARD LARYNGOSCOPE

The Bullard laryngoscope is available in an adult and pediatric size (see Fig. 16-16B). The fiberoptic bundles are on the posterior aspect of the blade, 26 mm from the distal tip, and create a 55-degree field of vision. This laryngoscope has an adjustable focus on the eyepiece. The laryngoscope blade contains a 3.7-mm channel for drug injection or oxygen insufflation.

The Bullard laryngoscope can be used with a battery pack handle or a fiberoptic light cable. There are several interchangeable stylets for the laryngoscope. The laryngoscope, with an endotracheal tube loaded on the stylet, is advanced in the midline of the patient's pharynx until the glottic opening is brought into view, and the endotracheal tube is then advanced under direct visualization. As a result of the stylet's position on the right side of the device, the right arytenoid cartilage may inhibit passage of the endotracheal tube. When this occurs, the laryngoscope and stylet position needs to be adjusted to better align the endotracheal tube with the patient's airway.[17]

UPSHERSCOPE

The blade of the UpsherScope has a semicircular design that serves as an endotracheal tube guide and allows for easy removal of the scope after tracheal intubation (see Fig. 16-16C). It can be used with a battery-powered handle or a fiberoptic light cable. There is an adjustable-diopter eyepiece that can be immersed during cleaning. The technique for using the UpsherScope is similar to that described for the Bullard laryngoscope.[17]

III

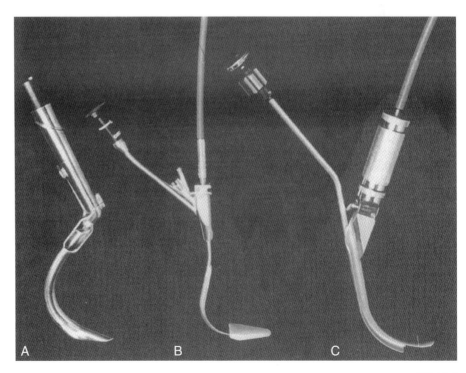

Figure 16-16 Rigid fiberoptic laryngoscopes. **A,** WuScope. **B,** Bullard laryngoscope. **C,** UpsherScope. (From Stackhouse RA, Bainton CR. Difficult airway management. *In* Hughes SC, Levinson G, Rosen MA [eds]: Shnider and Levinson's Anesthesia for Obstetrics, 4th ed. Philadelphia: Lippincott Williams & Wilkins 2001, pp 375-389.)

GLIDESCOPE

The GlideScope is an anatomically shaped, fixed-angle laryngoscope blade made of medical-grade plastic. It has a miniature fog-resistant video camera embedded in the undersurface of the blade that transmits the image to a 17.5-cm monitor screen that can be mounted on a pole. The laryngoscope blade has red and blue diodes at the tip to illuminate and provide contrast to the black and white picture produced. The system is now available with color imaging. The maximum diameter of the scope is 18 mm. As with the other rigid laryngoscopes, it does not require line of sight and can be inserted from the side or in the midline. The tip of the laryngoscope blade may be placed in the vallecula or be used to lift the epiglottis directly. An endotracheal tube with a stylet angled to mimic that of the distal tip of the GlideScope is advanced blindly until it can be visualized on the monitor, after which the tube is advanced into the trachea based on the image on the monitoring screen.

RETROGRADE TRACHEAL INTUBATION

Retrograde tracheal intubation has been used in cases of difficult airway management, particularly when there is bleeding, limited mouth opening, or neck movement. It should not be used when the patient's cricothyroid membrane is not identifiable or there is pathology of the anterior aspect of the neck (tumors, infection, stenosis) or coagulopathy.[18]

Technique

Placing the patient in the sniffing position optimizes the ability to identify the cricothyroid membrane. Kits for performing retrograde intubation are commercially available. The cricothyroid membrane is punctured with a needle while aspirating with an attached syringe. A change in resistance is felt as a pop when the needle enters the trachea and air can be aspirated. The syringe is detached and a wire is threaded through the needle in a cephalad direction and retrieved from the mouth or nose. An endotracheal tube, with or without a fiberoptic laryngoscope, is threaded over the wire until it stops on impact with the anterior wall of the trachea. Tension on the guidewire can be relaxed to allow the endotracheal tube to pass further into the trachea before removing the wire. Commercially available kits have improved this technique by adding a guiding catheter that fits over the wire and under the endotracheal tube.

BLIND NASOTRACHEAL INTUBATION

The use of blind nasotracheal intubation has decreased over the years with the introduction of other devices for difficult airway management. However, there are still clinical situations in which it can be lifesaving.

Technique

If time permits, the nasal mucosa should be anesthetized and vasoconstricted to minimize discomfort and bleeding. A 6.0- to 7.0-mm ID endotracheal tube is generally chosen for an adult. An Endotrol tube, with a pulley to adjust the angle of curvature of the tube, can facilitate blind nasotracheal intubation. The endotracheal tube is advanced through the nose and into the pharynx while listening to breath sounds at the distal end of the endotracheal tube. Alternatively, the endotracheal tube can be attached to an anesthesia breathing circuit, and reservoir bag movement and carbon dioxide can be monitored to verify that the endotracheal tube is advancing into the trachea. If tugging is seen on the anterior surface of the patient's neck, the endotracheal tube is lodging in the vallecula. When this occurs, rotating the tube to free it from the epiglottis before advancing can be advantageous. If evidence of breathing through the endotracheal tube disappears, the endotracheal tube has advanced into the esophagus because it is not traversing anterior enough to enter the trachea. When this occurs, the endotracheal tube should be withdrawn back to a depth where breathing again occurs through the endotracheal tube. If a standard endotracheal tube has been used, the cuff can be inflated with air to lift it off the posterior pharyngeal wall. The endotracheal tube is then advanced until slight resistance is felt, the cuff is deflated, and then the tube is advanced further into the trachea.

SUPRAGLOTTIC AIRWAY DEVICES

Classic Laryngeal Mask Airway

The LMA has become an invaluable supraglottic airway device for routine and difficult airway management. Factors related to difficult tracheal intubation on direct laryngoscopy do not correlate with those that make LMA placement difficult. Therefore, the incidence of experiencing difficulty with both endotracheal intubation and LMA placement is very low.[19] The ASA guidelines for management of a difficult airway include the use of an LMA.[1] The difficult airway algorithm shifts back to the non-emergency pathway if an adequate airway and ventilation can be established with an LMA.

An LMA consists of a 12-mm ID flexible shaft connected to a silicone rubber mask that seals with the airway in the hypopharynx (Fig. 16-17). The distal tip of the cuff should be against the upper esophageal sphincter (cricopharyngeus muscle), the lateral edges rest in the piriform sinuses, and the proximal end seats under the base of the tongue. LMA size selection is determined by the patient's weight (Table 16-8).

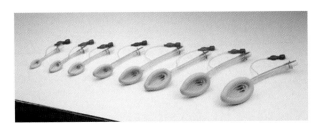

Figure 16-17 Classic laryngeal mask airways.

Table 16–8 Appropriate-Size Laryngeal Mask Airway Based on Patient Weight

LMA Size	Weight (kg)	Cuff Inflation Volume (mL of Air)
1	<5	4
1.5	5-10	7
2	10-20	10
2.5	20-30	14
3	30-50	20
4	50-70	30
5	70-100	40

LMA Fastrach

The LMA Fastrach (Intubating LMA, ILMA) was designed to obviate the problems encountered when attempting to blindly intubate the trachea through a classic LMA.[20] The ILMA consists of an anatomically shaped stainless steel tube connected to a laryngeal mask. It has an attached handle to aid insertion of the device and to facilitate optimization of its positioning to increase the likelihood of successful blind tracheal intubation through the device. A 15-mm connector allows for ventilation of the patient's lungs (Fig. 16-18).[19] The ILMA is designed to be used with silicone Euromedical endotracheal tubes (size 7.0 ID, 7.5 ID, or 8.0 ID). These tracheal tubes exit the laryngeal mask at a different angle than standard endotracheal tubes do and result in better alignment with the airway. The ILMA is advanced into the pharynx by following the natural curvature of the patient's upper airway.

TECHNIQUE

With the patient breathing oxygen, the Chandy maneuver (lift and posterior rotation) is used to optimize the position of the ILMA before attempting tracheal intubation. A lubricated endotracheal tube is inserted into the ILMA. Because Euromedical tubes have low-volume, high-pressure cuffs, it is recommended that the largest size that is appropriate for the patient be used to minimize mucosal pressure from the cuff.

Slight resistance to advancing the endotracheal tube may be felt as the horizontal marking on the tube aligns with the proximal end of the ILMA. This position marks

Figure 16-18 LMA Fastrach. (From Bogetz MS. Using the laryngeal mask airway to manage the difficult airway. Anesthesiol Clin North Am 2002;20:863-870.)

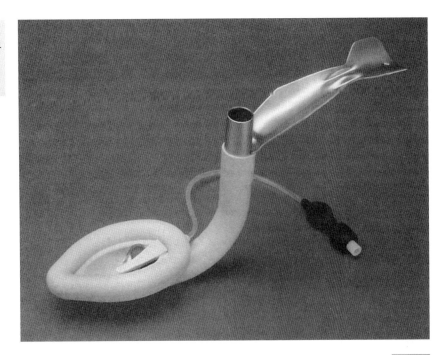

III

the depth at which the endotracheal tube impacts the epiglottic elevating bar in the bowl of the mask. The endotracheal tube should advance without resistance toward the glottic opening and the trachea. If resistance is felt beyond the point where the horizontal line passes into the ILMA, the cause depends on the depth that the tube has advanced. Immediate resistance indicates that the ILMA is too large. Resistance that is encountered 2 cm distal to the horizontal line may be secondary to a down-folded epiglottis. If the ILMA is too small, resistance is felt 3 cm distal. Resistance at 4 to 5 cm generally indicates that too large an ILMA has been selected. After verification of endotracheal intubation, the cuff of the ILMA is deflated, the 15-mm endotracheal tube connector is disconnected, and the ILMA is removed by using the stabilizer bar to push the endotracheal tube through the ILMA. The 15-mm connector is reattached to the anesthesia breathing circuit, and the patient's lungs are ventilated.

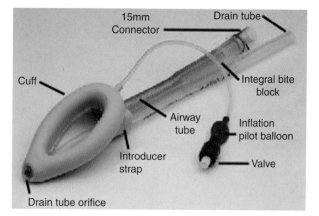

Figure 16-19 ProSeal LMA. (From Brimacombe J, Keller C: The ProSeal laryngeal mask airway. Anesthesiol Clin North Am 2002;20:871-891.)

LMA CTrach

The LMA CTrach is a modified LMA Fastrach. It has the same anatomically curved stainless steel tube and is available in three mask sizes (3, 4, and 5). The epiglottic elevating bar has been modified to allow for visualization of the larynx by means of fiberoptic bundles located within the bowl of the mask. A lightweight viewer attaches magnetically after the device has been inserted.[19] Size selection, insertion (no cricoid pressure), and ventilation are as with the LMA Fastrach. The LMA Fastrach has been demonstrated to have a high first-attempt success rate for achieving ventilation; however, there have been widely disparate reports (25% to 98%) on successful first-attempt blind tracheal intubation.[20] The LMA CTrach is intended to be more rapid and less cumbersome technically than the LMA Fastrach.

ProSeal LMA

The ProSeal LMA is a modification of the classic LMA (Fig. 16-19).[19] The cuff of the ProSeal LMA extends onto the back of the mask, which results in an improved airway seal without increasing mucosal pressure. It has a second lumen that parallels the one for the airway but opens at the distal tip of the mask to act as an esophageal vent. When optimally seated, the ProSeal LMA effectively isolates the trachea from the esophagus, thus protecting the lungs from aspiration when a minimum of 10 mL of air has been placed in the LMA cuff.[21]

Successful first-attempt placement of the ProSeal LMA varies with the insertion technique (84% with an introducer tool, 88% with digital insertion, and 100% with a bougie technique).[22] It is likely that cricoid pressure, as with the classic LMA, will interfere with proper placement of the ProSeal LMA. Specifically, cricoid pressure will prevent the LMA from seating distally at the cricopha-

ryngeus muscle because the esophagus is occluded at the level of the cricoid cartilage. The ProSeal LMA protects against aspiration only if it is optimally seated.

Esophageal-Tracheal Combitube

The Esophageal-Tracheal Combitube (ETC) is a double-lumen device that can function as either an endotracheal device or an esophageal obturator (Fig. 16-20).[23] Two sizes are available. The 37-French small adult ETC can be used in patients who are between 120 and 180 cm tall, and the 41-French ETC is for patients taller than 180 cm.

TECHNIQUE

The ETC is passed blindly while lifting the patient's mandible with the other hand. Alternatively, a laryngoscope may be used to aid insertion. Whichever technique is used, the ETC should be inserted without force (could result in esophageal tear or rupture) by following the natural curvature of the patient's upper airway. The oropharyngeal cuff is inflated first with the prefilled syringe attached to the blue pilot balloon. This seats and anchors the ETC. The distal cuff is then inflated and ventilation begun through the longer (blue) lumen, which ends in fenestrations between the two cuffs. If no breath sounds are heard, ventilation should be attempted through the other lumen.[24] If ventilation is still not detected, the tube is probably placed too deeply in the esophagus and should be pulled back and ventilation attempted through the blue lumen again.

CLINICAL USES

The ETC has been used successfully in emergency medical management and requires minimal training. Positive-pressure ventilation can be used with this device. It is recommended that airway reflexes not be intact during ETC use. The ETC protects against aspiration when

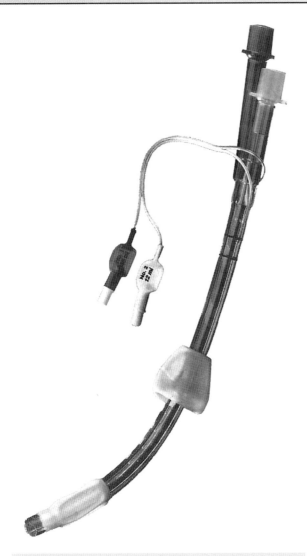

Figure 16-20 Esophageal-Tracheal Combitube. (From Gaitni LA, Vaida SJ, Agro F. The Esophageal-Tracheal Combitube. Anesthesiol Clin North Am 2002;20:893-906.)

properly positioned. This device is not intended for long-term airway management, however, and should be removed within a few hours to decrease the risk of ischemia of the tongue and subsequent edema formation.[24]

Laryngeal Tube

The laryngeal tube is a multiuse single-lumen silicone tube with a dual cuff system (a pharyngeal cuff and a blind distal esophageal cuff) (Fig. 16-21).[17] Ventilation of the patient's lungs is through a fenestration between the two cuffs. The cuffs connect to a single pilot balloon. The laryngeal tube is available in sizes 1 to 5. It is passed blindly into the pharynx.

Pharyngeal Airway Xpress

The Pharyngeal Airway Xpress is a disposable device with a rigid curved tube and a terminal end with gills that seats at the cricopharyngeus muscle (Fig. 16-22).[17] It has a high-volume, low-pressure pharyngeal cuff and is inserted blindly. The lumen is large enough to accommodate a 7.5-mm endotracheal tube if tracheal intubation is desired.

Glottic Aperture Seal Airway

The Glottic Aperture Seal Airway is a disposable single-lumen tube that forms an airway seal with a sponge-like distal tip. A plastic insertion blade lifts the epiglottis as the tube is inserted.

Cuffed Oropharyngeal Airway

The cuffed oropharyngeal airway consists of a modified conventional oral airway with a cuff at its distal end. When the cuff is inflated, it displaces the base of the patient's tongue anteriorly and passively elevates the epiglottis away from the posterior pharyngeal wall. The proximal end of a cuffed oropharyngeal airway has a standard 15-mm connector that permits attachment to the anesthetic breathing circuit.

III

TRANSTRACHEAL TECHNIQUES

Cricothyrotomy

Cricothyrotomy can be performed in less than 30 seconds and has significant advantages over transtracheal jet ventilation because it establishes a definitive airway that can be used for up to 72 hours.[9] After this period, the incidence of vocal cord dysfunction and subglottic stenosis increases. The larger diameter of a cricothyrotomy tube allows both inhalation and exhalation to occur through the device, and it does not rely on a patent native airway, as does transtracheal jet ventilation. For this reason, laryngospasm during transtracheal jet ventilation can cause the patient's lungs to become rapidly overinflated and lead to pulmonary barotrauma.

The cricothyrotomy kit should require minimal or no assembly because this technique is almost always performed under emergency circumstances. The system should be designed such that if the airway is initially identified (generally by aspiration of air through a needle), the final device cannot then be forced into another tissue plane. The Seldinger technique is ideal for avoiding this problem. The final device left in the airway should be of adequate caliber (preferably >4 mm). If the cricothyrotomy kit has a cuffed tube, pulmonary compliance is less of an issue and the airway is protected against aspiration.

Transtracheal Jet Ventilation

Commercially available products for transtracheal jet ventilation obviate the need for self-assembled products

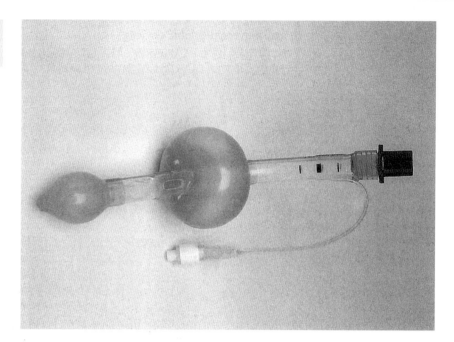

Figure 16-21 Laryngeal tube (courtesy of VBM Medizintechnik GmbH, Sulz).

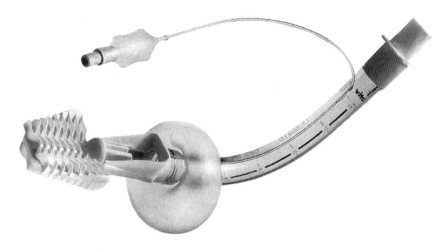

Figure 16-22 Pharyngeal Airway Xpress (courtesy of Vital Signs, Totowa, NJ).

that rely on friction connections and can easily become disconnected under high-pressure (50 psi) ventilation. The risk profile for transtracheal jet ventilation is similar to that for cricothyrotomy and includes pneumothorax, pneumomediastinum, bleeding, infection, and subcutaneous emphysema. As a result of the oxygen pressure used for transtracheal jet ventilation, these complications can become life threatening very quickly.[25] Absolute contraindications to transtracheal jet ventilation are upper airway obstruction or any disruption of the airway.

TRACHEAL EXTUBATION

Tracheal extubation after general anesthesia requires skill and judgment learned through experience. The patient must be either deeply anesthetized or fully awake at the time of tracheal extubation. Tracheal extubation during a light level of anesthesia (disconjugate gaze, breath-holding or coughing, but not responsive to command) increases the risk for laryngospasm. It should be realized that a patient reaching for the endotracheal tube might indicate a localizing response to noxious stimulation in the absence of sufficient awakening from anesthesia to follow commands.

Tracheal extubation before the return of protective airway reflexes (deep tracheal extubation) is generally associated with less coughing and attenuated hemodynamic effects on emergence. This may be preferred in patients at risk from increased intracranial or intraocular pressure, bleeding into the surgical wound, or wound dehiscence. However, previous difficult facemask ventilation or endotracheal intubation, risk of aspiration, and a surgical procedure that may have resulted in airway edema or increased airway irritability are contraindications to deep tracheal extubation.

Technique

Spontaneous ventilation breathing of pure oxygen is established before tracheal extubation. As with tracheal intubation, an FRC filled with oxygen allows for the longest safe period should breath-holding or laryngospasm occur immediately after tracheal extubation. The effects of neuromuscular blocking drugs should be fully reversed. The oropharynx is suctioned just before tracheal extubation. The endotracheal tube cuff is deflated and the tracheal tube rapidly removed from the patient's trachea and upper airway while a positive-pressure breath is delivered to help expel any secretions. The cuff should not remain deflated for any significant period before tracheal extubation because the vocal cords cannot effectively close around the endotracheal tube and supraglottic secretions can be aspirated. Timing tracheal extubation at the peak of inspiration is intended for the following exhalation or cough to eliminate any aspirated secretions from the trachea. After tracheal extubation, oxygen is delivered by facemask.

If tracheal intubation was difficult at the beginning of the procedure, awake extubation to ensure that the patient is capable of breathing spontaneously and maintaining oxygenation and ventilation is recommended. Tracheal extubation over a fiberoptic bronchoscope or an endotracheal tube exchange catheter so that immediate tracheal reintubation can be performed is also an option.

COMPLICATIONS OF TRACHEAL INTUBATION

Complications of tracheal intubation are rare and should not influence the decision to place a tracheal tube. Certainly, the benefits of a properly placed tracheal tube far exceed the risks of tracheal intubation. Complications of tracheal intubation may be categorized as those occurring (1) during direct laryngoscopy and tracheal intubation, (2) while the tracheal tube is in place, and (3) after tracheal extubation, either immediately or after a delay of several days (Table 16-9).

Complications during Direct Laryngoscopy and Tracheal Intubation

Dental trauma is the most serious and frequent type of damage related to direct laryngoscopy. It is estimated that 1 in every 4500 patients undergoing upper airway management during anesthesia sustains a dental injury that requires further treatment and/or extraction.[26] Patients at greatest risk for dental injury include those

with preexisting poor dentition and those who possess upper airway anatomy that makes direct laryngoscopy or tracheal intubation technically difficult. Use of a plastic shield placed over the patient's upper teeth and avoidance of using the laryngoscope blade as a lever on the teeth may minimize the likelihood of dental trauma. Should injury occur, prompt consultation with a dentist is often indicated. A dislodged tooth must be recovered, but if the

Table 16–9 Complications of Tracheal Intubation

During Direct Laryngoscopy and Tracheal Intubation
Dental and oral soft tissue trauma
Systemic hypertension and tachycardia
Cardiac dysrhythmias
Myocardial ischemia
Inhalation (aspiration) of gastric contents
While the Tracheal Tube Is in Place
Tracheal tube obstruction
Endobronchial intubation
Esophageal intubation
Tracheal tube cuff leak
Pulmonary barotrauma
Nasogastric distention
Accidental disconnection from the anesthesia breathing circuit
Tracheal mucosa ischemia
Accidental extubation
Immediate and Delayed Complications after Tracheal Extubation
Laryngospasm
Inhalation (aspiration) of gastric contents
Pharyngitis (sore throat)
Laryngitis
Laryngeal or subglottic edema
Laryngeal ulceration with or without granuloma formation
Tracheitis
Tracheal stenosis
Vocal cord paralysis
Arytenoid cartilage dislocation

search is unsuccessful, appropriate radiographs of the chest and abdomen should be obtained to ensure that the tooth has not passed through the glottic opening into the trachea or more distal airways.

Systemic hypertension and tachycardia frequently accompany direct laryngoscopy (regardless of the type of laryngoscope blade used) and tracheal intubation. These responses are usually transient and innocuous. In patients with preexisting systemic hypertension or ischemic heart disease, however, these changes may be exaggerated or may jeopardize the balance between myocardial oxygen requirements and delivery. In these patients, it is important to minimize the duration of direct laryngoscopy. Serious or persistent cardiac dysrhythmias during tracheal intubation are unlikely if apneic time is minimized and adequate preoxygenation and denitrogenation are performed.

Direct upper airway trauma is more likely to occur with difficult tracheal intubation because of the application of more physical force to the patient's airway than is normally applied, as well as the need for multiple attempts at intubation. The most common consequence is a chipped or broken tooth. Posterior pharyngeal and lip lacerations and bruises are more likely with difficult tracheal intubation. In extreme cases, prolonged interruption of oxygenation and ventilation may result in cardiac arrest and brain damage.

Complications While the Tracheal Tube Is in Place

Obstruction of the tracheal tube may occur as a result of inspissated secretions or kinking. The chance of endobronchial intubation can be minimized by calculating the proper endotracheal tube length for the patient and then noting the centimeter marking on the tube at the point of fixation at the patient's lips. In adults, taping the endotracheal tube at the patient's lips corresponding to the 21- to 23-cm markings on the tracheal tube usually places the distal end of the endotracheal tube in the midtrachea. Flexion of the patient's head may advance the tube up to 1.9 cm and convert a tracheal placement into an endobronchial intubation, especially in children. Conversely, extension of the head can withdraw the tube up to 1.9 cm and result in pharyngeal placement. Lateral rotation of the head moves the distal end of the tracheal tube approximately 0.7 cm.

Immediate and Delayed Complications after Tracheal Extubation

Laryngospasm and inhalation of gastric contents are the two most serious potential immediate complications after tracheal extubation. Laryngospasm is unlikely if the depth of anesthesia is sufficient during tracheal extubation (laryngeal reflexes suppressed) or the patient is allowed to awaken before tracheal extubation (laryngeal reflexes intact). A patient who is lightly anesthetized at the time of

tracheal extubation (laryngeal reflexes neither adequately suppressed nor recovered) is most at risk. If laryngospasm occurs, oxygen delivered with positive pressure through a facemask and forward displacement of the mandible with the anesthesiologist's index fingers to apply pressure at the temporomandibular joints may be sufficient treatment. Administration of succinylcholine (0.1 mg/kg IV) is indicated if laryngospasm persists.

Pharyngitis is the most frequent complaint after tracheal extubation, particularly in females, presumably because of thinner mucosal covering over the posterior vocal cords than in males. Skeletal muscle myalgia associated with the administration of succinylcholine may be manifested in the peripharyngeal muscles as postoperative "sore throat," which is often incorrectly attributed to prior tracheal intubation. Use of large (8.5 to 9.0 mm ID) versus small (6.5 to 7.0 mm ID) tracheal tubes may increase the likelihood of pharyngitis. Regardless of the mechanism, pharyngitis usually disappears spontaneously without any treatment in 48 to 72 hours. Some degree of laryngeal incompetence may be present in the first 4 to 8 hours after tracheal extubation.

The major complication of prolonged tracheal intubation (>48 hours) is damage to the tracheal mucosa, which may progress to destruction of cartilaginous rings and subsequent cicatricial scar formation and tracheal stenosis. Stenosis becomes symptomatic when the adult tracheal lumen is decreased to less than 5 mm.

AIRWAY MANAGEMENT IN INFANTS AND CHILDREN

Airway Differences between Infants and Adults

Understanding the anatomic differences between the infant airway and the adult airway is critical to proper airway management in infants and children (Table 16-10). All these differences between the infant airway and the adult airway resolve as the child grows, and usually by the time that the child is about 10 years old, the upper airway has taken on more adult-like characteristics.

Table 16–10 The Infant Airway versus the Adult Airway
Larynx positioned higher in the neck
Tongue larger relative to mouth size
Epiglottis larger, stiffer, and angled more posteriorly
Head and occiput larger relative to body size
Short neck
Narrow nares
Cricoid ring is the narrowest region

The infant larynx is located higher in the neck at the level of C3-4 than in adults, where the larynx is at the level of C4-5. This causes the tongue to shift more superiorly, closer to the palate. The tongue more easily apposes the palate, which can cause airway obstruction in situations such as the inhalation induction of anesthesia. An infant's tongue is also larger in proportion to the size of the mouth than in adults. The relatively large size of the tongue makes direct laryngoscopy more difficult and can contribute to obstruction of the upper airway during sedation, inhalation induction of anesthesia, or emergence from anesthesia. Anterior pressure on the angle of the mandible to shift the tongue to a more anterior position often solves this problem. An oral or nasal airway can also be beneficial in these situations.

The epiglottis in an infant's airway is often described as relatively larger, stiffer, and more omega shaped than an adult epiglottis. More importantly, an infant's epiglottis is typically angled in a more posterior position, thereby blocking direct visualization of the vocal cords during direct laryngoscopy. In infants and small children it is often necessary to lift the epiglottis with the tip of the blade of the laryngoscope to visualize the vocal cords and successfully intubate the trachea. This is an advantage of a straight laryngoscope blade, which often has a narrower tip than a curved laryngoscope blade does.

An infant's airway is often described as funnel shaped with a relatively large thyroid cartilage above and a relatively narrow cricoid cartilage below. The narrowest portion of an infant's airway is the cricoid cartilage, whereas the narrowest portion of an adult's airway is the vocal cords. Because the narrowest part of an infant's airway is the cricoid ring, uncuffed endotracheal tubes can successfully seal and protect the airway from aspiration if the endotracheal tube is the appropriate size when an air leak is noted around the endotracheal tube with the application of 20- to 25-cm H_2O positive pressure. Cuffed endotracheal tubes can be used in infants and children if the inflation of the cuff is carefully adjusted and monitored so that the leak pressure remains at 20 to 25 cm H_2O. If nitrous oxide is used during the anesthetic, the nitrous oxide will diffuse into the air-filled cuff increasing both its volume and the pressure transmitted to the underlying tracheal mucosa. If the leak pressure is too high with either an uncuffed endotracheal tube or a cuffed one, the tracheal mucosa will be compressed causing subglottic edema either at the level of the cricoid cartilage or below. This complication can result in postextubation croup or stridor in mild cases and tracheal stenosis in more severe cases involving prolonged tracheal intubation.

An infant's head and occiput are relatively larger than an adult's. The proper position for direct laryngoscopy and tracheal intubation in an adult is often described as the sniffing position with the head elevated and the neck flexed at C6-7 and extended at C1-2. An infant, on the other hand, requires a shoulder roll or neck roll to establish an optimal position for facemask ventilation and direct laryngoscopy. An infant's nares are relatively smaller than an adult's and can offer significant resistance to airflow and increase the work of breathing, especially when secretions, edema, or bleeding narrow them.

Managing the Normal Airway in Infants and Children

A complete history plus physical examination is the first step in managing infant and pediatric airways.

HISTORY

The history should include whether there were any problems with previous anesthetics, and previous anesthetic records should be obtained if necessary. A history of snoring should prompt additional questioning about whether the child has obstructive sleep apnea and should alert the anesthesiologist that respiratory obstruction may develop during the induction and emergence phases of anesthesia, as well as in the postoperative period especially if opioids are given for pain management.

PHYSICAL EXAMINATION

It is often difficult to perform a complete physical examination on infants and children. Asking a child to look up at the sky and then down at the floor is one way of assessing neck extension and flexion, respectively. If there are any masses, tumors, or abscesses in the neck or upper airway that compromise neck flexion, extension, or breathing function, further evaluation is important and should include computed tomography to evaluate the location and degree of any airway compromise. Children will often voluntarily open their mouths to enable determination of a Mallimpati classification. If an infant or child is uncooperative, external examination of the airway often reveals enough information to determine whether it is a normal or a potentially difficult airway. Examining the profile of an infant or child can indicate whether the thyromental distance is short and whether the patient has micrognathia or a hypoplastic mandible. Difficult airway management can be expected if the infant's chin is posterior to the upper lip. If the chin is neutral to the upper lip, the infant or child probably has a normal airway.

It is important to ask the parents and the child directly whether there are any loose teeth. If loose teeth are present, they should be identified and care taken to avoid traumatizing the tooth during direct laryngoscopy and tracheal intubation. If the tooth is very loose, it should be removed before proceeding with direct laryngoscopy to prevent the possibility of aspirating the tooth.

Preanesthetic Medication

Preanesthetic medication can facilitate separation of the infant or child from the parents before the induction of

III

anesthesia. Preanesthetic medication is not necessary in infants younger than 6 months because stranger anxiety does not usually develop until 6 to 9 months of age. Midazolam can be administered in small doses and titrated to effect if the infant or child has an intravenous catheter in place. If the child does not have an intravenous catheter in place, midazolam syrup can be given orally (2 mg/mL) in a dose of about 0.5 mg/kg up to a maximum dose of about 20 mg. If the child is uncooperative with taking oral midazolam and preanesthetic medication is essential, midazolam can also be given intranasally, intramuscularly, or rectally. One approach to minimizing the need for preanesthetic medication is allowing the parents to be present for the induction of anesthesia.

Induction of Anesthesia

If the infant or child has an intravenous catheter, induction of anesthesia with thiopental or propofol is usually safer and quicker than inhalation induction of anesthesia. Advantages of thiopental are its relatively low cost and lack of pain on intravenous administration. Propofol is more quickly metabolized and eliminated than thiopental, but intravenous administration of propofol is painful and this pain is not routinely eliminated by the prior intravenous administration of lidocaine. After the infant or child loses consciousness and the ability to ventilate with a facemask is demonstrated, an LMA can be inserted or a neuromuscular blocking drug can be given to facilitate direct laryngoscopy and tracheal intubation.

Inhalation induction of anesthesia can be performed if the infant or child does not have an intravenous catheter in place. Beginning the induction of anesthesia with the odorless mixture of nitrous oxide and oxygen through a facemask and then slowly increasing the concentration of inhaled drug such as sevoflurane is the best approach in a cooperative child. When the infant or child becomes unconscious, the nitrous oxide is discontinued and the patient breathes oxygen and the vapor of the potent volatile anesthetic. The increasing level of anesthesia will decrease skeletal muscle tone and may cause airway obstruction in certain infants and children. If airway obstruction does occur, it can usually be relieved by opening the mouth, extending the neck, and pushing anteriorly on the angle of the jaw. Occasionally, an oral or nasal airway may need to be inserted at this point. An intravenous catheter should be placed, and once the ability to ventilate the patient has been confirmed, either an LMA can be inserted or a neuromuscular blocking drug can be given to facilitate direct laryngoscopy and tracheal intubation.

Direct Laryngoscopy and Tracheal Intubation

When performing direct laryngoscopy and tracheal intubation in infants and children it is important to appropriately position the infant or child with a roll under the neck or shoulders. Ideally, the mouth should be viewed as being divided into three compartments, with the tongue on the left, the laryngoscope blade in the midline, and the endotracheal tube entering from the right corner of the mouth. Gentle, external posterior pressure applied with the fingers of the anesthesiologist's right hand at the level of the thyroid or cricoid cartilage is sometimes necessary to bring the vocal cords into view.

Once the patient's trachea is intubated, correct positioning of the endotracheal tube should be confirmed by capnography, by watching the chest rise and fall, and by auscultation. Because the trachea in infants and children is short, it is easy to accidentally intubate a main stem bronchus. The correct depth of a cuffed endotracheal tube can be estimated by detecting endotracheal tube cuff inflation in the suprasternal notch during external palpation. The correct tracheal depth of an uncuffed endotracheal tube can be estimated by placing the double line at the distal end of the endotracheal tube at the vocal cords while performing direct laryngoscopy. In infants and children it is important to reconfirm that the endotracheal tube is correctly positioned by listening for equal bilateral breath sounds after securing the endotracheal tube and at any later time when there is a change in the patient's position.

Although it is possible to accomplish tracheal intubation without the use of neuromuscular blocking drugs, these drugs will make it easier to perform direct laryngoscopy and intubation and will decrease the incidence of laryngospasm. In nonemergency situations in infants and children, the use of a nondepolarizing neuromuscular blocking drug such as rocuronium (0.5 to 1 mg/kg IV) is recommended.

Airway Equipment

NASAL AND ORAL AIRWAYS

Nasal airways and oral airways can sometimes be useful in infants and pediatric patients to relieve airway obstruction, especially during facemask ventilation at the beginning or end of anesthesia. The nasal airway is usually made of soft plastic and is carefully placed through one of the nares after lubricating its exterior. The nasal airway must be long enough to pass through the nasopharynx, but short enough that it still remains above the glottis. Nasal airways should be placed as gently as possible to minimize the possibility of bleeding or laceration of adenoidal tissue.

Oral airways are also plastic and relieve airway obstruction by displacing the tongue anteriorly. Too large an oral airway will either obstruct the glottis or may cause coughing, gagging, or laryngospasm in a patient who is not deeply anesthetized. Too small an oral airway will push the tongue posteriorly and make the airway obstruction worse. Oral airways should be placed with care to prevent trauma to the oropharynx.

LARYNGEAL MASK AIRWAYS

The classic LMA is ideally suited for situations in which the patient is breathing spontaneously, but it can also be used to deliver positive-pressure ventilation.[27] Care must be taken when using positive-pressure ventilation with an LMA to minimize peak inspiratory pressure. Patients who have lung disease or any other patient whose peak inspiratory pressures required for ventilation are higher than normal are poor candidates for an LMA because air may leak into the esophagus and result in distention of the stomach and an increased risk for emesis and aspiration. An LMA does not protect the airway from aspiration and should not be routinely used in patients with full stomachs or those at increased risk for aspiration.

Selection of Proper Size

Determining the appropriate size of LMA to use is most easily done by using the weight of the infant or child (see Table 16-8). An LMA that is too large will be difficult to place. An LMA that is too small will not form as good a seal, and it may be difficult to ventilate the patient's lungs with positive airway pressure. A slightly smaller LMA will seat better than a slightly larger LMA and may be beneficial in cases in which the operative site will be near or around the LMA. The LMA Flexible has a wire-reinforced airway tube that resists kinking and can be positioned in such a way that interference with surgical procedures involving the head and neck is minimized.

Technique

There are numerous methods for placing an LMA in infants and children. One method is with the LMA deflated and placed in its normal orientation. Alternatively, an LMA can be both placed and removed while inflated. Placing the LMA already inflated is associated with a higher success rate and less oral trauma than placing it deflated.[28] An LMA can also be rotated 90 degrees in the lateral oropharynx to bypass the base of the tongue and then rotated 90 degrees back to its correct position. It can also be turned backward to facilitate its placement posterior to the base of the tongue and then rotated 180 degrees into its correct position.[29] Both the lateral and the backward approaches can be used with the LMA either deflated or inflated.

ENDOTRACHEAL TUBES

The appropriately sized endotracheal tube for infants and children can be estimated by using the following formula:

$$(\text{Age} + 16)/4 = \text{Endotracheal tube (ID) size}$$

It is important to remember that this formula is for uncuffed endotracheal tubes. Because the cuff is located on the outside of the endotracheal tube, to adapt this formula to cuffed endotracheal tubes it is necessary to subtract half a size from the calculated size. An endotracheal tube a half size larger and a half size smaller than calculated should always be available. Endotracheal tube size may also be based on patient age and body weight (see Table 16-6). An appropriately sized suction catheter should also always be available to suction secretions, blood, or fluid from the endotracheal tube.

Cuffed or Uncuffed Endotracheal Tube

In general, uncuffed endotracheal tubes are used in infants and smaller children because the appropriately sized cuffed endotracheal tube would be smaller and this would increase resistance and the work of breathing. Cuffed endotracheal tubes can be used in infants and small children only if the inflation of the cuff is carefully adjusted and monitored, which may be difficult if nitrous oxide is used. Regardless of whether an uncuffed or cuffed endotracheal tube is chosen, it is important to maintain leak pressure around the tracheal tube no greater than 20 to 25 cm H_2O to decrease the likelihood of postextubation croup and the possibility of subsequent tracheal stenosis.

Stylet

Using a stylet stiffens the endotracheal tube and makes it easier to manipulate during direct laryngoscopy and tracheal intubation. The trachea of infants and small children can often be intubated without using a stylet, but a stylet may be useful for whenever a difficult tracheal intubation is anticipated. When intubating without a stylet, the appropriately sized stylet should always be immediately available (see Table 16-6).

LARYNGOSCOPES

In general, a straight-blade laryngoscope is easier to use in infants and small children than a curved blade. The disadvantage of a straight blade is that it does not retract the tongue as well to the left side of the mouth. A curved blade has a larger flange that retracts the tongue to the left more effectively and may be useful in certain patient populations in which the tongue is larger than normal (Beckwith-Wiedemann syndrome, trisomy 21).

In infants younger than 1 year, a Miller 1 straight laryngoscope blade is most useful. In children between 1 and 3 years of age, a 1½ straight laryngoscope blade, such as a Wis-Hipple, is often useful. A longer straight laryngoscope blade such as a Miller 2 is appropriate for most children between 3 and 10 years of age. The tracheas of children older than 11 years are often more easily intubated with a curved laryngoscope blade such as a Macintosh 3. Both straight and curved laryngoscope blades of various sizes should always be available.

Managing Difficult Airways in Infants and Children

The same general principles as outlined for managing a normal pediatric airway apply to managing either an unexpected or an expected difficult pediatric airway. It is unlikely that infants and children will cooperate with procedures such as awake fiberoptic tracheal intubation, so it is necessary to induce anesthesia and manage the airway with the patient asleep.

UNEXPECTED DIFFICULTY

When one encounters an unexpected difficult airway in pediatric patients, the most important first step is to call for an additional anesthesia colleague to help (Fig. 16-23). It is critical to not persist with repeated attempts at direct laryngoscopy, which can result in trauma to the upper airway, edema, and bleeding. In most situations, an LMA should be inserted to provide an airway to oxygenate and ventilate the patient and allow time to obtain additional personnel and airway equipment. An LMA may be the only way to maintain an airway until the patient wakes up or a surgical airway is established. An LMA is also an excellent conduit for fiberoptic intubation.[30]

EXPECTED DIFFICULTY

An expected difficult airway in pediatric patients should be approached with caution. Only preanesthetic medications that have minimal ventilatory depressant effects, such as midazolam, should be used. Preanesthetic medications should be administered in a location with appropriate airway equipment, including suction and a method of delivering oxygen with positive pressure. Pulse oximetry monitoring may be initiated at this time.

An additional anesthesia colleague should be available for help during the induction of anesthesia, inserting an intravenous line, and securing the airway. A surgeon capable of establishing a surgical airway and emergency airway equipment should be in the operating room before beginning the induction of anesthesia. The most difficult decision in managing an expected difficult pediatric airway is whether to attempt direct laryngoscopy or to proceed directly with an alternative strategy for managing the airway (fiberoptic, lighted stylet, surgical airway). It is often reasonable to make one attempt at direct laryngoscopy. Alternatively, the history and physical examination may indicate situations in which direct laryngoscopy will be unsuccessful (halo traction preventing neck movement, unable to open the mouth), and one should proceed directly to an alternative strategy for managing the airway.

LIGHTED STYLETS

A lighted stylet (lightwand) can be a useful adjunct for managing both an unexpected and an expected difficult airway in infants and children.[31] A lighted stylet can be used in patients who have limited mouth opening or limited neck flexion or extension. Tracheal intubation with the use of a lighted stylet may be much simpler and quicker than intubation with a fiberoptic bronchoscope. A lighted stylet can be used successfully in the presence of secretions or bleeding when the fiberoptic bronchoscope has failed. Disadvantages of a lighted stylet include the need for the operating room lights to be dimmed, and this technique is more difficult to use when the anatomy of the airway is distorted such that the laryngeal structures are not midline.

Technique

The lighted stylet is placed through the endotracheal tube (smaller tubes are more likely to be successfully placed) so that the tip of the stylet is several millimeters

Figure 16-23 A suggested simplified algorithm for management of a difficult airway in infants and children. LMA, laryngeal mask airway.

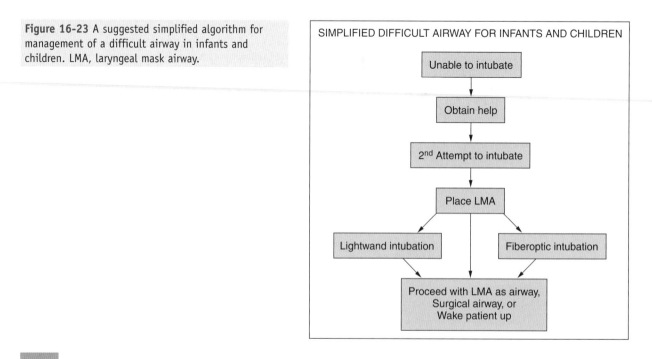

SIMPLIFIED DIFFICULT AIRWAY FOR INFANTS AND CHILDREN

proximal to the distal tip of the endotracheal tube (see Table 16-7). The lighted stylet with the loaded endotracheal tube is manually angled to between 90 and 120 degrees. The key to the successful use of a lighted stylet is to stay midline and anterior. The light should remain bright red as it passes from the supraglottic area into the trachea. Once the lighted stylet is in the trachea, the endotracheal tube should be advanced further into the trachea and the stylet removed. A lighted stylet can also be used for nasotracheal intubation after appropriate vasoconstriction of the nasal mucosa to minimize bleeding.

FIBEROPTIC BRONCHOSCOPE
A flexible fiberoptic bronchoscope is another tool for managing a difficult pediatric airway. It is particularly valuable when the patient's mouth opening or neck mobility is limited. Disadvantages of a fiberoptic bronchoscope include a limited field of vision and interference from bleeding, secretions, or both. Fiberoptic bronchoscopes as small as 2.2 mm in outside diameter are available and can be used for endotracheal tubes as small as 3.0 mm ID. These small bronchoscopes, however, do not have a suction channel and have optics that are inferior to those of larger scopes. In general, the fiberoptic bronchoscope should be at least 1 mm smaller in outside diameter than the ID of the endotracheal tube (Table 16-11).

Technique
Successful use of a fiberoptic bronchoscope as a tool to intubate the trachea in infants and children depends on several factors. Infants and children are unlikely to be able to cooperate with an awake fiberoptic intubation, and it is easier to perform an asleep fiberoptic intubation. Some anesthesiologists prefer to maintain spontaneous ventilation during fiberoptic laryngoscopy and tracheal intubation, especially if there is concern about the ability to ventilate the patient's lungs with a facemask. Frequently, it is easier to administer neuromuscular blocking drugs to a pediatric patient to provide better viewing conditions with less movement, less fogging of the bronchoscope, and less chance of laryngospasm. Using an elbow with a port that permits insertion of the fiberoptic bronchoscope allows for either continued spontaneous ventilation or assisted positive-pressure ventilation through the facemask.

For nasal fiberoptic laryngoscopy and tracheal intubation, a vasoconstrictor (phenylephrine [Neo-Synephrine]) should be administered to prevent bleeding, which will make visualization difficult. For oral fiberoptic laryngoscopy and tracheal intubation, an LMA can provide an excellent channel directly to the vocal cords while allowing for either spontaneous or controlled ventilation and oxygenation and shielding the bronchoscope from secretions and bleeding. It is useful to select the largest endotracheal

LMA Size	Largest ETT inside the LMA (ID, mm)	Largest FOB inside the ETT (OD, mm)	Compatible FOB Models with OD (mm)
1	3.0 uncuffed	2.2	Olympus LF-P (2.2)
1.5	4.0 uncuffed	3.0	Olympus LF-P (2.2) Pentax FI-9BS/RBS (3.0)
	3.5 cuffed	2.4	Olympus LF-P (2.2) Pentax FI-7P/BS/RBS (2.4)
2	4.5 uncuffed	3.4	Olympus LF-DP (3.1) Pentax FI-10BS/RBS (3.4)
	4.0 cuffed	3.0	Olympus LF-P (2.2) Pentax FI-9BS/RBS (3.0)
2.5	5.0 uncuffed	4.0	Olympus LF-2 (4.0) Pentax FI-10BS/RBS (3.4)
	4.5 cuffed	3.4	Olympus LF-DP (3.1) Pentax FI-10P2/BS/RBS (3.4)
3	5.5 cuffed	4.2	Olympus LF-2/GP (4.0/4.1) Pentax FI-13P/BS/RBS (4.2/4.1/4.1)
4	5.5 cuffed	4.2	Olympus LF-2/GP (4.0/4.1) Pentax FI-13P/BS/RBS (4.2/4.1/4.1)
5	6.5 cuffed	5.2	Olympus LF-TP (5.2) Pentax FI-16BS/RBS (5.1)

Table 16–11 The Laryngeal Mask Airway as a Conduit for Tracheal Intubation with a Fiberoptic Bronchoscope

ETT, endotracheal tube; FOB, fiberoptic bronchoscope; ID, internal diameter; LMA, laryngeal mask airway; OD, outside diameter.

III

tube that will easily fit through the LMA and the largest bronchoscope that will fit through the endotracheal tube (see Table 16-11). If an LMA is used as a conduit for oral fiberoptic laryngoscopy and tracheal intubation, it is simplest to leave the LMA in place until the end of the procedure while remembering to partially deflate the cuff of the LMA to prevent unnecessary pressure in the oropharynx.

Tracheal Extubation in Infants and Children

CROUP OR STRIDOR

Infants and small children are at higher risk than adults for croup or stridor after tracheal extubation. Croup occurs most commonly when either a cuffed or uncuffed endotracheal tube is used that is too large or when the cuff is inflated with too much air. The resulting mechanical pressure on the tracheal mucosa causes venous congestion and edema and in severe cases can even compromise the arterial blood supply and give rise to mucosal ischemia. The resulting edema can narrow the tracheal lumen, especially in infants and small children. Because resistance to flow in an endotracheal tube is inversely proportional to the radius of the lumen to the fourth power, 1 mm of edema in an infant airway is much more significant than 1 mm of edema in an adult airway. Other risk factors for croup include multiple tracheal intubation attempts, unusual positioning of the head during surgery, increased duration of surgery, and procedures involving the upper airway, such as rigid bronchoscopy.

Manifestations

An infant or child with postextubation croup usually has respiratory distress in the postanesthesia care unit. Nasal flaring, retractions, an increased respiratory rate, audible stridor, and decreased oxygen saturation are common clinical findings.

Treatment

Treatment of postextubation croup or stridor depends on the degree of respiratory distress. Mild symptoms can be managed with humidified oxygen and prolonged observation in the postanesthesia care unit. More severe cases may require aerosolized racemic epinephrine and postoperative observation in an intensive care unit. Patients whose respiratory distress is severe and not relieved with these measures may need to be reintubated with an endotracheal tube smaller than previously used. Steroids administered intravenously for preventing upper airway edema are more beneficial when given before the airway is instrumented and should be administered before procedures such as rigid bronchoscopy.

OBSTRUCTIVE SLEEP APNEA

Infants and children with obstructive sleep apnea are at significant risk for airway obstruction, respiratory distress, and the potential for apnea in the postoperative period. At baseline these infants and children hypoventilate, which results in hypercapnia and often arterial hypoxemia when they are asleep. Residual inhaled anesthetics or residual neuromuscular blockade can depress airway reflexes, skeletal muscle tone and strength, and respiratory drive and result in significant airway compromise in infants and children with obstructive sleep apnea. Opioids must be very carefully titrated both intraoperatively and postoperatively because they can depress the ventilatory drive and contribute to significant hypercapnia and arterial hypoxemia in these infants and children.

Tracheal extubation in patients with obstructive sleep apnea should be considered only when these infants and children are fully awake. All infants and children with obstructive sleep apnea should be monitored postoperatively with pulse oximetry and apnea monitoring. High-risk patients should be monitored postoperatively in an intensive care unit setting.

EXTUBATION AFTER A DIFFICULT INTUBATION

Tracheal extubation of an infant or child after a difficult intubation is considered carefully because reintubation can be more difficult than the initial intubation. The tracheas of infants and children with difficult airways should be extubated only when they are fully awake and there is no residual neuromuscular blockade.

Postoperative factors that can further compromise respiratory function must also be considered when extubating the trachea of an infant or child with a difficult airway. For example, postoperative pain, especially if there is splinting from an abdominal or thoracic incision, may compromise respiratory function. Postoperative pain requiring significant opioid use will also compromise breathing by decreasing the respiratory drive. The use of regional anesthesia, such as an epidural, may hasten the ability to extubate the trachea of these infants and children.

Edema of the airway from surgical trauma, positioning, or excessive fluid administration can significantly affect the ability to extubate the tracheas of infants and children with difficult airways and can make emergency reintubation more difficult. Infants and children with postoperative airway edema and difficult airways should remain intubated until the edema has resolved. An infant or child with a difficult airway should be extubated only when appropriate equipment and personnel are available for urgent reintubation.

REFERENCES

1. Caplan RA, Benumof JL, Berry FA, et al. Practice guidelines for management of the difficult airway. Anesthesiology 2003;98:1269-1277.
2. Langeron O, Masso E, Huraux C, et al. Prediction of difficult mask ventilation. Anesthesiology 2000;92:1229-1236.
3. Hawthorne L, Wilson R, Lyons G, et al. Failed intubation revisited: 17-year experience in a teaching maternity unit. Br J Anaesth 1996;76:680-684.
4. Ovassapian A. Fiberoptic Endoscopy in Anesthesia and Critical Care. New York: Raven Press, 1990, pp 57-79.
5. Stackhouse RA. Fiberoptic airway management. Anesthesiol Clin North Am 2002;20:933-951.
6. Patil VU, Stehling LC, Zauder HL. Fiberoptic Endoscopy in Anesthesia. St Louis: CV Mosby, 1983.
7. Isaacs RS, Sykes JM. Anatomy and physiology of the upper airway. Anesthesiol Clin North Am 2002;20:733-745.
8. Stackhouse RA, Bainton CR. Difficult airway management. *In* Hughes SC, Levinson G, Rosen MA (eds): Shnider and Levinson's Anesthesia for Obstetrics. Philadelphia: Lippincott Williams & Wilkins, 2001, pp 375-389.
9. Mallampati SR, Gatt SP, Gugino LD, et al. A clinical sign to predict difficult tracheal intubation: A prospective study. Can Anaesth Soc J 1985;32:429-434.
10. Samsoon GLT, Young JRB. Difficult tracheal intubation: A retrospective study. Anaesthesia 1987;42:487-490.
11. Cormack RS, Lehane J. Difficult tracheal intubation in obstetrics. Anaesthesia 1984;39:1105-1111.
12. Williams KN, Carli F, Cormack RS. Unexpected, difficult laryngoscopy: A prospective survey in routine general surgery. Br J Anaesth 1991;66:38-44.
13. Harmer M. Difficult and failed intubation in obstetrics. Int J Obstet Anesth 1997;6:25-31.
14. Tournadre J-P, Chassard D, Berrada KR, et al. Cricoid cartilage pressure decreases lower esophageal sphincter tone. Anesthesiology 1997;86:7-9.
15. Brimacombe JR, Berry AM. Cricoid pressure. Can J Anaesth 1997;44:414-425.
16. Owen RL, Cheney RW. Endobronchial intubation: A preventable complication. Anesthesiology 1987;67:255-257.
17. Hagberg CA. Special devices and techniques. Anesthesiol Clin North Am 2002;20:907-932.
18. Behringer EC. Approaches to managing the upper airway. Anesthesiol Clin North Am 2002;20:813-832.
19. Bogetz MS. Using the laryngeal mask airway to manage the difficult airway. Anesthesiol Clin North Am 2002;20:863-870.
20. Brain AIJ, Verghese C, Addy EV, et al. The intubating laryngeal mask. II: A preliminary clinical report of a new means of intubating the trachea. Br J Anaesth 1997;79:704-709.
21. Keller C, Brimacombe J, Kleinsasser A, et al. Does the ProSeal laryngeal mask airway prevent aspiration of regurgitated fluid? Anesth Analg 2000;91:1017-1020.
22. Brimacombe J, Keller C, Judd DV. Gum elastic bougie-guided insertion of the ProSeal laryngeal mask airway is superior to the digital and introducer tool techniques. Anesthesiology 2004;100:25-29.
23. Gaitni LA, Vaida SJ, Agro F. The Esophageal-Tracheal Combitube. Anesthesiol Clin North Am 2002;20:894.
24. Agro F, Frass M, Benumof JL, et al. Current status of the Combitube: A review of the literature. J Clin Anesth 2002;14:307-314.
25. Stackhouse RA. Transtracheal oxygenation. Int Anesthesiol Clin 1994;32:85-94.
26. Warner ME, Benenfeld SM, Warner MA, et al. Perianesthetic dental injuries. Frequency, outcomes, and risk factors. Anesthesiology 1999;90:1302-1305.
27. O'Neill B, Templeton J, Camarico L, Schreiner M: The laryngeal mask airway in pediatric patients: Factors affecting ease of use during insertion and emergence. Anesth Analg 1994;78:659-662.
28. Wakeling H, Butler P, Baxter P. The laryngeal mask airway: A comparison between two insertion techniques. Anesth Analg 1997;85:687-690.
29. Pennant J, White P. The laryngeal mask airway: Its uses in anesthesiology. Anesthesiology 1993;79:144-163.
30. Benumof J: Laryngeal mask airway and the ASA difficult airway algorithm. Anesthesiology 1996;84:686-699.
31. Holzman R, Nargozian C, Florence F: Lightwand intubation in children with abnormal upper airways. Anesthesiology 1988;69:784-787.

III

SPINAL AND EPIDURAL ANESTHESIA

Kenneth Drasner and Merlin D. Larson

Collectively referred to as central neuraxial block, spinal anesthesia and epidural anesthesia represent a subcategory of regional or conduction anesthesia. In addition to their current widespread use in the operating room for surgical anesthesia and as an adjunct to general anesthesia, neuraxial techniques are effective means for controlling obstetric and postoperative pain.

COMPARISON OF SPINAL AND EPIDURAL ANESTHESIA

Spinal anesthesia is accomplished by injecting local anesthetic solution into the cerebrospinal fluid (CSF) contained within the subarachnoid (intrathecal) space. In contrast, epidural anesthesia is achieved by injection of local anesthetic solution into the space that lies within the vertebral canal but outside or superficial to the dural sac. Caudal anesthesia represents a special type of epidural anesthesia in which local anesthetic solution is injected into the caudal epidural space through a needle introduced through the sacral hiatus. Although epidural anesthesia is routinely performed at various levels along the neuraxis, subarachnoid injections are limited to the lumbar region below the termination of the spinal cord.

When compared with epidural anesthesia, spinal anesthesia takes less time to perform, causes less discomfort during placement, requires less local anesthetic, and produces more intense sensory and motor block. In addition, correct placement of the needle in the subarachnoid space is confirmed by a clearly defined end point (appearance of CSF).

Advantages of epidural anesthesia include a decreased risk for post–dural puncture headache (assuming a negligible incidence of inadvertent dural puncture), a lower incidence of systemic hypotension, the ability to produce a segmental sensory block, and greater control over the intensity of sensory anesthesia and motor block achieved by adjustment of the local anesthetic concentration. The routine placement of catheters for epidural anesthesia imparts additional benefit by allowing titration of the block to the duration of surgery. Perhaps even more important, a catheter provides a means for long-term administration of local anesthetics or opioid-containing solutions (or both), which are highly effective for control of postoperative or obstetric pain.

Patients may remain completely awake during surgery performed under neuraxial block, but more commonly they are sedated with various combinations of intravenous drugs, including sedative-hypnotics, opioids, and anesthetics (propofol). Skeletal muscle relaxation is profound in the presence of neuraxial anesthesia and thus obviates the need for neuromuscular blocking drugs. However, despite potential advantages, patients may be reluctant to accept neuraxial anesthesia for fear of permanent nerve damage. Although there does exist the rare possibility of neural injury as a result of neuraxial anesthesia, patient concerns generally far exceed the clinical reality and at times are based on undocumented and unfounded stories of paralysis.[1]

As with other regional techniques, central neuraxial techniques require an understanding of the underlying anatomy and physiologic principles.

ANATOMY

Vertebral Canal

The spinal cord and its nerve roots are contained within the vertebral (spinal) canal, a bony structure that extends from the foramen magnum to the sacral hiatus (Fig. 17-1).[2] On a lateral view the vertebral canal exhibits four curvatures, of which the thoracic convexity (kyphosis) and the lumbar concavity (lordosis) are of major importance to the distribution of local anesthetic solution in the subarachnoid space. In contrast, these curves have little effect on the spread of local anesthetic solutions in the epidural space.

In addition to structural support, the vertebral canal provides critical protection to vulnerable neural structures. Unfortunately, this bony canal also creates a barrier to an advancing spinal or epidural needle seeking to trespass this space. Successful neuraxial block is thus critically dependent on the anesthesiologist's appreciation of the anatomy of this structure.

ARCHITECTURE

The building blocks of the vertebral canal are the vertebrae, which are stacked to form the tubular column (Figs. 17-2 and 17-3; also see Fig. 17-1).[2,3] This complex architecture is best appreciated by examination of a skeleton or a three-dimensional model. Although the structure of the vertebrae varies considerably, depending on their location and function, each consists of an anterior vertebral body and a posterior arch. The posterior arch is created by fusion of the lateral cylindrical pedicles with the two flattened

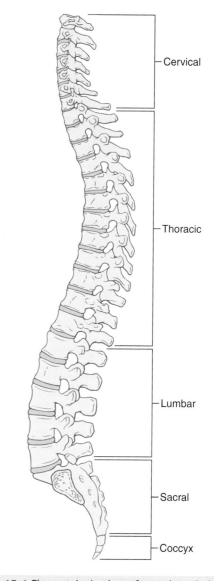

Figure 17-1 The vertebral column from a lateral view exhibits four curvatures. (From Covino BG, Scott DB, Lambert DH. Handbook of Spinal Anaesthesia and Analgesia. Philadelphia: WB Saunders, 1994, pp 12-24.)

posterior laminae. A transverse process extends out laterally at each junction of the pedicle and laminae, whereas a single spinous process projects posteriorly from the junction of the two laminae. Each pedicle is notched on its superior and inferior surface, and when two adjacent vertebrae are articulated, these notches form the intervertebral foramina through which the spinal nerves emerge.

NOMENCLATURE AND FEATURES

Of the 24 true vertebrae, the first 7, located in the neck, are called cervical vertebrae, the next 12 are attached to

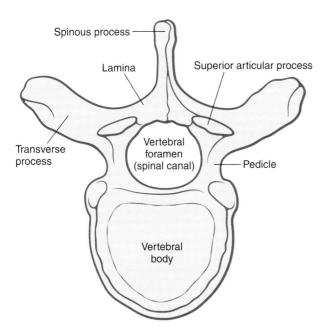

Figure 17-2 Typical thoracic vertebra. (From Covino BG, Scott DB, Lambert DH. Handbook of Spinal Anaesthesia and Analgesia. Philadelphia: WB Saunders, 1994.)

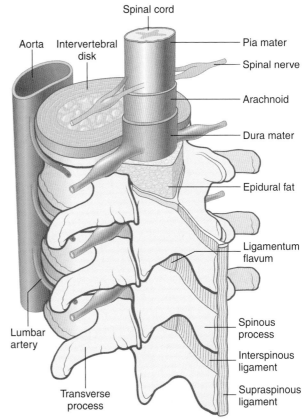

Figure 17-3 The spine in an oblique view. (From Afton-Bird G. Atlas of regional anesthesia. *In* Miller RD [ed]: Miller's Anesthesia. Philadelphia: Elsevier, 2005.)

the ribs and are called thoracic (or dorsal) vertebrae, and the remaining 5 are the lumbar vertebrae. Another five vertebrae, called false or fixed vertebrae, are fused to form the bony sacrum (Fig 17-4).[4] Thus, the sacrum and coccyx are distal extensions of the vertebral column, and the sacral canal is a continuation of the vertebral canal through the sacrum.

The features of the midthoracic and lumbar vertebrae can ideally be represented by two articulated vertebrae (Fig. 17-5).[5] The nearly perpendicular orientation of the spinous process in the lumbar area and the downward angular orientation in the thoracic area define the angle required for placement and advancement of a needle intended to access the vertebral canal. The wide interlaminar space in the lumbar spine reflects the fact that the lamina occupies only about half the space between adjacent vertebrae. In contrast, the interlaminar space is just a few millimeters wide at the level of the thoracic vertebrae.

SACRUM AND SACRAL HIATUS

The sacrum is a large curved wedge-shaped bone whose dorsal surface is convex and gives rise to the powerful sacrospinalis muscle. The opening between the unfused lamina of the fourth and fifth sacral vertebrae is called the sacral hiatus. There is considerable anatomic variability in the features of the dorsal surface of the sacrum. Indeed, the sacral hiatus is absent in nearly 8% of adult subjects, thereby preventing entry through the sacrococcygeal

ligament into the sacral canal and performance of caudal anesthesia independent of the experience and skills of the anesthesiologist.

SURFACE LANDMARKS

Surface landmarks are used to identify specific spinal interspaces (Fig. 17-6).[4] The most important of these landmarks is a line drawn between the iliac crests. This line generally traverses the body of the L4 vertebra and is the principal landmark used to determine the level for insertion of a needle intended to produce spinal anesthesia. The C7 spinous process can be appreciated as a bony knob at the lower end of the neck. The T7-8 interspace is identified by a line drawn between the lower limits of the scapulae and is often used to guide needle placement for passage of a catheter into the thoracic epidural space. The terminal portion of the 12th rib intersects the L2 vertebral body, whereas the posterior iliac spines indicate the level of the S2 vertebral body, which is the caudal limit of the dural sac in most adults. Other interspaces are identified by counting up or down along the spinous processes from these major landmarks.

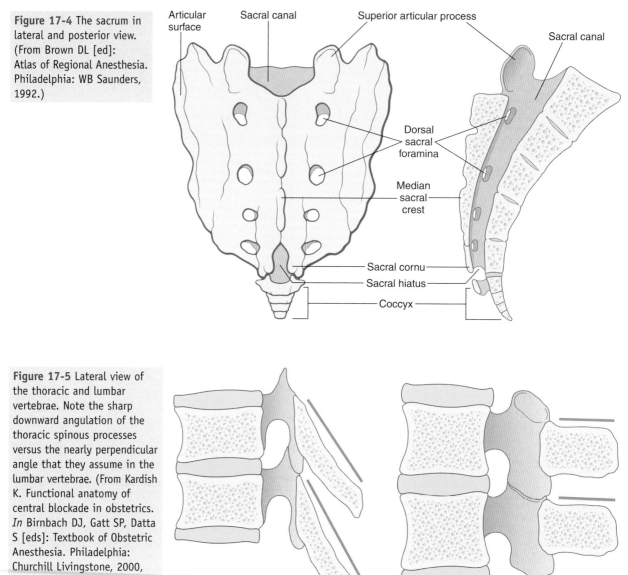

Figure 17-4 The sacrum in lateral and posterior view. (From Brown DL [ed]: Atlas of Regional Anesthesia. Philadelphia: WB Saunders, 1992.)

Articular surface

Sacral canal

Superior articular process

Sacral canal

Dorsal sacral foramina

Median sacral crest

Sacral cornu

Sacral hiatus

Coccyx

Figure 17-5 Lateral view of the thoracic and lumbar vertebrae. Note the sharp downward angulation of the thoracic spinous processes versus the nearly perpendicular angle that they assume in the lumbar vertebrae. (From Kardish K. Functional anatomy of central blockade in obstetrics. *In* Birnbach DJ, Gatt SP, Datta S [eds]: Textbook of Obstetric Anesthesia. Philadelphia: Churchill Livingstone, 2000, pp 121-156.)

Ligaments

The vertebral column is stabilized by several ligaments (Figs. 17-7 and 17-8).[2] Adjacent vertebral bodies are joined by anterior and posterior spinal ligaments, the latter forming the anterior border of the vertebral canal. The ligamentum flavum is composed of thick plates of elastic tissue that connect the lamina of adjacent vertebrae. The supraspinous ligament runs superficially along the spinous processes, which makes it the first ligament that a needle will traverse when using a midline approach to the vertebral canal.

Spinal Cord

The spinal cord begins at the rostral border of the medulla and, in the fetus, extends the entire length of the vertebral canal. However, because of disproportionate growth of neural tissue and the vertebral canal, the spinal cord generally terminates around the third lumbar vertebra at birth and at the lower border of the first lumbar vertebra in adults. As a further consequence of this differential growth, the spinal nerves become progressively longer and more closely aligned with the longitudinal axis of the vertebral canal. Below the conus, the roots are oriented

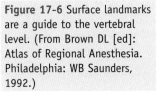

Figure 17-6 Surface landmarks are a guide to the vertebral level. (From Brown DL [ed]: Atlas of Regional Anesthesia. Philadelphia: WB Saunders, 1992.)

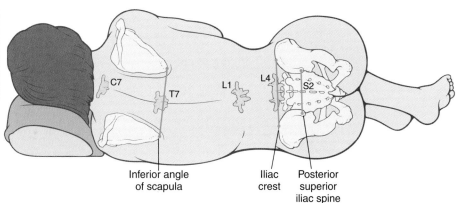

Inferior angle of scapula

Iliac crest

Posterior superior iliac spine

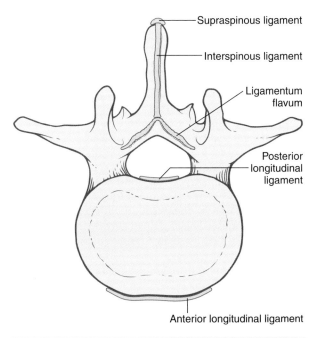

Supraspinous ligament

Interspinous ligament

Ligamentum flavum

Posterior longitudinal ligament

Anterior longitudinal ligament

Figure 17-7 Cross section of a lumbar vertebra showing the attachment of the spinal ligaments. 1, Supraspinous ligament; 2, interspinous ligament; 3, ligamentum flavum; 4, posterior longitudinal ligament; 5, anterior longitudinal ligament. (From Covino BG, Scott DB, Lambert DH. Handbook of Spinal Anaesthesia and Analgesia. Philadelphia: WB Saunders, 1994, p 15.)

Meninges

In addition to the CSF, the spinal cord is surrounded and protected by three layers of connective tissue known as the meninges.

DURA MATER

The outermost layer, the dura mater, originates at the foramen magnum as an extension of the inner (meningeal) layer of cranial dura and continues caudally to terminate

III

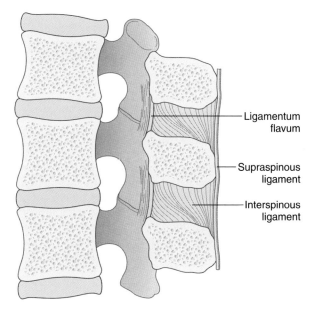

Ligamentum flavum

Supraspinous ligament

Interspinous ligament

Figure 17-8 Sagittal section through adjacent lumbar vertebrae showing the attachment of the spinal ligaments. 1, Supraspinous ligament; 2, interspinous ligament; 3, ligamentum flavum. (From Covino BG, Scott DB, Lambert DH. Handbook of Spinal Anaesthesia and Analgesia. Philadelphia: WB Saunders, 1994, p 15.)

parallel to this axis and resemble a horse's tail, from which the name cauda equina is derived (Fig. 17-9).[6] The nerve roots of the cauda equina move relatively freely within the CSF, a fortunate arrangement that permits them to be displaced rather than pierced by an advancing needle.

a spinal needle that penetrates the dura will generally pass through the arachnoid membrane. However, "subdural" injections can occur in clinical practice and result in a "failed spinal" because of the relative impermeability of the arachnoid membrane.

PIA

The innermost layer of the spinal meninges, the pia is a highly vascular structure closely applied to the cord that forms the inner border of the subarachnoid space. Along the lateral surface between the dorsal and ventral roots, an extension of this membrane forms the denticulate ligament—a dense serrated longitudinal projection that provides lateral suspension through its attachment to the dura. As the spinal cord tapers to form the conus medullaris, the pia continues interiorly as a thin filament, the filum terminale. Distally, the filum terminale becomes enveloped by the dura at the caudal termination of the dural sac (generally around S2) and continues inferiorly to attach to the posterior wall of the coccyx.

Spinal Nerves

Along the dorsolateral and ventrolateral aspect of the spinal cord, rootlets emerge and coalesce to form the dorsal (afferent) and ventral (efferent) spinal nerve roots (Fig. 17-10).[2] Distal to the dorsal root ganglion, these nerve roots merge to form 31 pairs of spinal nerves (8 cervical, 12 thoracic, 5 lumbar, 5 sacral, and 1 coccygeal). Because the sensory fibers traverse the posterior aspect of the subarachnoid space, they tend to lie dependent in a supine patient, thus making them particularly vulnerable to hyperbaric (heavier than CSF) solutions containing local anesthetic.

As the nerves pass through the intervertebral foramen, they become encased by the dura, arachnoid, and pia, which form the epineurium, perineurium, and endoneurium, respectively. The dura becomes thinned as it traverses this area (often called the dural sleeve), thereby facilitating penetration of local anesthetic. The onset of epidural block by local anesthetics thus occurs by blockade of sodium ion conductance in this region. With time, epidural local anesthetics transfer into the subarachnoid space, and the nerve roots and spinal cord tracts are variably affected. This accounts for the observation that the onset of an epidural block spreads rostrally and caudally from the point of injection, but the pattern of recession is not a strict reversal of the onset.

PREGANGLIONIC SYMPATHETIC NERVE FIBERS

Preganglionic sympathetic nerve fibers originating in the intermediolateral gray columns of the thoracolumbar cord leave with the ventral nerve roots passing into the spinal nerve trunks (Fig. 17-11). They then leave the nerve via the white rami communicantes and project to the paravertebral sympathetic ganglia or more distant sites (adrenal

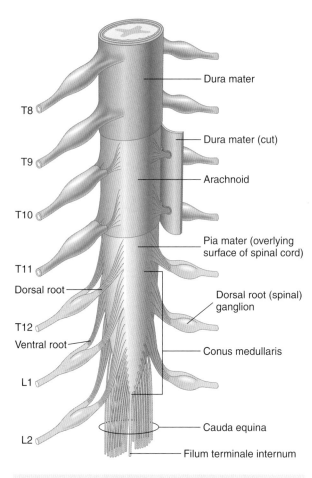

Figure 17-9 Terminal spinal cord and cauda equina. (From Bridenbaugh PO, Greene NM, Brull SJ. Spinal [subarachnoid] blockade. *In* Cousins MJ, Bridenbaugh PO [eds]: Neural Blockade in Clinical Anesthesia and Management of Pain. Philadelphia: Lippincott-Raven, 1998, pp 203-242.)

between S1 and S4. It is a tough fibroelastic membrane that provides structural support and a fairly impenetrable barrier that normally prevents displacement of an epidural catheter into the fluid-filled subarachnoid space. Although cases of epidural catheter migration into the subarachnoid space occur clinically, it has been well established in cadaver studies that catheters cannot penetrate an intact dura.[7]

ARACHNOID MEMBRANE

Closely adherent to the inner surface of the dura lies the arachnoid membrane. Though far more delicate than the dura, the arachnoid serves as the major pharmacologic barrier preventing movement of drug from the epidural to the subarachnoid space. Conceptually, the dura provides support and the arachnoid membrane imparts impermeability. Because the dura and arachnoid are closely adherent,

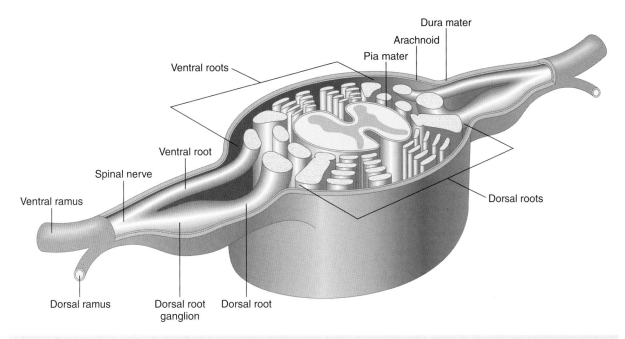

Figure 17-10 The spinal cord and nerve roots. (From Covino BG, Scott DB, Lambert DH. Handbook of Spinal Anaesthesia and Analgesia. Philadelphia: WB Saunders, 1994, p 19.)

medulla, mesenteric and celiac plexus). After a cholinergic synapse (nicotinic) in the autonomic ganglia, the postsynaptic sympathetic nerve fibers join the spinal nerves via the gray rami communicantes and innervate diverse adrenergic effector sites.

CERVICAL NERVES

The first cervical nerve passes between the occipital bone and the posterior arch of the first cervical vertebra (atlas), and this relationship continues, with the seventh cervical nerve passing above the seventh cervical vertebra. However, because there are eight cervical nerves but only seven cervical vertebrae, the eighth cervical nerve passes between the seventh cervical vertebra and the first thoracic vertebra. Below this point, each spinal nerve passes through the inferior notch of the corresponding vertebra. For example, the T1 spinal nerve passes through the notch formed by the first and second thoracic vertebrae.

DERMATOME

The area of skin innervated by each spinal nerve is called a dermatome (Fig. 17-12).[8] Because the lower nerve roots descend before exiting the intervertebral foramen, the spinal cord terminations of the afferent fibers from each dermatome are more rostral than their corresponding vertebral level. For example, the sensory fibers from the L4 dermatome enter the spinal canal below the L4 vertebral body. However, primary afferent terminals for the L4 dermatome are located anterior to the T11-12 interspace.

Subarachnoid Space

Between the arachnoid and the pia lies the subarachnoid space, which contains the CSF formed mainly by the choroid plexus of the lateral, third, and fourth ventricles. Because the spinal and cranial arachnoid spaces are continuous, cranial nerves can be blocked by local anesthetics migrating into the CSF above the foramen magnum.

Epidural Space

The epidural space lies between the dura and the wall of the vertebral canal, an irregular column of fat, lymphatics, and blood vessels. It is bounded cranially by the foramen magnum, caudally by the sacrococcygeal ligament, anteriorly by the posterior longitudinal ligament, laterally by the vertebral pedicles, and posteriorly by both the ligamentum flavum and vertebral lamina. The epidural space is not a closed space but communicates with the paravertebral spaces by way of the intervertebral foramina. The depth of the epidural space is maximal (about 6 mm) in the midline at L2 and is 4 to 5 mm in the midthoracic region. It is minimal where the lumbar and cervical enlargements of the spinal cord (T9-T12 and C3-T2, respectively) encroach on the epidural space, with roughly 3 mm left between the ligamentum flavum and the dura. There are subcompartments in the epidural space at each vertebral level, but injected fluid communicates freely throughout the space from the rostral limit at the foramen magnum to the sacral hiatus caudally. There is contro-

Figure 17-11 Cell bodies in the thoracolumbar portion of the spinal cord (T1-L2) give rise to the peripheral sympathetic nervous system. Efferent fibers travel in the ventral root and then via the white ramus communicans to paravertebral sympathetic ganglia or more distant sites such as the celiac ganglion. Afferent fibers from the paravertebral sympathetic ganglia travel via the gray ramus communicans to join somatic nerves, which pass to the dorsal root and spinal cord.

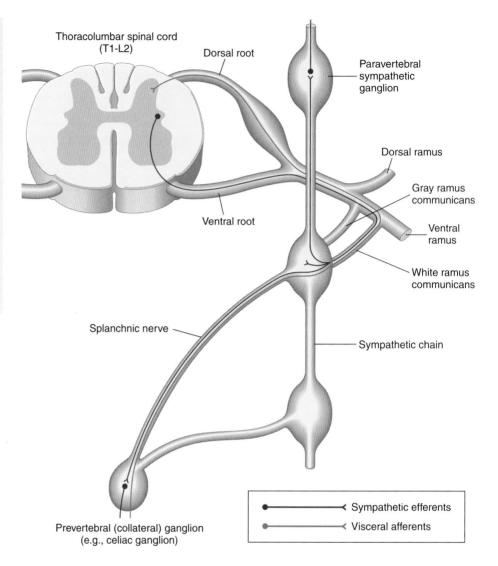

Thoracolumbar spinal cord (T1-L2)
Dorsal root
Paravertebral sympathetic ganglion
Dorsal ramus
Gray ramus communicans
Ventral root
Ventral ramus
White ramus communicans
Splanchnic nerve
Sympathetic chain
Prevertebral (collateral) ganglion (e.g., celiac ganglion)

Sympathetic efferents
Visceral afferents

versy regarding the existence and clinical significance of a connective tissue band (plica mediana dorsalis) extending from the dura mater to the ligamentum flavum and hence dividing the posterior epidural space into two compartments. Anatomic studies have suggested the presence of this structure and have led to the speculation that this tissue band may be responsible for the occasional difficulty threading a catheter into the epidural space or the unexplained occurrence of a unilateral sensory block. Nevertheless, others are unable to confirm the presence of this structure.[9]

Blood Vessels

ARTERIAL

The blood supply of the spinal cord arises from a single anterior and two paired posterior spinal arteries (Fig. 17-13).[2]

The posterior spinal arteries emerge from the cranial vault and supply the dorsal (sensory) portion of the spinal cord. Because they are paired and have rich collateral anastomotic links from the subclavian and intercostal arteries, this area of the spinal cord is relatively protected from ischemic damage. This is not the case with the single anterior spinal artery that originates from the vertebral artery and supplies the ventral (motor) portion of the spinal cord. The anterior spinal artery receives branches from the intercostal and iliac arteries, but these branches are variable in number and location. The largest anastomotic link, the radicularis magna (artery of Adamkiewicz), arises from the aorta in the lower thoracic or upper lumbar region.

Artery of Adamkiewicz

The vessel is highly variable but, most commonly, is on the left and enters the vertebral canal through the L1 inter-

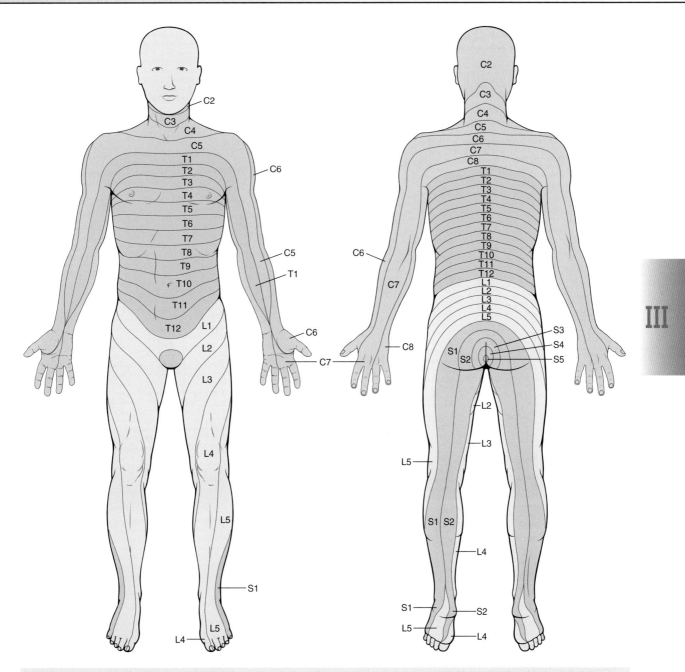

Figure 17-12 Areas of sensory innervation by spinal nerves. Note that the thoracic nerves innervate the thorax and abdomen and the lumbar and sacral nerves innervate the leg. (From Cousins MJ, Bromage PR. Epidural neural blockade. *In* Cousins MJ, Bridenbaugh PO [eds]: Neural Blockade in Clinical Anesthesia and Management of Pain. Philadelphia: Lippincott-Raven, 1998, pp 243-321.)

vertebral foramen. The artery of Adamkiewicz is critical to the blood supply of the lower two thirds of the spinal cord, and damage to this artery during surgery on the aorta (aortic aneurysm resection) or by a stray epidural needle will produce characteristic bilateral lower extremity motor loss (anterior spinal artery syndrome).

VENOUS

The internal vertebral venous plexus drains the contents of the vertebral canal. These veins are prominent in the lateral epidural space and ultimately empty into the azygos venous system. The azygos vein enters the chest, arches over the right lung, and then empties into the superior vena

III

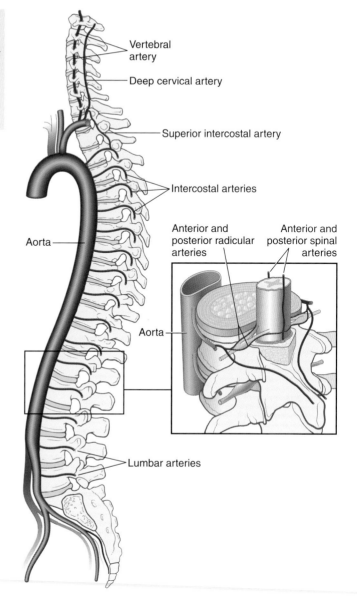

Figure 17-13 Arterial blood supply to the spinal cord. 1, Vertebral artery; 2, deep cervical artery; 3, superficial intercostal artery; 4, intercostal artery; 5, anterior spinal artery; 6, posterior spinal artery; 7, anterior and posterior radicular arteries; 8, spinal branch of the intercostal artery; 9, artery of Adamkiewicz. (From Covino BG, Scott DB, Lambert DH. Handbook of Spinal Anaesthesia and Analgesia. Philadelphia, WB Saunders 1994, p 24.)

cava. The internal vertebral venous plexus communicates above with the basilar sinuses of the brain and below with the pelvic connections to the inferior vena cava.

The anatomy of the venous plexus assumes additional importance in patients with increased intra-abdominal pressure or those with tumors or masses that compress the vena cava. In these patients, blood is diverted from the inferior vena cava and engorges veins in the epidural space, which increases the likelihood of accidental vascular cannulation during attempted epidural anesthesia. In addition, because the vertebral veins are enlarged, the effective volume of the epidural space is reduced, thereby resulting in greater longitudinal spread of injected local anesthetic solutions.

PREOPERATIVE PREPARATION

Preoperative preparation for regional anesthesia does not differ from that for general anesthesia (see Chapter 13). However, as with any regional anesthetic, a discussion with the patient regarding the specific benefits and potential complications should precede the block. Relevant complications include (1) those that are rare but serious, including nerve damage, bleeding, and infection, and (2) those that are common but of relatively minor consequence, such as post–dural puncture headache. There are no common serious complications (if there were, these techniques would not be used in clinical practice), and the infrequent minor problems are of little clinical significance. The possibility of a failed block should be discussed, and the patient should be reassured that in such circumstances, alternative anesthetic techniques will be provided to ensure their comfort.

Indications for Spinal Anesthesia

Spinal anesthesia is generally used for surgical procedures involving the lower abdominal area, perineum, and lower extremities. Although the technique can also be used for upper abdominal surgery, most consider it preferable to administer a general anesthetic to ensure patient comfort. In addition, the extensive block required for upper abdominal surgery and the nature of these procedures may have a negative impact on breathing (oxygenation and ventilation).

Indications for Epidural Anesthesia

Epidural anesthesia, like spinal anesthesia, is often used as the primary anesthetic for surgeries involving the abdomen or lower extremities. However, because of its segmental nature, anesthesia provided by lumbar epidural anesthesia may be suboptimal for procedures involving the lower sacral roots. Epidural anesthesia is also frequently used as a supplement to general anesthesia, particularly for thoracic and upper abdominal procedures. In such cases, significant benefit derives from the ability to provide continuous epidural anesthesia postoperatively to facilitate effective treatment of postoperative pain. Similarly, continuous epidural anesthesia is very effective and widely used for the control of labor pain. Cervical epidural anesthesia is rarely, if ever used for operative surgery, but injections of dilute solutions of corticosteroids and local anesthetics into the cervical epidural space are sometimes used to treat chronic pain.

Absolute and Relative Contraindications to Neuraxial Anesthesia

Absolute contraindications to neuraxial anesthetic techniques include patient refusal, infection at the site of planned needle puncture, elevated intracranial pressure, and bleeding diathesis. Patients should never be encouraged against their wishes to accept a regional anesthetic technique.

BACTEREMIA

Bacteremia does not necessarily mitigate against performance of a regional anesthetic technique. Although concern that an epidural abscess or meningitis might result from the introduction of infected blood during the procedure, clinical experience suggests that the risk is small and can be weighed against the potential benefit. In such cases, there is evidence to suggest that institution of appropriate antibiotic therapy before the block may decrease the risk for infection.[10]

PREEXISTING NEUROLOGIC DISEASE

The significance of any preexisting neurologic disease should be considered relative to its underlying pathophysiology. For example, patients with multiple sclerosis experience exacerbations and remissions of symptoms reflecting demyelination of peripheral nerves. Local anesthetic toxicity, when it occurs, can be associated with similar histopathology.[11] Although neuraxial anesthetic techniques have been viewed as acceptable for patients with multiple sclerosis, in the absence of compelling benefit, neuraxial techniques would be best avoided in these patients.

Chronic back pain does not represent a contraindication to neuraxial anesthetic techniques, although they may be avoided because patients may perceive a relationship between postoperative exacerbation of pain and the block, even though they are not causally related.

CARDIAC DISEASE

Patients with mitral stenosis, idiopathic hypertrophic subaortic stenosis, and aortic stenosis are intolerant of acute decreases in systemic vascular resistance. Thus, though not a contraindication, neuraxial block should be used cautiously in such cases.

ABNORMAL COAGULATION

The decision to use a neuraxial block in patients with abnormal coagulation, either endogenous or produced by the administration of anticoagulants, must be based on a risk-benefit assessment and include discussion with the patient and the surgical team. Guidelines developed by the American Society of Regional Anesthesia provide guidance in the management of these patients (www.asra.com) (see Chapter 22).

SPINAL ANESTHESIA

An intravenous infusion is started before performance of the anesthetic, and all of the equipment, drugs, and monitors normally present for a general anesthetic are also required for neuraxial anesthesia. Supplemental oxygen is commonly administered. Although accurate end-tidal carbon dioxide monitoring may not always be feasible, a capnograph is often used to monitor breathing. For example, the gas sampling line may be attached to a specially designed nasal cannula.

To decrease the discomfort associated with needle insertions, inclusion of an opioid in the preoperative medication should be considered. However, in selected patients premedication can be withheld, provided that there is adequate attention to infiltration of the skin and subcutaneous tissues with local anesthetic solution.

Sterile technique with hat, mask, and gloves is mandatory, and in modern practice, the required equipment is obtained from prepackaged sterile kits. Antiseptic prepa-

III

ration of the skin is performed, but contact with gloves and needles should be avoided because of the potential neurotoxicity of these antiseptic solutions.

Patient Positioning

Spinal anesthesia can be performed with the patient in the lateral decubitus, sitting, or less commonly, the prone position. To the extent possible, the spine should be flexed by having the patient bend at the waist and bring the chin toward the chest, which will optimize the interspinous space and the interlaminar foramen.

LATERAL POSITION

The lateral decubitus position is more comfortable and more suitable for the ill or frail. It also enables the anesthesiologist to safely provide greater levels of sedation.

SITTING POSITION

The sitting position encourages flexion and facilitates recognition of the midline, which may be of increased importance in an obese patient. Because lumbar CSF is elevated in this position, the dural sac is distended, thus providing a larger target for the spinal needle. This higher pressure also facilitates recognition of the needle tip within the subarachnoid space, as heralded by the free flow of CSF. When combined with a hyperbaric anesthetic, the sitting position favors a caudal distribution, the resultant anesthesia commonly being referred to as a "saddle block." However, in addition to being poorly suited for a heavily sedated patient, vasovagal syncope can occur.

PRONE POSITION

The prone position is rarely used except for perineal procedures performed in the "jackknife" position. Performance of spinal anesthesia in this position is more challenging because of the limited flexion, the contracted dural sac, and the low CSF, which generally requires aspiration with the plunger of the syringe to achieve backflow of CSF through the spinal needle.

Selection of Interspace

Several factors influence the selection of the interspace to be used for spinal anesthesia. The most obvious is the specific anatomy of the patient's spine and the likelihood that a needle can be successfully passed into the subarachnoid space. A second and often underappreciated consideration is that the interspace selected for spinal anesthesia has considerable impact on the distribution of anesthetic within the subarachnoid space. This, in turn, will affect the success or failure of the technique. For example, the likelihood of a "failed spinal" increases as interspaces that are more caudal are used,

with up to a 7% incidence occurring when the L4-5 interspace is selected.[12]

Although more rostral interspaces are associated with higher success rates, this benefit must be balanced against the potential for traumatic injury to the spinal cord while keeping in mind that the caudal limitation of the spinal cord in an adult usually lies between the L1 and L2 vertebrae. For this reason, spinal anesthesia is not ordinarily performed above the L2-3 interspace. Nevertheless, some risk remains because the spinal cord extends to the third lumbar vertebra in approximately 2% of adults. Furthermore, the use of a conceptual line across the iliac crests to identify the body of the L4 vertebra often results in selection of an interspace that is one or more levels higher than believed.[13] For this reason and the risk of traumatic injury to the spinal cord when a higher lumbar interspace is selected, it has been suggested that the anesthesiologist should not intentionally attempt spinal anesthesia cephalad to the L3-4 interspace.[14]

Spinal Needles

A variety of needles are available for spinal anesthesia and are generally classified by their size (most commonly 22 to 25 gauge) and the shape of their tip (Fig. 17-14).[15] The two basic designs of spinal needles are (1) an open-ended (beveled or cutting) needle and (2) a closed tapered-tip pencil-point needle with a side port. The incidence of post–dural puncture headache varies directly with the size of the needle, and it is also lower when a pencil-point (Whitacre or Sprotte) rather than a beveled-tip (Quincke) needle is used.[16] Consequently, a 24- or 25-gauge pencil-point needle is usually selected when spinal anesthesia is performed on younger patients, in whom post–dural puncture headache is more likely to develop. The design of the tip also affects the "feel" of the needle because a pencil-point needle requires more force to insert than a beveled-tip needle does but provides better tactile feel of the various tissues encountered as the needle is advanced.

Approach

Local anesthetic solution is infiltrated to anesthetize the skin and subcutaneous tissue at the anticipated site of cutaneous needle entry, which will be determined by the approach (midline or paramedian) to the subarachnoid space. The midline approach is technically easier, and the needle passes through less sensitive structures, thus requiring less local anesthetic infiltration to ensure patient comfort. However, the paramedian approach is better suited to challenging circumstances when there is narrowing of the interspace or difficulty in flexion of the spine. This can be readily appreciated by examination of a skeleton, which shows that the interlaminar space is largest when viewed from a slightly caudad and lateral vantage point.

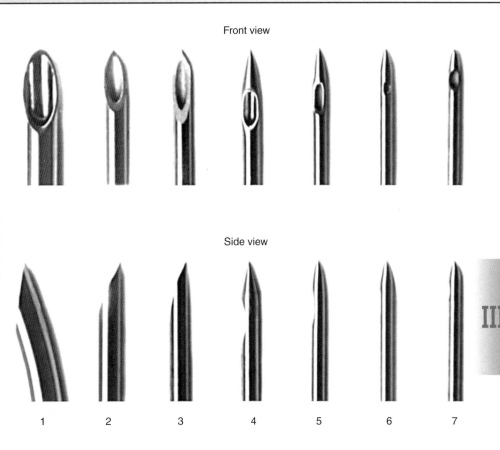

Front view

Side view

1   2   3   4   5   6   7

Figure 17-14 Comparative needle configuration for (1) 18-gauge Tuohy, (2) 20-gauge Quincke, (3) 22-gauge Quincke, (4) 24-gauge Sprotte, (5) 25-gauge Polymedic, (6) 25-gauge Whitacre, and (7) 26-gauge Gertie Marx. (From Schneider MC, Schmid M. Post–dural puncture headache. *In* Birnbach DJ, Gatt SP, Datta S [eds]: Textbook of Obstetric Anesthesia. Philadelphia: Churchill Livingstone, 2000, pp 487-503.)

III

MIDLINE TECHNIQUE

When using the midline approach, the needle is inserted at the top margin of the lower spinous process of the selected interspace. This point is generally easily identified by visual inspection and palpation. However, palpation of the spinous process and even identification of the midline become progressively more challenging with increasing obesity. In such circumstances, it may be helpful to ask whether the patient perceives the needle to be midline or off to one side. After passage through the skin, the needle is progressively advanced with a slight cephalad orientation because of the fact that even in the lumbar area where the spinous processes are relatively straight, the interlaminar space is slightly cephalad to the interspinous space. There is a tendency for small needles to deflect or bend during insertion. Consequently, it is common practice when using 24-gauge or smaller needles to pass them through a larger-gauge introducer needle placed in the interspinous ligament, which serves to guide and stabilize their path. This is particularly important when a beveled needle is used because the angle of the bevel displaces the needle from its path and causes it to veer in a direction opposite the bevel as it is being advanced.

As the spinal needle progresses toward the subarachnoid space, it passes through the skin, subcutaneous tissue, supraspinous ligament, interspinous ligament, ligamentum flavum, and the epidural space to reach and pierce the dura/arachnoid. Although some controversy exists, the dural fibers appear to be largely oriented along the longitudinal axis of the dural sac. Thus, orienting the bevel of a cutting needle parallel to this axis tends to spread rather than cut the fibers, which may reduce the risk for post–dural puncture headache.[17]

PARAMEDIAN TECHNIQUE

The point of cutaneous needle insertion for the paramedian technique is typically 1 cm lateral to the midline but varies in the rostral-caudal plane according to the patient's anatomy and the anesthesiologist's preference. Success depends on an appreciation of the anatomy and appropriate angulation of the needle and not on the precise location of needle insertion. The most common error is to underestimate the distance to the subarachnoid space and direct the needle too medially, with resultant passage across the midline. With the paramedian technique, the needle bypasses the supraspinous and interspinous ligaments, and the ligamentum flavum will be the first resistance encountered.

Taylor Approach

The Taylor approach (first described by Dr. John A. Taylor, a urologist) describes the paramedian technique to access the L5-S1 interspace (Fig. 17-15). Though generally the widest interspace, it is often inaccessible from the midline because of the acute downward orientation of the L5 spinous process. The spinal needle is passed from a point 1 cm caudad and 1 cm medial to the posterior superior iliac spine and advanced cephalad at a 55-degree angle with a medial orientation based on the width of the sacrum. The Taylor approach is technically challenging but very useful because it is minimally dependent on patient flexion for successful passage of the needle into the subarachnoid space.

Anesthetic Injection

After penetration of the dura by the spinal needle (can often be felt by the anesthesiologist's fingers as a rather

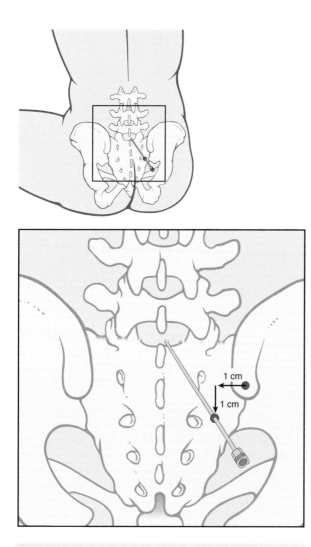

Figure 17-15 The L5-S1 paramedian (Taylor) approach. (From Brown DL [ed]: Atlas of Regional Anesthesia. Philadelphia: WB Saunders, 1992.)

distinct pop), the needle is further advanced a short distance to ensure that the bevel or side port rests entirely within the subarachnoid space. Free flow of CSF from the hub of the needle confirms correct placement of the distal end of the spinal needle. Occasionally, blood-tinged CSF initially appears at the hub of the needle. If clear CSF is subsequently seen, the spinal anesthetic can be completed. Conversely, if blood-tinged CSF continues to flow, the needle should be removed and reinserted at a different interspace. Should blood-tinged CSF still persist, the attempt to induce spinal anesthesia should be terminated. Similarly, spinal anesthesia should never be administered in the presence of a paresthesia. The occurrence of a paresthesia during needle placement mandates withdrawal of the needle.

If using a pencil-point needle, the side port should be positioned to encourage the desired distribution of local anesthetic solution within the subarachnoid space, which is generally cephalad. However, the orientation of the bevel of a cutting needle has no effect on the trajectory of the anesthetic stream emerging from the tip. The needle is secured by holding the hub between the thumb and index finger, with the dorsum of the anesthesiologist's hand resting against the patient's back; the syringe is then attached to the needle, and CSF is again aspirated to reconfirm placement. Care should be taken to ensure that CSF can be easily withdrawn and flows freely into the syringe. With the syringe firmly attached to the needle to prevent loss of local anesthetic solution, the contents of the syringe are delivered into the subarachnoid space over approximately a 3- to 5-second period. Aspiration plus reinjection of a small quantity of CSF again at the conclusion of the injection confirms the needle position and verifies subarachnoid delivery of the local anesthetic solution. Finally, the needle and syringe are withdrawn as a single unit and the antiseptic wiped from the patient's back. The patient is then placed in a position that will encourage the desired distribution of local anesthetic solution or positioned for surgery.

Level and Duration

The distribution of local anesthetic solution in CSF is influenced principally by (1) the baricity of the solution, (2) the contour of the spinal canal, and (3) the position of the patient in the first few minutes after injection of local anesthetic solution into the subarachnoid space. Assuming that an appropriate dose is selected, the duration of spinal anesthesia depends on the drug selected and the presence or absence of a vasoconstrictor (epinephrine or phenylephrine) in the local anesthetic solution (Table 17-1). During recovery, anesthesia regresses from the highest dermatome in a caudad direction.

BARICITY AND PATIENT POSITION

Local anesthetic solutions are classified as hypobaric, isobaric, and hyperbaric based on their density relative to

Table 17–1 Local Anesthetics Used for Spinal Anesthesia

		Dose (mg)			Duration (min)	
	Concentration (%)	T10	T4	Onset (min)	Plain	Epinephrine (0.2 mg)
Lidocaine	5*	40-50	60-75	2-4	45-75	†
Tetracaine	0.5	8-10	12-15	4-6	60-120	120-180
Bupivacaine	0.5-0.75	8-10	12-15	4-6	60-120	†
Ropivacaine	0.5-0.75	10-14	15-20	4-6	60-90	†
Chloroprocaine	2-3	40-50	60	2-4	30-60	†

*Must be diluted to 2.5% or less before administration.
†Not recommended.

the density of CSF. Baricity is an important consideration because it predicts the direction that local anesthetic solution will move after injection into CSF. Consequently, by selecting a local anesthetic solution of appropriate density relative to the position of the patient and the contour of the subarachnoid space, the anesthesiologist seeks to control both the direction and the extent of local anesthetic movement in the subarachnoid space and the resultant distribution of anesthesia.

Hyperbaric Solutions

The most commonly selected local anesthetic solutions for spinal anesthesia are hyperbaric (achieved by the addition of glucose [dextrose]), and their principal advantage is the ability to achieve greater cephalad spread of anesthesia. Commercially available hyperbaric local anesthetic solutions include 0.75% bupivacaine with 8.25% glucose and 5% lidocaine with 7.5% glucose. Tetracaine is formulated as a 1% plain solution and is most often used as a 0.5% solution with 5% glucose, which is achieved by dilution of the anesthetic with an equal volume of 10% glucose.

The contour of the vertebral canal is critical to the subarachnoid distribution of hyperbaric local anesthetic solutions. For example, in the supine horizontal position, the patient's thoracic and sacral kyphosis will be dependent relative to the peak created by the lumbar lordosis (see Fig. 17-1).[2] Anesthetic delivered cephalad to this peak will thus move toward the thoracic kyphosis, which is normally around T6. Placing the patient in a head-down (Trendelenburg) position will further accentuate this cephalad spread of local anesthetic solution and help ensure an adequate level of spinal anesthesia for abdominal surgery.

Hyperbaric local anesthetic solutions can also be administered caudad to the lumbosacral peak to encourage restricted sacral anesthesia (referred to as a saddle block reflecting sensory anesthesia of the area that would be in contact with a saddle). The spinal is performed with the patient seated.

At times it may be desirable to minimize the impact of the lumbosacral lordosis. In such cases, a pillow can be placed under the patient's knees, which will tend to flatten this curve. Even more effective, the patient can be maintained in the lateral position, which will effectively eliminate the influence of the lumbosacral curvature on the distribution of local anesthetic solution in the subarachnoid space. Movement of hyperbaric local anesthetic solution will now be directly influenced by the patient's position on the operating table (the Trendelenburg position promoting cephalad spread and the reverse Trendelenburg position encouraging a restricted block).

Hypobaric Solutions

Hypobaric local anesthetic solutions find limited use in clinical practice and are generally reserved for patients undergoing perineal procedures in the "prone jackknife" position or undergoing hip arthroplasty where anesthetic can "float up" to the nondependent operative site. A common technique is to use a 0.1% solution (1 mg/mL) of tetracaine by diluting the commercial 10% solution with sterile water. However, although these solutions have been used in clinical practice for many years, they are extremely hypotonic, and alternative solutions prepared with third- or half-normal saline will still permit gravitational control but will present far less osmotic stress to neural tissue.

Isobaric Solutions

Isobaric local anesthetic solutions undergo limited spread in the subarachnoid space, which may be considered an advantage or disadvantage depending on the clinical circumstances. A potential advantage of isobaric local anesthetic solutions is a more profound motor block and more prolonged duration of action than that achieved with equivalent hyperbaric local anesthetic solutions. Because the distribution of local anesthetic solutions is not affected by gravity, spinal anesthesia can be performed without concern that the resultant block might be influenced by patient position. Commercially prepared "epidural" anesthetic solutions, which are generally formulated in saline, are commonly used for isobaric spinal anesthesia. However, although these solutions are considered isobaric, they actually behave clinically as though they were slightly hyperbaric, due to the effect of their low temperature relative to the cerebrospinal fluid.

Isobaric spinal anesthesia is particularly well suited for perineal or lower extremity procedures, as well as surgery involving the lower part of the trunk (hip arthroplasty, inguinal hernia repair). Although spread of local anesthetic solution may be limited caudally, subarachnoid injection does not produce segmental anesthesia because the nerves innervating more caudad structures are vulnerable to block as they pass through the region of high local anesthetic concentration.

Adjuvants

VASOCONSTRICTORS

Vasoconstrictors are frequently added to local anesthetic solutions to increase the duration of spinal anesthesia. This is most commonly achieved by the addition of epinephrine (0.1 to 0.2 mg, which is 0.1 to 0.2 mL of a 1:1000 solution) or phenylephrine (2 to 5 mg, which is 0.2 to 0.5 mL of a 1% solution). Increased duration of spinal anesthesia is believed to result from a reduction in spinal cord blood flow, which decreases loss of local anesthetic from the perfused areas and thus increases the duration of exposure to local anesthetic. However, with epinephrine, there may be a small contribution as a result of its α_2-adrenergic analgesic activity.

The effect of vasoconstrictors is not equivalent for all local anesthetics, with tetracaine-induced spinal anesthesia exhibiting the greatest prolongation. This distinction appears to result from the differential effects of the local anesthetics on spinal cord blood flow. Tetracaine produces intense vasodilatation; the effect of lidocaine is more modest, whereas bupivacaine actually decreases both spinal cord and dural blood flow.

The addition of vasoconstrictors to local anesthetic solutions containing lidocaine has been questioned because of reports of nerve injury attributed to spinal lidocaine and experimental evidence showing that epinephrine increases lidocaine neurotoxicity.[18] Adding a vasoconstrictor to other local anesthetic solutions may also produce adverse effects. Epinephrine has been associated with significant "flulike" side effects when coadministered with spinal chloroprocaine, whereas adding epinephrine or phenylephrine to tetracaine has been associated with an increased risk for transient neurologic symptoms.[19,20]

OPIOIDS AND OTHER ANALGESIC AGENTS

Opioids may be added to local anesthetic solutions to enhance surgical anesthesia and provide postoperative analgesia. This effect is mediated at the dorsal horn of the spinal cord, where opioids mimic the effect of endogenous enkephalins. Commonly, fentanyl (25 µg) is used for short surgical procedures, and its administration does not preclude discharge home on the same day. The use of morphine (0.1 to 0.5 mg) can provide effective control of postoperative pain for roughly 24 hours, but it necessitates in-hospital monitoring for respiratory depression. Clonidine, an α_2-adrenergic drug, is not as effective as opioids, and its addition to the local anesthetic solution augments the sympatholytic and hypotensive effects of the local anesthetics.[21]

Choice of Local Anesthetic

Although there are differences among the local anesthetics with respect to the relative intensity of sensory and motor block, selection is based largely on the duration of action and potential adverse side effects.

LIDOCAINE FOR SHORT-DURATION SPINAL ANESTHESIA

Lidocaine has been the most popular short-acting local anesthetic for spinal anesthesia. It has a duration of action of 60 to 90 minutes, and it produces excellent sensory anesthesia and a fairly profound motor block. These features, in conjunction with a favorable recovery profile, make lidocaine particularly well suited for brief surgical procedures, particularly in the ambulatory setting.

Neurotoxicity

Unfortunately, despite a long history of apparent safe use, recent reports of major and minor complications associated with spinal lidocaine have tarnished its reputation and jeopardize its continued clinical use. Initial reports of permanent neurologic deficits were restricted to its use for continuous spinal anesthesia, where extremely high doses were administered.[22] However, other reports suggest that injury may occur even with the administration of a dose historically recommended for single-injection spinal anesthesia.[1,23] These injuries have led to suggested modifications in practice that include a reduction in the lidocaine dose from 100 mg to 60 to 75 mg and dilution of the commercial formulation of 5% lidocaine with an equal volume of saline or CSF before subarachnoid injection.[23]

Transient Neurologic Symptoms

Lidocaine has been linked to the development of transient neurologic symptoms (pain and/or dysesthesia in the back, buttocks, and lower extremities) in up to a third of patients receiving lidocaine for spinal anesthesia.[24] Factors that increase the risk for transient neurologic symptoms in association with lidocaine-induced spinal anesthesia include patient positioning (lithotomy, knee arthroscopy) and outpatient status.[19,25]

ALTERNATIVE LOCAL ANESTHETICS FOR SHORT-DURATION SPINAL ANESTHESIA

The etiology of transient neurologic symptoms is not established, but their occurrence has reinforced dissatisfaction with lidocaine and generated interest in alternative local anesthetics for short-duration spinal anesthesia. Mepivacaine appears to have an incidence of transient neurologic symptoms that is intermediate and may offer some limited benefit. Although procaine has a very short duration of action, its use is associated with a fairly high incidence of nausea, and the incidence of transient neurologic symptoms is probably only marginally better.

Chloroprocaine

Chloroprocaine appears to have promise as a spinal anesthetic.[26,27] Although this local anesthetic was linked to neurologic injuries in the 1980s, it appears that these injuries were due either to excessively high epidural doses that were accidentally injected into the subarachnoid space or to the preservative contained in the commercial anesthetic solution.[28] In any event, recent studies of low-dose (40 to 60 mg) preservative-free chloroprocaine suggest that chloroprocaine can produce excellent short-duration spinal anesthesia with little, if any, risk for transient neurologic symptoms. If additional studies confirm its safety, chloroprocaine will likely replace lidocaine for short-duration spinal anesthesia. The addition of epinephrine to chloroprocaine solutions for spinal anesthesia has been associated with side effects, and vasoconstrictors should not be used to prolong or enhance chloroprocaine spinal anesthesia. In contrast, both fentanyl and clonidine have been shown to provide the expected enhancement of chloroprocaine spinal anesthesia without apparent ill effects.

LONG-DURATION SPINAL ANESTHESIA

Bupivacaine and tetracaine are the local anesthetics most frequently used for long-duration spinal anesthesia. Although ropivacaine has been used as a spinal anesthetic, it is not clear that this drug offers any advantage over bupivacaine. Spinal bupivacaine is available as a 0.75% solution with 8.25% glucose for hyperbaric anesthesia. Tetracaine is prepared as 1% plain solution, which can be diluted with glucose, saline, or water to produce a hyperbaric, isobaric, or hypobaric solution, respectively. The recommended doses (5 to 20 mg) and reported durations of action (90 to 120 minutes) of bupivacaine and tetracaine are similar. However, bupivacaine produces slightly more intense sensory anesthesia (as evidenced by a lower incidence of tourniquet pain), whereas motor block with tetracaine appears to be slightly more pronounced. The more important distinction between these local anesthetics is that the duration of tetracaine spinal anesthesia is more variable and more profoundly affected by the addition of a vasoconstrictor. Consequently, tetracaine remains the most useful spinal anesthetic in circumstances in which a prolonged block is sought. The inclusion of a vasoconstrictor with tetracaine results in a significant incidence of transient neurologic symptoms, as opposed to the rarity of these symptoms when tetracaine is used alone.

Documentation of Anesthesia

Within 30 to 60 seconds after subarachnoid injection of local anesthetic solutions, an attempt should be made to determine the developing level of spinal anesthesia. The desired level of spinal anesthesia is dependent on the type of surgery (Table 17-2). Because nerves of the sympathetic nervous system are usually the first to be blocked, an early indication of the level of a spinal anesthetic can be obtained by evaluating the patient's ability to discriminate temperature changes as produced by "wetting" the skin with an alcohol sponge. In the area blocked by the spinal anesthetic, the alcohol produces a warm or neutral sensation rather than the cold perceived in the unblocked areas. It is important to remember that the level of sympathetic nervous system anesthesia usually exceeds the level of sensory block, which in turn exceeds the level of motor block. The level of sensory anesthesia is often evaluated by the patient's ability to discriminate sharpness as produced by a needle. Skeletal muscle strength is tested by asking the patient to dorsiflex the foot (S1-2), raise the knees (L2-3), or tense the abdominal rectus muscles (T6-12). The first 5 to 10 minutes after the administration of hyperbaric or hypobaric local anesthetic solutions is the most critical time for adjusting the level of anesthesia (Table 17-3). The first 5 to 10 minutes are critical for assessing cardiovascular responses (systemic blood pressure and heart rate) to the evolving spinal anesthesia. Delayed bradycardia and cardiac asystole mandate continuous vigilance beyond early attainment of anesthesia.

Continuous Spinal Anesthesia

Inserting a catheter into the subarachnoid space increases the utility of spinal anesthesia by permitting repeated drug administration as necessary to maintain the level and duration of sensory and motor block (Table 17-4).[22]

Table 17-2   Sensory Level Necessary for Surgical Procedures

Sensory Level	Type of Surgery
S2-S5	Hemorrhoidectomy
L2-L3 (knee)	Foot surgery
L1-L3 (inguinal ligament)	Lower extremity
T10 (umbilicus)	Hip surgery Transurethral resection of the prostate Vaginal delivery
T6-T7 (xiphoid process)	Lower abdominal surgery Appendectomy
T4 (nipple)	Upper abdominal surgery Cesarean section

III

Table 17-3 Levels and Significance of Sensory Block

Cutaneous Level	Segmental Level	Significance
Fifth digit	C8	All cardioaccelerator fibers blocked
Inner aspect of the arm and forearm	T1-2	Some degree of cardioaccelerator block
Apex of the axilla	T3	Easily determined landmark
Nipple	T4-5	Possibility of cardioaccelerator block
Tip of the xiphoid	T7	Splanchnics (T5-L1) may be blocked
Umbilicus	T10	Sympathetic nervous system block limited to the legs
Inguinal ligament	T12	No sympathetic nervous system block
Outer side of the foot	S1	Confirms block of the most difficult root to anesthetize

Table 17-4 Continuous Spinal Anesthesia: Guidelines for Anesthetic Administration

Insert the catheter just far enough to confirm and maintain placement.

Use the lowest effective local anesthetic concentration.

Place a limit on the dose of local anesthetic to be used.

Administer a test dose and assess the extent of any sensory and motor block.

If maldistribution is suspected, use maneuvers to increase the spread of local anesthetic (change the patient's position, alter the lumbosacral curvature, switch to a solution with a different baricity).

If well-distributed sensory anesthesia is not achieved before the dose limit is reached, abandon the technique.

Adapted from Rigler ML, Drasner K, Krejcie TC, et al: Cauda equina syndrome after continuous spinal anesthesia. Anesth Analg 1991;72:275-281.

Anesthesia can be provided for prolonged operations without delaying recovery. An added benefit is the possibility of using lower doses of anesthetic. With the single-injection technique, relatively high doses must be administered to all patients to ensure successful anesthesia in a large percentage of cases. With a catheter in place, smaller doses can be titrated to the patient's response.

TECHNIQUE

After inserting the needle and obtaining free flow of CSF, the catheter is advanced through the needle into the subarachnoid space. Care must be exercised to limit the catheter insertion distance to 2 to 4 cm because unlike placement in the epidural space, further advancement of a subarachnoid catheter runs the risk of impaling the spinal cord. The use of large-bore epidural needles and catheters introduces a significant risk for post–dural puncture headache.

Microcatheters

Microcatheters (27 gauge and smaller) for continuous spinal anesthesia were withdrawn from clinical practice after reports of cauda equina syndrome associated with their use.[22] It is likely that the injury associated with the use of microcatheters resulted from the combination of maldistribution and repetitive injection of local anesthetic solution. It is speculated that pooling of local anesthetic solution in the dependent sacral sac produced a restricted block that was inadequate for surgery. In response to inadequate anesthesia, injections were repeated and ultimately achieved adequate sensory anesthesia, but not before neurotoxic concentrations were reached in the caudal region of the subarachnoid space.[29] It is possible that the microcatheter contributed to this problem because the long narrow-bore tubing creates resistance to injection and thereby results in a low flow rate that can encourage a restricted distribution. However, removal of microcatheters from clinical practice has not eliminated the risk. The problem of maldistribution is not restricted to microcatheters, and the same injuries have occurred with larger "epidural" catheters and other local anesthetics.

Failed Spinal Anesthesia and Repetitive Subarachnoid Injections

Spinal anesthesia is not uniformly successful, and failure may derive from technical considerations such as an inability to identify the subarachnoid space or failure to inject all or part of the local anesthetic solution into the subarachnoid space. A second and generally underappreciated cause of failure is local anesthetic maldistribution. In support of this mechanism is the correlation of success rate with the vertebral interspace, the more caudad interspaces being more prone to failure.[12] This issue becomes important when considering whether to repeat a "failed" spinal and, if so, the dose of anesthetic that should be used for the second injection. In the past, it was considered acceptable to readminister a "full dose." However, if failure derives from maldistribution of the local anesthetic solution, this strategy may introduce a risk of injury.[30] If a spinal anesthetic is to be repeated, it should be assumed that the first injection was delivered in the subarachnoid space as intended, and the combination of the two doses should not exceed that considered reasonable as a single injection for spinal anesthesia.

Physiology

Spinal anesthesia interrupts sensory, motor, and sympathetic nervous system innervation. Local anesthetic solutions injected into the subarachnoid space produce a conduction block of small-diameter, unmyelinated (sympathetic) fibers before interrupting conduction in larger myelinated (sensory and motor) fibers. The sympathetic nervous system block typically exceeds the somatic sensory block by two dermatomes. This estimate may be conservative, with sympathetic nervous system block sometimes exceeding somatic sensory block by as many as six dermatomes, which explains why systemic hypotension may accompany even low sensory levels of spinal anesthesia.

Spinal anesthesia has little, if any effect on resting alveolar ventilation (arterial blood gases unchanged), but high levels of motor anesthesia that produce paralysis of abdominal and intercostal muscles can lead to a decreased ability to cough and expel secretions. Additionally, patients may complain of difficulty breathing (dyspnea) despite adequate ventilation because of inadequate sensation of breathing from loss of proprioception in the abdominal and thoracic muscles.

Spinal anesthesia above T5 inhibits sympathetic nervous system innervation to the gastrointestinal tract, and the resulting unopposed parasympathetic nervous system activity results in contracted intestines and relaxed sphincters. The ureters are contracted, and the ureterovesical orifice is relaxed. Block of afferent impulses from the surgical site by spinal anesthesia is consistent with the absence of an adrenocortical response to painful stimulation. Decreased bleeding during regional anesthesia and certain types of surgery (hip surgery, transurethral resection of the prostate) may reflect a decrease in systemic blood pressure, as well as a reduction in peripheral venous pressure, whereas increased blood flow to the lower extremities after sympathetic nervous system block appears to be a major factor in the decreased incidence of thromboembolic complications after hip surgery. There is no difference in perioperative mortality between regional anesthesia and general anesthesia administered to relatively healthy patients scheduled for elective surgery.

Side Effects and Complications

Side effects associated with spinal anesthesia can usually be predicted from the physiologic effects of the block. Persistent neurologic complications are rare and can be minimized by an appreciation of the factors that can contribute to injury.

NEUROLOGIC COMPLICATIONS

Neurologic complications after spinal anesthesia may result from trauma, either directly provoked by a needle or catheter or indirectly by compression from hematoma or abscess. The occurrence of a paresthesia can, on occasion, be associated with postoperative neurologic findings, which generally resolve. Such injuries will occur with greater frequency and will be more profound if injection of anesthetic is made in the presence of a paresthesia, thus emphasizing the importance of stopping local anesthetic injection should a paresthesia occur. Local anesthetics, if administered in sufficient quantity (particularly within restricted areas of the subarachnoid space), can induce permanent injury.[22,30] Transient neurologic symptoms are a common occurrence after the subarachnoid administration of certain local anesthetics, particularly lidocaine.[19,24,25] Despite the designation as "neurologic," the cause and significance of this self-limited condition remain to be determined.

HYPOTENSION

Hypotension (systolic blood pressure <90 mm Hg) is estimated to occur in about a third of patients receiving spinal anesthesia.[31] This hypotension results from a sympathetic nervous system block that (1) decreases venous return to the heart and decreases cardiac output and/or (2) decreases systemic vascular resistance. Modest decreases in systemic blood pressure are most likely due to decreases in systemic vascular resistance, whereas large decreases in systemic blood pressure are believed to be the result of decreases in venous return and cardiac output. The degree of hypotension often parallels the sensory level of spinal anesthesia and the intravascular fluid volume of the patient. Indeed, the magnitude of hypotension produced by spinal anesthesia is greatly exaggerated by coexisting hypovolemia.

Treatment

Spinal anesthesia–induced hypotension is treated physiologically by restoration of venous return to increase cardiac output. In this regard, the internal autotransfusion produced by a modest head-down position (5 to 10 degrees) will facilitate venous return without greatly exaggerating cephalad spread of the spinal anesthetic. Adequate hydration before the institution of spinal anesthesia is important for minimizing the effects of venodilation from sympathetic nervous system block. However, excessive hydration may be detrimental, particularly in a patient with limited cardiac function or ischemic heart disease, in whom volume load or hemodilution may be poorly tolerated.

Sympathomimetics with positive inotropic and veno-constrictor effects, such as ephedrine (5 to 10 mg IV), are often chosen as first-line drugs to maintain perfusion pressure during the first few minutes after the institution of spinal anesthesia. Phenylephrine (50 to 100 µg IV) and other sympathomimetics that increase systemic vascular resistance may decrease cardiac output and do not specifically correct the decreased venous return contributing to the spinal anesthesia–induced hypotension. Nevertheless, anesthesiologists have long used phenylephrine successfully to treat decreases in systemic blood pressure associated with spinal anesthesia. Furthermore, this drug is of particular value when administration of ephedrine is associated with significant increases in heart rate. In the past, phenylephrine was thought to be contraindicated in parturients because of possible detrimental effects on uterine blood flow, but recent data do not support this proscription (see Chapter 32). In the rare instance when hypotension does not promptly respond to ephedrine or phenylephrine, it is critical to immediately administer epinephrine to avoid progression to cardiac arrest.

BRADYCARDIA AND ASYSTOLE

The heart rate does not change significantly in most patients during spinal anesthesia. However, in an estimated 10% to 15% of patients, significant bradycardia occurs. As with hypotension, the risk for bradycardia increases with increasing sensory levels of anesthesia. Speculated mechanisms for this bradycardia include block of cardioaccelerator fibers originating from T1 through T4 and decreased venous return (Bezold-Jarisch reflex).

Although bradycardia is usually of moderate severity and promptly responsive to atropine or ephedrine, there are reports of precipitous bradycardia and asystole in the absence of any preceding event (Fig. 17-16).[32,33] This catastrophic event can probably be prevented through maintenance of preload and reversal of bradycardia by aggressive stepwise escalation of treatment (ephedrine, 5 to 50 mg IV, atropine, 0.4 to 1.0 mg IV; epinephrine, 0.05 to 0.25 mg IV), whereas the development of profound bradycardia or asystole mandates immediate treatment with full resuscitation doses of epinephrine (1.0 mg IV).

POST–DURAL PUNCTURE HEADACHE

Post–dural puncture headache is a direct consequence of the puncture hole in the dura, which results in loss of CSF at a rate exceeding production. Loss of CSF causes downward displacement of the brain and resultant stretch on sensitive supporting structures (Fig. 17-17).[34] Pain also results from distention of the blood vessels, which must compensate for the loss of CSF because of the fixed volume of the skull.

Manifestations

The pain associated with post–dural puncture headache generally begins 12 to 48 hours after transgression of the

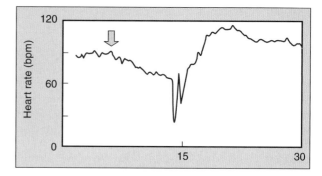

Figure 17-16 Recording of heart rate over time from a single patient who received a spinal anesthetic at the *arrow*, followed by a subsequent gradual decrease in heart rate that culminated in precipitous bradycardia that was unresponsive to atropine and ephedrine. Immediate institution of external cardiac compressions was promptly followed by sinus rhythm (85 beats/min). The precipitous bradycardia occurred while the patient was conversing with the anesthesiologist and in the presence of normal vital signs (oxygen saturation, 98%; systemic blood pressure, 120/50 mm Hg; heart rate, 68 beats/min). (From Mackey DC, Carpenter RL, Thompson GE, et al. Bradycardia and asystole during spinal anesthesia: A report of three cases with morbidity. Anesthesiology 1989;70:866-868, with permission.)

dura, but it can occur immediately and has been reported to occur up to several months after the event. The characteristic feature of post–dural puncture headache is its postural component: it appears or intensifies with sitting or standing and is partially or completely relieved by recumbency. This feature is so distinctive that it is difficult to consider the diagnosis in its absence. Post–dural puncture headache is typically occipital or frontal (or both) and is usually described as dull or throbbing. Associated symptoms such as nausea, vomiting, anorexia, and malaise are common. Ocular disturbances, manifested as diplopia, blurred vision, photophobia, or "spots," may occur and are believed to result from stretch of the cranial nerves, most commonly cranial nerve VI, as the brain descends because of the loss of CSF. Although symptomatic hearing loss is unusual, formal auditory testing will routinely reveal abnormalities.

Though generally a transient problem, loss of CSF may rarely result in significant morbidity because caudal displacement of the brain can result in tearing of bridging veins with the development of a subdural hematoma. Concern should be raised if post–dural puncture headache is progressive or refractory or loses its postural component.

Risk Factors

Age is one of the most important factors affecting the incidence of post–dural puncture headache. Children are

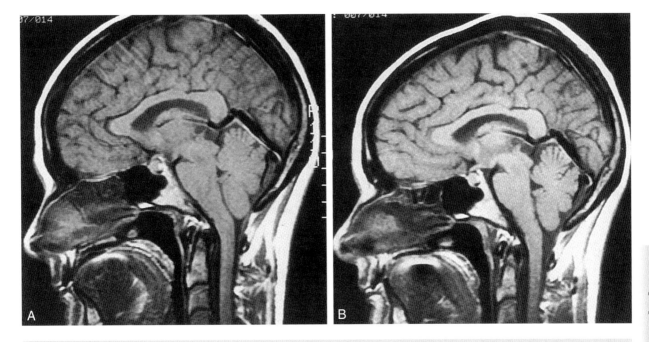

Figure 17-17 A, Anatomy of a "low-pressure" headache. **A,** A T1-weighted sagittal magnetic resonance image demonstrates a "ptotic brain" manifested as tonsillar herniation below the foramen magnum, forward displacement of the pons, absence of the suprasellar cistern, kinking of the chiasm, and fullness of the pituitary gland. **B,** A comparable image of the same patient after an epidural blood patch and resolution of the symptoms demonstrates normal anatomy. (From Drasner K, Swisher JL. *In* Brown DL [ed]: Regional Anesthesia and Analgesia. Philadelphia: WB Saunders, 1996.)

at low risk, but after puberty, risk increases substantially and then slowly declines with advancing age. Although females have been considered more susceptible, this may reflect the marked vulnerability of pregnant women.[35]

A previous history of post–dural puncture headache places one at increased risk for the development of this complication after a subsequent spinal anesthetic.

The incidence of post–dural puncture headache varies directly with the diameter of the needle that has pierced the dura. However, the benefit of a smaller needle with respect to post–dural puncture headache must be balanced against the technical challenge that it may impose. The common use of 24- and 25-gauge needles represents a balance between these two considerations. The shape of the hole created by the needle also has an impact on loss of CSF; this has led to the development of "pencil-point" needle tips, which appear to spread the dural fibers and produce less tear and a smaller hole for a given diameter needle.

Treatment

Initial treatment of post–dural puncture headache is usually conservative and consists of bed rest, fluids, analgesics, and possibly caffeine (500 mg IV). More definitively, a blood patch can be performed, in which 15 to 20 mL of the patient's blood, aseptically obtained, is injected into the epidural space. The injection should be made near or preferably below the site of initial puncture because there is preferential cephalad spread. The patient should remain supine for at least 1 hour and relief should be immediate. The immediate effect is related to the volume effect of the injected blood, whereas long-term relief occurs from sealing or "patching" of the dural tear.

HIGH SPINAL ANESTHESIA

Systemic hypotension frequently accompanies high spinal anesthesia, and patients will become nauseated and agitated. Total spinal anesthesia is the term applied to excessive sensory and motor anesthesia associated with loss of consciousness. Apnea and loss of consciousness are often attributed to ischemic paralysis of the medullary ventilatory centers because of profound hypotension and associated decreases in cerebral blood flow. However, loss of consciousness may also be the direct consequence of local anesthetic effect above the foramen magnum inasmuch as patients may lose or fail to regain consciousness despite restoration of systemic blood pressure. Lesser degrees of excessive spinal anesthesia may warrant conversion to a general anesthetic because of patient distress or ventilatory failure. Total spinal anesthesia is typically manifested soon after injection of the local anesthetic solution into the subarachnoid space.

Treatment

Treatment of high or total spinal anesthesia consists of maintenance of the airway and ventilation, as well as support of the circulation with sympathomimetics and intravenous fluid administration. Patients are placed in a head-down position to facilitate venous return. An attempt to limit the cephalad spread of local anesthetic solution in CSF by placing patients in a head-up position is not recommended because this position jeopardizes cerebral blood flow and thus may contribute to medullary ischemia. Tracheal intubation is usually warranted and is mandated for patients at risk of aspiration (pregnant women). It may be appropriate to administer an intravenous induction drug before tracheal intubation if consciousness is retained and cardiovascular status is acceptable.

NAUSEA

Nausea occurring after the initiation of spinal anesthesia must alert the anesthesiologist to the possibility of systemic hypotension sufficient to produce cerebral ischemia. In such cases, treatment of hypotension with a sympathomimetic should eliminate the nausea. Alternatively, nausea may occur because of a predominance of parasympathetic activity as a result of selective block of sympathetic nervous system innervation to the gastrointestinal tract. Similar to bradycardia, the incidence of nausea and vomiting parallels the sensory level of spinal anesthesia.

URINARY RETENTION

Because spinal anesthesia interferes with innervation of the bladder, administration of large amounts of intravenous fluids can cause bladder distention, which may require catheter drainage. For this reason, it seems prudent to avoid overhydrating patients undergoing minor surgery with spinal anesthesia. However, adequate intravascular fluid replacement must be administered to maintain effective preload and reduce the degree of hypotension and possible progression to bradycardia and asystole.[1,33] Inclusion of epinephrine in the local anesthetic solution may be associated with a prolonged time to voiding.

BACKACHE

Minor, short-lived back pain frequently follows spinal anesthesia and is more likely with multiple attempts at correct advancement of the spinal needle. Backache may also be related to the position required for surgery. Ligament strain may occur when anesthetic-induced sensory block and skeletal muscle relaxation permit the patient to be placed in a position that would normally be uncomfortable or unobtainable. Backache can be confused with transient neurologic symptoms.

HYPOVENTILATION

Decreases in vital capacity can occur if the motor block extends into the upper thoracic and cervical dermatomes. Loss of proprioception from the intercostal musculature can produce subjective feelings of dyspnea. Exaggerated hypoventilation may accompany the intravenous administration of drugs intended to produce a sleeplike state during spinal anesthesia. Constant vigilance of ventilatory status is enhanced by monitors, which must include pulse oximetry and may include capnography.

EPIDURAL ANESTHESIA

Epidural anesthesia, like spinal anesthesia, can be instituted with the patient in the sitting or lateral decubitus position, whereas the prone position is generally selected for caudal blocks. Patients typically receive drugs to produce sedation, except when epidural catheters are placed for labor analgesia in pregnant women.

Timing of Catheter Placement

Controversy exists regarding the wisdom of placing lumbar epidural catheters after induction of general anesthesia. Although there is concern that an inability to elicit a patient response might increase the risk for neural injury, a retrospective review challenges this assertion.[36] Nonetheless, many anesthesiologists believe that lumbar epidural anesthesia and catheter placement are best performed in a communicative patient.[37] Performance of thoracic epidural anesthesia in an anesthetized patient should be avoided.[38] However, the same considerations do not apply to pediatric anesthesia, where a conscious patient would probably impart no benefit but instead add substantial risk. Consequently, it is standard practice to place caudal, lumbar, and even thoracic epidural catheters in children after induction of general anesthesia.

Epidural Needles

The most commonly used epidural needle (Tuohy needle) was originally designed and first used for continuous spinal anesthesia and only later adapted for epidural use. The modern Tuohy needle has a blunt tip so that it might rest against the dura without penetration, but the tip has retained its gentle curve, which serves to guide the catheter's exit obliquely from the needle. Other epidural needles represent modifications of this basic design. For example, the Weiss needle has prominent wings to help stabilize the anesthesiologist's grip, and the Crawford needle has a straighter tip that may be better suited to the steep approach of a midline thoracic epidural or to passage of a catheter into the sacral canal.

Epidural Catheters

Like needles, catheter designs vary (Fig. 17-18).[39] For example, some catheters have an inner stainless steel wire coil to impart flexibility and prevent kinking. This charac-

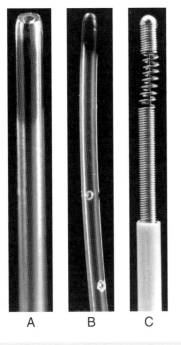

A   B   C

Figure 17-18 A-C, Epidural catheters may have an open end or several openings proximal to the tip. (From Brown DL. Spinal, epidural and caudal anesthesia. *In* Miller RD [ed]: Miller's Anesthesia. Philadelphia: Elsevier, 2005, pp 1653-1683.)

teristic makes them less likely to (1) find false passage into a fascial plane, (2) be advanced out of the epidural space through the intervertebral foramen, and (3) pierce an epidural vessel. However, their flexibility also makes them more difficult to thread into the epidural space. The tip of the catheter may be open or have a closed "bullet" tip with proximal ports. Bullet-tipped or multiorifice catheters tend to produce more uniform distribution of local anesthetic solution, but they have the disadvantage of requiring greater insertion depth to ensure complete delivery of local anesthetic solution into the epidural space.

Epidural Kit

As with spinal anesthesia, epidural anesthesia is performed with equipment obtained from prepackaged sterile epidural kits. Most epidural kits contain a 17- or 18-gauge needle, which permits passage of a 19- or 20-gauge catheter, respectively. Both the needles and the catheters have calibrated markings so that the anesthesiologist can determine the depth of insertion from the skin, as well as the distance that the catheter has advanced past the tip of the needle.

Each epidural kit has one or two needles for infiltration of the skin and for probing the intervertebral space

before insertion of the larger epidural needle. The length of this "finder needle" is usually 3.8 cm, which is sufficient to reach the subarachnoid space in some patients, although the depth of the epidural space is generally 4 to 6 cm. The distance to the epidural space will be affected by body weight and by the angulation of the needle (insertion depth is obviously greater with marked cephalic angulation).

Technique

LUMBAR AND LOW THORACIC EPIDURAL

The technique for a lumbar epidural and low thoracic epidural is similar because the anatomic features of the spine are similar at these vertebral levels. Both midline and paramedian approaches can be used successfully, but the midline is more popular. Advantages of the midline approach include (1) simpler anatomy because there is no need to determine the appropriate lateral orientation of the needle and (2) passage of the needle through less sensitive structures and less probability of contacting facet joints or large spinal nerves that innervate the leg. However, some anesthesiologists prefer to use a paramedian approach based on the unproven concept that needle passage through the interspinous ligament increases the risk for postoperative back pain. The paramedian approach is better suited when challenging circumstances such as hypertrophied bony spurs, spinal abnormalities, or failure to adequately flex create obstacles to needle advancement.

THORACIC EPIDURAL

In contrast to procedures performed in the lumbar area, thoracic epidural anesthesia is generally accomplished through a paramedian approach. In this region the spinous processes are angulated and closely approximated, which makes it difficult to avoid bony obstruction when approaching from the midline. Identification of the lamina is the initial step. If the spinous process can be identified, a skin wheal is raised 0.5 to 1 cm off midline at the caudad tip of the spinous process. The finder needle is then directed at a right angle to the skin and the needle advanced until the lamina is contacted. Local anesthetic is deposited, the needle is withdrawn, and the longer epidural needle is positioned and advanced in a similar manner. After the lamina is contacted, the needle is repeatedly retracted and advanced in a slightly more medial and cephalad direction until it fails to make bony contact at the depth anticipated by previous insertions. If contact with bone continues to occur, the needle is retracted and positioned at a slightly different angle and the process repeated. If success is not obtained, the process is repeated at an insertion site that is slightly (about 1 cm) cephalad or caudad. The midline approach to the thoracic epidural space is similar to that described for lumbar epidurals except that the needle must be advanced cephalad at an acute angle to pass between the steep down-sloping spinous processes (see Fig. 17-5).[5]

Identification of the Epidural Space

Firm engagement of the needle tip in the ligamentum flavum is the most critical step in identification of the epidural space when using either a paramedian or midline approach.

LOSS-OF-RESISTANCE TECHNIQUE

With the loss-of-resistance technique, a syringe containing saline, air, or both is attached to the needle, and the needle is slowly advanced while assessing resistance to injection (Fig. 17-19).[3] One method is to use a syringe containing 2 to 3 mL of saline with a small air bubble (0.1 to 0.3 mL). If the needle is properly seated in the ligamentum flavum, it will be difficult to inject the saline or the air bubble, and the plunger of the syringe will "spring back" to its original position. If the air bubble cannot be compressed without injecting the saline, the needle is most likely not in the ligamentum flavum. In this case, the needle tip may still be in the interspinous ligament, or it may be off the midline in the paraspinous muscles. After proper positioning in the ligamentum flavum, the needle is advanced while continuous pressure is exerted on the plunger of the syringe. An abrupt loss of resistance to injection signals passage through the ligamentum flavum and into the epidural space, at which point the contents of the syringe are delivered. An often-cited advantage of this method is that the dura tends to be forced away from the advancing needle by the saline ejected from the syringe.

HANGING-DROP TECHNIQUE

The "hanging-drop" technique is an alternative method for identifying the epidural space. With this technique, a small drop of saline is placed at the hub of the epidural needle. As the needle passes through the ligamentum flavum into the epidural space, the saline drop is retracted into the needle by the negative pressure in the epidural space. Interestingly, the hanging-drop technique can be used in the lumbar region despite the lack of negative pressure in the lumbar epidural space. In this region, the needle pushing the dura away from the ligamentum flavum creates negative pressure. This technique is likely to be associated with a higher incidence of accidental dura penetration (wet taps).

Administration of Local Anesthetic

As with spinal anesthesia, epidural anesthesia can be performed by injection of local anesthetic solution through the needle (single shot) or through a catheter threaded into and maintained in the epidural space (continuous).

SINGLE-SHOT EPIDURAL ANESTHESIA

The advantage of the single-injection technique is its simplicity, and the distribution of local anesthetic solution tends to be more uniform than when administered through an indwelling catheter. Achievement of anesthesia

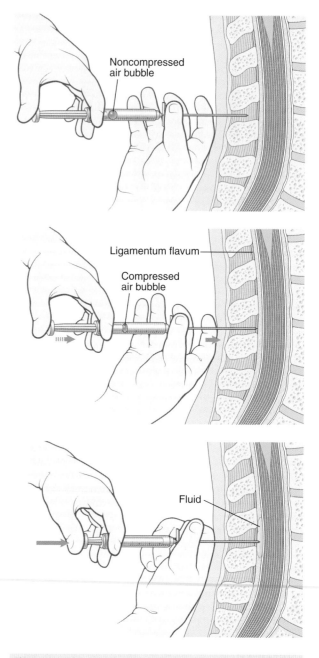

Figure 17-19 Loss-of-resistance technique. The needle is inserted into the ligamentum flavum, and a syringe containing saline and an air bubble is attached to the hub. After compression of the air bubble is obtained by applying pressure on the syringe plunger, the needle is carefully advanced until its entry into the epidural space is confirmed by the characteristic loss of resistance to syringe plunger pressure, and the fluid enters the space easily. (From Afton-Bird G. Atlas of regional anesthesia. *In* Miller RD [ed]: Miller's Anesthesia. Philadelphia: Elsevier, 2005.)

with the single-injection technique begins with administration of a test dose of local anesthetic solution (3 mL of 1.5% lidocaine with 1:200,000 epinephrine). Failure of the test dose to produce sensory and motor anesthesia is assessed after 3 minutes to rule out accidental subarachnoid injection (spinal anesthesia has a rapid onset of sensory and motor block, in contrast to epidural anesthesia). If epinephrine has been included in the test dose, the heart rate is carefully monitored to detect an increase that may signal accidental intravascular injection. The local anesthetic solution is then injected in fractionated doses (multiple injections of 5-mL aliquots) over a 1- to 3-minute period at an appropriate volume and concentration (dose) for the planned surgical procedure. Intermittent dosing is critical because a negative test result does not conclusively rule out intravascular placement. Moreover, the needle's position may have changed during or between injections.

CONTINUOUS EPIDURAL ANESTHESIA

With the continuous epidural technique, a catheter is advanced 3 to 5 cm beyond the tip of the needle positioned in the epidural space. Further advancement increases the risk that the catheter might enter an epidural vein, exit an intervertebral foramen, or wrap around a nerve root. The epidural needle is withdrawn over the catheter, with care taken to not move the catheter. No attempt should be made to withdraw a catheter back through the needle because shearing (transection) of the catheter might result, with retention of the transected tip of the catheter in the epidural space. The catheter is taped to the patient's back, and an empty 3-mL syringe is attached to the distal end of the catheter. Negative pressure is applied to the syringe, and failure to aspirate CSF or blood helps rule out accidental subarachnoid or intravascular placement. After negative aspiration and a negative test dose, epidural anesthesia is initiated by the administration of local anesthetic solution in fractionated doses (multiple injections of 5-mL aliquots). It is important to reconfirm negative aspiration of CSF or blood from the catheter before any subsequent dose of local anesthetic is administered. Documentation of the level of sympathetic nervous block and sensory anesthesia is determined as described for spinal anesthesia (see the section "Documentation of Anesthesia").

CAUDAL ANESTHESIA

Caudal anesthesia in an adult is performed with the patient in either the prone or the lateral position. The sacral area is prepared and draped and the sacral cornu (typically 3 to 5 cm above the coccyx) identified by the anesthesiologist's palpating fingers. The depression between the cornu is the sacral hiatus, and a skin wheal is raised. The needle is introduced perpendicular to the skin through the sacrococcygeal ligament (generally felt as a rather distinct pop) and advanced until the sacrum is

contacted. The needle is then slightly withdrawn, the angle is reduced, and the needle is advanced about 2 cm into the epidural caudal canal (Fig. 17-20).[3] Confirmation that the needle is properly positioned can be obtained by rapidly injecting 5 mL of air or saline through the needle while palpating the skin directly covering the caudal canal. Subcutaneous crepitus or midline swelling indicates that the needle is positioned posterior to the bony sacrum and requires replacement.

Although infection is rare, the nearness of this approach to the rectum mandates particular attention to sterile technique. Subarachnoid injection may occur if the needle is advanced too far cephalad in the sacral canal, or it may result from anatomic variation (the dural sac extends beyond S2 in approximately 10% of individuals). Anatomic variation may also hinder success inasmuch as the sacral hiatus is absent in nearly 10% of patients.

In contrast to adults, location of the sacral hiatus and performance of caudal anesthesia are technically easy in children. After induction of general anesthesia, the child is placed in the lateral position and a needle or catheter is

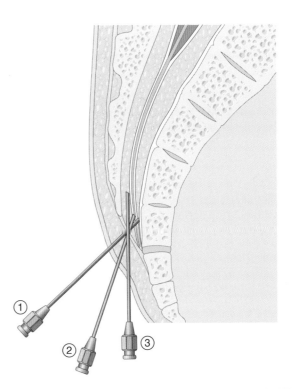

Figure 17-20 Caudal anesthesia. (1) Skin penetration at a 60- to 90-degree angle, (2) redirection of the needle, and (3) slight penetration (1 to 2 mm) within the spinal canal. (From Afton-Bird G. Atlas of regional anesthesia. *In* Miller RD [ed]: Miller's Anesthesia. Philadelphia: Elsevier, 2005.)

III

advanced into the sacral canal. A long-acting local anesthetic will limit general anesthetic requirements and produce effective postoperative analgesia for procedures involving the perineum or lower lumbar dermatomes.

Level of Anesthesia

The principal factors affecting the spread of epidural anesthesia are dose (volume times concentration) and site of injection. However, administration of an equivalent dose (mass) at lower concentration may foster greater spread, particularly with lower concentrations of local anesthetic. Cephalad-to-caudad extension of epidural anesthesia depends on the site of administration of the local anesthetic solution into the epidural space. Lumbar epidural injections produce preferential cephalad spread because of negative intrathoracic pressure transmitted to the epidural space, whereas resistance to caudad spread of local anesthetic solution is created by narrowing of the space at the lumbosacral junction. In contrast, thoracic injections tend to produce symmetric anesthesia and result in greater dermatomal spread for a given dose of local anesthetic. This latter effect results from the comparative volumes of the epidural space, which is smaller in the thoracic region. The site of placement of the local anesthetic solution in the epidural space also defines the area of peak anesthetic effect, which decreases with increasing distance from the injection site.

Spread of anesthesia may vary directly with age and inversely with height, although these effects are likely to be overshadowed by interpatient variability. Achievement of anesthesia is not equivalent at all dermatomes. For example, anesthesia in the L5-S1 distribution may be relatively spared, an effect believed to result from the large diameter of these nerve roots. In contrast to spinal anesthesia, the baricity of local anesthetic solutions does not influence the level of epidural anesthesia. Likewise, patient position during performance of an epidural block is less important, but the dependent portion of the body may still manifest more intense anesthesia than the nondependent side. This effect is most noticeable in a pregnant woman who has remained in a specific lateral position for a prolonged period during labor.

Duration of Anesthesia

The duration of epidural anesthesia, as with spinal anesthesia, is principally affected by the choice of local anesthetic and whether a vasoconstrictor drug is added to the local anesthetic solution. Because achievement of epidural anesthesia is delayed relative to spinal anesthesia, onset time is an additional consideration in selection of the local anesthetic. In this regard, the local anesthetics most commonly selected for epidural anesthesia are (1) chloroprocaine (rapid onset and short duration), (2) lidocaine (intermediate onset and duration), and (3) bupivacaine, levobupivacaine, and ropivacaine (slow onset and prolonged duration of action) (Table 17-5). Tetracaine and procaine have long latency times, which makes them unsuitable for epidural use. Levobupivacaine is clinically similar to bupivacaine, whereas ropivacaine is less potent and often used at higher concentrations.

Adjuvants

EPINEPHRINE

The addition of epinephrine (generally 1:200,000; 5 µg/mL) to local anesthetic solutions decreases vascular absorption of the local anesthetic from the epidural space, thus maintaining effective anesthetic concentrations at the nerve roots for more prolonged periods. Decreased vascular absorption also serves to limit systemic uptake and reduce the risk for systemic toxicity from the local anesthetic. These effects are far more pronounced when epinephrine is coadministered with chloroprocaine or lidocaine than with bupivacaine. The low plasma concentrations of epinephrine that result from epidural injection produce mild β-adrenergic stimulation, which may accentuate the decrease in systemic blood pressure resulting from the epidural block.

OPIOIDS

Similar to spinal anesthesia, opioids are often administered with epidural local anesthetic solutions to enhance surgical anesthesia and to provide postoperative pain control. However, in contrast to spinal administration, lipid solubility of the opioid is a critical factor in determining the selection and appropriate use of epidural opioids. For

Table 17–5	Local Anesthetics Used for Epidural Anesthesia			
			Duration	
	Concentration (%)	Onset (min)	*Plain (min)*	*Epinephrine (1:200,000)*
Chloroprocaine	2-3	5-10	45-60	60-90
Lidocaine	1-2	10-15	60-120	90-180
Bupivacaine	0.25-0.5	15-20	120-200	150-240
Ropivacaine	0.25-1.0	10-20	120-180	150-200

example, morphine, which is relatively hydrophilic, spreads rostrally within the CSF and can produce effective analgesia for thoracic surgery, even when administered into the lumbar epidural space. In contrast, a lipophilic opioid such as fentanyl is rapidly absorbed into the systemic circulation and exhibits little rostral spread. Consequently, the lipophilic opioids demonstrate limited selective spinal activity when administered in the lumbar epidural region because their site of action, the dorsal horn of the spinal cord, rests several segments rostral to the site of administration.

SODIUM BICARBONATE

Local anesthetic effect requires transfer across the nerve membrane. Because local anesthetics are weak bases, they exist largely in the ionic form in commercial preparations. Adding sodium bicarbonate to the solution favors the nonionized form of the local anesthetic and promotes more rapid onset of epidural anesthesia. Most commonly, 1 mL of 8.4% sodium bicarbonate is added to 10 mL of a solution containing lidocaine or chloroprocaine. Alkalinization of a bupivacaine solution is not recommended because this local anesthetic precipitates at alkaline pH.

Failed Epidural Anesthesia

Failed epidural anesthesia may occur when local anesthetic solution is not delivered into the epidural space or because spread of the local anesthetic solution is inadequate to cover the relevant dermatomes. A false loss of resistance can occur in the interspinous ligament before entry into the ligamentum flavum or as the needle passes through fascial planes. For example, the paramedian approach in the thoracic region requires the needle to pass through the latissimus dorsi and trapezius muscles as they insert onto the thoracic vertebrae. It is conceivable that a needle passing through these fascial coverings could transmit a feeling of loss of resistance to the fingers of the anesthesiologist. In some cases, failure results from advancement of the catheter through an intervertebral foramen, which generally gives rise to a limited unilateral block. Fortunately, these blocks can often be salvaged by retracting the catheter a few centimeters. Opinion varies on the presence of a midline barrier to diffusion of local anesthetics.

If epidural anesthesia is nearly adequate and there are concerns that additional local anesthetic would create a risk for systemic toxicity, small doses of chloroprocaine, which are rapidly hydrolyzed in plasma, may provide adequate extension to permit surgery.[40] At other times, failure of epidural anesthesia may be managed by replacement of the epidural catheter or abandonment of the technique in favor of a general or spinal anesthetic. However, subarachnoid injection after a failed epidural produces unpredictable and often excessive spinal anesthesia.[41] This effect probably results from compression of the dural sac by the volume of anesthetic solution in the epidural space.

Physiology

The major site of action of local anesthetic solutions placed in the epidural space appears to be the spinal nerve roots, where the dura is relatively thin. A spinal nerve root site of action is consistent with the often-observed delayed onset or absence of anesthesia in the S1-2 region, presumably reflecting the covering of these nerve roots with connective tissue. To a lesser extent, anesthesia results from diffusion of local anesthetic solutions from the epidural space into the subarachnoid space.

Because the epidural space ends at the foramen magnum, the cranial nerves cannot be blocked by epidural injection of local anesthetics. Even with very high sensory blocks there are areas of sensation that will be unaffected by local epidural anesthetics because they are innervated by afferent fibers in the cranial nerves. The oculomotor nerve contains the pupilloconstrictor fibers that induce miosis after opioid administration. Preservation of this response may provide a potential clue to distinguish high epidural anesthesia from total spinal anesthesia in that the latter may induce pupillary dilatation and loss of the light reflex even in the presence of opioids. It is theoretically possible to completely block the motor breathing apparatus by high epidural anesthesia without loss of consciousness because the phrenic nerve, which innervates the diaphragm, arises from C3 to C5.

SYMPATHETIC NERVOUS SYSTEM BLOCK

As with spinal anesthesia, the most important physiologic alteration produced by an epidural block is sympathetic nervous system block leading to pooling of blood in the large capacitance venous system of the visceral compartment. The result is a reduction in preload and a decrease in cardiac output and systemic blood pressure. As the sympathetic nervous system block extends into the higher T1 through T4 spinal nerves, there is interruption of the cardioaccelerator fibers that control myocardial contractility and heart rate. Because of the sympatholytic effects of epidural anesthesia, patients with low blood volume or other causes of reduced venous return such as pregnancy, ascites, or vena cava obstruction are prone to exaggerated decreases in systemic blood pressure. Additionally, parasympathetic nervous system innervation of the heart is not impaired. Vagal reflexes can therefore produce significant bradycardia and even sinus arrest during epidural anesthesia.

In contrast to spinal anesthesia, the onset of sympathetic nervous system block produced by epidural anesthesia is generally slower, and the likelihood of abrupt hypotension is less. β-Agonist effects from the systemic absorption of epinephrine in the local anesthetic solution produce sufficient vasodilation to accentuate systemic blood pressure decreases when compared with those produced by local anesthetics alone.

Opinions vary regarding whether sympathetic nervous system block from epidural anesthesia is advantageous or deleterious in a normovolemic patient. Sympathetic nervous system denervation of the bowel increases mucosal blood flow and peristalsis, which may hasten the return of bowel function.[42] Thoracic epidural anesthesia with selective block of cardiac sympathetic fibers favorably alters myocardial oxygen supply, reduces cardiac ischemic events, decreases myocardial infarct size after coronary artery occlusion, and improves functional recovery from myocardial stunning in experimental animals.[43] In contrast, lumbar epidural anesthesia results in compensatory sympathetic nervous system activation of the upper thoracic sympathetic segments and may place a marginally perfused myocardium at risk.

Surgical bleeding is less for some procedures during the hypotension produced by epidural anesthesia. Disadvantages of sympathectomy include loss of the body's compensatory mechanisms in response to surgical bleeding and the risk for stroke, spinal cord ischemia, or myocardial infarction if systemic blood pressure is persistently or dangerously low. Additionally, compression of the dural sac by the large volume of epidural fluid may increase pressure in the subarachnoid space and elevate the systemic blood pressure required for adequate perfusion of the spinal cord.

MOTOR BLOCK
Motor block results in difficulty with ambulation after lumbar epidural anesthesia. This complication can impede recovery by restricting the patient to bed rest. Diaphragm function is unaffected by epidural anesthesia unless the motor block rises into the upper cervical nerve roots. With surgery in the thorax and upper abdominal region, epidural anesthesia has favorable effects on respiratory function because it prevents pain-induced splinting and permits uninhibited coughing and deep breathing.

CATABOLISM
Surgery is associated with increased catabolism that results in loss of muscle protein and negative nitrogen balance. Adequate epidural anesthesia can prevent this catabolic response after surgical procedures on the lower abdominal region and lower extremity. The overall stress reduction may result in decreased morbidity and a faster return to normal daily activity.[44]

Side Effects and Complications

Side effects of epidural anesthesia resemble those described for spinal anesthesia, with the added risks of accidental dural puncture, accidental subarachnoid injection, and local anesthetic systemic toxicity, the latter attributable to the high doses of local anesthetic required for the epidural anesthetic. Additional potential complications include epidural hematoma and epidural abscess, particularly in patients with preexisting coagulopathy or infection.

EPIDURAL HEMATOMA
Although potentially attributed to bleeding from vascular trauma during placement of the epidural needle or catheter (or both), it is recognized that both epidural hematoma and epidural abscess may occur spontaneously. When an epidural hematoma is suspected, urgent performance of magnetic resonance imaging is needed because recovery of motor function correlates inversely with the time until surgical decompression of the epidural hematoma.[45]

ACCIDENTAL DURAL PUNCTURE ("WET TAP") AND HEADACHE
Theoretically, epidural anesthesia, which avoids dural puncture, should circumvent the problem of post–dural puncture headache. Unfortunately, inadvertent trespass of the dura does occur, with the incidence greatly affected by the experience of the anesthesiologist. Moreover, if a "wet tap" does occur during attempted performance of epidural anesthesia, the risk for post–dural puncture headache is far greater than after deliberate dural puncture with a small pencil-point needle. Post–dural puncture headache that occurs in the absence of a recognized dural puncture probably reflects the fact that the CSF leak may be too small to be detectable through the epidural needle. When fluid appears at the hub of the epidural needle, it may be difficult to distinguish between CSF or saline used in the syringe to determine loss of resistance. A method to determine the source of fluid is to allow some of it to drip on the anesthesiologist's forearm. The saline, having been administered at room temperature, will be cool and thus easily distinguished from warm CSF (concern for infections such as human immunodeficiency virus, which is concentrated in CSF, detracts from this technique).

Management
Accidental dural puncture may be managed by converting to single-injection or continuous spinal anesthesia, or epidural anesthesia can be attempted at a different lumbar interspace. Placement of an epidural catheter at another interspace, or passage of a subarachnoid catheter, may decrease the risk for post–dural puncture headache.

SYSTEMIC HYPOTENSION
As with spinal anesthesia, systemic hypotension parallels the degree of sympathetic nervous system block. However, because the onset of sympathetic nervous system block is slower, excessive decreases in systemic blood pressure do not usually accompany epidural anesthesia administered to normovolemic patients. Treatment of hypotension is as described for spinal anesthesia.

SYSTEMIC ABSORPTION AND INTRAVASCULAR INJECTION
The high doses of local anesthetics required for epidural anesthesia plus the presence of numerous venous plexuses in the epidural space increase the likelihood of substantial

systemic absorption of local anesthetic. Nevertheless, the resulting blood concentrations of local anesthetics are rarely sufficient to produce systemic toxicity, especially if epinephrine is added to the local anesthetic solution. However, accidental intravascular injection of local anesthetic will produce high blood levels and predictable toxicity ranging from mild central nervous system symptoms (restlessness, slurred speech, tinnitus) to loss of consciousness, seizures, and cardiovascular collapse. Cardiac toxicity is of particular concern with the use of bupivacaine and related anesthetic compounds (see Chapter 11).

ACCIDENTAL SUBARACHNOID INJECTION

Accidental subarachnoid injection of the large volumes of local anesthetic solution used for epidural anesthesia may produce rapid progression to total spinal anesthesia. Immediate treatment is focused on supporting ventilation and restoring or maintaining hemodynamics. However, in contrast to an excessive block produced during spinal anesthesia, the large epidural doses of local anesthetics injected into the subarachnoid space can result in permanent neurologic deficits because of the neurotoxic effects of these agents. In the past, such concerns were limited to chloroprocaine. However, reports of injury establish the potential for neurotoxic injury with the subarachnoid administration of epidural doses of lidocaine and probably any local anesthetic.[46] Consequently, consideration should be given to irrigation of the subarachnoid space with saline, particularly if CSF can be readily aspirated from the misplaced catheter. This maneuver may circumvent or minimize neurologic injury.

Although readily diagnosed in an awake patient, subarachnoid injection may go unrecognized when epidural anesthesia is used in conjunction with a general anesthetic. An unexpected dilated nonreactive pupil after local anesthetic injection into an epidural catheter may indicate migration of the catheter into the subarachnoid space.

SUBDURAL INJECTION

The subdural space is difficult to enter deliberately because the arachnoid is generally closely adherent to the overlying dura. The rare occurrence of subdural injection is difficult to detect because CSF cannot be aspirated through the catheter and the usual test dose is negative. Subdural injection of a local anesthetic solution produces an unusual block characterized by patchy sensory anesthesia and often unilateral dominance. Subdural placement of an epidural catheter is dangerous because the catheter can abruptly pierce the thin arachnoid membrane and thereby enter the subarachnoid space.

NEURAL INJURY

Neural injury after an epidural anesthetic is very rare but seems to be more likely if a paresthesia occurs during performance of this technique. The development of paresthesia as a result of the advancing epidural needle reflects stimulation of a nerve root and is a signal to the anesthesiologist that the needle is not in the midline and needs to be redirected. As with spinal anesthesia, injection of local anesthetic solution in the presence of a paresthesia is contraindicated because nerve damage may be induced or enhanced by the injection. Nevertheless, occurrence of paresthesia is an inherent risk of epidural anesthesia, and neurologic changes attributed to the development of a paresthesia reflect injury that is almost always transient.

COMBINED SPINAL-EPIDURAL ANESTHESIA

Combined spinal-epidural anesthesia is a technique in which a spinal anesthetic and an epidural catheter are placed concurrently. This approach combines the rapid onset and intense sensory anesthesia of a spinal anesthetic with the ability to supplement and extend the duration of the block afforded by an epidural catheter. The technique is commonly used in obstetric anesthesia (see Chapter 32), as well as orthopedic procedures such as hip and knee replacement.

Technique

Combined spinal-epidural anesthesia is performed by placing a needle in the epidural space, followed by passage of a small spinal needle into the subarachnoid space through the lumen of the epidural needle. After injection of the local anesthetic solution, the spinal needle is removed and a catheter is threaded into the epidural space through the epidural needle. Although standard spinal and epidural equipment may be used, there are commercially available needles specifically designed for combined spinal-epidural anesthesia (Fig. 17-21).[6]

An undocumented concern associated with combined spinal-epidural anesthesia is that the meningeal puncture site may permit high concentrations of subsequently administered epidural local anesthetics to enter the subarachnoid space or facilitate passage of the epidural catheter through the dura.

COMBINED EPIDURAL-GENERAL ANESTHESIA

Advantages of epidural block during general anesthesia include less need for opioids, pain-free emergence from anesthesia, and block of the stress response that is nearly complete for most surgical procedures performed below the umbilicus. Various modifications of the combined epidural-general anesthetic are used, but if the administration of general anesthesia is not altered by limiting the use of volatile anesthetics and opioids, there is little advantage to the technique. Combined epidural-general anesthesia requires strict attention to fluid management and

Figure 17-21 A, A spinal needle and epidural needle are used for the combined spinal-epidural technique. **B,** Tuohy needle with a "back eye" that permits placement of the spinal needle directly into the subarachnoid space (*left panel*) and subsequent threading of the epidural catheter into the epidural space after removal of the spinal needle. (From Bridenbaugh PO, Greene NM, Brull SJ. Spinal [subarachnoid] blockade. *In* Cousins MJ, Bridenbaugh PO [eds]: Neural Blockade in Clinical Anesthesia and Management of Pain. Philadelphia: Lippincott-Raven, 1998, pp 203-242.)

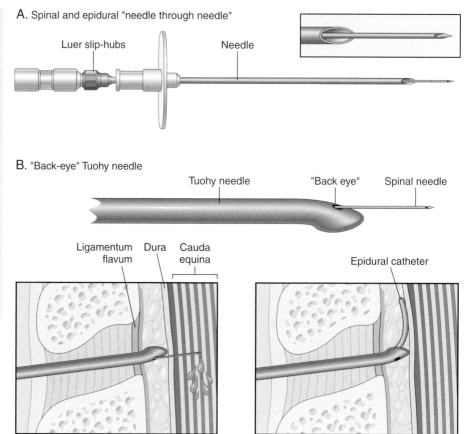

A. Spinal and epidural "needle through needle"

Luer slip-hubs   Needle

B. "Back-eye" Tuohy needle

Tuohy needle   "Back eye"   Spinal needle

Ligamentum flavum   Dura   Cauda equina   Epidural catheter

blood pressure. Sympathomimetics with α-adrenergic activity, such as phenylephrine, dopamine, or epinephrine, can be used to counteract the consequences of afterload reduction, especially in patients at risk for stroke or myocardial ischemia. Excessive fluid administration to treat hypotension is discouraged because it is often not effective and can lead to fluid overload as the block recedes.

REFERENCES

1. Auroy Y, Narchi P, Messiah A, et al. Serious complications related to regional anesthesia: Results of a prospective survey in France. Anesthesiology 1997;87:479-486.
2. Covino BG, Scott DB, Lambert DH. Handbook of Spinal Anaesthesia and Analgesia. Philadelphia: WB Saunders, 1994, pp 12-24.
3. Afton-Bird G. Atlas of regional anesthesia. *In* Miller RD (ed): Miller's Anesthesia. Philadelphia: Elsevier, 2005.
4. Brown DL (ed): Atlas of Regional Anesthesia. Philadelphia: WB Saunders, 1992.
5. Kardish K. Functional anatomy of central blockade in obstetrics. *In* Birnbach DJ, Gatt SP, Datta S (eds): Textbook of Obstetric Anesthesia. Philadelphia: Churchill Livingstone, 2000, pp 121-156.
6. Bridenbaugh PO, Greene NM, Brull SJ. Spinal (subarachnoid) blockade. *In* Cousins MJ, Bridenbaugh PO (eds): Neural Blockade in Clinical Anesthesia and Management of Pain. Philadelphia: Lippincott-Raven, 1998, pp 203-242.
7. Hardy PA. Can epidural catheters penetrate dura mater? An anatomical study. Anaesthesia 1986;41:1146-1147.
8. Cousins MJ, Bromage PR. Epidural neural blockade. *In* Cousins MJ, Bridenbaugh PO (eds): Neural Blockade in Clinical Anesthesia and Management of Pain. Philadelphia: Lippincott-Raven, 1998, pp 243-321.
9. Harrison GR. Topographical anatomy of the lumbar epidural region: An in vivo study using computerized axial tomography. Br J Anaesth 1999;83:229-234.
10. Carp H, Bailey S. The association between meningitis and dural puncture in bacteremic rats. Anesthesiology 1992;76:739-742.
11. Hashimoto K, Sakura S, Bollen AW, et al. Comparative toxicity of glucose and lidocaine administered intrathecally in the rat. Reg Anesth Pain Med 1998;23:444-450.
12. Munhall RJ, Sukhani R, Winnie AP. Incidence and etiology of failed spinal anesthetics in a university hospital: A prospective study. Anesth Analg 1988;67:843-848.
13. Broadbent CR, Maxwell WB, Ferrie R, et al. Ability of anaesthetists to identify a marked lumbar interspace. Anaesthesia 2000;55:1122-1126.

14. Reynolds F. Damage to the conus medullaris following spinal anaesthesia. Anaesthesia 2001;56:238-247.

15. Schneider MC, Schmid M. Post–dural puncture headache. *In* Birnbach DJ, Gatt SP, Datta S (eds): Textbook of Obstetric Anesthesia. Philadelphia: Churchill Livingstone, 2000, pp 487-503.

16. Buettner J, Wresch KP, Klose R. Postdural puncture headache: Comparison of 25-gauge Whitacre and Quincke needles. Reg Anesth 1993;18:166-169.

17. Mihic DN. Postspinal headaches, needle surfaces and longitudinal orientation of the dural fibers. Results of a survey. Reg Anaesth 1986;9:54-56.

18. Hashimoto K, Hampl KF, Nakamura Y, et al. Epinephrine increases the neurotoxic potential of intrathecally administered lidocaine in the rat. Anesthesiology 2001;94:876-881.

19. Freedman JM, Li DK, Drasner K, et al. Transient neurologic symptoms after spinal anesthesia: An epidemiologic study of 1,863 patients. Anesthesiology 1998;89:633-641.

20. Smith KN, Kopacz DJ, McDonald SB. Spinal 2-chloroprocaine: A dose-ranging study and the effect of added epinephrine. Anesth Analg 2004;98:81-88.

21. Eisenach JC, De Kock M, Klimscha W. Alpha2-adrenergic agonists for regional anesthesia. A clinical review of clonidine (1984-1995). Anesthesiology 1996;85:655-674.

22. Rigler ML, Drasner K, Krejcie TC, et al. Cauda equina syndrome after continuous spinal anesthesia. Anesth Analg 1991;72:275-281.

23. Drasner K. Lidocaine spinal anesthesia: A vanishing therapeutic index? Anesthesiology 1997;87:469-472.

24. Hampl KF, Schneider MC, Ummenhofer W, Drewe J. Transient neurologic symptoms after spinal anesthesia. Anesth Analg 1995;81:1148-1153.

25. Pollock JE, Neal JM, Stephenson CA, Wiley CE. Prospective study of the incidence of transient radicular irritation in patients undergoing spinal anesthesia. Anesthesiology 1996;84:1361-1367.

26. Kouri ME, Kopacz DJ. Spinal 2-chloroprocaine: A comparison with lidocaine in volunteers. Anesth Analg 2004;98:75-80.

27. Drasner K. Chloroprocaine spinal anesthesia: Back to the future? Anesth Analg 2005;100:549-552.

28. Taniguchi M, Bollen AW, Drasner K. Sodium bisulfite: Scapegoat for chloroprocaine neurotoxicity? Anesthesiology 2004;100:85-91.

29. Rigler ML, Drasner K. Distribution of catheter-injected local anesthetic in a model of the subarachnoid space. Anesthesiology 1991;75:684-692.

30. Drasner K, Rigler ML. Repeat injection after a "failed spinal": At times, a potentially unsafe practice. Anesthesiology 1991;75:713-714.

31. Carpenter RL, Caplan RA, Brown DL, et al. Incidence and risk factors for side effects of spinal anesthesia. Anesthesiology 1992;76:906-916.

32. Mackey DC, Carpenter RL, Thompson GE, et al. Bradycardia and asystole during spinal anesthesia: A report of three cases with morbidity. Anesthesiology 1989;70:866-868.

33. Caplan RA, Ward RJ, Posner K, Cheney FW. Unexpected cardiac arrest during spinal anesthesia: A closed claims analysis of predisposing factors. Anesthesiology 1988;68:5-11.

34. Drasner K, Swisher JL. Delayed complications and side effects. *In* Brown DL (ed): Regional Anesthesia and Analgesia. Philadelphia: WB Saunders, 1996.

35. Lybecker H, Moller JT, May O, Nielsen HK. Incidence and prediction of postdural puncture headache. A prospective study of 1021 spinal anesthesias. Anesth Analg 1990;70:389-394.

36. Horlocker TT, Abel MD, Messick JM Jr, Schroeder DR. Small risk of serious neurologic complications related to lumbar epidural catheter placement in anesthetized patients. Anesth Analg 2003;96:1547-1552.

37. Rosenquist RW, Birnbach DJ. Epidural insertion in anesthetized adults: Will your patients thank you? Anesth Analg 2003;96:1545-1546.

38. Drasner K. Thoracic epidural anesthesia: Asleep at the wheal? Anesth Analg 2004;99:578-579.

39. Brown DL. Spinal, epidural and caudal anesthesia. *In* Miller RD (ed): Miller's Anesthesia. Philadelphia: Elsevier, 2005, pp 1653-1683.

40. Crosby E, Read D. Salvaging inadequate epidural anaesthetics: "The chloroprocaine save." Can J Anaesth 1991;38:136-137.

41. Mets B, Broccoli E, Brown AR. Is spinal anesthesia after failed epidural anesthesia contraindicated for cesarean section? Anesth Analg 1993;77:629-631.

42. Liu SS, Carpenter RL, Mackey DC, et al. Effects of perioperative analgesic technique on rate of recovery after colon surgery. Anesthesiology 1995;83:757-765.

43. Rolf N, Van de Velde M, Wouters PF, et al. Thoracic epidural anesthesia improves functional recovery from myocardial stunning in conscious dogs. Anesth Analg 1996;83:935-940.

44. Carli F, Mayo N, Klubien K, et al. Epidural analgesia enhances functional exercise capacity and health-related quality of life after colonic surgery: Results of a randomized trial. Anesthesiology 2002;97:540-549.

45. Groen RJ, van Alphen HA. Operative treatment of spontaneous spinal epidural hematomas: A study of the factors determining postoperative outcome. Neurosurgery 1996;39:494-508.

46. Drasner K, Rigler ML, Sessler DI, Stoller ML. Cauda equina syndrome following intended epidural anesthesia. Anesthesiology 1992;77:582-585.

III

Chapter 18

PERIPHERAL NERVE BLOCKS

Andrew T. Gray, Adam B. Collins, and Helge Eilers

Peripheral nerve blocks are used for anesthesia, post-operative analgesia, and diagnosis and treatment of chronic pain syndromes (see Chapter 43). Advantages and disadvantages of peripheral nerve blocks for anesthesia must be considered when advising patients about anesthetic options (see Chapter 14). Peripheral nerve blocks may improve acute pain management and patient disposition even when used only as adjunct techniques. Patients are often more receptive to peripheral nerve blocks when they are reassured that supplemental sedation can be administered intravenously to reduce awareness or if they become uncomfortable during surgery. During the preoperative evaluation the potential sites for peripheral nerve blocks should be examined. The presence of a skin infection in the area to be used for needle insertion must be recognized preoperatively. Confirmation of normal coagulation (history of bleeding or bruising and possibly specific coagulation tests) is generally recommended before performance of peripheral nerve blocks. The presence of a preexisting neuropathy, especially in the area involving the proposed operation, may deter the anesthesiologist from selecting peripheral nerve block anesthesia.

PREPARATION FOR NERVE BLOCKS

Patients scheduled for peripheral nerve block anesthesia are evaluated medically in the same way as patients scheduled for general or neuraxial anesthesia (see Chapter 13). Preoperative medication is useful for decreasing apprehension and providing analgesia during the needle insertions necessary to perform the block. A holding area ("block room") for performing peripheral nerve blocks may be useful for minimizing any delay once the operating room becomes available. Increasing the efficiency of block administration and operating room turnover through the use of a block room will greatly improve acceptance of regional anesthesia techniques. The block room must have appropriate monitors, equipment, and drugs available should adverse reactions to local anesthetics occur. Also for this reason, an intravenous catheter should be in place before performance of a peripheral nerve block. In the operating room, the anesthesiologist must be prepared to provide appropriate supplemental intravenous sedation or induce general anesthesia if necessary.

Prepackaged sterile trays are often used for performance of peripheral nerve blocks. Syringes may include control rings to facilitate delivery of local anesthetic solution and aspiration by the anesthesiologist with one hand. Organic iodine solutions are useful for skin preparation.

The choice of local anesthetic agent for peripheral nerve blockade depends on a number of factors, including the desired onset, duration, and degree of conduction block (see Chapter 11). Lidocaine and mepivacaine, 1% to 1.5%, produce surgical anesthesia in 10 to 20 minutes that lasts 2 to 3 hours. Ropivacaine, 0.5%, and bupivacaine, 0.375% to 0.5%, have a slower onset and produce less motor blockade, but the effect lasts for 6 to 8 hours. The addition of epinephrine, 1:200,000 (5 µg/mL), can serve as a marker for intravascular injection and can substantially increase the duration of a conduction block. In addition, through a decrease in the rate of systemic absorption, epinephrine can reduce peak plasma levels of local anesthetic. Considerations for the choice of local anesthetic solution for intravenous regional neural anesthesia are different from those for peripheral nerve blocks (see the section "Intravenous Regional Neural Anesthesia").

SPECIFIC BLOCK TECHNIQUES

A number of methods can be used to locate peripheral nerves and guide the injection of local anesthetic solutions, including paresthesias, nerve stimulation, and ultrasound.

Paresthesias

Paresthesias are radiating electric shock–like sensations that can occur during regional anesthetic procedures. Historically, practitioners were instructed to remember the dictum "no paresthesias, no anesthesia," which indicates that paresthesias are necessary for a successful block because the needle must be in close proximity to the nerve. Today, although paresthesias remain a standard for block success, they also may indicate the likelihood of nerve injury and are therefore not usually intentionally elicited.[1] Local anesthetic solution should not be injected in the presence of a persistent paresthesia because intraneural injection is accompanied by intense pain and a high likelihood of permanent nerve injury. When paresthesias occur, the block needle should be slightly repositioned before injection of local anesthetic solution.

Nerve Stimulation

Nerve stimulation to evoke a motor response is a common way of identifying peripheral nerves that carry a mixed population of sensory and motor fibers. For nerve stimulation, the block needle is used as a stimulating cathode and another lead on the body serves as the anode to complete the electrical circuit (Fig. 18-1). Cathodal stimulation is more efficient than anodal stimulation, so it is important to not reverse the leads during nerve stimulation–guided block procedures. The location of the surface anode (usually an electrocardiographic pad) on the patient does not alter the stimulation.[2]

A motor response evoked with currents of approximately 0.5 mA indicates sufficient proximity of the block needle to the nerve for success of the block after the injection of local anesthetic solution.[3] Some authors have suggested that the threshold stimulating current (the lowest current that produces a motor response) should be greater than 0.2 mA to ensure that the tip of the needle is not intraneural.[4] Injection of small amounts of local anesthetic solution (1 to 2 mL, the "Raj test") will eliminate the motor response, probably by reducing current density near the tip of the needle rather than by physical separation of the block needle and nerve.[5,6] Recent concerns have been raised that nerve stimulation may fail to produce a motor response in some subjects, even when paresthesias occur.[7]

Nerve stimulation–based approaches may fail to produce plexus anesthesia if the nerves of the plexus are not in sufficient proximity to each other. Longer pulse widths (0.3 msec rather than 0.1 msec) can be used for

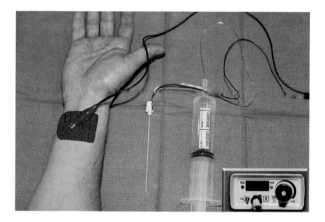

Figure 18-1 Setup for nerve stimulation. The block needle is connected to a stimulator with adjustable current (*inset*) and to extension tubing for injection of local anesthetic solution. An electrocardiographic pad can be used to complete the electrical circuit by functioning as a surface anode (shown in *red*). The shaft of the block needle is coated with insulation.

the stimulation of pure sensory nerves. Nerve stimulators for monitoring neuromuscular blockade are not recommended for peripheral nerve localization because they can deliver large currents (>50 mA) and may not accurately deliver the small currents used for peripheral nerve blocks (range, 0.4 to 2.0 mA).

Ultrasound

High-resolution ultrasound imaging allows direct visualization of peripheral nerves, block needle placement, and the distribution of local anesthetic solution and thereby improves block success and minimizes local anesthetic volume (Fig. 18-2). In addition, ultrasound can also be used to visualize adjacent structures, such as blood vessels or pleura, and may therefore reduce the risk for complications from peripheral nerve blocks. A major advantage of ultrasound imaging is that variability in surface landmarks, body habitus, and patient positioning can be appreciated.

Peripheral nerves can be round, oval, or triangular in transverse cross section (short-axis view) and can change shape along their nerve path.[8] About a third of the fascicles within a peripheral nerve can be seen with high-resolution ultrasound. Though usually considered static structures within the body, peripheral nerves can change position in response to extremity movement.[9]

Ultrasound frequencies of 10 MHz or higher are required to distinguish tendons from nerves based on sonographic appearance. Fortunately, most blocks are performed in regions where this distinction is not a diagnostic issue. High-frequency ultrasound provides better resolution but poor penetration into deeper tissue because of attenuation of the sound beam. Ultrasound visibility of needles for a regional block primarily depends on the gauge and insertion angle.

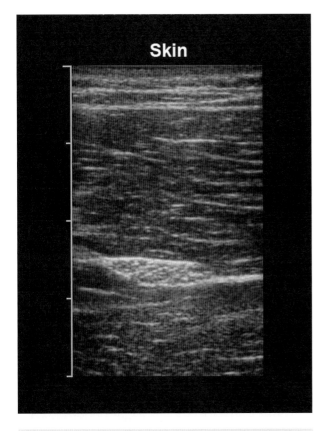

Figure 18-2 Ultrasound can be used to image peripheral nerves. In this example the common peroneal (lateral) and tibial (medial) nerves are seen adjoining each other in the posterior aspect of the thigh. These nerves form the common sciatic nerve, which is approximately 15 mm in mediolateral dimension and 3.5 mm in anteroposterior dimension. Peripheral nerves have a fascicular architecture ("honeycomb" appearance). The *tick marks* are spaced 10 mm apart.

PERIPHERAL NERVE CATHETERS

Catheters can be placed adjacent to peripheral nerves for postoperative analgesia by infusion of dilute local anesthetic solutions. For placement of these catheters, the peripheral nerve is first located in a fashion similar to that for single-injection blocks (typically nerve stimulation or ultrasound guidance with a large-bore needle), and then the catheter is threaded. Some practitioners prefer to first inject local anesthetic solution to create more space adjacent to the nerve before catheter placement. Catheters capable of nerve stimulation can also be used. Peripheral nerve catheters are more prone to dislodgment than epidural catheters because movement of skin near the catheter entry point is usually greater.

CERVICAL PLEXUS BLOCK

The cervical plexus is formed by the first four cervical nerves.[10] With the patient's head turned to the opposite side, the superficial cervical plexus can be blocked by infiltration of local anesthetic solution just deep to the platysma and investing fascia of the neck along the posterior lateral border of the sternocleidomastoid muscle (Fig. 18-3). The anesthesia produced by a cervical plexus block includes the area from the inferior surface of the mandible to the level of the clavicle. A cervical plexus block is used most often to provide anesthesia in conscious patients undergoing carotid endarterectomy. Although combined superficial and deep cervical plexus blocks have traditionally been used for this surgical procedure, studies have demonstrated that a superficial block alone is sufficient.[11]

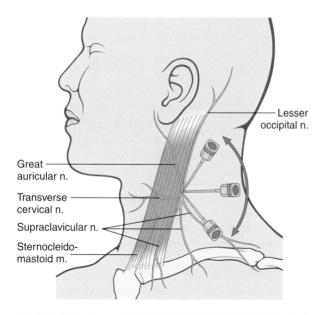

Figure 18-3 Anatomic landmarks and method of needle placement for a superficial cervical plexus block. With the patient's head turned to the side, local anesthetic is infiltrated along the posterolateral border of the sternocleidomastoid muscle. (Adapted from Brown DL, Factor DA [eds]: Regional Anesthesia and Analgesia. Philadelphia: WB Saunders, 1996, p 245.)

BRACHIAL PLEXUS ANATOMY

The brachial plexus arises from the anterior rami of C5 through C8 and T1 (Fig. 18-4). These rami unite to form three trunks in the space between the anterior and middle scalene muscles and then pass over the first rib and under the clavicle to enter the axilla. The trunks form three anterior and three posterior divisions, which recombine to create three cords. These cords divide into terminal branches that supply all the motor and sensory innervation of the upper extremity, with the exception of the skin over the shoulders, which is supplied by the cervical plexus, and the medial aspect of the arm, which is supplied by the intercostobrachial branch of the second intercostal nerve (Fig. 18-5).

Brachial Plexus Block

Although nerves can be anesthetized anywhere along their path, four anatomic locations (interscalene, supraclavicular, infraclavicular, and axillary) are commonly used to place local anesthetic solutions to block the brachial plexus (Table 18-1).

INTERSCALENE BLOCK

An interscalene block of the brachial plexus is achieved by injecting 25 to 40 mL of local anesthetic solution into the interscalene groove adjacent to the transverse process

Figure 18-4 Roots, trunks, divisions, cords, and branches of the right brachial plexus. (Adapted from Wedel DJ, Horlocker TT. Nerve blocks. *In* Miller RD [ed]: Miller's Anesthesia, 6th ed. Philadelphia: Elsevier, 2005.)

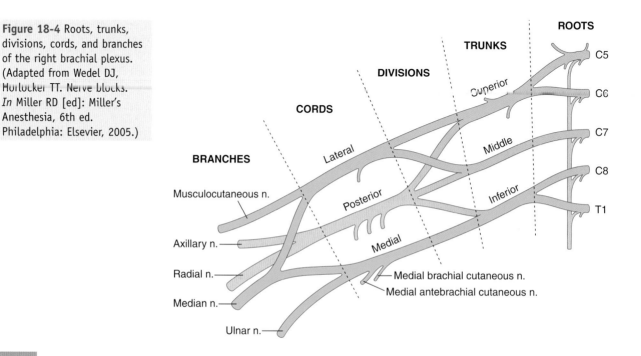

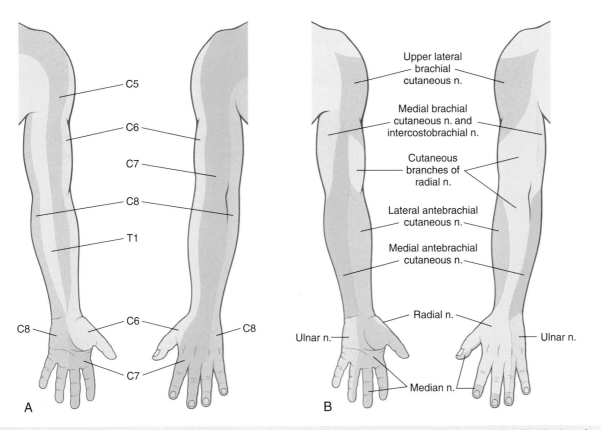

Figure 18-5 A, Cutaneous distribution of the cervical and thoracic roots of the upper extremity. **B,** Cutaneous distribution of the peripheral nerves of the upper extremity. (Adapted from Wedel DJ, Horlocker TT. Nerve blocks. *In* Miller RD [ed]: Miller's Anesthesia, 6th ed. Philadelphia: Elsevier, 2005.)

Table 18–1   Techniques for Brachial Plexus Block

Brachial Plexus Block	Level	Potential Drawback
Interscalene	Roots/trunks	Spares the inferior trunk
Supraclavicular	Trunks/divisions	Risk for pneumothorax
Infraclavicular	Cords	Pectoral discomfort
Axillary	Branches	Spares the musculocutaneous nerve

of C6 (the external jugular vein often overlies this area) (Fig. 18-6). A line extended laterally from the cricoid cartilage intersects the interscalene groove at the level of C6. Paresthesias or a nerve stimulation–evoked motor response of the upper extremity can be elicited before the injection of local anesthetic solutions, while keeping in mind that the brachial plexus is superficial (1 to 2 cm from the skin surface). Although a paresthesia in the shoulder may not reflect stimulation of the brachial plexus, such a paresthesia is associated with the anesthesia necessary for shoulder surgery. Injection of 40 mL of local anesthetic solution will anesthetize the cervical plexus and brachial plexus and thus permit surgery on the acromioclavicular joint, although fibers that innervate the ulnar side of the forearm and hand (C8-T1, inferior trunk) may be spared (see Fig. 18-5) (Table 18-2). An interscalene block of the brachial plexus should be performed with the arm at the patient's side to relax the shoulder.

Complications

Although the risk for pneumothorax is remote, the diagnosis should be considered if cough or chest pain is produced while exploring for the location of the brachial plexus. An ipsilateral phrenic nerve block with associated hemiparesis of the diaphragm is an expected side effect of the interscalene approach to the brachial plexus. Because the phrenic nerve lies on the anterior scalene muscle, the

Figure 18-6 Interscalene block of the brachial plexus. With the patient's head turned to the opposite side and the shoulders relaxed, the interscalene groove is palpated with the fingers of the nondominant hand. The block needle is inserted at the level of the cricoid cartilage in a slight caudad and posterior direction. For convenience of injection and minimal displacement of the needle from its correct position, the needle can be connected with extension tubing to a syringe containing the local anesthetic solution. (Adapted from Wedel DJ, Horlocker TT. Nerve blocks. *In* Miller RD [ed]: Miller's Anesthesia, 6th ed. Philadelphia: Elsevier, 2005.)

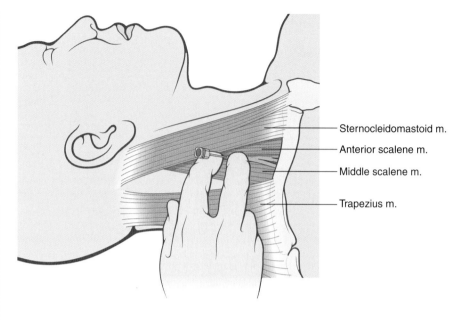

- Sternocleidomastoid m.
- Anterior scalene m.
- Middle scalene m.
- Trapezius m.

Table 18–2 Examples of Peripheral Nerve Blocks
Cervical plexus
Brachial plexus
Interscalene
Supraclavicular
Infraclavicular
Axillary
Wrist block
Median
Ulnar
Radial
Intercostal
Ilioinguinal and iliohypogastric
Femoral
Saphenous
Lateral femoral cutaneous
Obturator
Sciatic
Popliteal
Ankle
Intravenous regional neural anesthesia (Bier block)

incidence of diaphragmatic paralysis after an interscalene block is nearly 100%.[12] Although the resultant unilateral phrenic nerve block is asymptomatic in normal subjects at rest, patients with respiratory insufficiency or contralateral phrenic nerve palsy will tolerate this condition poorly.[13]

Blockade of the recurrent laryngeal nerve can also occur, but much less commonly. It can cause complete airway obstruction in patients with contralateral vocal cord palsy. A preoperative history of hoarseness or neck surgery should alert the practitioner to this possibility. A slight caudad direction of the needle will reduce the chance of an epidural block, subarachnoid block, and injection into a vertebral artery. With this caudad approach the needle will be more likely to contact a transverse process than pass between adjacent ones. If local anesthetics are accidentally injected into a vertebral artery, convulsions will immediately follow. Therefore, meticulous aspiration technique during the procedure is advised.

SUPRACLAVICULAR BLOCK

Supraclavicular block of the brachial plexus is achieved by injecting 25 to 40 mL of local anesthetic solution.[14] Pneumothorax is the most common serious complication of a supraclavicular block (about a 1% incidence) and can be manifested initially as cough, dyspnea, or pleuritic chest pain. Block of the phrenic nerve occurs frequently (50% of procedures) but generally causes no clinically significant symptoms. Bilateral supraclavicular blocks are not recommended for fear of bilateral pneumothorax or phrenic nerve paralysis. Likewise, patients with chronic obstructive pulmonary disease may not be ideal candidates for a supraclavicular block. Advantages of a supraclavicular block are rapid onset and ability to perform the block with the arm in any position. The increased risk for pneumothorax may limit the use of supraclavicular block for outpatients. Because of these risks, many practitioners have advocated the use of ultrasound imaging to guide supraclavicular blocks.

For the "plumb bob" approach to a supraclavicular block the patient should be in the supine position with the arm at the side and the head turned slightly to the side opposite the intended block. The needle is inserted at the point at which the lateral edge of the sternocleidomastoid muscle inserts on the clavicle. The block needle is then advanced in an anterior-to-posterior direction (true vertical, as would be determined by a plumb bob weight suspended from a cord) until it encounters the trunks of the brachial plexus as they course between the anterior and middle scalene muscles to join the subclavian artery. If the brachial plexus is not encountered on the first pass, the needle is redirected in a parasagittal plane (first cephalad and then caudad) on subsequent passes.

INFRACLAVICULAR BLOCK

An infraclavicular block is a versatile procedure that can provide excellent anesthesia and analgesia for procedures on the hand, forearm, and elbow. Blockade of the cords of the brachial plexus occurs in the axilla, just distal to the clavicle (Fig. 18-7). The needle path is remote from the lung and neuraxis, and conduction block occurs at the point where the cords of the brachial plexus tightly surround the axillary artery. Arm abduction is not required but can facilitate assessment of the surface anatomy.

With the patient supine and the arm abducted to 90 degrees, a line is drawn between the ipsilateral Chassaignac tubercle (C6 transverse process) and the axillary artery pulsation in the axilla (Fig. 18-8). A mark is made 2.5 cm distal to the location where this line crosses the clavicle. The skin, underlying subcutaneous tissue, and pectoral muscles are infiltrated with a lidocaine-containing solution, and an 18- to 22-gauge needle is advanced toward the underlying course of the axillary artery. When paresthesia or nerve stimulation indicates proximity to the brachial plexus, 30 to 40 mL of local anesthetic solution is incrementally injected.

When the block is facilitated with a stimulating needle, an evoked motor response below the elbow is most consistent with favorable spread of local anesthetic solution because it suggests that one of the three cords has been identified rather than a nerve branch that may have already left the fascial compartment of the neurovascular bundle. Ultrasound has been used successfully to guide

III

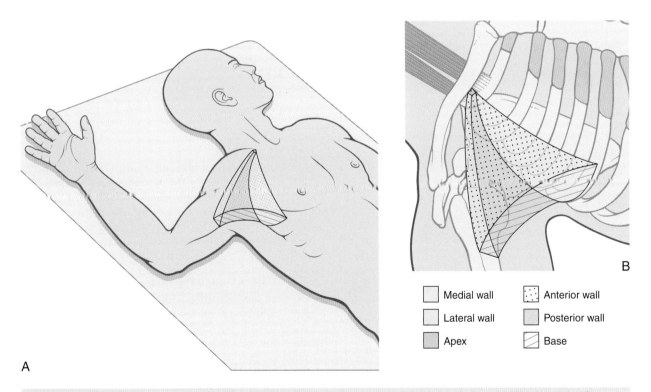

	Medial wall		Anterior wall
	Lateral wall		Posterior wall
	Apex		Base

B

A

Figure 18-7 Surface anatomy of an infraclavicular block (**A**) and the concept of the pyramid-shaped axilla, important for an infraclavicular block (**B**). (Adapted from Brown DL, Factor DA [eds]: Regional Anesthesia and Analgesia. Philadelphia: WB Saunders, 1996.)

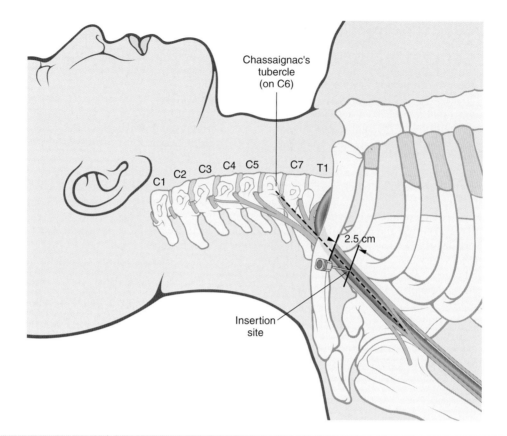

Chassaignac's
tubercle
(on C6)

C1 C2 C3 C4 C5 C7 T1

2.5 cm

Insertion
site

Figure 18-8 Technique of infraclavicular block. **A,** Surface markings for the block. **B,** Parasagittal view showing the arc of needle redirection. (Adapted from Brown DL, Factor DA [eds]: Regional Anesthesia and Analgesia. Philadelphia: WB Saunders, 1996.)

needle placement and shows promise for improving efficacy and safety.[15]

The infraclavicular site is an excellent choice for the insertion of a continuous brachial plexus catheter because it is a secure, clean site that is comfortable for the patient.[16]

Disadvantages

Disadvantages of an infraclavicular block include the risk of vascular puncture and patient discomfort associated with traversing the pectoralis major and minor muscles with the block needle. Appropriate levels of sedation and adequate infiltration of local anesthetic along the needle path are required.

AXILLARY BLOCK

An axillary brachial plexus block is achieved by injecting 30 to 40 mL of local anesthetic solution around the nerves that lie in close proximity to the axillary artery (Fig. 18-9). At the level of the axilla, the terminal branches of the brachial plexus reside within the axillary sheath and in the tissue that immediately surrounds it (Fig. 18-10). An

axillary block can be used for anesthesia of the hand, forearm, and elbow.[17]

The patient is positioned supine with the arm abducted to 90 degrees and externally rotated to gain access to the axilla. For the transarterial approach, a 2.5- to 3.75-cm needle is advanced into and through the axillary artery, as confirmed by aspiration of arterial blood, which stops as the needle exits the vessel on the opposite side. The needle tip is now within the potential space of the axillary sheath. Half the local anesthetic volume is injected in divided doses on the far side of the artery with frequent aspiration. The needle is then withdrawn through the axillary artery until blood return stops, which indicates that the needle is now just superficial to the axillary artery, but still within the sheath. The other half of the local anesthetic solution is deposited to complete the two-point injection. An additional 5 mL of local anesthetic solution is injected in a fanning pattern into the coracobrachialis muscle to block the musculocutaneous nerve. A final 5 mL of local anesthetic solution is infiltrated into the subcutaneous tissue immediately superficial to the axillary

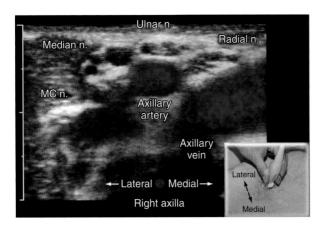

Figure 18-9 Key structures in the right axilla as visualized with a high-frequency ultrasound transducer. The ultrasound image shows superficial structures at the *top* of the image, lateral structures on the *left*, and medial on the *right*. The axillary artery is depicted in *red* and the axillary vein in *blue*. The median, ulnar, radial, and musculocutaneous (MC) nerves are distributed around the periphery of the axillary artery. Large *tick marks* are spaced 10 mm apart. The *inset* shows the corresponding surface anatomy.

artery to block the intercostobrachial, medial brachial cutaneous, and medial antebrachial cutaneous nerves.

Advantages and Complications

An axillary perivascular block has the advantage of being remote from the lung and neuraxis and can therefore be performed with relative safety. Potential complications include systemic local anesthetic toxicity as a result of intravascular injection and nerve injury from needle trauma, intraneural injection, or hematoma.[18]

DISTAL NERVE BLOCKS OF THE UPPER EXTREMITY—WRIST BLOCK

Anesthesia of the hand can be achieved by injecting local anesthetic solution at the wrist to block the median, ulnar, and radial nerves (Fig. 18-11). This anesthetic technique can be useful for hand surgery when a tourniquet is not used for surgical hemostasis. Nerve blocks at the level of the wrist can also be very helpful to supplement a brachial plexus block with incomplete sensory distribution. Blockade at the elbow does not produce more extensive anesthesia than blockade at the wrist does.

Median Nerve Block

The median nerve provides most of the sensory inner-vation to the palm of the hand. At the wrist the median

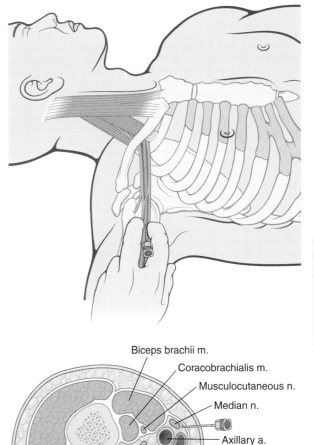

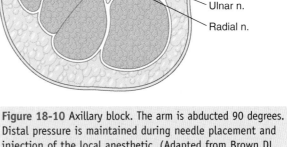

Biceps brachii m.
Coracobrachialis m.
Musculocutaneous n.
Median n.
Axillary a.
Axillary v.
Ulnar n.
Radial n.

Figure 18-10 Axillary block. The arm is abducted 90 degrees. Distal pressure is maintained during needle placement and injection of the local anesthetic. (Adapted from Brown DL, Factor DA [eds]: Regional Anesthesia and Analgesia. Philadelphia: WB Saunders, 1996.)

nerve can be blocked by injecting 3 to 5 mL of local anesthetic solution between the palmaris longus and flexor carpi radialis tendons.

Ulnar Nerve Block

The ulnar nerve provides sensation to the dorsal and palmar sides of the ulnar aspect of the hand. The ulnar nerve is blocked by injecting local anesthetic solution

Figure 18-11 Transverse cross section through the arm at the wrist showing the position of the median, radial, and ulnar nerves, as well as related structures.

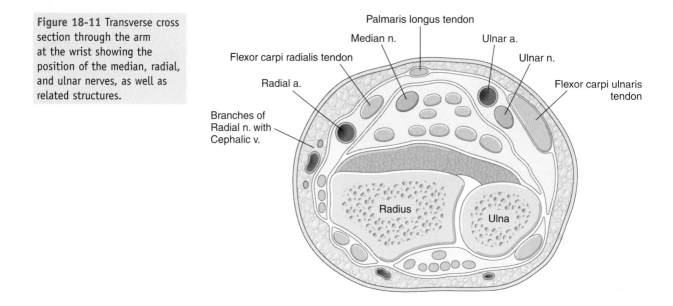

medial to the ulnar artery, between the flexor carpi ulnaris and ulna. Because the dorsal cutaneous branch of the ulnar nerve frequently arises proximal to the wrist, additional local anesthetic solution should be infiltrated in a subcutaneous ring on the dorsal aspect of the wrist.

Radial Nerve Block

Most patients have radial dominance of sensation on the dorsal aspect of the hand. The superficial radial nerve can be blocked by subcutaneous infiltration of local anesthetic solution within the anatomic snuffbox.

INTERCOSTAL NERVE BLOCK

Block of the intercostal nerves provides sensory and motor anesthesia of the chest wall in a dermatomal distribution and without associated sympathetic nervous system blockade. Intercostal nerve blocks are rarely sufficient to perform surgical interventions, but they may provide postoperative analgesia after thoracic and breast surgery or relieve pain after pulmonary contusions or rib fractures. These blocks may also be helpful in the differential diagnosis of somatic and autonomic pain conditions.

Anatomy

The 12 pairs of intercostal nerves lie within the inferior groove of each rib and supply the skin and chest wall skeletal muscles. An intercostal artery and vein accompany each nerve and lie superior to the nerve (Fig. 18-12). Each intercostal nerve has an anterior and lateral cutaneous branch.

Performance of the Block

Although intercostal nerve blocks are optimally performed with the patient in the prone position, they can also be done in almost any other position. To mark needle insertion points, parallel lines are drawn about 5 to 7 cm from the midline on the back where the sharp posterior angulation of the 6th through 11th ribs can be easily palpated, and the ribs are marked on the lines. A short-bevel needle is advanced through a skin wheal at an angle of about 80 degrees until the rib is contacted (see Fig. 18-12, needle position 1). At that point the needle and skin are pushed caudally so that the needle slides under the inferior edge of the rib (Fig. 18-12, needle position 2). The needle is then advanced only 3 to 5 mm, and 3 to 5 mL of local anesthetic solution is injected with frequent aspiration to minimize the likelihood of inadvertent intravascular injection. Ribs above the fifth rib are difficult to palpate because of the overlying scapula and paraspinous muscles. The intercostal nerves at these levels are more easily blocked through a paravertebral approach. Because the lateral cutaneous branches of the intercostal nerves arise at the midaxillary line, they may not be blocked if the needle is inserted too far anteriorly.

Complications

The principal risks of intercostal nerve blocks are pneumothorax and inadvertent intravascular injection of local anesthetic solution. Careful attention should be paid to the total dose of local anesthetic used because systemic absorption is very high after intercostal nerve blocks (see Chapter 11). If multiple levels need to be blocked, alternative techniques such as a thoracic epidural block or

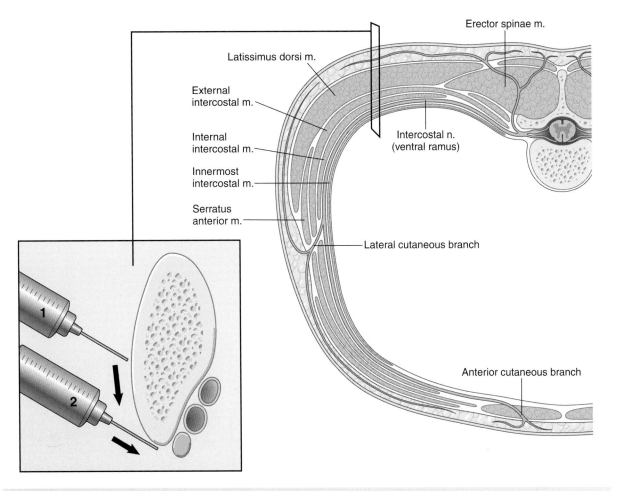

Figure 18-12 Anatomy and technique for an intercostal nerve block. A cross-sectional view shows the course of the intercostal nerve with its cutaneous branches. The *inset* demonstrates the technique of the block. (Adapted from Brown DL, Factor DA [eds]: Regional Anesthesia and Analgesia. Philadelphia: WB Saunders, 1996.)

thoracic paravertebral block with a single injection or continuous infusion should be considered to limit the total dose of local anesthetic used.

ILIOINGUINAL AND ILIOHYPOGASTRIC NERVE BLOCKS

A field block that includes the ilioinguinal and iliohypogastric nerves can provide anesthesia for surgery in the inguinal and genital region, such as inguinal herniorrhaphy or orchiopexy. The ilioinguinal and iliohypogastric nerves are terminal branches of the lumbar plexus and recruit fibers mainly from the L1 root with some contribution from T12. A lateral cutaneous branch of the iliohypogastric nerve innervates the skin of the anterolateral gluteal region. Both the iliohypogastric and ilioinguinal nerves penetrate the transverse abdominal as well as the internal and external oblique muscles and run parallel to the inguinal ligament. The ilioinguinal nerve then enters the inguinal canal and provides sensory innervation to the medial aspect of the thigh and the scrotum and penis in males or part of the labia and mons pubis in females.

Performance of the Block

The needle insertion point is marked 3 cm medial and 3 cm inferior to the anterior superior iliac spine (Fig. 18-13). A 22-gauge short-bevel or pencil-point spinal needle is inserted cephalolaterally through the abdominal muscles to contact the iliac bone on its inner surface (Fig. 18-14, needle position 1; also see Fig. 18-13). While the needle is slowly withdrawn, local anesthetic solution is injected (see Figs. 18-13 and 18-14, needle position 2). This is repeated one or two times with the needle directed more medially to cover a fan-shaped area. A total of 10 to 20 mL

Figure 18-13 Anatomy and surface landmarks for ilioinguinal and iliohypogastric block. (Adapted from Brown DL, Factor DA [eds]: Regional Anesthesia and Analgesia. Philadelphia: WB Saunders, 1996.)

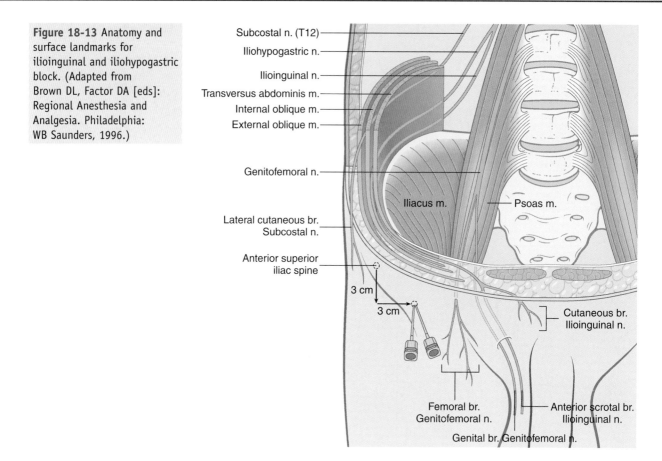

of local anesthetic solution should be sufficient. In some cases, the ilioinguinal and iliohypogastric blocks have to be supplemented by a genitofemoral nerve block.

BLOCKS OF THE LOWER EXTREMITY

Unlike the compactness of the brachial plexus, the lower extremity is supplied by nerves that are widely separated from each other as they enter the thigh (Fig. 18-15). Major nerves to the lower extremity include the sciatic, posterior femoral cutaneous, femoral, lateral femoral cutaneous, and obturator nerves. For many operations, it is easier to perform an epidural or spinal anesthetic than to attempt the same extent of anesthesia with multiple peripheral nerve blocks. However, reports of epidural hematomas in patients being treated with low-molecular-weight heparin and receiving neuraxial anesthesia have raised interest in peripheral nerve blocks of the lower extremity. Even when these lower extremity blocks do not serve as definitive anesthetics, they can improve patient disposition by providing superior postoperative pain relief.

Femoral Nerve Block

A femoral nerve block provides anesthesia to the anterior aspect of the thigh and knee, as well as the medial aspect of the leg. It is a definitive anesthetic only for superficial surgical procedures such as muscle biopsy and is therefore typically combined with other blocks such as a sciatic nerve block. A femoral nerve block alone or in combination with other peripheral nerve blocks is very useful for postoperative analgesia and provides a good alternative when contraindications to neuraxial blockade are present.

ANATOMY

Arising from lumbar segments L2 through L4, the femoral nerve reaches the thigh by passing underneath the inguinal ligament just lateral to the femoral artery and vein. Along its course, the femoral nerve divides into multiple anterior cutaneous branches of the thigh and gives rise to the saphenous nerve of the medial aspect of the leg.

PERFORMANCE OF THE BLOCK

A femoral nerve block is performed with the patient in the supine position and the thigh slightly abducted and

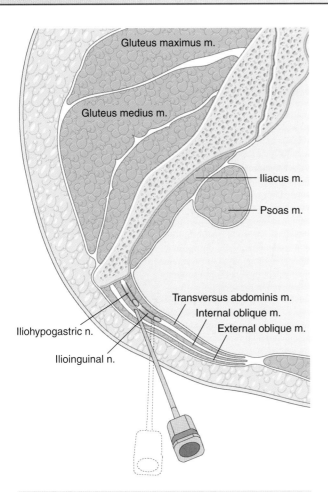

Figure 18-14 Cross-sectional anatomy of the ilioinguinal and iliohypogastric nerves. (Adapted from Brown DL, Factor DA [eds]: Regional Anesthesia and Analgesia. Philadelphia: WB Saunders, 1996.)

externally rotated for easier palpation of the femoral artery (Fig. 18-16). The use of a nerve stimulator is helpful, but not essential. A line is drawn between the anterior superior iliac spine and the pubic tubercle to indicate the inguinal ligament. The pulse of the femoral artery is palpated and marked 1 to 2 cm caudal to the ligament. Through a skin wheal 1 cm lateral to this mark a 22-gauge, 40-mm needle is inserted perpendicular to the skin to a depth of approximately 2 to 3 cm until the nerve is identified by paresthesia or stimulation of quadriceps muscle contraction. With intermittent aspiration, 20 mL of local anesthetic solution is injected to produce blockade of the nerve. This is best done in a fan-shaped pattern in the mediolateral dimension, especially if no nerve stimulation was used and no paresthesias elicited. Because of the close proximity of the femoral artery and vein, vascular puncture is possible and associated with a risk for hematoma or intravascular injection.

Saphenous Nerve Block

The saphenous nerve is the only branch of the femoral nerve to contribute to innervation below the knee. The saphenous nerve follows the course of the saphenous vein along the medial aspect of the leg. Anesthesia in this distribution can be achieved by infiltrating local anesthetic solution around the saphenous vein at the level of the tibial tuberosity. Because the saphenous vein can be difficult to palpate, ultrasound can be used to guide this block.[19] This block is often combined with a popliteal nerve block for ankle anesthesia.

Lateral Femoral Cutaneous Nerve Block

The lateral femoral cutaneous nerve (LFCN) is a sensory nerve that innervates the lateral aspect of the thigh. This nerve is highly variable in its course and number of branches. The LFCN can be blocked by infiltrating 5 to 10 mL of local anesthetic solution at a point 2 cm medial and 2 cm distal to the anterior superior iliac spine. This block may provide suitable anesthesia for superficial interventions such as removal of small skin grafts or biopsies, but it can also be used to supplement other lower extremity nerve blocks for surgery on or above the knee. A large-volume femoral nerve block usually blocks the LFCN, and therefore this additional procedure may not be necessary.

Obturator Nerve Block

The obturator nerve provides variable cutaneous innervation of the thigh and can be medial (20%), posterior (23%), or absent (57%).[20] An obturator nerve block is performed by introducing the needle 1 to 2 cm distal and lateral to the pubic tubercle. When the pubic bone is reached, the needle is withdrawn and redirected cephalad to identify the obturator canal, where 10 to 15 mL of local anesthetic solution is injected. Contraction of the adductor muscles with nerve stimulation indicates proximity of the block needle to the obturator nerve. Because this nerve is frequently missed after 3-in-1 blocks, it is a valuable supplement to sciatic, femoral, and LFCN blocks for surgery on or above the knee.[21]

Sciatic Nerve Block (Classic Approach of Labat)

The sacral plexus (L4-5, S1-3) gives rise to the sciatic nerve, which is nearly 2 cm wide as it leaves the pelvis. The classic approach to a sciatic nerve block is with the patient lying on the side opposite the nerve to be blocked (Fig. 18-17). A line is drawn between the posterior superior iliac spine and the greater trochanter of the femur. The needle is inserted about 5 cm caudad from the midpoint of this line. Foot movement evoked by nerve stimulation is a satisfactory end point for needle placement before the injection of local anesthetic

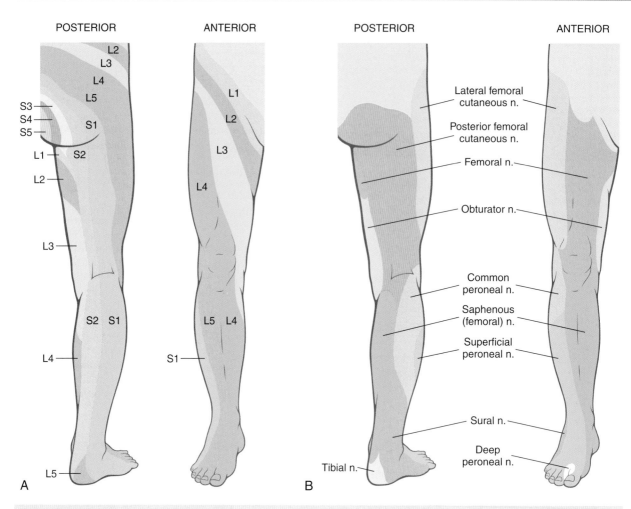

Figure 18-15 A, Cutaneous distribution of the lumbosacral nerves. **B**, Cutaneous distribution of the peripheral nerves of the lower extremity. Note that the cutaneous distribution of the obturator nerve is highly variable, but shown here on the medial aspect of the thigh. (Adapted from Wedel DJ, Horlocker TT. Nerve blocks. *In* Miller RD [ed]: Miller's Anesthesia, 6th ed. Philadelphia: Elsevier, 2005.)

solution (about 25 to 30 mL is typically used). This block provides nearly complete anesthesia of the foot and lower part of the leg. More often, a sciatic nerve block is combined with a femoral nerve block to provide more extensive anesthesia.

Popliteal Nerve Block

A popliteal nerve block provides sciatic nerve anesthesia just proximal to the point where the sciatic nerve divides into its common peroneal and tibial nerve components in the popliteal fossa (Fig. 18-18). It is most commonly used for foot and ankle surgery, but supplementation with a femoral or saphenous nerve block may be necessary for surgery on the medial aspect of the leg or if a tourniquet is used. The block can be performed with the patient prone (posterior approach) or supine (lateral approach). For the posterior approach, the block needle is inserted just lateral to the midline. For the lateral approach, the block needle is inserted just anterior to the tendon of the biceps femoris muscle. With either approach the block needle is inserted 5 to 10 cm proximal to the knee crease to help ensure that both the tibial and common peroneal nerves are blocked. As with a sciatic nerve block, nerve stimulation that evokes foot movement can be used as an end point before injecting 20 to 30 mL of local anesthetic solution for a popliteal block.

One problem with this block is biologic variability in the point of division of the sciatic nerve.[22] Ultrasound is useful for guiding injections of local anesthetic solution into the popliteal fossa to ensure complete block in both the tibial and common peroneal distributions.[23]

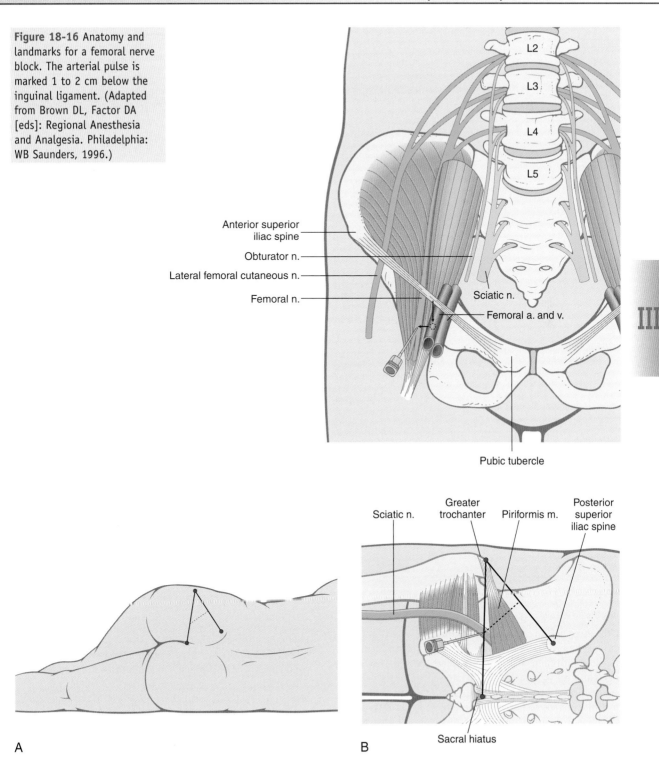

Figure 18-16 Anatomy and landmarks for a femoral nerve block. The arterial pulse is marked 1 to 2 cm below the inguinal ligament. (Adapted from Brown DL, Factor DA [eds]: Regional Anesthesia and Analgesia. Philadelphia: WB Saunders, 1996.)

Anterior superior iliac spine

Obturator n.

Lateral femoral cutaneous n.

Femoral n.

Sciatic n.

Femoral a. and v.

Pubic tubercle

Sciatic n.

Greater trochanter

Piriformis m.

Posterior superior iliac spine

Sacral hiatus

A

B

Figure 18-17 Posterior approach to a sciatic nerve block. **A**, Patient positioning. **B**, Anatomic landmarks. The sciatic nerve lies beneath a point 5 cm caudad along a perpendicular line that bisects a line joining the posterior iliac spine and the greater trochanter of the femur. This point is also usually the intersection of that perpendicular line with a line joining the greater trochanter and the sacral hiatus. (Adapted from Wedel DJ, Horlocker TT. Nerve blocks. *In* Miller RD [ed]: Miller's Anesthesia, 6th ed. Philadelphia: Elsevier, 2005.)

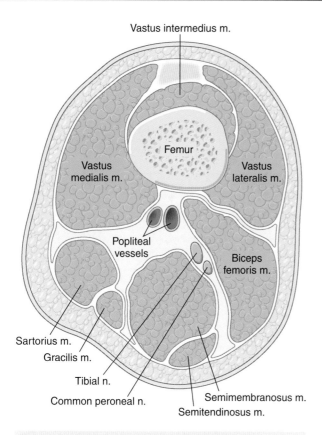

Figure 18-18 Anatomic section of the leg within the popliteal fossa just distal to where the sciatic nerve divides into the common peroneal nerve and tibial nerve. (From Hahn MB, McQuillan PM, Sheplick GJ. Regional Anesthesia: An Atlas of Anatomy and Techniques. St Louis: CV Mosby, 1996.)

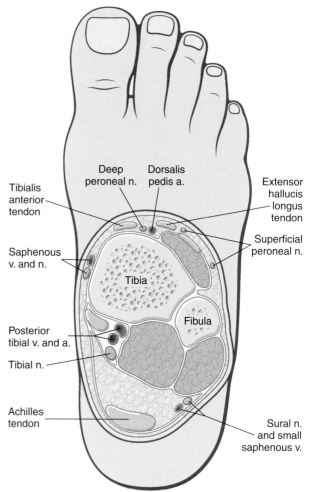

Figure 18-19 Cross-sectional anatomy for an ankle block. An ankle block is performed by injecting local anesthetic solution at five separate nerve locations. The superficial peroneal nerve, sural nerve, and saphenous nerve are usually blocked by subcutaneous infiltration because they may have already branched as they cross the ankle joint. The tibial and deep peroneal nerves require deeper injection adjacent to the accompanying blood vessels (the posterior tibial and anterior tibial arteries, respectively). Because the block needle approaches the ankle from many angles, it is convenient to elevate the foot by supporting the calf. (Adapted from Brown DL, Factor DA [eds]: Regional Anesthesia and Analgesia. Philadelphia: WB Saunders, 1996.)

Ankle Block

All five peripheral nerves that supply the foot can be blocked (ankle block) at the level of the malleoli (Fig. 18-19). The tibial nerve is the major nerve to the sole of the foot. This nerve lies on the heel side of the posterior tibial artery and can be blocked by infiltrating 3 to 5 mL of local anesthetic solution in a fanning pattern around this artery. The sural nerve innervates the lateral side of the foot and can be blocked by injecting 5 mL of local anesthetic solution in the groove between the lateral malleolus and the calcaneus near the small saphenous vein. The saphenous nerve innervates the medial aspect of the foot. Infiltration of 5 mL of local anesthetic solution anterior to the medial malleolus near the great saphenous vein blocks this nerve. The deep peroneal nerve innervates the webbing between the first and second toes and is blocked by injecting 5 mL of local anesthetic solution adjacent to the anterior tibial artery. Alternatively, if arterial pulsation is absent, the deep peroneal nerve can also be blocked deep to the extensor

hallucis longus tendon and extensor retinaculum. The dorsum of the foot is innervated by the superficial peroneal nerve. The superficial branches of this nerve are blocked by injecting a subcutaneous ridge of local anesthetic between the medial and lateral malleoli over the anterior surface of the foot. Because the foot does not have a generous blood supply, systemic toxicity after an ankle block is rare.

INTRAVENOUS REGIONAL NEURAL ANESTHESIA

Intravenous regional neural anesthesia (Bier block, named after August Bier) is a simple method of producing anesthesia of the arm or leg. This technique involves the intravenous injection of large volumes of dilute local anesthetic solutions into an extremity after occlusion of the circulation by a tourniquet. A Bier block is an alternative method of producing extremity anesthesia without blocking individual peripheral nerves. A Bier block can be used for surgical procedures with a duration of 2 hours or less. Severe tourniquet pain and the maximum allowable tourniquet time limit the practical duration of the block. Because the duration of postoperative analgesia is also limited, this procedure is not usually performed when postoperative pain is a significant issue.

Contraindications

Contraindications to a Bier block are essentially contraindications to tourniquet application (sickle cell disease, infection, ischemic vascular disease). Pain limits the effectiveness of exsanguination of extremities with fractures. Traumatic lacerations may allow escape of local anesthetic from the extremity.

Performance of the Block

A small intravenous catheter is placed in the distal portion of the involved extremity. The arm or leg is then exsanguinated by wrapping with an Esmarch bandage (Fig. 18-20). The tourniquet is inflated to 250 to 275 mm Hg, or about 100 mm Hg above the patient's systolic blood pressure. Plain (without epinephrine) local anesthetic solution (40 to 50 mL for the upper extremity) is injected for a 70-kg adult patient. The intravenous catheter is normally removed after this injection. Beyond 45 minutes of surgery, many patients experience pain at the site of tourniquet placement. A double-tourniquet technique can be used to reduce tourniquet pain. With this technique the proximal cuff is initially inflated, and when the patient subsequently experiences pain, the more distal cuff over anesthetized skin is inflated and the proximal cuff is then deflated. Blockade of the intercostobrachial nerve by local anesthetic infiltration proximal to the tourniquet on the medial aspect of the arm can also be used to reduce pain from tourniquet inflation.

Selection of Local Anesthetic

Commonly used local anesthetic solutions for intravenous regional neural anesthesia are 0.5% lidocaine or prilocaine (plain solutions without epinephrine). Racemic bupivacaine is avoided because of potential systemic toxicity, most notably malignant ventricular cardiac dysrhythmias

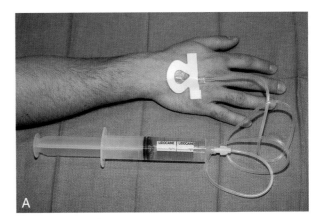

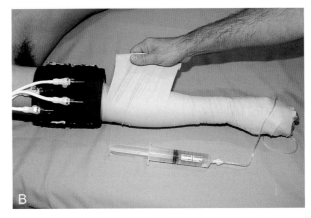

Figure 18-20 A, Placement and securing of a small intravenous catheter. **B,** Exsanguination of the arm with an Esmarch bandage before inflation of the tourniquet and injection of the local anesthetic solution through the catheter.

leading to refractory cardiac arrest. Ropivacaine (1.2 to 1.8 mg/kg in 40 mL) and levobupivacaine (40 mL of 0.125% solution) have been used for intravenous regional neural anesthesia in adult patients because they are associated with less cardiovascular and central nervous system toxicity than racemic bupivacaine is.[24,25] Preservative-free solutions of local anesthetic are recommended for intravenous regional anesthesia because preservatives have been associated with thrombophlebitis.

Characteristics of the Block

The onset of anesthesia rapidly follows the intravenous administration of local anesthetic solution into the isolated extremity. The duration of surgical anesthesia depends on the time that the tourniquet is inflated and not on the local anesthetic selected. When compared with lidocaine, the intravenous regional neural anesthesia produced by ropivacaine and levobupivacaine appears to be comparable but has slightly longer-lasting residual effects.[24,25] Technically, a regional intravenous neural block is easier and faster to perform than a brachial plexus block or lower extremity block and is readily applicable to all age groups, including pediatric patients.

Risks

The principal risk associated with intravenous regional neural anesthesia is the potential systemic toxicity that may occur when the tourniquet is deflated and large amounts of local anesthetic solution from the previously isolated part of the extremity enter the systemic circulation. Local anesthetic levels peak approximately 2 to 5 minutes after tourniquet deflation when an intravenous regional block is used. In this regard, one recommendation is to keep the tourniquet inflated for at least 20 minutes, even if the surgical procedure is completed in less time. If 40 minutes has elapsed, the tourniquet can be deflated in a single maneuver. Between 20 and 40 minutes, the tourniquet can be deflated, reinflated immediately, and finally deflated after 1 minute. This method will reduce the peak plasma level of local anesthetic. Limitation of extremity movement after release of the tourniquet is also useful for minimizing local anesthetic blood levels. The rapid metabolism of prilocaine is advantageous for decreasing the likelihood of systemic toxicity after deflation of the tourniquet. Significant methemoglobinemia is unlikely to accompany metabolism of prilocaine when the total dose of this local anesthetic administered to adults is less than 600 mg (see Chapter 11).

If the extremity is not adequately exsanguinated, the skin will have a blotchy appearance after injection of the local anesthetic. In this situation, the quality of the block and surgical field will be poor. Intravenous regional sympathetic blocks with guanethidine, reserpine, or bretylium are sometimes used for chronic pain management.

REFERENCES

1. Selander D, Edshage S, Wolff T. Paresthesiae or no paresthesiae? Nerve lesions after axillary blocks. Acta Anaesthesiol Scand 1979;23:27-33.
2. Hadzic A, Vloka JD, Claudio RE, Hadzic N, et al. Electrical nerve localization: Effects of cutaneous electrode placement and duration of the stimulus on motor response. Anesthesiology 2004;100:1526-1530.
3. Carles M, Pulcini A, Macchi P, et al. An evaluation of the brachial plexus block at the humeral canal using a neurostimulator (1417 patients): The efficacy, safety, and predictive criteria of failure. Anesth Analg 2001;92:194-198.
4. Hadzic A. Peripheral nerve stimulators: Cracking the code—one at a time. Reg Anesth Pain Med 2004;29:185-188.
5. Montgomery SJ, Raj PP, Nettles D, Jenkins MT. The use of the nerve stimulator with standard unsheathed needles in nerve blockade. Anesth Analg 1973;52:827-831.
6. Tsui BC, Wagner A, Finucane B. Electrophysiologic effect of injectates on peripheral nerve stimulation. Reg Anesth Pain Med 2004;29:189-193.
7. Mulroy MF, Mitchell B. Unsolicited paresthesias with nerve stimulator: Case reports of four patients. Anesth Analg 2002;95:762-763.
8. Schafhalter-Zoppoth I, Gray AT. The musculocutaneous nerve: Ultrasound appearance for peripheral nerve block. Reg Anesth Pain Med 2005;30:385-390.
9. Schafhalter-Zoppoth I, Younger SJ, Collins AB, Gray AT. The "seesaw" sign: Improved sonographic identification of the sciatic nerve. Anesthesiology 2004;101:808-809.
10. Pandit JJ, Dutta D, Morris JF. Spread of injectate with superficial cervical plexus block in humans: An anatomical study. Br J Anaesth 2003;91:733-735.
11. Pandit JJ, Bree S, Dillon P, et al. A comparison of superficial versus combined (superficial and deep) cervical plexus block for carotid endarterectomy: A prospective, randomized study. Anesth Analg 2000;91:781-786.
12. Urmey WF, Talts KH, Sharrock NE. One hundred percent incidence of hemidiaphragmatic paresis associated with interscalene brachial plexus anesthesia as diagnosed by ultrasonography. Anesth Analg 1991;72:498-503.
13. Hashim MS, Shevde K. Dyspnea during interscalene block after recent coronary bypass surgery. Anesth Analg 1999;89:55-56.
14. Brown DL, Cahill DR, Bridenbaugh LD. Supraclavicular nerve block: Anatomic analysis of a method to prevent pneumothorax. Anesth Analg 1993;76:530-534.
15. Sandhu NS, Capan LM. Ultrasound-guided infraclavicular brachial plexus block. Br J Anaesth 2002;89:254-259.
16. Ilfeld BM, Morey TE, Enneking FK. Continuous infraclavicular brachial plexus block for postoperative pain control at home: A randomized, double-blinded, placebo-controlled study. Anesthesiology 2002;96:1297-1304.
17. Schroeder LE, Horlocker TT, Schroeder DR. The efficacy of axillary block for surgical procedures about the elbow. Anesth Analg 1996;83:747-751.
18. Hebl JR, Horlocker TT, Sorenson EJ, Schroeder DR. Regional anesthesia does not increase the risk of postoperative neuropathy in patients undergoing ulnar nerve transposition. Anesth Analg 2001;93:1606-1611.
18. Gray AT, Collins AB. Ultrasound-guided saphenous nerve block. Reg Anesth Pain Med 2003;28:148, author reply 148.
20. Bouaziz H, Vial F, Jochum D, et al. An evaluation of the cutaneous distribution after obturator nerve block. Anesth Analg 2002;94:445-449.
21. Macalou D, Trueck S, Meuret P, et al. Postoperative analgesia after total knee replacement: The effect of an obturator nerve block added to the femoral 3-in-1 nerve block. Anesth Analg 2004;99:251-254.
22. Vloka JD, Hadzic A, April E, Thys DM. The division of the sciatic nerve in the popliteal fossa: Anatomical implications for popliteal nerve blockade. Anesth Analg 2001;92:215-217.
23. Gray AT, Huczko EL, Schafhalter-Zoppoth I. Lateral popliteal nerve block with ultrasound guidance. Reg Anesth Pain Med 2004;29:507-509.
24. Atanassoff PG, Aouad R, Hartmannsgruber MW, Halaszynski T. Levobupivacaine 0.125% and lidocaine 0.5% for intravenous regional anesthesia in volunteers. Anesthesiology 2002;97:325-328.
25. Chan VW, Weisbrod MJ, Kaszas Z, Dragomir C. Comparison of ropivacaine and lidocaine for intravenous regional anesthesia in volunteers: A preliminary study or anesthetic efficacy and blood level. Anestheology 1999;90:1602-1608.

Chapter 19

POSITIONING AND ASSOCIATED RISKS

Jae-Woo Lee and Lydia Cassorla

Anesthesiologists share a critical responsibility in the proper positioning of patients for surgery in the operating room. Positions deemed necessary for surgery often result in undesirable physiologic changes such as hypotension from impaired venous return to the heart or oxygen desaturation as a result of ventilation-to-perfusion mismatching. In addition, peripheral nerve injuries during surgery remain a significant source of perioperative morbidity.[1-3] Proper positioning requires the cooperation and participation of the anesthesiologist, surgeon, and nursing staff to ensure patient comfort and safety while optimizing surgical exposure.

CARDIORESPIRATORY RESPONSES TO POSITIONING

Patient positioning must take into account the dramatic effects of general or regional anesthesia (or both) on cardiovascular and respiratory reserve. Normally, as a person moves from the standing to the supine position, venous return to the heart initially increases as pooled blood from the lower extremities redistributes toward the heart. The initial increase in cardiac output and arterial blood pressure activates afferent baroreceptors from the aorta (via the vagus nerve) and within the walls of the carotid sinuses (via the glossopharyngeal nerve) to increase parasympathetic nervous system impulses to the sinoatrial node and myocardium. The result is a decrease in heart rate, stroke volume, and cardiac output. Low-pressure mechanoreceptors from the atria and ventricle are also activated to decrease sympathetic nervous system outflow to the skeletal muscles and splanchnic vascular beds. Finally, atrial reflexes are activated to regulate renal sympathetic nerve activity, plasma renin concentrations, and atrial natriuretic peptide and arginine vasopressin levels.[4] Consequently, systemic blood pressure is maintained within a narrow range during postural changes.

Impact of Anesthesia

General anesthesia that includes positive-pressure ventilation of the patient's lungs and drug-induced skeletal muscle relaxation blunts the compensatory sympathetic nervous system cardiovascular responses to postural changes and diminishes venous return to the heart. The use of spinal or epidural anesthesia causes a significant sympathectomy across all affected dermatomes, independent of the presence of general anesthesia, thereby further reducing preload. Consequently, systemic blood pressure is often particularly labile immediately following the induction of anesthesia and during patient positioning. Frequent blood pressure measurements should be made, as well as appropriate adjustments in intravenous fluid administration and the delivered anesthetic concentrations, until systemic blood pressure reaches a new level of homeostasis. Vasopressors may be required during this hemodynamic transition.

General anesthesia and patient positioning also affect both ventilation and perfusion to the lungs. The normal distribution of ventilation is determined by the excursion of the diaphragm, movement of the chest wall, and compliance of the lung. Normal diaphragmatic excursion helps enhance ventilation in the dependent portions of the lung where perfusion is maximal. In assuming the supine position, the distribution of ventilation is a function of abdominal and diaphragmatic movement, with less contribution from the rib cage/chest wall. Anesthetized patients breathing spontaneously have reduced tidal volume and functional residual capacity and increased closing volume. In addition, any position that limits movement of the diaphragm or chest wall may also increase atelectasis and create intrapulmonary shunts. Positive-pressure ventilation with skeletal muscle relaxation may blunt the ventilation-to-perfusion mismatches induced by general anesthesia by maintaining adequate minute ventilation and preventing the development of atelectasis.

SPECIFIC POSITIONS

Supine

The supine position is the most common surgical position and produces the least hemodynamic and ventilatory changes (Fig. 19-1A). Several variations of the supine position exist. The lawn-chair position, in which the hips and knees are slightly flexed, is better tolerated by patients undergoing monitored anesthesia care (Fig. 19-1B). In addition, venous drainage from the lower extremity is facilitated and the xiphoid-to-pubic distance is decreased, thereby reducing tension on the ventral abdominal musculature and easing closure of laparotomy incisions. The frog-leg position, in which the hips and knees are flexed and the hips are externally rotated with the heels in apposition, allows access to the perineum, medial aspect of the thighs, genitalia, and rectum.

COMPLICATIONS

Patients in the supine position are susceptible to several complications. Pressure alopecia is often related to prolonged immobilization of the head with its full weight falling on a limited area, thus rendering the hair follicles ischemic. Hypothermia and hypotension during surgery, such as during cardiopulmonary bypass, may increase the incidence of this complication. Consequently, when possible, during prolonged surgery, it is prudent to cushion and periodically rotate the head to redistribute the weight. Backache may occur because the normal lumbar lordotic curvature and tone of the paraspinal musculature are lost during general anesthesia with skeletal muscle relaxation or a neuraxial block. Accordingly, patients with extensive kyphoscoliosis or a previous history of back pain may require extra padding of the spine or slight flexion at the hip. Finally, tissues overlying all bony prominences, such as the heels and sacrum, must be padded to prevent ischemia due to pressure, especially during long procedures.[5]

Positioning the Upper Extremities

Peripheral nerve injuries are often attributed to errors in positioning and padding, but in fact they most often have a complex and multifactorial etiology (see the section "Peripheral Nerve Injury"). The American Society of Anesthesiologists (ASA) published a practice advisory in 2000 that is intended to help prevent perioperative peripheral neuropathy.[6] In a supine patient, one or both arms may be abducted to the side or adducted (tucked) alongside the body. To minimize the likelihood of injury to the ulnar nerve, it is recommended that upper extremity abduction be limited to less than 90 degrees, with the hand and forearm either supinated or kept in a neutral position to reduce external pressure from the supporting surface (padded arm board) on the spiral groove of the humerus and the ulnar nerve (Fig. 19-1C).

In surgeries in which the arms are adducted, the arms are secured with a "draw sheet" that passes around the patient's arm and is tucked under the patient (not the mattress) to ensure that the arm remains properly placed next to the patient's body. Patients' palms are placed in a neutral position, facing the body. The elbows, as well as any sharp object such as intravenous fluid lines and stopcocks, are padded (Fig. 19-1D).

TRENDELENBURG POSITION

Tilting a supine patient head down (Trendelenburg position) is often used to increase venous return during hypotension, improve exposure during lower abdominal surgery, and prevent air emboli during central venous line placement (Fig. 19-1E). Nonsliding mattresses are recommended to keep the patient from sliding cephalad. Shoulder braces to keep the patient from moving are not recommended because the risk of compressive injury to the brachial plexus is significant.

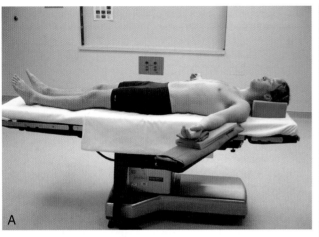

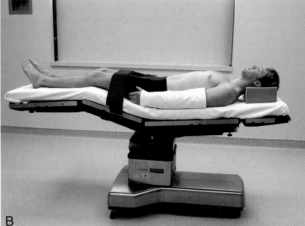

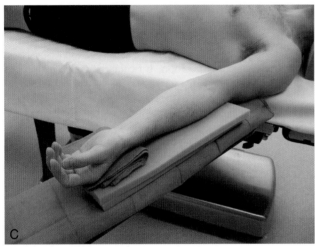

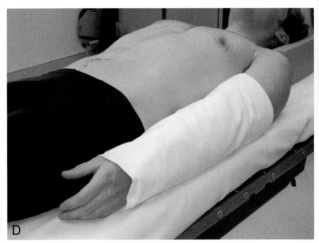

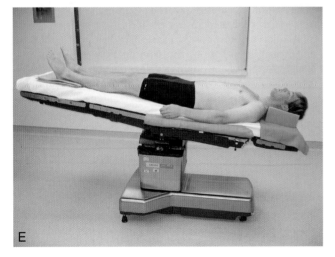

III

Figure 19-1 **A**, Supine position. **B**, Lawn-chair position. Flexion of the hips and knees decreases tension on the back. **C**, Arm position on an arm board. Limit abduction of the arm to less than 90 degrees whenever possible. Supinate the arm and pad the elbow. **D**, The arm is tucked at the patient's side in a neutral position with the palm to the hip. Pad the elbow and ensure that the arm is supported. **E**, Trendelenburg position. Avoid shoulder braces.

Complications

The Trendelenburg position causes significant cardio-vascular and respiratory consequences. The head-down position increases central venous, intracranial, and intraocular pressure. Prolonged head-down positioning can lead to swelling of the face, conjunctiva, larynx, and tongue with an increased potential for postoperative upper airway obstruction. The cephalad movement of abdominal viscera against the diaphragm also decreases functional residual capacity and pulmonary compliance. Therefore, endotracheal intubation is often preferred to protect the airway from pulmonary aspiration and to prevent hypoxia as a result of atelectasis and ventilation-to-perfusion mismatches. Air leaks around the endotracheal tube are confirmed before extubation in surgeries in which patients are in the Trendelenburg position for prolonged periods (risk for edema of the trachea and laryngeal structures).

Lithotomy

The classic lithotomy position is frequently used during gynecologic and urologic surgery. The hips are flexed 80 to 100 degrees from the trunk and the legs are abducted 30 to 45 degrees from the midline. The knees are flexed until the legs are parallel to the torso, and the legs are held in this configuration with stirrups ("candy cane," knee crutch, or calf support) (Fig. 19-2A).

Initiation and discontinuation of the lithotomy position require coordinated positioning of the lower extremities by two assistants. Both legs should be raised together while flexing the hips and knees simultaneously to prevent torsion of the lumbar spine. The lower extremities should be padded to prevent compression against the stirrups. After the surgery, the patient must also be placed in a supine position in a coordinated manner. The legs should be removed from the holders simultaneously, the knees brought together in the midline, and the legs slowly unflexed to the supine position.

COMPLICATIONS

With the legs elevated, venous return (preload) increases and causes a transient rise in cardiac output and intracranial pressure in otherwise healthy patients. In addition, the lithotomy position causes the abdominal viscera to displace the diaphragm cephalad, which can potentially result in decreased tidal volume. When a large abdominal mass is present (tumor, gravid uterus), abdominal pressure may increase sufficiently to obstruct venous return to the heart. Finally, the normal lordotic curvature of the lumbar spine is lost in the lithotomy position, thereby potentially aggravating any previous lower back pain.[7] In the lithotomy position, the hands and fingers often lie near the edge of the lowered foot section of the operating room table. When raising the foot of the table at the end of surgery, strict attention must be paid to the position of the fingers to avoid a potential crush injury. For this reason, arm boards are recommended to keep the hands far from the table hinge point when patients are in the lithotomy position (Fig. 19-2C).

Injury to the Common Peroneal Nerve

In a retrospective review of 198,461 patients undergoing surgery in the lithotomy position from 1957 to 1991, it was found that injury to the common peroneal nerve was the most common lower extremity motor neuropathy and accounted for 78% of nerve injuries.[8] A potential cause of the injury was compression of the nerve between the lateral head of the fibula and the bar holding the legs, especially when "candy cane" stirrups were used (Fig. 19-2B). The injury was more common in patients who had a low body mass index, recent cigarette use, or prolonged duration of surgery.[8]

Duration of the Lithotomy Position

In a prospective review of 991 patients undergoing surgery in the lithotomy position from 1997 to 1998, the incidence of lower extremity neuropathy was infrequent, and when it did occur, the most predictable risk factor was duration of the lithotomy position (>2 hours).[9] These findings suggest that reducing the time spent in the lithotomy position may decrease the risk for lower extremity neuropathy.

Compartment Syndrome

Compartment syndrome is a rare complication associated with the lithotomy position. It occurs when perfusion to an extremity is inadequate and results in ischemia, edema, and extensive rhabdomyolysis from increased tissue pressure within a fascial compartment. In a retrospective review of 572,498 surgeries, the incidence of compartment syndrome was higher in the lithotomy (1 in 8720) and lateral decubitus (1 in 9711) positions than in the supine (1 in 92,441) position.[10] Long surgical procedure time was the only distinguishing characteristic of the surgeries in which lower extremity compartment syndrome developed.

Lateral Decubitus

The lateral decubitus position (surgery on the chest, retroperitoneal structures, or hip) is associated with pulmonary compromise (Fig. 19-3A). In the presence of mechanical ventilation, the combination of the lateral weight of the mediastinum and disproportionate cephalad pressure of the abdominal contents on the dependent lung favors overventilation of the nondependent lung. At the same time, pulmonary blood flow goes preferentially to the underventilated dependent lung because of gravity. Consequently, ventilation-to-perfusion mismatch increases and can potentially affect gas exchange and ventilation.

PLACEMENT IN THE LATERAL DECUBITUS POSITION

The act of moving a patient into the lateral decubitus position requires participation of the entire operating room staff to prevent potential injuries. The patient's head must be kept in a neutral position to prevent excessive lateral rotation of the neck and stretch injuries to the brachial plexus. This may require additional head support (Fig. 19-3B). The dependent eye must be checked frequently for external compression to avoid corneal abrasion and retinal artery thrombosis. It should be verified that the patient's eyelids are taped closed before repositioning if the patient is asleep.

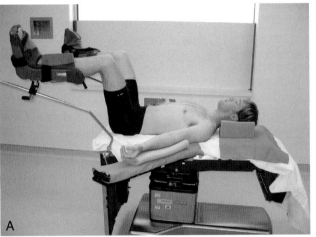

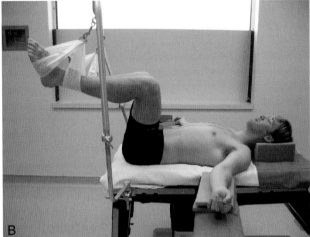

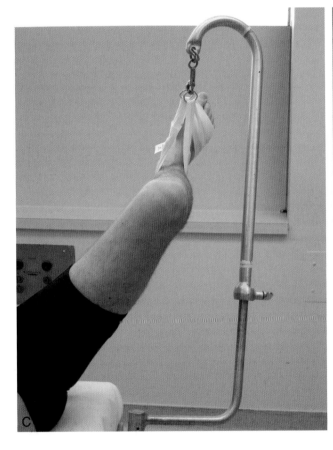

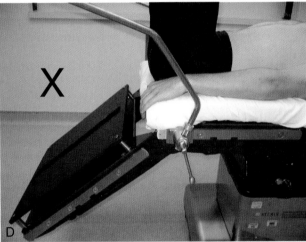

III

Figure 19-2 A, Lithotomy position. The hips are flexed 80 to 100 degrees with the lower part of the leg parallel to the body. The arms are on armrests. **B,** Lithotomy position with candy cane stirrups. **C,** Lithotomy position with correct positioning of the candy cane stirrup well away from the lateral head of the fibula. **D,** Illustration of an improper position of the arms with the fingers at risk for compression when the lower section of the bed is raised.

Chest Roll

To avoid compression injuries to the brachial plexus, an "axillary roll" (more correctly described as a "chest roll") is placed just caudad to the dependent axilla while the dependent arm is placed perpendicular to the torso on a padded arm board (Fig. 19-3C). The axillary roll should *never* be placed in the axilla. Its purpose is to ensure that

the weight of the thorax is borne by the chest wall caudad to the axilla rather than by the axilla itself. It may be helpful to monitor the pulse in the dependent arm for early detection of compression of axillary neurovascular structures. Hypotension detected in the dependent arm must be differentiated from axillary compression by comparison with the nondependent arm. The nondependent

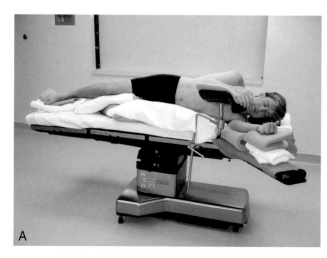

A

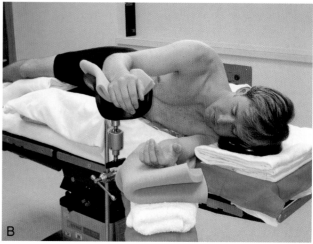

B

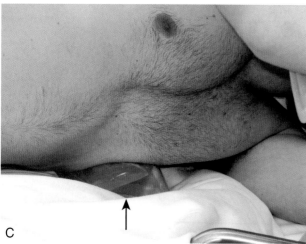

C

Figure 19-3 A, Lateral decubitus position. Note the flexion of the lower part of the leg, padding between the legs, and proper support of both arms. **B**, Note the additional padding under the headrest to ensure alignment of the head with the spine. Keep the headrest away from the dependent eye. **C**, "Axillary" roll. The roll, in this case a bag of intravenous fluid, is placed well away from axilla to prevent compression of the axillary artery and brachial plexus.

arm is often wrapped around a pillow or suspended with an armrest or foam cradle. Again, the arm should be checked periodically for any external compression of the vascular structures. For some high thoracotomies, the nondependent arm may be elevated above the shoulder plane for exposure. If possible, the arm should not be abducted greater than 90 degrees. When a kidney rest is used, it must be properly placed under the dependent iliac crest to prevent inadvertent compression of the inferior vena cava. Finally, a pillow or other padding is generally placed between the knees with the dependent leg flexed to minimize excessive pressure on bony prominences and stretch of the lower extremity nerves.

Prone

The prone position is used primarily for surgical access to the posterior fossa of the skull, the posterior aspect of the spine, the buttocks and perirectal area, and the lower extremities (Fig. 19-4A).

PLACEMENT IN THE PRONE POSITION

When general anesthesia is planned, the patient's trachea is first intubated on the stretcher, and all intravenous or arterial access is obtained. The endotracheal tube is securely taped to prevent dislodgment and loosening of the tape from drainage of saliva when prone. With the coordination of the entire operating room staff, the patient is then turned prone onto the operating room table while keeping the neck in line with the spine. The anesthesiologist is primarily responsible for coordinating the move and for maintaining the position of the patient's head.

Positioning the Head

The patient's head may be turned to the side once prone if neck mobility is adequate. However, as in the lateral decubitus position, the dependent eye must be checked frequently for the absence of external compression. In addition, in certain patient populations with cervical arthritis or cerebrovascular disease, lateral rotation of the neck may compromise carotid or vertebral arterial blood

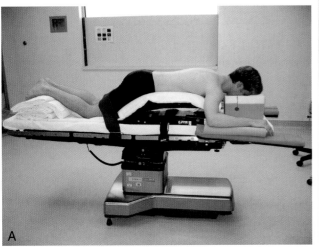

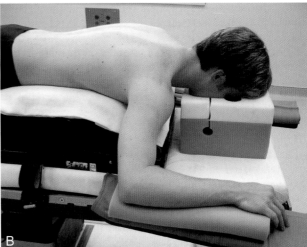

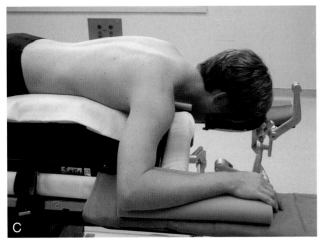

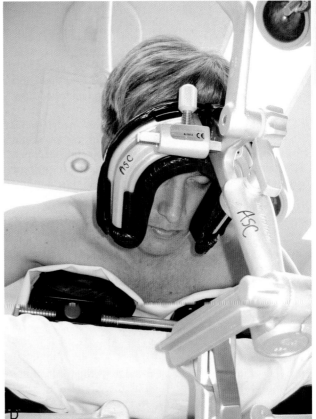

Figure 19-4 A, Prone position with a Wilson frame. The arms are extended less than 90 degrees whenever possible. Pressure points are padded, and the chest is supported away from the bed to preserve pulmonary compliance. **B,** Foam pillow designed to permit endotracheal tube exit. The eyes must be checked frequently. **C,** Horseshoe adapter. **D,** Face seen from below. The horseshoe adapter permits superior access to the airway and visualization of the eyes. The width may be adjusted to ensure proper support by bony facial structures.

flow or jugular venous drainage. In most cases, the head is kept in a neutral position by using a surgical pillow, horseshoe headrest, or Mayfield pins. Most specially designed foam pillows support the forehead, malar regions, and the chin with cutouts for the eyes, nose, and mouth (Fig. 19-4B). The horseshoe headrest supports only the forehead and malar regions and allows excellent access to the airway (Fig. 19-4C). Mayfield pins support the head without any direct pressure on the face, allow access to the airway, and hold the head firmly in one position.

Regardless of the device used, the eyes and the airway must be checked periodically to ensure that pressure is placed only on the bony structures of the face (Fig. 19-4D). Verification of proper position is noted on the anesthetic record. Because of special risks associated with facial and eye pressure, the face should be rechecked if any patient motion occurs during surgery or if the table is repositioned significantly.

Supporting the Thorax

The thorax is generally supported by firm rolls or bolsters placed under the patient's sides from the clavicle to the iliac crest. Multiple commercial rolls/bolsters are available, including the Wilson frame (see Fig. 19-4A), Jackson table, Relton frame, and the Mouradian/Simmons modification of the Relton frame. All devices serve to relieve abdominal compression by the operating room table and maintain normal pulmonary compliance. If uncorrected, the pressure of the mattress on the abdomen may push the diaphragm cephalad and thereby decrease functional residual capacity and pulmonary compliance and increase peak airway pressure. Abdominal pressure may also impede venous return through compression of the inferior vena cava and aorta and increase surgical bleeding during spine surgery as a result of engorgement of epidural veins. It is recommended that female breasts be placed medial to the bolsters to prevent postoperative tenderness or actual tissue injury. The lower portion of the rolls/bolsters must be placed over its respective iliac crest to prevent pressure injury to the genitalia and the femoral vasculature.[11]

Obesity

The prone position presents special risks for morbidly obese patients, whose respiration is already compromised and who may be difficult to reposition quickly. At times it may be necessary to discuss alternative position options with the surgeon to ensure patient safety.

Placement of the Arms

The patient's arms may be placed either at the sides or alongside the head on padded arm boards. Additional padding of the elbow may be added to further protect the ulnar nerve from compression at the elbow. The arms should not be abducted greater than 90 degrees in order to prevent excessive stretching of the brachial plexus, especially in patients with lateral placement of the head. Elastic stockings will be needed for the lower extremities to minimize pooling of blood, especially with any flexion of the body.

Sitting

The sitting position, though rarely used, offers advantages to the surgeon in approaching the posterior cervical spine and the posterior fossa. A variation of the sitting position is used for shoulder surgery (Fig. 19-5A and B).

ADVANTAGES AND DISADVANTAGES

Advantages of the sitting position over the prone position are excellent surgical exposure, decreased blood loss in the operative field, and possibly, reduced perioperative blood loss. Advantages to the anesthesiologist are superior access to the airway, reduced facial swelling, and improved ventilation, particularly in obese patients.

HEMODYNAMIC EFFECTS

The hemodynamic effects of placing a supine patient in the sitting position are dramatic. Because of pooling of blood in the lower part of the body during general anesthesia, patients are particularly prone to hypotensive episodes. The degree and duration of hypotension can be reduced by incremental positioning, administering intravenous fluids and vasopressors, and adjusting the depth of anesthesia appropriately until homeostasis is achieved and a surgical incision is imminent. Compression stockings that incorporate sequential inflation characteristics are a consideration to facilitate venous return.

COMPLICATIONS

Potential complications can occur during posterior spine and skull surgery when the patient is placed in the sitting position. Excessive flexion of the neck can impede both arterial and venous blood flow and cause hypoperfusion and inadequate drainage of the brain. Excessive flexion can also obstruct (kink) the endotracheal tube and place significant pressure on the tongue leading to macroglossia. In general, at least two fingerbreadths distance is required between the chin and the sternum for a safe degree of neck flexion. Arm support and mild flexion of the knees are maintained to prevent excessive stretching of the brachial plexus and sciatic nerve, respectively.[12]

Venous Air Embolism

Because of elevation of the surgical field above the heart and the lack of valves in the cerebral venous circulation, the risk for venous air embolism is constant. Venous air embolism may be manifested as cardiac dysrhythmias, arterial oxygen desaturation, pulmonary hypertension, or cardiac arrest, depending on the volume of air entrained. If the foramen ovale is patent, even small amounts of venous air may result in stroke or myocardial infarction as a result of paradoxical embolism. Even in the absence of a patent foramen ovale, it is possible for air to traverse the lungs (transpulmonary passage in the pulmonary circulation) and produce effects related to the presence of air in the cerebral or coronary circulation.[13] Adequate hydration and early detection with the use of precordial Doppler ultrasound may decrease the incidence and severity of venous air embolism.

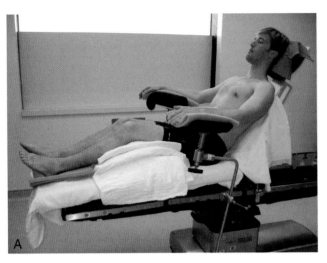

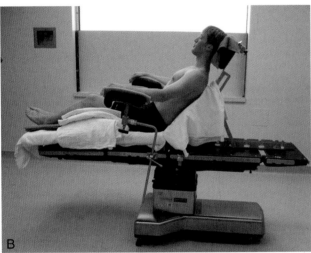

Figure 19-5 A, Sitting position adapted for shoulder surgery. **B,** Note the absence of pressure over the ulnar area of the elbow.

PERIPHERAL NERVE INJURY

Despite its rare incidence—approximately 0.11% of 81,765 anesthetic procedures reviewed from 1987 to 1993—peripheral nerve injuries remain a serious perioperative complication and a significant source of professional liability.[14] In 1984, the ASA developed a Closed Claims Project to evaluate adverse anesthetic outcomes from the closed claims files of 35 U.S. liability insurance companies. Since the initial report in 1990, the incidence of nerve injury has remained essentially constant and accounted for 18% of all claims during 1990 to 1994, second only to death (22%).[1-3] Among the total 670 claims filed, ulnar neuropathy remained the most frequent site (28%) of

injury, followed by the brachial plexus (20%), lumbosacral nerve root (16%), and spinal cord (13%). However, the distribution of nerve injuries by time of occurrence has changed. Ulnar neuropathy decreased from 37% in 1980 to 1984 to 17% in the 1990s, and spinal cord injury increased from 8% in 1980 to 1984 to 27% in the 1990s. Spinal cord injury and lumbosacral nerve root neuropathy were predominantly associated with regional anesthesia. Epidural hematoma and chemical injury represented 29% of the known mechanisms of injury among the claims filed. The injuries were probably related to the use of neuraxial blockade in anticoagulated patients, particularly patients receiving low-molecular-weight heparin, and the increased use of blocks for chronic pain management (Table 19-1).[3,15,16]

Etiology

With the exception of spinal cord injury, the mechanism of peripheral nerve injury has remained largely unknown. Most injuries, particularly those to the ulnar nerve and brachial plexus, have occurred in the presence of proper positioning and adequate padding. Because of the significant morbidity associated with peripheral nerve injury, in 2000 the ASA published a practice advisory for the prevention of peripheral neuropathies.[6] This report was not based on scientific literature (only 6 of the 509 positioning studies reviewed demonstrated a relationship between intervention and outcomes) but rather represented the consensus of a consultant expert group.

Ulnar Neuropathy

The etiology of perioperative ulnar neuropathy is complex. The ulnar nerve lies in a superficial position at the elbow. Previously, the injury was thought to be associated with hyperflexion of the elbow and compression of the nerve at the condylar groove and the cubital tunnel against the posterior aspect of the medial epicondyle of the humerus by the firm edge of the operating room table. The neuropathy resulted in an inability to abduct or oppose the fifth finger, diminished sensation in the fourth and fifth fingers, and eventual atrophy of the intrinsic muscles of the hands with the creation of a "claw"-like hand.

CURRENT UNDERSTANDING

Current consensus is that the cause of ulnar nerve palsy is multifactorial and not always preventable despite the routine use of padded arm boards. In a large retrospective review of perioperative ulnar neuropathy lasting longer than 3 months, it was found that the onset of symptoms occurred more than 24 hours postoperatively in 57% of patients undergoing general anesthesia, 70% were male, and 9% experienced bilateral symptoms.[17] The Closed Claims Project also demonstrated that peri-

Table 19-1 Nerve Injuries and Recommendations for Prevention

Most Common Nerve Injuries in the 1990s[1-3]	Recommendations for Prevention
Ulnar nerve (25%)	Avoid excessive pressure on the postcondylar groove of the humerus
	Limit abduction of the arm to less than 90 degrees in the supine position
	Keep the hand and forearm either supinated or in a neutral position
Brachial plexus (19%)	Avoid the use of shoulder braces in patients in the Trendelenburg position (use nonsliding mattresses)
	Avoid excessive lateral rotation of the head in either the supine or prone position
	Limit abduction of the arm to less than 90 degrees in the supine position
	Avoid the placement of a high "axillary" roll in the decubitus position—keep the roll out of the axilla
	Use ultrasound to find the internal jugular vein for central line placement
Spinal cord (16%) and lumbosacral nerve root (15%)	Follow current guidelines for regional anesthesia in anticoagulated patients*
Sciatic (also peroneal) (5%)	Minimize the time of surgery in the lithotomy position
	Use two assistants to coordinate the simultaneous movement of both legs to and from the lithotomy position
	Avoid excessive flexion of the hips, extension of the knees, or torsion of the lumbar spine
	Avoid excessive pressure on the peroneal nerve at the fibular head
Median (4%) and radial (3%)	Be aware that 25% of injuries to the median and radial nerves were associated with an axillary block and 25% were associated with traumatic insertion or infiltration of an intravenous line

*Horlocker TT, Wedel DJ, Benon H, et al. Regional anesthesia in the anticoagulated patient: Defining the risks (the second ASRA Consensus Conference on Neuraxial Anesthesia and Anticoagulation). Reg Anesth Pain Med 2003;28:172–197.

operative ulnar neuropathy occurred predominantly in males, in an older population, and with a delayed onset (median of 3 days).[3] Although most injuries occurred during general anesthesia, payment was also made for ulnar damage claims when the patient was awake or sedated during regional anesthesia involving the lower extremity. Interestingly, in a prospective study of medical patients who did not undergo surgical procedures, ulnar neuropathy developed in 2 of 986 patients.[18]

RISK FACTORS

The preponderance of males with injury may be due to anatomic differences. Males have a more developed and thickened flexor retinaculum with less protective adipose tissue and a larger (1.5×) tubercle of the coronoid process, which can predispose to compression of the nerve in the cubital tunnel.[19,20] Other risk factors such as diabetes mellitus, vitamin deficiency, alcoholism, cigarette smoking, and cancer await validation.

ASSOCIATED MORBIDITY

Although the incidence is low, the morbidity associated with ulnar neuropathy can be severe. In a prospective study of 1502 patients undergoing noncardiac surgery, it was found that perioperative ulnar neuropathy developed in 7 patients, 3 of whom had residual symptoms after 2 years.[21] In this same report, the symptoms attributed to ulnar nerve compression in many patients reflected compression of the median nerve at the wrist (carpal tunnel syndrome).

Brachial Plexus Injury

The brachial plexus is susceptible to injury from stretching or compression as a result of its long superficial course in the axilla between two points of fixation, the vertebra and axillary fascia, in association with the mobile clavicle and humerus. The patient often complains of sensory deficit in the distribution of the ulnar nerve.

ETIOLOGY

The injury is most commonly associated with arm abduction greater than 90 degrees, lateral rotation of the head, asymmetric retraction of the sternum for internal mammary artery dissection, and direct trauma. Ideally, to avoid brachial plexus injury, patients should be placed with the head midline, arms kept at the sides, and the elbows mildly flexed. Brachial plexus injury, specifically to the C8-T1 nerve roots, often occurs with cardiac surgery requiring median sternotomy.[22] In noncardiac surgery, the incidence is reported to be 0.02%.[23]

Brachial plexus injury is also associated with direct compression, particularly with the use of shoulder braces in patients undergoing surgery in the Trendelenburg position. Medial placement of the braces can compress the proximal roots, and lateral placement of the braces can stretch the plexus by displacing the shoulders. Consequently, nonsliding mattresses should be used in place of shoulder braces.

Radial and Median Nerve Injury

Though quite rare, the radial nerve can be injured from direct pressure as it traverses the spiral groove of the humerus in the lower third of the arm. The injury is often manifested as wristdrop with an inability to abduct the thumb or extend the metacarpophalangeal joints. Isolated median nerve injury may follow the insertion of an intravenous needle into the antecubital fossa in an anesthetized patient at the point where the nerve is adjacent to the medial cubital and basilic veins. Patients with injury are unable to oppose the first and fifth digits and have decreased sensation over the palmar surface of the lateral three and a half fingers.

Lower Extremity Nerve Injury

Injury to the sciatic and common peroneal nerves most often occurs in the lithotomy position. Because of its fixation between the sciatic notch and the neck of the fibula, the sciatic nerve can be stretched with external rotation of the leg. Hyperflexion of the hips or extension of the knees can also aggravate stretch of the sciatic nerve in this position. The common peroneal nerve, a branch of the sciatic, can be damaged by the compression of the nerve between the head of the fibula and the metal frame of the stirrups used to support the legs in the lithotomy position. Most often, patients who suffer injury will complain of footdrop and an inability to extend the toes in a dorsal direction or evert the foot.

RISK RELATED TO THE LITHOTOMY POSITION

In a prospective study of 991 patients undergoing surgery under general anesthesia in the lithotomy position, the incidence of lower extremity neuropathy was 1.5%, with injuries to the sciatic and peroneal nerves representing 40%

of the cases.[9] Interestingly, symptoms were predominantly paresthesias that occurred within 4 hours of surgery and generally resolved within 6 months. No motor deficits were noted. In a previous retrospective study, the incidence of severe motor disability in patients undergoing surgery in the lithotomy position was 1 in 3608.[8]

INJURY TO THE FEMORAL AND OBTURATOR NERVES

Injury to the femoral or obturator nerves generally occurs during lower abdominal surgical procedures with excessive retraction. The obturator nerve can also be injured during a difficult forceps delivery or by excessive flexion of the thigh to the groin. A femoral neuropathy is characterized by decreased flexion of the hip, decreased extension of the knee, or loss of sensation over the superior aspect of the thigh and medial/anteromedial side of the leg. An obturator neuropathy is manifested as an inability to adduct the leg with decreased sensation over the medial side of the thigh.

EVALUATION AND TREATMENT OF PERIOPERATIVE NEUROPATHIES

When a nerve injury becomes apparent postoperatively, it is essential to perform a directed physical examination and correlate the extent of sensory or motor deficits to the preoperative examination, as well as the intraoperative position. Regardless of whether a particular cause is suspected, it is prudent to seek neurologic consultation. Sensory neuropathies are generally transient and require only reassurance to the patient with follow-up. For motor neuropathy, an electromyogram can be performed to determine the exact location of the injury. An electromyogram can also suggest whether a neuropathy was present preoperatively; signs of denervation resulting from acute injury do not appear until 18 to 21 days after the inciting event. Regardless, most motor neuropathies include demyelination of the peripheral fibers of a nerve trunk (neurapraxia) and generally take 4 to 6 weeks for recovery. Injury to the axon within an intact nerve sheath (axonotmesis) or complete nerve disruption (neurotmesis) can cause severe pain and disability. When reversible, recovery frequently takes 3 to 12 months. Interim physical therapy is recommended to prevent contractures and muscle atrophy.

PERIOPERATIVE EYE INJURY AND VISUAL LOSS

Though quite rare (incidence of 0.056%) perioperative eye injuries are a source of significant morbidity and liability.[24] In the ASA Closed Claims Database, eye complications represented 3% of all claims and were associated with greater monetary settlements than nonocular injuries were.[3]

Corneal Abrasion

Corneal abrasion continues to be the most common type of perioperative eye injury. It is associated with direct trauma to the cornea from facemasks, surgical drapes, or other foreign objects. It can also be associated with decreased basal tear production or swelling of the dependent eye in patients in the prone position. Patients who suffer a corneal abrasion complain of pain associated with a foreign body sensation in the eye on awakening from surgery. Symptoms are generally transient, and treatment includes supportive care and antibiotic ointment to prevent bacterial infection. In a prospective study of 671 patients undergoing nonocular surgery, it was found that 4.2% of patients reported a new onset of blurred vision lasting at least 3 days after surgery.[25] For most patients, the symptoms resolved within 2 months without complication. Precautionary measures to reduce the incidence of corneal abrasion include taping the eyelids closed after induction of anesthesia, care regarding dangling objects when leaning over patients, and close observation as patients awaken (patients often try to rub their eye or nose as they recover from the effects of anesthesia).

Postoperative Blindness

Postoperative blindness is a devastating complication that has been associated with specific types of surgery and patient risk factors. The incidence varies from 1 in 60,965 to 1 in 125,234 for patients undergoing noncardiac, nonocular surgery, from 0.06% to 0.113% in patients undergoing cardiac surgery with cardiopulmonary bypass, and 0.09% in patients undergoing spine surgery in the prone position.[24,26-29] Ischemic optic neuropathy (ION) and to a lesser extent central retinal arterial occlusion from direct retinal pressure are the conditions most cited as potential causes.

RISK FACTORS FOR ISCHEMIC OPTIC NEUROPATHY

Potential perioperative factors associated with ION include prolonged hypotension, long duration of surgery, especially in the prone position, excessive blood loss, excessive crystalloid use, anemia or hemodilution, and increased intraocular or venous pressure from the prone position.[30] Patient risk factors associated with ION include systemic hypertension, diabetes mellitus, atherosclerosis, morbid obesity, and tobacco use. However, in the absence of obvious external compression of the eyes, the cause of perioperative visual loss secondary to ION appears to be multifactorial with no consistent underlying mechanism.

POSTOPERATIVE VISUAL LOSS REGISTRY

In 1999, the ASA Committee on Professional Liability established the ASA Postoperative Visual Loss Registry to better understand the complication. Among the 79 cases reported to the registry by 2003, 67% involved patients undergoing spine surgery and 10% involved cardiopulmonary bypass. Of the 53 cases involving spine surgery, 81% were diagnosed with ION (predominantly posterior) and 13% with central retinal artery occlusion. In patients in whom ION was diagnosed after spine surgery, more than 58% of cases were bilateral. Surprisingly, 44% of the patients with ION eventually recovered their vision.[31] Based on the literature as well as case reports, several recommendations have been made for patients undergoing complex spine surgery:

1. Re-evaluate the protocols for management of blood pressure (deliberate hypotension), hematocrit, and fluid replacement in consultation with the surgeons.
2. Avoid excessive increases in intraocular pressure as a result of head position below the body, as well as external compression of the abdomen or chest.
3. Discuss the possibility of staging the spine surgery in consultation with the surgeon.[31,32]

REFERENCES

1. Cheney FW. The American Society of Anesthesiologists Closed Claims Project: What have we learned, how has it affected practice, and how will it affect practice in the future. Anesthesiology 1999;91:552-556.
2. Kroll DA, Caplan RA, Posner K, et al. Nerve injury associated with anesthesia. Anesthesiology 1990;73:202-207.
3. Cheney FW, Domino KB, Caplan RA, Posner KL. Nerve injury associated with anesthesia: A closed claim analysis. Anesthesiology 1999;90:1062-1069.
4. O'Brien TJ, Ebert TJ. Physiologic changes associated with the supine position. In Martin JT, Warner MA (eds): Positioning in Anesthesia and Surgery, 3rd ed. Philadelphia: WB Saunders, 1997, pp 27-36.
5. Warner MA. Supine positions. In Martin JT, Warner MA (eds): Positioning in Anesthesia and Surgery, 3rd ed. Philadelphia: WB Saunders, 1997, pp 39-46.
6. ASA Task Force on Prevention of Perioperative Peripheral Neuropathies. Practice advisory for the prevention of perioperative peripheral neuropathies. Anesthesiology 2000;92:1168-1182.
7. Martin JT. Lithotomy. In Martin JT, Warner MA (eds): Positioning in Anesthesia and Surgery, 3rd ed. Philadelphia: WB Saunders, 1997, pp 47-70.
8. Warner MA, Martin JT, Schroeder DR, et al. Lower-extremity motor neuropathy associated with surgery performed on patients in a lithotomy position. Anesthesiology 1994;81:6-12.
9. Warner MA, Warner DO, Harper CM, et al. Lower extremity neuropathies associated with lithotomy positions. Anesthesiology 2000;93:938-942.
10. Warner ME, LaMaster LM, Thoeming AK, et al. Compartment syndrome in surgical patients. Anesthesiology 2001;94:705-708.

11. Martin JT. The ventral decubitus (prone) positions. *In* Martin JT, Warner MA (eds): Positioning in Anesthesia and Surgery, 3rd ed. Philadelphia: WB Saunders, 1997, pp 155-195.

12. Newberg Milde L. The head-elevated positions. *In* Martin JT, Warner MA (eds): Positioning in Anesthesia and Surgery, 3rd ed. Philadelphia: WB Saunders, 1997, pp 1-93.

13. Edmonds CR, Barbut D, Hager D, Sharrock NE. Intraoperative cerebral arterial embolization during total hip arthroplasty. Anesthesiology 2000;93:315-318.

14. Blitt CD, Kaufer-Bratt C, Ashby J, Caillet JR. QA program reveals safety issues, promotes development of guidelines. Anesthesia Patient Safety Foundation Newsletter 1994;9:17. Available at http://www.apsf.org.

15. Lee LA, Posner KL, Domino KB, et al. Injuries associated with regional anesthesia in the 1980s and 1990s. A closed claim analysis. Anesthesiology 2004;101:143-152.

16. Fitzgibbon DR, Posner KL, Domino KB, et al. Chronic pain management. American Society of Anesthesiologists Closed Claims Project. Anesthesiology 2004;100:98-105.

17. Warner MA, Warner ME, Martin JT. Ulnar neuropathy: Incidence, outcome, and risk factors in sedated or anesthetized patients. Anesthesiology 1994;81:1332-1340.

18. Warner MA, Warner DO, Harper CM, et al. Ulnar neuropathy in medical patients. Anesthesiology 2000;92:614-615.

19. Contreras MG, Warner MA, Charboneau WJ, Cahill DR. Anatomy of the ulnar nerve at the elbow: Potential relationship of acute ulnar neuropathy to gender differences. Clin Anat 1998;11:372-378.

20. Morell RC, Prielipp RC, Harwood TN, et al. Men are more susceptible than women to direct pressure on unmyelinated ulnar nerve fibers. Anesth Analg 2003;97:1183-1188.

21. Warner MA, Warner DO, Matsumoto JY, et al. Ulnar neuropathy in surgical patients. Anesthesiology 1999;90:54-59.

22. Hanson MR, Breuer AC, Furlan AJ, et al. Mechanism and frequency of brachial plexus injury in open-heart surgery: A prospective analysis. Ann Thorac Surg 1983;36:675-679.

23. Cooper DE, Jenkins RS, Bready L, Rockwood CA Jr. The prevention of injuries to the brachial plexus secondary to malposition of the patient during surgery. Clin Orthop Relat Res 1988; Mar (228):33–41.

24. Roth S, Thisted RA, Erickson JP, et al. Eye injuries after nonocular surgery: A study of 60,965 anesthetics from 1988 to 1992. Anesthesiology 1996;85:1020-1027.

25. Warner ME, Fronapfel PJ, Hebl JR, et al. Perioperative visual changes. Anesthesiology 2002;96:855-859.

26. Warner ME, Warner MA, Garrity JA, et al. The frequency of perioperative vision loss. Anesth Analg 2001;93:1417-1421.

27. Kalyani SD, Miller NR, Dong LM, et al. Incidence of and risk factors for perioperative optic neuropathy after cardiac surgery. Ann Thorac Surg 2004;78:34-37.

28. Nuttall GA, Garrity JA, Dearnani JA, et al. Risk factors for ischemic optic neuropathy after cardiopulmonary bypass: A matched case/control study. Anesth Analg 2001;93:1410-1416.

29. Roth S, Barach P. Postoperative visual loss: Still no answers—yet. Anesthesiology 2001;95:575-577.

30. Hunt K, Bajekal R, Calder I, et al. Changes in intraocular pressure in anesthetized prone patients. J Neurosurg Anesthesiol 2004;16:287-290.

31. Lee LA. ASA Postoperative Visual Loss Registry: Preliminary analysis of factors associated with spine operations. ASA Newsletter 2003;67:7-8.

32. Ho V, Newman NJ, Song S, et al. Ischemic optic neuropathy following spine surgery. J Neurosurg Anesthesiol 2005;17:38-44.

III

ANESTHETIC MONITORING

Anil de Silva

Monitoring of anesthetized patients is designed to collect data that reflect (1) physiologic homeostasis, thereby allowing prompt recognition of adverse changes; (2) responses to therapeutic interventions; and (3) proper functioning of anesthetic equipment. Monitoring provides an early warning of adverse changes or trends before irreversible damage occurs. The most important monitor in the operating room is a vigilant anesthesiologist who continually obtains subjective and objective information from the anesthetized patient. This continual vigilance (awareness) on the part of the anesthesiologist is enhanced by the use of monitoring equipment designed to provide objective data relevant to the anesthetized patient's well-being. Indeed, human vigilance is not infallible, which emphasizes the importance of using monitors beyond the anesthesiologist's subjective observations.

Standards for basic anesthetic monitoring have been adopted by the American Society of Anesthesiologists (see Appendix 2). For example, these standards either encourage or mandate the use of pulse oximetry, capnography, an oxygen analyzer, disconnect alarms, measurement of body temperature, and a visual display of the electrocardiogram (ECG) during the intraoperative period in all patients undergoing anesthesia. Systemic blood pressure and heart rate must be evaluated every 5 minutes. As with all such policy statements, however, the anesthesiologist must exercise medical judgment in the application of these standards as dictated by extenuating circumstances. Depending on the patient's medical conditions and the complexity of the surgery, intraoperative monitoring may be expanded to include more technologically sophisticated and often invasive monitors (Table 20-1). The inherent risk in the use of all monitors, especially invasive monitors, must be weighted against the potential benefits in selecting their use for individual patients (Fig. 20-1).[1] Monitoring devices should not be selected or denied on the basis of cost.

Table 20–1 Measured and Calculated Hemodynamic Variables

	Normal Value	Range
Systolic blood pressure (mm Hg)	120/80	90-140/70-90
Mean arterial pressure (mm Hg)	93	77-97
Heart rate (beats/min)	72	60-80
Mean right atrial pressure (mm Hg)	5	0-10
Right ventricular pressure (mm Hg)	25/5	15-30/0-10
Pulmonary artery pressure (mm Hg)	23/10	15-30/5-15
Mean pulmonary artery pressure (mm Hg)	15	10-20
Pulmonary artery occlusion pressure (mm Hg)	10	5-15
Mean left atrial pressure (mm Hg)	8	4-12
Cardiac output (L/min)	5	4-6
Stroke volume (mL/beat)	70	60-90
Systemic vascular resistance (dynes/sec/cm^5)	1200	900-1500
Pulmonary vascular resistance (dynes/sec/cm^5)	100	50-150

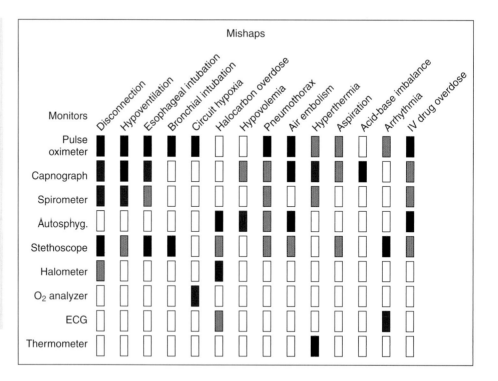

Figure 20-1 Estimate of the relative value of several monitors for detection of a variety of potential intraoperative mishaps. Most mishaps can be detected to some degree with the pulse oximeter or capnograph (or both). Dark red, high value; black, moderate value; light red, low value; white, no value. ECG, electrocardiogram. (From Whitcher C, Ream AK, Parsons D, et al. Anesthetic mishaps and the cost of monitoring: A proposed standard for monitoring equipment. J Clin Monit 1988;4:5-15, with permission.)

ELECTROCARDIOGRAPHY

The ECG is used to measure cardiac rhythm and rate and can also detect cardiac ischemia. The standard bipolar limb leads I, II, and III and the augmented unipolar leads aVR, aVL, and aVF provide the clinician with important, though limited views of the myocardium. Because the electrical vector of lead II parallels the atrial and ventricular depolarization waves, one can normally obtain large P waves and QRS complexes when using this limb lead.

However, monitoring of cardiac ischemia is significantly enhanced by the use of precordial leads V_1 through V_6.

Normal Electrocardiogram

A normal ECG is composed of a P wave, PR interval, QRS complex, ST segment, and T wave, perhaps followed by a U wave (Fig. 20-2). The P wave is created by a wave of depolarization generated by the sinoatrial node, which is normally situated in the right atrium. The impulse travels through the atrioventricular node through the bundle of His down the Purkinje fibers to the ventricle. The QRS complex ensues when the ventricle contracts in response to electrical stimulation. Commencement of repolarization is reflected by the T wave that follows the QRS complex.

Evidence of Myocardial Ischemia

The ECG displays ischemia by means of changes in the rate of repolarization of ischemic myocardial tissue. Thus, the ST-segment and T-wave portions of the ECG signal are primarily affected. Generally, the T wave is affected initially, followed by ST-segment changes as the ischemia worsens. Myocardial necrosis is displayed by the production of Q waves.

Use of lead V_5 alone results in the ECG detection of 75% of ischemic episodes in men aged 40 to 60.[1] The addition of lead V_4 increases the sensitivity of the ECG to 90%. The combination of leads II, V_4, and V_5 results in detection of up to 96% of ischemic episodes.[2]

SYSTEMIC BLOOD PRESSURE

The most common techniques of measuring systemic blood pressure involve variations of the Riva-Rocci method.[3] The Riva-Rocci method entails the placement of an inflatable cuff around a limb. The cuff is inflated until the pulse distal to the cuff disappears. It is then deflated until the pulse reappears—this point is considered the patient's systolic blood pressure (Table 20-2).

Korotkoff Method

It is generally accepted that systolic blood pressure is consistent with the blood pressure when the sound (Korotkoff technique) is first heard (phase 1) during deflation of the blood pressure cuff (Fig. 20-3). As the cuff is further deflated, the sound changes in quality (phases 2 and 3). Phase 4 occurs with the sudden onset of a muffled sound, followed by phase 5, which is the absence of any sort of sound. Diastolic blood pressure is considered to be either phase 4 or 5. The American Heart Association recommends using phase 5 as diastolic blood pressure, except in cases in which the sound may not dependably disappear.

It is important to realize that the size of the blood pressure cuff influences the measurement of blood pressure. A cuff that is too small results in a reading that is too high; a larger cuff than indicated may show a decreased blood pressure reading. The cuff is appropriately sized when its width is 40% the circumference of the arm.[3] Variations in blood pressure may also result with changes in posture. Diastolic blood pressure is routinely somewhat higher in sitting patients.

Oscillometric Method

The oscillometric method may be used to determine systemic blood pressure. The cuff is inflated until oscillations on the blood pressure gauge are no longer seen; this point is considered systolic blood pressure. The cuff

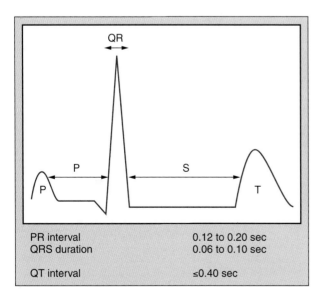

PR interval	0.12 to 0.20 sec
QRS duration	0.06 to 0.10 sec
QT interval	≤0.40 sec

Figure 20-2 A normal electrocardiogram is composed of a P wave, PR interval, QRS complex, ST segment, and T wave.

Table 20–2 Recommendations for the Use of Noninvasive Blood Pressure Devices
Do not wrap the cuff tightly
Do not apply the cuff across a joint, bony prominence, or superficial nerve (ulnar nerve, peroneal nerve)
Select the maximum cycle time consistent with safe monitoring
Inspect the cuff site periodically during prolonged cuff application
Record cuff location and cycle time
Keep alarms enabled

III

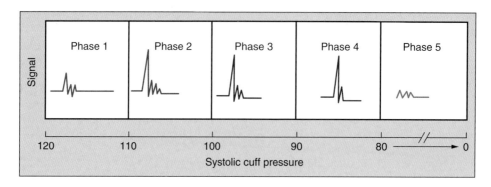

Figure 20-3 Phases of Korotkoff sounds during deflation of the blood pressure cuff.

is then further deflated until the point of maximum oscillations occurs; this point is thought to correlate with mean blood pressure. Diastolic blood pressure cannot be measured with this technique.

Dinamap Method

The Dinamap (device for indirect noninvasive automatic mean arterial pressure) is an automated blood pressure measurement device that uses the oscillometric method to determine systemic blood pressure. The oscillometric variation is compared at each reduction in cuff pressure. Automated blood pressure measurements generally correlate well with systolic and mean blood pressure as measured with an intra-arterial catheter. However, diastolic pressure is usually about 10 mm Hg higher with automated devices than with direct arterial measurements. Automated oscillometry has replaced auscultatory and palpatory techniques for routine intraoperative and early postoperative monitoring of systemic blood pressure.

Finometer

The Finometer uses the principle of the "unloaded arterial wall." A cuff is placed on a finger and inflated until transmural pressure across the digital arteries is equal to zero. The magnitude of the plethysmograph is maximized at this point because arterial wall compliance is greatest. Blood pressure is measured by the photoplethysmographic detection of changes in light intensity transmitted through the finger. The Finometer is quite accurate when compared with direct arterial blood pressure measurements.[3]

Direct Arterial Pressure Monitoring

Continuous blood pressure monitoring is accomplished by placement of a catheter in a peripheral artery connected to a transducer system and display. Direct blood pressure monitoring is indicated (1) during cardiopulmonary bypass, (2) when wide swings in blood pressure are expected, (3) when rigorous control of blood pressure is necessary, and (4) when there is a need for analysis of multiple blood gas samples. Complications resulting from arterial cannulation include distal ischemia, infection, and hemorrhage, but they are quite rare. In particular, numerous clinical studies have shown that the rate of distal ischemia after radial artery catheterization is less than 0.1%.[4]

CANNULATION SITE

The most frequently chosen site for arterial cannulation is the radial artery, which is close to the skin surface and relatively easily palpable in comparison to some deeper arterial possibilities, and the extensive collateral circulation minimizes complications (Table 20-3). Other acceptable sites for arterial pressure monitoring are the brachial, axillary, dorsalis pedis, and femoral arteries.

The site of placement of the catheter in various arterial systems determines the shape of the systemic blood pressure wave (Table 20-4). As the pressure wave is measured at sequentially further distances from the heart, one notices that high-frequency components such as the dicrotic notch

Table 20-3 Sites for Monitoring Systemic Blood Pressure with an Indwelling Catheter

Arterial Cannulation Site	Clinical Considerations
Radial artery	Most commonly selected site
Ulnar artery	Principal source of blood flow to the hand
Brachial artery	Near the median nerve
Femoral artery	Accessible in low-flow states Risk for local and retroperitoneal hematoma
Dorsalis pedis artery	Higher systolic blood pressure displayed

Table 20-4 Central Venous Pressure Catheter Placement Sites

	Advantages	Disadvantages
Right internal jugular vein	Good landmarks Predictable anatomy Accessible from the head of the operating room table	Carotid artery puncture Trauma to the brachial plexus
Left internal jugular vein	Same as above	Same as above Thoracic duct damage
Subclavian vein	Good landmarks Remains patent despite hypovolemia Patient comfort when awake	Pneumothorax
External jugular vein	Superficial location	Often difficult to thread the catheter into the central circulation
Antecubital vein	Safety	Often difficult to thread the catheter into the central circulation

III

begin to disappear. There is more resonance such that the systolic peak is higher and the diastolic measurement is lower as the blood pressure wave travels distally from the heart (Fig. 20-4). Mean arterial pressure remains about the same at all measurement sites.

TECHNIQUE OF MEASUREMENT

The transducer is the hardware essential for direct pressure monitoring. All pressure transducers use a diaphragm with low compliance characteristics that will bend and cause a volume change in response to an applied pressure. The most commonly used types of transducers are the Wheatstone bridge and the unbonded strain gauge. The transducer must be zeroed at whatever level is most appropriate for the patient. Although there may be certain inaccuracies, many clinicians place the transducer at a level corresponding to the center of the heart. Zeroing exposes the transducer system to ambient atmospheric pressure. Once the transducer system is isolated from atmospheric pressure, all subsequent pressure changes will be considered to be changes in physiologic pressure.[5] It is sometimes useful to know that for every 15 cm in height that the transducer is moved up or down, there is a corresponding change of 10 mm Hg in the pressure reading.

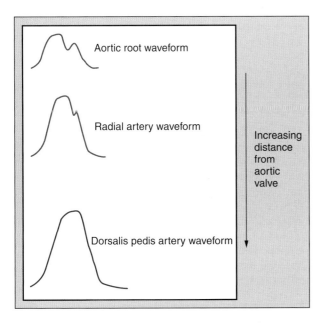

Figure 20-4 The shape of the arterial pulse wave changes as the waveform progresses distally from the central aorta.

CENTRAL VENOUS PRESSURE

Central venous pressure (CVP) monitoring is used to evaluate right ventricular function or to reflect left ventricular function when there is a correlation between left and right ventricular function. The CVP waveform consists of three positive waveforms called a, c, and v and two negative slopes called the x and y depressions (Fig. 20-5). The "a" wave represents the increase in right atrial pressure during the phase of atrial contraction. The "c" wave is caused by bulging of the closed tricuspid valve into the right atrium during the beginning of ventricular systole. The "x" descent occurs during ventricular systole and corresponds to atrial relaxation. The "v" wave descent represents filling of the atrium while the tricuspid valve is closed. The "y" wave descent occurs when the tricuspid valve opens and the atrium starts to empty.

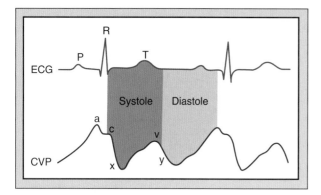

Figure 20-5 Central venous pressure (CVP) waveforms in relation to electrical events on the electrocardiogram (ECG). (From Mark JB. Central venous pressure monitoring: Clinical insights beyond the numbers. J Cardiothoracic Vasc Anesth 1991;5:164.)

Table 20–5 Possible Clinical Indications for Insertion of a Pulmonary Artery Catheter

Poor left ventricular function (ejection fraction, <0.4; cardiac index, <2 L/min/m²)
Assessment of intravascular fluid volume
Evaluation of the response to fluid administration or administration of drugs (vasopressors, vasodilators, inotropes)
Valvular heart disease
Recent myocardial infarction
Adult respiratory distress syndrome
Massive trauma (shock, hemorrhage)
Major vascular surgery (cross-clamping of the aorta, large fluid shifts)

Clinical Uses

CVP is typically used to help in the assessment of a patient's intravascular volume status (see Table 20-4). In addition, CVP may be helpful for assessing atrial cardiac dysrhythmias, right-sided cardiac valvular defects, cardiac tamponade, and myocardial ischemia.[6] In particular, in the case of atrial fibrillation, the "a" wave will vanish and be replaced by a more discernible "c" wave. Tricuspid regurgitation can be diagnosed by noticing a prominent "c-v" wave. Tamponade will exhibit an elevated CVP waveform and loss of the "y" descent.

PULMONARY ARTERY CATHETER

The pulmonary artery (PA) catheter is a 110-cm plastic tube containing four separate lumens. The tip of the catheter has a distal balloon with a volume capacity of 1.5 mL. A PA catheter may be used to measure cardiac output, mixed venous oxygen partial pressure, PA and right atrial pressure, and indirectly, left ventricular end-diastolic pressure (LVEDP) (Table 20-5). Complications from placement of a PA catheter are infrequent (<0.5% of insertions) but include cardiac dysrhythmias, catheter knotting, cardiac valve injury, and pulmonary artery rupture.[7] The waveform displayed from the distal end of a PA catheter as it is advanced from its venous insertion site reflects the position of the distal catheter tip in the vascular system (Fig. 20-6).

Pulmonary Artery Occlusive Pressure

Pulmonary artery occlusive pressure (PAOP), or "wedge pressure," is used as a measure of LVEDP (Table 20-6). To measure PAOP, the distal balloon is inflated, thus isolating the distal lumen; theoretically, blood flow ceases

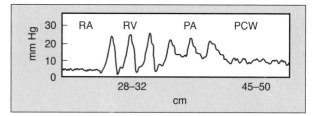

Figure 20-6 Schematic depiction of pressure waveforms as a pulmonary artery catheter passes through the right atrium (RA), right ventricle (RV), and pulmonary artery (PA). Note the narrowing of pulse pressure ("diastolic step-up") as the catheter enters the PA. Loss of a pulsatile trace as the catheter is advanced through the PA reflects pulmonary capillary wedge (PCW) pressure, which is also designated pulmonary artery occlusive pressure. Insertion of the pulmonary artery catheter through the right internal jugular vein should result in an RV tracing after the catheter has been advanced 28 to 32 cm and a PCW tracing at 45 to 50 cm.

between the tip of the catheter and the left atrium. During diastole, when the mitral valve is open, the pressure between the left atrium and left ventricle should equalize, thus allowing the tip of the catheter to reflect LVEDP.

Normal PAOP is 8 to 12 mm Hg, but higher cardiac output can often be obtained by increasing the pressure to 14 to 18 mm Hg. A PAOP higher than 18 mm Hg can result in dyspnea, whereas one greater than 20 mm Hg can cause the onset of fluid movement into alveoli. A PAOP greater than 30 mm Hg indicates frank pulmonary edema.

Measurement of Cardiac Output

Thermodilution cardiac output is measured by using a modification of the Stewart-Hamilton equation that takes

Table 20-6 Use of the Pulmonary Artery Catheter to Evaluate Hemodynamic Disorders

	Central Venous Pressure	Pulmonary Artery Occlusive Pressure (PAOP)	Pulmonary Artery End-Diastolic Pressure (PAEDP)
Hypovolemia	Decreased	Decreased	PAEDP = PAOP
Left ventricular failure	Increased	Increased	PAEDP = PAOP
Right ventricular failure	Increased	No change	PAEDP = PAOP
Pulmonary embolism	Increased	No change	PAEDP > PAOP
Cardiac tamponade	Increased	Increased	PAEDP = PAOP

into account temperature changes between the injectate and PA blood, which is proportional to pulmonary blood flow (cardiac output). The possibilities for inaccuracies in determination of cardiac output are multiple. An error of 0.5 mL out of a 10-mL injectate volume can alter the output by 5%. A 1°C increase in the temperature of the injectate can cause an error of 3% in cardiac output. In addition, a decrement in the volume of the injectate will increase the calculated cardiac output.

Measurement of Mixed Venous Oxygen Partial Pressure

The PA catheter is often used to measure the partial pressure of mixed venous oxygen (Pv_{O_2}). This value corresponds to a global representation of total-body oxygen supply and demand. Normal Pv_{O_2} is about 40 mm Hg with a saturation of 75%. A reduction in Pv_{O_2} may be attributed to a reduction in oxygen delivery (secondary to a reduction in the oxygen content of blood or a decrease in cardiac output) or an increase in oxygen consumption (secondary to an increased metabolic state).

ECHOCARDIOGRAPHY

Conventionally, hemodynamic monitoring of the cardiovascular system has been accomplished by the use of intravascular catheters. However, the advent of echocardiography has revolutionized the field (Table 20-7).[8]

Technology

Echocardiography uses ultrasound waves emitted by a piezoelectric crystal to penetrate tissue. This high-frequency sound is inaudible. The sound energy strikes various tissue planes and is subsequently reflected back to the crystal. The energy striking the crystal is analyzed with regard to attenuation, time delay, and frequency change, and the results are displayed in a format that gives the clinician information regarding velocity, distance, and density.

M-MODE ECHOCARDIOGRAPHY

M-mode echocardiography offers a unidimensional view of the myocardium. It represents the tissue densities and velocities encountered by a thin beam of ultrasound energy that is directed at the heart. M-mode echocardiography is best used for determining velocities.

B-MODE ECHOCARDIOGRAPHY

Two-dimensional echocardiography, also called B-mode echocardiography, displays a two-dimensional image of the myocardium. The ultrasound energy is swept through the heart in a planar fashion, thus providing a cross-sectional view of the heart. The cross section is updated every few milliseconds, and therefore it is possible to view changes in myocardial performance immediately.

Velocity

Velocity is monitored in echocardiography by using the principle of the Doppler shift in sound wave frequencies. When the emitted ultrasound strikes moving erythrocytes, the shift in the frequency of the reflected sound energy represents the velocity of the erythrocyte.

PULSED-WAVE DOPPLER

Pulsed-wave Doppler uses one crystal for both emission and reception of the ultrasound energy (Fig. 20-7). The

Table 20-7 Clinical Information Derived from Intraoperative Transesophageal Echocardiography

Regional (segmental) wall motion abnormalities (myocardial ischemia)
Stroke volume (ejection fraction)
Cardiac valve function (aortic, mitral)
Intracardiac air
Effects of anesthesia and surgery on cardiac function
Adequacy of intravascular fluid volume

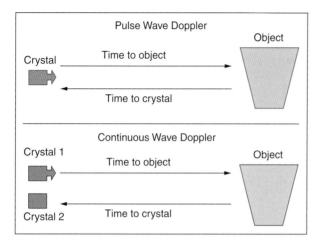

Pulse Wave Doppler

Crystal

Time to object

Time to crystal

Object

Continuous Wave Doppler

Crystal 1

Time to object

Object

Crystal 2

Time to crystal

Figure 20-7 Timing differences between Doppler modalities.

crystal emits ultrasound for a specified period and then waits for the reflected energy to return. The number of ultrasound emissions per minute is defined as the "pulse repetition frequency." Because the crystal will not emit another sound until the reflected sound energy returns, the velocities that it can measure with this technique are necessarily slow. The advantage, however, is that the location of the tissue with the velocity being measured is known. The maximal Doppler shift measurable is limited to half the pulse repetition frequency, which is known as the Nyquist limit. Velocities that produce a Doppler shift higher than the Nyquist limit are inaccurate. This phenomenon is known as "aliasing."

CONTINUOUS-WAVE DOPPLER

Continuous-wave Doppler differs from pulsed-wave Doppler by virtue of its use of two crystals—one for ultrasound emission and one for detection of the returning energy. The continuous production of sound energy permits measurement of high-velocity Doppler shifts and thus yields information on higher velocities.[9]

Color Doppler Imaging

Color Doppler imaging is a technology based on pulsed-wave Doppler. However, color Doppler overlays a color grid on the traditional gray-scale cross-sectional view seen for pulsed-wave Doppler. Blood flowing toward the transducer head is seen as a shade of red, and flow away from the transducer is seen as blue. The velocity of the flow is characterized by deeper shades of blue and red. With the interposition of color on the image, the clinician is able to better correlate blood flow with the structural elements of the heart.

PULSE OXIMETRY

Pulse oximetry is based on an application of the Beers-Lambert law, which relates the concentration of a solute (hemoglobin) to the intensity of light transmitted through the solution. The typical pulse oximeter illuminates the tissue sample with two wavelengths of light—660-nm red light and 940-nm infrared light (Fig. 20-8). An increased absorbance of red light transmitted through tissue during cardiac systole is related to arterial hemoglobin saturation. The pulse oximeter determines the amount of absorbance that is attributed to the pulsatile arterialized blood and then divides it by the nonpulsatile baseline absorbance, which is attributed to capillary and venous blood. The amount of increased absorbance seen in the pulsatile component is a measure of arterial oxygen saturation.[10]

Measurement Errors

Most pulse oximeters are two-wavelength devices that measure light absorbance only from oxyhemoglobin and deoxyhemoglobin. Thus, any other substance that also absorbs light at the same wavelengths will lead to measurement errors (Table 20-8).

METHEMOGLOBIN

Methemoglobin absorbs light almost equally well in both the red and infrared wavelengths. Consequently, a large quantity of methemoglobin will force the ratio between pulse-added absorbance and baseline absorbance toward unity, which conforms to an arterial saturation of 85%.

CARBOXYHEMOGLOBIN

Carboxyhemoglobin absorbs red light but not infrared light. As a result, pulse oximeter–reported arterial oxygen saturation values will vary widely.

INTRAVASCULAR DYES

Intravascular dyes injected into the vascular tree will also cause errors in pulse oximeter–measured arterial oxygen saturation. Methylene blue forces the reported arterial oxygen saturation to decrease to about 65%. Other dyes, including indigo carmine and indocyanine green, will cause spurious drops in measured saturation as well.

EVOKED POTENTIALS

Evoked potentials (visual, auditory, somatosensory, motor) are the electrical signals produced by the nervous system in response to various stimuli. Certain changes in the potentials can indicate neuronal pathway dysfunction. Evoked potentials are generally described in terms of latency, amplitude, and site of the stimulus. The potentials are displayed as a plot of voltage changes versus time (Fig. 20-9).[11] Latency describes the time between the

Figure 20-8 Light emission and absorbance in the pulse oximeter.

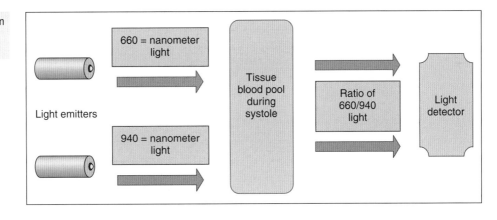

| 660 = nanometer light |
| 940 = nanometer light |

Light emitters

Tissue blood pool during systole

Ratio of 660/940 light

Light detector

Table 20–8 Factors That Influence the Accuracy of Pulse Oximetry

Low–blood flow conditions

Patient movement

Ambient light

Dysfunctional hemoglobin (carboxyhemoglobin, methemoglobin)

Methylene blue

Altered relationship between $Paco_2$ and Sao_2 (shift in the oxyhemoglobin dissociation curve)

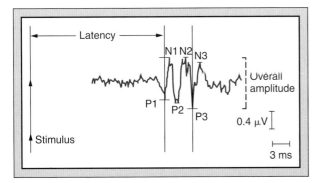

Figure 20-9 A typical somatosensory evoked potential consisting of three positive peaks (P1, P2, and P3) and three negative peaks (N1, N2, N3). More than a 50% decrease in the amplitude of the positive peaks or loss of one or more of the negative peaks, or both, may indicate the effects of volatile anesthetics or interference with the transmission of sensory nerve signals. (From Loghnan BA, Hall GM. Spinal cord monitoring 1989. Br J Anaesth 1989;63:587-594, with permission.)

stimulus and the subsequently generated potential. Amplitude is a measure of the peak of the displayed waveform from its baseline.

Somatosensory Evoked Potentials

Somatosensory evoked potentials (SSEPs) are generally monitored by placing surface or subcutaneous stimulating electrodes near the median or ulnar nerves of the arms or the posterior tibial nerves of the legs. The recording electrodes are placed on the scalp or close to the spinal cord. Lower limb SSEPs generally monitor the integrity of the dorsal columns of the spinal cord (sensory pathways) and are often used during surgery on the spinal cord or vertebral column. The vascular supply of the dorsal columns is obtained from the posterior spinal arteries, and thus the SSEP serves to warn against posterior spinal cord ischemia.

TECHNOLOGY

A square-wave signal with a time interval between 0.2 and 2 msec is applied to the peripheral nerve. The electrical signal then enters the dorsal root ganglia, traverses the posterior columns of the spinal cord, and continues on to the dorsal column nuclei at the cervical medullary junction. Second-order fibers then cross the midline and travel to the thalamus through the medial lemniscus. Third-order fibers continue from the thalamus to the frontoparietal sensorimotor cortex.

INTERPRETATION

Volatile anesthetics cause a dose-related decrease in SSEP amplitude and an increase in latency. Nitrous oxide increases this tendency. In general, SSEP recording can be performed with a 0.5 to 0.75 minimum alveolar concentration (MAC) of the volatile anesthetic with up to 60% nitrous oxide. If nitrous oxide were to be discontinued, even higher volatile anesthetic concentrations may be used. Barbiturates have a variable effect on the SSEP, depending on the dosage. Benzodiazepines administered as preanesthetic medication appear to cause only a slight change in the SSEP. Opioids such as fentanyl may also interfere with SSEPs, whereas neuromuscular blocking drugs do not affect SSEPs.

CLINICAL USES

SSEP monitoring is essential when surgery is performed in the region of major peripheral nerves, plexuses, or the spinal cord. Although serious neurologic injury may result when SSEPs show a prolonged increase in latency and a decrease in amplitude, the extent of the change required remains unclear.[12]

Motor Evoked Potentials

Motor pathways located within the corticospinal tracts are not monitored by SSEPs, and monitoring of motor evoked potentials has not been widely practiced. The stimulating electrode must be placed on the scalp, or perhaps lower down the motor pathway, and the recording electrode placed on the contracting muscle. Motor evoked potentials are generally difficult to obtain and are prone to inaccuracy. Their sensitivity to anesthetics and muscle relaxants (in contrast to SSEPs) increases the difficulty of clinical interpretation.

CAPNOGRAPHY

The carbon dioxide waveform is helpful (1) in determining that the patient is in fact being ventilated, (2) as an estimate of $PaCO_2$, and (3) as an evaluation of dead space (Table 20-9). The carbon dioxide waveform itself is characterized by four phases: (1) an inspiratory baseline, (2) an expiratory upstroke, (3) an expiratory plateau, and (4) an inspiratory downstroke (Fig. 20-10). A sustained carbon dioxide waveform (>30 mm Hg) confirms that an

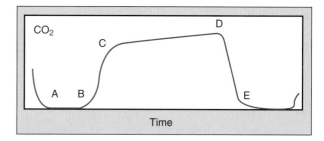

Figure 20-10 The capnogram is divided into four distinct phases. Phase A-B represents the exhalation of anatomic dead space, which is normally devoid of carbon dioxide. Phase B-C is present on the capnogram as a sharp upstroke that is determined by the evenness of ventilation and alveolar emptying. A slow rate of rise in this phase may reflect chronic obstructive pulmonary disease or acute airway obstruction, including bronchospasm. Phase C-D reflects the exhalation of alveolar gas, with point D being designated the end-tidal carbon dioxide concentration. Phase D-E reflects the beginning of inspiration and entrainment of gases lacking carbon dioxide. Normally, unless rebreathing of carbon dioxide occurs, the baseline approaches zero.

endotracheal tube is placed in the trachea, although a tube placed in the pharynx can occasionally exhibit a carbon dioxide waveform. However, an endotracheal tube placed in the esophagus should be distinguishable from tracheal intubation because any carbon dioxide present in the stomach will quickly vanish (usually within three "tidal volumes") and the waveform will become essentially flat line. Healthy, conscious people exhale gas from alveoli that are all essentially well perfused and ventilated; therefore, dead space ranges from 2% to 3%, and the differential between arterial and end-tidal carbon dioxide is about 0.6 mm Hg.

BRAIN ELECTRICAL ACTIVITY MONITORING

Most of the devices designed to monitor brain electrical activity for the purpose of assessing anesthetic effect record electroencephalographic (EEG) activity from electrodes placed on the patient's forehead. Systems may be subdivided into those that process spontaneous EEG and electromyographic (EMG) activity (bispectral index [BIS], entropy, Narcotrend, Patient State Analyzer) and those that acquire evoked responses to auditory stimuli (auditory evoked potentials).

Bispectral Index

The BIS monitor attempts to measure the effects of anesthesia on a patient's level of consciousness by algorithmi-

Table 20-9 Causes of Changes in the Exhaled Concentration of Carbon Dioxide

Increase	Decrease
Hypoventilation	Hyperventilation
Malignant hyperthermia	Hypothermia
Sepsis	Low cardiac output
Rebreathing	Pulmonary embolism
Administration of bicarbonate	Accidental disconnection or tracheal extubation
Insufflation of carbon dioxide during laparoscopy	Cardiac arrest

cally processing the patient's EEG activity and converting it to a single number, which is thought to represent the patient's state of awareness (Fig. 20-11).[13] A BIS number lower than 60 is thought to represent a state in which the patient is unable to respond to verbal commands. A BIS number higher than 70 is believed to correspond to a higher likelihood of awareness. A BIS reading of 100 represents the awake state. BIS numbers between 45 and 60 are, in general, considered to be optimal for a relatively healthy patient undergoing routine general anesthesia and surgery.

CLINICAL USES

The problem of awareness during surgery is significantly greater than most anesthesiologists realize. Awareness with recall during anesthesia is thought to occur in up to 1 in 500 cases. It is quite possible that the incidence is much higher in obstetric, cardiac, and trauma patients.[14] Therefore, if the BIS monitor can be shown to be exceedingly effective in reducing the incidence of awareness, the monitor would probably be very useful.

The BIS monitor has been shown to allow clinicians to use reduced amounts of anesthetic for light sedation cases and may enable anesthesiologists to modify their anesthetics to allow for faster wake-up. However, if the BIS monitor is used primarily to decrease the amount of anesthetic administered for reasons of cost and efficiency, it is possible that an even higher incidence of recall might result.[15]

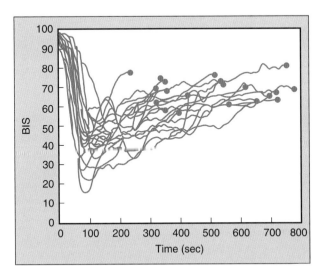

Figure 20-11 Plot of the bispectral index (BIS) against time from induction of anesthesia to recovery of consciousness after the administration of propofol. (From Flaishon RI, Windsor A, Sigl J, et al. Recovery of consciousness after thiopental or propofol: Bispectral index and the isolated forearm technique. Anesthesiology 1997;86;613-619, with permission.)

DISADVANTAGES

The BIS monitor is subject to artifact. For example, it is unclear whether a patient with head trauma can reliably be assumed to be adequately sedated despite low BIS numbers. Factors such as hypothermia and EMG contamination of the EEG signal can also degrade the utility of BIS. Physiologic conditions that may result in central nervous system effects (such as hepatic failure) may also affect the BIS number.

TEMPERATURE MONITORING

Thermal perturbations are frequent intraoperative events during surgical procedures. The exposed state of the patient causes the skin to cool, and even more importantly, the general anesthetics administered cause a decline in thermoregulatory functioning. Most general anesthetics have vasodilatory properties, which cause a flow of thermal energy from core areas of the body to more peripheral areas. In general, core temperatures decline by approximately 1°C to 1.5°C in the first hour after anesthetic induction. After the initial hour, body heat continues to decrease secondary to factors such as initial body thermal content, environmental temperature, and the size of the surgical incision. Core heat loss continues from redistributive effects, whereas peripheral heat loss persists through radiation, conduction, convection, and evaporation.[16]

Hypothermia

Hypothermia cannot be considered a benign condition. Mild hypothermia can delay recovery from anesthesia. Shivering can increase oxygen utilization, systemic blood pressure, and heart rate and can result in myocardial ischemia in elderly or physiologically weakened patients. More profound hypothermia may be directly related to myocardial dysrhythmias. Coagulation times and wound healing are also impaired.[16]

Body Temperature Monitoring Sites

The body temperature monitoring site must be chosen for the accuracy with which it registers the central thermal content.[17] The best core temperature monitors are the PA catheter, which measures blood temperature within the PA, and the tympanic membrane monitor, which measures blood temperature in the carotid artery. Bladder fluid temperature is close to core temperature, whereas rectal temperature is a relatively poor substitute. Many anesthesiologists use an esophageal temperature monitor, but it may be better used to indicate the trend of heat gain or loss. Axillary and skin temperature monitors are highly prone to artifact.

ANESTHETIC AGENT MONITORING

Monitoring concentrations of inhaled anesthetic drugs is important for determining levels or confirming the identification of the anesthetic drug or drugs and the amount present in the gases being inhaled or exhaled by the patient. Several different technologies may be used for the identification and determination of inhaled anesthetic drug levels, and each has its own strengths and limitations.

Monochromatic Infrared Spectrometry

In monochromatic infrared spectrometry, an infrared beam of light with a wavelength of 3.3 µm is passed through a representative gas sample. Because the absorption spectrum of halogenated agents is very similar at this wavelength of light, it is critically important to program the correct inhaled drug into the monitor.

Polychromatic Infrared Spectrometry

The polychromatic infrared spectrometer emits an infrared beam of light with a wavelength of 7 to 13 µm. The absorption spectrum of inhaled anesthetic drugs is relatively different at this wavelength. As a result, this monitor can automatically identify the inhaled anesthetic drug, as well as describe the concentration of gas being delivered. Should the anesthesiologist switch from one to another inhaled anesthetic drug, this monitor can measure the concentrations of both drugs simultaneously.[18]

Mass Spectrometry

Mass spectrometers ionize the gas sample and then allow the ionized particles to fall on a magnetized plate. Because of the differing atomic weights of the ionized particles, it is possible to identify the type of particles and the concentration of anesthetic drug. This technology uses a central machine that draws gases from multiple operating rooms simultaneously. The system analyzes the gas from each room sequentially, thus providing continuous, but not completely constant, gas monitoring. This type of centralized monitoring is quite expensive and is infrequently used in today's operating rooms.

Raman Scattering Spectrometry

The Raman scattering spectrometer emits an intense beam of light into a sample of gas. Collision of a photon and a gas molecule causes the photon to change its energy characteristics and emerge at a substantially different wavelength typical for the particular gas. The change in frequency allows the Raman monitor to identify the type and concentration of the specific inhaled anesthetic drug.

REFERENCES

1. Whitcher C, Ream AK, Parsons D, et al. Anesthetic mishaps and the cost of monitoring: A proposed standard for monitoring equipment. J Clin Monit 1988;4:5-15.
2. Slogoff S, Keats AS. Does perioperative myocardial ischemia lead to postoperative myocardial infarction? Anesthesiology 1985;73:1074-1081.
3. Pickering TG. Principles and techniques of blood pressure measurement. Card Clin 2002;20:207-223.
4. Slogoff S, Keats AS, Arlund C. On the safety of radial artery cannulation. Anesthesiology 1983;59:42-47.
5. Courtois M, Fattal P, Kovacs S, et al. Anatomically and physiologically based reference level for measurement of intracardiac pressures. Circulation 1995;92:1994-2000.
6. Mark JB. Central venous pressure monitoring: Clinical insights beyond the numbers. J Cardiothorac Vasc Anesth 1991;5:163-173.
7. Roizen M, Berger D, Gabel R, et al. Practice guidelines for pulmonary artery catheterization. Anesthesiology 2003;99:988-1014.
8. Sutton DC, Cahalan MK. Pro: TEE is a routine monitor. J Cardiothorac Vasc Anesth 1993;7:357-360.
9. Cahalan M. Intraoperative Transesophageal Echocardiography. An Interactive Text and Atlas. New York: Churchill Livingstone, 1997.
10. Severinghaus JW, Kehheher JF. Recent developments in pulse oximetry. Anesthesiology 1992;76:1018-1038.
11. Loghnan BA, Hall GM. Spinal cord monitoring 1989. Br J Anaesth 1989;63:587-594.
12. Kumar AB, Makhija NA. Evoked potential monitoring in anaesthesia and analgesia. Anaesthesia 2001;55:225-241.
13. Flaishon RI, Windsor A, Sigl J, et al. Recovery of consciousness after thiopental or propofol: Bispectral index and the isolated forearm technique. Anesthesiology 1997;86:613-619.
14. Ghoneim NM. Learning and consciousness during general anesthesia. Anesthesiology 1992;76:279-305.
15. O'Connor MF, Daves SM. BIS monitoring to prevent awareness during general anesthesia. Anesthesiology 2000;94:520-522.
16. Sessler D. Perioperative heat balance. Anesthesiology 2000;92:578-600.
17. Cereda Maurizio MG. Intraoperative temperature monitoring. Int Anesthesiol Clin 2004;42:41-54.
18. Walder BLR, Zbinden AM. Accuracy and cross-sensitivity of 10 different anesthetic gas monitors. J Clin Monit 1993;9:364-373.

Chapter 21

ACID-BASE BALANCE AND BLOOD GAS ANALYSIS

Joseph F. Cotten

The concentrations of hydrogen and bicarbonate ions in plasma must be precisely regulated to optimize enzyme activity, hemoglobin saturation with oxygen, myocardial contractility, and rates of chemical reactions within cells. Hydrogen ions are continuously being produced as substrates and oxidized during the production of adenosine triphosphate and therefore must be continuously eliminated, ultimately by the lungs and kidneys.

At 37°C, the normal hydrogen ion concentration in arterial blood and extracellular fluid is 35 to 45 nmol/L, which is equivalent to an arterial pH (pHa) of 7.45 to 7.35, respectively (Fig. 21-1). The normal plasma bicarbonate ion concentration is 24 ± 2 mEq/L. Venous blood tends to be slightly more acidic than arterial blood, with normal venous pH values being 7.3 to 7.4. The intracellular hydrogen ion concentration is approximately 160 nmol/L, which is equivalent to a pH of 6.8.

TERMINOLOGY

Acidosis and alkalosis refer to acid-base disorders in which blood is overly acidic or overly alkaline, respectively. However, a patient with either disorder may have a nearly normal pHa secondary to renal or pulmonary compensatory responses, or both. Additionally, patients may be afflicted with a mixed disorder characterized by both acidosis and alkalosis. In a mixed disorder the more dominant disorder dictates the pHa. Acidemia refers simply to a pHa less than 7.35 and alkalemia to a blood pHa greater than 7.45, regardless of the mechanism.

Base excess, a number frequently provided on arterial blood gas studies, refers to the nonrespiratory or metabolic component of an acid-base disturbance. When determined experimentally, base excess is the amount of strong acid (hydrochloric acid for base excess greater than zero) or strong base (sodium hydroxide for base excess less than zero) titrated to normalize the pHa of a blood sample under standardized conditions (37°C and PaCO$_2$ of 40 mm Hg).

$$\text{Arterial hydrogen ion concentration} = [H^+]_a$$
$$\text{Arterial pH} = pH_a = -\log_{10}([H^+]_a)$$

Figure 21-1 Arterial hydrogen ion concentration ($[H^+]_a$).

In practice, however, blood gas machines estimate base excess with algorithms that use measured pH_a, Pa_{CO_2}, Pa_{O_2}, and hemoglobin concentration data as parameters. Base excess has a normal value of zero. A value significantly less than zero (negative) suggests the presence of a metabolic acidosis, and a value significantly greater than zero (positive) suggests the presence of a metabolic alkalosis.

REGULATION OF THE HYDROGEN ION CONCENTRATION

Three basic systems are in place to prevent changes in pH_a: (1) buffer systems, (2) the ventilatory response, and (3) the renal response. Buffer systems resist changes in pH_a after the introduction of small amounts of acids or bases and represent the first line of defense in maintaining pH_a homeostasis. However, when the buffer systems are overwhelmed and pH_a deviates from normalcy, first ventilatory responses (in minutes) and, later, renal responses (in hours to days) provide nearly complete restoration of pH_a.

Buffer Systems

A buffer system is composed of a base molecule (bicarbonate) and its weak conjugate acid (carbonic acid). The base molecules of the buffer system bind excess hydrogen ions, and the weak acid protonates excess base molecules, each acting to maintain a constant pH_a. The term pKa indicates the strength of an acid and is derived from the classic Henderson-Hasselbalch equation (Fig. 21-2). pKa indicates the pH at which an acid is 50% protonated and 50% deprotonated such that a smaller pKa value indicates a stronger acid. The most important buffer systems in blood, in order of importance, are the (1) bicarbonate buffer system, (2) hemoglobin buffer system, (3) other protein buffer systems, and (4) phosphate buffer system.

BICARBONATE BUFFER SYSTEM

The five components of the bicarbonate buffer system are (1) carbon dioxide, (2) water, (3) carbonic anhydrase, (4) carbonic acid, and (5) bicarbonate (Fig. 21-3). Carbon dioxide is generated through aerobic metabolism and reacts with water to form carbonic acid, which spontaneously and rapidly deprotonates to form bicarbonate. The formation of carbonic acid from carbon dioxide and water is relatively slow; however, the enzyme carbonic anhydrase, present in the endothelium, erythrocytes, and kidneys, catalyzes this reaction to accelerate the formation of carbonic acid. Carbon dioxide permeates freely through the plasma membrane of cells.

A buffer system functions most effectively at a pH near its pKa. The bicarbonate system has a pKa of 6.1, which is significantly different from physiologic pH_a. However, the relatively high concentration of bicarbonate in blood, combined with renal and pulmonary regulation of bicarbonate and carbon dioxide levels, respectively, makes this the most important buffering system.

HEMOGLOBIN BUFFER SYSTEM

The hemoglobin protein is the second most important buffering system. Erythrocytes are packed with hemoglobin protein, which contains multiple protonatable sites created by the imidazole side chains of histidine residues (pKa 6.8). Because hemoglobin is sequestered in erythrocytes, buffering by hemoglobin depends on the bicarbonate system. Carbon dioxide freely diffuses into erythrocytes down a concentration gradient and combines with water and carbonic anhydrase to form carbonic acid, which rapidly deprotonates. The protons generated are bound up by hemoglobin, and the bicarbonate anions are exchanged electroneutrally back into plasma with extracellular chloride ("chloride shift"). This process allows the plasma bicarbonate pool to make use of intraerythrocyte carbonic anhydrase. The reverse of this process occurs in the pulmonary capillaries, with return of carbon dioxide into plasma and the lung alveoli for ventilatory elimination. This process allows a large fraction of extrapulmonary carbon dioxide to be transported back to the lungs as plasma bicarbonate. Hemoglobin also buffers and trans-

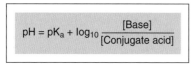

$$pH = pK_a + \log_{10}\frac{[Base]}{[Conjugate\ acid]}$$

Figure 21-2 Henderson-Hasselbalch equation. [Base], concentration of base; [Conjugate acid], concentration of conjugate acid.

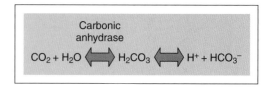

Figure 21-3 Hydration of carbon dioxide results in carbonic acid, which dissociates into bicarbonate and hydrogen ions.

ports carbon dioxide by reacting directly with it to form carbaminohemoglobin. Deoxyhemoglobin has higher affinity for carbon dioxide (Haldane effect), which facilitates removal of carbon dioxide from peripheral tissues and release into the lungs.

Ventilatory Response

Chemoreceptors in the carotid bodies and to a lesser extent the aortic arch and in the ventral surface of the medulla oblongata in the brainstem respond in minutes to changes in carbon dioxide or pHa by increasing or decreasing alveolar ventilation to change $PaCO_2$ in blood, which in turn changes pHa. There is an inverse relationship between $PaCO_2$ and alveolar minute ventilation (Fig. 21-4). The carotid bodies are peripheral chemosensing organs located at the bifurcation of bilateral carotid arteries in the neck; carotid body afferents travel centrally via the glossopharyngeal cranial nerve. The stimulus from central and peripheral chemoreceptors to either increase or decrease alveolar ventilation diminishes as the pHa approaches 7.4 such that complete correction or overcorrection is not possible. The central chemoreceptor accounts for approximately 85% of the ventilatory response to elevated $PaCO_2$. For example, after bilateral carotid endarterectomy, a procedure that unintentionally ablates the carotid body organ, patients have almost no hypoxic ventilatory drive, only a slightly elevated resting $PaCO_2$, and a blunted ventilatory response to increased $PaCO_2$.[1]

Renal Response

The proximal tubules of the kidney regulate plasma bicarbonate levels by nearly complete reabsorption of bicarbonate from the glomerular filtrate and by secretion of hydrogen ions into the tubular lumen with concomitant intracellular bicarbonate production. Under normal conditions, urine is virtually free of bicarbonate secondary to proximal tubule reabsorption. Secreted hydrogen ions, with the assistance of luminal, membrane bound carbonic anhydrase, convert virtually all the filtered bicarbonate into carbon dioxide for reabsorption; any additional secreted hydrogen ions are trapped by water-soluble urinary buffers (ammonia and phosphate) for excretion in urine. This process is regulated by a multitude of factors, including

$PaCO_2$, bicarbonate levels, and urinary ammonia buffer production. A defect in proximal tubule bicarbonate absorption results in bicarbonate-wasting disease (proximal renal tubular acidosis). Acetazolamide, a carbonic anhydrase inhibitor, similarly impairs bicarbonate absorption and production in the proximal tubules and causes a normal–anion gap metabolic acidosis. This drug may be administered to reverse iatrogenic chloride-resistant metabolic alkalosis.

DIFFERENTIAL DIAGNOSIS OF ACID-BASE DISTURBANCES

Acid-base disturbances are categorized as respiratory or metabolic acidosis (pHa lower than 7.35) or alkalosis (pHa higher than 7.45) (Table 21-1).[2,3] These disorders are further stratified into acute versus chronic based on their duration, which is gauged clinically by the patient's compensatory responses. It must be kept in mind that a patient may have a mixed acid-base disorder. To provide appropriate treatment and diagnosis, rapid, systematic, and accurate interpretation of a patient's acid-base status through analysis of arterial blood gas data, electrolyte data, and patient history is essential.

Adverse Responses to Acidemia and Alkalemia

Predictable adverse responses accompany acidemia and alkalemia. The direct effects of alkalemia on myocardial contractility are less striking than those of acidemia. Although acidemia decreases myocardial contractility, little clinical effect occurs until the pHa is below 7.2. Because acidemia also induces the release of catecholamines, most of the direct myocardial depressant effects are mitigated in mild acidemia. When the pHa is lower than 7.1, however, myocardial responsiveness to catecholamines decreases and the compensatory increases in myocardial contractility are

III

Table 21–1 Stepwise Approach for Interpreting Acid-Base Status
Is the pH value life threatening (<7.1 requires immediate intervention)?
Does the pH value reflect acidosis or alkalosis?
Could an acute increase in $PaCO_2$ explain the entire blood gas picture?
Is there evidence of a chronic respiratory disturbance?
Is there evidence of an acute metabolic disturbance?
Are compensatory changes present?
Does the clinical history fit the acid-base picture?

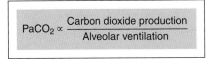

$$PaCO_2 \propto \frac{\text{Carbon dioxide production}}{\text{Alveolar ventilation}}$$

Figure 21-4 The partial pressure of arterial carbon dioxide is proportional to carbon dioxide production and inversely proportional to alveolar ventilation.

diminished (Fig. 21-5).[4] Respiratory acidosis may produce more rapid and profound myocardial dysfunction than metabolic acidosis does because of the ability of carbon dioxide to freely diffuse across cell membranes and exacerbate intracellular acidosis to a greater extent than metabolic acidosis. The detrimental effects of acidemia may be accentuated in the presence of ischemic heart disease or in patients in whom sympathetic nervous system activity may be impaired, as by β-blockade or general anesthesia.

Respiratory Acidosis

Respiratory acidosis is caused by a mismatch between carbon dioxide production and ventilatory elimination (alveolar ventilation) (Table 21-2). Respiratory acidosis occurs when drug- or disease-induced decreases in alveolar ventilation result in an increased $PaCO_2$, which in turn leads to the formation of carbonic acid and hydrogen ions and a pHa less than 7.35 (see Fig. 21-4). A patient with normal or even elevated total minute ventilation may experience respiratory acidosis as a result of diseased lungs with markedly increased dead space ("wasted ventilation" reflecting aeration of lung regions not participating in gas exchange). Volatile and intravenous anesthetics and opioids cause respiratory acidosis by blunting the existing peripheral and central chemosensory ventilatory response to carbon dioxide. Increased carbon dioxide production or increased systemic carbon dioxide absorption, particularly in a patient who is mechanically ventilated or has limited ventilatory reserve, can result in respiratory acidosis.

COMPENSATORY RESPONSES TO RESPIRATORY ACIDOSIS

Over the course of hours to days the kidneys compensate for respiratory acidosis by increased hydrogen ion secretion and bicarbonate reabsorption and production (Table 21-3). After a few days, the pHa will be near normal despite the persistence of increased $PaCO_2$. A nearly normal pHa despite an increased $PaCO_2$ (greater than 40 mm Hg) confirms that the respiratory acidosis is chronic rather than acute.

TREATMENT OF RESPIRATORY ACIDOSIS

Respiratory acidosis with a pHa below 7.1 indicates the need for tracheal intubation and increased ventilatory support. Ventilatory parameters should be guided by arterial or venous blood gas data to avoid overventilation, particularly in patients with chronic respiratory acidosis. Metabolic alkalosis from overventilation can result in central nervous system (CNS) irritability, and the vasoconstrictive effects of hypocapnia have the potential to cause CNS and cardiac ischemia. Metabolic alkalosis associated with chronic respiratory acidosis is treated by avoidance of mechanical hyperventilation and careful intravenous administration of potassium chloride or acetazolamide.

Respiratory Alkalosis

Respiratory alkalosis occurs when there is increased alveolar ventilation relative to carbon dioxide production (Table 21-4). $PaCO_2$ is diminished relative to bicarbonate levels, thereby resulting in a pHa greater than 7.45. In normal circumstances, decreased $PaCO_2$ and increased pHa decrease the stimulus to breathe, which is normally mediated by peripheral and central chemoreceptors. During prolonged respiratory alkalosis, active transport of bicarbonate ions out of cerebrospinal fluid (CSF) causes the central chemoreceptors to reset to a lower $PaCO_2$ level. By the same mechanism, mechanical hyperventilation of the lungs during anesthesia results in the initiation of spontaneous ventilation at a lower $PaCO_2$ than was present before hyperventilation. Likewise, continued hyperventilation after returning to sea level from altitude reflects the effect of central chemoreceptors exposed to bicarbonate-depleted CSF.

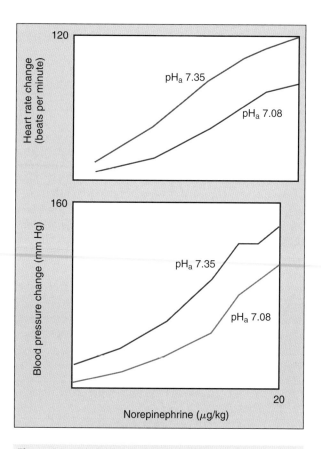

Figure 21-5 Diminished hemodynamic response to intravenously administered norepinephrine in a canine model of lactic acidosis. (From Ford GD, Cline WH, Fleming WW. Am J Physiol 1968;215:1123-1129, with permission.)

Table 21–2 Causes of Respiratory Acidosis

Decreased Carbon Dioxide Elimination (Hypoventilation)

Upper or lower airway obstruction (asthma, chronic obstructive pulmonary disease, sleep apnea, tumor)

Central nervous system depression (anesthetics, opioids, neurologic injury)

Lung or chest wall restriction (scoliosis, obesity, extreme ascites, pneumothorax, pleural effusion)

Decreased skeletal muscle strength (residual effects of neuromuscular blocking drugs, myopathy, neuropathy, spinal cord injury, botulinum toxin)

Intrinsic pulmonary disease (pneumonia, pulmonary edema, fibrosis, sarcoidosis)

Increased Carbon Dioxide Production/Reabsorption

Increased metabolic production of carbon dioxide (malignant hyperthermia, hyperthyroidism, hyperalimentation with a high carbohydrate content)

Rebreathing of exhaled gases (exhausted soda lime, incompetent one-way valve in the anesthetic breathing system)

Carbon dioxide absorption from pneumoperitoneum (laparoscopic surgery)

Metabolic Compensation

$\Delta pHa = 0.008 \times \Delta Pa_{CO_2}$ (acute)

$\Delta pHa = 0.003 \times \Delta Pa_{CO_2}$ (chronic)

III

Table 21–3 Guidelines to Estimate Impact of Changes in Pa_{CO_2} on pH and Bicarbonate Measurements

pH will decrease 0.08 unit for every acute 10–mm Hg increase in Pa_{CO_2}

pH will return toward normal if elevated Pa_{CO_2} is sustained

Bicarbonate will increase 1 mEq/L for every acute 10–mm Hg increase in Pa_{CO_2}

Bicarbonate will increase 4 mEq/L for every chronic 10–mm Hg increase in Pa_{CO_2}

COMPENSATORY RESPONSES TO RESPIRATORY ALKALOSIS

Respiratory alkalosis is compensated for by decreased reabsorption of bicarbonate ions from renal tubules. The subsequent increased urinary excretion of bicarbonate ions in association with sodium and potassium ions returns the pHa to nearly normal in patients with chronic decreases in Pa_{CO_2}. In addition, alkalosis stimulates the activity of phosphofructokinase, which results in glycolysis and the generation of lactic acid. The tetany that may accompany respiratory alkalosis reflects hypocalcemia secondary to the greater affinity of plasma proteins for calcium ions in an alkaline pHa.

TREATMENT OF RESPIRATORY ALKALOSIS

Treatment of chronic respiratory alkalosis is directed at correcting the underlying disorder responsible for the

Table 21–4 Causes of Respiratory Alkalosis

Increased Carbon Dioxide Elimination (Hyperventilation)

Iatrogenic (mechanical or self-induced)

Drugs (doxapram, salicylates)

Pregnancy

Pain or anxiety

Decreased barometric pressure

Central nervous system injury (central neurogenic hyperventilation)

Arterial hypoxemia

Pulmonary vascular disease (pulmonary embolism)

Cirrhosis of the liver

Sepsis

Hyperthermia-induced hyperventilation

Decreased Carbon Dioxide Production

Hypothermia

Hypothyroidism

Skeletal muscle paralysis by a neuromuscular blocking drug

Metabolic Compensation

$\Delta pHa = 0.008 \times \Delta Pa_{CO_2}$ (acute)

$\Delta pHa = 0.017 \times \Delta Pa_{CO_2}$ (chronic)

increased elimination of carbon dioxide by the lungs or decreased metabolic production of carbon dioxide. During anesthesia, acute respiratory alkalosis is easily remedied by decreasing total minute ventilation.

Metabolic Acidosis

Metabolic acidosis is present when accumulation of any acid in the body other than carbon dioxide results in a pHa lower than 7.35 (Table 21-5). An increase in ventilatory elimination of carbon dioxide starts in minutes after the development of metabolic acidosis to provide near normalization of pHa. One must keep in mind, however, that some patients may be physically unable to evoke or sustain a compensatory ventilatory response. Measurement of $PaCO_2$ will clarify whether the acidosis is primary or compensatory as in response to respiratory alkalosis.

ANION GAP

For diagnostic reasons, metabolic acidosis is divided into that with an increased anion gap or a normal anion gap. The anion gap is the measured concentration difference between sodium cations and the sum of chloride and bicarbonate anions and represents the concentration of anions (known and unknown) in serum that are unaccounted for in this equation. A normal anion gap value is 3 to 11 mEq/L and is contributed primarily by anionic serum albumin. A patient with a low serum albumin concentration is anticipated to have a lower anion gap value. Metabolic acidosis with an elevated anion gap (greater than 11, or less in hypoalbuminemic patients) suggests the accumulation of unmeasured anions (lactic acid or ketoacids); metabolic acidosis with a normal anion gap suggests a bicarbonate-wasting process in the kidneys or gastrointestinal tract (renal tubular acidosis or diarrhea). Overzealous fluid resuscitation with 0.9% normal saline (>30 mL/kg/hr) will induce an iatrogenic normal-gap metabolic acidosis secondary to excessive chloride administration, which impairs bicarbonate reabsorption in the kidneys.[5]

COMPENSATORY RESPONSES TO METABOLIC ACIDOSIS

The compensatory responses initiated by metabolic acidosis include increased alveolar ventilation as a result of stimulation of the carotid bodies by hydrogen ions and renal tubule secretion of hydrogen ions into urine (Table 21-6). As with respiratory acidosis, volatile anesthetics blunt the carotid body–mediated response to metabolic acidosis. Another compensatory mechanism is the use of buffers present in bone to neutralize nonvolatile acids present in the circulation. Chronic metabolic acidosis, as seen with chronic renal failure, is commonly associated with loss of bone mass.

TREATMENT OF METABOLIC ACIDOSIS

Management of metabolic acidosis is guided by diagnosis and treatment of the underlying cause (intravenous fluid and insulin therapy in the setting of diabetic ketoacidosis). Minute ventilation can be increased in a patient who is mechanically ventilated to compensate until more definitive treatment takes effect. Additionally, though controversial, intravenous administration of sodium bicarbonate may be considered in the setting of extreme metabolic acidosis (pHa less than 7.1) as a temporizing measure, particularly when a patient is deteriorating. Sodium bicarbonate administration generates carbon dioxide, which unless eliminated by ventilation, can worsen any intracellular and extracellular acidosis.[6] Therefore, sodium

Table 21-5   Causes of Metabolic Acidosis
Increased Anion Gap (>11 mEq/L)
Drugs (methanol, ethanol, salicylate)
Ketoacidosis (alcohol, diabetes mellitus, starvation)
Lactic acidosis (anaerobic glycolysis because of underperfusion of tissue during hypovolemia, heart failure, or cardiac arrest; cyanide toxicity; sepsis)
Renal failure (accumulation of organic acids)
Liver failure/cirrhosis (decreased conversion of lactate to glucose)
Normal Anion Gap (3-11 mEq/L)
Administration of 0.9% normal saline or hyperalimentation
Gastrointestinal bicarbonate losses (diarrhea, ileostomy, pancreatic fistula, neobladder)
Renal bicarbonate losses (renal tubular acidosis)
Drugs (acetazolamide)
Ventilatory Compensation
Expected $PaCO_2 = 1.5 \times HCO_3^- + 8 \ (\pm 2)$

Table 21-6   Adverse Effects of Respiratory or Metabolic Acidosis
Hyperkalemia
Central nervous system depression
Cardiovascular depression (offset by increased secretion of catecholamines)
Cardiac dysrhythmias
Hypovolemia (as a result of decreased precapillary and increased postcapillary sphincter tone)

bicarbonate should be given only to a patient with adequate ventilatory support and never in the setting of respiratory acidosis. Because it is of questionable benefit and has the potential to adversely affect a patient, it should be administered on a trial basis. A common approach is to slowly administer about half the calculated dose of sodium bicarbonate and then repeat the pHa measurement and monitor hemodynamics to determine the impact of treatment. Calculation of the dose of sodium bicarbonate is based on deviation of the plasma bicarbonate concentration from normal (Table 21-7). An infusion is prepared by diluting three ampules of sodium bicarbonate in a 1-L bag of 5% dextrose in water. This yields a solution with a sodium concentration of approximately 150 mEq/L, similar to that of 0.9% normal saline (154 mEq/L). One ampule of sodium bicarbonate contains 50 mEq of sodium. Newer alkalinizing agents that do not generate carbon dioxide have been developed but have not yet been shown to reduce mortality in patients with severe metabolic acidosis. Such agents include Carbicarb, which is equimolar sodium carbonate and sodium bicarbonate, and THAM, which is tris(hydroxymethyl)aminomethane. Alkalinizing agents, because of their osmotic properties, introduce the risk of causing hypervolemia and hypertonicity.

Metabolic Alkalosis

Metabolic alkalosis is present when the pHa is higher than 7.45 because of gain of bicarbonate ions or loss of hydrogen ions (Table 21-8). For example, conversion of citrate to lactate by the liver after the administration of large volumes of stored whole blood can result in metabolic alkalosis.[7] Citrate, a calcium chelator, is used as an anticoagulant for stored blood. Depletion of intravascular fluid volume is often the most important factor in maintenance of metabolic alkalosis. In this regard, hypovolemia

Table 21-8 Causes of Metabolic Alkalosis

Excessive loss of hydrogen ions (vomiting, gastric suction)
Chloride and/or potassium loss (diuretics)
Excessive production of bicarbonate ions (metabolism of lactate in lactated Ringer's solution, citrate in stored blood, acetate in hyperalimentation solutions)
Hypovolemia
Hyperaldosteronism
Permissive hypercapnia
Ventilatory Compensation (Variable)
Expected $Pa_{CO_2} = 0.7 \times HCO_3^- + 20 \, (\pm1.5)$

should be considered in postoperative patients in whom metabolic alkalosis develops. Metabolic alkalosis also correlates with decreases in the total-body concentration of chloride and potassium ions, as may accompany diuretic therapy. With the adoption of smaller tidal volumes (5 to 7 mL/kg) and requisite underventilation in the long-term ventilatory management of patients with adult respiratory distress syndrome, a compensatory metabolic alkalosis secondary to "permissive hypercapnia" is a common finding that is relatively well tolerated.

COMPENSATORY RESPONSES TO METABOLIC ALKALOSIS

Compensatory responses initiated by metabolic alkalosis include increased reabsorption of hydrogen ions by renal tubule cells, decreased secretion of hydrogen ions by renal tubule cells, and alveolar hypoventilation (Table 21-9). The efficiency of the renal compensatory mechanism is dependent on the presence of cations (sodium, potassium) and chloride. Depletion of these ions, as occurs with vomiting, impairs the ability of the kidneys to excrete excess bicarbonate ions and thereby results in incomplete renal compensation for metabolic alkalosis. Hypoventilation in an attempt to compensate for metabolic alkalosis will initially stimulate the medullary chemoreceptors and thus offset the compensatory effect of decreased alveolar ventilation. With time, CSF pH is normalized by active transport of bicarbonate ions into CSF, and the volume of ventilation decreases despite the persistence of a compensatory increase in Pa_{CO_2}. If Pa_{CO_2} increases again, however, CSF pH will decrease and the same sequence will be repeated. Of note, respiratory compensation for pure metabolic alkalosis, in contrast to metabolic acidosis, is never more than 75% complete. As a result, the pHa remains increased in patients with primary metabolic alkalosis. Furthermore, a Pa_{CO_2} value greater than 55 mm Hg is beyond the normal compensatory mechanism for metabolic alkalosis and reflects concomitant respiratory acidosis.

Table 21-7 Calculation of Sodium Bicarbonate Dosing for Metabolic Acidosis

Sodium bicarbonate dose = Body weight (kg) × Deviation of plasma bicarbonate from 24 mEq/L × Extracellular fluid volume as a fraction of body mass (0.3)
Administer half the calculated dose and repeat the measurement of pHa to determine the impact of treatment
Example
A 70-kg patient with a plasma bicarbonate concentration of 12 mEq/L would require (70)(24 − 12)(0.3) = 252 mEq sodium bicarbonate. Half of this is 126 mEq

III

Table 21-9 Adverse Effects of Respiratory or Metabolic Alkalosis

Hypokalemia

Hypocalcemia (manifested as decreased myocardial contractility and tetany)

Central nervous system excitation

Decreased cerebral blood flow

Coronary artery vasoconstriction

Leftward shift of the oxyhemoglobin dissociation curve (Bohr effect)

Cardiac dysrhythmias

Increased airway resistance

TREATMENT OF METABOLIC ALKALOSIS

Treatment of metabolic alkalosis is directed at resolution of the process responsible for the acid-base derangement and, in most cases (chloride-sensitive alkalosis), intravenous infusion of saline plus potassium chloride, which allows the kidneys to excrete excess bicarbonate ions. On occasion (chloride-resistant alkalosis), intravenous infusion of hydrogen ions in the form of ammonium chloride or hydrochloric acid or the diuretic acetazolamide is used to facilitate the return of pHa to near normal. Administration of acid requires the insertion of a central venous catheter because peripheral injections can cause sclerosis of veins and hemolysis. Life-threatening metabolic alkalosis is rarely encountered.

MEASUREMENT OF ARTERIAL BLOOD GASES

Technologic advances that permit analysis of arterial and mixed venous blood gases, as well as pH, have contributed greatly to patient management during anesthesia and in the intensive care unit. Moreover, small blood volume requirements (as little as 0.1 mL) extend blood gas analysis to the care of premature infants, as well as children and adults. Arterial blood gas measurements serve to verify the adequacy of oxygenation and alveolar ventilation as continuously monitored by pulse oximetry and capnography.

Sampling

Arterial blood is most often obtained percutaneously from the radial, brachial, or femoral artery. Peripheral venous blood may be an alternative when arterial sampling is not possible. Venous blood from the dorsum of the hand, which becomes somewhat arterialized under the vasodilating effects of general anesthetics, can be used for PCO_2, pH, and base excess measurements. Venous PCO_2 is only 4 to 6 mm Hg higher and pH only 0.03 to 0.04 lower than arterial values.[8] Venous blood, however, cannot be used for estimation of PaO_2 because venous PO_2 is variably and significantly lower than PaO_2. Nonetheless, venous PO_2 may be high enough to rule out arterial hypoxemia (venous PO_2 greater than 60 mm Hg).

Blood is drawn into a plastic or glass syringe that contains sufficient heparin to fill the dead space of the syringe. Heparin is acidic, and excessive amounts of this anticoagulant in the sampling syringe could falsely lower the measured pHa. Elimination of air bubbles from the syringe after obtaining the sample is important because equilibration of oxygen and carbon dioxide in the blood with the corresponding partial pressures in the air bubble could influence the measured results. Unlike mature red blood cells, white blood cells in an arterial blood gas sample are metabolically active and as such consume oxygen and generate carbon dioxide despite being removed from the body. Prompt analysis or placing the sample on ice helps minimize the small error introduced by the continued metabolic activity of leukocytes. A large decrease in oxygen content does occur, however, when the white blood cell count is markedly elevated, as during leukemia, and it can cause arterial blood samples to "reflect" a hypoxemic value even though the patient's oxygenation is acceptable. This phenomenon is often referred to as "leukocyte larceny."[9]

Temperature Correction

Cooling blood causes it to become more alkaline by increasing carbon dioxide solubility, which decreases $PaCO_2$, and by decreasing H_2O dissociation into H^+ and OH^-. This raises the issue of how to best manage pHa in patients under extreme hypothermia. For example, a patient cooled to 25°C and undergoing cardiopulmonary bypass, if left untreated, will have a pHa of 7.6. However, warming the blood sample to 37°C, as arterial blood gas machines do, will decrease the measured pHa to 7.4. The concept of alpha stat and pH stat describes two schools of thought regarding temperature correction of arterial blood gas values.[10]

ALPHA STAT

Alpha refers to the protonation state of the α-imidazole side chain of histidine. Interestingly, the pKa of histidine changes with temperature such that its protonation state is relatively constant regardless of temperature. Consequently, by allowing a patient's pHa to drift with temperature, you are in fact allowing the protonation state of the histidine residues to remain "static," hence the term alpha stat. This concept arose from the observation that "cold-blooded" poikilothermic animals, which rely on a relatively similar complement of enzymes as "warm-blooded" homeothermic animals do, function well over a wide range of body temperatures.

pH STAT

pH stat is a more involved technique than alpha stat in that it requires keeping a patient's pHa static at 7.4 (through modification of $PaCO_2$) regardless of the core temperature (similar to that of a hibernating, homeothermic animal). The lower pHa maintained during pH stat may improve cerebrovascular perfusion during hypothermia; however, there is still debate about which method provides better outcomes, neurologic or otherwise.

ROUTINE ANALYSIS

Most routine arterial blood gas samples are analyzed at a temperature of 37°C, regardless of the patient's actual body temperature. This provides standardization for these studies, particularly when viewed by multiple independent practitioners, and bypasses the need for accurate body temperature assessment, which can be fraught with error. Temperature correction of PO_2 remains relatively important, however, for assessing oxygenation. As a guideline, the measured PO_2 should be decreased 6% for every 1°C that the patient's body temperature is below the temperature of the measuring electrode (37°C). PO_2 is increased 6% for every 1°C that the body temperature exceeds 37°C. Furthermore, calculation of the alveolar-to-arterial difference for oxygen ($A\text{-}aDO_2$) requires a temperature correction of PaO_2 (Table 21-10).

Blood Gas and pH Electrodes

OXYGEN ELECTRODE

The oxygen electrode (Clark electrode) used to measure PO_2 is a polarographic cell consisting of a silver reference anode and a platinum cathode charged to 0.5 V. The platinum surface is covered with an oxygen-permeable membrane (polyethylene), on the other side of which is placed the unknown sample. The electric current passing through the polarographic cell is directly proportional to the PO_2 outside the membrane.

CARBON DIOXIDE ELECTRODE

The carbon dioxide electrode (Severinghaus electrode) used to measure PCO_2 has a carbon dioxide–permeable membrane (Teflon) that permits carbon dioxide to diffuse from the unknown sample into a buffer solution containing bicarbonate ions bathing a conventional glass pH electrode. The measured pH in the bathing solution is altered in direct proportion to PCO_2.

pH ELECTRODE

Measurement of pH involves a glass electrode that senses the concentration of hydrogen ions in the unknown sample. This hydrogen ion concentration produces a proportional change in voltage between the glass and reference electrode.

Table 21–10 Alveolar Gas Equation and Calculation of the Alveolar-to-Arterial Oxygen Gradient

Alveolar gas equation: $PAO_2 = (PB - PH_2O)FIO_2 - PaCO_2/RQ$
Alveolar-to-arterial oxygen gradient: $A\text{-}aDO_2 = PAO_2 - PaO_2$

$A\text{-}aDO_2$ = alveolar-to-arterial oxygen gradient (mm Hg)
PAO_2 = alveolar partial pressure oxygen (mm Hg)
PaO_2 = measured arterial partial pressure oxygen (mm Hg)
PB = barometric pressure (mm Hg) (760 mm Hg at sea level)
PH_2O = partial pressure of water vapor (47 mm Hg at 37°C)
FIO_2 = inspired oxygen concentration
$PaCO_2$ = arterial partial pressure of carbon dioxide (mm Hg)
RQ = respiratory quotient (relative carbon dioxide produced per mL oxygen consumed) = 0.8

Example

Arterial blood gas analysis reveals a PaO_2 of 310 mm Hg and a $PaCO_2$ of 40 mm Hg while breathing 100% oxygen ($FIO_2 = 1.0$). PB is 760 mm Hg, and PH_2O is 47 mm Hg

$PAO_2 = (760 - 47)1.0 - 40/0.8$
$PAO_2 = 713 - 50$
$PAO_2 = 663$ mm Hg
$A\text{-}aDO_2 = 663 - 310$
$A\text{-}aDO_2 = 353$ mm Hg (normal, <60 mm Hg)

Each 20 mm Hg of $A\text{-}aDO_2$ represents venous admixture equivalent to 1% of cardiac output; 353/20 = 18% of cardiac output shunted past the lungs

INFORMATION PROVIDED BY BLOOD GASES AND pH

Assessment of oxygenation and ventilation includes the measurement of pHa, PaO_2, and $PaCO_2$. Additional measurements and calculations that further define the efficiency of oxygenation and ventilation include (1) $A\text{-}aDO_2$, (2) the arterial-to-alveolar PO_2 ratio (a/A), (3) mixed venous PO_2, (4) arterial and mixed venous content of oxygen, (5) position of the oxyhemoglobin dissociation curve, and (6) the dead space–to–tidal volume ratio (VD/VT). These measurements and calculations facilitate the rapid diagnosis and management of hypoxia and hypercapnia.

III

Oxygenation

Oxygenation is assessed by measurement of PaO_2. Arterial hypoxemia, as reflected by a decrease in PaO_2 to less than 60 mm Hg, may be caused by (1) a low PO_2 in the inhaled gases (altitude, accidental occurrence during anesthesia), (2) hypoventilation, and (3) venous admixture with or without decreased mixed venous oxygen content.

LOW PO_2

Atmospheric oxygen is a constant 21% of barometric pressure; however, barometric pressure diminishes with altitude such that the partial pressure of inspired oxygen decreases with altitude. Additionally, the water vapor pressure generated by humidification of gases in the lungs assumes a greater partial pressure fraction at altitude, thus making "less room" for oxygen. The alveolar gas equation for estimating the partial pressure of alveolar oxygen accounts for both these variables, barometric pressure and water vapor pressure, as well as the inspired oxygen concentration (see Table 21-10).

HYPOVENTILATION

Decreases in PaO_2 as a result of hypoventilation reflect encroachment of carbon dioxide on the space available in the alveolus for oxygen. With hypoventilation, the carbon dioxide concentration in alveoli increases and dilutes the oxygen concentration. The decrease in alveolar oxygen concentration is estimated by the alveolar gas equation, and decreases in PaO_2 are roughly equivalent to increases in alveolar PCO_2 ($PACO_2$) (see Table 21-10).

VENOUS ADMIXTURE

Venous admixture refers to deoxygenated venous blood mixing with oxygenated arterial blood through shunting. Shunting is blood circulating from the right side of the heart to the left side via the lungs (intrapulmonary) or other routes (ventricular septal defect in the heart) without becoming oxygenated. For anatomic reasons, a small fraction of venous blood is always shunted (usually less than 1% through the pleural, thebesian, and bronchial veins). Venous admixture as a cause of decreased PaO_2 may reflect right-to-left intrapulmonary shunts (atelectasis, pneumonia, endobronchial intubation) or intracardiac shunts (congenital heart disease). A right-to-left shunt causes arterial hypoxemia by diluting oxygenated arterial blood with deoxygenated venous blood. With significant shunting (greater than 50%), inhalation of 100% oxygen produces minimal, if any effect on PaO_2. Anemic blood (with diminished oxygen-carrying capacity) and increased oxygen consumption (or extraction as during a low–cardiac output state) will deplete mixed venous blood of oxygen content and thus amplify the oxygen-diluting effects of venous admixture.

$A-aDO_2$

The magnitude of venous admixture or shunting may be estimated in the clinical setting by calculating $A-aDO_2$ (see Table 21-10). This calculation estimates the difference in oxygen partial pressure between alveoli (PAO_2) and arterial blood (PaO_2). There is always a small difference (5 to 10 mm Hg while breathing room air) expected because of shunting via the thebesian and other veins, even in a young, healthy individual. However, greater differences suggest the presence of pathologic shunting, either intrapulmonary or extrapulmonary. It must be kept in mind that $A-aDO_2$ normally increases with age, elevated inspired oxygen concentration ($A-aDO_2$ up to 60 mm Hg while breathing 100% oxygen), and vasodilating drugs (nitroglycerin, nitroprusside), which impair hypoxic pulmonary vasoconstriction.

Pulse oximetry, which measures hemoglobin saturation, may provide a false sense of reassurance in patients breathing a high inspired oxygen concentration. For example, significant shunting secondary to a pulmonary process can be ongoing despite an oxygen saturation of 100%. This problem is best identified by determining the patient's $A-aDO_2$. The shunt fraction of a patient's cardiac output is roughly estimated from $A-aDO_2$. When PaO_2 is higher than 150 mm Hg such that hemoglobin is completely saturated with oxygen, the magnitude of venous admixture is approximately 1% of the cardiac output for every 20 mm Hg of $A-aDO_2$. Below a PaO_2 of 150 mm Hg or when cardiac output is increased relative to metabolism, this guideline will underestimate the actual amount of venous admixture.

a/A RATIO

A disadvantage of $A-aDO_2$ is that the normal range changes with varying concentrations of inspired oxygen. For this reason, the a/A ratio may be more useful because it remains relatively constant regardless of the inspired concentration of oxygen (Table 21-11).[11] For example, a patient with an

---

Table 21–11 Calculation of the Arterial-to-Alveolar Oxygen Ratio

Alveolar-to-arterial oxygen ratio: $a/A = PaO_2/PAO_2$

Example

Arterial blood gas values are a PaO_2 of 310 mm Hg and a $PaCO_2$ of 40 mm Hg while breathing 100% oxygen ($FIO_2 = 1.0$). PB is 760 mm Hg, and PH_2O is 47 mm Hg

$PAO_2 = (760 - 47)1.0 - 40/0.8$
$PAO_2 = 713 - 50$
$PAO_2 = 663$ mm Hg
$a/A = 310/663$
$a/A = 0.47$ (normal, >0.75)

a/A ratio of 0.5 will have a PaO_2 equal to 50% of the PAO_2, regardless of the inspired concentration of oxygen.

PaO_2/FIO_2

The PaO_2/FIO_2 ratio is a simple alternative to the a/A ratio that also remains relatively constant over a range of inspired oxygen concentrations. Hypoxemia is defined as a ratio less than 300; a ratio less than 200 suggests a shunt fraction greater than 20%.[13]

Mixed Venous PO_2

A mixed venous blood sample is obtained from the distal port of an unwedged pulmonary artery catheter. Mixed venous blood PO_2 is a function of both cardiac output and tissue oxygen consumption, with a normal value being approximately 40 mm Hg. In the presence of unchanging tissue oxygen consumption, mixed venous PO_2 varies directly with changes in cardiac output. The Fick equation allows estimation of cardiac output by using PaO_2, mixed venous PO_2, and hemoglobin concentration data. When cardiac output is decreased, less blood flow is available for tissue oxygen extraction. Therefore, continued extraction of the same amount of oxygen from a decreased blood flow will result in a decreased mixed venous PO_2. A mixed venous PO_2 less than 30 mm Hg is suggestive of tissue hypoxia; however, disease states associated with arterial-venous admixture through peripheral shunting (sepsis, portal hypertension) or impaired oxygen use (cyanide toxicity) may result in a high mixed venous PO_2 despite inadequate tissue oxygenation.

ARTERIAL AND MIXED VENOUS CONTENT OF OXYGEN

The vast majority of the oxygen content in blood is bound to hemoglobin. The difference between the arterial and mixed venous oxygen content is an estimate of the adequacy of cardiac output relative to tissue oxygen consumption (Table 21-12). The normal difference in the oxygen content of arterial and mixed venous blood is 4 to 6 mL/dL of blood. When tissue oxygen consumption is constant, a decreased cardiac output is accompanied by increased oxygen extraction from mixed venous blood, thereby increasing the difference between arterial and mixed venous blood. When assumptions are made about oxygen consumption, cardiac output is estimated with the Fick Equation (see Table 21-12).

OXYHEMOGLOBIN DISSOCIATION CURVE

The oxyhemoglobin dissociation curve describes the saturation of hemoglobin with oxygen relative to PO_2 (Fig. 21-6). A normal oxyhemoglobin dissociation curve is characterized by 50% saturation of hemoglobin with oxygen at a PO_2 of 26 mm Hg. The PO_2 that results in 50% saturation is referred to as the P_{50}. Events that shift the oxyhemoglobin dissociation curve to the left (P_{50} lower than 26 mm Hg) may jeopardize tissue oxygenation because oxygen is more tightly bound to hemoglobin and PaO_2 must decrease to a lower than normal level before oxygen is released from hemoglobin and becomes available to tissues. Events that shift the oxyhemoglobin dissociation curve to the right (P_{50} higher than 26 mm Hg) facilitate tissue oxygen availability by permitting the unloading of oxygen from hemoglobin at an increased PaO_2 (see Fig. 21-6).

Table 21-12 Arterial and Venous Oxygen Content

Arterial oxygen content (mL/dL): $CaO_2 = (Hb \times 1.39)Sat + PO_2(0.003)$

Venous oxygen content (mL/dL): $CvO_2 = (Hb \times 1.39)Sat + PaO_2(0.003)$

Hb = hemoglobin (g/dL)

1.39 = oxygen bound to hemoglobin (mL/g)

Sat = percent oxygen saturation of hemoglobin

PaO_2 = arterial partial pressure of oxygen (mm Hg)

PvO_2 = mixed venous partial pressure of oxygen (mm Hg)

0.003 = dissolved oxygen (mL/dL × mm Hg)

Fick Equation: $VO_2 = CO \times (CaO_2 - CvO_2)$

VO_2 = oxygen consumption (approximately 3.5 mL/kg/min)

CO = cardiac output

Example

Hb = 15 g/dL, PaO_2 = 100 mm Hg (resulting in nearly 100% saturation), PvO_2 = 40 mm Hg (resulting in 75% saturation)

$CaO_2 = (15 \times 1.39)1.00 + 100(0.003) = 20.85 + 0.3 = 21.15$ mL/dL

$CvO_2 = (15 \times 1.39)0.75 + 40(0.003) = 15.63 + 0.12 = 15.75$ mL/dL

$CaO_2 - CvO_2 = 5.4$ mL/dL

Oxygen consumption = 250 mL/min = CO × 5.4 mL/dL

CO = 250/5.4 = 46 dL/min = 4.6 L/min

III

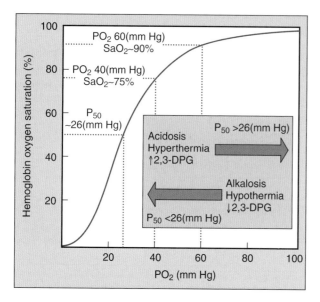

Figure 21-6 The oxyhemoglobin dissociation curve describes the relationship between hemoglobin saturation with oxygen (%) and PO_2. P_{50} is the PO_2 that results in 50% saturation (normally 26 mm Hg at 37°C and pH 7.4). Events that shift the oxyhemoglobin dissociation curve to the left (P_{50} less than 26 mm Hg) (alkalosis, hypothermia, decreased 2,3-diphosphoglycerate [2,3-DPG]) may impair oxygen release to tissues. Conversely, events that shift the oxyhemoglobin dissociation curve to the right (P_{50} greater than 26 mm Hg) (acidosis, hyperthermia, increased 2,3-DPG) permit oxygen unloading to tissues at a higher PO_2, thus favoring tissue oxygenation. Mixed venous PO_2 is normally 40 mm Hg (75% saturation), and a PO_2 of 60 mm Hg is 90% saturation. Saturation is 100% when the PO_2 is greater than 150 mm Hg.

	Normoxia	Hypoxia
V_E, L/min	6.0	49.7
MAP, mm Hg	109	121
TPR, dyn·s·cm^{-5}	2335	1707

Figure 21-7 Ventilatory and hemodynamic response to isocapnic hypoxia in a canine model. Hypoxia, PaO_2 of 30 mm Hg; MAP, mean arterial pressure; normoxia, PaO_2 of 78 mm Hg; TPR, total peripheral resistance; V_E, minute ventilation. (Adapted from Rose CE, Althous JA, Kaiser DL, et al. Acute hypoxemia and hypercapnia: Increase in plasma catecholamines in conscious dogs. Am J Physiol 1983;245:H924-H929, with permission.)

oxygen consumption by respiratory muscles may offset the gain in oxygenation produced by hyperventilation. Compensation for acute hypoxia, both cardiovascular and ventilatory, is initiated by chemosensors in the carotid bodies, and this response is blunted by volatile anesthetics.

VENTILATION

$PaCO_2$ reflects in part the adequacy of ventilation for removing carbon dioxide from pulmonary capillary blood. In the steady state, $PaCO_2$ is directly proportional to the metabolic production of carbon dioxide and inversely proportional to alveolar ventilation (see Fig. 21-4). The production of carbon dioxide depends on the metabolic state of the individual and parallels tissue oxygen consump-

COMPENSATION FOR ARTERIAL HYPOXEMIA

Acute hypoxia causes activation of the sympathetic nervous system with endogenous catecholamine release, which augments blood pressure and cardiac output despite the vasodilating effects of hypoxemia (Fig. 21-7).[12] The increased cardiac output will increase oxygen delivery from the lungs to peripheral tissues, and if tissue oxygen consumption is unchanged, the oxygen content of returned mixed venous blood will be higher. A given fraction of mixed venous blood is always shunted (less than 1%), and because the shunted venous blood has a higher oxygen content, it will produce less dilution of the oxygen content of arterial blood after shunting. A less efficient compensatory mechanism to offset arterial hypoxemia is hyperventilation, which increases the alveolar oxygen concentration and PaO_2 by lowering the alveolar and arterial carbon dioxide concentration. However, the increased

Table 21-13 Calculation of the Dead Space–to–Tidal Volume Ratio

$V_D/V_T = (PaCO_2 - PECO_2)/PaCO_2$

V_D/V_T = ratio of dead space to tidal volume

$PaCO_2$ = arterial partial pressure of carbon dioxide (mm Hg)

$PECO_2$ = mixed exhaled partial pressure of carbon dioxide (mm Hg)

Example

$PaCO_2$ is 40 mm Hg and $PECO_2$ is 20 mm Hg during controlled ventilation of the lungs. $V_D/V_T = (40 - 20)/40 = 0.5$ (normal, <0.3)

tion. Under normal conditions, only 80% as much carbon dioxide is produced as oxygen is consumed (respiratory quotient of 0.8). Assuming a tissue oxygen consumption of 250 mL/min (approximately 3.5 mL/kg/min), the production of carbon dioxide would be 200 mL/min. A measured $PaCO_2$ above 45 mm Hg suggests that a patient is hypoventilating relative to carbon dioxide production, whereas a $PaCO_2$ below 35 mm Hg suggests that a patient is hyperventilating. Increased dead space ventilation ("wasted ventilation") markedly decreases the efficiency of ventilation. The V_D/V_T ratio is the fraction of each tidal volume that aerates regions of the lung and respiratory tract not involved in blood-gas exchange. This value should not exceed 0.3 in the upright position (Table 21-13). Unlike problems with oxygenation, increased alveolar ventilation can completely overcome increased dead space. In contrast to PaO_2, venous admixture has little to no impact on $PaCO_2$ because of the extreme diffusibility of carbon dioxide relative to that of oxygen.

REFERENCES

1. Wade JG, Larson CP Jr, Hickey RF, et al. Effect of carotid endarterectomy on carotid chemoreceptor and baroreceptor function in man. N Engl J Med 1970;282:823-829.
2. Gluck SL. Acid-base. Lancet 1998;352:474-479.
3. Adrogue HJ, Madias NE. Management of life-threatening acid-base disorders. N Engl J Med 1998;338:26-34, 107-111.
4. Ford GD, Cline WH, Fleming WW. Influence of lactic acidosis on cardiovascular response to sympathomimetic amines. Am J Physiol 1968;215:1123-1129.
5. Scheingraber S, Rehm M, Schmisch C, et al. Rapid saline infusion produces hyperchloremic acidosis in patients undergoing gynecologic surgery. Anesthesiology 1999;90:1265-1270.
6. Hindman BJ. Sodium bicarbonate in the treatment of subtypes of acute lactic acidosis: Physiologic considerations. Anesthesiology 1990;72:1064-1076.
7. Barcenas CG, Fuller TJ, Knochel JP. Metabolic alkalosis after massive blood transfusion. Correction by hemodialysis. JAMA 1976;236:953-954.
8. Williamson DC, Munson ES. Correlation of peripheral venous and arterial blood gas values during general anesthesia. Anesth Analg 1982;61:950-952.
9. Fox MJ, Brody JS, Weintraub LR. Leukocyte larceny: A cause of spurious hypoxemia. Am J Med 1979;67:742-746.
10. Reves RB. An imidazole alpha stat hypothesis for vertebrate acid-base regulation: Tissue carbon dioxide content and body temperature in bullfrogs. Respir Physiol 1972;14:219-236.
11. Doyle JD. Arterial/alveolar oxygen tension ratio. A critical appraisal. Can Anaesth Soc J 1986;33:471-474.
12. Rose CE, Althous JA, Kaiser DL, et al. Acute hypoxemia and hypercapnia: Increase in plasma catecholamines in conscious dogs. Am J Physiol 1983;245:H924-H929.
13. Marino PL. The ICU Book, 2nd ed. Philadelphia: Lippincott Williams & Wilkins, 1998.

III

Chapter 22

HEMOSTASIS

Elizabeth Donegan, Greg Stratmann, and Tin-Na Kan

Interdependent, often competing physiologic systems in blood and in tissue both maintain intravascular fluidity and isolate, plug, and resolve endovascular interruptions. Trauma, surgery, and hereditary or spontaneous disease may favor one system over others and lead to either hemorrhage or thrombosis. New therapeutic agents and perioperative practices have been introduced to prevent or normalize hemostatic imbalance, halt hemorrhage, and inhibit thrombosis.

COAGULATION

Mechanisms of Coagulation

At one time, hemostasis was viewed as a stepwise process beginning with a vascular phase, during which arteries and arterioles constricted, activated platelets aggregated at sites of injury, and platelets released cytoplasmic granules to form a primary vascular plug. The coagulation phase followed and was viewed as a cascading system of sequentially activated enzymes culminating in the generation of cross-linked fibrin. Two separate systems of coagulation were proposed—an intravascular (intrinsic) and an extravascular (extrinsic) system. Activation of either system culminates in a common pathway leading to the generation of thrombin, which converts fibrinogen to fibrin. Two laboratory tests, the prothrombin time (PT) and the partial thromboplastin time (PTT), have been used to distinguish between abnormalities in the intrinsic and extrinsic systems. Clinically, the PT and PTT remain useful for diagnostic and therapeutic purposes, but coagulation is now understood to be a cell-based process occurring on the surface of endothelial cells, subendothelial cells, and platelets rather than a plasma-based process initiated by two separate initiators/mechanisms of coagulation (Fig. 22-1).[1-3]

Protection against Spontaneous Thrombus Formation

Normally, endothelium is protected from spontaneous thrombus formation by the constitutive expression of

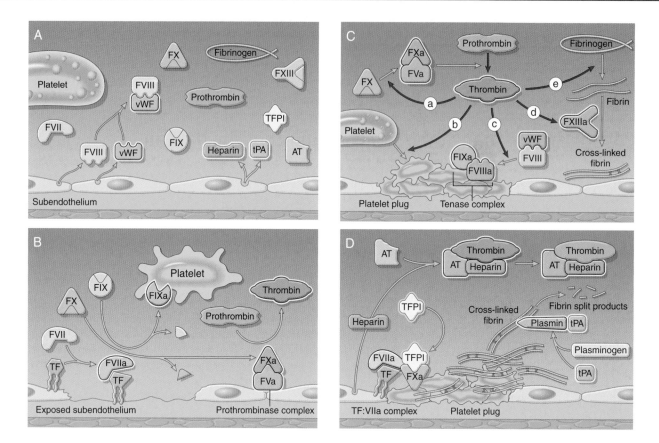

Figure 22-1 A, Normal endothelium. Procoagulants (factors [F] VII, VIII, IX, X, XIII, prothrombin), fibrinogen, and platelets circulate in their inactive forms. Anticoagulants (tissue factor pathway inhibitor [TFPI], heparin, and tissue plasminogen activator [tPA]) actively prevent endothelial spontaneous thrombus formation. **B,** Vascular injury, initial phase. Subendothelial tissue factor (TF) exposed to circulating FVII forms a TF:VII complex. TF:VII activates FIX and FX. FIXa binds to platelets. FXa activates FV to form prothrombinase complex, which converts localized, small amounts of prothrombin to thrombin. **C,** Vascular injury, role of thrombin. Thrombin (a) activates FX and FV to form prothrombinase complexes that generate the secondary thrombin burst, (b) activates platelets, (c) separates FVIII from von Willebrand factor (vWF) and activates FVIII, (d) converts fibrinogen to fibrin, and (e) activates FXIII, the stabilizer of cross-linked fibrin. Stable clot is formed. **D,** Control of coagulation and fibrin clot dissolution. Antithrombin (AT) binds heparin and potently inhibits thrombin activity. TFPI binds to FXa to inhibit the TF:VIIa complex. Plasminogen is activated to plasmin by tPA and cleaves fibrin into soluble fibrin split products.

native anticoagulants such as heparin sulfate proteoglycans. Heparin's anticoagulant effect comes from its ability to increase the activity of antithrombin and thrombomodulin. Endothelium also releases nitric oxide, prostacyclin, and tissue plasminogen activator intravascularly to enhance blood flow. Physical (surgery or trauma), chemical, or cellular damage to the vascular lining activates the local endothelium. Once activated, these anticoagulant molecules are removed and downregulated, whereas procoagulant molecules are expressed and upregulated.

Events at the Site of Vascular Injury

At the site of vascular injury, tissue factor on the surface of perivascular subendothelial cells is exposed to circulating blood.[4] The extracellular portion of tissue factor (a transmembrane protein) undergoes conformational change when exposed to circulating factor VII. The transformed tissue factor binds with circulating factor VII and forms an active catalytic tissue factor–factor VIIa complex. This tissue factor–factor VIIa complex rapidly cleaves amino acid sequences from factors IX and X and thereby converts each factor from the inactive to the active form (factor

IXa and factor Xa). Factor Xa remains localized and activates factor V to form a factor Xa–factor Va complex (prothrombinase complex) on tissue factor–bearing cells. The prothrombinase complex catalyzes the conversion of small amounts of prothrombin to thrombin. This localized thrombin serves as a priming mechanism for the clotting process. It rapidly catalyzes the activation of additional factor Xa and factor IXa. Local thrombin also separates factor VIII from von Willebrand factor (vWF) and catalyzes the activation of factor VIII. This localized process then triggers a wide burst of thrombin generation that initiates a potent feed-forward loop. Thrombin also activates platelets at the site of injury. In contrast to factor Xa, factor IXa does not remain localized to tissue factor–bearing cells but binds to the surface of activated platelets.

Role of Activated Platelets

Coagulation becomes more generalized as activated platelets form an initial vascular plug at the injury site and release vasoconstrictive substances such as thromboxane to limit blood flow and contain thrombus formation. Activated platelets play an important role in bringing factor VIIIa and factor Va together with their coenzymes to produce additional prothrombinase and tenase (factor IXa–factor VIIIa) complexes. Tenase complexes recruit and activate more factor X from plasma. Platelet membrane–bound prothrombinase complexes convert large amounts of prothrombin to thrombin. Sufficient thrombin is now formed to generate fibrin from fibrinogen and activate factor XIII to cross-link fibrin. The cross-linked fibrin meshwork shrinks and traps activated platelets and red blood cells to form a strong blood clot.

Physiologic Control of Coagulation

Potent feedback loops limiting clot formation are initiated as coagulation continues. Coagulation is terminated mainly by the action of inhibitor proteins and anticoagulant proteases. The three major categories of regulatory molecules are (1) serine protease inhibitors (serpins), (2) heparins, and (3) anticoagulant proteases.

Serpins are described as (1) antithrombin (once called antithrombin III), (2) heparin cofactor II, (3) α_2-macroglobulins, and (4) tissue factor pathway inhibitor. Antithrombin inhibits thrombin and factors VIIa, IXa, Xa, and XIa. Endogenous heparin found on the endothelial cell surface speeds the action of antithrombin 1000-fold, and this serves to protect normal endothelium from spontaneous thrombus formation and localizes the coagulation process to activated endothelium. α_2-Macroglobulins trap, inactivate, and rapidly clear circulating activated coagulation factors, thereby contributing to systemic control of generalized activation states such as disseminated intravascular coagulation (DIC). Tissue factor pathway inhibitor is a kunin protein that regulates the tissue

factor–factor VIIa complex and becomes more potent after binding factor Xa. Thrombomodulin is a membrane protein receptor that binds thrombin and alters the thrombin molecule. Altered thrombin activates protein C. Activated protein C inactivates factor Va and factor VIIIa. Protein S accelerates the action of protein C.

Fibrin Clot Dissolution (Fibrinolysis)

Normally, plasmin circulates in the blood in the inactive plasminogen form, and normal endothelium secretes plasminogen activator inhibitor type 1 to inhibit the activation of plasminogen. When endothelium is activated by injury, tissue plasminogen activator is secreted and plasminogen is activated to plasmin. The plasmin formed is now able to degrade fibrin to soluble products (D-dimers, fibrin degradation products), and these products inhibit thrombin activity. Because tissue plasminogen activator also binds to plasmin's substrate (fibrin), conversion of plasminogen to plasmin remains localized to areas of thrombus. Circulating plasmin, in comparison, is inhibited by a much more powerful (100×) second inhibitor, α_2-antiplasmin. Generally, surgery and massive trauma induce a hypercoagulable state with elevation of acute-phase reactants that also retard the normal process of fibrinolysis.

Rarely, uncontrolled systemic fibrinolysis is activated in the setting of surgery, cardiopulmonary bypass, or massive trauma by unknown mechanisms. Plasmin activity becomes systemic and degrades both local fibrin and circulating fibrinogen. Systemic antifibrinolytics such as ε-aminocaproic acid and aprotinin have been useful in the setting of systemic fibrinolysis.

COMMON LABORATORY TESTS OF HEMOSTASIS (TABLE 22-1)

Tests of Platelet Function

PLATELET COUNT
Platelet levels are quantified by optical or impedance measurements on automated instruments as part of the complete blood count. Even minimal platelet activation, as with a difficult blood draw, can cause platelet clumping and result in artifactually decreased counts on automated analyzers. Most clinical laboratories examine stained blood films for clumping if the platelet count is less than 100,000 cells/μL.

BLEEDING TIME
To calculate the bleeding time, a standardized incision 9 mm long and 1 mm deep is made on the volar surface of the forearm, with backpressure maintained by inflating a blood pressure cuff on the upper part of the arm to 40 mm Hg of pressure. Excess blood is blotted away every 30 seconds with filter paper without disturbing the wound edge. Although this test is the single best predictor of func-

Table 22–1 Common Laboratory Tests of Hemostasis and Normal Ranges

Platelet Tests	Coagulation Tests	Fibrinolysis Tests
Platelet count (140,000-450,000 cells/μL)	Prothrombin time (11.5-14.5 sec)*	Thrombin time (22.1-31.2 sec)
Bleeding time (<11 min)	Partial thromboplastin time (24.5-35.2 sec)*	Fibrinogen–fibrin degradation products (>5 μg/dL)
Platelet function analysis	Thrombin time (22.1-31.2 sec)*	Fibrin D-dimer assay (<250 μg/mL)
Collagen/epinephrine (94-193 sec)	Fibrinogen (175-433 mg/dL)	
Collagen/adenosine diphosphate (71-118 sec)	Activated coagulation time (70-180 sec)	
Platelet aggregation (response to aggregating agents: collagen, adenosine diphosphate, epinephrine, and ristocetin)		

*The normal range varies with reagent lots.

tional platelet disorders, the test must be performed in a standardized controlled setting, is difficult to control, and is often not readily available. Bleeding as a consequence of a platelet abnormality is best predicted by a prolonged bleeding time, but it is a poor predictor of perioperative bleeding because it is independent of plasma coagulation factor levels. The bleeding time is prolonged with platelet counts less than 100,000 cells/μL. Scarring at the test site may result.

PLATELET FUNCTION ANALYSIS

The presence of dysfunctional platelets is assessed with this assay, provided that the hematocrit is greater than 35% and the platelet count is normal. Anticoagulated whole blood is exposed to high–shear flow conditions, and membrane-bound collagen coated with either adenosine diphosphate (ADP) or epinephrine initiates the release of platelet granules and membrane adhesion. The time to instrument aperture occlusion as a result of platelet thrombus formation is measured. Common causes of platelet dysfunction such as uremia, antiplatelet medications, von Willebrand's disease, other hereditary platelet disorders, and post–cardiopulmonary bypass platelet dysfunction can be documented but not distinguished with this test.

PLATELET AGGREGATION STUDIES

Platelet aggregation studies are not performed intraoperatively and are infrequently performed perioperatively. Preoperative evaluation of patients with potential platelet disorders may include measurement of the response of platelets to aggregating agents (collagen, ADP, epinephrine, and ristocetin). Platelet aggregometers measure increasing plasma clarity as platelets aggregate and decrease light scatter. Low ADP concentrations induce a biphasic aggregation pattern. Samples from individuals with

Glanzmann's thrombasthenia do not aggregate with ADP, epinephrine, or collagen. Patient's with von Willebrand's disease and Bernard-Soulier syndrome have a normal response to epinephrine, collagen, and ADP but do not respond to ristocetin. Aspirin ingestion, uremia, liver disease, and myeloproliferative syndromes can also be differentiated with this test.

Tests of Coagulation

PROTHROMBIN TIME

Citrated plasma is recalcified, and tissue thromboplastin is added to activate factor X in the presence of factor VII. The time until clot formation is measured in seconds. Low levels of factors VII, X, and V, prothrombin, and fibrinogen prolong the PT. Factor VII deficiency is the only cause of a prolonged PT with a normal PTT. The international normalized ratio (INR) standardizes reagent differences between PT results across laboratories and is useful in monitoring oral anticoagulant treatment.

PARTIAL THROMBOPLASTIN TIME

Citrated plasma is recalcified, and phospholipids are added to initiate coagulation. Plasma activators such as kaolin, celite, ellagic acid, or silica speed the reaction by providing the surface for contact activation of factor XII. The time to clot formation is measured in seconds. Low levels of factors VIII, IX, XI, and XII prolong the PTT. Adequate amounts of factor X, factor V, prothrombin, and fibrinogen must also be present. Factor VII is not required for a normal PTT.

THROMBIN TIME

Citrated plasma is recalcified, and thrombin is added. The time until clot formation is measured in seconds. This test measures thrombin-fibrinogen interaction and is prolonged with low levels of fibrinogen (<100 mg/dL), in the presence of abnormal fibrinogen, and in the presence of circulating anticoagulants such as heparin. The PT and PTT will both be prolonged in all conditions in which the thrombin time is prolonged.

FIBRINOGEN LEVELS

Several types of tests are available to quantify fibrinogen in milligrams per deciliter. Classic methods add thrombin to recalcified plasma to convert all fibrinogen to fibrin and measure the amount of clot protein or the time until clot formation. The amount of fibrinogen is extrapolated. Immunologic methods are useful when dysfibrino-genemia is suspected.

ACTIVATED CLOTTING TIME

The activated clotting time (ACT) measures the amount of time in seconds required for whole blood to clot in a test tube. Finely divided clay (celite or kaolin) shortens the time until clotting and reduces test variability. The ACT is used to monitor heparin therapy in the operating room. Heparin therapy can also be monitored in central laboratories with the PTT.

THROMBOELASTOGRAPHY

Causes of abnormal coagulation are determined by using viscoelastic measures of the time until blood clot formation, consolidation, and lysis in this system. Measures include (1) the time until initial clot formation (r value), which is dependent on the clotting factor concentration or anticoagulant medication; (2) the time until clot formation (α-angle), which is dependent on fibrinogen and platelets; (3) the absolute clot strength (maximum amplitude [MA]), for which sufficient platelets and normal platelet aggregation are needed; and (4) the degree of clot lysis (the amplitude 60 minutes after MA or A60), with high A60 being indicative of hyperfibrinolysis or antifibri-nolytic therapy. Thromboelastography does not assess platelet adhesion or the effects of aspirin, uremia, or von Willebrand's disease. Thromboelastography is time consuming for the operator and difficult to maintain as a routine point-of-care testing.

Tests of Fibrinolysis

The plasmin released during fibrinolysis cleaves fibrin and fibrinogen. Decreased amounts of fibrinogen and increased amounts of fibrin degradation products prolong the thrombin time.

FIBRINOPEPTIDES AND FIBRIN MONOMER LEVELS

Thrombin releases two peptides (fibrinopeptides A and B) from fibrinogen to generate fibrin monomer. Fibrin monomers polymerize and cross-link in the presence of factor XIII. Elevated levels of fibrinopeptide or fibrin monomer suggest intravascular coagulation.

FIBRIN DEGRADATION PRODUCTS

Normally, plasmin degrades fibrin, but excessive plasmin activity also cleaves fibrinogen. Fibrin degradation products cannot clot and interfere with clotting of the remaining fibrinogen. High concentrations of fibrin degradation products also inhibit platelet plug formation. Elevated levels suggest conditions of intravascular fibrin deposition with resultant secondary fibrinolysis, such as DIC.

D-DIMER LEVELS

This monoclonal antibody test measures blood levels of D-dimer fragments that are released when plasmin cleaves cross-linked fibrin. Elevated D-dimer levels are present with fibrinolytic states and in more than 90% of patients with thrombotic or thromboembolic disorders. D-dimer levels are not elevated in primary fibrinolysis because the fibrin is not cross-linked.

DISORDERS ASSOCIATED WITH ALTERED HEMOSTASIS DURING SURGERY

III

Disorders Favoring Bleeding

Hereditary and acquired coagulation factor and platelet disorders, some systemic diseases, and certain environmental conditions can lead to excessive bleeding in the operating room. In general, levels of coagulation factors of less than 20% to 30% of normal or platelet counts of less than 50,000 cells/μL are associated with uncontrolled intraoperative bleeding. Severe congenital coagulation factor deficiency leads to impaired conversion of fibrinogen to fibrin. These diseases typically become manifested in early childhood as subcutaneous, intramuscular, and intra-articular hemorrhage after minor trauma. Congenital platelet disorders are associated with mucosal bleeding, epistaxis, prolonged bleeding after dental procedures, and menorrhagia in women (Table 22-2).

Hereditary Coagulation Factor and Platelet Disorders

Hemophilia A (factor VIII deficiency), hemophilia B (Christmas disease or factor IX deficiency), and von Willebrand's disease account for the majority of perioperative bleeding secondary to hereditary diseases (Table 22-3). Of the three diseases, von Willebrand's disease is the most common, with a prevalence as high as 1% to 2% in some populations. The prevalence of hemophilia A is estimated to be 1 per 10,000 persons, with hemophilia B being less frequent (1 per 100,000 persons). Factor XII deficiency is associated with clotting rather than bleeding. Factor VIII and IX deficiencies are inherited on the X chromosome. The other factor deficiencies are autosomal recessive inherited diseases.

TREATMENT

Deficiencies in both factor VIII and factor IX are treated with specific factor concentrate (recombinant, intermediate

Table 22–2 Diseases Associated with Altered Hemostasis during Surgery

Increased Incidence of Bleeding	Increased Incidence of Thrombosis	Initiators of Disseminated Intravascular Coagulation
Hereditary coagulation factor deficiency	Blood stasis	Crush injury
Factors I, II, VII, IX, X, XI, XII	Vascular damage	Acute hemolytic transfusion reaction
Hereditary platelet disorders	Hereditary hypercoagulable states	Abruptio placentae
von Willebrand's disease	Procoagulant mutations	Cardiopulmonary bypass
Bernard-Soulier syndrome	Antithrombin deficiency	Intravascular emboli (fat, air)
Glanzmann's thrombasthenia	Protein C deficiency	Sepsis
Storage pool disease	Protein S deficiency	Liver disease
Spontaneous coagulation factor disorders	Anticoagulant mutations	Arterial hypoxemia
Liver disease	Factor V Leiden	Acidosis
Drugs (warfarin)	Homocystinemia	Acute pancreatitis
Coagulation factor inhibitors	Mutant factor II or VIII	Immune complex disease
Spontaneous platelet disorders	Factor XII deficiency (rare)	Allergic reactions
Renal disease	Dysfibrinogenemia	Transplant rejection
HELLP syndrome	Increased platelet turnover	Cancer (pancreas, prostate)
Acute immune thrombocytopenia	Prosthetic heart valves	
Drugs	Valvular heart disease	
Heparin, aspirin, nonsteroidal anti-inflammatory drugs, digitalis, thiazide diuretics, abciximab, ethyl alcohol	Spontaneous hypercoagulable states	
Elevated plasma proteins	Antiphospholipid antibody	
Multiple myeloma	Lupus anticoagulant	
Dysproteinurias	Anticardiolipin antibody	
Myeloproliferative disorders		
Hypothermia		

HELLP, hemolysis, elevated liver function tests, low platelet count.

purity, or ultrahigh purity) replacement. Mild forms of factor VIII deficiency can be treated with cryoprecipitate and adjuvant therapy as needed. Perioperatively, coagulant activity is maintained by replacement therapy at 50% to 100% of normal levels until wound healing is complete. Adjuvant therapy consists of the intravenous infusion of desmopressin (DDAVP) and antifibrinolytics. DDAVP (0.3 µg/kg IV) induces the release of stored vWF and factor VIII into plasma. Antifibrinolytics (tranexamic acid, 10 to 15 mg/kg IV every 8 to 12 hours, or ε-aminocaproic acid, 50 to 60 mg/kg IV every 4 to 6 hours) retard clot resolution.

von Willebrand's Disease

Considered a platelet disorder, von Willebrand's disease is characterized by uncontrolled mucosal bleeding and is the most common cause of unsuspected hereditary bleeding in the operating room.[5] Individuals with von Willebrand's disease display the clinical features of both defective platelet plug formation and defective fibrin formation. Synthesized in vascular endothelial cells and megakaryocytes, vWF is stored in platelet Weibel-Palade bodies and secreted into plasma and the subendothelial matrix. vWF functions as an adhesion protein that diverts circulating platelets to sites of vascular injury, and it complexes

Table 22–3 Coagulation Factor Synthesis and Disorders Associated with Coagulation Factor Deficiencies

Coagulation factors synthesized in the liver	Fibrinogen (factor II); factors VII, IX, X; protein C; protein S
Coagulation factors synthesized in endothelial cells	Factor VIII, von Willebrand factor
Coagulation factor with the shortest half-life	Factor VII (2.5 hours)
Vitamin K–dependent factors	Factors VII, IX, X
Most common inherited bleeding disorder	von Willebrand's disease
Level of circulating coagulant factor below which bleeding occurs	Plasma levels ≤30%
Hemophilia A	Factor VIII deficiency
Hemophilia B (Christmas disease)	Factor IX deficiency

with plasma factor VIII to protect it from inactivation and clearance. When sufficient effective vWF is unavailable to carry and stabilize factor VIII, factor VIII levels are decreased.

PHENOTYPES

Three phenotypes of von Willebrand's disease are recognized (Table 22-4). Types 1 and 2 are transmitted predominantly as autosomal dominant traits, and type 3, the least frequent and most severe form, is transmitted as an autosomal recessive trait. Type 1 accounts for 60% to 80% of cases and is a mild to moderate quantitative deficiency of vWF, with factor VIII levels being decreased to 5% to 30% of normal. Type 2 accounts for 20% to 30% of cases and is a qualitative vWF deficiency with several subtypes. Type 3 accounts for 1% to 5% of cases and is characterized by very low to undetectable levels of vWF and very low levels of factor VIII. The symptoms of type 3 von Willebrand's disease are similar to those of moderately severe factor VIII deficiency. An abnormal bleeding time (normal bleeding time with factor VIII deficiency), ristocetin cofactor, von Willebrand antigen level, or platelet function analysis distinguishes between the two diseases (see Table 22-1).

TREATMENT

Episodes of spontaneous or perioperative bleeding associated with von Willebrand's disease can be treated with DDAVP (with the exception of platelet types), fresh frozen plasma (20 to 25 mL/kg IV), or intermediate-purity factor VIII concentrates (Humate-P and Profilate), which contain large amount of vWF, antifibrinolytics, and platelets. Recombinant factor VIII is not used because it does not contain vWF. DDAVP is contraindicated for the treatment of type 2B von Willebrand's disease because of transient thrombocytopenia after its administration. It is also not recommended in patients with unstable coronary artery disease because the ultralarge vWF multimers released by DDAVP can aggregate platelets at

sites of high fluid shear stress and increase the risk for myocardial infarction.

Spontaneous Coagulation Factor Disorders

Vitamin K deficiency, liver disease, antibody to coagulation factors, and some therapeutic drugs cause acquired coagulation disorders.

VITAMIN K DEFICIENCY

Vitamin K is fat soluble with limited tissue storage. A dietary source or bacterial synthesis of vitamin K in the intestine is needed to make functional factors VII, IX, and X, prothrombin, protein C, and protein S. Fasting patients or patients with diseases involving impaired intestinal absorption (obstructive jaundice, sprue, or regional ileitis) are vulnerable to vitamin K deficiency when intestinal bacterial flora is compromised by antibiotic therapy.

LIVER DISEASE

With the exception of factor VIII, plasma clotting factors are synthesized in the liver. Therefore, liver disease that is severe enough to cause decreased synthetic function will lead to decreased factor levels and an increased risk for uncontrolled bleeding. PT is often used as a surrogate test of hepatic synthetic capability. Fibrinolysis is also increased in liver disease as a result of impaired clearance of plasminogen activators and impaired synthesis of plasmin, fibrin degradation products, and tissue plasminogen inhibitors.

ACQUIRED COAGULATION DEFECTS

Antibodies to coagulation factors develop in some patients with autoimmune disease and occasional hemophiliac patients treated with factor replacement therapy. These antibodies usually act as inhibitors neutralizing factor activity. Clinically, patients will have severe bleeding after minor injury. Less commonly, antibody may bind to factor without neutralizing factor activity but create a deficiency

Table 22-4   Classification of von Willebrand's Disease

Type	Characteristic	Frequency	Inheritance	Treatment Options
1	Quantitative deficiency of vWF and factor VIII	70% to 80%	Autosomal dominant	Desmopressin (first choice) Factor VIII/vWF concentrate (alternative choice)
2	Qualitative defect in vWF	15% to 20%	Autosomal dominant	
[A]	Defective platelet-dependent vWF function (no large multimers)	Common		Factor VIII/vWF concentrates (first choice) Desmopressin (alternative choice)
[B]	Heightened platelet-dependent vWF; no large multimers			Factor VIII/vWF concentrates (best choice)
[M]	Defective platelet-dependent vWF function; normal multimers	Rare		Factor VIII/vWF concentrates (first choice) Desmopressin (alternative choice)
[N]	Defective vWF binding to factor VIII	Rare		Factor VIII/vWF concentrates (first choice) Desmopressin (alternative choice)
3	Severe or complete vWF deficiency and moderately severe factor VIII deficiency	Very rare	Autosomal recessive	Factor VIII/vWF concentrates (first choice if alloantibodies absent) Platelet concentrates (alternative choice if alloantibodies absent) Recombinant factor VIII (first choice if alloantibodies present)

vWF, von Willebrand factor.

by rapidly clearing antigen-antibody complexes. Factor VIII inhibitors may be present in patients with rheumatoid arthritis or ulcerative colitis and in older persons with no known cause. Patients with factor VIII inhibitors have a prolonged PTT and a normal PT, thrombin time, and bleeding time. Acquired inhibitors to factors VIII, IX, or XI, as detected by an isolated prolonged PTT, are associated with significant intraoperative bleeding.

Systemic Lupus Erythematosus

Lupus anticoagulant is an antiphospholipid antibody that is present in 5% to 10% of patients with systemic lupus erythematosus. It is also found in patients with other immunologic disorders and after treatment with certain drugs (chlorpromazine, procainamide, quinidine). Laboratory findings consist of a prolonged PTT, normal to slightly prolonged PT, and normal thrombin time. Patients with lupus anticoagulant without the rare associated acquired hypoprothrombinemia and with normal platelet counts do not bleed abnormally postoperatively. In fact, lupus anticoagulant is more likely to be associated with thrombosis requiring anticoagulation as long as the antibody persists.

Spontaneous Platelet Disorders

Bleeding as a result of platelet disorders is characterized by a prolonged bleeding time (>11 minutes). Poor

platelet function may be due to thrombocytopenia (<100,000 cells/μL) or to qualitative platelet disorders. Both these conditions result in a prolonged bleeding time and abnormal findings on platelet function analysis (see Table 22-1).

THROMBOCYTOPENIA

Thrombocytopenia is caused by either insufficient platelet production or peripheral platelet destruction/sequestration (Table 22-5). Heparin-induced thrombocytopenia occurs in 5% of treated patients and is the most common cause of drug-induced thrombocytopenia and thrombosis. Thrombocytopenia during pregnancy is associated with a spectrum of disorders, including gestational thrombocytopenia, preeclampsia, and pregnancy-associated hypertensive disorders, of which the HELLP syndrome (hemolysis, elevated liver function test results, low platelet count) is the most severe form. Normally, a third of peripheral platelets sequester in the spleen, with a portion of these platelets released into circulation at times of vascular stress. Splenic sequestration of platelets increases with splenomegaly, and these platelets are not available for release.

QUALITATIVE PLATELET DISORDERS

Despite adequate numbers, poor platelet function increases bleeding risk, prolongs the bleeding time, and variably

Table 22-5 Causes of Peripheral Platelet Destruction
Idiopathic antiplatelet antibody formation
Viral infection
Human immunodeficiency virus
Cytomegalovirus
Hepatitis B
Malignancy
Chronic lymphocytic leukemia
Lymphoma
Colon cancer
Collagen vascular disease
Drugs
Heparin
Quinine
Quinidine
Digitoxin
Thiazide
Multiple blood transfusions

affects measures of platelet aggregation. Drugs such as alcohol, aspirin, and nonsteroidal anti-inflammatory drugs (NSAIDs) commonly impair platelet function. Impaired platelet granule release is seen in severe uremia. Treatment with transfused platelets is not effective because both the patient's native platelets and the transfused platelets function abnormally. High levels of circulating fibrin-fibrinogen split products inhibit platelet aggregation and thereby lead to impaired hemostatic plug formation. Increased fibrin-fibrinogen split products are present in hepatic failure as a result of decreased clearance of these fibrin split products, in DIC, and with conditions of therapeutically induced fibrinolysis such as treatment with streptokinase or urokinase. High levels of abnormal serum proteins (multiple myeloma, dysproteinemias, or transfused dextran solutions) also inhibit normal platelet function.

Intraoperative Conditions Facilitating Bleeding

Systemic hypotension, hypothermia, acidosis, and anemia contribute to intraoperative bleeding (see Table 22-2). Hypothermia with temperatures of 34°C or less is associated with poor platelet function and decreased procoagulant activity. The formation and strength of hemostatic plugs are impaired in the presence of low plasma viscosity. Plasma viscosity decreases with increasing anemia.

Aggressive intravenous fluid resuscitation can dilute plasma coagulation factors and platelet numbers below amounts needed for effective hemostasis.

DISORDERS FAVORING THROMBOSIS

Hereditary Hypercoagulable States

Inherited deficiency of antithrombin, protein C, or protein S and qualitative abnormalities in factor V (factor V Leiden) or prothrombin (prothrombin 20210) and MTHFR mutation with elevated homocysteine are the commonly recognized conditions leading to intraoperative deep vein thrombosis and pulmonary embolism (see Table 22-2).[6] Individuals with factor V Leiden are resistant to activated protein C and may constitute as many as 4% to 8% of the normal population. Hyperhomocysteinemia (tetramethylhydrofolate reductase deficiency) treated with folate is also associated with hypercoagulability. Hereditary conditions should be suspected in patients with a positive family history, recurrent thromboembolic disease, or thromboemboli at a young age without predisposing factors or at an unusual site. Optimally, laboratory tests to aid in diagnosis should be performed after resolution of the episode and in the absence of anticoagulation.

Spontaneous Hypercoagulable States

A diverse group of conditions are associated with perioperative thrombosis. Venous thrombosis is associated with venous stasis, hypercoagulable states, and vascular damage. Acquired antiphospholipid antibodies are associated with thrombosis. Venous blood flow is impaired in pregnancy and with abdominal tumors, varicose veins, or conditions involving vascular damage such as vasculitis. Common hypercoagulable states include coronary artery disease, diabetes mellitus, malignancy, nephritic syndrome, prolonged bed rest, postoperative status, and sepsis. Patients with artificial heart valves, atrial fibrillation, and certain types of valvular heart disease have an increased risk for the development of arterial thrombosis.

Disseminated Intravascular Coagulation: Systemic Bleeding and Thrombosis

DIC is an acquired disorder characterized by uncontrolled intravascular activation of coagulation and fibrinolysis with bleeding and thrombosis. Generalized intravascular thrombin generation and fibrin deposition in small blood vessels lead to the formation of microvascular thrombi. Tissue hypoxia and multiorgan failure follow. Normal regulatory control of thrombin and plasmin is impaired, thereby allowing these proteolytic enzymes to activate and consume circulating coagulation factors, fibrinogen, and platelets.

III

DIAGNOSIS

DIC should not be thought of as a disease but rather as a syndrome with variable severity and chronicity that is initiated by multiple different stimuli (see Table 22-2). No single laboratory test definitively identifies DIC. The combination of a decreased platelet count, decreased fibrinogen, prolonged PT and PTT, and elevated fibrin degradation products or D-dimers is present in DIC. Once elevated, D-dimers remain increased for days, thus making serial test measurements more sensitive and specific than single measurements. Both fibrin degradation products and D-dimers are elevated with trauma or recent surgery and with liver and kidney disease. Coagulation test results in patients with severe liver disease may be similar to those in patients with DIC, although D-dimer levels may not be as high and platelet counts not as low. Factor VIII activity is helpful in discriminating between these conditions because factor VIII is consumed in DIC and factor VIII levels are normal in liver disease.

TREATMENT

Definitive treatment consists of removing the inciting stimulus when possible. Patients with active bleeding should be supported with platelet, plasma, cryoprecipitate, and red blood cell transfusion as needed. There is no evidence that transfusion of these products worsens DIC. Heparin treatment has little role unless the thrombosis is profound. The role of recombinant factor VIIa in halting uncontrolled bleeding in patients experiencing DIC is unclear. Theoretically, factor VIIIa is contraindicated in a condition such as DIC, which is characterized, in part, by systemic thrombosis.

ANTICOAGULANTS, THROMBOLYTICS, AND ANTIPLATELET DRUGS

Anticoagulants (coumarin derivatives, heparin, low-molecular-weight heparin [LMWH], fondaparinux, direct thrombin inhibitors), antiplatelet drugs (aspirin, ADP receptor antagonists [clopidogrel and ticlopidine], glycoprotein IIb/IIIa [GPIIb/IIIa] antagonists [abciximab, eptifibatide, tirofiban], dipyridamole), and thrombolytics are used for the prevention and treatment of stroke, myocardial infarction, and deep vein thrombosis/pulmonary embolism in many patients undergoing surgery. Perioperative use of these drugs has an impact on the risk-benefit ratio of spinal, epidural, and regional anesthetic techniques. Intraoperative anticoagulation of varying degrees is required during certain operations and procedures, with the anesthesiologist administering, monitoring, and at times reversing the anticoagulant effect.

Coumarin Derivatives

Vitamin K antagonists such as warfarin (Coumadin) inhibit vitamin K epoxide reductase, an intracellular enzyme that recycles vitamin K. Oral warfarin reaches effective plasma concentrations in 90 minutes, with the full anticoagulant effect developing over a period of several days. Several factor half-times are required to deplete normal factor to the 20% to 30% level needed for effective anticoagulation. Initiation of the anticoagulant and antithrombotic effects of warfarin depends on the plasma factor VII concentration because factor VII has the shortest half-time (6 hours). Heparinization during the initial phase of warfarin therapy serves two purposes. Insufficient antithrombotic activity during the time required to lower plasma prothrombin levels and the initial warfarin-induced hypercoagulable state caused by early reductions in the anticoagulant proteins C and S are avoided.

MONITORING

Warfarin effect is monitored in the laboratory by using the PT (INR standardized). Because pharmacokinetic and pharmacodynamic factors vary widely from patient to patient, frequent PT determination is necessary. Warfarin has a very narrow therapeutic window between bleeding and prevention/treatment of thrombosis, and drugs, foods, and alcohol can profoundly alter the pharmacokinetic profile of warfarin. Warfarin is contraindicated in pregnancy because fetal exposure can lead to embryopathy.

Heparin

Heparin is the most commonly used anticoagulant drug in the operating room. It is a highly negatively charged sugar that is extracted from mast cells, pig intestinal mucosa, or bovine lung. Saccharide units of very different size are stripped from the proteoglycan skeleton, which accounts for the large variation in size of unfractionated heparin (5000 to 30,000 kd). Advantages of unfractionated heparin over LMWH or pentasaccharide drugs are its immediate onset, short half-time of 30 to 60 minutes, and reversibility with protamine, a highly positively charged protein isolated from salmon. The need for close monitoring of heparin therapy reflects its unpredictable pharmacokinetics caused by heparin binding to plasma proteins, macrophages, endothelial cells, and proteins released from activated platelets and endothelial cells.

CLINICAL USES

Heparin is the anticoagulant of choice for cardiac surgery, vascular surgery, and neurointerventional procedures. Full-dose heparin for cardiac surgery is administered as an intravenous bolus of 300 to 400 U/kg. An ACT greater than 400 seconds is usually considered safe for initiation of cardiopulmonary bypass. The concomitant use of aprotinin artificially shortens the kaolin-activated ACT and thus necessitates an ACT greater than 600 seconds for safe initiation of bypass. The celite-activated ACT is not affected. Protamine at approximately 1 mg to 100 units of heparin is commonly used to reverse the activity of heparin at the conclusion of cardiopulmonary bypass. Most vascular and neurointerventional procedures require lower levels of anticoagulation, and intravenous doses of 3000 to 5000 units of heparin are administered to achieve an ACT of twice baseline or less. Protamine reversal of anticoagulation is not usual with this low level of anticoagulation. Bolus heparin can cause a moderate decrease in systemic vascular resistance and systemic blood pressure, for unclear reasons.

HEPARIN RESISTANCE

Heparin resistance is present when the usual heparin doses do not result in adequate prolongation of the PTT or ACT. Insufficient antithrombin or excessive heparin-binding proteins (factor VIII, fibrinogen, and other acute-phase proteins) are thought to be the cause. If insufficient anticoagulation persists after the administration of additional heparin, fresh frozen plasma may be used in an attempt to increase antithrombin plasma concentrations.

COMPLICATIONS

The major complications of heparin therapy include heparin-induced thrombocytopenia types 1 and 2 and osteopenia (Table 22-6). Heparin-induced thrombocytopenia type 1 is not mediated by immunoglobulin G (IgG), is self-limited, and does not require intervention. Heparin-induced thrombocytopenia type 2 is the most feared nonhemorrhagic complication of heparin treatment and is usually due to antiplatelet factor 4 antibodies causing platelet aggregation. The diagnosis of heparin-induced thrombocytopenia type 2 is recognized by a decrease in the platelet count to less than 100,000 cells/μL or less than 50% of baseline 5 to 10 days after the initiation of heparin therapy and recovery of the platelet count after discontinuation of heparin. Heparin-induced thrombocytopenia type 2 has a mortality of 20% to 30%. Heparin (including heparin flushes or heparin-coated central venous catheters) should be avoided once the diagnosis is suspected and alternative anticoagulants used. Heparin-induced thrombocytopenia antibody testing confirms the diagnosis.

Low-Molecular-Weight Heparin

LMWH is produced by cleaving heparin into shorter fragments. The pentasaccharide unit binds to and activates antithrombin, but the shorter saccharide units make LMWH ineffective in inhibiting thrombin directly. Instead, the LMWH/antithrombin complex binds to and inactivates factor Xa and indirectly inhibits thrombin production. LMWH has a delayed onset of 20 to 60 minutes and a longer half-time than heparin and can be administered subcutaneously either once or twice daily. The predictable anticoagulant effect obviates the need for regular monitoring, thus making it a better choice for outpatient therapy, except in some clinical situations (obese patients, patients with renal disease, or neonates) in which anti–factor Xa levels are monitored. Most LMWH preparations are eliminated by the kidneys. Disadvantages of LMWH are that it cannot be reversed and the risk of bleeding exceeds that of unfractionated heparin during long-term use.

Pentasaccharides (Fondaparinux)

Pentasaccharides (fondaparinux) contain only the pentasaccharide unit necessary for binding and activation of antithrombin. Its longer half-life as compared with LMWH allows once-daily subcutaneous administration. Like LMWH, therapy does not require laboratory monitoring. LMWH derivatives are not associated with osteopenia and have a much lower risk of heparin-induced thrombocytopenia. The risk of bleeding during long-term therapy with pentasaccharides exceeds that of LMWH.

Direct Thrombin Inhibitors

Direct thrombin inhibitors are the most important alternative anticoagulants available. When used perioperatively, direct thrombin inhibitors all share a high risk of bleeding and cannot be reversed. Direct thrombin inhibitors are classified as parenteral (argatroban, melagatran, hirudin, and bivalirudin) or oral (ximelagatran).

Table 22-6 Heparin-Induced Thrombocytopenia (HIT)	
HIT Type 1	**HIT Type 2**
Not immunoglobulin G mediated	Immunoglobulin G mediated
Self-limited	Progressive (mortality 20% to 30%)
Onset 1 to 2 days after the start of heparin	Onset 5 to 10 days after the start of heparin
Platelet count usually >100,000 cells/μL	Platelet count often <100 cells/mL
Incidence, 20% to 25% of heparin-treated patients	Incidence, 1% to 3% of heparin-treated patients
No treatment necessary	Stop heparin therapy and use an alternative anticoagulant Measure platelet factor 4 antibodies Perform serotonin release assay

XIMELAGATRAN

Ximelagatran is converted to melagatran (the active form) after oral ingestion and is a potential alternative to warfarin. At doses of 24 to 36 mg twice daily, it has been shown to be at least as effective and as safe as warfarin for the prevention of deep vein thrombosis/pulmonary embolism and arterial embolism from atrial fibrillation. Ximelagatran therapy does not necessitate laboratory monitoring. Interactions with other drugs, foods, or alcohol are absent. Ximelagatran may elevate liver enzymes with unknown clinical significance.

ARGATROBAN, HIRUDIN, AND BIVALIRUDIN

Argatroban and hirudin are licensed for use in patients with heparin-induced thrombocytopenia. Bivalirudin is used for anticoagulation during percutaneous coronary intervention and as an adjunct to thrombolytics in patients with acute myocardial infarction. All three have been used for intraoperative anticoagulation, including surgery involving cardiopulmonary bypass. The relatively long half-life of hirudin (2.8 hours) makes this drug a poor choice for intraoperative use. Bivalirudin, with a half-life of 30 minutes, is a more attractive choice. Argatroban, with a half-life of 45 minutes, is an alternative direct thrombin inhibitor in patients with renal insufficiency because both bivalirudin and hirudin are excreted by the kidneys and argatroban is eliminated by the liver. Argatroban anticoagulation is monitored with either the ACT or PTT. Neither the ACT nor the PTT is reliable for monitoring either bivalirudin or hirudin therapy because of falsely elevated readings. Bleeding remains a major concern with the use of direct thrombin inhibitors, including the drugs with a short half-life. To avoid using direct thrombin inhibitors in patients with confirmed antibody-positive heparin-induced thrombocytopenia type 2, surgeons can delay surgery for 3 months (to allow spontaneous disappearance of antibodies) or use plasmapheresis (for rapid antibody clearance).

Thrombolytics

Thrombolytics are classified as native tissue plasminogen activators, streptokinase and urokinase, or as exogenous tissue plasminogen activator formulations, alteplase and tenecteplase. Native tissue plasminogen activators are potent activators of plasmin and act by cleaving a single bond from plasminogen to form plasmin. Exogenous tissue plasminogen activator formulations are more fibrin selective, with less of an effect on circulating plasminogen. Tissue plasminogen activators are both thrombolytics and anticoagulants because fibrinolysis generates increased amounts of circulating fibrin degradation products. Increased fibrin degradation product levels inhibit platelet aggregation by binding to platelet surfaces without participating in the process of coagulation. Surgery or puncture of noncompressible vessels is contraindicated within a 10-day period after the use of thrombolytic drugs.

Antiplatelet Drugs

Antiplatelet drugs include cyclooxygenase (COX) inhibitors, thienopyridine derivatives, and platelet GPIIb/IIIa antagonists.

CYCLOOXYGENASE INHIBITORS

COX inhibitors include (1) nonselective inhibitors (aspirin and NSAIDs) and (2) selective agents inhibiting only COX-2. Aspirin irreversibly inhibits COX-1–mediated platelet granule release over the platelet's lifetime. NSAIDs (naproxen, piroxicam, and ibuprofen) reversibly inhibit platelet COX and prevent thromboxane A_2 synthesis. Platelet function normalizes 3 days after discontinuing the use of NSAIDs. Platelet function is not affected by COX-2–specific inhibitors because platelets do not express COX-2.

THIENOPYRIDINE DERIVATIVES

The thienopyridine derivatives ticlopidine and clopidogrel interfere with platelet function by inhibiting ADP-induced primary and secondary platelet aggregation and by interfering with fibrinogen binding to platelets. Platelet functions normalize 7 days after discontinuing clopidogrel and 14 to 21 days after discontinuing ticlopidine.

GPIIB/IIIA ANTAGONISTS

Available GPIIb/IIIa platelet receptor antagonists include abciximab, eptifibatide, and tirofiban. These drugs are potent inhibitors of platelet aggregation because binding of fibrinogen and vWF to platelet GPIIb/IIIa receptors is blocked. Platelet aggregation normalizes 8 hours after discontinuing eptifibatide and tirofiban and 24 to 48 hours after discontinuing abciximab.

AN APPROACH TO ANTICOAGULATED PATIENTS

Patients who are chronically anticoagulated present a particular challenge in the perioperative setting. Therapeutic levels of warfarin can result in excessive bleeding, and reversing the action of warfarin is associated with perioperative thromboembolism. The risk for a thrombotic complication after stopping warfarin therapy depends on the original indication for therapy. Long-term anticoagulation is recommended for patients who experience recurrent venous thrombosis or those at risk for arterial embolic disease. The highest risk for perioperative recurrence exists for patients who have experienced thromboemboli during the previous month. Elective surgery in these patients should be deferred until a 3-month course of warfarin is completed. The risk for perioperative recurrence can be considered intermediate for patients who have experienced thromboemboli during the previous 30 and 90 days and low when the event dates back past 3 months (Fig. 22-2).

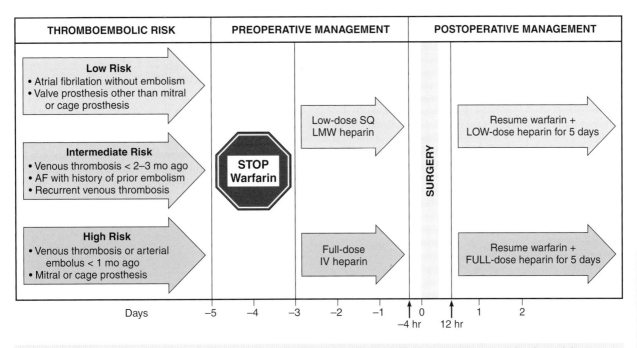

THROMBOEMBOLIC RISK	PREOPERATIVE MANAGEMENT	POSTOPERATIVE MANAGEMENT

Low Risk
- Atrial fibrillation without embolism
- Valve prosthesis other than mitral or cage prosthesis

Intermediate Risk
- Venous thrombosis < 2–3 mo ago
- AF with history of prior embolism
- Recurrent venous thrombosis

High Risk
- Venous thrombosis or arterial embolus < 1 mo ago
- Mitral or cage prosthesis

STOP Warfarin

Low-dose SQ LMW heparin

Full-dose IV heparin

SURGERY

Resume warfarin + LOW-dose heparin for 5 days

Resume warfarin + FULL-dose heparin for 5 days

Days   −5   −4   −3   −2   −1   0   1   2
−4 hr   12 hr

Figure 22-2 Perioperative management of an anticoagulated patient. AF, atrial fibrillation; LWM, low molecular weight.

Hypercoagulable State

Thrombin formation is abnormally high 2 to 7 days after the cessation of warfarin therapy and precedes normalization of coagulation factor concentrations and INR values. Postoperative increases in plasminogen activator inhibitor type 1 concentrations add to the temporary hypercoagulable state. Surgery increases the risk for venous thrombosis but not for arterial embolism unless the procedure involves the artery directly. If the original indication for warfarin therapy was prevention of arterial emboli, the perioperative risk for thromboemboli is considered low. Generally, patients at risk for arterial emboli are chronically anticoagulated to prevent the relatively high risk and devastating consequences of recurrent arterial embolization. When warfarin therapy is discontinued 4 days before surgery, some anticoagulant effect, as measured by an INR value greater than 1.5, probably persists until 1 day before surgery, and therapeutic levels of warfarin can be reestablished 1 day after reinitiation of warfarin. The antithrombotic effect of warfarin, conferred by reduced prothrombin plasma concentrations, persists longer than normalization of the INR because prothrombin with its long half-time is slow to recover after discontinuation of warfarin therapy. From a stable baseline INR of 2.0 to 3.0, most patients will have an INR less than 1.5 within roughly 4 days after discontinuation of the drug. Older patients eliminate warfarin less effectively. INR values are poor predictors of postoperative bleeding. Many experts recommend a target INR value of 1.3 to 1.5, but others consider INR values less than 2.0 to be safe.

RISK ASSESSMENT AND PROPHYLAXIS FOR PERIOPERATIVE VENOUS THROMBOEMBOLISM IN ADULTS

For unknown reasons, orthopedic surgery is associated with a higher incidence of venous thrombosis than other major surgical procedures are. Cardiothoracic and major abdominal surgeries have the highest risk for venous thrombosis after warfarin reversal.

Preoperative Therapeutic Heparinization

In patients with a high perioperative thrombotic risk, preoperative therapeutic heparinization, either with intravenous unfractionated heparin or with LMWH, is indicated as a bridge between discontinuation of oral anticoagulation therapy and surgery. Intravenous heparin should be discontinued 6 hours before the surgical procedure, and the last dose of LMWH should be given 12 hours before the procedure. Heparin should not be restarted until 12 hours after the surgical procedure, even in high-risk patients, because the risk for severe hemorrhage is significant. Preoperative heparinization is avoided in patients with a high likelihood of perioperative bleeding, such as elderly patients or those with known risk factors (thrombocytopenia, concurrent aspirin or NSAID therapy, recent history of bleeding in the gastrointestinal, genitourinary, or central nervous system).

Postoperative Therapeutic Heparinization

When restarted postoperatively, intravenous heparin is initiated at the maintenance dose, with a loading dose omitted, and is discontinued when the warfarin-induced INR is greater than 2.0 for more than 24 hours. In high-risk patients a more careful approach is to continue heparin for a full 5 days. Therapeutic doses of LMWH and fondaparinux are at least as effective as full-dose unfractionated heparin and allow subcutaneous administration without laboratory monitoring. This is an advantage in patients who can be discharged within 5 days of surgery because it allows reinitiation of warfarin therapy to be accomplished as an outpatient.

INTERMEDIATE OR LOW RISK

Patients at intermediate or low risk for perioperative thrombosis require only postoperative pharmacologic therapy. In patients at low risk, prophylactic subcutaneous unfractionated heparin, LMWH, or fondaparinux is probably all that is required to supplement physical means of deep vein thrombosis prophylaxis (pneumatic compression devices, early ambulation) while anticoagulation is reestablished. It is unclear whether prophylactic or therapeutic dosing of these drugs is more appropriate for patients at intermediate risk.

Restoration of Vitamin K Activity

In emergency circumstances, vitamin K activity can be restored by the transfusion of fresh frozen plasma (10 to 15 mL/kg IV). Prothrombin complex concentrate (25 to 50 IU/kg), a highly thrombogenic factor IX concentrate that contains variable concentrations of vitamin K–dependent coagulation factors, is also effective. The risk-benefit ratio of treatment with prothrombin complex, however, must be considered when the risk for perioperative thrombosis is high.

Although vitamin K–dependent coagulation factors are quickly restored with these products, the factor half-life is only 4 to 6 hours, thus necessitating the concomitant oral administration of vitamin K (1 mg). Intravenous administration of vitamin K carries a higher risk for anaphylaxis. Larger doses of vitamin K should be avoided because of postoperative warfarin resistance.

NEURAXIAL INTERVENTIONS IN PATIENTS BEING TREATED WITH ANTICOAGULANT DRUGS

The introduction of potent antithrombotic drugs to prevent and treat perioperative thrombosis has raised awareness about the risks of bleeding and neurologic injury with neuraxial interventions. Developing definitive recommendations that improve patient safety is complicated by the low incidence of untoward outcomes, including epidural hematoma leading to paralysis. Current consensus conference recommendations on neuraxial anesthesia and anticoagulation by the American Society of Regional Anesthesia are continually updated as additional information becomes available (Table 22-7).[7]

AN INTRAOPERATIVE APPROACH TO UNCONTROLLED BLEEDING

Laboratory tests (platelet count, PT, PTT, fibrinogen) are indicated to aid in diagnosis and to determine appropriate replacement therapy in the presence of uncontrolled

Table 22–7 American Association of Regional Anesthesia Guidelines for Neuraxial Anesthesia in Anticoagulated Patients

Medication	Event	Recommendation*
Antiplatelet medications	Neuraxial interventions	
Nonsteroidal anti-inflammatory drugs		No contraindication
Aspirin		No contraindication
Ticlopidine		Discontinue 14 days preoperatively
Clopidogrel		Discontinue 7 days preoperatively
GPIIb/IIIa inhibitors		
Abciximab		Discontinue 7 days preoperatively
Eptifibatide		Discontinue 4 to 8 hours preoperatively
Tirofiban		Discontinue 14 days preoperatively

Table 22-7 American Association of Regional Anesthesia Guidelines for Neuraxial Anesthesia in Anticoagulated Patients—cont'd

Medication	Event	Recommendation*
Dipyridamole		Discontinue
Unfractionated heparin		
Subcutaneous	Neuraxial interventions	No contraindication; measure platelet count if >4 days of heparin treatment
	After intervention	If >4 days of heparin treatment, measure platelet count before removing catheter
Intravenous	Vascular surgery and neuraxial interventions	Avoid in presence of other coagulopathies
		Delay heparin for 1 hour after catheter placement
		No restrictions before procedure with dosing every 12 hours; delay if difficult catheter placement is anticipated
	After intervention	Catheter removal 2 to 4 hours after heparin dosing and normal PTT or ACT
		No mandatory delay if traumatic, but wait 1 hour after catheter removal to administer repeat heparin dose
	Cardiac surgery with full heparinization and neuraxial interventions	No data
Warfarin	Neuraxial interventions	Stop warfarin 4 to 5 days preoperatively
		Document normal INR before intervention
	After intervention	Remove catheter when INR <1.5
Low-molecular-weight heparin	Neuraxial interventions	Delay 10 to 12 hours after dose
		Delay 24 hours after traumatic (bloody) tap or with twice-daily dosing
	After intervention	Once-daily dosing: remove catheter 10 to 12 hours after last dose and start next dose 2 hours later
		Twice-daily dosing: remove catheter 2 hours before first dose
Thrombolytics	Neuraxial interventions	No safety data; avoid for first 10 days if possible
	After intervention	Remove catheter when fibrinogen levels normalize
		Frequent neurologic checks (minimize degree of sensory and motor blockade)

*Antiplatelet medications combined with unfractionated heparin, low-molecular-weight heparin, oral anticoagulants, and thrombolytics increase the frequency of bleeding.

ACT, activated clotting time; GPIIb, glycoprotein IIb; INR, international normalized ratio; PTT, partial thromboplastin time.

Adapted from Horlocker TT, Wedel DJ, Benzon H, et al. Regional anesthesia in the anticoagulated patient: Defining the risks (The Second ASRA Consensus Conference on Neuraxial Anesthesia and Anticoagulation). Reg Anesth Pain Med 2003;28:172-197.

intraoperative bleeding without apparent surgical cause (Fig. 22-3). Estimates of circulating levels of either coagulation factors or platelets based on the estimated blood loss during surgery are often inaccurate but necessary under circumstances in which laboratory testing is not available. In the absence of coagulation test results, fresh frozen plasma is often transfused after blood loss equivalent to one blood volume, and platelets are transfused after blood loss equivalent to two blood volumes.

Coagulation Factor Deficiency

Blood loss caused by a low level of one or more coagulation factors (PT or PTT prolonged to 1.5 times the normal range) is replaced with fresh frozen plasma (10 to 15 mL/kg IV). Platelet counts lower than 50,000 to 80,000 cells/μL are increased by administering concentrated platelets. One platelet pheresis unit contains a minimum of 6×10^6 cells/μL and generally raises the platelet count by 30,000 to 60,000 cells/μL in a 70-kg patient.

	Dilution	DIC	Fibrinolysis
PT/PTT High = >1.5 x normal	↑	↑	↑
Platelet count Low = < 50,000-80,000 cells =μL	↓	↓	↔
Fibrinogen Low = < 80 mg/dL	↓	↓	↓
D-Dimers High = >1:2	↔	↑	↔

Figure 22-3 An intraoperative laboratory approach to uncontrolled bleeding. DIC, disseminated intravascular coagulation; PT, prothrombin time; PTT, partial thromboplastin time.

Cryoprecipitate (1 concentrate per 10-kg body weight) can be used to augment fibrinogen levels less than 125 mg/dL. Each fresh frozen plasma and platelet pheresis unit has approximately twice the amount of fibrinogen contained in 1 cryoprecipitate concentrate.

Recombinant Factor Concentrates

Although designed and licensed for the treatment of bleeding in hemophilia patients with inhibitors to factor concentrates, prothrombin complex and recombinant factor VIIa have been found to be useful, but expensive treatments of uncontrolled intraoperative bleeding that is unresponsive to replacement of blood components. Prothrombin complex concentrate contains variable concentrations of coagulation factors and may include proteins C and S, thus making it highly thrombogenic. Factor VIIa is less thrombogenic. At doses of 30 to 90 μg/kg, factor VIIa may be effective as rapid rescue treatment of uncontrolled bleeding that is unresponsive to conventional replacement therapy in trauma and surgery. Redosing may be needed after 2 hours if bleeding recurs.

Other Hemostatic Drugs

Other hemostatic drugs useful perioperatively include DDAVP and the antifibrinolytics aprotinin, ε-aminocaproic acid, and tranexamic acid. DDAVP (0.3 μg/kg IV) releases vWF from endothelial cells, with maximum effect occurring within 30 minutes. DDAVP has proved useful for the prevention of bleeding in some forms of von Willebrand's disease and in mild forms of factor VIII deficiency and for bleeding associated with uremia. Aprotinin, a serine protease inhibitor extracted from bovine lung, inactivates plasminogen and plasmin and inhibits several enzymatic activators of coagulation when infused intravenously at 2×10^6 kallikrein inhibitory units (KIU), followed by 5×10^5 KIU. There is a risk of anaphylaxis if aprotinin is reinfused within 6 months. By blocking plasminogen from binding to fibrin through the lysine receptor, plasmin formation is impaired and fibrinolysis inhibited. Aprotinin may be useful perioperatively to decrease bleeding caused by increased fibrinolysis (liver disease, prostate surgery, cardiopulmonary bypass).

REFERENCES

1. Colman RW, Clowes AW, George JN, et al. Overview of hemostasis. In Colman RW, Hirsh J, Marder VJ, et al (eds): Hemostasis and Thrombosis, 4th ed. Philadelphia: Lippincott Williams & Wilkins, 2001, pp 3-16.
2. Robers HR, Monroe DM, Escobar MA. Current concepts of hemostasis. Anesthesiology 2004;100:722-730.
3. Schenone M, Furie B, Furie B. The blood coagulation cascade. Curr Opin Hematol 2004;11:272-277.
4. Hathcock J. Vascular biology: The role of tissue factor. Semin Hematol 2004;41:30-34.
5. Mannucci M. Treatment of von Willebrand's disease. N Engl J Med 2004;35:683-694.
6. Edmonds MJ, Crichton TJ, Runciman WB, Pradhan M. Evidence-based risk factors for postoperative deep vein thrombosis. Aust N Z J Surg 2004;74:1082-1097.
7. Horlocker TT, Wedel DJ, Benzon H, et al. Regional anesthesia in the anticoagulated patient. Defining the risks (The Second ASRA Consensus Conference on Neuraxial Anesthesia and Anticoagulation). Reg Anesth Pain Med 2003;28:172-197.

FLUID MANAGEMENT

Alicia G. Kalamas

The goal of perioperative fluid management is to provide the appropriate amount of parenteral fluid to maintain adequate intravascular fluid volume, left ventricular filling pressure, cardiac output, systemic blood pressure, and ultimately, oxygen delivery to tissues. In addition to surgical considerations (blood loss, evaporative loss, third spacing), certain conditions and changes that occur during the perioperative period can make the management of fluid balance a challenge, including preoperative fluid volume status, preexisting disease states, and the effect of anesthetic drugs on normal physiologic functions. All these factors must be considered when devising a rational approach to fluid management for patients during the perioperative period.

Management of fluid therapy may influence intraoperative and postoperative morbidity and mortality. Providing sufficient intravascular fluid volume is essential for adequate perfusion of vital organs. Although quantitative considerations are of primary concern, oxygen-carrying capacity, coagulation, and electrolyte and acid-base balance are also of critical importance. A definitive answer regarding the best solution (crystalloid versus colloid) for resuscitation and maintenance does not exist; sound clinical judgment remains the cornerstone of optimizing fluid management.

PREOPERATIVE CONSIDERATIONS

Preoperative assessment of intravascular fluid volume is important before induction of anesthesia. Bowel preparations, vomiting, diarrhea, diaphoresis, hemorrhage, burns, and inadequate intake are all common causes of preoperative hypovolemia. Redistribution of intravascular fluid volume without evidence of external loss is another important cause of preoperative volume depletion that is generally encountered in patients with sepsis, adult respiratory distress syndrome, ascites, pleural effusions, and bowel abnormalities. Often, these processes are accompanied by increased capillary permeability resulting in loss of intravascular fluid volume to interstitial and other fluid compartments.

Evaluation of Intravascular Fluid Volume

Evaluation of intravascular fluid volume relies on indirect measurements such as systemic blood pressure, heart rate, and urine output because measurements of fluid compartments are not readily available. Unfortunately, these measurements provide only a gross estimate of organ perfusion. Furthermore, even with sophisticated monitoring techniques (pulmonary artery catheters, arterial oxygen saturation), the adequacy of intravascular fluid volume replacement and tissue oxygen delivery to individual vital organs cannot be precisely determined.[1] For these reasons, clinical evaluation of intravascular fluid volume is necessary.

PHYSICAL EXAMINATION AND LABORATORY MEASUREMENTS

Physical examination and laboratory measurements are needed to guide preoperative fluid therapy. Clues to intravascular fluid volume depletion include skin turgor, hydration of mucous membranes, palpation of peripheral pulses, resting heart rate, systemic blood pressure (including orthostatic changes), and urine output (Table 23-1).[2] Laboratory measurements that are useful indices of intravascular fluid volume include serial hematocrit, arterial blood gas analysis and base deficit, urine specific gravity or osmolality, serum sodium, and the serum creatinine–to–blood urea nitrogen ratio. Physical examination and laboratory tests are indirect, nonspecific measures of intravascular fluid volume, and no single parameter can be relied on to the exclusion of other observations.

Table 23-1 Estimation of Intravascular Fluid Volume
Patient's history
Systemic blood pressure (supine and standing)
Heart rate
Urine output
Hematocrit
Blood urea nitrogen
Electrolytes
Arterial blood gases and pH
Central venous pressure

INTRAVASCULAR FLUID VOLUME STATUS AND ANESTHETIC TECHNIQUE

Both general anesthesia and regional anesthesia have indirect effects on fluid requirements.

Intravenous Induction Drugs

Induction of anesthesia with thiopental leads to a decrease in venous return, whereas induction with propofol produces a decrease in systemic vascular resistance, cardiac contractility, and preload. Though normally producing small perturbations in systemic blood pressure in euvolemic patients, induction of anesthesia with these drugs in intravascularly depleted patients can lead to undesirable decreases in systemic blood pressure and perfusion of vital organs.

Ketamine produces increases in systemic blood pressure, heart rate, and cardiac output through stimulation of the sympathetic nervous system and inhibition of norepinephrine reuptake. The direct myocardial depressant effects of ketamine may be unmasked by exhaustion of catecholamine stores (congestive heart failure, end-stage shock) and result in paradoxical decreases in blood pressure when ketamine is administered to these patients for induction of anesthesia.

Neuromuscular Blocking Drugs

Neuromuscular blocking drugs, though generally devoid of direct cardiovascular effects, can lead to histamine release (atracurium) and decreased systemic vascular resistance or produce venous pooling because of loss of muscle tone.

Inhaled Anesthetic Drugs

Isoflurane, desflurane, and sevoflurane all decrease systemic vascular resistance and mildly depress myocardial contractility. In addition, institution of positive pressure ventilation of the patient's lungs reduces preload and is particularly likely to decrease systemic blood pressure in hypovolemic patients.

Regional Anesthesia

Neuraxial blockade, by blocking sympathetic nervous system fibers innervating arterial and venous vascular smooth muscle, causes vasodilatation, pooling of blood, and decreased venous return to the heart. Though producing significant perturbations in systemic blood pressure in intravascularly depleted patients, these effects are often mitigated by fluid administration before the institution of regional anesthesia.

PERIOPERATIVE FLUID THERAPY: QUANTITATIVE CONSIDERATIONS

Perioperative fluid therapy includes (1) replacement of preexisting fluid deficits, (2) replacement of normal losses (maintenance requirements), and (3) replacement of surgical wound ("third-space") losses (including blood loss) (Tables 23-2 to 23-4).

Preexisting Fluid Deficits

Patients undergoing surgery after an overnight fast have preexisting fluid deficits proportionate to the duration of the fast. This deficit can be estimated by multiplying the normal maintenance rate (see Table 23-2) by the length of the fast. Although hypotonic fluids such as 0.5 normal

Table 23-2	Estimating Maintenance Fluid Requirements
Up to 10 kg	4 mL/kg/hr
11-20 kg	Add 2 mL/kg/hr
21 kg and above	Add 1 mL/kg/hr

Table 23-3 Redistributive and Evaporative Surgical Fluid Losses

Degree of Tissue Trauma	Additional Fluid Requirement
Minimal (herniorrhaphy)	2-4 mL/kg/hr
Moderate (cholecystectomy)	4-6 mL/kg/hr
Severe (bowel resection)	6-8 mL/kg/hr

Table 23-4 Guidelines for Intraoperative Maintenance and Replacement Crystalloid Therapy

Isotonic electrolyte-containing solution (sodium and potassium) at 2 mL/kg/hr to replace insensible losses

Isotonic electrolyte-containing solution to replace third-space losses

   Minimal surgical trauma (herniorrhaphy), 2-4 mL/kg/hr

   Moderate surgical trauma (cholecystectomy), 4-6 mL/kg/hr

   Severe surgical trauma (bowel resection), 6-8 mL/kg/hr

Replace 1 mL of blood loss with 3 mL crystalloid solution

Monitor vital signs and maintain urine output at 0.5 mg/kg/hr

saline can be administered to correct this fluid deficit, isotonic crystalloids are generally favored (Tables 23-5 and 23-6).[2]

ABNORMAL FLUID LOSSES

Abnormal fluid losses (vomiting, diarrhea, preoperative bleeding), occult losses (ascites, infected tissues), and insensible losses (fever, sweating, hyperventilation) must not be overlooked in the preoperative correction of fluid deficits so that the hypotension and hypoperfusion that can occur during induction of anesthesia can be minimized. The fluid used for replacement should be similar in composition to the fluid lost (see Tables 23-5 and 23-6).[2]

Maintenance Requirements

Maintenance fluid is required in fasting adults as a result of continued urine formation, gastrointestinal secretions, and insensible losses from the skin and respiratory tract. Maintenance fluid requirements are calculated and replaced with crystalloid solutions during the intraoperative period (see Table 23-2).

III

Surgical Fluid Losses

BLOOD LOSS

The anesthesiologist must continually record ongoing estimates of surgical blood loss. Measurement of blood in the surgical suction container is only one component; occult bleeding into the wound or under surgical drapes may complicate such estimates. Additionally, blood on surgical sponges and laparotomy pads ("laps") must be accounted for. A fully soaked sponge ("4 × 4") holds 10 mL of blood, whereas a soaked "lap" holds 100 to 150 mL. The use of irrigating solutions may also complicate the estimate. Serial hematocrit values reflect the ratio of blood cells to plasma, not blood loss. Typically, both surgeons and anesthesiologists tend to underestimate actual blood loss, and clinical signs such as tachycardia are insensitive and nonspecific. Furthermore, decreasing urine output, a decline in arterial pH, and a rising base deficit may be manifested only when tissue hypoperfusion has become moderate to severe. Therefore, visual estimation of continual blood loss is mandatory to guide fluid therapy and transfusion.

In replacing blood loss with isotonic crystalloid solutions, a 3:1 ratio of crystalloid administration to blood loss is often required to maintain intravascular fluid volume, whereas milliliter-per-milliliter replacement with colloid or blood is generally sufficient (see Table 23-4).

OTHER LOSSES

Less obvious than hemorrhage but of great import are fluid shifts or loss from the operative site. Evaporative

Table 23-5 Composition of Crystalloid Solutions

	Dextrose (mg/dL)	Sodium (mEq/L)	Chloride (mEq/L)	Potassium (mEq/L)	Magnesium (mEq/L)	Calcium (mEq/L)	Lactate (mEq/L)	Approximate pH	mOsmol/L (Calculated)
ECF	90–110	140	108	4.5	2.0	5.0	5.0	7.3	290
5% Dextrose in water	5000							4.3	253
5% Dextrose in 0.45% NaCl	5000	77	77					4.3	406
5% Dextrose in 0.9% NaCl	5000	154	154					4.2	561
0.9% NaCl		154	154					5.6	308
Lactated Ringer's solution		130	109	4.0		3.0	28	6.6	273
5% Dextrose in lactated Ringer's solution	5000	130	109	4.0		3.0	28	4.9	525
Plasma-Lyte		140	98	5.0	3.0		*	7.4	295
5% NaCl		855	855					5.6	1171

*Contains acetate 27 mEq/L and gluconate 23 mEq/L.
ECF, extracellular fluid.

Table 23-6 Electrolyte Content of Body Fluids

Fluid	Sodium (mEq/L)	Potassium (mEq/L)	Chloride (mEq/L)	Bicarbonate (mEq/L)
Sweat	30-50	5-15	45-55	
Saliva	2-40	10-30	6-30	30
Gastric	20-80	5-20	50-150	5-25
Pancreatic	120-140	5-15	50-90	60-110
Biliary	120-150	5-15	80-120	30-40
Ileal	40-130	5-15	20-100	20-30
Diarrhea	20-140	10-60	20-120	30-50

losses are most apparent with large wounds, but a considerable amount of fluid can be lost through the lungs during mechanical ventilation unless a humidifier is used.

Internal Redistribution of Fluids

Internal redistribution of fluids, or "third spacing," can cause large fluid shifts and severe intravascular fluid volume depletion, especially during major abdominal or thoracic procedures. In addition, traumatized, inflamed, or infected tissue can sequester large amounts of fluid in the interstitial space. Replacement of evaporated and "third-spaced" fluid is necessary to avoid organ hypoperfusion, especially renal insufficiency (see Table 23-3).

PERIOPERATIVE FLUID THERAPY: QUALITATIVE CONSIDERATIONS

Intravenous fluids are classified as crystalloid or colloid solutions. Crystalloids are solutions of inorganic and small organic molecules dissolved in water. The main solute is either glucose or saline, and these solutions may be isotonic, hypotonic, or hypertonic (see Table 23-5). Crystalloid solutions have the advantage of being safe, nontoxic, reaction free, and inexpensive. The major disadvantage of hypotonic and isotonic crystalloids is their limited ability to remain within the intravascular space. Edema formation is not uncommon if large volumes of crystalloid solutions are needed to maintain intravascular fluid volume.

Crystalloid Solutions

Isotonic crystalloid solutions are favored intraoperatively because hypotonic solutions generally have an insufficient intravascular half-life and tend to promote hyponatremia. The most commonly used solutions are normal saline, lactated Ringer's solution, and Plasma-Lyte (see Table 23-5).

The major consideration in selecting one solution over another is its effect on the sodium-to-chloride ratio and acid-base balance. Administration of large volumes of saline solution can lead to a hyperchloremic-induced non-gap metabolic acidosis, whereas administration of large volumes of lactated Ringer's solution may result in metabolic alkalosis because of increased bicarbonate production from the metabolism of lactate. Although assessment and correction of abnormalities in calcium, magnesium, and phosphate must be part of the complete evaluation, sodium, potassium, and chloride are the principal electrolytes affecting the choice of crystalloid solution. Both lactated Ringer's solution and Plasma-Lyte contain potassium and should be used with caution in hyperkalemic patients. The calcium present in lactated Ringer's solution prohibits its use in the presence of citrated blood products.

In the absence of disease states affecting glucose metabolism, dextrose-containing solutions should be avoided because hyperglycemic-induced hyperosmolality, osmotic diuresis, and cerebral acidosis are known complications. Hypoglycemia is a risk with abrupt discontinuation of glucose-containing total parenteral nutrition solutions during the intraoperative period. For this reason, infusions of total parenteral nutrition solutions should be continued during anesthesia and surgery; alternatively, a dextrose-containing infusion can be substituted, with frequent monitoring of the patient's blood glucose concentration.

Colloids

Colloids are homogeneous noncrystalline substances consisting of large molecules dissolved in a solute. Most colloid solutions are dissolved in isotonic saline, but isotonic glucose, hypertonic saline, and isotonic "physiologic" solutions are available. Colloids have much greater capacity than crystalloids to remain within the intra-

III

vascular space and therefore are more efficient volume expanders. Clinically used colloids include albumin, hydroxyethyl starch, and dextran.

ALBUMIN

Albumin is purified from human plasma and is commercially available as either a 5% or 25% solution. Because it is pasteurized at 60°C for 10 hours, there is no known risk of transmission of hepatitis B or C or human immunodeficiency virus. However, because albumin is a blood product, Jehovah's Witnesses may object to its use for religious reasons. The half-life of albumin in plasma is approximately 16 hours, with about 90% of the dose remaining in the intravascular space 2 hours after administration.

HYDROXYETHYL STARCH

Hydroxyethyl starch (hetastarch) is a semisynthetic colloid synthesized from amylopectin, a branching D-glucose polymer. Examples of commercially available starches are 6% high-molecular-weight hetastarch in saline (Hespan) and 6% high-molecular-weight hetastarch in balanced electrolytes (Hextend). The half-life for 90% of hydroxyethyl starch particles is 17 days.

DEXTRAN

Dextran is a semisynthetic colloid that is biosynthesized commercially from sucrose by the bacterium *Leuconostoc mesenteroides*. Based on differing molecular weights, the two frequently selected dextrans are dextran 40 and dextran 70. Smaller dextran particles are rapidly cleared in the urine in a matter of hours, but larger particles have half-lives on the order of several days. Therefore, dextran 70 is generally preferred for volume expansion, whereas dextran 40 is thought to improve blood flow in the microcirculation, presumably by decreasing blood viscosity. Indeed, dextran 40 is frequently used by vascular and plastic surgeons to assist in maintaining the patency of microvascular anastomoses.

A 6% solution of dextran 70 has a volume-expanding capacity similar to that of 6% hetastarch, with approximately 80% of a 1-L dextran infusion remaining in the intravascular space at the completion of the infusion. In contrast, an estimated 80% of a 1-L infusion of lactated Ringer's solution will have entered the interstitial space at the completion of the infusion.[3]

SAFETY PROFILES

Even though the clinically available colloids exhibit similar effectiveness in maintaining colloid oncotic pressure, differences in safety profiles are well recognized. Hypersensitivity reactions, including anaphylaxis, have been reported with albumin, hydroxyethyl starch, and dextran, although allergic reactions to albumin are

rare. Dextran 1 (Promit) may be administered before dextran 40 or dextran 70 to prevent severe anaphylactic reactions; it acts as a hapten and binds any circulating dextran antibodies. Pruritus is seen with hydroxyethyl starch in a dose-dependent fashion; it is typically delayed in onset and unresponsive to currently available forms of therapy.[5]

COAGULATION ABNORMALITIES

Bleeding associated with the use of the synthetic colloids has been widely reported. Dextran 70 and, to a lesser extent, dextran 40 produce a dose-related reduction in platelet aggregation and adhesiveness, whereas hydroxyethyl starch can lead to a reduction in factor VIII and von Willebrand factor, impairment of platelet function, and prolongation of the partial thromboplastin time.[5] Coagulation studies and bleeding times are not generally significantly affected after infusions of up to 1 L; however, these colloids are best avoided in patients with a known coagulopathy.

Colloid versus Crystalloid Solutions

For many years, controversy has existed over the relative merits of colloid versus crystalloid solutions for the resuscitation of surgical patients. Despite numerous studies comparing crystalloid with colloids, none has unequivocally demonstrated a distinct advantage in terms of pulmonary complications or survival with either therapy.[6] Because colloids are more expensive and do not enjoy the same safety profile as crystalloids, it is hard to justify their use outside situations in which rapid intravascular fluid volume expansion is needed.

Transfusion Considerations

Blood loss should be replaced with crystalloid or colloid solutions to maintain intravascular fluid volume until the danger of anemia or depletion of coagulation factors necessitates the administration of blood products. Below a hemoglobin level of 7 g/dL, resting cardiac output has to increase greatly to maintain normal oxygen delivery to tissues. Therefore, blood loss should be replaced with transfusion of erythrocytes to maintain a hemoglobin concentration between 7 and 8 g/dL. A level of 10 g/dL is generally desired for patients with significant cardiac or pulmonary disease.

The most common intraoperative coagulopathy is dilutional thrombocytopenia, which occurs with either large-volume blood product transfusion or crystalloid/colloid administration. Factor deficiency is less common in the absence of hepatic dysfunction because stored blood retains 20% to 30% activity of factors VII and VIII, which is sufficient for coagulation.

REFERENCES

1. Gold MS. Perioperative fluid management. Crit Care Clin 1992;8:409-421.
2. Rosenthal MH. Intraoperative fluid management—what and how much? Chest 1999;115:106S-112S.
3. Ratner LE, Smith GW: Intraoperative fluid management. Surg Clin North Am 1993;73:229-241.
4. Grocott MP, Mythen MG, Gan TJ. Perioperative fluid management and clinical outcomes in adults. Anesth Analg 2005;100:1093-1106.
5. Barron ME, Wilkes MM, Navickis RJ. A systematic review of the comparative safety of colloids. Arch Surg 2004; 139:552-563.
6. Roberts I, Alderson P, Bunn F, et al. Colloids versus crystalloids for fluid resuscitation in critically ill patients. Cochrane Database Syst Rev 2004;(4): CD000567.

III

BLOOD THERAPY

Ronald D. Miller

Allogeneic blood transfusions are given for inadequate oxygen-carrying capacity/delivery and correction of coagulation deficits. Blood transfusion can secondarily provide additional intravascular fluid volume. "Practice Guidelines for Perioperative Blood Transfusions and Adjuvant Therapies" provide information and recommendations regarding blood therapy from the American Society of Anesthesiologists.[1]

BLOOD THERAPY

Determination of the blood types of the recipient and donor is the first step in selecting blood for transfusion therapy. Routine typing of blood is performed to identify the antigens (A, B, Rh) on the membranes of erythrocytes (Table 24-1). Naturally occurring antibodies (anti-B, anti-A) are formed whenever erythrocyte membranes lack A or B antigens (or both). These antibodies are capable of causing rapid intravascular destruction of erythrocytes that contain the corresponding antigens.

Cross-Match

The major cross-match occurs when the donor's erythrocytes are incubated with the recipient's plasma. Incubation of the donor's plasma with the recipient's erythrocytes constitutes a minor cross-match. Agglutination occurs if either the major or minor cross-match is incompatible. The major cross-match also checks for immunoglobulin G antibodies (Kell, Kidd). Type-specific blood means that only the ABO-Rh type has been determined. The chance of a significant hemolytic reaction related to the transfusion of type-specific blood is about 1 in 1000.

Emergency Transfusion

In an emergency situation that requires transfusion before compatibility testing is completed, the most desirable

Table 24-1 Blood Groups and Cross-Match Blood

Blood Group	Antigen on Erythrocyte	Plasma Antibodies	Incidence (%) White	African American
A	A	Anti-B	40	27
B	B	Anti-A	11	20
AB	AB	None	4	4
0	None	Anti-A, anti-B	45	40
Rh	Rh		42	17

approach is to transfuse type-specific, partially cross-matched blood. The donor erythrocytes are mixed with recipient plasma, centrifuged, and observed for macroscopic agglutination. If the time required to complete this examination (should require <5 minutes) is not acceptable, the second option is to administer type-specific, non–cross-matched blood. The least attractive option is to administer O-negative packed red blood cells. O-negative whole blood is not selected because it may contain high titers of anti-A and anti-B hemolytic antibodies. Even if the patient's blood type becomes known and available, after 2 units of type O-negative packed red blood cells have been transfused, subsequent transfusions should continue with O-negative blood.

Type and Screen

Type and screen denotes blood that has been typed for A, B, and Rh antigens and screened for common antibodies. This approach is used when the scheduled surgical procedure is unlikely to require transfusion of blood (hysterectomy, cholecystectomy) but is one in which blood should be available. Use of type and screen permits more cost-efficient use of stored blood because it is available to more than one patient. The chance of a significant hemolytic reaction related to the use of type and screen is approximately 1 in 10,000 units transfused.

Blood Storage

Blood can be stored in a variety of solutions that contain phosphate, dextrose, and possibly adenine at temperatures of 1°C to 6°C. Storage time (70% viability of transfused erythrocytes 24 hours after transfusion) is 21 to 35 days, depending on the storage media. Adenine increases erythrocyte survival by allowing the cells to resynthesize the adenosine triphosphate needed to fuel metabolic reactions. Changes that occur in blood during storage reflect the length of storage and the type of preservative used. Recently, fresher blood (<5 days of storage) has been recommended for critically ill patients in an effort to improve the delivery of oxygen (2,3-

diphosphoglycerate [2,3-DPG] concentrations better maintained).

DECISION TO TRANSFUSE

The decision to transfuse should be based on a combination of (1) monitoring for blood loss, (2) monitoring for inadequate perfusion and oxygenation of vital organs, and (3) monitoring for transfusion indicators, especially the hemoglobin concentration.

Monitoring for Blood Loss

Visual estimation is the simplest technique for quantifying intraoperative blood loss. The estimate is based on blood on sponges and drapes and in suction devices.

Monitoring for Inadequate Perfusion and Oxygenation of Vital Organs

Standard monitors, including arterial blood pressure, heart rate, urine output, electrocardiogram, and oxygen saturation, are commonly used. Analysis of arterial blood gases, mixed venous oxygen saturation, and echocardiography may be useful in selected patients. Tachycardia is an insensitive and nonspecific indicator of hypovolemia, especially in patients receiving a volatile anesthetic. Maintenance of adequate systemic blood pressure and central venous pressure (6 to 12 mm Hg) suggests adequate intravascular blood volume.[2] Urinary output usually declines during moderate to severe hypovolemia and the resulting tissue hypoperfusion. Arterial pH may decrease only when tissue hypoperfusion becomes severe.

Monitoring for Transfusion Indicators (Especially Hemoglobin)

The decision to transfuse is based on the risk that anemia poses to an individual patient and the patient's ability to compensate for decreased oxygen-carrying capacity, as well as the inherent risks associated with transfusion. Otherwise, healthy patients with hemoglobin values greater than 10 g/dL rarely require transfusion, whereas those with hemoglobin values less than 6 g/dL almost always require transfusion, especially when anemia or surgical bleeding (or both) is acute and continuing. Determination of whether intermediate hemoglobin concentrations (6 to 10 g/dL) justify or require transfusion should be based on the patient's risk for complications of inadequate oxygenation. For example, certain clinical situations (coronary artery disease, chronic lung disease, surgery associated with large blood loss) may warrant transfusion of blood at a higher hemoglobin value than in otherwise healthy patients. A hemoglobin concentration of 8 g/dL may be an appropriate threshold for transfusion in surgical patients with no risk factors for ischemia, whereas a transfusion threshold of 10 g/dL may be justified in patients who are considered to be at risk (emphysema, coronary artery disease).

Controlled studies to determine the hemoglobin concentration at which blood transfusion improves outcome in a surgical patient with acute blood loss are few; most studies have been conducted in nonsurgical patients.[3-6] Furthermore, there is no evidence that mild to moderate anemia impairs wound healing, increases bleeding, or alters the patient's length of stay in the hospital.

Transfusion of packed red blood cells in patients with hemoglobin concentrations higher than 10 to 12 g/dL does not substantially increase oxygen delivery. Further decreases in the hemoglobin concentration can sometimes be offset by increases in cardiac output. The exact hemoglobin value at which cardiac output increases varies among individuals and is influenced by age, whether the anemia is acute or chronic, and sometimes anesthesia. The focus on hemoglobin has existed for many years and is still contemporary.[1,7-9] Perhaps the development of a more sensitive indication of tissue oxygenation will provide better indicators for transfusion in the future.[10]

BLOOD COMPONENTS

Packed Red Blood Cells

Packed red blood cells (250- to 300-mL volume with a hematocrit of 70% to 80%) are used for treatment of the anemia usually associated with surgical blood loss. The major goal is to increase the oxygen-carrying capacity of blood. Although packed red blood cells can increase intravascular fluid volume, nonblood products, such as crystalloids and colloids, can also achieve that end point. A single unit of packed red blood cells will increase adult hemoglobin concentrations about 1 g/dL. Administration of packed red blood cells can be facilitated by reconstituting them in crystalloid solutions, such as 50 to 100 mL of saline. The use of hypotonic glucose solutions may theoretically cause hemolysis, whereas the calcium present in lactated Ringer's solution may cause clotting if mixed with packed red blood cells.

COMPLICATIONS

Complications associated with packed red blood cells are similar to those of whole blood. An exception would be the chance for development of citrate intoxication, which would be less with packed red blood cells than with whole blood because less citrate is infused. Removal of plasma decreases the concentration of factors I (fibrinogen), V, and VIII as compared with whole blood.

DECISION TO ADMINISTER PACKED RED BLOOD CELLS

The decision to administer packed red blood cells should be based on measured blood loss and inadequate oxygen-carrying capacity.

Acute Blood Loss

Acute blood loss in the range of 1500 to 2000 mL (approximately 30% of an adult patient's blood volume) may exceed the ability of crystalloids to replace blood volume without jeopardizing the oxygen-carrying capacity of the blood. Hypotension and tachycardia are likely, but these compensatory responses may be blunted by anesthesia or other drugs (β-adrenergic blocking drugs). Compensatory vasoconstriction may conceal the signs of acute blood loss until at least 10% of the blood volume is lost, and healthy patients may lose up to 20% of their blood volume before signs of hypovolemia occur. To ensure an adequate oxygen content in blood, packed red blood cells should be administered when blood loss is sufficiently large. When available, whole blood may be preferable to packed red blood cells when replacing blood losses that exceed 30% of the blood volume.

With acute blood loss, interstitial fluid and extravascular protein are transferred to the intravascular space, which tends to maintain plasma volume. For this reason, when crystalloid solutions are used to replace blood loss, they should be given in amounts equal to about three times the amount of blood loss, not only to replenish intravascular fluid volume but also to replenish the fluid lost from interstitial spaces. Albumin and hetastarch are examples of solutions that are useful for acute expansion of the intravascular fluid volume. In contrast to crystalloid solutions, albumin and hetastarch are more likely to remain in the intravascular space for prolonged periods (about 12 hours). These solutions avoid complications associated with blood-containing products but do not improve the oxygen-carrying capacity of the blood and, in large volumes (>20 mL/kg), may cause coagulation defects.

Platelet Concentrates

Platelet concentrates allow specific treatment of thrombocytopenia without the infusion of unnecessary blood

III

components. During surgery, platelet transfusions are probably not required unless the platelet count is less than 50,000 cells/mm^3 as determined by laboratory analysis. One unit of platelet concentrate will increase the platelet count 5000 to 10,000 cells/mm^3 as documented by platelet counts obtained 1 hour after infusion.

COMPLICATIONS

The risks associated with platelet concentrate infusions are (1) sensitization reactions because of human leukocyte antigens on the cell membranes of platelets and (2) transmission of infectious diseases. One of the leading causes of transfusion-related fatalities in the United States is bacterial contamination, which is mostly likely to occur in platelet concentrates (Table 24-2). Platelet-related sepsis can be fatal and occurs as frequently as 1 in 5000 transfusions; it is probably under-recognized because of the many other confounding variables present in critically ill patients. When donor platelets are cultured before infusion, the incidence of sepsis may be reduced to less than 1 in 50,000. The fact that platelets are stored at 20°C to 24°C instead of 4°C probably accounts for the greater risk of bacterial growth than with other blood products.[11,12] As a result, any patient in whom a fever develops within 6 hours of receiving platelet transfusions should be considered to possibly be manifesting platelet-induced sepsis, and empirical antibiotic therapy should be instituted.

Fresh Frozen Plasma

Fresh frozen plasma (FFP) is the fluid portion obtained from a single unit of whole blood that is frozen within 6 hours of collection. All coagulation factors, except platelets, are present in FFP, which explains the use of this component for the treatment of hemorrhage from presumed coagulation factor deficiencies. FFP transfusions during surgery are probably not necessary unless the prothrombin time (PT) or partial thromboplastin time (PTT), or both, are at least 1.5 times longer than normal. Other indications for FFP are urgent reversal of warfarin and management of heparin resistance.

Cryoprecipitate

Cryoprecipitate is the fraction of plasma that precipitates when FFP is thawed. This component is useful for treating hemophilia A (contains high concentrations of factor VIII in a small volume) that is unresponsive to desmopressin. Cryoprecipitate can also be used to treat hypofibrinogenemia (as induced by packed red blood cells) because it contains more fibrinogen than FFP does.

Albumin

Albumin is available as 5% and 25% solutions. The 5% solution is isotonic with pooled plasma and is most often used when rapid expansion of intravascular fluid volume is indicated. Hypoalbuminemia is the most frequent indication for the administration of 25% albumin. It must be recognized that albumin solutions do not provide coagulation factors. Increased mortality has been described in critically ill patients receiving albumin.[13] Therefore, the overall efficacy of albumin administration may be questioned.[14] Plasma protein fractions (Plasmanate) are 5% solutions of plasma proteins in saline. The risk for transmission of hepatitis with all protein solutions is eliminated by heat treatment at 60°C for 10 hours.

Hydroxyethyl Starch

Hetastarch is a synthetic colloid that is a 6% solution in 0.9% saline (Hespan).[15] Its osmolarity is about 310 mOsm/L. When doses in excess of 20 mL/kg are given, factor VIII can be reduced with prolongation of the PTT.

Hextend is a colloid with smaller molecules. It is 6% hetastarch in a solution that contains physiologic concentrations of electrolytes. Whether it has a lesser effect on factor VIII remains to be determined. Pentastarch is another lower-molecular-mass hetastarch that is under study.

COMPLICATIONS OF BLOOD THERAPY

Complications of blood therapy, like an adverse effect of any therapy, must be considered when evaluating the risk-to-benefit ratio for treatment of individual patients with blood products. The risk of having a fatal outcome from blood transfusion is remote but possible. The leading causes of a fatal outcome from blood transfusion are bacterial contamination, transfusion-related acute lung injury (TRALI), and ABO mismatch (see Table 24-2).

Anesthesiologists are among the most likely physicians to administer blood products to patients; therefore, it is imperative that complications of this therapy be fully appreciated. Transmission of infectious diseases, hepatitis,

Table 24-2 Transfusion-Related Fatalities in the United States, 2001-2002

Cause of Fatalities	Number of Fatalities
Bacterial contamination	17
Transfusion-related acute lung injury	16
Mistransfusion: ABO mismatch	14

Data from the Food and Drug Administration, October 1, 2001, to September 30, 2002.

and human immunodeficiency virus (HIV) and hemolytic transfusion reactions are probably the most feared complications of transfusion therapy, but they are now not the most common. These fears have even raised the concern that transfusions are sometimes underused.[16]

Transmission of Infectious Diseases

The incidence of infection from blood transfusions has markedly decreased. For example, in 1980, the incidence of hepatitis was as high as 10%. Improved donor blood testing has dramatically decreased the risk of transmission of hepatitis C and HIV to less than 1 in 1 million transfusions (Table 24-3).[11] Although many factors account for the marked decreased incidence of transmission of infectious agents by blood transfusion, the most important one is improved testing of donor blood. Currently, hepatitis C, HIV, and West Nile virus (WNV) are tested by nucleic acid technology. In 2002, more than 30 cases of transfusion-transmitted WNV occurred. By 2003, nearly universal screening of donor blood by nucleic acid technology has reduced the incidence to that of HIV.[11]

Other less commonly transmitted infectious agents include hepatitis B, human T-cell lymphotropic virus, cytomegalovirus, malaria, Chagas' disease, and possibly variant Creutzfeldt-Jakob disease.

Transfusion-Related Acute Lung Injury (TRALI)

Although bacterial contamination of blood was the leading cause of transfusion-induced fatalities in 2001-2002 (see Table 24-2), TRALI has become number 1 in 2005. TRALI is respiratory distress syndrome that occurs within 6 hours after transfusion of a blood product such as packed red blood cells or FFP. It is characterized by dyspnea and arterial hypoxemia secondary to noncardiogenic pulmonary edema. The diagnosis of TRALI is confirmed when pulmonary edema occurs in the absence of left atrial hypertension and the pulmonary edema fluid has a high protein content. Immediate actions to take when TRALI is suspected include (1) stopping the trans-

fusion, (2), supporting the patient's vital signs, (3) determining the protein concentration of the pulmonary edema fluid via the endotracheal tube, (4) obtaining a complete blood count and chest radiograph, and (5) notifying the blood bank of possible TRALI so that other associated units can be quarantined.

Because the diagnosis is sometimes difficult to make, follow-up paperwork is especially important, including sending a blood specimen and bags of units of blood given to the blood bank. All copies of transfusion forms and anesthetic records will be required by the blood bank.

Transfusion-Related Immunomodulation

Blood transfusion suppresses cell-mediated immunity, which when combined with similar effects produced by surgical trauma, may place patients at risk for postoperative infection.[17,18] The association with long-term prognosis in cancer surgery is unclear, but there is a suggestion of a correlation between tumor recurrence and blood transfusions. Conversely, patients who receive blood transfusions may have more extensive disease and a poorer prognosis independent of the administration of blood. As such, the role of blood transfusions in postoperative infections and cancer is difficult to ascertain. Packed red blood cells, which contain less plasma than whole blood does, may produce less immunosuppression, thus suggesting that plasma contains an undefined immunosuppressive factor.

Removing most of the white blood cells from blood and platelets (leukoreduction) is becoming increasingly common. This practice reduces the incidence of nonhemolytic febrile transfusion reactions and the transmission of leukocyte-associated viruses. Other possible benefits (reduction of cancer recurrence and postoperative infections) are more speculative.

Metabolic Abnormalities

Metabolic abnormalities that accompany the storage of whole blood include accumulation of hydrogen ions and potassium and decreased 2,3-DPG concentrations. The citrate present in the blood preservative may produce changes in the recipient.

HYDROGEN IONS

The addition of most preservatives promptly increases the hydrogen ion content of stored whole blood. Continued metabolic function of erythrocytes results in additional production of hydrogen ions. Despite these changes, metabolic acidosis is not a consistent occurrence in recipients of blood products, even with rapid infusion of large volumes of stored blood. Therefore, intravenous administration of sodium bicarbonate to patients receiving transfusions of whole blood should be determined by measurement of pH and not be based on arbitrary regimens.

Table 24-3 Estimated Risk of Infection Transmitted by Blood Transfusion	
Hepatitis B	1 in 220,000
Hepatitis C	1 in 1.6 million
HIV	1 in 1.8 million
HTLV-I	1 in 640,000
West Nile virus	1 in >1 million

HIV, human immunodeficiency virus; HTLV-I, human T-cell lymphotropic virus type I.

POTASSIUM

The potassium content of stored blood increases progressively with the duration of storage, but even massive transfusions rarely increase plasma potassium concentrations. Failure of plasma potassium concentrations to increase most likely reflects the small amount of potassium actually present in 1 unit of stored blood. For example, because 1 unit of whole blood contains only 300 mL of plasma, a measured potassium concentration of 21 mEq/L would represent the administration of less than 7 mEq of potassium to the patient.

Decreased 2,3-Diphosphoglycerate

Storage of blood is associated with a progressive decrease in concentrations of 2,3-DPG in erythrocytes, which results in increased affinity of hemoglobin for oxygen (decreased P_{50} values). Conceivably, this increased affinity could make less oxygen available for tissues and jeopardize tissue oxygen delivery. There is speculation that fresh blood (with more oxygen available for tissues) should be used for critically ill patients. Despite these observations, the clinical significance of the 2,3-DPG oxygen affinity changes remains unconfirmed.

Citrate

Citrate metabolism to bicarbonate may contribute to metabolic alkalosis, whereas binding of calcium by citrate could result in hypocalcemia. Indeed, metabolic alkalosis rather than metabolic acidosis can follow massive blood transfusions. Hypocalcemia as a result of citrate binding of calcium is rare because of mobilization of calcium stores from bone and the ability of the liver to rapidly metabolize citrate to bicarbonate. Therefore, arbitrary administration of calcium in the absence of objective evidence of hypocalcemia (prolonged QT intervals on the electrocardiogram, measured decrease in plasma ionized calcium concentrations) is not indicated. Supplemental calcium may be needed when (1) the rate of blood infusion is more rapid than 50 mL/min, (2) hypothermia or liver disease interferes with the metabolism of citrate, or (3) the patient is a neonate. Patients undergoing liver transplantation are the most likely to experience citrate intoxication, and these patients may require calcium administration during a massive transfusion of stored blood.

Hypothermia

Administration of blood stored at below 6°C can result in a decrease in the patient's body temperature, with the possible development of cardiac irritability. Even a decrease in body temperature as small as 0.5°C to 1°C may induce shivering postoperatively, which in turn may increase oxygen consumption by as much as 400%. To meet the demands of increased oxygen consumption, cardiac output must be increased. Passage of blood through specially designed warmers greatly decreases the likelihood of transfusion-related hypothermia. Unrecognized malfunction of these warmers, causing them to overheat, may result in hemolysis of the blood being transfused.

Coagulation

The conclusion that excessive microvascular bleeding is occurring should be the combined judgment of both the surgical and anesthesia teams. Laboratory tests are only a supplement to clinically determined excessive microvascular bleeding. Blood loss should be determined by checking suction canisters, surgical sponges, and drains. A decision needs to be made regarding whether the blood loss is from inadequate surgical control of vascular bleeding or a coagulopathy. A platelet count, PT or international normalized ratio (INR), PTT, and fibrinogen level can confirm both the presence and type of coagulopathy. Platelet concentrates may be administered if the platelet count is less than 50,000 cells/mm³. A qualitative platelet defect (antiplatelet drugs, cardiopulmonary bypass) may require platelet concentrates to be given even with a normal platelet count.

TREATMENT OF EXCESSIVE MICROVASCULAR BLEEDING

Administration of FFP should be considered when the PT is greater than 1.5 times normal or the INR more than 2.0 and if laboratory tests are unavailable, more than one blood volume (about 70 mL/kg) has been given, and excessive microvascular bleeding is present. The dose of FFP (10 to 15 mL/kg) should achieve at least 30% of most plasma factor concentrations.

Cryoprecipitate should be considered if fibrinogen levels are less than 150 mg/dL. In addition, desmopressin or a topical hemostatic (fibrin glue) may be used for excessive bleeding. Recombinant activated factor VII may be considered as a "rescue" drug when standard therapy has failed to successfully treat a coagulopathy (microvascular bleeding).[18] It apparently enhances thrombin generation on already activated platelets.

Transfusion Reactions

Although transfusion reactions are traditionally categorized as febrile, allergic, and hemolytic, anesthesia, especially general anesthesia, may mask the signs and symptoms of all types of transfusion reactions.[19] The possibility of a transfusion reaction during anesthesia should be suspected in the presence of hyperthermia, increased peak airway pressure, or an acute change in urine output or color.

In considering the occurrence of transfusion reactions, it is important to periodically check for signs and symptoms of bacterial contamination, TRALI, and hemolytic transfusion reactions, including urticaria, hypotension, tachycardia, increased peak airway pressure, hyperthermia, decreased urine output, hemoglobinuria, and microvascular bleeding.[1] Before instituting therapy for transfusion reactions, stop the blood transfusion and order appropriate diagnostic testing.[1]

FEBRILE REACTIONS

Febrile reactions are the most common adverse nonhemolytic response to the transfusion of blood, and they accompany 0.5% to 1% of transfusions. The most likely explanation for febrile reactions is an interaction between recipient antibodies and antigens present on the leukocytes or platelets of the donor. The patient's temperature rarely increases above 38°C, and the condition is treated by slowing the infusion and administering antipyretics. Severe febrile reactions accompanied by chills and shivering may require discontinuation of the blood transfusion.

ALLERGIC REACTIONS

Allergic reactions to properly typed and cross-matched blood are manifested as increases in body temperature, pruritus, and urticaria. Treatment often includes intravenous administration of antihistamines and, in severe cases, discontinuation of the blood transfusion. Examination of plasma and urine for free hemoglobin is useful to rule out hemolytic reactions.

HEMOLYTIC REACTIONS

Hemolytic reactions occur when the wrong blood type is administered to a patient. The common factor in the production of intravascular hemolysis and the development of spontaneous hemorrhage is activation of the complement system. With the exception of hypotension, the immediate signs (lumbar and substernal pain, fever, chills, dyspnea, skin flushing) of hemolytic reactions are masked by general anesthesia. Even hypotension may be attributed to other causes in an anesthetized patient. The appearance of free hemoglobin in plasma or urine is presumptive evidence of a hemolytic reaction. Acute renal failure reflects precipitation of stromal and lipid contents (not free hemoglobin) of hemolyzed erythrocytes in distal renal tubules. Disseminated intravascular coagulation causing a coagulopathy is initiated by material released from hemolyzed erythrocytes.

Treatment

Treatment of acute hemolytic reactions is immediate discontinuation of the incompatible blood transfusion and maintenance of urine output by infusion of crystalloid solutions and administration of mannitol or furosemide. The use of sodium bicarbonate to alkalinize the urine and improve the solubility of hemoglobin degradation products in the renal tubules is of unproven value, as is the administration of corticosteroids.

AUTOLOGOUS BLOOD

Types of autologous blood transfusion are (1) predeposited (preoperative) autologous donation (PAD), (2) intraoperative and postoperative blood salvage, and (3) normovolemic hemodilution. Two primary reasons for the use of autologous blood are to decrease or eliminate complications from allogeneic blood transfusions and to conserve blood resources. In the 1980s, both patient and physician fear escalated because of a legitimate concern regarding infectious diseases, especially hepatitis C and HIV. Although there is still an inherent belief that PAD blood is safer, the markedly reduced rate of infectious disease transmission from allogeneic blood makes that view difficult to prove. Furthermore, PAD blood is more expensive and not very effective in reducing allogeneic blood transfusion. Therefore, PAD is not generally a cost-effective alternative to allogeneic blood.

Predeposited Autologous Donation

Patients scheduled for elective surgery that may require transfusion of blood may choose to predonate (predeposit) blood for possible transfusion in the perioperative period. Patient-donors must have a hemoglobin concentration of at least 11 g/dL. Most patients can donate 10.5 mL/kg of blood approximately every 5 to 7 days (maximum, 2 to 3 units), with the last unit collected 72 hours or more before surgery to permit restoration of plasma volume. Oral iron supplementation is recommended when blood is withdrawn within a few days preceding surgery. Treatment with recombinant erythropoietin is very expensive, but it increases the amount of blood that patients can predeposit by as much as 25%.

Intraoperative and Postoperative Blood Salvage

Intraoperative blood salvage for reinfusion into the patient decreases the amount of allogeneic blood needed. Typically, semiautomated systems are used in which the red blood cells are collected and washed and then delivered to a reservoir for future administration either intraoperatively or postoperatively. The presence of infection or malignant disease at the operative site is considered a contraindication to blood salvage. Complications of intraoperative salvage include dilutional coagulopathy, reinfusion of excessive anticoagulant (heparin), hemolysis, air embolism, and disseminated intravascular coagulation. A documented quality assurance program, as recommended by the American Association of Blood Banks, is required for those who use intraoperative salvage techniques.

Normovolemic Hemodilution

Normovolemic hemodilution consists of withdrawing a portion of the patient's blood volume early in the intra-

III

operative period and concurrent infusion of crystalloids or colloids to maintain intravascular volume. The end point is a hematocrit of 27% to 33%, depending on the patient's cardiovascular and respiratory status. By initially hemodiluting the patient, fewer red blood cells will be lost per millimeter of blood loss during surgery. At the conclusion of surgery, the patient's blood, with its enhanced oxygen-carrying capacity by virtue of a higher hematocrit and its greater clotting ability by virtue of platelets and other coagulation factors, is reinfused. Whether the use of this technique actually decreases allogeneic blood administration is questionable. The survival of recovered red blood cells appears to be similar to that of transfused allogeneic cells.

REFERENCES

1. ASA Task Force. Practice guidelines for blood therapy. Anesthesiology (in press).
2. Stoneham MD. Less is more: Using systolic blood pressure variation to assess hypovolemia. Br J Anaesth 1999;83:550.
3. Hebert PC, Fergusson DA. Red blood cell transfusion in critically ill patients. JAMA 2002;288:1525.
4. Vincent JL, Baron JF, Reinhart K, et al. Anemia and blood transfusion in critically ill patients. JAMA 2002; 288:1499.
5. Walsh TS, McClelland DBL. When should we transfuse critically ill and perioperative patients with coronary artery disease? Br J Anaesth 2003; 90:709.
6. Ely EW, Bernard GR. Transfusion in critically ill patients. N Engl J Med 1999;340:467.
7. Miller RD, Von Ehrenberg W. Should the same indication be used for autologous and homologous transfusions? Transfusion 1995;35:703.
8. Miller RD, Stehling L. What is the transfusion trigger? What is the message? Anesthesiology 1997;86:750.
9. Thurer RL. Evaluating transfusion triggers. JAMA 1998;279:238.
10. Sehgal LR, Zebala LP, Takagi I, et al. Evaluation of oxygen extraction ratio as a physiologic transfusion trigger in coronary artery bypass graft surgery patients. Transfusion 2001;41:591.
11. Busch MP, Kleinman SH, Nemo GJ. Current and emerging infectious risks of blood transfusions. JAMA 2003; 289:959.
12. Snyder EL, Rinder HM. Platelet storage—time to come in from the cold? N Engl J Med 2003;348:2032.
13. Vincent JL, Wilkes NM, Navickis RJ. Safety of human albumin—serious adverse events reported world wide in 1998-2002. Br J Anaesth 2003;91:625.
14. Offringa M. Excess mortality after human albumin administration in critically ill patients: Clinical and pathophysiological evidence suggests albumin is harmful. BMJ 1998;317:223.
15. Friedman Z, Berkenstadt H, Preisman S, et al. A comparison of lactated Ringer's solution to hydroxy ethyl starch 6% in bleeding in dogs. Anesth Analg 2003;96:39.
16. Sexena S, Wehrli G, Markarewicz K, et al. Monitoring for underutilization of RBC components and platelets. Transfusion 2001;41:587.
17. Corwin HL, AuBuchon JP. Is leukoreduction of blood components for everyone? JAMA 2003;289:1993.
18. Weiskopf RB. Intraoperative use of recombinant activated coagulation factor VII. Anesthesiology 2002; 96:1287.
19. Kopke PM, Holland PV. Mechanisms of severe transfusion reaction. Transfus Clin Biol 2001;8:278.

SPECIAL ANESTHETIC CONSIDERATIONS

CARDIOVASCULAR DISEASE

Art Wallace

Cardiovascular disease is the leading cause of death in the United States, Canada, Europe, and Japan.[1] It is estimated that 8 of every 1000 live births are associated with some form of congenital heart disease (see Chapter 26). Many of the risk factors identified to predict perioperative mortality reflect cardiac disease. Recent myocardial infarction, the presence of congestive heart failure, and aortic stenosis are the highest risk factors. Coronary artery disease (ischemic heart disease), peripheral vascular disease, and risk for coronary artery disease increase operative risk. Management of anesthesia in patients with cardiovascular disease requires (1) an understanding of the pathophysiology of the disease process; (2) appropriate preoperative testing; (3) application of perioperative risk reduction strategies; (4) careful selection of anesthetic, analgesic, and neuromuscular and autonomic blocking drugs; and (5) monitors to match the needs created by this disease.

CORONARY ARTERY DISEASE

Coronary artery disease (ischemic heart disease) is often asymptomatic and is a common accompaniment of aging in the American population. Of the adult patients who undergo surgery annually in the United States, it is estimated that 40% will either have or be at risk for coronary artery disease.[1] The presence of coronary artery disease in patients who undergo anesthesia for noncardiac surgery may be associated with increased morbidity and mortality. The history and physical examination with specific attention to cardiac and pulmonary disease and risks, as well as evaluation of the patient's electrocardiogram (ECG), are important components of routine preoperative cardiac evaluation. Ultimately, the history and physical examination with specific attention to signs and symptoms of new onset of angina, change in angina pattern, unstable angina, recent myocardial infarction, congestive heart failure, or aortic stenosis determine whether patients are in the best medical condition possible before elective cardiac or noncardiac surgery.[2]

Specialized Procedures to Evaluate Cardiac Function

Specialized procedures, such as ambulatory ECG monitoring (Holter monitoring), exercise stress testing, transthoracic or transesophageal echocardiography, radionuclide ventriculography (determination of ejection fraction), dipyridamole-thallium scintigraphy (mimics the coronary vasodilator response but not the heart rate response associated with exercise), cardiac catheterization, and angiography, are performed on selected patients. There is no evidence that echocardiography adds appreciably to the information provided by routine clinical and ECG data for predicting adverse outcomes.[1] Likewise, determination of the ejection fraction does not seem to provide information that improves on the ability to predict the presence of a preoperative myocardial infarction beyond that provided by a careful preoperative clinical evaluation. Thallium scintigraphy, which evaluates the adequacy of coronary blood flow, does not predict patients at risk for perioperative cardiac events.

Patient History

Important aspects of the history taken from patients with coronary artery disease before noncardiac surgery include (1) evaluation of cardiac reserve (exercise tolerance), (2) characteristics of their angina pectoris, (3) previous occurrence of myocardial infarction, and (4) medical, interventional cardiology, and cardiac surgical therapy for these conditions. Potential interactions of medications used in the treatment of coronary artery disease with drugs used to produce anesthesia must also be considered. Coexisting noncardiac diseases that are often present in these patients include systemic hypertension, peripheral vascular disease, chronic obstructive pulmonary disease from cigarette smoking, renal dysfunction associated with chronic hypertension, and diabetes mellitus.

CARDIAC RESERVE

Limited exercise tolerance in the absence of significant pulmonary disease is the most striking evidence of decreased cardiac reserve. Inability to lie flat, awakening from sleep with angina or shortness of breath, or angina at rest or with minimal exertion is evidence of significant cardiac disease. If a patient can climb two to three flights of stairs without symptoms, cardiac reserve is probably adequate.

ANGINA PECTORIS

Angina pectoris is considered to be stable when no change in precipitating factors, frequency, and duration has occurred for at least 60 days. Chest pain produced with less than normal activity and lasting for increasingly

longer periods is considered characteristic of unstable angina pectoris and may signal an impending myocardial infarction. Dyspnea after the onset of angina pectoris may be indicative of acute left ventricular dysfunction secondary to myocardial ischemia. Angina pectoris caused by spasm of the coronary arteries (variant or Prinzmetal's angina) differs from classic angina pectoris in that it may occur at rest and then be absent during vigorous exertion. Silent myocardial ischemia does not evoke angina pectoris (asymptomatic) and usually occurs at a heart rate and systemic blood pressure lower than that present during exercise-induced myocardial ischemia. It is estimated that about 70% of ischemic episodes are not associated with angina pectoris and as many as 15% of acute myocardial infarctions are silent. Females and individuals with diabetes mellitus are more likely to have painless myocardial ischemia and infarctions.

The heart rate or systolic blood pressure (or both) at which angina pectoris or evidence of myocardial ischemia is indicated on the ECG is useful preoperative information. An increased heart rate is more likely than systemic hypertension to produce signs of myocardial ischemia (Fig. 25-1).[3] Tachycardia increases myocardial oxygen requirements while at the same time decreasing the duration of diastole, thereby reducing coronary blood flow and delivery of oxygen to the left ventricle. Conversely, increased systolic and diastolic blood pressure, though increasing oxygen consumption, simultaneously increases coronary perfusion through pressure-dependent atherosclerotic coronary arteries.

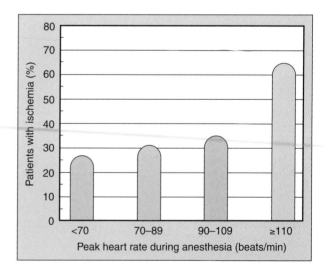

Figure 25-1 The incidence of myocardial ischemia rises with increases in heart rate, with the greatest effect at heart rates greater than 110 beats/min. (From Slogoff S, Keats AS. Does chronic treatment with calcium entry blocking drugs reduce perioperative myocardial ischemia? Anesthesiology 1988;68:676-680, with permission.)

PREVIOUS MYOCARDIAL INFARCTION

The incidence of myocardial reinfarction in the perioperative period is related to the time elapsed since the previous myocardial infarction (Table 25-1).[4-7] The incidence of perioperative myocardial reinfarction generally does not stabilize at 5% to 6% until 6 months after the previous myocardial infarction. Thus, a common recommendation is to delay elective surgery, especially thoracic, upper abdominal, or other major procedures, for a period (2 to 6 months) after a myocardial infarction, but the exact period of suggested delay is not clear. Even after 6 months, the 5% to 6% incidence of myocardial reinfarction is about 50 times greater than the 0.13% incidence of perioperative myocardial infarction in patients undergoing similar operations but in the absence of a previous myocardial infarction. Most perioperative myocardial reinfarctions occur in the first 48 to 72 hours postoperatively. However, if myocardial ischemia is initiated by the stress of surgery, there can be an increased risk for myocardial infarction for several months after surgery.

FACTORS THAT INCREASE THE RISK FOR PERIOPERATIVE MYOCARDIAL INFARCTION

Factors that predispose to myocardial reinfarction include (1) the site of the previous myocardial infarction, (2) a history of prior coronary artery bypass graft (CABG) surgery, (3) intrathoracic or intra-abdominal operations lasting longer than 3 hours, (4) the site of the operative procedure if the duration of the surgery is less than 3 hours, and (5) techniques used to produce anesthesia. Perioperative β-blockade started 7 to 30 days before surgery and continued for 30 days postoperatively has been shown to reduce the risk for cardiac morbidity (myocardial infarction or cardiac death) by 90%.[8] Perioperative β-blockade started just before surgery and continued for 7 days reduces the risk for mortality by 50%.[9] Perioperative clonidine administration reduces the risk for 30-day and 2-year mortality.[10] Close hemodynamic monitoring with an intra-arterial and pulmonary artery catheter (alternatively, transesophageal echocardiography) and prompt pharmacologic intervention with fluid infusion to treat physiologic hemodynamic alterations from the normal range may decrease the risk for perioperative cardiac morbidity in high-risk patients (see Table 25-1).[4-7]

CURRENT MEDICATIONS

Drugs most likely to be encountered in patients with coronary artery disease are β-antagonists, nitrates, calcium channel blockers, angiotensin-converting enzyme inhibitors, lipid-lowering agents, diuretics, and platelet inhibitors. Knowledge of the pharmacology of these drugs and potential adverse interactions with anesthetics is an important preoperative consideration. All patients with known coronary artery disease, known peripheral vascular disease, or two risk factors for coronary artery disease (age ≥60 years, systemic hypertension, diabetes mellitus, significant smoking history, or cholesterol >240 mg/dL) should receive perioperative β-blockers unless there is a specific contraindication. Reactive asthma, but not chronic obstructive pulmonary disease is a contraindication to perioperative β-blockade. In patients who cannot tolerate β-blockers, the α_2-agonist clonidine may be used.[10] Despite the potential for adverse drug interactions, cardiac medications being taken preoperatively should be continued without interruption through the perioperative period. Discontinuation of β-blockers, calcium channel blockers, nitrates, or angiotensin-converting enzyme inhibitors in the perioperative period increases perioperative morbidity and mortality and should be avoided.

Electrocardiogram

The preoperative ECG should be examined for evidence of (1) myocardial ischemia, (2) previous myocardial infarction, (3) cardiac hypertrophy, (4) abnormal cardiac rhythm or conduction disturbances (or both), and (5) electrolyte abnormalities. The exercise ECG simulates sympathetic nervous system activity, as may accompany perioperative events such as direct laryngoscopy, tracheal intubation, and surgical incision. The resting ECG in the absence of angina pectoris may be normal despite extensive coronary artery disease. Nevertheless, an ECG demonstrating ST-segment depression greater than 1 mm, particularly during angina pectoris, confirms the presence of myocardial ischemia. Furthermore, the ECG lead demonstrating changes of myocardial ischemia can help determine the specific diseased coronary artery (Table 25-2). It should be remembered that a previous myocar-

IV

Table 25-1 Incidence of Perioperative Myocardial Infarction

Time Elapsed Since Previous Myocardial Infarction	Tarhan et al[4]	Steen et al[5]	Rao et al[6]	Shah et al[7]
0-3 months	37%	27%	5.7%	4.3%
4 to 6 months	16%	11%	2.3%	0
>6 months	5%	6%		5.7%

Table 25-2 Area of Myocardial Ischemia as Reflected by the Electrocardiogram

Electrocardiogram Lead	Coronary Artery Responsible for Myocardial Ischemia	Area of Myocardium That May Be Involved
II, III, aVF	Right coronary artery	Right atrium Sinus node Atrioventricular node Right ventricle
V_3-V_5	Left anterior descending coronary artery	Anterolateral aspects of the left ventricle
I, aVL	Circumflex coronary artery	Lateral aspects of the left ventricle

dial infarction, especially if subendocardial, may not be accompanied by persistent changes on the ECG. The preoperative presence of ventricular premature beats may signal their probable occurrence intraoperatively. A prolonged PR interval (>0.2 second) on the ECG may be related to digitalis therapy. Conversely, block of conduction of cardiac impulses below the atrioventricular node (right bundle branch block, left bundle branch block, intraventricular conduction delay) most likely reflects pathologic changes rather than drug effect.

Risk Stratification versus Risk Reduction

One of the standard approaches to the perioperative care of patients with cardiac disease is risk stratification. Risk stratification consists of a preoperative history and physical examination, followed by a series of tests thought to predict perioperative cardiac morbidity and mortality. The results of these tests (Persantine thallium scintigraphy, echocardiography, Holter monitoring, dobutamine stress echocardiography, angiography) can justify subsequent angioplasty with or without an intracoronary stent or CABG surgery. However, there is no evidence suggesting that preoperative risk stratification with invasive testing is superior to a careful history and physical examination, followed by prophylactic medical therapy.[3,8-10] Furthermore, no evidence exists that combining the risk of angiography and an intracoronary stent or CABG with a surgical procedure reduces total risk. The combined risk of two procedures exceeds that of the original operation.[11] Perioperative risk reduction therapy with β-blockers and clonidine may be superior to risk stratification with invasive testing, angioplasty, and CABG.[11,12]

PERIOPERATIVE CARDIAC RISK REDUCTION THERAPY

Recommendations have been established for the administration of prophylactic medical therapy to stable patients with known coronary artery disease or at risk for such disease (Fig. 25-2).[8-10] All patients who either have coronary artery disease, peripheral vascular disease, or two risk factors for coronary artery disease should receive perioperative β-blockers unless they have a specific intolerance to these drugs (see the section "Current Medications"). If a patient has an absolute contraindication to perioperative β-blockers, clonidine may be used as an alternative.

Management of Anesthesia

Intraoperative anesthetic management, as well as postoperative pain management in patients with coronary artery disease, should permit modulation of sympathetic nervous system responses and provide for rigorous control of hemodynamic variables.[1] In this regard, management of anesthesia in these patients is based on preoperative evaluation of left ventricular function and maintenance of a favorable balance between myocardial oxygen requirements and myocardial oxygen delivery so that myocardial ischemia is prevented (Tables 25-3 and 25-4). Any event associated with persistent tachycardia, systolic hypertension, arterial hypoxemia, or diastolic hypotension can adversely influence this delicate balance.

It is critical that persistent and excessive changes in heart rate and systemic blood pressure be minimized (see Fig. 25-1).[3] A common recommendation is to maintain heart rate and systemic blood pressure within 20% of awake values. Monitoring with an intra-arterial catheter greatly improves the ability to maintain stable systemic blood pressure. Nevertheless, an estimated half of all new perioperative ischemic episodes are not preceded by or associated with significant changes in heart rate or systemic blood pressure. A single 1-minute episode of myocardial ischemia detected by 1-mm ST-segment elevation or depression on the ECG increases the risk for cardiac events 10-fold and for death 2-fold.[13] Tachycardia (>105 beats/min) for 5 minutes in the postoperative period can increase the risk for death 10-fold. The only clinically proven method to reduce the risk for perioperative myocardial ischemia and associated death is perioperative β-blocker (atenolol or metoprolol) or α_2-agonist (clonidine) therapy. Vasoconstrictors, β-agonists, β-blockers, anticholinergics, and vasodilators should be immediately available.

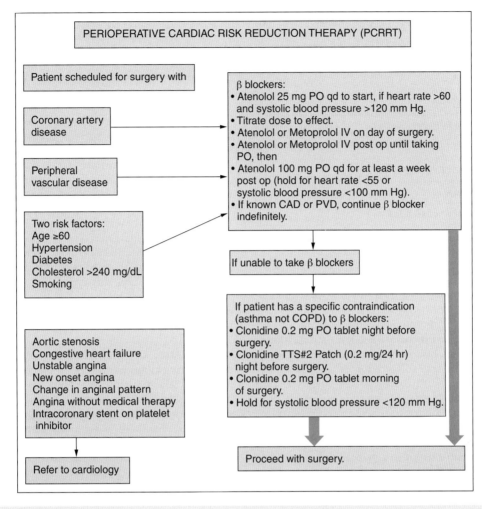

Figure 25-2 Protocol for perioperative cardiac risk reduction therapy with β-blockers and clonidine. All patients with known coronary artery disease (CAD), vascular disease, or two risk factors for CAD should receive prophylactic anti-ischemic therapy with a long-acting β-blocker unless there is a specific contraindication. In patients with a contraindication to β-blockade, prophylactic therapy with clonidine is an alternative.[9-13] COPD, chronic obstructive pulmonary disease; PVD, peripheral vascular disease.

Table 25-3   Evaluation of Left Ventricular Function

	Good Function	Impaired Function
Previous myocardial infarction	No	Yes
Evidence of congestive heart failure	No	Yes
Ejection fraction	>0.55	<0.4
Left ventricular end-diastolic pressure	<12 mm Hg	>18 mm Hg
Cardiac index	>2.5 L/min/m²	<2 L/min/m²
Areas of ventricular dyskinesia	No	Yes

Table 25-4 Determinants of Myocardial Oxygen Requirements and Delivery
Myocardial Oxygen Requirements
Heart rate
Systolic blood pressure
Myocardial contractility
Ventricular volume
Myocardial Oxygen Delivery
Coronary blood flow
Oxygen content of arterial blood

PREOPERATIVE MEDICATION

Preoperative anxiety can lead to preoperative myocardial ischemia. Preoperative β-blocker therapy or clonidine reduces the incidence of myocardial ischemia. Patients should receive their routine medications except for oral hypoglycemic agents. Preoperative sedative medication is intended to produce sedation and reduce anxiety, which if unopposed, could lead to secretion of catecholamines and an increase in myocardial oxygen requirements because of an increase in heart rate and systemic blood pressure. Oral administration of benzodiazepines is an effective pharmacologic approach that is frequently selected to allay anxiety. Supplemental oxygen may be useful, especially if opioids are combined with benzodiazepines for sedation.

INDUCTION OF ANESTHESIA

Induction of anesthesia is acceptably accomplished with the intravenous administration of rapidly acting drugs. Etomidate is a popular induction drug because of its limited inhibition of the sympathetic nervous system and minimal hemodynamic effects. Propofol is popular because of its antiemetic effects and rapid recovery, but the dose should be reduced to avoid undesirable degrees of hypotension. Fentanyl plus midazolam in combination with an infusion of phenylephrine and a nondepolarizing neuromuscular blocking drug produces minimal changes in systemic blood pressure and heart rate. Ketamine is not popular as an induction drug for patients with coronary disease because of the drug-induced increase in heart rate and systemic blood pressure, which may increase myocardial oxygen requirements. If desflurane is chosen, care should be taken to not increase the dose rapidly to avoid sympathetic nervous system stimulation and associated tachycardia, pulmonary hypertension, and myocardial ischemia.[14]

TRACHEAL INTUBATION

Tracheal intubation is facilitated by the administration of succinylcholine or a nondepolarizing neuromuscular blocking drug. Myocardial ischemia may accompany the tachycardia and hypertension that result from the stimulation induced by direct laryngoscopy before tracheal intubation. A brief duration of direct laryngoscopy (preferably <15 seconds) is important for minimizing the magnitude of these circulatory changes. When the duration of direct laryngoscopy is not likely to be brief or when systemic hypertension coexists, the addition of other drugs to minimize the pressor response produced by direct laryngoscopy and tracheal intubation may be a consideration. For example, laryngotracheal lidocaine (2 mg/kg) administered just before placing the tube in the trachea produces rapid topical anesthesia of the tracheal mucosa and minimizes the magnitude and duration of the systemic blood pressure increase. Likewise, lidocaine (1.5 mg/kg IV) administered just before initiating direct laryngoscopy is efficacious. Opioids (fentanyl, sufentanil, alfentanil, or remifentanil) before initiating direct laryngoscopy reduce the circulatory responses associated with tracheal intubation. β-Blockers are effective in attenuating the heart rate increases associated with tracheal intubation.

MAINTENANCE OF ANESTHESIA

The choice of anesthesia is often based on the patient's left ventricular function (see Table 25-3). For example, in patients with coronary artery disease but normal left ventricular function, tachycardia and systemic hypertension are likely to develop in response to intense stimulation. Controlled myocardial depression produced by a volatile anesthetic, with or without nitrous oxide, may be appropriate if the primary goal is to prevent increased myocardial oxygen requirements. Equally acceptable for maintenance of anesthesia is the use of a nitrous oxide–opioid technique with the addition of a volatile anesthetic as necessary to treat acute increases in systemic blood pressure produced by a change in the level of surgical stimulation. When hypertension is treated with a volatile anesthetic (isoflurane, desflurane, or sevoflurane), the drug-induced decrease in systemic vascular resistance is more responsible for decreases in systemic blood pressure than drug-induced myocardial depression is. The ability to rapidly increase the alveolar concentration of sevoflurane makes this drug uniquely efficacious for treating sudden increases in systemic blood pressure. Abrupt and large increases in the delivered concentration of desflurane may be accompanied by stimulation of the sympathetic nervous system, transient increases in systemic blood pressure, heart rate, and pulmonary artery pressure, and the appearance of myocardial ischemia.[14]

Volatile anesthetics (halothane, isoflurane, sevoflurane, and desflurane) to varying degrees have been shown to induce ischemic preconditioning and may protect the myocardium from subsequent ischemia.[15] All facts considered, volatile anesthetics may either be beneficial in patients with coronary artery disease because they decrease myocardial oxygen requirements and induce ischemic preconditioning or be detrimental because they lower systemic blood pressure and coronary perfusion pressure. A large clinical trial in patients undergoing cardiac surgery failed to demonstrate a difference between halothane, enflurane, isoflurane, or opioid-based anesthetics.[16] Avoiding tachycardia with the use of long-acting β-blockers (metoprolol or atenolol) is more important than the choice of anesthetic.[8-10] Intraoperative bolus doses of short-acting β-blockers (esmolol) have not been shown to be effective in reducing perioperative cardiac risk, thus emphasizing that prophylactic perioperative administration of long-acting β-blockers is needed to produce a beneficial effect in the perioperative period.[10]

Patients with impaired left ventricular function, as associated with a previous myocardial infarction, may not tolerate the direct myocardial depression produced by volatile anesthetics. In such patients, short-acting opioids with nitrous oxide may be a more acceptable selection. It must be remembered that nitrous oxide, when administered to patients who have received opioids for anesthesia, may produce undesirable decreases in systemic blood pressure and cardiac output. High-dose fentanyl (50 to 100 μg/kg IV) or an equivalent dose of sufentanil or alfentanil as the primary anesthetic, with benzodiazepines added to ensure amnesia, has been advocated for patients who cannot tolerate even minimal anesthetic-induced myocardial depression. Nevertheless, there is no evidence to support the superiority of this technique over moderate-dose opioids with an inhaled agent or intravenous anesthetics.[16]

A regional anesthetic may be an appropriate technique in selected patients with coronary artery disease. It is important to realize, however, that flow through critically narrowed coronary arteries is pressure dependent. Therefore, decreases in systemic blood pressure associated with a regional anesthetic that are greater than 20% of the preblock value should probably be treated by the intravenous infusion of crystalloid solutions or a vasoconstrictor (phenylephrine), or both. Phenylephrine improves coronary perfusion pressure, but at the expense of increasing afterload and myocardial oxygen requirements. Nevertheless, the increase in coronary perfusion pressure is likely to more than offset any increase in myocardial oxygen requirements. Perioperative β-blockers or clonidine should be administered to patients with known cardiac risk factors who are undergoing surgery with regional anesthesia.

NEUROMUSCULAR BLOCKING DRUGS

The choice of nondepolarizing neuromuscular blocking drugs during maintenance of anesthesia in patients with coronary artery disease may be influenced by the circulatory effects of these drugs and the probable impact of these changes on myocardial oxygen requirements and myocardial oxygen delivery (see Chapter 12). Vecuronium, rocuronium, and cisatracurium do not evoke histamine release and associated decreases in systemic blood pressure, even with the rapid intravenous administration of large doses. Likewise, the systemic blood pressure–lowering effects of atracurium and mivacurium are usually modest, especially if these drugs are injected over a period of 30 to 45 seconds to minimize the likelihood of drug-induced histamine release. It is unlikely that any of these neuromuscular blocking drugs will adversely alter myocardial oxygen requirements.

Pancuronium increases the heart rate and systemic blood pressure, but these changes are usually less than 15% above predrug values, thus making this drug a possible choice for administration to patients with coronary artery disease. Furthermore, the circulatory changes produced by pancuronium can be used to offset the negative inotropic and chronotropic effects of drugs being used for anesthesia. For example, pancuronium might offset decreases in systemic blood pressure or heart rate associated with the administration of high doses of opioids.

Nondepolarizing neuromuscular blockade in patients with coronary artery disease can be safely antagonized with anticholinesterase drugs combined with an anticholinergic drug. Glycopyrrolate has more titratable chronotropic effects than atropine does. Nevertheless, undesirable increases in heart rate may occur with drug-assisted antagonism of nondepolarizing neuromuscular blocking drugs. One of the common causes of postoperative myocardial ischemia and infarction is tachycardia after emergence, which may be the result of the combination of emergence, surgical pain, and reversal of nondepolarizing neuromuscular blocking drugs. Long-acting intravenous β-blockers may be added to decrease the incidence of tachycardia, which may lead to myocardial ischemia in this period.

MONITORING

The intensity of monitoring in the perioperative period is influenced by the complexity of the operative procedure and the severity of the coronary artery disease. The five-lead ECG serves as a noninvasive monitor of the balance between myocardial oxygen requirements and myocardial oxygen delivery in unconscious patients. When this balance is unfavorably altered, myocardial ischemia occurs, as evidenced on the ECG by at least 1-mm downsloping of the ST segment from baseline. A precordial V_5 lead is a useful selection for detecting ST-segment changes characteristic of ischemia of the left ventricle during anesthesia. Intra-arterial pressure monitoring can speed the identification and treatment of hemodynamic changes. Monitoring should be continuous if possible. Ventricular wall motion abnormalities observed by transesophageal echocardiography may be the most

IV

sensitive indicator of myocardial ischemia, but this monitor is expensive and invasive and requires additional training before use. Indeed, the evidence suggests that intraoperative monitoring of pulmonary artery pressure or the use of transesophageal echocardiography should be reserved for selected high-risk patients (cardiac surgery, recent myocardial infarction, current congestive heart failure, unstable angina).[1]

The appearance of signs of myocardial ischemia on the ECG supports the need for aggressive treatment of adverse changes in heart rate, systemic blood pressure, or both. Tachycardia is treated by the administration of atenolol, metoprolol, propranolol, or esmolol. Excessive increases in systemic blood pressure may respond to the administration of opioids, β-blockers, vasodilators (nitroglycerin, nitroprusside), or increased delivered concentrations of volatile anesthetics.

Nitroglycerin is a more appropriate choice than nitroprusside when myocardial ischemia is associated with normal systemic blood pressure. Hypotension may be treated with a phenylephrine infusion to rapidly restore pressure-dependent perfusion through atherosclerotic coronary arteries. In addition to drugs, the intravenous infusion of fluids to restore systemic blood pressure is useful because myocardial oxygen requirements for volume work of the heart are lower than those for pressure work. A disadvantage of this approach is the time necessary for fluid treatment to be effective.

In selected patients, a pulmonary artery catheter may be helpful for monitoring responses to intravenous fluid replacement and the therapeutic effects of drugs on left ventricular function. Right atrial (central venous) pressure may not reliably reflect left heart filling pressure in the presence of left ventricular dysfunction secondary to coronary artery disease if the ejection fraction is less than 0.5. Right atrial pressure is more likely to correlate with pulmonary artery occlusion pressure in patients with coronary artery disease when the ejection fraction is greater than 0.5 and there is no evidence of left ventricular dysfunction.[17] Abrupt increases in pulmonary artery pressure may also reflect acute myocardial ischemia. When compared with transesophageal echocardiography, monitoring with a pulmonary artery catheter is not a highly sensitive approach for detecting myocardial ischemia. Indeed, transesophageal echocardiography also provides an assessment of regional wall motion, global ventricular function, valvular function, intravascular fluid volume, and associated ventricular filling. Transesophageal echocardiography is more accurate and useful than monitoring with a pulmonary artery catheter. Any sudden change in the pulse oximeter reading or tone is a signal to the anesthesiologist to search for correctable causes (arterial hypoxemia, hypotension, decreased cardiac output).

Decreases in body temperature that occur intraoperatively may predispose to shivering on awakening and lead to abrupt increases in myocardial oxygen requirements. Attempts to minimize decreases in body temperature and provision of supplemental oxygen are of obvious importance. Postoperative pain relief is important because pain-induced activation of the sympathetic nervous system can increase myocardial oxygen requirements.

Postoperative Care

Postoperative care of patients with coronary artery disease is based on provision of perioperative anti-ischemic drugs (β-blockers, clonidine), analgesia, and if needed, sedation to blunt excessive sympathetic nervous system activity and facilitate rigorous control of hemodynamic variables. Intensive and continuous postoperative monitoring is useful for detecting myocardial ischemia, which is often asymptomatic. However, it is more effective to prevent the occurrence of myocardial ischemia than to detect it. Reducing the incidence of episodes of myocardial ischemia with β-blockers or clonidine reduces 30-day and 2-year mortality.

The major determinant of pulmonary complications (atelectasis, pneumonia) after cardiac surgery is poor cardiac function. Early mobilization and pain control are likely to minimize the incidence of clinically significant pulmonary complications.

VALVULAR HEART DISEASE

The most frequently encountered forms of valvular heart disease produce pressure overload (mitral stenosis, aortic stenosis) or volume overload (mitral regurgitation, aortic regurgitation) of the left ventricle.[18] The net effect of valvular heart disease is interference with forward flow of blood from the heart to the systemic circulation. Transesophageal echocardiography has revolutionized the evaluation and intraoperative management of valvular heart disease (Table 25-5). Selection of anesthetic drugs and neuromuscular blocking drugs for patients with valvular heart disease is often based on the probable effects of drug-induced changes in cardiac rhythm, heart rate, systemic blood pressure, systemic vascular resistance,

Table 25-5 Transesophageal Echocardiography and Valvular Heart Disease

Determine the significance of cardiac murmurs (most often aortic stenosis)

Identify hemodynamic abnormalities associated with physical findings (most often mitral regurgitation)

Determine the transvalvular pressure gradient

Determine cardiac valve regurgitation

Evaluate prosthetic valve function

and pulmonary vascular resistance relative to maintenance of cardiac output in these patients. Although no specific type of general anesthetic has been shown to be superior, when cardiac reserve is minimal, an anesthetic combination that includes a high dose of a short-acting opioid, an amnestic benzodiazepine, and a low dose of a volatile anesthetic is common. Prophylactic infusion of a vasoconstrictor (phenylephrine) may reduce hemodynamic changes. Patients with valvular heart disease should receive antibiotics in the perioperative period for protection against infective endocarditis. Monitoring intra-arterial pressure is helpful in patients with clinically significant valvular heart disease.

Mitral Stenosis

Mitral stenosis is characterized by mechanical obstruction to left ventricular diastolic filling secondary to a progressive decrease in the orifice of the mitral valve. The obstruction produces an increase in left atrial and pulmonary venous pressure. Increased pulmonary vascular resistance is likely when left atrial pressure is chronically higher than 25 mm Hg. Distention of the left atrium predisposes to atrial fibrillation, which can result in stasis of blood, the formation of thrombi, and systemic emboli. Chronic anticoagulation or antiplatelet therapy (or both) can reduce the risk for systemic embolic events in patients with atrial fibrillation.

Mitral stenosis is almost always due to fusion of the mitral valve leaflets during the healing process of acute rheumatic carditis. Symptoms of mitral stenosis do not usually develop until about 20 years after the initial episode of rheumatic fever. A sudden increase in the demand for cardiac output as produced by pregnancy or sepsis, however, may unmask previously asymptomatic mitral stenosis. In addition, patients with mitral stenosis may be more susceptible than normal individuals to the ventilatory depressant effects of the sedative drugs used for preoperative medication. If patients are given sedative drugs, supplemental oxygen may increase the margin of safety.

Most medications that patients are receiving, except anticoagulants, antiplatelet drugs, and oral hypoglycemic drugs, should be continued throughout the preoperative period. Patients with mitral stenosis who are being chronically treated with digitalis for control of their heart rate should continue to receive this drug until surgery. Adequate digitalis effect for heart rate control is generally reflected by a ventricular rate less than 80 beats/min. Because diuretic therapy is common in these patients, the serum potassium concentration is often measured preoperatively.

Management of anticoagulant or antiplatelet therapy should be discussed with the surgeon and cardiologist. Patients should be switched from warfarin (Coumadin) to heparin therapy preoperatively, depending on the type

of surgery. Patients with diabetes may benefit from an intravenous infusion of insulin with frequent glucose monitoring.[19]

MANAGEMENT OF ANESTHESIA

Intra-arterial pressure monitoring can speed the identification and treatment of hemodynamic changes in patients with clinically significant valvular disease. Induction of anesthesia in the presence of mitral stenosis can be achieved with intravenous drugs, with the possible exception of ketamine, which may be avoided because of its propensity to increase the heart rate. Tracheal intubation is facilitated by the administration of a neuromuscular blocking drug. Neuromuscular blocking drugs with minimal effects on heart rate are commonly chosen. Drugs used for maintenance of anesthesia should cause minimal changes in heart rate and systemic and pulmonary vascular resistance. Furthermore, these drugs should not greatly decrease myocardial contractility. No one anesthetic has been proved to be superior.

Goals for the management of anesthesia can be achieved with combinations of an opioid and low concentrations of volatile anesthetics or intravenous anesthetics, with or without nitrous oxide. Although nitrous oxide can increase pulmonary vascular resistance, this increase is not sufficiently great to justify avoiding this drug in all patients with mitral stenosis.[20] The effect of nitrous oxide on pulmonary vascular resistance, however, seems to be accentuated when coexisting pulmonary hypertension is severe. Avoiding the use of nitrous oxide allows the administration of higher inspired oxygen concentrations and may reduce pulmonary vasoconstriction. Rapid increases in the concentration of desflurane may cause stimulation of the sympathetic nervous system with accompanying tachycardia and pulmonary hypertension.

Nondepolarizing neuromuscular blocking drugs with minimal circulatory effects are useful in patients with mitral stenosis. Pancuronium is less appropriate because of its ability to increase the speed of transmission of cardiac impulses through the atrioventricular node, which could lead to excessive increases in heart rate. Such increases may be problematic in the presence of atrial fibrillation because the ventricular response to atrial impulses is determined by the degree of atrioventricular conduction. Although there is no reason to avoid drug-assisted antagonism of nondepolarizing neuromuscular blocking drugs, it is desirable to avoid the adverse effects of drug-induced tachycardia (Table 25-6). In this regard, an option may be to allow the neuromuscular blockade to wane spontaneously with metabolism of the drug.

Intraoperative fluid therapy must be carefully titrated because these patients are susceptible to intravascular volume overload and the development of left ventricular failure and pulmonary edema. Likewise, the head-down position may not be well tolerated because pulmonary blood volume is already increased. Monitoring intra-

Table 25-6 Anesthetic Considerations in Patients with Mitral Stenosis

Avoid sinus tachycardia or a rapid ventricular response rate during atrial fibrillation

Avoid marked increases in central blood volume associated with overtransfusion or the head-down position

Avoid drug-induced decreases in systemic vascular resistance

Avoid events that may exacerbate pulmonary hypertension and evoke right ventricular failure, such as arterial hypoxemia or hypoventilation

arterial pressure and possibly right atrial pressure is a helpful guide to the adequacy of intravascular fluid replacement. An increase in right atrial pressure could also reflect pulmonary vasoconstriction and thus suggests the need to check for causes, which may include nitrous oxide, desflurane, acidosis, arterial hypoxemia, increased mitral regurgitation, or light anesthesia.

Postoperatively, patients with mitral stenosis are at high risk for pulmonary edema and right heart failure. Mechanical support of ventilation of the lungs may be necessary, particularly after major thoracic or abdominal surgery. The shift from positive-pressure ventilation to spontaneous ventilation with weaning and extubation of the patient's trachea may lead to increased venous return and increased central venous pressure with worsening of congestive heart failure.

Mitral Regurgitation

Mitral regurgitation is characterized by left atrial volume overload and decreased left ventricular forward stroke volume as a result of the backflow of part of each stroke volume through the incompetent mitral valve back into the left atrium. This regurgitant flow is responsible for the characteristic V waves seen on the recording of pulmonary artery occlusion pressure.[21] Mitral regurgitation secondary to rheumatic fever usually has a component of mitral stenosis. Dilated cardiomyopathy resulting from chronic myocardial ischemia, repeated myocardial infarctions, or viral infections may cause mitral regurgitation. Isolated mitral regurgitation may be acute and reflect papillary muscle dysfunction after a myocardial infarction or rupture of the chordae tendineae secondary to infective endocarditis.

MANAGEMENT OF ANESTHESIA

Management of anesthesia in patients with mitral regurgitation should be designed to reduce the likelihood of decreases in forward left ventricular stroke volume. Conversely, cardiac output can be improved by mild increases in heart rate and mild decreases in systemic vascular resistance (Table 25-7). Intra-arterial pressure monitoring can speed the identification and treatment of hemodynamic changes in patients with clinically significant valvular disease.

A general anesthetic is the usual choice for patients with mitral regurgitation. Although decreases in systemic vascular resistance are theoretically beneficial, the uncontrolled nature of this response with a regional anesthetic may detract from the use of this technique. Regional anesthesia may be used safely for surgery on peripheral body sites. Maintenance of general anesthesia can be provided with volatile anesthetics, with or without nitrous oxide, or a continuous intravenous infusion of drugs. The delivered concentration of volatile anesthetics can be adjusted to attenuate the undesirable increases in systemic blood pressure and systemic vascular resistance that can accompany surgical stimulation. Avoiding the use of nitrous oxide allows the administration of higher inspired oxygen concentrations and may reduce pulmonary vasoconstriction. Rapid increases in the delivered concentration of desflurane may evoke sympathetic nervous system stimulation (tachycardia, pulmonary hypertension) and should be avoided.

Nondepolarizing neuromuscular blocking drugs that lack significant circulatory effects are useful. Pancuronium is acceptable because the increase in heart rate produced by this drug could increase forward left ventricular stroke volume. Intravascular fluid volume must be maintained by prompt replacement of blood loss to ensure adequate venous return and ejection of an optimal forward left ventricular stroke volume.

Aortic Stenosis

Aortic stenosis is characterized by increased left ventricular systolic pressure to maintain the forward stroke volume through a narrowed aortic valve. The magnitude of the pressure gradient across the valve serves as an estimate of the severity of valvular stenosis. Hemodynamically significant aortic stenosis is associated with pressure gradients less than 50 mm Hg or valve areas less than 1.2 cm². A peak systolic gradient higher than 50 mm Hg in the presence of normal cardiac output or an effective

Table 25-7 Anesthetic Considerations in Patients with Mitral or Aortic Regurgitation

Avoid sudden decreases in heart rate

Avoid sudden decreases in systemic vascular resistance

Minimize drug-induced myocardial depression

Monitor the magnitude of the V wave as a reflection of mitral regurgitant flow

aortic orifice less than 0.75 cm^2 in an average-sized adult is generally considered to represent critical aortic stenosis. The combination of clinical symptoms (angina, congestive failure, fainting), signs (left ventricular dysfunction, progressive cardiomegaly), and reduced valve area suggests the presence of critical aortic stenosis requiring surgical replacement. Increased intraventricular pressure is accompanied by compensatory increases in the thickness of the left ventricular wall. Angina pectoris often occurs in these patients in the absence of coronary artery disease and reflects increased myocardial oxygen demand because of the increased amounts of ventricular muscle associated with myocardial hypertrophy in combination with high intraventricular pressure. There is a decrease in oxygen delivery secondary to the aortic valve pressure gradient along with an increase in oxygen requirements from the increase in left ventricular pressure.

Isolated nonrheumatic aortic stenosis usually results from progressive calcification and stenosis of a congenitally abnormal (usually bicuspid) valve. Aortic stenosis secondary to rheumatic fever almost always occurs in association with mitral valve disease. Likewise, aortic stenosis is usually accompanied by some degree of aortic regurgitation. Regardless of the cause of aortic stenosis, the natural history of the disease includes a long latent period, often 30 years or more, before symptoms occur. Because aortic stenosis may be asymptomatic, it is important to listen for this cardiac murmur (systolic murmur in the second right intercostal space that may radiate to the right carotid) in patients scheduled for surgery. The incidence of sudden death is increased in patients with aortic stenosis.

MANAGEMENT OF ANESTHESIA

Goals during management of anesthesia in patients with aortic stenosis are maintenance of normal sinus rhythm and avoidance of extreme and prolonged alterations in heart rate, systemic vascular resistance, and intravascular fluid volume (Table 25-8). Preservation of normal sinus rhythm is critical because the left ventricle is dependent on properly timed atrial contractions to ensure optimal left ventricular filling and stroke volume. Increases in heart rate (>100 beats/min) can decrease the time for left ventricular filling and ejection, whereas bradycardia (<60 beats/min) can lead to acute overdistention of the left ventricle. Tachycardia may lead to myocardial ischemia and ventricular dysfunction. In view of the obstruction to left ventricular ejection, it must be appreciated that decreases in systemic vascular resistance may be associated with large decreases in systemic blood pressure and coronary blood flow and thus with myocardial ischemia. Intra-arterial pressure monitoring is helpful and can speed identification and treatment of hemodynamic changes.

The most important technique for the management of patients with aortic stenosis is intra-arterial pressure monitoring with careful avoidance of hypotension. A general anesthetic may be preferred over a regional anesthetic because sympathetic nervous system blockade can lead to undesirable decreases in systemic vascular resistance. However, if the surgical site is on an extremity, a regional anesthetic with intra-arterial pressure monitoring can be equally successful. Maintenance of general anesthesia can be achieved with volatile anesthetics, with or without nitrous oxide, or with intravenous drugs. A potential disadvantage of volatile anesthetics is depression of sinus node automaticity, which may lead to junctional rhythm and decreased left ventricular filling because of loss of properly timed atrial contractions. Intravascular fluid volume must be maintained by prompt replacement of blood loss and liberal intravenous administration of fluids. If a pulmonary artery catheter is placed, it should be remembered that occlusion pressure may overestimate left ventricular end-diastolic volume as a result of the decreased compliance of the left ventricle that accompanies chronic aortic stenosis. A cardiac defibrillator should be promptly available when anesthesia is administered to patients with aortic stenosis because external cardiac compressions are unlikely to generate an adequate stroke volume across a stenosed aortic valve.

Aortic Regurgitation

Aortic regurgitation is characterized by decreased forward left ventricular stroke volume as a result of regurgitation of part of the ejected stroke volume from the aorta back into the left ventricle through an incompetent aortic valve. A gradual onset of aortic regurgitation results in marked left ventricular hypertrophy. Increased myocardial oxygen requirements secondary to left ventricular hypertrophy, plus a characteristic decrease in aortic diastolic pressure that decreases coronary blood flow, can be manifested as angina pectoris in the absence of coronary artery disease. Coronary blood flow to the left ventricle occurs during ventricular diastole. In severe or acute aortic regurgitation with low diastolic pressure and elevated end-diastolic

---

Table 25-8 Anesthetic Considerations in Patients with Aortic Stenosis

Intra-arterial pressure monitoring

Rapid availability or prophylactic administration of intravenous vasoconstrictors (phenylephrine)

Maintenance of normal sinus rhythm

Avoidance of bradycardia

Avoidance of sudden decreases in systemic vascular resistance

Optimization of intravascular fluid volume

IV

ventricular pressure, coronary blood flow can be severely compromised. The combination of low diastolic pressure as a result of aortic regurgitation plus an increase in left ventricular diastolic pressure substantially decreases the coronary perfusion pressure gradient. Acute aortic regurgitation is most often due to infective endocarditis, trauma, or dissection of a thoracic aneurysm. Chronic aortic regurgitation is usually due to previous rheumatic fever. In contrast to aortic stenosis, the occurrence of sudden death in patients with aortic regurgitation is rare.

MANAGEMENT OF ANESTHESIA

Management of anesthesia for noncardiac surgery in patients with aortic regurgitation is the same as described for patients with mitral regurgitation (see Table 25-7). Intra-arterial pressure monitoring can speed the identification and treatment of hemodynamic changes and is often recommended for patients with significant aortic regurgitation.

Mitral Valve Prolapse

Mitral valve prolapse (click-murmur syndrome, Barlow's syndrome) is characterized by an abnormality of the mitral valve support structure that permits prolapse of the valve into the left atrium during contraction of the left ventricle.[22] Previous estimates that mitral valve prolapse was present in 5% to 15% of individuals are most likely erroneously high.[23] Transesophageal or transthoracic echocardiography is helpful in confirming the diagnosis of mitral valve prolapse, particularly in the absence of the characteristic systolic murmur. There seems to be an increased incidence of mitral valve prolapse in patients with musculoskeletal abnormalities, including Marfan's syndrome, pectus excavatum, and kyphoscoliosis.

Despite the prevalence of mitral valve prolapse, most patients are asymptomatic, thus emphasizing the usually benign course of this abnormality. Nevertheless, serious complications may accompany mitral valve prolapse (Table 25-9). For example, mitral valve prolapse is probably the most common cause of pure mitral regurgitation, which may progress to the need for surgical intervention. Infective endocarditis is a potential complication, and transient ischemic attacks in patients younger

Table 25-9 Complications Associated with Mitral Valve Prolapse
Mitral regurgitation
Infective endocarditis
Transient ischemic events
Cardiac dysrhythmias
Sudden death (extremely rare)

than 45 years are often associated with mitral valve prolapse. Sudden death is an extremely rare complication of mitral valve prolapse and, when it occurs, is presumed to be due to a ventricular cardiac dysrhythmia.

MANAGEMENT OF ANESTHESIA

The important principle in the management of anesthesia in patients with mitral valve prolapse is avoidance of events that can increase cardiac emptying and subsequently accentuate prolapse of the mitral valve into the left atrium.[22] Perioperative events that can increase cardiac emptying include (1) sympathetic nervous system stimulation, (2) decreased systemic vascular resistance, and (3) performance of surgery with patients in the head-up or sitting position. With this in mind, it is important to optimize intravascular fluid volume in the preoperative period. Induction of anesthesia in patients with mitral valve prolapse can be achieved with most of the available intravenous drugs if one keeps in mind the need to avoid sudden prolonged decreases in systemic vascular resistance. Intra-arterial pressure monitoring can speed the identification and treatment of hemodynamic changes and is often recommended for patients with clinically significant mitral valve prolapse. Ketamine and pancuronium are not recommended because of their ability to increase cardiac contractility and heart rate. Nevertheless, it is likely that these drugs are often administered without incident to patients with undiagnosed and asymptomatic mitral valve prolapse.

Maintenance of anesthesia is most often achieved with a volatile anesthetic, with or without nitrous oxide, and an opioid to minimize sympathetic nervous system activation as a result of noxious intraoperative stimulation. The dose of volatile anesthetic is titrated to avoid excessive decreases in systemic vascular resistance. A regional anesthetic could also produce undesirable decreases in systemic vascular resistance, but it can be used with appropriate monitoring and rapid hemodynamic therapy if needed. Prompt replacement of blood loss and generous intravenous administration of fluids will contribute to maintenance of an optimal intravascular fluid volume and decrease the potential adverse effects of positive-pressure ventilation on the patient's lungs. Lidocaine, amiodarone, and esmolol should be available to treat cardiac dysrhythmias. If a sympathomimetic is needed to treat hypotension, an α-agonist such as phenylephrine is useful.

DISTURBANCES IN CARDIAC CONDUCTION AND RHYTHM

The ECG is a valuable tool for diagnosing disturbances in cardiac conduction and rhythm. Ambulatory ECG monitoring (Holter monitoring) is useful in documenting the occurrence of life-threatening cardiac dysrhythmias and assessing the efficacy of antidysrhythmic drug therapy. The incidence of intraoperative cardiac dysrhythmia depends on the definition (benign versus life-threatening), patient characteristics, and the type of surgery (high incidence during cardiothoracic surgery).[24] The following questions should be asked when interpreting the ECG:

1. What is the heart rate?
2. Are P waves present, and what is their relationship to the QRS complexes?
3. What is the duration of the PR interval (normal, 0.12 to 0.2 second)?
4. What is the duration of the QRS complex (normal, 0.05 to 0.11 second)?
5. Is the ventricular rhythm regular?
6. Are there early cardiac beats or abnormal pauses after a preceding QRS complex?
7. Is there evidence of previous myocardial infarction or ventricular hypertrophy?
8. Is there evidence of myocardial ischemia?
9. Is there a conduction disturbance such as left bundle branch block, right bundle branch block, or intraventricular conduction delay?

Heart Block

Disturbances in conduction of cardiac impulses can be classified according to the site of the conduction block relative to the atrioventricular node (Table 25-10). Heart block occurring above the atrioventricular node is usually benign and transient, whereas heart block occurring below the atrioventricular node tends to be progressive and permanent.

Table 25-10   Classification of Heart Block
First-degree atrioventricular heart block
Second-degree atrioventricular heart block
Mobitz type I (Wenckebach)
Mobitz type II
Unifascicular heart block
Left anterior hemiblock
Left posterior hemiblock
Right bundle branch block
Left bundle branch block
Bifascicular heart block
Right bundle branch block plus anterior hemiblock
Right bundle branch block plus posterior hemiblock
Third-degree (trifascicular, complete) atrioventricular heart block

A theoretical concern in patients with bifascicular heart block is that perioperative events, such as alterations in systemic blood pressure, arterial oxygenation, or electrolyte concentrations, might compromise conduction in the one remaining intact fascicle and lead to the acute intraoperative onset of third-degree atrioventricular heart block. There is no evidence, however, that surgery performed during general or regional anesthesia predisposes to the development of third-degree atrioventricular heart block in patients with coexisting bifascicular block. Therefore, placement of a prophylactic artificial cardiac pacemaker is not required before anesthesia and surgery, but it should be available.

Third-degree atrioventricular heart block is treated by placement of an artificial cardiac pacemaker. A pacemaker can be inserted intravenously (endocardial lead) or by the subcostal approach (epicardial or myocardial lead). An alternative to emergency transvenous artificial cardiac pacemaker placement is noninvasive transcutaneous cardiac pacing. A continuous intravenous infusion of isoproterenol acting as a pharmacologic cardiac pacemaker may be necessary to maintain an adequate heart rate until artificial electrical cardiac pacing can be established.

Sick Sinus Syndrome

Sick sinus syndrome is characterized by inappropriate sinus bradycardia along with degenerative changes in the sinoatrial node. Frequently, the bradycardia associated with this syndrome is complicated by episodes of supraventricular tachycardia. Artificial cardiac pacemakers may be indicated when therapeutic plasma concentrations of drugs necessary to control tachycardia result in bradycardia. The increased incidence of pulmonary embolism in these patients may be a reason to initiate anticoagulation.

Ventricular Premature Beats

Ventricular premature beats are recognized on the ECG by (1) premature occurrence, (2) the absence of a P wave preceding the QRS complex, (3) a wide and often bizarre QRS complex, (4) an inverted T wave, and (5) a compensatory pause that follows the premature beat. Ventricular premature beats are often treated with lidocaine (1 to 2 mg/kg IV followed by 1 to 2 mg/min infusion) when they (1) are frequent (more than six premature beats/min), (2) are multifocal, (3) occur in salvos of three or more, or (4) take place during the ascending limb of the T wave (R on T phenomenon), which corresponds to the relative refractory period of the ventricle. The primary goal should be to identify the underlying cause (myocardial ischemia, arterial hypoxemia, hypercapnia, hypertension, hypokalemia, mechanical irritation of the ventricles) if possible and correct it.

IV

Ventricular Tachycardia

Ventricular tachycardia is defined as the appearance of at least three consecutive wide QRS complexes (>0.12 second) on the ECG occurring at an effective heart rate greater than 120 beats/min. Ventricular tachycardia not associated with hypotension is initially treated by the intravenous administration of lidocaine, amiodarone, or procainamide. Symptomatic ventricular tachycardia is best treated by external electrical cardioversion.

Pre-excitation Syndromes

Pre-excitation syndromes are characterized by activation of a portion of the ventricles by cardiac impulses that travel from the atria via accessory (anomalous) conduction pathways. These pathways bypass the atrioventricular node such that activation of the ventricles occurs earlier than it would if impulses reached the ventricles by normal pathways.

WOLFF-PARKINSON-WHITE SYNDROME

Wolff-Parkinson-White syndrome is the most common of the pre-excitation syndromes, with an incidence that may approach 0.3% of the general population. The lack of physiologic delay in transmission of cardiac impulses along the Kent fibers results in the characteristic short PR interval (<0.12 second) on the ECG. The wide QRS complex and delta wave on the ECG reflect the composite of cardiac impulses conducted by normal and accessory pathways. Paroxysmal atrial tachycardia is the most frequent cardiac dysrhythmia associated with this syndrome. Treatment of this syndrome often involves catheter ablation of accessory pathways as identified by electrophysiologic mapping. Supraventricular tachycardias such as atrial fibrillation or atrial flutter with one-to-one conduction may lead to hemodynamic collapse in patients with Wolff-Parkinson-White syndrome.

Management of Anesthesia

The goal during management of anesthesia in a patient with a pre-excitation syndrome is to avoid events (anxiety) or drugs (anticholinergics, ketamine, pancuronium) that might increase sympathetic nervous system activity and predispose to tachydysrhythmias.[24] All cardiac antidysrhythmic drugs should be continued throughout the perioperative period. Induction of anesthesia can be acceptably achieved with intravenous drugs, with the possible exception of ketamine. Tracheal intubation should be performed only after a sufficient concentration of anesthetic drugs (intravenous drugs, opioids, or volatile anesthetics, with or without nitrous oxide, or any combination of these drugs) has been achieved so that the sympathetic nervous system stimulation evoked by instrumentation of the upper airway is reliably blunted. β-Blockers (atenolol, metoprolol, propranolol, or esmolol) administered intravenously can be used to avoid tachy-

cardia during induction of anesthesia. Succinylcholine or a nondepolarizing neuromuscular blocking drug with minimal effects on heart rate is useful to facilitate tracheal intubation or to provide skeletal muscle paralysis during surgery.

The onset of paroxysmal atrial tachycardia or fibrillation in the perioperative period can be treated by the intravenous administration of drugs that abruptly prolong the refractory period of the atrioventricular node (adenosine) or lengthen the refractory period of accessory pathways (procainamide). Digitalis and verapamil may decrease the refractory period of the accessory pathways responsible for atrial fibrillation and thereby result in an increase in the ventricular response rate during this dysrhythmia and thus should be avoided. Electrical cardioversion is indicated when tachydysrhythmias are life-threatening.

Prolonged QT Interval Syndrome

Prolonged QT interval syndrome (>0.44 second on the ECG) is associated with ventricular dysrhythmias, syncope, and sudden death. Treatment of these patients is often empirical but may include β-antagonists or left stellate ganglion block. The effectiveness of left stellate ganglion block supports the hypothesis that this syndrome results from a congenital imbalance of autonomic innervation to the heart produced by decreases in right cardiac sympathetic nerve activity. Management of anesthesia includes avoidance of events or drugs that are likely to activate the sympathetic nervous system and the availability of β-antagonists (metoprolol, atenolol, propranolol, or esmolol) or electrical cardioversion (or both) to treat life-threatening ventricular dysrhythmias.[24]

Inhaled and injected anesthetics administered to normal patients often prolong the QT interval on the ECG. Nevertheless, the same drugs administered to patients with known prolonged QT interval syndrome do not predictably further prolong this interval.[25] However, drugs that have the potential to prolong the QT interval (droperidol) are likely to be avoided in patients with prolonged QT syndrome.

ARTIFICIAL CARDIAC PACEMAKERS

Preoperative Evaluation

Preoperative evaluation of a patient with an artificial cardiac pacemaker includes determination of the reason for placing the pacemaker and assessment of its present function, as well as the brand, model, magnet mode, and availability of a programmer for this specific device.[26] There are a large number of implanted electrical devices (deep brain stimulators, automatic implantable cardiac defibrillators, intravenous pumps, spinal stimulators for chronic pain, bladder stimulators for neurogenic bladder, gastric stimulators for the treatment of obesity, intravenous ports, and vagal stimulators for sleep), and one cannot always assume that the subcutaneous device is a cardiac pacemaker.

If the device is a cardiac pacemaker placed for third-degree atrioventricular heart block, special considerations for continuous operation of the device and monitoring of its operation should be taken. If a pacemaker implanted for third-degree atrioventricular heart block is to be disconnected to change the stimulator, transvenous pacing may be needed. If the device is an automatic defibrillator, it will need to be inactivated during electrosurgical cautery to avoid the device erroneously sensing ventricular dysrhythmias and defibrillating, which would waste battery life and possibly cause R on T phenomena and ventricular fibrillation.

The magnet mode of many implanted devices is programmable, but one cannot assume that the magnet mode is "safe." The magnet mode for many pacemakers is asynchronous at 99 beats/min. If the patient has a spontaneous heart rate of 60 to 80 beats/min, the asynchronous mode at 99 beats/min would be safe. However, in some devices, the magnet mode shifts to asynchronous at 50 beats/min at the end of battery life. Asynchronous pacing at 50 beats/min may lead to R on T phenomena if the patient has a spontaneous heart rate greater than 50 beats/min. It is best to know what the specific magnet mode is for the device in question and set it to the needs of the patient for the procedure.

Management of Anesthesia

Selection of drugs or techniques for anesthesia is not influenced by the presence of artificial cardiac pacemakers because there is no evidence that the threshold and subsequent response of these devices are altered by drugs administered in the perioperative period. Insertion of a pulmonary artery catheter will not disturb epicardial electrodes but might dislodge recently placed (<2 weeks' duration) transvenous endocardial electrodes.[27]

INTRAOPERATIVE MONITORING
Intraoperative monitoring of patients with artificial cardiac pacemakers includes the ECG and possible intra-arterial pressure monitoring to promptly detect the appearance of asystole. Atropine, isoproterenol, and an external pacemaker should be available if artificial cardiac pacemaker function ceases. If electrocautery interferes with the ECG, monitoring intra-arterial pressure or arterial oxygenation, auscultation through an esophageal stethoscope, or a palpable pulse confirms continued cardiac activity. Monitoring systemic blood pressure with an intra-arterial catheter provides immediate evidence of loss of pacemaker function and should be considered in patients with third-degree atrioventricular heart block. Inhibition of pulse generator activity by electromagnetic interference, most commonly from electrosurgical cautery,

which is interpreted as spontaneous cardiac activity by the artificial cardiac pacemaker, is most likely when the ground plate for electrocautery is placed too near the pulse generator or unipolar cautery is used. For this reason, the ground plate should be placed as far as possible from the pulse generator. Bipolar electrocautery may also reduce interference between electrosurgical cautery and the pacemaker. If surface pads are used for external pacing or defibrillation, they should be placed away from the implanted device to reduce current passing down the pacing lead and hyperpolarizing a small segment of myocardium, which could interfere with pacemaker capture after defibrillation.

Artificial implantable cardioversion devices sense ventricular fibrillation or ventricular tachycardia. They provide a cardioversion shock through implanted cardiac leads. Electrocautery signals can be misinterpreted as ventricular dysrhythmias, thus triggering unnecessary shocks and decreasing battery life. These devices should be reprogrammed to the standby mode before elective surgery and returned to full function postoperatively with interrogation of proper function.

ESSENTIAL HYPERTENSION

Essential hypertension is arbitrarily defined as sustained increases in systemic blood pressure (>160 mm Hg) or diastolic blood pressure (>90 mm Hg), or both, independent of any known cause. Treatment of essential hypertension with appropriate drug therapy decreases the incidence of stroke and congestive heart failure. Systemic hypertension is a risk factor for coronary artery disease, and the longer the patient has hypertension, the higher the risk for end-organ damage. Patients with two risk factors (age ≥65 years, systemic hypertension, smoking, diabetes mellitus, cholesterol >240 mg/dL) for coronary artery disease should be treated as though they have coronary artery disease.

Management of Anesthesia

Management of anesthesia for patients with essential hypertension includes preoperative evaluation of drug therapy and extent of the disease plus a consideration of the implications of exaggerated systemic blood pressure responses elicited by painful intraoperative stimulation.[28] Anesthesia care for patients with cardiac disease needs to be perioperative for optimal outcomes.

PREOPERATIVE EVALUATION
Preoperative evaluation of patients with essential hypertension begins with a determination of the adequacy of systemic blood pressure control and a review of the pharmacology of the antihypertensive drugs being used for therapy. It is important to maintain current therapy

IV

with antihypertensive drugs throughout the perioperative period. Evidence of major organ dysfunction (congestive heart failure, coronary artery disease, cerebral ischemia, renal dysfunction) must be sought. Patients with essential hypertension have an increased risk for coronary artery disease. Evidence of peripheral vascular disease should be recognized inasmuch as all patients with peripheral vascular disease have coronary artery disease. It can be assumed that nearly half of patients with evidence of peripheral vascular disease will have greater than 50% stenosis of one or more coronary arteries, even in the absence of angina pectoris and in the presence of a normal resting ECG.

Essential hypertension is associated with a shift of the curve for the autoregulation of cerebral blood flow to the right, thus emphasizing that these patients are more vulnerable to cerebral ischemia should perfusion pressure decrease. Detection of renal dysfunction secondary to chronic hypertension may influence the selection of drugs, particularly if elimination from plasma depends on renal clearance or if metabolites of the drugs are known potential nephrotoxins (fluoride from the metabolism of sevoflurane).

The value of treating essential hypertension before an elective operation is suggested by the observation that the incidence of hypotension and evidence of myocardial ischemia on the ECG during maintenance of anesthesia are increased in patients who remain hypertensive before induction of anesthesia.[28] Perioperative therapy with β-blockers for at least 7 days and continued for 30 days postoperatively reduces the risk for cardiac morbidity and death in patients at risk.[8,9] Perioperative therapy with clonidine started the night before surgery and continued for 4 days reduces the risk for 30-day and 2-year mortality.[10]

Despite antihypertensive therapy, increases in systemic blood pressure during the intraoperative period are more likely to occur in patients with a history of essential hypertension regardless of the degree of pharmacologic control of systemic blood pressure established preoperatively. Furthermore, there is no evidence that the incidence of postoperative cardiac complications is increased when hypertensive patients undergo elective operations, as long as preoperative diastolic blood pressure is not higher than 110 mm Hg and the heart rate is controlled.

The night before surgery is stressful, and prophylactic β-blockade or clonidine can reduce the risk of sympathetic nervous system stimulation resulting in tachycardia and subsequent myocardial ischemia. There is the erroneous belief that minor surgery causes minor stress. Patients scheduled for ophthalmic surgery, a minor outpatient procedure, commonly experience sympathetic nervous system stimulation resulting in preoperative hypertension. Prophylactic therapy with β-blockers or clonidine can reduce the preoperative hypertensive episodes and myocardial ischemia.

INDUCTION OF ANESTHESIA

Induction of anesthesia with intravenous drugs is acceptable if one remembers that an exaggerated decrease in systemic blood pressure may occur, particularly if systemic hypertension is present preoperatively. Thiopental, propofol, midazolam, opioids (fentanyl, sufentanil, alfentanil, remifentanil), and etomidate have all been used as intravenous induction drugs. Etomidate or combinations of midazolam and fentanyl are frequently used for induction because of their limited hemodynamic effects. Ketamine is rarely selected for induction of anesthesia in patients with essential hypertension because of its circulatory effects, which can increase systemic blood pressure and cause tachycardia, potentially leading to myocardial ischemia. Hemodynamic changes with induction of anesthesia most likely reflect unmasking of decreased intravascular fluid volume as a result of chronic hypertension combined with stiffening of the arterial vasculature.

Exaggerated increases in systemic blood pressure during direct laryngoscopy for tracheal intubation are predictable in patients with the preoperative diagnosis of essential hypertension, but such increases may be reduced with the prior administration of opioids or β-blockers. Tachycardia may lead to episodes of myocardial ischemia. A single 1-minute episode of myocardial ischemia increases the risk for perioperative cardiac morbidity 10-fold and the risk for death 2-fold.

It is important to ensure maximal attenuation of the sympathetic nervous system responses evoked during direct laryngoscopy by selected pharmacologic interventions (inhaled and intravenous anesthetics, β-blockers). If the patient has a recognized difficult airway precluding direct laryngoscopy, hemodynamic control with specific attention to heart rate control must be sought while securing the airway with alternative approaches (fiberoptic intubation). Regardless of the drugs administered before tracheal intubation, it is important to recognize that an excessive concentration of anesthetic drugs can produce decreases in systemic blood pressure that are as undesirable as hypertension. An important concept for limiting the pressor responses elicited by tracheal intubation is to limit the duration of direct laryngoscopy to less than 15 seconds if possible. In addition, the administration of laryngotracheal lidocaine immediately before placement of the tube in the trachea will minimize any additional pressor response.

MAINTENANCE OF ANESTHESIA

The goal during maintenance of anesthesia is to adjust the concentrations of anesthetic drugs so that tachycardia is prevented and wide fluctuations in systemic blood pressure are minimized (Table 25-11). No anesthetic technique has been shown to be superior. Combinations of volatile anesthetics with or without nitrous oxide and an opioid are commonly used. Changes in the concentration of volatile anesthetic allow rapid adjustments in the

Table 25-11 Management of Anesthesia for Patients with Essential Hypertension

Preoperative evaluation

Determine the adequacy of systemic blood pressure control

Review the pharmacology of antihypertensive drugs

Evaluate associated organ dysfunction (cardiac, central nervous system, renal)

Consider the administration of prophylactic anti-ischemic therapy (perioperative β-blockade or clonidine)

Choose appropriate monitors and consider intra-arterial pressure monitoring

Consider initiation of prophylactic infusion of phenylephrine to reduce homodynamic perturbation with induction

Induction of anesthesia and tracheal intubation

Anticipate exaggerated systemic blood pressure changes

Minimize the pressor response during tracheal intubation by limiting the duration of direct laryngoscopy to <15 seconds

Maintenance of anesthesia

Use a volatile anesthetic and vasoconstrictors to control systemic blood pressure

Monitor the electrocardiogram for evidence of myocardial ischemia (avoidance is better than detection)

Anticipate excessive increases in systemic blood pressure with emergence

Postoperative management

Ensure effective pain control

Continue perioperative anti-ischemic therapy for at least a week for low-risk patients, 30 days for higher risk, and permanently in patients with known coronary artery or vascular disease

depth of anesthesia in response to increases or decreases in systemic blood pressure. Changes in surgical stimulation may lead to changes in blood pressure and heart rate. Additional doses of opioids and β-blockers and changes in the dose of volatile anesthetic can be used to control hemodynamics. Heart rate control is the most critical element for preventing cardiac morbidity and mortality.

Volatile anesthetics are useful for attenuating sympathetic nervous system activity and associated pressor responses. The ability to rapidly increase the alveolar concentration of sevoflurane (low blood solubility) makes this volatile anesthetic uniquely efficacious for treating sudden increases in systemic blood pressure. Rapid increases in desflurane concentration may lead to sympathetic nervous system stimulation and myocardial ischemia. A positive feedback situation can occur during desflurane anesthesia; specifically, a surgical stimulus can raise blood pressure, and in response the anesthesiologist increases the desflurane concentration, which stimulates the sympathetic system and causes the blood pressure to further increase.

A nitrous oxide–opioid technique is also acceptable for maintenance of anesthesia, but the addition of a volatile anesthetic is often necessary to control undesirable increases in systemic blood pressure, particularly during periods of maximal surgical stimulation. Total intravenous anesthesia (combinations of dexmedetomidine, propofol, opioids, and benzodiazepines) can also be selected. Continuous intravenous infusions of phenylephrine, nitroprusside, nitroglycerin, carvedilol, or esmolol can be used to maintain normotension during the intraoperative period. Hypotension that occurs during maintenance of anesthesia is often treated by decreasing the concentration of volatile anesthetic while infusing fluids to increase intravascular fluid volume. Sympathomimetics, such as ephedrine, or vasoconstrictors, such as phenylephrine, may be necessary to restore perfusion pressure until the underlying cause of the hypotension can be corrected.

The choice of intraoperative monitors for patients with coexisting essential hypertension is influenced by the complexity of the surgery. The ECG is monitored with the goal of recognizing changes suggestive of myocardial ischemia. Intra-arterial pressure is commonly monitored. A pulmonary artery catheter may be indicated if major surgery is planned and there is evidence preoperatively of left ventricular dysfunction, although it is difficult to demonstrate improved outcomes with pulmonary artery catheter monitoring. Monitoring with transesophageal echocardiography is an alternative to placement of a pulmonary artery catheter.

There is no evidence that a specific neuromuscular blocking drug is the best selection in patients with essential hypertension. Pancuronium can induce tachycardia and increase systemic blood pressure, although no data suggest that this mild pressor response is exaggerated by coexisting hypertension.

POSTOPERATIVE MANAGEMENT

Hypertension in the early postoperative period is a frequent occurrence in patients with a preoperative diagnosis of essential hypertension. Prophylactic or therapeutic administration of β-blockers or clonidine can decrease these episodes of hypertension and reduce perioperative ischemia and mortality. If hypertension persists despite β-blockers and adequate analgesia, it may be necessary to pharmacologically decrease systemic blood pressure by using a continuous infusion of nitroprusside

IV

or nitroglycerin or intermittent injections of labetalol (0.1 to 0.5 mg/kg IV). Tachycardia in the postoperative period must be actively avoided.

CONGESTIVE HEART FAILURE

Elective surgery should not be performed on patients with congestive heart failure, except when the congestive heart failure is optimally treated. The preoperative presence of congestive heart failure is often associated with significant postoperative morbidity or mortality. Cardiology consultation is frequently helpful in patients with congestive failure because consideration of surgical or interventional revascularization and optimization of medical therapy can improve cardiac function. Preoperative initiation of β-blockers and vasodilator therapy with angiotensin-converting enzyme inhibitors can improve ventricular function and reduce operative risk.

When surgery cannot be delayed, the drugs and techniques chosen to provide anesthesia must be selected with the goal of optimizing cardiac output. Regional anesthesia should be considered for patients with congestive heart failure who require peripheral or minor surgery. Etomidate may be useful for the induction of anesthesia in the presence of congestive heart failure because of its limited effect on the sympathetic nervous system. Volatile anesthetics in low doses are acceptable for maintenance of anesthesia but must be used carefully to avoid excessive cardiac depression. In the presence of severe congestive heart failure, the use of opioids in high doses in combination with amnestic doses of benzodiazepines (midazolam) may be justified, although no evidence supports the benefit of high-dose opioid anesthesia over a volatile anesthetic combined with opioids. Positive-pressure ventilation of the lungs may be beneficial by decreasing pulmonary congestion, improving arterial oxygenation, and eliminating the work of breathing. Care must be taken during tracheal extubation of patients with congestive failure because the resumption of negative intrathoracic pressure with spontaneous ventilation can lead to increased filling pressure and worsening heart failure. Intra-arterial blood pressure monitoring is helpful for the hemodynamic management of patients undergoing both regional and general anesthesia. Maintenance of blood pressure with vasoconstrictors (phenylephrine) should precede increasing myocardial contractility with continuous infusions of dopamine or dobutamine, or both, because administration of β-agonists to patients with congestive heart failure may decrease survival.

HYPERTROPHIC CARDIOMYOPATHY

Hypertrophic cardiomyopathy (idiopathic hypertrophic subaortic stenosis) is characterized by obstruction to left ventricular outflow produced by asymmetric hypertrophy of the intraventricular septal muscle.[29] The associated left ventricular hypertrophy in an attempt to overcome the obstruction may be so massive that the volume of the left ventricular chamber is decreased. Despite these adverse changes, stroke volume remains normal or increased because of the hypercontractile state of the myocardium. This disease is often hereditary, and the genetic defect seems to be an increased density of calcium channels manifested as myocardial hypertrophy.

Management of Anesthesia

The goal during management of anesthesia for patients with hypertrophic cardiomyopathy is to decrease the pressure gradient across the left ventricular outflow obstruction (Table 25-12). Decreases in myocardial contractility and increases in preload (ventricular volume) and afterload will decrease the magnitude of left ventricular outflow obstruction. With this in mind, volatile anesthetics are useful for maintenance of anesthesia because they provide mild depression of myocardial contractility. Theoretically, isoflurane, desflurane, and sevoflurane would be less ideal choices than halothane because these drugs decrease systemic vascular resistance more than halothane does. In practice, halothane is rarely used as a result of its dysrhythmogenic potential and concerns regarding halothane hepatitis. Rapid increases in the delivered concentration of desflurane may cause undesirable sympathetic nervous system stimulation. Opioids as the primary anesthetic may not be optimal because they do not produce myocardial depression and can decrease systemic vascular resistance. Combinations of volatile anesthetics (sevoflurane, isoflurane) with an opioid are commonly selected. Nondepolarizing neuromuscular blocking drugs with minimal circulatory effects (vecuronium, rocuronium, cisatracurium) are most often

Table 25-12 Events That Decrease Left Ventricular Outflow Obstruction in the Presence of Hypertrophic Cardiomyopathy

Decreased Myocardial Contractility

β-Adrenergic blockade (atenolol, metoprolol, propranolol, esmolol)

Volatile anesthetic (sevoflurane or isoflurane)

Increased Preload

Increased intravascular fluid volume

Bradycardia (fentanyl or sufentanil)

Increased Afterload

α-Adrenergic stimulation (phenylephrine infusions)

selected. Pancuronium is not a likely choice because its drug-induced increases in heart rate and systemic blood pressure are undesirable.

Intraoperative hypotension is generally treated with intravenous fluids or an α-agonist such as phenylephrine, or with both. Drugs with β-agonist activity are not likely to be used to treat hypotension because any increase in cardiac contractility or heart rate could increase left ventricular outflow obstruction. When systemic hypertension occurs, an increased delivered concentration of the volatile drug (isoflurane, sevoflurane) is a useful treatment. Vasodilators, such as nitroprusside or nitroglycerin, should be used only with great care when needed for lowering systemic blood pressure because decreases in systemic vascular resistance can increase left ventricular outflow obstruction.

COR PULMONALE

Cor pulmonale is the designation for the right ventricular hypertrophy and eventual cardiac dysfunction that occurs secondary to chronic pulmonary hypertension. Elective operations in patients with cor pulmonale should not be performed until reversible components of the coexisting pulmonary vascular disease have been treated.

Goals during management of anesthesia in patients with cor pulmonale are to avoid events or drugs that could increase pulmonary vascular resistance. Volatile anesthetics are useful for relaxing vascular smooth muscle and attenuating airway responsiveness to stimuli produced by a tracheal tube. Nitrous oxide may increase pulmonary vascular resistance and should probably be avoided.[20] Another disadvantage of nitrous oxide is the associated decrease in the inspired concentration of oxygen necessitated by administration of this drug. Intra-arterial pressure monitoring is very helpful for hemodynamic management. Monitoring of pulmonary arterial or right atrial pressure (or both) may be helpful to detect any adverse effect on the pulmonary vasculature. Transesophageal echocardiographic monitoring can be very helpful in blood volume management. In severe cor pulmonale, inotropic support with β-agonists can improve cardiac function. β-Agonists must be used carefully to avoid myocardial ischemia. In severe right ventricular failure, combinations of β-agonists and phosphodiesterase inhibitors (amrinone, milrinone) can provide synergistic improvement in ventricular function and vasodilation.

CARDIAC TAMPONADE

Cardiac tamponade is characterized by (1) decreases in diastolic filling of the ventricles, (2) reductions in stroke volume, and (3) decreases in systemic blood pressure because of increased intrapericardial pressure from accumulation of fluid in the pericardial space (Table 25-13). Diastolic dysfunction from increased pericardial pressure and not systolic dysfunction is the primary problem. Decreased stroke volume from inadequate ventricular filling results in activation of the sympathetic nervous system (tachycardia, vasoconstriction) in an attempt to maintain cardiac output. Cardiac output and systemic blood pressure are maintained only as long as pressure in the central veins exceeds right ventricular end-diastolic pressure.

Management of Anesthesia

Institution of general anesthesia and positive-pressure ventilation of the patient's lungs in the presence of cardiac tamponade can lead to profound hypotension or death as a result of anesthetic-induced peripheral vasodilation, direct myocardial depression, and decreased venous return. When percutaneous pericardiocentesis cannot be performed under local anesthesia, induction plus maintenance of general anesthesia is dangerous but may be achieved with ketamine while carefully maintaining spontaneous respiration in recognition of the potential adverse effects of positive-pressure ventilation (increased intrathoracic pressure) on venous return. If possible, positive-pressure ventilation of the lungs should be avoided until drainage of the pericardial space is imminent. In this regard, tracheal intubation with topical anesthesia has been suggested.

Before induction of general anesthesia in a patient with significant cardiac tamponade, the patient should be positioned on the operating room table. Intra-arterial monitoring is helpful if time permits. The chest and abdomen should be prepared and draped for surgery. The surgeons should be prepared to make the incision immediately after induction of anesthesia. It is optimal if anesthetic induction, tracheal intubation, surgical incision, and drainage of the pericardial tamponade can occur in rapid succession. Although continuous infusions of catecholamines (epinephrine, norepinephrine, dopamine, dobutamine, or isoproterenol) and vasoconstrictors may be necessary to maintain cardiac output and systemic

Table 25-13 Manifestations of Cardiac Tamponade
Hypotension
Tachycardia
Vasoconstriction
Equalization of diastolic filling pressures
Fixed and reduced stroke volume (cardiac output and systemic blood pressure dependent on heart rate)
Primary diastolic dysfunction from increased pericardial pressure

blood pressure, the definitive therapy is pericardial drainage. Once the pericardium is drained, venous return and hemodynamics will rapidly normalize.

ANEURYSMS OF THE AORTA

Aneurysms of the aorta most often involve the abdominal aorta. Most patients are hypertensive, and many have associated atherosclerosis. A dissecting aneurysm denotes a tear in the intima of the aorta that allows blood to enter and penetrate between the walls of the vessel, thereby producing a false lumen. Ultimately, the dissection may reenter the lumen through another tear in the intima or rupture through the adventitia.

Elective resection of an abdominal aneurysm is often recommended when the estimated diameter of the aneurysm is larger than 5 cm. The incidence of spontaneous rupture increases dramatically when the size of the aneurysm exceeds this diameter. Extension of the abdominal aneurysm to include the renal arteries occurs in about 5% of patients.

Preoperative Preparation

Perioperative administration of β-blockers reduces perioperative mortality 50% to 90%.[8] β-Blockers should be started as soon as patients are identified as needing surgery. Starting β-blockers 7 to 30 days preoperatively and continuing these drugs for at least 30 days postoperatively is considered desirable. Alternatively, β-blockers are initiated on the day of surgery and continued for 7 days postoperatively. Clonidine reduces 30-day and 2-year mortality and may be used in patients with specific contraindications to β-blockade.[10]

Management of Anesthesia

Patients undergoing anesthesia for resection of an abdominal aortic aneurysm should have continuous monitoring of intra-arterial pressure. Patients with coexisting coronary artery disease are likely to demonstrate increases in pulmonary artery occlusion pressure and evidence of myocardial ischemia during cross-clamping of the abdominal aorta. Nevertheless, the use of pulmonary artery pressure monitoring is controversial and not supported by improved survival data.[17] Transesophageal echocardiography may be useful in evaluating the adequacy of intravascular volume replacement and recognizing cardiac wall motion abnormalities associated with myocardial ischemia. Intraoperatively, myocardial ischemia is treated by decreasing the heart rate with β-blockers and maintaining systemic blood pressure and ventricular filling pressure at acceptable levels with specific pharmacologic interventions (phenylephrine, nitroprusside, nitroglycerin).

Preoperative hydration with a balanced salt solution and prompt intraoperative replacement of blood loss as guided by data obtained from the pulmonary artery catheter or echocardiography are considered useful for maintaining intravascular fluid volume and thus renal function. Diuresis is often facilitated by the intraoperative administration of a diuretic (mannitol or furosemide, or both), with or without dopamine. Despite these interventions, the glomerular filtration rate and renal blood flow are not predictably improved.[30]

The exact cause of hypotension and vasodilation after removal of the aortic cross-clamp is unclear. Decreases in systemic blood pressure can be minimized by intravenously infusing fluids to maintain pulmonary artery occlusion pressure between 10 and 20 mm Hg before removal of the aortic cross-clamp. Gradual removal of the aortic cross-clamp minimizes decreases in systemic blood pressure by allowing time for return of pooled venous blood to the circulation.

CARDIOPULMONARY BYPASS

Cardiopulmonary bypass (CPB) entails gravity drainage of blood from the vena cava into a reservoir, followed by pumping of the blood through a heat exchanger, oxygenator, and filter and then return of the blood to the arterial system, usually the ascending aorta, by means of a centrifugal or roller pump (see Chapter 33) (Fig. 25-3). In the presence of a competent aortic valve, the heart is excluded from the patient's circulation either by a single venous cannula inserted into the right atrium or by dual catheters placed into the superior and inferior venae cavae so that all returning blood enters the large cannulas in these vessels (see Fig. 25-3). If the aortic valve is not competent, venting of the left ventricle may be necessary (1) through a drain placed from the right superior pulmonary vein into the left ventricle, (2) by aspirating from the antegrade cardioplegia line placed in the proximal ascending aorta, or (3) via a pulmonary venous drain. Otherwise, retrograde blood flow through the incompetent aortic valve could cause distention of the left ventricle and damage ventricular function. Venting of blood returning through the thebesian or bronchial veins may also be necessary.

An aortic cross-clamp is placed between the antegrade cardioplegia catheter and the arterial inflow catheter to separate the heart from the circulation and allow cardioplegic arrest. It is important to observe the ventricle for overdistention in any situation in which it is not pumping. If the aortic cross-clamp is removed and ventricular contraction has not returned, the ventricle may become overdistended in situations involving aortic valve insufficiency. When the heart is isolated from the circulation, total CPB is present, and ventilation of the lungs is no longer necessary to maintain oxygenation. However, in

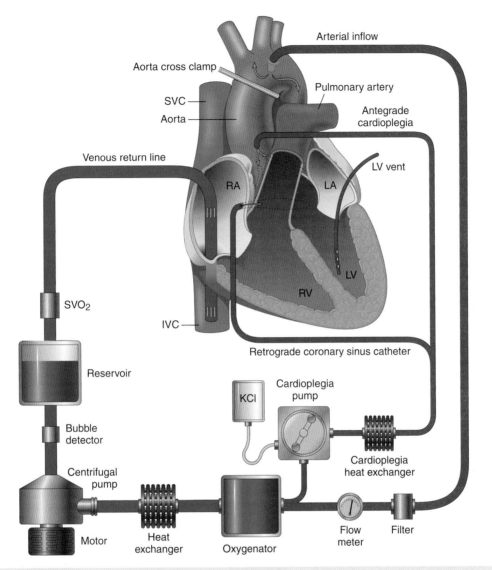

Figure 25-3 Schematic diagram of a cardiopulmonary bypass circuit. Blood from cannulas placed through the right atrium and into the inferior vena cava drains by gravity into a reservoir and is then pumped by a centrifugal pump through a heat exchanger, oxygenator, and filter before returning to the ascending aorta. Blood mixed with cardioplegia solution is pumped alternatively into the proximal ascending aorta or into the coronary sinus. Venting can be accomplished with a cannula placed through the right superior pulmonary vein into the left ventricle or from the ascending aorta antegrade cardioplegia cannula or the pulmonary artery. Cx, circumflex; IVC, inferior vena cava; LAD, left anterior descending; LM, left main; LV, left ventricular; OM, obtuse marginal; RCA, right coronary artery; SVC, superior vena cava.

any situation in which there is a pulsatile pulmonary pressure detected by pulmonary artery catheter monitoring, there is partial CPB, and the lungs should be ventilated to avoid delivering desaturated blood systemically. Gravity-dependent venous drainage to the CPB machine can be improved by raising the level of the operating table or placing a small vacuum on the cardiotomy reservoir. Before initiating CPB it is important to review a checklist (Table 25-14).

Components of the Cardiopulmonary Bypass Circuit

The CPB machine produces nonpulsatile flow into the patient's aorta by either a centrifugal or a roller pump. A centrifugal pump has three disks rotating at 3000 to 4000 rpm to pump blood. Centrifugal pumps are superior to roller pumps because they (1) cause less trauma to blood cells, (2) do not pump air bubbles because of air being less dense than blood, and (3) are afterload dependent,

Table 25-14	Checklist before Initiating Cardiopulmonary Bypass (HADDSUE)
Heparin	Was it administered?
	When the surgeon is placing sutures in the aorta for aortic cannulation, ask about heparin.
	Do not allow a surgeon to initiate cardiopulmonary bypass without prior heparin administration or an alternative anticoagulant.
ACT	Did the heparin increase the activated coagulation time to ≥450 seconds?
	Were antifibrinolytics given?
Drugs	Were additional nondepolarizing neuromuscular blocking drugs and/or anesthetics administered to prevent spontaneous respiratory efforts (risk of air aspiration) during placement of the venous cannula?
Drips	Did you discuss infusions with the perfusionist that may interfere with hemodynamic management during cardiopulmonary bypass?
	Blood pressure during cardiopulmonary bypass depends on flow and resistance.
	Drugs that affect resistance will affect blood pressure.
	Drugs that affect venous capacity will reduce venous return to the reservoir and force a reduction in pump flow.
Swan	Pull the pulmonary artery catheter back 5 cm to avoid pulmonary arterial injury or pulmonary infarction during bypass.
Urine	Measure the total urine output so that the urine produced during cardiopulmonary bypass can be tabulated.
	Urine output can be quite variable during cardiopulmonary bypass, depending on the extracorporeal circulatory prime, volume administered, intrinsic hormonal response to cardiopulmonary bypass, and renal function.
Emboli	Check the aortic cannula visually to detect any emboli.

ACT, activated clotting time.

thereby avoiding the risk of line rupture with clamping of the arterial inflow circuit. The necessary cardiac index delivered by the CPB pump is determined by the patient's body temperature and oxygen consumption. For normothermia or mild hypothermia, a cardiac index of 2 to 4 L/min/m^2 is satisfactory, although flows of about half these levels have been used successfully. Low flow has the advantage of less blood trauma and less non-coronary collateral blood flow, which might result in better myocardial protection.

MEMBRANE OXYGENATORS

Blood is oxygenated by a membrane (most commonly used) or bubble oxygenator. Membrane oxygenators use a blood-membrane-gas interface rather than a blood-gas interface and produce less trauma to blood cells than bubble oxygenators do. With either form of oxygenator, PaO_2 is maintained by adjusting the concentration of oxygen (air-oxygen mixing may be used to avoid hyperoxia) flowing into the oxygenator. Carbon dioxide levels are controlled between 35 and 45 mm Hg by controlling the total free gas flow through the oxygenator. Carbon dioxide is no longer added to CPB circuits to maintain blood gases.

HEAT EXCHANGERS

Heat exchangers are incorporated into bypass circuits to control the patient's body temperature by heating or cooling blood as it circulates. Hot or cold water entering the unit at one end with blood entering at the other provides an efficient countercurrent flow system. Metabolic requirements are decreased about 8% for every degree Celsius decrease in body temperature below 37°C. The optimal temperature management for CPB is not entirely clear (18°C is used before circulatory arrest and 28°C is common during aortic cross-clamping with rewarming to 37°C before weaning from bypass).[31]

CARDIOTOMY RESERVOIR

Blood from the pericardial cavity and the opened heart, as during valve replacement, is returned to a cardiotomy reservoir, where it is filtered, defoamed, and pumped to the oxygenator for recirculation. The cardiotomy suction may be a major cause of hemolysis and emboli during CPB. Filters are incorporated in the cardiotomy reservoir and the arterial circuit to serve as traps for particulate debris (blood clot, latex, talc, fat, Silastic, polyethylene) that could act as systemic emboli.

PUMP PRIME

The tubing used for the CPB circuit is flushed with carbon dioxide and then filled (primed) with crystalloid. Additives to the crystalloid pump prime may include albumin, hetastarch, blood, bicarbonate, heparin, and antibiotics. The goal is a predetermined solution that is calculated to produce a specific hematocrit with the institution of total CPB. Because whole-body hypothermia (18°C to 28°C) may be used, the pump prime often contains little or no blood such that the hematocrit of blood during cardiopulmonary bypass is 20% to 30%. Hemodilution is important for decreasing viscosity during hypothermia. It is mandatory that all air be cleared from the arterial side of the circuit before the institution of CPB. Indeed, pumping of air into the patient by the CPB machine is an ever-present hazard. Continuous flushing of the pericardium with carbon dioxide is intended to reduce the risk for gas emboli.

ANTICOAGULATION

Heparin-induced anticoagulation of the patient is mandatory before placement of the venous and aortic cannulas used for CPB. The usual initial intravenous dose of heparin is 300 to 400 units/kg. The adequacy of anticoagulation is subsequently confirmed by determination of the activated coagulation time, which is typically maintained at greater than 450 seconds (normal is 90 to 120 seconds) during CPB.[32]

Monitoring during Cardiopulmonary Bypass

Institution of CPB is often associated with decreases in mean arterial pressure, presumably reflecting the dramatic decreases in blood viscosity that result from the infusion of prime solutions and activation of systemic inflammatory responses. In addition, peripheral vasodilation may accompany the decreased oxygen delivery that occurs in the early period of hemodilution. Administration of an α-agonist such as phenylephrine to increase perfusion pressure to greater than 40 mm Hg in the early period after institution of CPB may be recommended on the assumption that perfusion pressure is important for maintenance of cerebral blood flow. The desirable blood pressure during bypass is debatable. Lower pressures may reduce cerebral blood flow, but they also reduce the embolic load to the brain. Higher pressures may improve cerebral blood flow and reduce the risk for watershed infarction, but they introduce the risk of more emboli per unit time. Pressures lower than 40 mm Hg are avoided if possible in adults. Pressures higher than 60 mm Hg are used during rewarming. Pressures up to 80 to 90 mm Hg may be used in patients with cerebral vascular disease, although evidence to support these recommendations is limited.

After the initial decrease, mean arterial pressure during CPB often begins to increase spontaneously, perhaps reflecting activation of the renin-angiotensin system or sympathetic nervous system. Mean arterial pressure higher than 100 mm Hg can lead to impairment of tissue perfusion, as well as a risk for hemorrhage. Furthermore, noncoronary collateral blood flow is likely to be increased as mean arterial pressure increases and could result in perfusion of the heart with blood at higher temperatures than desired for optimal cellular protection. Systemic hypertension is often treated by decreasing systemic vascular resistance with volatile anesthetic agents administered through the oxygenator or the continuous administration of nitroprusside.

An increasing central venous pressure with or without facial edema (eyelids and sclera) may reflect improper placement of the vena cava cannula and result in obstruction to venous drainage. For example, insertion of a cannula too far into the superior vena cava can obstruct the right innominate vein and lead to an increase in cerebral venous pressure with associated cerebral edema. Placement of a cannula too far into the inferior vena cava results in abdominal vascular distention. Confirmatory evidence of misplacement of a vena cava cannula is inadequate venous return from the patient to the CPB machine. Prompt withdrawal of the vena cava cannula to a more proximal position should immediately improve venous drainage.

A pulmonary artery catheter detects increases in pulmonary artery pressure caused by malfunction of the left ventricular vent and associated inadequate decompression of the left ventricle. Persistent left ventricular distention can result in damage to the contractile elements of the myocardium.

Blood gases and pH are monitored frequently during CPB. A mixed venous P_{O_2} lower than 30 mm Hg associated with metabolic acidosis suggests inadequate tissue perfusion. Temperature correction of Pa_{CO_2} and pH is probably not necessary. Urine output may serve as a guide to the adequacy of renal perfusion, with an output of 1 mL/kg/hr being a common expectation.

During total CPB, the lungs are left quiescent, with or without moderate continuous positive airway pressure. The best composition of gases in the lungs during this period is unsettled. Continued ventilation of the lungs with oxygen may be appropriate when there is some pulmonary blood flow, as evidenced by a pulsatile pulmonary artery trace. If there is a pulsatile pulmonary arterial pressure or systemic arterial pressure, the lungs should be ventilated because the CPB is only partial.

Esophageal, rectal, bladder, or blood temperature (or any combination) is monitored routinely. Rapid rewarming caused by a high blood-to-body temperature gradient is avoided to reduce the risk for gas emboli. Drug-induced vasodilation as produced by a volatile anesthetic or nitroprusside may speed the rewarming process, as reflected by a more rapid approach of rectal (core) to

IV

esophageal (blood) temperature. Measurement of urinary bladder temperature may reflect core temperatures better than rectal temperature does.

Myocardial Preservation

The goal of myocardial preservation is to decrease the myocardial damage induced by the period of ischemia associated with CPB. This goal is achieved through decreases in myocardial oxygen consumption by infusing cardioplegia solutions containing potassium into the aortic root, which in the presence of a distally cross-clamped aorta and competent aortic valve ensures diversion of the solution into the coronary arteries. Alternatively, the cardioplegia solution may be administered retrogradely through a cannula placed in the coronary sinus. Monitoring of coronary sinus pressure during retrograde administration is used to assess catheter placement. If the pressure at the distal tip of the coronary sinus catheter during cardioplegia administration at 200 mL/min is equal to central venous pressure, the catheter is not in the coronary sinus but is most likely in the right atrium. If the pressure is very high (>100 mm Hg), the coronary sinus catheter is up against a vascular wall. If the pressure in the coronary sinus catheter is 40 to 60 mm Hg during a 200-mL/min infusion, the catheter is correctly positioned. Proper positioning of the coronary sinus catheter may be confirmed by transesophageal echocardiography and manual palpation by the surgeon. If the catheter is placed too distally, delivery of cardioplegia solution to the right ventricle will be compromised and result in poor right ventricular protection. An additional route for infusion of cardioplegia solutions is directly into newly placed bypass grafts.

Potassium in the cardioplegia solution blocks the initial phase of myocardial depolarization and thereby results in cessation of electrical and mechanical activity. The cold solution produces selective hypothermia of the cardiac muscle. At 30°C, the normally contracting heart muscle consumes oxygen at a rate of 8 to 10 mL/100 g/min. Oxygen consumption in the fibrillating ventricle at 22°C is 2 mL/100 g/min. An electromechanically quiet heart at 22°C consumes oxygen at a rate of 0.3 mL/100 g/min. The effectiveness of cold cardioplegia is monitored by measuring heart temperature with a temperature probe placed in the left ventricular muscle, plus the absence of any visible electrical activity on the ECG. Cold cardioplegia infusions are supplemented by total-body hypothermia and localized epicardial surface cooling with ice or cold irrigation solutions placed in the pericardial space. Adequate myocardial preservation is suggested by good myocardial contractility without the use of inotropic drugs at the conclusion of CPB.

A side effect of cardioplegia solutions is an increased incidence of atrioventricular heart block as a result of intramyocardial hyperkalemia. This heart block usually resolves in 1 to 2 hours and can be treated temporarily by the use of an artificial cardiac pacemaker. Intramyocardial hyperkalemia also produces decreased myocardial contractility. Systemic hyperkalemia is likely to occur when coronary sinus blood containing cardioplegia solution is returned to the oxygenator for subsequent circulation. Decreased renal function during CPB will also contribute to hyperkalemia. If hyperkalemia persists at the conclusion of CPB, it may be necessary to administer regular insulin (10 to 20 units IV, often in combination with glucose, 25 to 50 mg IV) in an attempt to shift potassium into the cells. Perfusionists can also add crystalloid solutions to the bypass circuit and then use a hemoconcentrator to ultrafiltrate the blood and thereby eliminate potassium.

Maintenance of Anesthesia

Drugs selected for maintenance of anesthesia in patients undergoing CPB are determined by the patient's cardiac disease. Institution of CPB, however, produces a sudden dilution of circulating drug concentrations. For this reason, supplemental anesthetics, such as benzodiazepines or opioids, may be administered intravenously at this time. Likewise, skeletal muscle paralysis may be supplemented with additional nondepolarizing neuromuscular blocking drugs. An additional dose of nondepolarizing muscle relaxant should be administered just before placement of the venous cannula to avoid entraining air secondary to inspiratory efforts. Anesthetic depth can also be increased by delivery of volatile anesthetics from vaporizers incorporated into the CPB circuit. It must be appreciated that the impact of hemodilution on drug concentrations is likely to be offset by a decreased need for drugs during hypothermia. For reasons that are not clear, anesthetic requirements seem to be minimal after rewarming to a normal body temperature at the conclusion of CPB. Therefore, additional anesthesia is not routinely required during rewarming or the early period after the conclusion of CPB. However, additional anesthetic (propofol, dexmedetomidine) may be needed to maintain tracheal intubation for transfer and postoperative ventilation in the intensive care unit.

Discontinuation of Cardiopulmonary Bypass

A checklist for weaning from CPB consists of the mnemonic WRMVP (Table 25-15). When the left side of the heart has been opened, as during valve replacement surgery, it is mandatory to remove all air from the cardiac chambers and pulmonary veins before permitting the heart to eject blood into the aorta. Otherwise, systemic air emboli could occur, with disastrous cardiac and central nervous system effects. The presence of air can be determined by transesophageal echocardiography. Unrecognized air in the coronary arteries may be a cause of sudden

Table 25-15 Checklist for Weaning from Cardiopulmonary Bypass (WRMVP)

<u>W</u>arm (37°C; body temperature is likely to decrease rapidly after cardiopulmonary bypass if not adequately rewarmed, with resultant metabolic acidosis and poor myocardial contractility)

<u>R</u>hythm

<u>M</u>onitors (confirm that they are turned on; pulse oximeter for arterial oxygen saturation and cardiac output)

<u>V</u>entilator (confirm that it is turned on)

<u>P</u>erfusion (heart beating, presence of vasodilation)

onset of poor myocardial contractility after discontinuation of CPB. Measurement of cardiac filling pressure, determination of thermodilution cardiac output, and calculation of systemic and pulmonary vascular resistance are helpful for guiding intravenous fluid replacement and the appropriate selection of drugs in the early period after CPB (Table 25-16). Alternatively, transesophageal echocardiography can be used to estimate the adequacy of intravascular fluid volume and myocardial contractility. Transesophageal echocardiography is also useful for evaluating cardiac valve function and intracardiac blood flow patterns, particularly after surgical repair or replacement.

SYSTEMIC VASCULAR RESISTANCE
The most common hemodynamic abnormality after CPB is low systemic vascular resistance (driving pressure divided by flow). It is very difficult to wean from CPB when systemic vascular resistance is low. Systemic vascular resistance can be normalized by the administration of a vasoconstrictor before weaning from CPB. It is much easier to adjust the peripheral vasculature to match the

heart than to force the heart to tolerate a dilated vasculature. On occasion, an inotrope (dopamine, epinephrine, norepinephrine, dobutamine) is needed. In severe cases a combination of drugs (epinephrine or norepinephrine and amrinone or milrinone), with or without an intra-aortic balloon pump, is necessary to maintain optimal cardiac output. If β-agonists are needed, frequent attention must be paid to measurement and control of potassium, glucose, calcium, pH, and the presence of cardiac dysrhythmias.

Gas emboli passing into the coronary arteries may suddenly and profoundly reduce ventricular function. Posterior papillary muscle dysfunction at the conclusion of CPB may result in mitral regurgitation, as evidenced by the presence of prominent V waves on the pulmonary artery occlusion pressure tracing. This dysfunction may reflect less than optimal cardioplegic protection of the posterior myocardium, which is most vulnerable to warming effects from blood in the adjacent descending aorta, as well as perfusion with warm blood representing noncoronary collateral circulation.

High resistance to blood flow in the arm induced by vasoconstriction may result in a falsely low systemic blood pressure reading from the radial artery in the early period after CPB. If there is a question of inadequate arterial blood pressure, direct pressure measurement from the ascending aorta can be instantly obtained. Any gradient between central aortic and radial artery blood pressure usually disappears within 60 minutes. Placement of a femoral arterial catheter is needed if there is a persistent gradient between central and radial pressure.

INTRA-AORTIC BALLOON PUMP
A mechanical alternative to inotropic support of cardiac output is an intra-aortic balloon pump. An intra-aortic balloon pump is a 25-cm-long balloon mounted on a 90-cm stiff plastic catheter that is typically inserted

IV

Table 25-16 Diagnosis and Treatment of Cardiovascular Dysfunction after Cardiopulmonary Bypass

Systemic Blood Pressure	Atrial Pressure	Cardiac Output	Diagnosis	Therapy
Decreased	Decreased	Decreased	Hypovolemia	Administer volume
Decreased	Decreased	Increased	Vasodilation Low blood viscosity	Vasoconstrictor Erythrocyte transfusion
Decreased	Increased	Decreased	Left ventricular dysfunction	Inotrope Inodilator Vasodilator Mechanical assistance
Increased	Increased	Decreased	Vasoconstriction Left ventricular dysfunction	Vasodilator Inotrope
Increased	Decreased	Increased	Hyperdynamic	Volatile anesthetic β-Antagonist

percutaneously through the femoral artery and advanced so that the tip is just distal to the left subclavian artery. The balloon is timed to inflate during diastole to augment diastolic blood pressure and increase the gradient for coronary perfusion. The balloon deflates immediately before systole, thus decreasing afterload and lowering oxygen requirements. Coronary blood flow is increased, with little or no increase in cardiac work, which may result in improvements in cardiac output. Rapid heart rates and cardiac dysrhythmias interfere with proper balloon timing and optimal augmentation of cardiac output.

REVERSAL OF ANTICOAGULATION

When adequate systemic blood pressure and cardiac output have been maintained for several minutes, the vena cava cannulas are removed and protamine administration is begun to reverse heparin anticoagulation. Protamine administration may be associated with hypotension from histamine release. Occasionally, pulmonary hypertension accompanies the administration of protamine. Protamine should be administered slowly intravenously after a test dose. Simultaneous infusion of phenylephrine can be used to maintain systemic blood pressure. In cases of hemodynamic collapse, even epinephrine boluses may be inadequate, and return to CPB, after emergency reheparinization, can be lifesaving. Diabetics who use NPH insulin (contains protamine) may be at increased risk for protamine reactions. Protamine allergic reactions may be reduced by prior administration of H_1 blockers (diphenhydramine), H_2 blockers (cimetidine), and corticosteroids. The aortic cannula is removed after protamine administration is safely concluded. Pharmacologic measures to decrease bleeding include the administration of antifibrinolytics (aminocaproic acid, tranexamic acid, aprotinin) and desmopressin (improves platelet function in patients with von Willebrand's disease). Blood loss throughout the procedure, as well as blood in the bypass tubing, can be salvaged, washed, and retransfused with the use of "cell saver" devices.

CONCLUSION OF SURGERY

Administration of nitrous oxide after CPB is not recommended because this gas could accentuate the effects of air in the heart or coronary arteries. For this reason, anesthesia is most often supplemented, when necessary, by the intravenous administration of propofol, dexmedetomidine, opioids, benzodiazepines, or alternatively, low inhaled concentrations of volatile anesthetics. Administration of these drugs may be continued in the intensive care unit to provide sedation until tracheal extubation. Tracheal extubation can be considered when the patient is awake and oxygenation is stable (PaO_2 >80 mm Hg with an FIO_2 of 0.4), bleeding is controlled, and neuromuscular function has recovered. There is no benefit from prolonged postoperative ventilation after cardiac surgery.

DURATION OF INTENSIVE CARE UNIT OBSERVATION

The high financial cost of cardiac surgery is due in part to the duration of intensive care required for these patients. Improvements in anesthetic, surgical, and perfusion techniques serve to decrease the need for prolonged care of these patients in an intensive care unit. The concept known as "fast track" as applied to cardiac surgical patients includes early postoperative awakening and tracheal extubation.[33]

Off-Pump Coronary Artery Bypass Graft Surgery

In an effort to minimize postoperative morbidity, CABG may be accomplished in selected patients without the institution of CPB and in the presence of a spontaneously beating heart and normothermia. Off-pump CABG ("beating heart surgery") was developed to reduce the sequelae of CPB, which may include stroke, global encephalopathy, renal failure, pulmonary injury, and mortality. The ability to immediately institute CPB support must be available. The presence of a beating heart makes suture placement for the distal anastomosis difficult. In this regard, a silicon stent can be placed in the target coronary artery during the anastomosis to maintain coronary flow. The silicon stent is removed just before completing the anastomosis. Stopping coronary blood flow in the target coronary may cause myocardial ischemia, ventricular dysrhythmias, ventricular dysfunction, heart block, hemodynamic collapse, and cardiac arrest. Prophylactic antidysrhythmic therapy (magnesium, lidocaine, or amiodarone) is often administered before off-pump CABG. Anticoagulation with heparin is achieved and the activated coagulation time measured. Antifibrinolytics (aprotinin, aminocaproic acid, tranexamic acid) are not used if CPB is not going to be instituted.

MANAGEMENT OF ANESTHESIA

Anesthesia for off-pump CABG is very similar to anesthesia for CPB. All preoperative medications with the exception of oral hypoglycemic agents should be continued in the perioperative period. Patients with diabetes mellitus may be managed with insulin infusions and frequent blood glucose determinations. Coumadin therapy should be stopped at least 7 days before planned surgery. Platelet inhibitors, with the exception of aspirin, should be discontinued preoperatively. Preoperative heparin infusions can be continued in the operating room and discontinued after full heparinization.

Induction of anesthesia follows the same goals as for patients who will be placed on CPB. Maintenance of anesthesia is usually achieved with a volatile anesthetic (isoflurane, sevoflurane) in combination with an opioid (fentanyl, sufentanil). Nitrous oxide is avoided to maximize delivered oxygen concentrations and minimize the possible impact of air bubble expansion should venous air embolism occur. Maintenance infusions of propofol, dexmedetomidine, or remifentanil are also commonly used.

Hemodynamic stability during the distal graft anastomosis is achieved with careful surgical manipulation and retraction of the heart, table positioning, infusions of vasoconstrictors, and volume. Inotropic stimulation with β-agonists has the potential to raise the heart rate and thus make completion of the distal anastomosis more difficult and lower the threshold for ventricular dysrhythmias. If β-agonists are needed to support cardiac output during conduct of the distal anastomosis, the use of CPB should be considered.

Heparin anticoagulation is reversed with protamine after completion of the proximal and distal anastomoses and is confirmed by return of the activated coagulation time to near baseline (120 to 140 seconds). The requirement for postoperative ventilation and sedation may be reduced with off-pump CABG. Postoperative β-blockade may decrease the incidence of atrial fibrillation and myocardial ischemia. Aspirin therapy should be resumed once bleeding is controlled.

REFERENCES

1. Mangano DT, Goldman L. Preoperative assessment of patients with known or suspected coronary disease. N Engl J Med 1995; 333:1750-1756.
2. Fleisher LA, Barash PG. Preoperative cardiac evaluation for noncardiac surgery: A functional approach. Anesth Analg 1992; 74:586-598.
3. Slogoff S, Keats AS. Does chronic treatment with calcium entry blocking drugs reduce perioperative myocardial ischemia? Anesthesiology 1988;68:676-680.
4. Tarhan S, Moffitt EA, Taylor WF, Giuliani ER. Myocardial infarction after general anesthesia. Anesth Analg 1977;56:455-461.
5. Steen PA, Tinker JH, Tarhan S. Myocardial reinfarction after anesthesia and surgery. JAMA 1978; 239:2566-2570.
6. Rao TL, Jacobs KH, El-Etr AA. Reinfarction following anesthesia in patients with myocardial infarction. Anesthesiology 1983;59:499-505.
7. Shah KB, Kleinman BS, Sami H, et al. Reevaluation of perioperative myocardial infarction in patients with prior myocardial infarction undergoing noncardiac operations. Anesth Analg 1990;71:231-235.
8. Poldermans D, Boersma E, Bax JJ, et al. Bisoprolol reduces cardiac death and myocardial infarction in high-risk patients as long as 2 years after successful major vascular surgery. Eur Heart J 2001;22:1353-1358.
9. Wallace A, Layug B, Tateo I, et al. Prophylactic atenolol reduces postoperative myocardial ischemia. McSPI Research Group. Anesthesiology 1998;88:7-17.
10. Wallace AW, Galindez D, Salahieh A, et al. Effect of clonidine on cardiovascular morbidity and mortality after noncardiac surgery. Anesthesiology 2004;101:284-293.
11. Hueb W, Soares PR, Gersh BJ, et al. The medicine, angioplasty, or surgery study (MASS-II): A randomized, controlled clinical trial of three therapeutic strategies for multivessel coronary artery disease: One-year results. J Am Coll Cardiol 2004; 43:1743-1751.
12. Kaluza GL, Joseph J, Lee JR, et al. Catastrophic outcomes of noncardiac surgery soon after coronary stenting. J Am Coll Cardiol 2000;35:1288-1294.
13. Mangano DT, Browner WS, Hollenberg M, et al. Association of perioperative myocardial ischemia with cardiac morbidity and mortality in men undergoing noncardiac surgery. The Study of Perioperative Ischemia Research Group. N Engl J Med 1990;323:1781-1788.
14. Helman JD, Leung JM, Bellows WH, et al. The risk of myocardial ischemia in patients receiving desflurane versus sufentanil anesthesia for coronary artery bypass graft surgery. The S.P.I. Research Group. Anesthesiology 1992;77:47-62.
15. Cason BA, Gamperl AK, Slocum RE, Hickey RF. Anesthetic-induced preconditioning: Previous administration of isoflurane decreases myocardial infarct size in rabbits. Anesthesiology 1997;87:1182-1190.
16. Slogoff S, Keats AS. Randomized trial of primary anesthetic agents on outcome of coronary artery bypass operations. Anesthesiology 1989; 70:179-188.
17. Practice guidelines for pulmonary artery catheterization: An updated report by the American Society of Anesthesiologists Task Force on Pulmonary Artery Catheterization. Anesthesiology 2003;99:988-1014.
18. Carabello BA, Crawford FA Jr. Valvular heart disease. N Engl J Med 1997;337:32-41.
19. van den Berghe G, Wouters P, Weekers F, et al. Intensive insulin therapy in the critically ill patients. N Engl J Med 2001;345:1359-1367.
20. Hilgenberg JC, McCammon RL, Stoelting RK: Pulmonary and systemic vascular responses to nitrous oxide in patients with mitral stenosis and pulmonary hypertension. Anesth Analg 1980;59:323-326.
21. Greenberg BH, Rahimtoola SH. Vasodilator therapy for valvular heart disease. JAMA 1981;246:269-272.
22. Hanson EW, Neerhut RK, Lynch C. Mitral valve prolapse. Anesthesiology 1996;85:178-195.
23. Freed LA, Levy D, Levine RA, et al. Prevalence and clinical outcome of mitral-valve prolapse. N Engl J Med 1999;341:1-7.
24. Atlee JL. Perioperative cardiac dysrhythmias: Diagnosis and management. Anesthesiology 1997;86:1397-1424.
25. Gallagher JD, Weindling SN, Anderson G, Fillinger MP. Effects of sevoflurane on QT interval in a patient with congenital long QT syndrome. Anesthesiology 1998; 89:1569-1573.
26. Kusumoto FM, Goldschlager N. Cardiac pacing. N Engl J Med 1996;334:89-97.
27. Zaidan JR. Pacemakers. Anesthesiology 1984;60:319-334.
28. Dagnino J, Prys-Roberts C. Studies of anaesthesia in relation to hypertension. VI: Cardiovascular responses to extradural blockade of treated and untreated hypertensive patients. Br J Anaesth 1984;56: 1065-1073.
29. Spirito P, Seidman CE, McKenna WJ, Maron BJ. The management of hypertrophic cardiomyopathy. N Engl J Med 1997;336:775-785.
30. Pass LJ, Eberhart RC, Brown JC, et al. The effect of mannitol and dopamine on the renal response to thoracic aortic cross-clamping. J Thorac Cardiovasc Surg 1988;95:608-612.

IV

31. Martin TD, Craver JM, Gott JP, et al. Prospective, randomized trial of retrograde warm blood cardioplegia: Myocardial benefit and neurologic threat. Ann Thorac Surg 1994;57:298-302.

32. Despotis GJ, Gravlee G, Filos K, Levy J. Anticoagulation monitoring during cardiac surgery: A review of current and emerging techniques. Anesthesiology 1999;91:1122-1151.

33. Engelman RM, Rousou JA, Flack JE, et al. Fast-track recovery of the coronary bypass patient. Ann Thorac Surg 1994;58:1742-1746.

Chapter 26

CONGENITAL HEART DISEASE

James E. Baker and Isobel A. Russell

Categorization of the many types of congenital heart disease (CHD) may be based on distinctive features of the pathophysiology of the cardiac and vascular defects (Table 26-1).

PATHOPHYSIOLOGY OF CONGENITAL HEART DISEASE

Shunts

Normally, pulmonary blood flow (Qp) and systemic blood flow (Qs) do not mix, and the entire cardiac output flows sequentially from one circulation to the other. Shunting occurs when a portion of the venous return of one circulation is redirected back to the arterial outflow of the same circulation.[1-3] Commonly, this occurs by way of an abnormal intracardiac channel (atrial or ventricular septal defect) or an abnormal communication between the systemic and pulmonary arterial vessels (patent ductus arteriosus). Anatomic lesions producing shunts may be *restrictive* or *nonrestrictive*.[1] Typically, smaller lesions behave as restrictive lesions, with limited shunt flow across the orifice. Larger defects may behave as nonrestrictive lesions, with unimpaired flow.

Table 26-1 Categorization of Congenital Heart Disease
Cyanotic (tricuspid atresia) versus acyanotic (ventricular septal defect)
Simple (atrial septal defect) versus complex (hypoplastic left heart syndrome)
Obstructive (congenital aortic stenosis, tetralogy of Fallot)
Restrictive versus nonrestrictive
Mixing lesions reflecting an admixture of systemic and pulmonary venous blood (common atrium, single ventricle, truncus arteriosus)

LEFT-TO-RIGHT SHUNT

A left-to-right shunt occurs when part of the pulmonary venous return is redirected toward the pulmonary arterial system.[3] Qp is the sum of the pulmonary blood flow that is redirected toward the pulmonary artery (*recirculated* pulmonary blood flow) and the flow that is appropriately directed toward the systemic circulation (*effective* pulmonary blood flow) (Figs. 26-1 and 26-2). Left-to-right shunts result in an effective systemic blood flow that is smaller than the *total* pulmonary blood flow. As a result, the effective circulation may be too low, and systemic hypotension or shock can ensue. Alternatively, total pulmonary blood flow may be too high, and pulmonary edema, long-term elevation of pulmonary vascular resistance, or abnormal cardiac chamber dilation can result.

RIGHT-TO-LEFT SHUNT

A right-to-left shunt occurs when a portion of the systemic venous return is redirected to the systemic arterial outflow without first circulating through the lungs.[2] The hallmark of lesions producing a right-to-left shunt is arterial oxygen desaturation. Because the pulmonary venous return mixes with recirculated systemic venous blood, the resulting arterial oxygen saturation will be low. The degree of desaturation depends on the magnitude of right-to-left shunting, as well as the degree of desaturation of the systemic venous return.

MIXING LESIONS

Whereas a shunt connotes *partial* mixing of the pulmonary and systemic venous circulation, many forms of CHD result in *complete* blending of the two circulations (see Table 26-1). As a result, oxygen content is equilibrated between the two circulations such that oxygen saturation is identical or nearly identical at both the pulmonary and systemic arterial level.[1] As with right-to-left shunts, one of the chief characteristics of mixing lesions is systemic arterial oxygen desaturation. A decrease in systemic venous oxygen saturation may result from either an increase in systemic oxygen consumption or a decrease in systemic oxygen delivery (low cardiac output, arterial oxygen desaturation, low hematocrit).

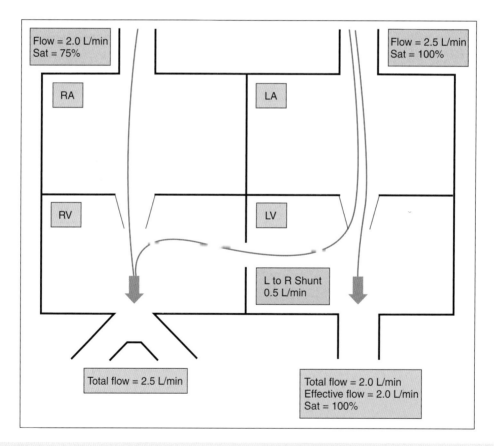

Figure 26-1 Schematic diagram of a simple shunt—ventricular septal defect. A left-to-right shunt occurs at a septal defect with 0.5-L/min flow. Thus, total systemic flow is 2.0 L/min, all of which is effective flow, and total pulmonary flow is 2.5 L/min, only 2.0 L of which is effective. LA, left atrium; LV, left ventricle; RA, right atrium; RV, right ventricle.

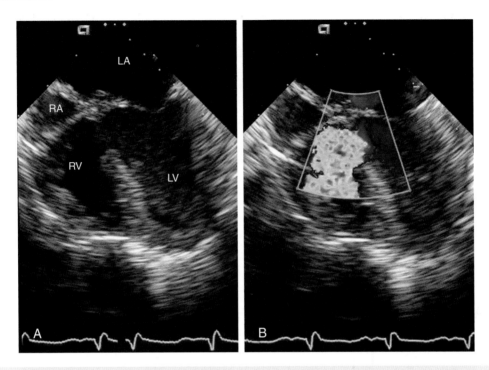

Figure 26-2 Transesophageal echocardiography of the heart. **A,** A four-chamber image demonstrates a 1.5- to 2.0-cm defect in the ventricular septum, just below the level of the atrioventricular valves. LA, left atrium; LV, left ventricle; RA, right atrium; RV, right ventricle. **B,** Color flow Doppler demonstrates abnormal left-to-right flow (shunting) across the defect. Also note in each figure that the right ventricle is abnormally thickened because of long-standing exposure to left ventricular pressure. The atrial septum bows toward the right atrium because of volume overload of the left atrium and ventricle.

IV

Relationship of Pulmonary Blood Flow to Systemic Blood Flow

The closer Qp can be maintained equal in magnitude to Qs, the less the pathophysiologic impact of the CHD lesion will be because equal blood flows tend to maximize the *effective* component of each circulation and minimize the wasteful *recirculated* component.[1] Any preferential flow toward the aorta will increase systemic blood flow, but at the expense of pulmonary blood flow, and the resulting mixed ventricular blood will have a lower oxygen saturation such that total tissue oxygen delivery will decrease. Any preferential flow toward the pulmonary artery will increase pulmonary blood flow and systemic oxygen saturation, but at the expense of systemic cardiac output and overall delivery of oxygen to tissues. Ultimately, the ratio of Qp to Qs is determined by the relative resistance to flow presented by each of the two circulations. If pulmonary vascular resistance (PVR) exceeds systemic vascular resistance (SVR), Qs will exceed Qp. Likewise, if SVR exceeds PVR, Qp will exceed Qs.

IMPACT OF ANESTHETIC MANAGEMENT

Anesthetic management of patients with CDH may affect the ratio of Qp to Qs (Table 26-2). For example, in a patient with a ventricular septal defect, intentionally keeping the PVR relatively high will decrease the amount of left ventricular blood that shunts through the defect toward the lungs. This will tend to keep the Qp/Qs ratio closer to 1:1. This concept is the basis of the terms *restrictive* and *nonrestrictive* as applied to shunting lesions. Generally, nonrestrictive lesions are larger and more susceptible to changes in the ratio of SVR to PVR. Restrictive lesions are smaller and less susceptible to changes in the ratio of SVR to PVR.

PVR may be lowered by means of hyperventilation and the attendant respiratory alkalosis, and incremental lowering may be achieved by decreasing $PaCO_2$ by as much as 20 mm Hg or increasing pH to as high as 7.6.[4] Likewise, hypercapnia and acidosis tend to increase PVR.[4] Some evidence, however, suggests that carbon dioxide per se is unimportant except to the extent that it creates the change in pH, which ultimately effects the change in PVR.

Effects of Congenital Heart Disease on Pulmonary Blood Flow and Pulmonary Vascular Resistance

CHD may subject the lungs to abnormal blood flow or pulmonary artery pressure (Table 26-3). Over time, the

Table 26-2 Impact of Anesthetic Management on the Ratio of Systemic to Pulmonary Blood Flow

Events That Increase Systemic Vascular Resistance
Light anesthesia
Sympathetic nervous system activation
Administration of α-agonists
Physical manipulations (compression of the femoral arteries by flexing the hips of infants and small children)
Events That Decrease Systemic Vascular Resistance
Deep anesthesia
Administration of vasodilating drugs (nitrates, intravenous and inhaled anesthetics)
Events That Increase Pulmonary Vascular Resistance
Alveolar hypoxemia (low inspired oxygen concentrations)
Hypercapnia
Acidosis
High lung volumes or pressures (tend to collapse pulmonary capillaries)
Low lung volumes with atelectasis (tend to collapse larger pulmonary blood vessels)
Light anesthesia
Sympathetic nervous system stimulation
Hypothermia

Table 26-3 Effect of Congenital Heart Disease on Pulmonary Blood Flow and Pulmonary Artery Pressure

Increased Pulmonary Blood Flow (Right-to-Left Shunt)
Atrial septal defect
Anomalous pulmonary venous return
Increased Pulmonary Artery Pressure (Right-to-Left Shunt)
Ventricular septal defect
Atrioventricular canal
Truncus arteriosus
Transposition of the great arteries
Double-inlet left ventricle

pulmonary vasculature may undergo a process of remodeling with a gradual increase in PVR that may result in pulmonary hypertension, even if the underlying hemodynamic problem is corrected.[4] When pulmonary hypertension becomes irreversible, blood is preferentially directed toward the systemic circulation and the direction of the shunt (ventricular septal defect) may change from left to right and become right to left (Eisenmenger's syndrome).

PREOPERATIVE ASSESSMENT AND PATIENT PREPARATION

Surgery for CHD should be planned with the cooperative input of a multidisciplinary team. Surgeons, cardiologists, critical care specialists, and anesthesiologists all play a very important role in preparing this highly complex patient population for surgery. It is important for anesthesiologists to identify aspects of the patient's condition that can or should be optimized before surgery. It is also important for the anesthesiologist to understand the physiology of the cardiac lesion and the subsequent effects of the planned surgical palliative or corrective procedure.

Review of the Patient's History

A review of the patient's history should include attention to details that are of importance to pediatric anesthetic care in general, such as pertinent pregnancy details, prematurity, and postnatal course. Patients with CHD frequently have associated syndromes (trisomy 21, DiGeorge's syndrome) or evidence of chronic illness (renal dysfunction, pulmonary edema, imbalances in electrolyte and glucose metabolism). Preoperative medications and laboratory studies (complete blood count, electrolytes, coagulation studies, indices of renal and hepatic function) are noted.

The anesthesiologist should review the available diagnostic studies that have been used to diagnose and characterize the cardiac lesion. In this regard, echocardiograms and cardiac catheterization studies will be most helpful. Likewise, electrocardiograms and chest radiographs may also provide important details. Medical interventions that have been instituted previously (therapy for congestive heart failure, previous palliative or corrective surgical procedures, percutaneous procedures such as balloon atrial septostomy) and any change or deterioration in the patient's status in the interim are evaluated. Previous cardiac surgery has implications for the anesthesiologist in terms of anticipating increased operative blood loss, as well as the potential for significant cardiac trauma during dissection as a result of adhesions to the sternum and chest wall. Many hospitalized neonates may be requiring continuous infusions of inotropes or other medications (prostaglandin E_1 to preserve patency of the ductus arteriosus) to maintain stability while awaiting surgery.

Physical Examination

Physical examination is important to assess for airway problems (trisomy 21), symptoms or signs of congestive heart failure, cyanosis, nutritional status, and any other coexisting conditions. Outpatients who have been scheduled for elective surgery should be evaluated on the day of surgery for the new onset of signs or symptoms of an intercurrent illness that may prompt delay of surgery, such as an upper respiratory tract infection. Examination of inpatients is beneficial for reviewing any intravenous or invasive catheters (arterial or central venous) that may be in place.

Preparation for Surgery

With the exception of intubated patients in a critical care setting, all patients (or their caregivers) should be given age-appropriate fasting instructions according to standard American Society of Anesthesiologists guidelines (see Appendix 1). Outpatients taking cardiac medications should generally be advised to continue therapy up to and including the day of surgery, although preference may vary among anesthesiologists regarding diuretics and angiotensin-converting enzyme inhibitors.

OPERATING ROOM SETUP

Preparation of the operating room should include readiness of age-appropriate airway equipment, intravenous equipment (Buretrol infusion sets and fluid warmers), and invasive monitors (catheters and transducers). All intravenous administration sets should be meticulously de-aired to prevent paradoxical arterial embolization of intravenous air bubbles. Any warming blankets or surface cooling equipment should be made available, and adjustment of the operating room temperature should precede entry of the patient (27°C for small or premature infants and 24°C for older children). Hemodynamic medications should be prepared in weight-appropriate dilutions before surgery. Preparation may include readiness of specialized equipment such as transesophageal echocardiography or nitric oxide delivery systems.

Induction of Anesthesia

Induction of anesthesia for patients with CHD may involve the use of inhaled or intravenous anesthetic drugs (Tables 26-4 and 26-5).[5]

INHALATION INDUCTION OF ANESTHESIA

Awake infants and children without intravenous access are frequently amenable to inhalation induction of anesthesia. This strategy is typically reserved for those with minimal or well-controlled congestive heart failure because a dose-dependent reduction in myocardial contractility occurs with volatile anesthetic drugs. Sevoflurane is the most likely drug selection as a result of its lack of pungency and airway irritant effect and the absence of cardiac sensitization to catecholamines. Nitrous oxide may be used to speed induction or limit the dose of sevoflurane. Concerns regarding the propensity of nitrous oxide to increase PVR have not been substantiated in patients with CHD, although it should be borne in mind that the use of nitrous oxide necessarily decreases Fi_{O_2}, which may be relevant in those who require protection against increased PVR. When used during induction, nitrous oxide is often discontinued thereafter because of its property of expanding intravascular air bubbles.

Placement of a pulse oximetry probe and a precordial stethoscope is minimally distressing to an anxious, awake child and provides ample monitoring for the initial stages of inhalation induction. Other noninvasive monitors may be placed in timely fashion once the patient achieves a light plane of anesthesia. Intravenous access is secured when anesthetic depth is adequate, at which time additional intravenous anesthetics (if needed), neuromuscular blocking drugs, and possibly anticholinergics may be given before laryngoscopy and intubation.

INTRAVENOUS INDUCTION OF ANESTHESIA

Patients with poorly controlled congestive heart failure, moderately impaired ventricular function, significant right-to-left shunting, or complete mixing lesions may benefit from the increased stability afforded by intravenous induction of anesthesia. Frequently, these patients

Table 26-4 Drugs for Induction of Anesthesia in Patients with Congenital Heart Disease

	Dose for Induction of Anesthesia	Predominant Hemodynamic Effects	Comments
Sevoflurane	1.5%-3.5% (ET)	↓SVR, ↓contractility	↓Dose if N$_2$O used; avoid if poorly controlled CHF, pronounced ventricular dysfunction, or right-to-left shunt
Halothane	0.8%-2.0% (ET)	↓Contractility, ↓HR, ↓CO, ?dysrhythmias	As above; more pronounced myocardial depression, bradycardia, and ventricular irritability
Fentanyl (IV, sole drug)	20-50 μg/kg	⇔Contractility, SVR, and PVR; ↓HR	Loss of sympathetic tone may ↓ SVR, PVR, or BP; chest wall rigidity with rapid or large doses
Sufentanil (IV, sole drug)	5-10 μg/kg	As above	As above
Ketamine (IV)	1-2 mg/kg	↑HR, ↑ or ⇔SVR, ⇔PVR, ↑ or preserved contractility	Actually a myocardial depressant with sympathetic stimulant properties; may ↓ contractility if no additional SNS recruitable; bronchorrhea may be prevented with atropine, 20 μg/kg
Ketamine (IM)	3-5 mg/kg		
Etomidate (IV)	0.2-0.3 mg/kg	⇔HR, SVR, PVR, contractility	May inhibit endogenous corticosteroid production; burning pain at the injection site

BP, blood pressure; CHF, congestive heart failure; CO, cardiac output; ET, end-tidal; HR, heart rate; IM, intramuscular; IV, intravenous; PVR, pulmonary vascular resistance; SVR, systemic vascular resistance; SNS, sympathetic nervous system.

Table 26-5 Common Congenital Cardiac Lesions—Summary of Anesthetic Goals and Induction Strategies

General Goals and Principles

Avoid air entrapment in intravenous and pressure tubing; meticulous clearing techniques

Avoid dehydration; careful orders regarding NPO status (following ASA guidelines)

Avoid myocardial depression

Maintain sinus rhythm whenever possible

Well-sedated, cooperative patient is ideal

Premedication for patients older than 1 year (oral midazolam, 1 mg/kg)

Close monitoring after sedation

Lesions Characterized by Excessive Pulmonary Blood Flow

Atrial Septal Defects
Avoid further decreases in pulmonary vascular resistance (hyperventilation, high Fio$_2$)

Consider early tracheal extubation

Ventricular Septal Defects
Avoid decreases in pulmonary vascular resistance

Avoid excessive myocardial depression, particularly in patients with congestive heart failure—inhaled induction may be rapid

Atrioventricular Septal Defects
Avoid decreases in pulmonary vascular resistance before cardiopulmonary bypass

Table 26-5 Common Congenital Cardiac Lesions—Summary of Anesthetic Goals and Induction Strategies—cont'd

Prepare to treat pulmonary hypertension (100% oxygen, hyperventilation, alkalinization, deep sedation)

Have nitric oxide available and ready

Inotropic support frequently required

Truncus Arteriosus
Neonates are critically ill; require close management of systemic and pulmonary vascular resistance

Addition of carbon dioxide or nitrogen may be needed to decrease inspired oxygen concentration to 17%

Hypoplastic Left Heart Syndrome (Surgical Correction Occurs in Three Stages)
Norwood procedure (the main pulmonary artery is used to reconstruct the hypoplastic aorta; pulmonary blood flow is provided by a Gore-Tex shunt from the subclavian artery or by a right ventricular–to–pulmonary artery conduit)

Anesthetic management includes prebypass PGE$_1$ infusion, maintenance of nearly equal pulmonary and systemic blood flow for adequate systemic perfusion, precautions against air embolism, maintenance of anesthesia with intravenous drugs, and postbypass maintenance of a high hematocrit and probably a need for inotropic support

Glenn procedure (creation of a direct connection between the superior vena cava and pulmonary artery)

Anesthetic management includes maintenance of a high hematocrit, elevation of the head of the bed to facilitate venous drainage, avoidance of central lines to reduce the risk for pulmonary artery thrombus, and recognition that positive-pressure ventilation of the patient's lungs may decrease pulmonary blood flow and cardiac output

Fontana procedure (rerouting of blood flow from the inferior vena cava into the above pulmonary circulation)

Anesthetic management includes the same principles as for the Glenn procedure

Lesions Characterized by Inadequate Pulmonary Blood Flow

Transposition of the Great Vessels
PGE$_1$ infusion maintained before cardiopulmonary bypass

Manipulation of pulmonary vascular resistance before cardiopulmonary bypass

Opioid-based anesthetic

Corrected Transposition of the Great Vessels
Avoid sudden systemic hypertension

Tetralogy of Fallot
Adequate preoperative hydration essential

Manipulations to decrease pulmonary vascular resistance and improve pulmonary blood flow

Hypercyanotic episodes treated by volume administration, sedation, and pharmacologically induced increases in systemic vascular resistance (phenylephrine)

Avoid increases in heart rate, which may worsen infundibular pulmonary stenosis

Rate of anesthetic induction may be slowed because of a right-to-left shunt

Tricuspid Atresia
Usually the right ventricle is diminutive or hypoplastic

Surgical approach involves an aortopulmonary shunt and subsequent Glenn and Fontan procedures

Anesthetic management as for the Glenn procedure

Total Anomalous Pulmonary Venous Return
Severe cyanosis treated by high inspired oxygen concentration

IV

Table 26-5 Common Congenital Cardiac Lesions—Summary of Anesthetic Goals and Induction Strategies—cont'd

Avoidance of acidosis and high hematocrit
Coarctation of the Aorta Arterial monitoring in the right arm
Ability to provide adequate ventilation in the thoracotomy position (tight-fitting endotracheal tube)
Inotropic support may be necessary in critically ill patients
Avoidance of acidosis
Aortic Stenosis Avoidance of tachycardia, dysrhythmias, hypotension
Decrease in myocardial oxygen demand and maintenance of preload and afterload

ASA, American Society of Anesthesiologists; PGE$_1$, prostaglandin E$_1$.

come to the operating room from a critical care setting and have intravenous access already available. Traditionally, intravenous opioids have been used in this setting because they produce little or no myocardial depression and also lack vasodilating properties in both the pulmonary and systemic vascular beds.[6] Other intravenous drugs that are used in patients with CHD include benzodiazepines, etomidate, and ketamine. Propofol is likely to result in hypotension or increased right-to-left shunting in all but the most hemodynamically robust patients.[7] Ketamine is notable for preserving or augmenting sympathetic nervous system tone and, in so doing, maintaining a high degree of circulatory stability. Concern regarding ketamine's propensity to increase PVR has not been substantiated in patients with CHD. Ketamine may be administered intramuscularly to achieve stable induction and allow subsequent vascular cannulation to proceed in an anesthetized patient. In this regard, anxiety, crying, coughing, or breath-holding may aggravate dynamic ventricular outflow obstruction or right-to-left shunting in susceptible patients. It is vital to avoid unintentional injection of air during the administration of all intravenous drugs because the presence of circulatory mixing or shunting in patients with CHD poses a real risk for paradoxical embolization.

AIRWAY MANAGEMENT

After induction of anesthesia and intravenous cannulation, airway management and tracheal intubation are usually facilitated by the administration of a neuromuscular blocking drug. The duration of action, hemodynamic properties, and mode of elimination each may affect the drug selected. Pancuronium may be desirable in some patients for its vagolytic effect in offsetting bradycardia. Succinylcholine is often preferred for its rapid onset, ability to be given intramuscularly (4 mg/kg), and short duration of action. However, succinylcholine may provoke untimely closure of the ductus arteriosus in patients who are

dependent on this anatomy. If desired, intravenous opioids may be used to supplement nonopioid induction techniques to minimize hemodynamic disturbances during laryngoscopy.

When planning induction of anesthesia it is important to consider how the circulatory system will be affected by changes in PVR, SVR, and the relative balance between them. This is particularly relevant during induction because the initial approach to ventilation of the patient's lungs may have an important effect on PVR (see Table 26-2). Induction drugs should cause minimal hemodynamic derangement, and the approach to ventilatory management should have minimal impact on blood flow across shunts or on tenuously balanced pulmonary-to-systemic flow ratios. In this regard, the anesthesiologist must understand the cardiac lesion in order to predict the effect of increasing or decreasing PVR. This understanding will help govern such parameters as F$_{IO_2}$, minute ventilation, use of positive end-expiratory pressure, and peak inspiratory airway pressure.

INVASIVE MONITORING

Invasive monitoring is usually established after induction of anesthesia, except in patients who may be cooperative enough for placement before induction. Patients undergoing cardiac surgery generally require arterial line placement, as well as some form of central venous access. When selecting the site for arterial line placement, the underlying cardiac lesion should be considered. For example, in a patient who has a Blalock-Taussig shunt (diversion of the subclavian artery to the ipsilateral pulmonary artery), the arterial line should be placed contralaterally. Similarly, patients with coarctation of the aorta may have unreliable pressure measurement in the left upper extremity either because of the location of the coarctation or because of aortic cross-clamp placement at or near the left subclavian artery during surgery. The internal jugular vein is a common choice for central pressure monitoring and infusion of medications intraoperatively, yet it is frequently acceptable to use right atrial catheters placed intraoperatively by the surgeon before separation from bypass.

BLOOD PRODUCTS

Many operations for CHD will require blood product administration, and the likelihood increases with smaller infants, lower preoperative hematocrit levels, repeat sternotomy incisions, and long cardiopulmonary bypass (CPB) times. Judgment and experience dictate how much and what type of blood products should be made available at the start of surgery, and many centers use standardized blood ordering schedules based on the surgical procedure and the child's age or weight. Generally, small infants are allocated the freshest blood available because older blood may become significantly hyperkalemic and develop leftward shifting of the oxygen-hemoglobin dissociation curve. Blood should be administered with the use of appropriate filters and warming devices because small infants are particularly susceptible to intraoperative hypothermia and even to bradydysrhythmias from boluses of hypothermic blood products. Having blood products available in the operating room before the skin incision is appropriate in cases of repeat sternotomy inasmuch as these patients may be at risk for severe bleeding from unintentional injury to major cardiac structures.

ANTIFIBRINOLYTIC DRUGS

Antifibrinolytic drugs reduce blood loss and transfusion requirements during surgery for CHD. A commonly used drug, aprotinin, is a serine protease inhibitor that is associated with a 1% incidence of anaphylaxis (up to 5% to 6% on re-exposure within 6 months), but it may have greater efficacy than lysine analog agents (ε-aminocaproic acid and tranexamic acid).[8] Other drugs commonly administered at or around the time of induction (before the skin incision) include antibiotics for the prevention of gram-positive mediastinitis or wound infection.

Maintenance of Anesthesia

Before cardiopulmonary bypass, anesthesia is maintained with a combination of intravenous opioids, volatile anesthetics (doses <1 minimum alveolar concentration [MAC]), and neuromuscular blocking drugs. Use of a low dose of a volatile anesthetic minimizes the myocardial depressant effects of the drug while also decreasing the total dose of opioids that would otherwise be necessary to ensure adequate anesthetic depth. It is not uncommon to administer high doses of opioids (fentanyl, 50 to 100 µg/kg IV, or sufentanil, 10 to 20 µg/kg IV) over the course of an operation.[6] These opioids may be administered in divided doses (fentanyl, 0.5 to 10 µg/kg, or sufentanil, 1 to 2 µg/kg) according to judgment of anesthetic depth or in anticipation of noxious surgical stimuli. Alternatively, opioids may be delivered as a continuous intravenous infusion. Patients who are critically ill or have complex cardiac anomalies may benefit from high-dose opioid techniques so that the hypotensive and myocardial depressant effects of the volatile agents may be avoided or minimized. In contrast, patients with good cardiac reserve who are undergoing procedures for simple defects (atrial septal defect, ventricular septal defect, patent ductus arteriosus, coarctation of the aorta) may benefit from limited opioid use (fentanyl, <20 µg/kg) and greater reliance on volatile drugs so that postoperative extubation is not delayed. Nitrous oxide is commonly omitted from balanced anesthesia techniques because of concern regarding expansion of unintentional intravascular air emboli.

MONITORING CHANGES IN SHUNT RATIOS

The potential for significant changes in the circulatory system after anesthetic induction warrant early and possibly repeated measurement of arterial blood gases to allow early correction or refinement of pulmonary ventilation parameters, as well as acid-base disorders, before the development of important circulatory derangements. In patients with shunts or mixing lesions, pulse oximetry also provides a continuous monitor of changes in the balance between pulmonary and systemic blood flow or changes in shunt direction or magnitude.

ANTICOAGULATION

Anticoagulation is achieved before cannulation for CPB. Heparin (3 mg/kg) is delivered via a central venous catheter (if available), and subsequent anticoagulation is assessed by measuring the activated clotting time (ACT). Target ACT values may vary with institutional preference, but 480 seconds is typical. Additional heparin is administered if target values are not initially obtained. Heparin concentration assays may also be used instead of or as a supplement to the ACT.

Cardiopulmonary Bypass

Most procedures for repair of congenital cardiac defects require that the patient be placed on CPB. As with adults, CPB for infants and children entails diversion of systemic venous return to the CPB machine and subsequent return of blood to the arterial system.[9] Venous blood is drained passively (by gravity) through two venous cannulas, one for each vena cava. The cannulas converge through a Y-connector to a *cardiotomy reservoir*, which allows rapid administration of blood products, crystalloid and colloid solutions, medications, and blood suctioned from the field by the surgeon ("pump suction"). The cardiotomy reservoir also provides a temporary buffer in the event that venous return is temporarily interrupted. Blood is next conducted to a pump mechanism, which is generally a centrifuge pump. This pump is adjustable and permits delivery of a specified rate of blood flow to the patient.

IV

Generally, flow rates are adjusted to maintain mean arterial pressure at or near 40 mm Hg (or other age-appropriate target values). Blood is then channeled through a membrane oxygenator, which equilibrates the blood with a supply of fresh gas; in this way, oxygen is added and carbon dioxide is removed. The perfusionist controls oxygenation and ventilation (carbon dioxide removal) by adjusting the blend (FIO_2) and flow rate of the fresh gas. Modern oxygenator circuits also allow rapid adjustment of blood temperature by running cooled or warmed water through a coil in contact with the blood path. Blood is then conducted back to the patient through tubing connected to a cannula positioned in the ascending aorta. An arterial filter is generally used downstream from the oxygenator to prevent micro-embolization of debris to the patient's arterial tree.

A still and bloodless heart is achieved by complete diversion of venous return to the CPB machine, subsequent aortic cross-clamping, and immediate administration of a cardioplegia solution. Because the act of aortic cross-clamping renders the heart ischemic, the cardioplegia solution has a dual purpose of providing both mechanical quiescence and myocardial protection. As with adults, these effects are achieved through the use of a cold (4°C) hyperkalemic crystalloid solution. Hypothermia and electromechanical arrest each contribute to minimizing myocardial oxygen requirements and lengthening the tolerable period of myocardial ischemia.

CALCULATION OF PHYSIOLOGIC PARAMETERS

Important parameters for the perfusionist and anesthesiologist to consider include the size of the patient so that the desired flow rate necessary to maintain metabolic function can be calculated (typically 2.2 to 2.6 L/min/m²). Equally important is the patient's estimated blood volume because it determines the degree of hemodilution that will be realized when the patient's blood mixes with the obligatory "priming volume" of fluid that occupies the CPB machine's tubing, oxygenator, and cardiotomy reservoir at the onset of CPB. Whereas adult patients frequently have acceptable degrees of anemia as a result of this hemodilution, infants and small children require smaller, shorter tubing and lower-volume cardiotomy reservoirs to minimize this effect. Most infants require some blood product to be mixed with the circuit prime to preserve adequate oxygen-carrying capacity while on CPB. The amount of blood product required is a function of the patient's starting hematocrit, estimated blood volume, circuit prime volume, and the lowest acceptable limit of anemia (institutional and physician preferences vary but are commonly in the range of a hematocrit of 20% to 30%).

BODY TEMPERATURE DURING CARDIOPULMONARY BYPASS

Institutional, surgeon, or anesthesiologist preference also provides the perfusionist with a target patient temperature to be achieved while on CPB. Mild (30°C to 35.5°C) to moderate (25°C to 30°C) systemic hypothermia reduces metabolic oxygen requirements (7% per °C) and provides protective effects on both cerebral and myocardial tissue.[9] Hypothermia is usually achieved by active cooling of CPB blood with a heat exchange device incorporated in the membrane oxygenator. Active rewarming is initiated toward the end of CPB. Deleterious effects of post-CPB hypothermia may include myocardial ischemia, cardiac dysrhythmias, elevated PVR, coagulation failure, or renal dysfunction.

DEEP HYPOTHERMIC CIRCULATORY ARREST

Deep hypothermic circulatory arrest is used in situations in which adequate surgical repair is precluded by CPB cannula placement or by the requirement to repair the aorta at or near the arch.[10-12] Sufficiently cooled, patients may safely undergo periods of complete circulatory arrest to permit surgical repair in a bloodless field unencumbered by CPB cannulas. Cardiac cannulation and active cooling by CPB are required to lower core temperature to approximately 18°C. After surgical repair, CPB is reestablished, and the patient is rewarmed.

Separation from Cardiopulmonary Bypass

Successful separation from CPB requires close communication between the anesthesiologist, the cardiac surgeon, and the perfusionist. Rewarming is effected via the CPB machine and is initiated at the request of the surgeon at an appropriate point during the surgical procedure. Pulmonary ventilation is commenced when the surgeon no longer requires the lungs to be collapsed in the surgical field.

CARDIAC RHYTHM

Ventricular fibrillation commonly occurs after removal of the aortic cross-clamp and reperfusion of the coronary arteries, especially when the hypothermia has not been fully corrected. It may revert spontaneously to a sinus rhythm but often requires electrical defibrillation. Acid-base or electrolyte disorders (hyperkalemia) may contribute to disturbances in cardiac rhythm. Relative bradycardia or atrioventricular node conduction failure can be corrected by means of temporary cardiac pacing. Many patients with good cardiac reserve who have endured relatively short periods (<1.5 hours) of aortic cross-clamping and the attendant myocardial ischemia may be able to separate from CPB without inotropic assistance. Many others will require infusion of inotropic drugs to achieve adequate cardiac output or systemic blood pressure before surgery. In particular, those with preexisting myocardial dysfunction, congestive heart failure, or hemodynamic instability are likely to require pharmacologic assistance for successful separation from CPB (Table 26-6).

Table 26-6 Inotropic Drugs Used in the Perioperative Management of Patients with Congenital Heart Disease

Drug	Dose Range	Comments
Dopamine	3-20 µg/kg/min	Lower maximum effect than with epinephrine and norepinephrine Tachycardia
Epinephrine	0.02-0.1 µg/kg/min	Drug of choice when maximum β effect is required Strong α effect at the medium to high dose range Tachycardia
Norepinephrine	0.02-0.1 µg/kg/min	Strong α, β effects, with α activity at lower doses than with epinephrine
Milrinone	Load: 25-50 µg/kg Infuse: 0.25-0.75 µg/kg/min	Can lower both PVR and SVR No tachycardia May need α-agonist to prevent hypotension
Dobutamine	1-20 µg/kg/min	Lower maximum effect than with epinephrine and norepinephrine May decrease SVR or BP because of peripheral β$_2$ vasodilation

BP, blood pressure; PVR, pulmonary vascular resistance; SVR, systemic vascular resistance

VENTILATION AND PULMONARY VASCULAR RESISTANCE

The approach to PVR and ventilation of the patient's lungs must be carefully considered before separation from CPB. Patients with simple defects that have been repaired are no longer at risk for shunting and unbalanced Qp/Qs ratios. For this reason, such patients are typically ventilated with maximum FiO$_2$ at the time of separation from CPB, with minute ventilation targeted to avoid respiratory acidosis. Patients with long-standing excessive pulmonary blood flow (PVR/SVR >1) may be at risk for elevated PVR from chronic volume or pressure overload of the pulmonary circulation. These patients may benefit from attempts to minimize PVR (see Table 26-2).

PRESENCE OF A RESIDUAL MIXING LESION

Difficulty arises when a palliative procedure has left the patient with a mixing lesion. This situation is exemplified by surgical treatment of hypoplastic left heart syndrome (Norwood procedure) that results in a single ventricle supplying blood flow to both the pulmonary and systemic circulation (see Table 26-5). In such circumstances it must be anticipated which circulation will be likely to receive most of the cardiac output and adjust so that PVR and SVR tend to yield a balanced circulation. Pulse oximetry is an invaluable tool in this particular situation because a patient with a complete mixing lesion will tend to have systemic oxygen saturation near 80% when the systemic and pulmonary circulations are balanced.[1] Systemic saturation greater than 85% to 90% indicates excessive pulmonary blood flow (possibly with resultant systemic hypoperfusion or hypotension), whereas saturation lower than 75% indicates inadequate pulmonary blood flow. The challenge for the anesthesiologist is to provide the best possible milieu (in the setting of the underlying defect) to promote satisfactory cardiac output, adequate oxygenation, and a balanced circulation.

DIFFICULTY IN SEPARATION FROM CARDIOPULMONARY BYPASS

Difficulty in separation from CPB may reflect multiple physiologic derangements but most often is due to inadequate pulmonary blood flow or inadequate systemic blood flow (Table 26-7). After separation from CPB, close attention should be paid to systemic blood pressure, as well as systemic oxygenation and acid-base status. Data derived from a central venous or pulmonary artery catheter may be helpful in diagnosing hemodynamic problems. Trans-

Table 26-7 Causes of Difficulty in Separation from Cardiopulmonary Bypass

Inadequate pulmonary blood flow (associated with arterial hypoxemia)

Inadequate systemic blood flow (associated with hypotension and metabolic acidosis

Valvular dysfunction

Dynamic outflow obstruction (decreases in cardiac output related to hyperdynamic or hypovolemic states)

Decreased systemic vascular resistance (associated with long cardiopulmonary bypass times)

Cardiac rhythm disturbances

Hypovolemia

esophageal echocardiography is useful in evaluating the surgical repair of CHD and cardiac function in the period after separation from CPB. In the event that pharmacologic support of cardiac contractility, vascular tone, and management of ventilation fails to achieve circulatory stability, patients may require resumption of CPB support. In some cases, a period of "rest" on CPB allows resolution of cross-clamp–related ischemic ventricular dysfunction, whereas in other situations, revision of the surgical repair may be indicated.

REVERSAL OF HEPARIN

Reversal of heparin is achieved with protamine (approximately 1 mg protamine per milligram of active heparin) by means of slow infusion (over at least a 10-minute period) after it has been ascertained that return to CPB will not be necessary. Like adults, pediatric patients are susceptible to important complications of protamine administration, including anaphylactic, anaphylactoid, hypotensive, or severe pulmonary hypertensive reactions.[13,14]

COAGULOPATHY

Although return of the ACT to baseline indicates successful reversal of heparin, residual elevation of the ACT may indicate coagulation factor or platelet deficiency. Hypothermia and hypocalcemia may contribute to in vivo coagulopathy but will not be reflected in the ACT or other laboratory tests of coagulation. Early measurement of the platelet count, prothrombin time, and partial thromboplastin time will facilitate appropriate blood product therapy in the event that hemostasis is not achieved with protamine. Often, however, the degree of clinical coagulopathy necessitates empirical administration of platelets, fresh frozen plasma, or other factor preparations before the results of such investigations become available.

BLOOD COMPONENT AND VOLUME THERAPY

Blood component and volume therapy must be administered very carefully to infants because their total intravascular volume is low (approximately 90 mL/kg in neonates) in comparison to adults. Unless critically hypovolemic, blood product or volume therapy should proceed in aliquots of approximately 5 mL/kg to prevent volume overload and possible ventricular dysfunction. Citrated blood products may cause important degrees of hypocalcemia, and calcium replacement may thus be necessary. Dilutional anemia should be borne in mind when administering platelet or plasma preparations. Fluid-warming devices prevent the delivery of cold fluid boluses to cardiac conduction tissue, as well as the development of systemic hypothermia.

POSTOPERATIVE CARE

Children undergoing surgery for CHD are managed in an intensive care setting, where continued invasive monitoring is possible along with direct nursing supervision. Mechanical ventilation of the patient's lungs is continued for variable intervals, depending on the type of surgery performed and the overall status of the patient. Sedation is maintained throughout the period of ongoing tracheal intubation. Critical care management entails the continuation of hemodynamic drug infusions and possibly electrical pacing of cardiac rhythm. Early postoperative management frequently involves correction of various electrolyte, glucose, and hematologic parameters. Mediastinal bleeding is assessed frequently. A high index of suspicion is always maintained for the possible requirement for revision of the surgical repair, and bedside echocardiography is frequently undertaken in the intensive care unit to clarify hemodynamic problems.

REFERENCES

1. DiNardo J. Anesthesia for congenital heart disease. *In* DiNardo J (ed): Anesthesia for Cardiac Surgery. Stamford, CT: Appleton & Lange, 1998, pp 141-200.
2. Andropoulos DB, Stayer SA, Skjonsby BS, et al. Anesthetic and perioperative outcome of teenagers and adults with congenital heart disease. J Cardiothorac Vasc Anesth 2002;16:731-736.
3. Mann D, Qu JZ, Mehta V. Congenital heart diseases with left-to-right shunts. Int Anesthesiol Clin 2004: 42:45-58.
4. Fischer LG, Van Aken H, Burkle H. Management of pulmonary hypertension: Physiological and pharmacological considerations for anesthesiologists. Anesth Analg 2003;96:1603-1616.
5. Andropoulos DB, Stayer SA, Russell IA. Anesthesia for Congenital Heart Disease. Malden, MA Futura, 2005, p 498.
6. Duncan HP, Cloote A, Weir PM, et al. Reducing stress responses in the pre-bypass phase of open heart surgery in infants and young children: A comparison of different fentanyl doses. Br J Anaesth 2000;84:556-564.
7. Williams GD, Jones TK, Hanson KA, et al. The hemodynamic effects of propofol in children with congenital heart disease. Anesth Analg 1999; 89:1411-416.
8. Carrel TP, Schwanda M, Vogt PR, et al. Aprotinin in pediatric cardiac operations: A benefit in complex malformations and with high-dose regimen only. Ann Thorac Surg 1998;66:153-158.
9. Vinas M. Extracorporeal circulation. *In* Kambam J (ed): Cardiac Anesthesia for Infants and Children. St Louis: Mosby–Year Book, 1994, pp 20-32.
10. Jonas RA. Deep hypothermic circulatory arrest: Current status and indications. Semin Thorac Cardiovasc Surg Pediatr Card Surg Annu 2002; 5:76-88.
11. Wypij D, Newburger JW, Rappaport LA, et al. The effect of duration of deep hypothermic circulatory arrest in infant heart surgery on late neurodevelopment: The Boston Circulatory Arrest Trial. J Thorac Cardiovasc Surg 2003;126:1397-1403.

12. Hickey PR. Neurologic sequelae associated with deep hypothermic circulatory arrest. Ann Thorac Surg 1998;65(6 Suppl):S65-S69, discussion S69-S70, S74-S76.

13. Hobbhahn J, Habazettl H, Conzen P, et al. Complications caused by protamine. 1: Pharmacology and pathophysiology. Anaesthesist 1991;40:365-374.

14. Hobbhahn J, Habazettl H, Conzen P, et al. Complications caused by protamine. 2: Therapy and prevention. Anaesthesist 1991; 40:421-428.

IV

Chapter 27

CHRONIC PULMONARY DISEASE

Anh L. Innes, Jeanine P. Wiener-Kronish, and Jeffrey A. Katz

Thoracic and upper abdominal operations are a particular risk for patients with chronic pulmonary disease. Anesthesia for thoracic surgery in these patients poses unique and significant risks.

OBSTRUCTIVE AIRWAY DISEASES

Asthma and chronic obstructive pulmonary disease (COPD), the two major categories of obstructive airway disease, affect millions of Americans and cause significant morbidity and mortality worldwide. Asthma is a chronic inflammatory disorder of the airways characterized by variable airflow obstruction, airway inflammation, and bronchial hyperresponsiveness.[1] In contrast, the airflow obstruction in COPD is defined as progressive and not fully reversible. The chronic inflammation of the airways and lung parenchyma in COPD is most often secondary to cigarette smoke exposure.[2] More than 10 million Americans suffer from asthma, which makes it one of the most common chronic diseases in the United States. It is estimated that COPD affects 14 million people in the United States alone, and the worldwide prevalence continues to increase because of exposure to cigarette smoke and environmental pollution in developing countries. Together, asthma and COPD constitute a major public health concern, and a basic understanding of these diseases is important when caring for patients who receive anesthesia.

ASTHMA

Asthma is a disease that is defined by the presence of (1) chronic inflammatory changes in the submucosa of the airways, (2) airway hyperresponsiveness, and (3) reversible expiratory airflow obstruction. Airway hyperresponsiveness characterizes this disease, even in asymptomatic patients, and is demonstrated by the development of bronchoconstriction in response to stimuli (allergens, exercise, mechanical airway stimulation) that have little or no effect on normal airways. Airway hyperresponsiveness elicited during methacholine bronchoprovocation and airway bronchodilation in response to inhaled albuterol help diagnose asthma.

Clinical Symptoms

The classic symptoms associated with asthma are cough, shortness of breath, and wheezing. However, symptoms of asthma may vary and range from cough with or without sputum production to chest pain or tightness. Chronic, nonproductive cough may be the sole initial complaint. Some asthmatics also experience symptoms exclusively with exertion ("exercise-induced asthma"), and this diagnosis is a consideration in the pediatric and young adult population. High-pitched, musical wheezes are characteristic of asthma, although they are not specific. In addition, the presence or absence of wheezing on physical examination is a poor predictor of the severity of airflow obstruction. Thus, the presence of wheezing suggests airway narrowing, which should be confirmed and quantified by spirometry. Pulmonary function studies demonstrate evidence of airflow obstruction, either by curvilin-

earity in the expiratory loop of the flow-volume curve for those with mild obstruction or by decreased forced expiratory volume in 1 second (FEV_1) in addition to curvilinearity (Fig. 27-1). Degrees of obstruction are defined according to the FEV_1 % predicted (Table 27-1). Reversibility of obstruction after the administration of a bronchodilator suggests a diagnosis of asthma. An increase in FEV_1 % predicted of more than 12% and an increase in FEV_1 of greater than 0.2 L suggest acute bronchodilator responsiveness and variability in airflow obstruction. In contrast, the airways of patients with COPD do not demonstrate reversibility of airflow obstruction to the same degree as do those with asthma, a characteristic that can help distinguish these two causes of airflow obstruction.

Treatment

Pharmacologic therapy is initiated by a stepwise approach according to guidelines set by the National Asthma Education and Prevention Program panel report (see Table 27-1).[3] Short-acting, inhaled beta agonists should be used to treat acute symptoms for all stages of severity. Inhaled corticosteroids are initiated in those meeting the criteria for mild persistent asthma.

IV

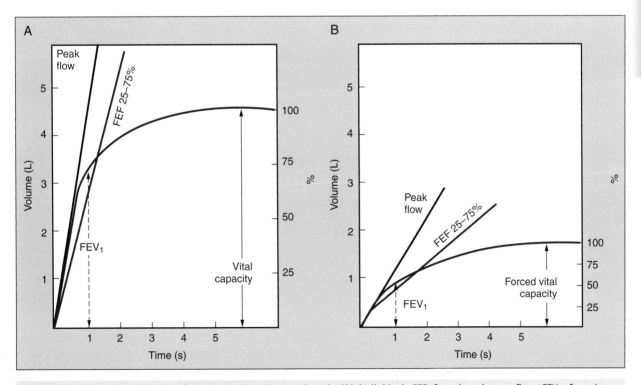

Figure 27-1 Flow-volume curves of a normal (**A**) and an asthmatic (**B**) individual. FEF, forced expiratory flow; FEV_1, forced expiratory volume in 1 second. (From Kingston HGG, Hirshman CA. Perioperative management of the patient with asthma. Anesth Analg 1984;63:844-855, with permission.)

Table 27-1 NAEPP Guidelines for a Stepwise Approach in Asthma Management

Severity (before Treatment)	Symptoms and Spirometry	Medications to Maintain Control
Severe persistent	Continual daytime, frequent nighttime $FEV_1 \leq 60\%$ of predicted	High-dose inhaled corticosteroids AND long-acting inhaled beta-agonist
Moderate persistent	Daily daytime, >1 night/week $60\% < FEV_1 < 80\%$	Low- to medium-dose inhaled corticosteroids AND long-acting inhaled beta-agonist
Mild persistent	>2/week daytime, >2 nights/month $FEV_1 \geq 80\%$	Low-dose inhaled corticosteroids
Mild intermittent	≤2 days/week, ≤2 nights/month $FEV_1 \geq 80\%$	No daily medication required

FEV_1, forced expiratory volume in 1 second.
Modified from National Asthma Education and Prevention Program. National Heart, Lung, and Blood Institute, 2002.

Bronchodilator therapy with a long-acting beta agonist is added to the treatment regimen for patients with moderate persistent asthma; these patients experience daytime as well as nocturnal symptoms more than once weekly. In addition, theophylline, leukotriene receptor antagonists, and cromolyn sodium can be added as adjunctive therapy.

During severe asthma exacerbations, intravenous therapy with glucocorticoids is the mainstay of therapy. In rare circumstances, when life-threatening status asthmaticus persists despite aggressive pharmacologic therapy, it may be necessary to consider general anesthesia (isoflurane or sevoflurane) in an attempt to produce bronchodilation.

Management of Anesthesia

Pulmonary function studies (especially FEV_1) obtained before and after bronchodilator therapy may be indicated in a patient with asthma who is scheduled for a thoracic or abdominal operation. Measurement of arterial blood gases before proceeding with elective surgery is a consideration if there are questions about the adequacy of ventilation or arterial oxygenation. All asthmatics who have persistent symptoms should be treated with either inhaled or systemic corticosteroids (depending on the severity of their airflow obstruction), in addition to scheduled doses of inhaled beta agonists.[4] Therapy should be continued throughout the perioperative period. Supplementation with cortisol may be indicated before major surgery for corticosteroid-dependent asthmatics because of suppression of the hypothalamic-pituitary-adrenal axis (see Chapter 29).

REGIONAL ANESTHESIA
Regional anesthesia may be preferred when the surgery is superficial or involves the extremities. Notably, however, bronchospasm has been reported in asthmatics who have received spinal anesthesia, although it is generally accepted that regional anesthesia is associated with lower complication rates related to bronchospasm in the asthmatic population.

GENERAL ANESTHESIA
The goal during induction and maintenance of general anesthesia in patients with asthma is to depress airway reflexes in order to avoid bronchoconstriction in response to mechanical stimulation of the airway. Before tracheal intubation, a sufficient depth of anesthesia should be established to minimize bronchoconstriction with subsequent stimulation of the airway. Rapid intravenous induction of anesthesia is most often accomplished with the administration of propofol or thiopental. Propofol may blunt tracheal intubation–induced bronchospasm in patients with asthma. Likewise, ketamine (1 to 2 mg/kg IV) is an alternative selection for rapid induction of anesthesia because its sympathomimetic effects on bronchial smooth muscle may decrease airway resistance. The increased secretions associated with the administration of ketamine, however, may limit the use of this drug in patients with asthma. Sevoflurane and isoflurane are potent volatile anesthetics that depress airway reflexes and do not sensitize the heart to the cardiac effects of the sympathetic nervous system stimulation produced by beta-agonists and aminophylline. Bronchodilation with sevoflurane and isoflurane depends on the ability of the normal airway epithelium to produce nitric oxide and prostanoids. Halothane is also an effective bronchodilator but may be associated with cardiac dysrhythmias in the presence of sympathetic nervous system stimulation. Desflurane may be accompanied by increased secretions, coughing, laryngospasm, and bronchospasm as a result of in vivo airway irritation.[5] Although case reports suggest that bronchodilation follows the intravenous administration of lidocaine, the clinical significance of this response is unclear and the data are equivocal. One prospective

study in humans in which the effects of intravenous lidocaine were compared with those of inhaled albuterol given before tracheal intubation reported blunted airway responses only in subjects who received inhaled albuterol.[6] Another study demonstrated a decreased reduction in FEV_1 in mild asthmatics undergoing tracheal intubation who had received an inhaled beta-agonist and topical lidocaine.[7] Thus, in asthmatic patients undergoing tracheal intubation, premedication with inhaled albuterol should be the first choice of therapy to prevent intubation-induced bronchoconstriction. Neuromuscular blocking drugs that are not associated with endogenous histamine release may also be used in patients with asthma (see Chapter 12). Although histamine release has been attributed to succinylcholine, there is no evidence that this drug is associated with increased airway resistance in patients with asthma.

Intraoperatively, PaO_2 and $PaCO_2$ can be maintained at normal levels by mechanical ventilation of the lungs at a slow breathing rate (6 to 10 breaths/min) to allow adequate time for exhalation, an important maneuver in patients with increased airway resistance. This slow breathing rate can usually be facilitated by the use of a high inspiratory flow rate to allow the longest possible time for exhalation. Positive end-expiratory pressure (PEEP) should be used cautiously because of the inherent, impaired exhalation in the presence of narrowed airways. At the conclusion of elective surgery, the trachea may be extubated while the depth of anesthesia is still sufficient to suppress airway reflexes. After the administration of anticholinesterase drugs to reverse the effects of nondepolarizing neuromuscular blocking drugs, bronchospasm may occur but is not usual, which may reflect the protective effects (decreased airway resistance) of simultaneously administered anticholinergics. When extubation is delayed for reasons of safety until the patient is awake (possible presence of gastric contents), intravenous administration of lidocaine may decrease the likelihood of airway stimulation as a result of the endotracheal tube in an awake patient.

Intraoperative Bronchospasm

Airway instrumentation can cause severe reflex bronchoconstriction and bronchospasm, especially in asthmatic patients with hyperactive airways. The bronchospasm that occurs intraoperatively is usually due to factors other than acute exacerbation of asthma. The frequency of perioperative bronchospasm in patients with asthma is low, especially if their asthma is asymptomatic at the time of surgery.[4] It is important to first consider mechanical causes of obstruction and inadequate levels of anesthesia before initiating treatment of intraoperative bronchospasm. Fiberoptic bronchoscopy may be useful to rule out mechanical obstruction in the tracheal tube. Asthma-related bronchospasm may respond to deepening of anesthesia with a volatile anesthetic. If the bronchospasm

is due to asthma and persists despite an increase in the concentration of delivered anesthetic drugs, albuterol should be administered by attaching a metered-dose inhaler to the anesthetic delivery system. When bronchospasm persists despite β_2-agonist therapy, it may be necessary to add intravenous corticosteroids.

CHRONIC OBSTRUCTIVE PULMONARY DISEASE: EMPHYSEMA AND CHRONIC BRONCHITIS

COPD consists of two entities, emphysema and chronic bronchitis. The **G**lobal Initiative for Chronic **O**bstructive **L**ung **D**isease (GOLD) guidelines provide criteria for diagnosis and classification of severity in patients with symptoms of chronic cough, sputum production, or exposure to cigarette smoke (Table 27-2).[8] Emphysema is characterized by loss of elastic recoil of the lungs, which results in collapse of the airways during exhalation and increased airway resistance. Chronic bronchitis is defined by the presence of cough and sputum production for 3 months in each of 2 successive years in a patient with risk factors, most commonly cigarette smoking. It has been estimated that 25% of surgical patients smoke and a further 25% are ex-smokers, thus making COPD an important diagnosis to consider in any patient undergoing anesthesia.

Prediction of Postoperative Outcome

The need for preoperative pulmonary function studies in patients with COPD is controversial because of the questionable correlation of these tests with postoperative outcome.[9] Although the FEV_1 % predicted has been used to grade the severity of airflow obstruction, data have shown that using a multidimensional grading system to assess the respiratory and systemic extent of COPD is a better predictor of mortality than using FEV_1 % alone. This grading system is based on four variables—body mass index (B), severity of airflow obstruction (O), functional dyspnea (D), and exercise capacity as assessed by the 6-minute walk test (E)—and is designated the BODE index (Table 27-3).[10] Patients with higher BODE scores were at higher risk for death. Hypercapnia and hypoxemia, as detected by arterial blood gas analysis, may also characterize patients with moderate to severe airflow obstruction. Chronic hypoxemia may lead to pulmonary hypertension and cor pulmonale. Preoperative detection plus treatment of hypoxemia-induced cor pulmonale with supplemental oxygen is an important part of preoperative management.

Management of Anesthesia

The presence of COPD does not dictate the use of specific drugs or techniques (regional or general) for the manage-

IV

Table 27-2 GOLD Guidelines: Classification of Severity (Based on Postbronchodilator FEV_1)

Stage	Characteristics
0: At risk	Normal spirometry Chronic symptoms (cough, sputum production)
I: Mild COPD	$FEV_1/FVC < 70\%$ $FEV_1 \geq 80\%$ of predicted With or without chronic symptoms (cough, sputum)
II: Moderate COPD	$FEV_1/FVC < 70\%$ $50\% \leq FEV_1 < 80\%$ of predicted With or without chronic symptoms (cough, sputum)
III: Severe COPD	$FEV_1/FVC < 70\%$ $30\% \leq FEV_1 < 50\%$ of predicted With or without chronic symptoms (cough, sputum)
IV: Very severe COPD	$FEV_1/FVC < 70\%$ $FEV_1 < 30\%$ of predicted or $FEV_1 < 50\%$ of predicted + chronic hypoxemia and hypercapnia

COPD, chronic obstructive pulmonary disease; FEV_1, forced expiratory volume in 1 second; FVC, forced vital capacity. Modified from Global Initiative for Chronic Obstructive Lung Disease. National Heart, Lung, and Blood Institute, World Health Organization, 2004.

Table 27-3 Variables and Point Values Used for the BODE Index: *B*ody Mass Index, Degree of Airflow *O*bstruction and *D*yspnea, and *E*xercise Capacity

Variable	Points on the BODE Index			
	0	1	2	3
FEV_1 (% predicted)	≥65	50-64	36-49	≤35
Distance walked in 6 min (m)	≥350	250-349	150-249	≤149
MMRC dyspnea scale	0-1	2	3	4
Body mass index	>21	≤21		

FEV_1, forced expiratory volume in 1 second; MMRC, Modified Medical Research Council. Modified from Celli BR, Cote CG, Marin JM, et al. The body-mass index, airflow obstruction, dyspnea, and exercise capacity index in chronic obstructive pulmonary disease. N Engl J Med 2004;350:1005-1012.

ment of anesthesia. If general anesthesia is selected, a volatile anesthetic with humidified inhaled gases and mechanical ventilation of the lungs is useful. Nitrous oxide may be used, but potential disadvantages include limitation of the inhaled concentrations of oxygen and passage of nitrous oxide into emphysematous bullae. Nitrous oxide could lead to enlargement and rupture of these bullae and result in the development of tension pneumothorax. Opioids are acceptable but are less ideal for maintenance of anesthesia because of the frequent need for high inhaled concentrations of nitrous oxide to ensure amnesia and associated decreases in inhaled concentrations of oxygen. To avoid this problem, administration of a volatile anesthetic at a low concentration may be substituted for nitrous oxide. Postoperative depression of ventilation may also reflect the residual effects of opioids administered intraoperatively.

MANAGEMENT OF VENTILATION

Patients with COPD are ventilated in a manner similar to those with asthma. Small tidal volumes may be delivered to decrease the likelihood of gas trapping and barotrauma. Slow breathing rates are used to permit maximal time for exhalation. Continued tracheal intubation and mechanical ventilation of the lungs in the postoperative period are often necessary after major surgery in patients with severe emphysema. Postoperative depression of ventilation may also reflect the residual effects of opioids administered intraoperatively. Hypercapnia secondary to chronic hypoventilation should not be corrected intraoperatively because it may then be difficult to wean the patient from mechanical ventilation as a result of the decreased respiratory drive in patients who chronically hypoventilate.

PULMONARY HYPERTENSION

Pulmonary hypertension is defined as an elevation in mean pulmonary artery pressure to levels higher than 25 mm Hg at rest or higher than 30 mm Hg with exercise. Most cases of pulmonary hypertension are secondary to cardiac or pulmonary disease; in a minority of cases, the etiology is unknown and the pulmonary hypertension is considered primary.

Classification

The World Health Organization has proposed a classification of pulmonary hypertension that includes pulmonary hypertension secondary to left heart disease, pulmonary disease, vascular disease, and primary pulmonary hypertension.[11] Indicators of disease severity include dyspnea at rest, hypoxemia, syncope, metabolic acidosis indicating low cardiac output, and signs of right heart failure on physical examination (elevated jugular venous pressure, hepatomegaly, and peripheral edema).

Diagnostic Evaluation

Diagnostic evaluation for pulmonary hypertension includes the electrocardiogram; echocardiogram; chest roentgenogram; assessment for secondary causes such as pulmonary embolism (computed tomographic angiography or ventilation/perfusion scanning), underlying pulmonary disease (pulmonary function testing), collagen vascular disease, or liver failure; and right heart catheterization. Right heart catheterization is the gold standard for diagnosis because it provides data on the severity of pulmonary artery hypertension, as well as pulmonary venous pressure and cardiac output, which have prognostic significance. In addition, right heart catheterization is a necessary part of testing for vasodilator response, the first step in the algorithm to determine appropriate therapy for pulmonary artery hypertension.

Pathophysiology

Chronic elevation of pulmonary artery pressure leads to elevated right ventricular systolic pressure, hypertrophy and dilatation of the right ventricle, and resultant right ventricular failure. Right ventricular preload and pulmonary blood flow are dependent on venous return in this setting. Maintaining balance between flow and pressure is crucial to keeping constant, forward flow from the systemic circulation through the pulmonary circulation, an important consideration when administering anesthetic agents.

Management of Anesthesia

Intraoperative considerations for a patient with severe pulmonary hypertension include maintaining adequate preload, minimizing tachycardia and cardiac dysrhythmias that may decrease cardiac output, and avoiding arterial hypoxemia and hypercapnia, which can increase pulmonary vascular resistance (PVR). Cardiac output from a failing right ventricle is critically dependent on filling pressure from venous return and pulmonary pressure. Options for treatment of pulmonary hypertension during surgery include inhaled nitric oxide (10 ppm), inhaled prostacyclin (either intermittent or continuous),[12] and phosphodiesterase inhibitors such as milrinone. Pulmonary artery catheters have been used for intraoperative monitoring.

PARTURIENTS
Mortality in pregnant patients undergoing vaginal delivery is near 50% and may be even higher when cesarean delivery is performed. Most often, vaginal deliveries are preferred, although regional anesthesia may be used successfully during cesarean sections. The danger of decreased venous return secondary to the sympathetic nervous system blockade produced by regional anesthesia should be considered.

POSTOPERATIVE PERIOD
In the postoperative period, care must be taken to avoid large-volume fluid shifts, arterial hypoxemia, systemic hypotension, and hypovolemia in patients with pulmonary hypertension. Morbidity and mortality in the postoperative period are significant concerns, with possible causes including pulmonary vasospasm, increases in pulmonary artery pressure, fluid shifts, cardiac dysrhythmias, and heightened sympathetic nervous system tone.

OBSTRUCTIVE SLEEP APNEA

Patients with obstructive sleep apnea (OSA) are at high risk for postoperative complications when undergoing general anesthesia. OSA is reported to occur in 2% of middle-aged women and 4% of middle-aged men. It is suspected, however, that up to 80% of cases of OSA are undiagnosed, thus suggesting that those with this disorder may be a significant portion of the surgical population.[13] Obesity is the most significant risk factor for the development of OSA, with a body mass index greater than 30 and a large neck circumference (>44 cm) being positively correlated with severe OSA.[14] Obese patients with OSA or suspected OSA are at risk for complications during tracheal intubation and extubation, as well as during the postoperative period. Comorbid medical illnesses such as hypertension, cardiovascular disease, and congestive heart

IV

failure are also more prevalent in patients with OSA than in the general population, a fact that contributes to their postoperative morbidity.[13,14] Systemic hypertension has been reported in up to 50% of patients with OSA and is independent of obesity, age, and gender.[14] Treatment of OSA by noninvasive ventilation results in better control of systemic hypertension. In addition to systemic hypertension, pulmonary hypertension is more prevalent in these patients than in the general population. One common mechanism that may explain both the systemic and pulmonary hypertension in patients with OSA is the chronic decrease in PaO_2 during apneic episodes.[14]

Management of Anesthesia

Evaluation of the oral cavity in patients with OSA may not reveal the true nature of their pharyngeal space because increased fat deposition in the lateral pharyngeal walls has been demonstrated in these patients and shown to correlate with the severity of OSA. Neck circumference reflects pharyngeal fat deposition and correlates more strongly with the incidence and severity of OSA than general obesity does.

IMPACT OF SEDATIVE DRUGS
Relaxation of the upper airway musculature in response to benzodiazepines may significantly reduce the pharyngeal space and result in longer periods of hypopnea, arterial hypoxemia, and hypercapnia in patients with OSA than in the general population. Any medications that depress the central nervous system must be administered carefully because airway patency and skeletal muscle tone, maintained in the awake state, may be lost at the onset of sleep. In addition, opioid analgesics may decrease the central respiratory drive and thus further add to the possible complications of sedation.

ANTICIPATION OF DIFFICULT AIRWAY MANAGEMENT
Full preparation for difficult airway management, including the availability of orotracheal tubes of various size, a Fastrach laryngeal mask, and a fiberoptic bronchoscope, should be made before initiating direct laryngoscopy for tracheal intubation. Adequate preoxygenation is necessary in obese patients with OSA because of their reduced functional residual capacity and risk for arterial hypoxemia with induction of anesthesia. Tracheal extubation should be performed only when the patient is breathing spontaneously with adequate tidal volumes, oxygenation, and ventilation.

MANAGEMENT IN THE POSTOPERATIVE PERIOD
Respiratory depression and repetitive apnea in the postoperative period can occur in patients with OSA, especially in the setting of opioid administration for pain control. It should also be noted that in patients with OSA who hypoventilate (obesity-hypoventilation syndrome), careful documentation of preoperative arterial blood gases is necessary to establish the baseline set point for ventilation, an important factor when considering the patient's respiratory drive after extubation. Relative hyperventilation intraoperatively to maintain a normal $PaCO_2$ in subjects who chronically hypoventilate may result in prolonged apnea when attempting extubation.

ANESTHESIA FOR THORACIC SURGERY

The major challenges in anesthesia for thoracic surgery are establishing adequate separation of the lungs, maintaining gas exchange, and ensuring circulatory stability during one-lung anesthesia. One-lung anesthesia involves lung separation and deliberate ventilation of the dependent lung by isolating its bronchus from that of the nondependent lung (the operative site) with specially designed endotracheal tubes. In addition, thoracic surgery often involves thoracotomy incisions, which are associated with severe pain and potentially deleterious changes in cardiopulmonary physiology after surgery. Some of these physiologic changes can be minimized by thoracic epidural analgesia for effective postoperative pain management (see Chapter 39).

Preoperative Evaluation and Preparation

Patients undergoing thoracic surgery are at high risk for postoperative pulmonary complications, particularly if coexisting chronic pulmonary disease is present. Risk factors associated with increased perioperative morbidity and mortality include the extent of lung resection (pneumonectomy > lobectomy > wedge resection), age older than 70 years, and inexperience of the operating surgeon.[15]

In patients with anatomically resectable lung cancer, pulmonary function testing, lung perfusion scanning, and exercise testing to measure maximum oxygen consumption may also predict postoperative pulmonary function, as well as increased mortality (Fig. 27-2). A decrease in FEV_1 to less than 70% of predicted and a reduction in diffusing capacity to less than 60% of predicted should prompt further testing with a quantitative lung perfusion scan. If postoperative FEV_1 or DLco are less than 40% as predicted by lung scan, an exercise study should be obtained. A significant decrease in oxygen consumption (<10 mL/kg/min) as measured by exercise testing predicts a postoperative mortality of 25% to 50% and should prompt discussion of alternatives to surgical resection.[15]

DISCONTINUATION OF SMOKING
Smoking increases airway irritability and secretions, decreases mucociliary transport, and increases the incidence of postoperative pulmonary complications. Cessation of smoking for 12 to 24 hours before surgery decreases the level of carboxyhemoglobin, shifts the oxyhemoglobin dissociation curve to the right, and increases the oxygen available to tissues. In contrast to these short-term effects,

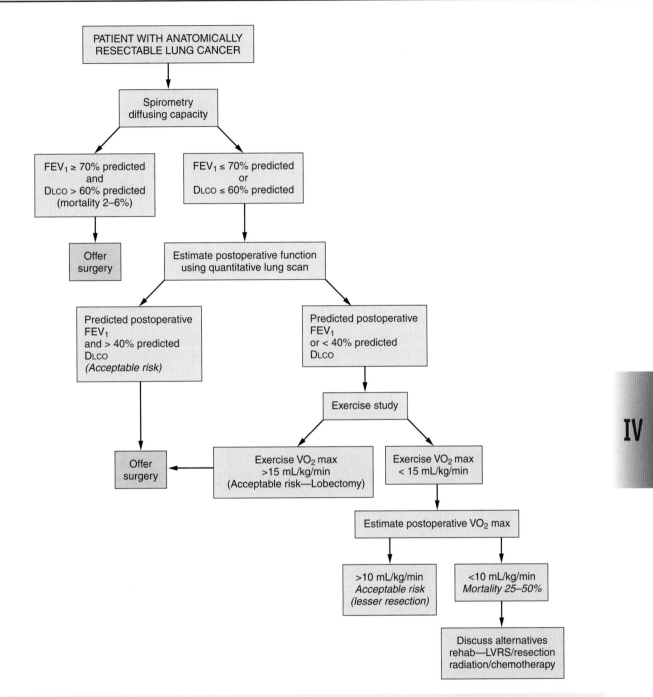

Figure 27-2 Algorithm for determining the resectability of lung carcinoma in patients with underlying lung disease. DLCO, diffusing capacity of the lung for carbon monoxide; FEV$_1$, forced expiratory volume in 1 second; LVRS, lung volume reduction surgery.

improvement in mucociliary transport and small airway function and decreases in sputum production require prolonged abstinence (8 to 12 weeks) from smoking. The incidence of postoperative pulmonary complications decreases with abstinence from cigarette smoking for more than 8 weeks in patients undergoing coronary artery bypass surgery (Fig. 27-3) and more than 4 weeks in patients undergoing pulmonary surgery.[16] Nevertheless, it is useful to encourage smoking abstinence in the perioperative period, especially because smoking shortly before surgery may be associated with an increased incidence of ST-segment depression on the electrocardiogram.

Management of Anesthesia

The five goals of anesthesia in thoracic surgery are to (1) produce controlled levels of narcosis and analgesia, (2) suppress cough and reflex airway activity, (3) minimize interference with protective reflexes such as hypoxic pulmonary vasoconstriction, (4) maintain satisfactory blood-gas exchange and cardiovascular stability, and (5) permit rapid recovery from anesthesia to avoid postoperative respiratory depression. A practical approach is to induce general anesthesia with intravenous propofol and maintain it with a potent volatile anesthetic supplemented with intravenous opioids and controlled ventilation of the patient's lungs. Depression of airway reflexes and rapid elimination allowing for rapid recovery are important benefits of volatile anesthetics. In addition, volatile anesthetics do not seem to inhibit regional hypoxic pulmonary vasoconstriction and thus aid in the maintenance of arterial oxygenation during one-lung anesthesia (Fig. 27-4).[17]

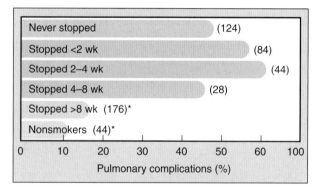

Figure 27-3 Preoperative duration of smoking cessation and pulmonary complication rates after cardiac surgery. The incidence of pulmonary complications begins to decrease only when abstinence from cigarette smoking is longer than 8 weeks. *$P < .001$ versus patients who never stopped smoking preoperatively. Numbers of patients studied are indicated in parentheses. (From Warner DO, Warner MA, Barnes RD, et al. Perioperative respiratory complications in patients with asthma. Anesthesiology 1996;85;460-467, with permission.)

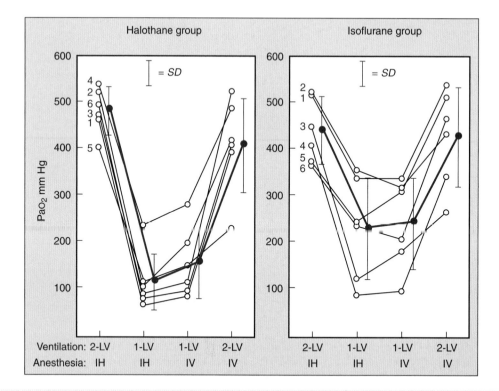

Figure 27-4 Pao_2 was measured during two-lung ventilation (2-LV) and then during one-lung ventilation (1-LV) with inhalation (IH) or intravenous (IV) anesthesia. The addition of halothane or isoflurane (about 1 minimum alveolar concentration) did not greatly alter Pao_2, thus suggesting that these anesthetics do not significantly inhibit regional hypoxic pulmonary vasoconstriction. *Open circles* indicate individual patient data; *solid circles* indicate mean ± SD for each group. (From Benumof JL, Augustine SD, Gibbons JA. Halothane and isoflurane only slightly impair arterial oxygenation during one-lung ventilation in patients undergoing thoracotomy. Anesthesiology 1987;67:910-915, with permission.)

If nitrous oxide is administered, the inhaled concentration is often limited to 50% until the adequacy of oxygenation can be confirmed by pulse oximetry or measurement of PaO_2. Caution must be used in patients with increased PVR because the addition of nitrous oxide to volatile anesthetics may exacerbate increased resistance of the pulmonary vasculature. In addition, nitrous oxide is contraindicated in situations in which it has the potential to expand within a closed air space, such as during closure of a thoracotomy after pneumonectomy when there is no thoracostomy drain. To decrease requirements for volatile anesthetics and facilitate controlled ventilation of the lungs, a nondepolarizing neuromuscular blocking drug is usually administered; these drugs also improve surgical exposure by maximizing mechanical separation of the ribs. Ketamine may likewise be useful for induction of anesthesia in patients undergoing emergency thoracotomy associated with hypovolemia (blunt trauma, gunshot wounds, and stab wounds).

For effective postoperative pain control, a thoracic epidural catheter is placed preoperatively while the patient is sedated but conscious. Patients undergoing thoracotomy usually have an intra-arterial catheter in place to permit continuous monitoring of systemic blood pressure and periodic measurement of arterial blood gases and pH. A central venous catheter may be helpful for guiding intravenous fluid replacement. Transesophageal echocardiography is also a useful intraoperative monitor for myocardial wall function, cardiac valve function, and any myocardial wall motion abnormalities that may reflect myocardial ischemia. A catheter should be inserted into the bladder of patients who are expected to undergo long operations associated with alterations in blood volume and thus the infusion of large amounts of intravenous fluids.

Separation of the Lungs (One-Lung Anesthesia)

Separation of the lungs is perhaps the most important anesthetic procedure in patients undergoing thoracic surgery (Table 27-4). Separation of the lungs permits intraoperative one-lung ventilation, which greatly facilitates the surgical procedure. Double-lumen endobronchial tubes (DLTs) and bronchial blockers (BBs) with single-lumen endotracheal tubes enable anatomic isolation of the lungs and facilitate lung separation.

ANATOMIC CONSIDERATIONS

The tracheobronchial anatomy should first be assessed by reviewing preoperative radiologic studies. In addition, bronchoscopy is helpful immediately before surgery for detecting abnormal anatomy that may complicate lung separation. For example, a markedly distorted carina or a proximal endobronchial tumor may necessitate fiberoptic-guided endobronchial intubation.

Tracheobronchial dimensions in general are approximately 20% larger in men than women. The right main

Table 27-4	Indications for Lung Separation
Prevent contamination or spillage	
Infection	
Hemorrhage	
Unilateral bronchopulmonary lavage	
Control of the distribution of ventilation and/or PEEP	
Bronchopleural fistula	
Unilateral lung cyst or bullous disease	
Severe hypoxemia as a result of asymmetric lung disease	
Enhance surgical exposure	
Pneumonectomy/lobectomy	
Thoracic aneurysm repair	
Esophageal resection	
Anterior mediastinal exploration with hilar extension	
Procedures on the thoracic spine	

PEEP, positive end-expiratory pressure.

bronchus diverges from the trachea at an angle of 25 degrees, whereas the left main bronchus diverges at 45 degrees. The right main bronchus is shorter but wider than the left (Fig. 27-5). Although there is variation in tracheal and bronchial width in the population, within individual

IV

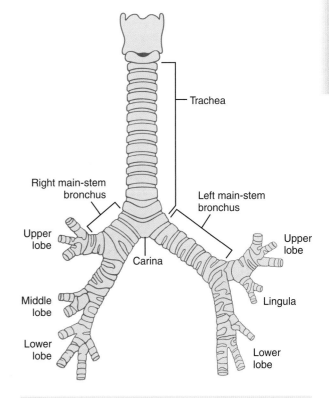

Figure 27-5 Tracheobronchial anatomy. (Right main-stem bronchus length, 1.8 ± 0.8 cm; width, 1.6 ± 0.2 cm. Left main-stem bronchus length, 4.8 ± 0.8 cm; width, 1.3 ± 0.2 cm.)

patients a significant correlation between tracheal and bronchial width has been determined (bronchial diameter is predicted to be 0.68 of tracheal diameter). Based on these dimensional relationships, a left-sided DLT is preferred because uniform ventilation to all lobes will most likely be achieved, and measurement of tracheal width from a posteroanterior chest roentgenogram can help select the size of a left-sided DLT.[18]

LEFT-SIDED DOUBLE-LUMEN TUBE
Placement of a left-sided DLT is the most reliable and widely used approach for endobronchial intubation in one-lung ventilation (Fig. 27-6). Several manufacturers such as Mallinckrodt, Rusch, and Sheridan produce clear, disposable polyvinyl chloride tubes with high-volume, low-pressure tracheal and bronchial cuffs. The BronchoCath by Mallinckrodt has been the most widely studied. In general, a 35- or 37-French tube can be used for most women and a 39-French tube for most men.

Insertion Technique for Placement of a Left-Sided Double-Lumen Tube
Endobronchial intubation is usually accomplished by direct laryngoscopy after induction of general anesthesia and neuromuscular blockade. The left-sided DLT tube is held so that the distal curve faces anteriorly while the proximal curve is to the right. The bronchial cuff is inserted through the vocal cords, and the stylet is removed. Next, the tube is rotated 90 degrees to the left (directing the bronchial lumen to the left main stem bronchus). The tube is advanced until moderate resistance to further passage is encountered. Force should never be used during advancement of the tube; resistance usually indicates impingement within the main stem bronchus. An estimate of the appropriate depth of placement of the DLT can be based on the patient's height. The average depth of insertion referenced to the corner of the mouth is 29 cm for patients 170 cm tall, and for each 10-cm increase or decrease in height, the average depth of placement correspondingly changes by 1 cm. Correct DLT position must be confirmed by fiberoptic bronchoscopy (Fig. 27-7). Dependence on physical examination to confirm proper position of a left-sided DLT is not reliable, with fiberoptic assessment showing malpositioning in 20% to 48% of placements considered to be appropriate on the basis of auscultation.[19]

Intraoperatively, if clamping of the left main stem bronchus is necessary, the DLT is withdrawn under fiber-

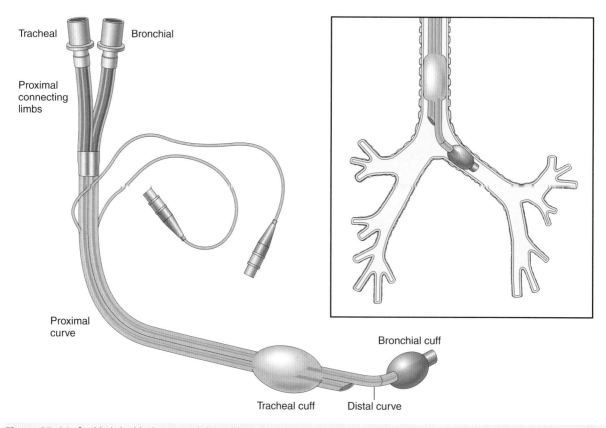

Tracheal

Bronchial

Proximal connecting limbs

Proximal curve

Bronchial cuff

Tracheal cuff   Distal curve

Figure 27-6 Left-sided double-lumen endobronchial tube.

optic guidance to just above the carina, and ventilation of the right lung is then continued through the bronchial lumen. This approach may be used effectively for lung separation during left pneumonectomy.

Fiberoptic Visualization of a Left-Sided Double-Lumen Tube

A 3.6-mm fiberscope is initially passed through the tracheal lumen. Correct position of the DLT is confirmed by visualization of the carina, a nonobstructed view of the right main stem bronchus, and the blue bronchial cuff below the carina (Fig. 27-8A). In addition, the line encircling the tube should be visualized. This line is 4 cm from the distal lumen, and it should ideally be positioned at or slightly above the carina. Fiberoptic visualization

through the bronchial lumen reveals the bronchial carina and the left lower and upper lobes (Fig. 27-8B).

Malpositioned Left-Sided Double-Lumen Tube

A malpositioned left-sided DLT may occur during initial placement, after surgical positioning, or during surgery. A malpositioned tube is usually detected by clinical signs and changes in lung mechanics. During initiation of one-lung ventilation, peak inspiratory airway pressure should increase by approximately 50% when compared with two-lung ventilation at the same tidal volume.[20] When the DLT is malpositioned, peak inspiratory airway pressure will increase by approximately 75%. Two algorithms define three types of malpositioned left-sided DLTs (Fig. 27-9A and B).

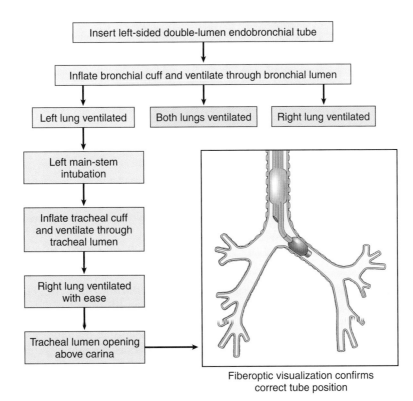

Fiberoptic visualization confirms correct tube position

Figure 27-7 Algorithm for determining the position for a left-sided double-lumen endobronchial tube. A sequence of cuff inflation and positive-pressure ventilation is performed to confirm tube position and functional isolation of the lungs. The sequence starts by inflating the bronchial cuff slowly with 0.5 to 1 mL of air. Initial ventilation through the bronchial lumen should produce left-lung ventilation. A malpositioned tube could result in either the right lung or both lungs being ventilated. Confirmation of ventilation of the left lung indicates that the bronchial lumen has entered the left main bronchus. Next, the tracheal cuff is inflated. Ventilation through the tracheal lumen should produce only right-lung ventilation, thus indicating that the tracheal lumen is above the carina.

IV

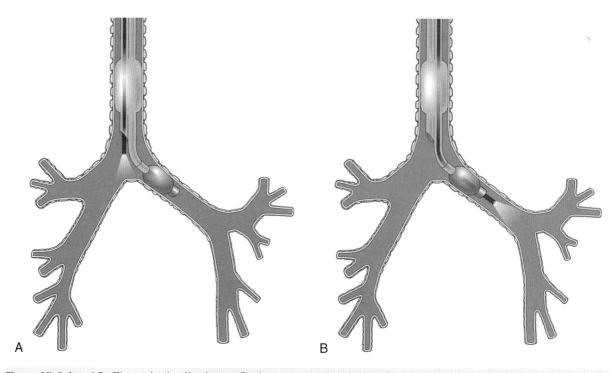

Figure 27-8 A and **B,** Fiberoptic visualization confirming correct position of a left-sided double-lumen tube.

RIGHT-SIDED DOUBLE-LUMEN TUBE

The short and variable distance of the right upper lobe orifice from the carina makes the use of a right-sided DLT undesirable for most procedures requiring lung separation. A small change in the position of the tube results in inadequate lung separation or collapse of the right upper lobe, or both. Nevertheless, in some situations it is best to avoid intubation of the left main stem bronchus (obstructed by tumor, disrupted after trauma, distorted secondary to a thoracic aortic aneurysm). Right-sided DLTs are designed to incorporate a separate opening in the bronchial lumen to allow ventilation of the right upper lobe (Fig. 27-10). Confirmation of correct right-sided DLT position by physical examination alone results in a 90% chance of malposition, with most being too deep. Proper positioning of a right-sided DLT must include fiberoptic guidance.[21]

Bronchial Blockers

Lung separation can also be effectively achieved with a single-lumen endotracheal tube and fiberoptically guided placement of a BB.[22] The BB technique can be useful if postoperative ventilation will be required because it eliminates the need to exchange the DLT for a single-lumen tube. Using a BB is especially helpful when managing a difficult airway. For example, in patients requiring an awake, fiberoptic intubation where DLT placement may be impossible, use of a BB may be the only practical approach to lung separation. Two BB systems are available, the Univent BB tube and the Arndt endobronchial blocker. Confirmation of proper BB position should include fiberoptic bronchoscopy.

UNIVENT BRONCHIAL BLOCKER TUBE

The Univent BB tube has two compartments: a large, main lumen for conventional air passage and a small lumen embedded in the anterior wall of the endotracheal tube that permits passage of the movable BB (Fig. 27-11). The BB is a relatively stiff catheter that has an internal channel measuring 2 mm through which oxygen may be insufflated. After tracheal intubation with the BB retracted, initial positioning is accomplished by the tube rotation method. Rotating the tube to the right or left positions the BB so that it may be advanced into the corresponding main stem bronchus. Fiberoptic visualization should be used to confirm appropriate main stem intubation and to guide the depth of insertion. For right-sided placement, the BB should be positioned so that inflation of the cuff will cause partial herniation into the right upper lobe (Fig. 27-12A). For left-sided placement, the BB should be inserted deep into the main stem bronchus to minimize dislodgment into the trachea with surgical manipulation (Fig 27-12B).

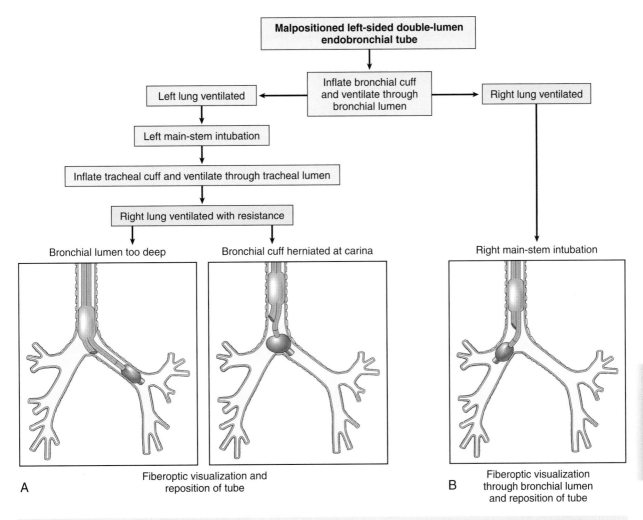

Figure 27-9 Malpositioned left-sided double-lumen endobronchial tube (DLT). **A,** Ventilation through the bronchial lumen results in left-lung ventilation, but ventilation of the right lung through the tracheal lumen results in increased resistance. Fiberoptic visualization through the tracheal lumen identifies either a bronchial lumen that is too deep in the left main stem bronchus or a bronchial cuff that has herniated over the carina. Repositioning is accomplished with fiberoptic guidance. **B,** The left-sided DLT is accidentally inserted into the right main bronchus. Ventilation through the bronchial lumen results in right-lung ventilation. Correction is accomplished by advancing the fiberscope through the bronchial lumen and identifying the bronchus intermedius. With both cuffs deflated, the DLT and fiberscope are withdrawn simultaneously until the carina comes into view. Next, the fiberscope is advanced into the left main bronchus and halted 1 cm above the bronchial carina. The tube is advanced until the rim of the bronchial lumen comes into view. The fiberscope is then advanced through the tracheal lumen, thus confirming correct tube position.

ARNDT ENDOBRONCHIAL BLOCKER

The Arndt endobronchial blocker consists of a 9-French, double-lumen, wire-guided endobronchial catheter and a multiairway adapter that allows independent passage of the BB and fiberscope (Fig 27-13).[22] The BB and a pediatric fiberscope are placed through a conventional endotracheal tube (8.0-mm internal diameter). The BB is coupled to the fiberscope through the guide loop (protruding at the distal end of the catheter). Once coupled, the fiberscope is advanced into the desired main stem bronchus. The BB is advanced while steadying the fiberscope until the guide loop is seen to exit at the end of the fiberoptic bronchoscope. The fiberscope is then retracted, and endobronchial placement of the BB is confirmed. After final positioning of the patient, endobronchial blockade is visualized by inflating the 3-cm-long elliptical cuff with approximately 6 mL of air, and the guide loop is removed.

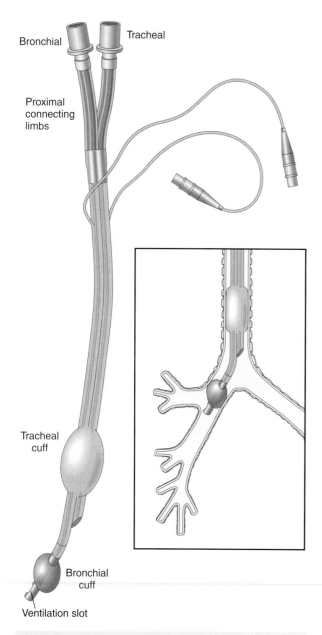

Bronchial

Tracheal

Proximal
connecting
limbs

Tracheal
cuff

Bronchial
cuff

Ventilation slot

Figure 27-10 Right-sided double-lumen endobronchial tube.

GAS EXCHANGE DURING THORACOTOMY AND ONE-LUNG VENTILATION

The intrapulmonary distribution of blood flow is regulated by gravity, lung volume, and regional PVR. As a result, in the lateral decubitus position, the dependent lung receives a greater proportion of the cardiac output (about 60%). During thoracotomy and mechanical ventilation, the proportion of tidal ventilation to the

operated (nondependent) lung increases because lung and thorax compliance in this hemithorax is greater once the chest is opened. In contrast, the dependent lung has low compliance and low ventilation per unit lung volume. Furthermore, the dependent lung is compressed because of pressure from the abdominal contents and the weight of the mediastinum, which is no longer offset by the subatmospheric pressure in the nondependent hemithorax. These factors, combined with the inhalation of soluble gases, promote atelectasis in the dependent lung. Thus, the nondependent lung is well ventilated but poorly perfused (high ventilation-to-perfusion [V/Q] ratio), and the dependent lung is well perfused but poorly ventilated (low V/Q ratio). These V/Q imbalances lead to altered pulmonary gas exchange.

Disadvantages of One-Lung Anesthesia

The major disadvantage of one-lung anesthesia is the introduction of an iatrogenic right-to-left intrapulmonary shunt by the continued perfusion of both lungs while only one lung, the dependent lung in the lateral decubitus position, is ventilated. After the initiation of one-lung ventilation, PaO_2 decreases progressively during the first 20 minutes and remains relatively constant thereafter.

The wide variability in PaO_2 and shunting during one-lung ventilation is the result of multiple factors affecting the distribution of blood flow between the lungs. Blood flow is decreased through the collapsed, nondependent lung by the effects of gravity, by hypoxic pulmonary vasoconstriction, and potentially, by surgical compression. In addition, blood flow diversion may have already occurred in the nondependent lung because of an increase in regional PVR as a result of the underlying pulmonary disease. Although gravity directs more than half the blood flow to the dependent lung, compensatory factors secondary to underlying disease may increase PVR in the dependent lung as well, thus preventing blood flow diversion from the collapsed, nondependent lung.

MANAGEMENT OF ONE-LUNG VENTILATION

An FIO_2 of nearly 1.0 is recommended during one-lung ventilation; nevertheless, arterial hypoxemia cannot be completely prevented (Table 27-5). In approximately 25% of patients, PaO_2 is ≤80 mm Hg, and in 10% of patients, ≤60 mm Hg.[23] The dependent lung should be ventilated with tidal volumes of 8 to 10 mL/kg. Ventilation with tidal volumes of 5 to 7 mL/kg may promote atelectasis in the dependent lung. The respiratory frequency is adjusted to maintain minute ventilation at the same level as during two-lung ventilation; $PaCO_2$ will be maintained at similar or slightly lower levels than those observed during two-lung ventilation.

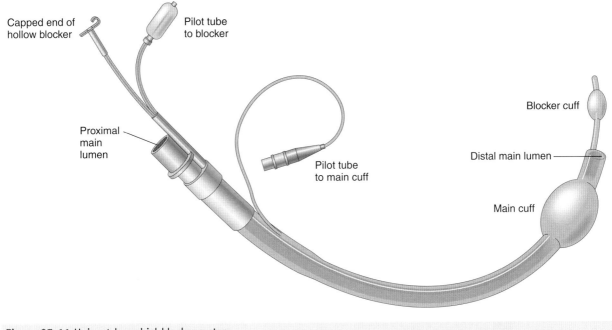

Figure 27-11 Univent bronchial blocker system.

IV

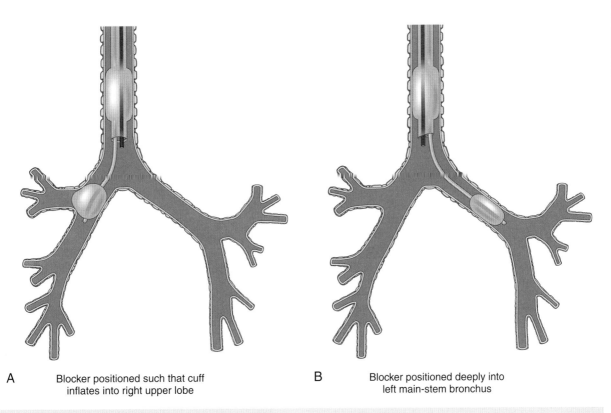

A   Blocker positioned such that cuff
     inflates into right upper lobe

B   Blocker positioned deeply into
     left main-stem bronchus

Figure 27-12 Positioning of the Univent bronchial blocker.

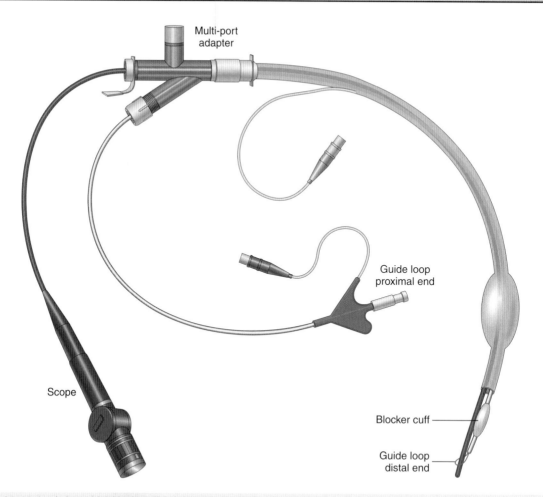

Multi-port adapter

Scope

Guide loop proximal end

Blocker cuff

Guide loop distal end

Figure 27-13 Arndt bronchial blocker. The Arndt endobronchial blocker and pediatric scope are connected through a multiport airway adapter. The blocker is coupled to the scope through the guide loop at the distal end of the blocker. Once coupled, the pediatric scope and blocker are advanced into the main bronchus of the lung to be blocked.

Approaches to Improve Oxygenation during One-Lung Ventilation

Proper positioning of the DLT should be confirmed with the fiberscope because dislodgment of the tube is not uncommon after positioning of the patient for surgery and again after surgical manipulation. The most effective approach to improve oxygenation is the application of 5 to 10 cm H_2O continuous positive airway pressure (CPAP) to the nondependent lung.[24] This level of CPAP results in minimal lung inflation and generally does not interfere with surgery. Nevertheless, discontinuing CPAP before lung stapling may be required to minimize postoperative air leaks. CPAP applied to the operative lung may not be helpful in certain conditions, such as thoracoscopy, bronchopleural fistula, sleeve resection, or massive pulmonary hemorrhage.

Because atelectasis in the dependent lung is an important factor causing arterial hypoxemia during one-lung ventilation, ventilation strategies applied to the dependent lung are often intended to improve arterial oxygenation. Initially, an alveolar recruitment maneuver (sustained increase in peak pressure [40 cm H_2O] for 5 to 10 breaths) may result in increased PaO_2 because of recruitment and expansion of atelectatic alveoli.[25] If the improvement in PaO_2 is not sustained, selective application of PEEP to the dependent lung is then initiated. In many circumstances, PEEP applied to the dependent lung may result in decreased PaO_2 because of the increased PVR of the dependent lung, which then diverts blood flow to the nondependent and atelectatic lung.[23,24] Nevertheless, in some circumstances, PEEP applied to the dependent lung may improve oxygenation because recruitment of atelectatic lung offsets the redistribution of pulmonary blood flow from the dependent to the nondependent lung. In addition, depending on the stage of surgery, clamping of the pulmonary artery will decrease the shunt fraction and thus improve oxygenation.

Table 27-5 Summary of the Approach to Management of One-Lung Ventilation

Deliver high F_{IO_2}

Initiate tidal ventilation with 8-10 mL/kg

Adjust respiratory frequency to maintain minute ventilation at the same level as during two-lung ventilation (Pa_{CO_2} = 40 mm Hg)

Continuous pulse oximetry and measurement of arterial blood gases after 15-20 minutes of one-lung ventilation and thereafter as indicated

Response to hypoxemia:
Reconfirm proper position of the double-lumen tube by fiberscope
Apply a recruitment maneuver to the dependent lung
Reinflate the nondependent lung and insufflate oxygen with CPAP (5-10 cm H_2O)
Titrate 5-10 cm H_2O PEEP to the dependent lung
Clamp or ligate the pulmonary artery or a segment of the pulmonary artery to the nondependent lung during pneumonectomy or lobectomy
Reposition to the semilateral decubitus position if surgery is in supine position
Resume two-lung ventilation if hypoxemia is uncorrected

CPAP, continuous positive airway pressure; PEEP, positive end-expiratory pressure.

CONCLUSION OF SURGERY

Hyperinflation of the lungs is an important maneuver to remove air from the pleural space at the conclusion of thoracic surgery. Furthermore, alveoli incised during segmental resection of the lungs continue to leak air into the pleural space, thus necessitating placement of chest tubes to minimize the air leak and promote continued expansion of the lung. Chest tubes should be set to continuous suction and must not be allowed to kink because sudden increases in intrathoracic pressure, as with coughing, may increase the air leak and cause tension pneumothorax if air cannot escape.

Placement of chest tubes is not necessary after pneumonectomy. Instead, intrapleural pressure on the operated side is adjusted by aspirating air to slightly below atmospheric pressure. Excessive negative pressure can cause hypotension by shifting the mediastinum and compromising cardiac output.

The trachea may be extubated when adequacy of spontaneous ventilation is confirmed and protective upper airway reflexes have returned. In otherwise healthy patients, extubation of the trachea may be performed at the conclusion of surgery, especially if pain relief (thoracic epidural analgesia) has been instituted (see Chapter 39). If mechanical ventilation of the lungs must be continued into the postoperative period, it will be necessary to replace the DLT with a single-lumen tube.

POSTOPERATIVE PULMONARY COMPLICATIONS

Postoperative pulmonary complications after thoracic surgery are often characterized by atelectasis, followed by pneumonia and arterial hypoxemia.[26] The severity of these complications parallels the magnitude of decrease in vital capacity and functional residual capacity. Presumably, decreases in these lung volumes interfere with the generation of an effective cough, as well as contribute to atelectasis. The net effect is decreased clearance of secretions from the airways and lungs leading to pneumonia and arterial hypoxemia. In addition, thoracotomy is known to produce intense postoperative pain as a result of skeletal muscle transection and rib removal during surgery.

Pain Management

Pain decreases respiratory effort, which results in atelectasis, contributes to development of the stress response with increased sympathetic nervous system activity, and increases cardiac morbidity. Thoracic epidural analgesia offers a unique opportunity for the anesthesiologist to improve postoperative recovery after thoracotomy. By delivering local anesthetics and opioids to a limited dermatomal distribution, thoracic epidural analgesia results in profound segmental analgesia, improved pulmonary function, earlier extubation of the trachea, and prompt mobility in the postoperative period. In addition, in patients with coronary artery disease, thoracic epidural analgesia may provide myocardial protection as a result of decreased sympathetic nervous system activity.

MEDIASTINOSCOPY

Mediastinoscopy is often performed before thoracotomy to establish the diagnosis or resectability of lung carcinoma. Hemorrhage and pneumothorax are the most frequently encountered complications of this procedure. If a thoracotomy is not subsequently performed, it is important to maintain a high index of suspicion for pneumothorax in the immediate postoperative period.

Positive-pressure ventilation of the lungs during mediastinoscopy is recommended to minimize the risk for venous air embolism. The mediastinoscope can also exert pressure against the right subclavian artery and cause loss of a pulse distal to the site of compression and an erroneous diagnosis of cardiac arrest. Likewise, unrecognized compression of the right carotid artery has been proposed as an explanation for the postoperative neurologic deficits that may occur after this procedure.

IV

Bradycardia may occur during mediastinoscopy and is due to stretching of the vagus nerve or trachea by the mediastinoscope. It is treated by repositioning the mediastinoscope, followed by the intravenous administration of atropine if the bradycardia persists.

THORACOSCOPY

Thoracoscopy is the insertion of an endoscope (thoracoscope) into the thoracic cavity and pleural space for the purpose of obtaining a lung biopsy and for the diagnosis of pleural disease. This procedure may be performed with local anesthetic infiltration or intercostal nerve blocks, which also anesthetize the parietal pleura. The addition of a stellate ganglion block helps suppress the cough reflex. When the thoracoscope enters the pleural cavity, the accompanying partial pneumothorax (limited by the seal between the thoracoscope and the skin and chest wall) permits surgical visualization. If general anesthesia is used, lung separation with a DLT is preferred because positive-pressure ventilation that includes both lungs would interfere with visualization. To negate the undesirable effects of pneumothorax, high inspired concentrations of oxygen are recommended, regardless of the anesthetic technique selected.

BRONCHOPLEURAL FISTULA

The priority in the management of anesthesia in patients with a bronchopleural fistula is isolation of the affected side with a DLT. The DLT may be placed during spontaneous breathing in an awake or anesthetized patient to avoid the development of tension pneumothorax. Chest tubes must also be left unclamped to avoid tension pneumothorax.

REFERENCES

1. Busse WW, Lemanske RF Jr. Asthma. N Engl J Med 2001;344:350-362.
2. Sutherland ER, Cherniack RM. Management of chronic obstructive pulmonary disease. N Engl J Med 2004;350:2689-2697.
3. National Asthma Education and Prevention Program. National Heart, Lung, and Blood Institute, 2002.
4. Warner DO, Warner MA, Barnes RD, et al. Perioperative respiratory complications in patients with asthma. Anesthesiology 1996;85:460-467.
5. Goff MJ, Arain SR, Ficke DJ, et al. Absence of bronchodilation during desflurane anesthesia: A comparison to sevoflurane and thiopental. Anesthesiology 2000;93:404-408.
6. Maslow AD, Regan MM, Israel E, et al. Inhaled albuterol, but not intravenous lidocaine, protects against intubation-induced bronchoconstriction in asthma. Anesthesiology 2000;93:1198-1204.
7. Groeben H, Schlicht M, Stieglitz S, et al. Both local anesthetics and salbutamol pretreatment affect reflex bronchoconstriction in volunteers with asthma undergoing awake fiberoptic intubation. Anesthesiology 2002;97:1445-1450.
8. Global Initiative for Chronic Obstructive Lung Disease. National Heart, Lung, and Blood Institute, World Health Organization, 2004.
9. De Nino LA, Lawrence VA, Averyt EC, et al. Preoperative spirometry and laparotomy: Blowing away dollars. Chest 1997; 111:1536-1541.
10. Celli BR, Cote CG, Marin JM, et al. The body-mass index, airflow obstruction, dyspnea, and exercise capacity index in chronic obstructive pulmonary disease. N Engl J Med 2004;350:1005-1012.
11. World Symposium on Primary Pulmonary Hypertension. Evian, France: World Health Organization, 1998.
12. Fiser SM, Cope JT, Kron IL, et al. Aerosolized prostacyclin (epoprostenol) as an alternative to inhaled nitric oxide for patients with reperfusion injury after lung transplantation. J Thorac Cardiovasc Surg 2001;121:981-982.
13. Hillman DR, Loadsman JA, Platt PR, Eastwood PR. Obstructive sleep apnoea and anaesthesia. Sleep Med Rev 2004;8:459-471.
14. Benumof JL. Obstructive sleep apnea in the adult obese patient: Implications for airway management. J Clin Anesth 2001;13:144-156.
15. Beckles MA, Spiro SG, Colice GL, Rudd RM. The physiologic evaluation of patients with lung cancer being considered for resectional surgery. Chest 2003;123:105S-114S.
16. Warner MA, Divertie MB, Tinker JH. Preoperative cessation of smoking and pulmonary complications in coronary artery bypass patients. Anesthesiology 1984;60:380-383.
17. Benumof JL, Augustine SD, Gibbons JA. Halothane and isoflurane only slightly impair arterial oxygenation during one-lung ventilation in patients undergoing thoracotomy. Anesthesiology 1987;67:910-915.
18. Brodsky JB, Macario A, Mark JB. Tracheal diameter predicts double-lumen tube size: A method for selecting left double-lumen tubes. Anesth Analg 1996;82:861-864.
19. Alliaume B, Coddens J, Deloof T. Reliability of auscultation in positioning of double-lumen endobronchial tubes. Can J Anaesth 1992;39:687-690.
20. Szegedi LL, Bardoczky GI, Engelman EE, d'Hollander AA. Airway pressure changes during one-lung ventilation. Anesth Analg 1997;84:1034-1037.
21. Campos JH, Massa FC. Is there a better right-sided tube for one-lung ventilation? A comparison of the right-sided double-lumen tube with the single-lumen tube with right-sided enclosed bronchial blocker. Anesth Analg 1998;86:696-700.
22. Campos JH. An update on bronchial blockers during lung separation techniques in adults. Anesth Analg 2003;97:1266-1274.
23. Katz JA, Laverne RG, Fairley HB, Thomas AN. Pulmonary oxygen exchange during endobronchial anesthesia: Effect of tidal volume and PEEP. Anesthesiology 1982; 56:164-171.
24. Capan LM, Turndorf H, Patel C, et al. Optimization of arterial oxygenation during one-lung anesthesia. Anesth Analg 1980; 59:847-851.
25. Tusman G, Bohm SH, Sipmann FS, Maisch S. Lung recruitment improves the efficiency of ventilation and gas exchange during one-lung ventilation anesthesia. Anesth Analg 2004; 98:1604-1609.
26. Weissman C. Pulmonary function after cardiac and thoracic surgery. Anesth Analg 1999;88:1272-1279.

Chapter 28

RENAL, LIVER, AND BILIARY TRACT DISEASE

C. S. Yost and Claus U. Niemann

RENAL DISEASE

The kidney has an important role in the excretion of all xenobiotics and is crucial in adjusting the composition and volume of the extracellular fluid compartment, maintaining acid-base balance, and regulating hemoglobin levels. Preoperatively, the three risk factors that most accurately predict the likelihood of acute renal failure in the postoperative period are (1) preexisting renal disease, (2) congestive heart failure, and (3) advanced age (Table 28-1).[1,2]

Renal Blood Flow

Although the kidneys represent only 0.5% of total body weight, their blood flow is equivalent to about 20% of cardiac output. Approximately two thirds of renal blood flow is distributed to the renal cortex. Renal blood flow and the glomerular filtration rate (GFR) remain relatively constant at mean arterial pressures in the range of

Table 28-1 Increased Risk for Acute Renal Failure
Preexisting renal disease
Advanced age
Congestive heart failure
Prolonged renal hypoperfusion (hypovolemia, hypotension)
High-risk surgery (abdominal aneurysm resection, cardiopulmonary bypass)
Extensive burns
Sepsis
Drug induced
End-stage liver disease

60 to 150 mm Hg. This ability to maintain renal blood flow at a constant rate despite changes in perfusion pressure is known as autoregulation. It is achieved by adjustment of afferent arteriolar tone, which alters the resistance to blood flow. Autoregulation is important because it acts to protect the glomerular capillaries from high systemic blood pressure during acute hypertensive episodes and maintains GFR and renal tubule function during modest decreases in systemic blood pressure. When mean arterial pressure is outside the autoregulatory range, renal blood flow becomes pressure dependent.

Renal blood flow is strongly influenced by the activity of the sympathetic nervous system and by release of renin and other hormones. Sympathetic nervous system stimulation can produce renal vasoconstriction and a marked decrease in renal blood flow even if systemic blood pressure is within the autoregulatory range. Any decrease in renal blood flow will initiate the release of renin, which can further decrease renal blood flow.

Glomerular Filtration Rate

Hydrostatic pressure within the glomerular capillaries is about 50 mm Hg. This pressure acts to force water and other low-molecular-weight substances such as electrolytes through the glomerular capillaries into Bowman's space. Plasma oncotic pressure is about 25 mm Hg at the afferent arteriole and with filtration increases to about 35 mm Hg at the efferent arteriole. Despite a relatively low net filtration pressure, the glomerular capillaries are able to filter plasma at a rate equivalent to about 125 mL/min. GFR is reduced by decreased mean arterial pressure or decreased renal blood flow. Ultimately, about 90% of the fluid filtered at the glomeruli is reabsorbed from renal tubules into peritubular capillaries and thus returned to the circulation (Fig. 28-1).

Humoral Substances

RENIN

Renin is a proteolytic enzyme secreted by the juxtaglomerular apparatus of the kidneys in response to (1) sympathetic nervous system stimulation, (2) decreased renal perfusion pressure, and (3) decreases in the delivery of sodium to the distal convoluted renal tubules. Renin acts on a circulating globulin in plasma (angiotensinogen) to form angiotensin I. Angiotensin I is split in the lungs by a converting enzyme to form angiotensin II. Angiotensin II is a potent vasoconstrictor and an important stimulus for the release of aldosterone from the adrenal cortex.

PROSTAGLANDINS

Prostaglandins are produced in the renal medulla and released in response to sympathetic nervous system stimulation and increased levels of angiotensin II. During periods of hemodynamic instability, prostaglandins act intrarenally to modulate the vasoconstrictive actions of catecholamines.

Drug Clearance

Excretion of drugs or their metabolites into urine depends on three mechanisms: (1) glomerular filtration, (2) active secretion by the renal tubules, and (3) passive reabsorption by the tubules. The net effect of these three processes is renal drug elimination from the body.

The glomerular filtration of small molecules characteristic of anesthetic drugs depends on the GFR and the fractional plasma protein binding. Drugs that are highly protein bound will be inefficiently filtered at the glomerulus. Un-ionized acidic and basic compounds undergo passive reabsorption by backdiffusion in the proximal and distal renal tubules. Ionized forms of these weak acids and bases are trapped within renal tubules, thus creating a mechanism to increase renal elimination by either alkalinization or acidification of urine.

Renal Function Tests

Renal function can be evaluated preoperatively by using several laboratory tests (Table 28-2).[3] These tests are not sensitive measurements, and significant renal disease (more than a 50% decrease in renal function) can exist while laboratory values remain normal. Furthermore, the normal values established in healthy individuals may not be adjusted for age or applicable during anesthesia. Trends are more useful for evaluating renal function than a single laboratory measurement is.

SERUM CREATININE

Serum creatinine concentrations are often used to indicate the GFR. In contrast to blood urea nitrogen (BUN) concentrations, serum creatinine levels are not influenced by protein metabolism or the rate of fluid flow through renal tubules. Serum creatinine concentrations are, however, influenced by skeletal muscle mass. Maintenance of normal serum creatinine concentrations in elderly patients with known decreases in GFR reflects decreased creatinine production because of the decreased skeletal muscle mass that frequently accompanies aging. Indeed, mild increases in the serum creatinine concentration in elderly patients may suggest significant renal disease. Likewise, in patients with chronic renal failure, serum creatinine concentrations may not accurately reflect the GFR because of (1) decreased creatinine production, (2) the presence of decreased skeletal muscle mass, or (3) nonrenal (gastrointestinal tract) excretion of creatinine.

BLOOD UREA NITROGEN

BUN concentrations, which are normally 10 to 20 mg/dL, vary with changes in GFR. The BUN concentration is

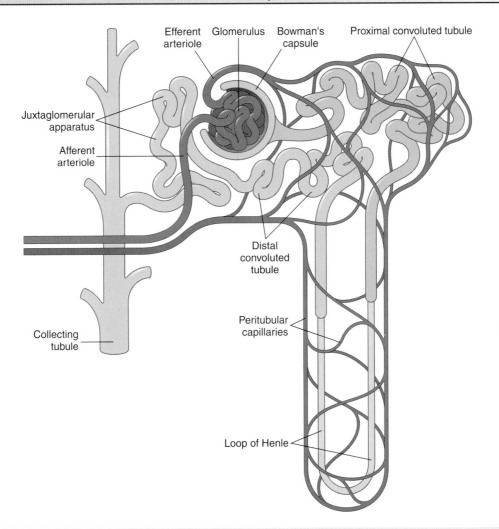

Figure 28-1 Anatomy of a nephron. The glomerulus is formed by the invaginated and blind end of the nephron known as Bowman's capsule. Hydrostatic pressure in these capillaries causes water and low-molecular-weight substances to filter through the glomerulus. Glomerular filtrate travels along the renal tubule (proximal convoluted tubule, loop of Henle, distal convoluted tubule), during which most of its water and various amounts of solutes are reabsorbed from the renal tubular lumen into peritubular capillaries. The remaining glomerular filtrate becomes urine.

a potentially misleading test of renal function because of the influence of dietary intake, coexisting illnesses, and intravascular fluid volume. For example, high-protein diets or gastrointestinal bleeding can increase the production of urea and thereby result in increased BUN concentrations (azotemia) despite a normal GFR. Other causes of increased BUN concentrations despite a normal GFR are increased catabolism during febrile illnesses and dehydration. Increased BUN concentrations in the presence of dehydration most likely reflect increased urea absorption because of the slow movement of fluid through the renal tubules, which results in a BUN-to-creatinine ratio greater than 20. When slow movement of fluid through the renal tubules is responsible for

increased BUN concentrations, serum creatinine levels remain normal. BUN concentrations can remain normal in the presence of low-protein diets despite decreases in GFR. Aside from these extraneous influences, BUN concentrations greater than 50 mg/dL almost always reflect a decreased GFR.

CREATININE CLEARANCE

Creatinine clearance (normal, 110 to 150 mL/min) is a measurement of the ability of the glomeruli to excrete creatinine into urine for a given serum creatinine concentration. Because creatinine clearance does not depend on corrections for age or the presence of a steady state, it is the most reliable measurement of GFR. The principal

Table 28-2   Tests Used for Evaluation of Renal Function

Test	Normal Value	Factors That Influence Interpretation
Glomerular Filtration Rate		
Blood urea nitrogen	8-20 mg/dL	Dehydration Variable protein intake Gastrointestinal bleeding Catabolism
Serum creatinine	0.5-1.2 mg/dL	Age Skeletal muscle mass Catabolism
Creatinine clearance Proteinuria	120 mL/min	Accurate urine volume measurement
Renal Tubular Function		
Urine specific gravity Urine osmolarity Urine sodium		

disadvantage of this test is the need for timed (2 hours may be as acceptable as 24 hours) urine collections.

PROTEINURIA

Small amounts of protein are normally filtered through glomerular capillaries and then reabsorbed in the proximal convoluted tubules. Proteinuria (excretion of more than 150 mg of protein per day) is most likely due to abnormally high filtration rather than impaired reabsorption by the renal tubules. Intermittent proteinuria occasionally occurs in healthy individuals when standing and disappears when supine. Other nonrenal causes of proteinuria include exercise, fever, and congestive heart failure.

URINE INDICES

Measurement of urine osmolality and urinary sodium and calculation of the fractional excretion of sodium can help differentiate between prerenal and renal tubular (intrarenal) causes of azotemia.

OTHER LABORATORY MEASUREMENTS

Measurement of serum calcium, uric acid, and creatinine kinase concentrations and serum osmolality may be useful in the differential diagnosis of acute renal failure secondary to conditions such as rhabdomyolysis, nephrotoxic drugs, or malignancy.

Pharmacology of Diuretics

THIAZIDE DIURETICS

Thiazide diuretics (hydrochlorothiazide, chlorthalidone) are generally administered for the treatment of essential hypertension and for mobilization of the edema fluid that is associated with renal, hepatic, or cardiac dysfunction. Diuresis occurs as a result of the inhibition of reabsorption of sodium and chloride ions from the early distal renal tubules. Side effects associated with diuretic-induced hypokalemia may include (1) skeletal muscle weakness, (2) increased risk for digitalis toxicity, and (3) potentiation of nondepolarizing neuromuscular blocking drugs (Table 28-3).[4]

LOOP DIURETICS

Loop diuretics (ethacrynic acid, furosemide, bumetanide) inhibit the reabsorption of sodium and chloride and augment the secretion of potassium, primarily in the loop of Henle. Intravenous administration of these drugs produces a diuretic response within minutes. Chronic administration of loop diuretics may result in hypochloremic, hypokalemic metabolic alkalosis and, in rare instances, deafness.

OSMOTIC DIURETICS

The most frequently administered osmotic diuretic is the six-carbon sugar mannitol. Mannitol produces diuresis because it is filtered by the glomeruli and not reabsorbed within the renal tubules. This leads to increased osmolarity of the renal tubule fluid and associated excretion of water. Another rationale for the administration of mannitol in low–urine output states is that it prevents renal tubular cell swelling and increases intratubular flow.

Mannitol increases fluid movement from intracellular spaces into extracellular spaces such that intravascular fluid volume expands acutely. This redistribution of fluid from intracellular to extracellular compartments decreases brain size and intracranial pressure. Mannitol may further

Table 28-3 Side Effects of Diuretics

	Hypokalemic, Hypochloremic Metabolic Alkalosis	Hyperkalemia	Hyperglycemia
Thiazide diuretics	Yes	No	Yes
Loop diuretics	Yes	No	Minimal
Osmotic diuretics	No	No	No
Aldosterone antagonists	No	Yes	No

diminish intracranial pressure by decreasing the rate of cerebrospinal fluid formation.

ALDOSTERONE ANTAGONISTS

Spironolactone blocks the renal tubular effects of aldosterone and offsets the loss of potassium that is associated with the administration of thiazide diuretics. Fluid overload secondary to cirrhosis of the liver is often treated with spironolactone. The most serious toxic effect of spironolactone is hyperkalemia. Preoperative measurement of the serum potassium concentration is indicated for patients taking spironolactone.

RENAL-DOSE DOPAMINE

Dopamine dilates renal arterioles, which increases renal blood flow and the GFR. Treatment with low-dose dopamine (0.5 to 3 µg/kg/min) may augment urine output but does not appear to alter the course of acute renal failure.[5] Dose-dependent side effects of dopamine include tachydysrhythmias, pulmonary shunting, and tissue ischemia (gastrointestinal tract, digits).

Pathophysiology of End-Stage Renal Disease

End-stage renal disease (ESRD) causes profound physiologic changes that affect several organs (Tables 28-4 and 28-5).

CARDIOVASCULAR DISEASE

Cardiovascular disease is the predominant cause of death in patients with ESRD. Acute myocardial infarction, cardiac arrest of unknown etiology, cardiac dysrhythmias, and cardiomyopathy account for more than 50% of deaths in patients maintained on dialysis. Fluid overload and systemic hypertension are frequently encountered in patients with ESRD. The accumulation of uremic toxins and metabolic acids may contribute to poor myocardial performance. The presence of ESRD with significantly depressed cardiac function does not necessarily contraindicate renal transplantation because cardiac ventricular function often improves after transplantation.

Uremia causes changes in lipid metabolism that lead to increased concentrations of serum triglycerides and reduced levels of protective high-density lipoproteins. Thus, ESRD accelerates the progression of atherosclerosis. Pericardial disease and cardiac dysrhythmias can also be encountered in patients with ESRD. Pericardial effusions are resolved when patients are adequately dialyzed.

METABOLIC DISEASE

A large number of patients with ESRD manifest diabetes mellitus. Kidney failure as a result of diabetes develops in nearly 30% to 40% of patients with ESRD, and these patients account for 30% of those on the waiting list for kidney transplantation. In fact, nephropathy develops in nearly 60% of insulin-dependent diabetic patients. Patients with ESRD and diabetes have a higher cardiovascular risk than do patients with renal failure alone.

Once patients are unable to excrete their dietary fluid and electrolyte loads, abnormalities in plasma electrolyte concentrations (sodium, potassium, calcium, magnesium, and phosphate) can develop. The most life-threatening electrolyte abnormality is hyperkalemia.

Table 28-4 Changes Characteristic of Chronic Renal Disease

Anemia
Depressed ejection fraction
Decreased platelet adhesiveness
Hyperkalemia
Unpredictable intravascular fluid volume
Metabolic acidosis
Systemic hypertension
Pericardial effusion
Decreased sympathetic nervous system activity

IV

Table 28-5 Stages of Chronic Renal Failure

Stage	Glomerular Filtration (mL/min/1.73 m²)
1	> 90
2	60-89
3	30-59
4	15-29
5	< 15

ANEMIA AND ABNORMAL COAGULATION

Patients with renal failure generally display a normochromic, normocytic anemia because of decreased erythropoiesis and retained toxins that are secondary to renal failure. Treatment with recombinant erythropoietin can frequently raise hemoglobin levels to 10 to 14 g/dL, which reduces symptoms of fatigue and improves both cerebral and cardiac function. Occasionally, recombinant erythropoietin therapy may exacerbate preexisting essential hypertension. Renal failure patients may also display uremia-induced defects in platelet function.

Management of Anesthesia in Patients with End-Stage Renal Disease

General endotracheal anesthesia provides acceptable hemodynamics, excellent skeletal muscle relaxation, and a predictable depth of anesthesia in patients with ESRD who are undergoing major operations.[6] Patients with advanced stages of comorbid conditions may require more extensive monitoring, such as continuous monitoring of systemic blood pressure and perhaps central venous pressure. Large swings in blood pressure may occur with hypotension being more likely than hypertension during maintenance of anesthesia. Those with the most severe comorbid conditions, such as symptomatic coronary artery disease or a history of congestive heart failure, may benefit from monitoring with a pulmonary artery catheter or transesophageal echocardiography. The status of hemodialysis shunts or fistulas should be monitored (presence of a thrill) during positioning and intraoperatively to confirm continued potency.

Patients with uremia and other comorbid conditions (diabetes mellitus) should be considered to be at risk for aspiration during induction of anesthesia and treated as though they have a "full stomach." The use of succinylcholine is not contraindicated in patients with ESRD. The increase in serum potassium concentration after an intubating dose of succinylcholine is approximately 0.6 mEq/L for patients both with and without ESRD. This increase can be tolerated without imposing a signifi-

cant cardiac risk, even in the presence of an initial serum potassium concentration higher than 5 mEq/L.

Several strategies have been successfully used to achieve adequate heart rate and blood pressure control during induction of anesthesia. Moderate to large doses of opioids such as fentanyl can blunt the response to laryngoscopy. However, systemic blood pressure is frequently more difficult to maintain after induction of anesthesia, and hypotension may require treatment with vasoconstrictors. The short-acting β-adrenergic blocker esmolol may be used to blunt the hemodynamic response to tracheal intubation and is ideally suited for patients with an adequate ejection fraction.

Drugs or their metabolites that depend on renal elimination (pancuronium, morphine, meperidine) should be used cautiously or avoided. Atracurium and cisatracurium are metabolized by spontaneous Hoffman degradation and plasma cholinesterase, which makes their duration of action independent of liver or kidney function. Similarly, fentanyl, sufentanil, alfentanil, and remifentanil are alternatives to morphine.

Choices of inhaled anesthetics include desflurane, isoflurane, and sevoflurane. The metabolism of sevoflurane to inorganic fluoride has been implicated in experimental studies of renal toxicity, although no controlled human studies are available to indicate either safety concerns or danger when using sevoflurane in the setting of ESRD.

Differential Diagnosis of Perioperative Oliguria

PRERENAL OLIGURIA

Prerenal oliguria is characterized by the excretion of concentrated urine that contains minimal amounts of sodium (Table 28-6). Excretion of highly concentrated and sodium-poor urine confirms that renal tubular function is intact and reflects an attempt by the kidneys to conserve sodium and restore intravascular fluid volume in response to decreased renal blood flow. The decreased renal blood flow most likely reflects an acute decrease in intravascular fluid volume or decreased cardiac output. Other causes of decreased renal blood flow are sepsis, liver failure, and congestive heart failure.

The initial management of patients with perioperative oliguria is influenced by their risk for the development of acute renal failure.[7] A brisk diuresis in response to a fluid challenge suggests that an acute decrease in intravascular fluid volume is the cause of the prerenal oliguria. When fluid replacement does not result in increased urine output, intrinsic renal disease or hemodynamic causes should be considered.

Administration of diuretics to maintain or stimulate urine flow in the perioperative period is controversial. Some believe that prevention of renal tubule urine stasis with diuretics can prevent prerenal oliguria from progressing to acute tubular necrosis. Nevertheless, urine output that is enhanced by the administration of a diuretic does

Table 28-6 Differential Diagnosis and Causes of Preoperative Oliguria

	Prerenal Oliguria	Acute Tubular Necrosis
Urine sodium (mEq/L)	<40	>40
Urine osmolarity (mOsm/L)	>400	<400
Causes	Decreased renal blood flow (hypotension, hypovolemia, decreased cardiac output)	Renal ischemia Nephrotoxins Free hemoglobin or myoglobin

not necessarily predict postoperative renal function. There is no evidence that drug-induced diuresis (dopamine, furosemide, mannitol) in the presence of low cardiac output or hypovolemia (or both) protects renal function. Likewise, there is no evidence that the incidence of acute renal failure is decreased when dopamine is administered to high-risk patients (abdominal aortic cross-clamping, cardiopulmonary bypass).

INTRINSIC RENAL DISEASE

Acute tubular necrosis, glomerulonephritis, and acute interstitial nephritis are intrinsic renal causes of oliguria. In contrast to oliguria secondary to hypovolemia, the urine of patients with acute tubular necrosis is poorly concentrated and contains excessive amounts of sodium (see Table 28-6). Hyperkalemia can accompany acute tubular necrosis.

POSTRENAL OLIGURIA

An obstruction that is distal to the renal collecting system usually involves a mechanical problem such as a blood clot in the ureter, bladder, or urethra. Surgical ligation and renal calculi are other postrenal causes of low urine output. Another common postrenal cause is bladder catheter obstruction.

LIVER DISEASE

The liver is responsible for the production of essential plasma proteins, the metabolism and detoxification of drugs and deleterious xenobiotics, the absorption of critical nutrients, and carbohydrate metabolism. Impaired liver function affects nearly every organ system in the body.

Hepatic Blood Flow

The liver is unique in that it receives a dual afferent blood supply that is equal to about 25% of cardiac output (Fig. 28-2). Approximately 70% of hepatic blood flow is supplied by the portal vein with the remainder supplied by the hepatic artery. Under normal conditions, each blood vessel contributes roughly 50% to the liver's oxygen supply. Decreases in systemic blood pressure and cardiac output result in decreased portal vein flow, which can be partially compensated by increased hepatic artery flow. In the presence of volatile anesthetics or cirrhosis of the liver, the reciprocal relationship between hepatic artery and portal vein blood flow (autoregulation) is not maintained and may expose the liver to an increased risk for ischemia. The relative inadequacy of blood flow to the liver can be even more pronounced in cirrhotic livers.

DETERMINANTS OF HEPATIC BLOOD FLOW

Hepatic perfusion pressure (mean arterial or portal vein pressure minus hepatic vein pressure) and splanchnic vascular resistance determine hepatic blood flow. The splanchnic vessels receive vasomotor innervation from the sympathetic nervous system. Splanchnic nerve stimulation (pain, arterial hypoxemia, surgical stress) can increase splanchnic vascular resistance and decrease hepatic blood flow. Blockade of β-adrenergic receptors by drugs such as propranolol is also associated with decreases in hepatic blood flow. Positive-pressure ventilation of the lungs, congestive heart failure, and fluid overload can decrease hepatic blood flow, presumably by causing increased central venous pressure (hepatic vein pressure) with resulting decreased hepatic perfusion pressure.

Glucose Homeostasis

The liver is the main organ for the storage and release of glucose. Glucose enters hepatocytes, where it can be stored as glycogen. Breakdown of glycogen (glycogenolysis) releases glucose back into the systemic circulation for maintenance of normal blood glucose concentrations. Surgical stress can cause increased sympathetic nervous system activity, which will stimulate glycogen breakdown with subsequent perioperative hyperglycemia.

Coagulation

Clotting abnormalities must be suspected in patients with liver disease because hepatocytes are responsible for the synthesis of most procoagulant proteins. The effectiveness of clotting is evaluated by measuring the

IV

Figure 28-2 Schematic depiction of the dual afferent blood supply to the liver provided by the portal vein and hepatic artery. About 70% of hepatic blood flow is via the portal vein, with the remainder via the hepatic artery. Total hepatic blood flow is directly proportional to perfusion pressure across the liver and inversely related to splanchnic vascular resistance. Cirrhosis of the liver increases resistance to blood flow through the portal vein and decreases hepatic blood flow.

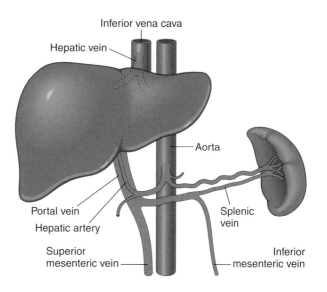

prothrombin time (international normalized ratio [INR]), partial thromboplastin time, and fibrinogen levels. Protein synthesis needs to be dramatically depressed before impaired coagulation develops because many coagulation factors require only 20% to 30% of their normal levels to prevent bleeding.

Acute liver dysfunction is likely to be associated with clotting abnormalities because the plasma half-times of hepatically produced clotting factors, such as the vitamin K–dependent factors II, VII, IX, and X, are relatively short.

Drug Metabolism

Drug metabolism is characterized by the conversion of lipid-soluble drugs to more water-soluble and pharmacologically less active substances. This metabolism is controlled by microsomal enzymes that are present in the smooth endoplasmic reticulum of hepatocytes. Chronic liver disease may interfere with the metabolism of drugs because of the decreased number of enzyme-containing hepatocytes or the decreased hepatic blood flow that typically accompanies cirrhosis of the liver. Prolonged elimination half-times for morphine, alfentanil, diazepam, lidocaine, pancuronium, and to a lesser extent, vecuronium have been demonstrated in patients with cirrhosis of the liver. Repeated injections of these drugs can produce cumulative effects in patients with severe liver disease. Enzyme induction/inhibition may also be a response to chronic drug therapy or alcohol abuse and can influence the metabolism of other administered drugs.

Bilirubin Formation and Excretion

Bilirubin is produced in the reticuloendothelial system from the breakdown of hemoglobin. This bilirubin is bound to albumin for transport to the liver. Because protein-bound bilirubin (unconjugated) is not water soluble, urinary excretion of it is minimal. Conjugation of bilirubin with glucuronic acid in the liver renders bilirubin water soluble.

Pathophysiology of End-Stage Liver Disease

HYPERDYNAMIC CIRCULATION
Severe parenchymal disease that has advanced to the point of cirrhosis usually results in a hyperdynamic circulation. Hemodynamic measurements generally reveal normal to low systemic blood pressure and increased cardiac output, which results in a very low calculated systemic vascular resistance. These hemodynamic changes reflect profound vasodilation and a heart that is pumping against a reduced afterload.

Low systemic vascular resistance in the presence of advanced cirrhosis of the liver arises from both vasodilation and abnormal anatomic and physiologic shunting. Physiologic shunting is the passage of blood from the arterial to the venous side of the circulation without effectively traversing a capillary bed. Abnormal blood vessels, such as those seen in the skin as spider angiomas, represent an anatomic shunt.

PORTAL HYPERTENSION
High resistance to blood flow through the liver causes an accumulation of blood in the vascular beds that are immediately upstream of the liver. Venous drainage of the esophagus, stomach, spleen, and intestines dilates and increases in capacity, which leads to the development of splenomegaly and esophageal, gastric, and intra-abdominal varices.

PULMONARY CIRCULATION

End-stage liver disease can be associated with the hepatopulmonary syndrome and portopulmonary hypertension. Hepatopulmonary syndrome is the pulmonary manifestation of physiologic shunting. The resulting arterial hypoxemia may improve somewhat with the supplemental oxygen provided by an increased F_{IO_2}.

Portopulmonary hypertension is an elevation in intrapulmonary vascular pressure in patients with portal hypertension. The cause is not well established, and fortunately this syndrome occurs in less than 5% of patients, even within the liver transplant population. Nevertheless, these patients are at increased risk for acute right heart failure if physiologic conditions that increase pulmonary vascular resistance (acidosis, arterial hypoxemia, hypercapnia) occur during anesthesia.

HEPATIC ENCEPHALOPATHY

An alteration in the mental state is a frequent complication of both acute and chronic liver failure and can range from minor changes in brain function to deep coma. One postulated explanation for hepatic encephalopathy is the passage of nitrogenous substances such as ammonia from the gut into the systemic circulation as a result of decreased hepatic function or portosystemic shunting. Other causes of altered mental status in patients with liver disease, such as intracranial bleeding or masses, hypoglycemia, or a postictal state, should be considered. Treatment generally involves reducing production and absorption of the nitrogenous load from the gastrointestinal tract with antibiotics such as neomycin or the administration of lactulose to increase bowel transit.

DRUG BINDING

When liver disease is so severe that albumin production is decreased, fewer sites are available for drug binding. This can increase levels of the unbound, pharmacologically active fraction of drugs such as thiopental. Increased drug sensitivity as a result of decreased protein binding is most likely to be manifested when plasma albumin concentrations are lower than 2.5 g/dL.

Effects of Anesthesia and Surgery on the Liver

IMPACT OF ANESTHETICS ON HEPATIC BLOOD FLOW

Inhaled anesthetics and regional anesthesia both typically decrease hepatic blood flow 20% to 30% in the absence of surgical stimulation. These changes reflect drug- or technique-induced effects on hepatic perfusion pressure or splanchnic vascular resistance, or both. For example, the various degrees of reduction in hepatic blood flow that are associated with volatile anesthetics, as well as regional anesthesia (T5 sensory level), are most likely due to decreased hepatic perfusion pressure. There is some experimental evidence that autoregulation (increased hepatic artery blood flow offsetting decreases in portal vein blood flow) of hepatic blood flow is best maintained with isoflurane. However, hepatic blood flow during the administration of desflurane and sevoflurane is maintained by a similar mechanism.[8]

IMPACT OF SURGICAL STIMULATION ON HEPATIC BLOOD FLOW

Surgical stimulation and the proximity of the operative site to the liver are important determinants of the magnitude of the decrease in hepatic blood flow seen during general anesthesia. The greatest decreases in hepatic blood flow occur when the operative site is near the liver.

DRUG-INDUCED HEPATIC DYSFUNCTION

A rare, but life-threatening form of hepatic dysfunction may reflect an immune-mediated hepatotoxicity caused by halothane.[9,10] The most compelling evidence for an immune-mediated mechanism is the presence of circulating immunoglobulin G antibodies in the majority of patients with the diagnosis of *halothane hepatitis*. These antibodies are directed against liver microsomal proteins on the surfaces of hepatocytes that have been covalently modified by the reactive oxidative trifluoroacetyl halide metabolite of halothane to form neoantigens. This acetylation of liver proteins in effect changes these proteins from self to nonself (neoantigens) and results in the formation of antibodies against this new protein. It is presumed that the subsequent antigen-antibody interaction is responsible for the rare (estimated to occur in 1 in 10,000 to 30,000 adult patients receiving halothane) liver injury that is characterized as halothane hepatitis. Isoflurane and desflurane are also capable of producing trifluoroacetyl metabolites, but the incidence of drug-induced hepatitis after exposure to these drugs is less because of the decreased magnitude of metabolism in comparison to halothane.

Management of Anesthesia in Patients with End-Stage Liver Disease

PREOPERATIVE EVALUATION OF LIVER DISEASE

Liver function tests (Table 28-7) are used to detect the presence of liver disease preoperatively and to establish the diagnosis when postoperative liver dysfunction occurs. A system for evaluating liver status is the Child-Pugh system (Table 28-8).[11] Patients with Child-Pugh class C liver dysfunction have a greatly increased risk for perioperative morbidity and mortality. Morbidity and mortality after elective operations are higher in patients with preexisting cirrhosis of the liver than in patients undergoing similar operations but in the absence of liver disease.[12]

It is important to recognize that liver function tests are rarely specific. Postoperative liver dysfunction is greater in the presence of coexisting liver disease. Furthermore, the large reserve of the liver means that considerable

Table 28-7 Liver Function Tests

Test	Normal Values*
Albumin	3.5-5.5 g/dL
Bilirubin	0.3-1.1 mg/dL
Unconjugated bilirubin (indirect reacting)	0.2-0.7 mg/dL
Conjugated bilirubin (direct reacting)	0.1-0.4 mg/dL
Aspartate aminotransferase (SGOT)	10-40 U/mL
Alanine aminotransferase (SGPT)	5-35 U/mL
Alkaline phosphatase	10-30 U/mL
Prothrombin time	12-14 sec

*Normal values for each individual laboratory should be considered when interpreting liver function test results.

hepatic damage can be present before liver function test results become altered. Indeed, cirrhosis of the liver may cause little alteration in liver function. It may take an additional stress, such as anesthesia and surgery, to reveal the underlying liver disease. Inadequate hepatocyte function during anesthesia and surgery will be manifested as metabolic acidosis intraoperatively.

INTRAOPERATIVE MANAGEMENT

Most major operations in patients with significant liver diseases involve the use of general anesthesia. Regional technique can be considered in selected patients with acceptable coagulation. The magnitude of the operation determines the extent of invasive monitoring that is required. Major operations during which blood loss is likely require continuous means of monitoring systemic blood pressure (arterial line) and filling pressure (central venous line). Correction of a severe coagulopathy before vascular line placement may be considered, whereas the use of ultrasound may facilitate central venous cannula-

tion. Communication with the blood bank before surgery is crucial to ensure adequate availability of red blood cells, platelets, and clotting factors, including fresh frozen plasma.

Induction and Maintenance of Anesthesia
Most patients have well-preserved cardiac function and no significant systemic or pulmonary hypertension. Induction of anesthesia can be achieved with an intravenous anesthetic such as propofol, thiopental, or etomidate, along with opioids and short- or intermediate-acting neuromuscular blocking drugs. A rapid-sequence or modified rapid-sequence induction of anesthesia is warranted if patients have significant ascites or delayed gastric emptying. Hypotension after induction of anesthesia may occur as a result of the low systemic vascular resistance and relative hypovolemia that may be present in these patients. This can usually be treated with small amounts of vasoconstrictors (phenylephrine). With the exception of halothane, all volatile anesthetics are suitable for patients with severe liver disease. No optimal anesthetic technique has been established for the maintenance of anesthesia.

Coagulopathy
Coagulopathy and surgical blood loss are treated by the administration of red blood cells, fresh frozen plasma, platelets, and cryoprecipitate. Pharmacologic treatment of hepatic-associated coagulopathy may include aprotinin, ε-aminocaproic acid, tranexamic acid, conjugated estrogen, and activated recombinant factor VII.

Postoperative Jaundice

Halothane or other volatile anesthetics are often implicated as the cause of postoperative jaundice, but there are many other and probably more likely causes (Table 28-9). A surgical cause of postoperative jaundice is likely if the operation involved the liver or biliary tract. Drugs, including antibiotics, and other metabolic or infectious causes must be considered.

Table 28-8 Child-Pugh Classification System for Liver Disease

	A	B	C
Serum bilirubin (mg/dL)	<2.0	2.0-3.0	>3.0
Serum albumin (g/dL)	>3.5	2.8-3.5	<2.8
Prothrombin time (seconds prolonged)	1-4 sec	4-6 sec	>6 sec
Ascites	None	Slight	Moderate
Encephalopathy	None	Minimal	Advanced

Data from Strunin L. Preoperative assessment of the patient with liver dysfunction. Br J Anaesth 1978;50:25-34.

Table 28-9   Classification and Causes of Postoperative Liver Dysfunction

	Prehepatic	**Intrahepatic**	**Posthepatic**
Bilirubin	Increased (unconjugated fraction)	Increased (conjugated fraction)	Increased (conjugated fraction)
Aminotransferase enzymes	No change	Markedly increased	Normal to slightly increased
Alkaline phosphatase	No change	No change to slightly increased	Markedly increased
Prothrombin time	No change	Prolonged	No change to prolonged
Albumin	No change	Decreased	No change to decreased
Causes	Hemolysis Hematoma reabsorption Bilirubin overload from whole blood	Viruses Drugs Sepsis Arterial hypoxemia Congestive heart failure Cirrhosis	Stones Cancer Sepsis

Management of Anesthesia in Intoxicated Patients

Acutely intoxicated patients require less anesthesia because there is an additive depressant effect between alcohol and anesthetics. Intoxicated patients are more vulnerable to regurgitation of gastric contents and aspiration pneumonia because alcohol slows gastric emptying and decreases the tone of the lower esophageal sphincter.

Alcohol Withdrawal Syndrome

Manifestations of severe alcohol withdrawal syndrome (delirium tremens) usually appear 48 to 72 hours after cessation of drinking.[13] This syndrome represents a medical emergency. Postoperatively, patients may manifest tremulousness and hallucinations. There is increased activity of the sympathetic nervous system with subsequent catecholamine release, which leads to diaphoresis, hyperpyrexia, tachycardia, and systemic hypertension. In some patients, grand mal seizures may be the first indication of alcohol withdrawal syndrome. When seizures occur, hypoglycemia should be ruled out as a possible cause.

TREATMENT
Treatment of delirium tremens must be aggressive and consists of the administration of midazolam, lorazepam, or diazepam (every 5 minutes until the patient becomes sedated but remains awake). A β-antagonist (propranolol or esmolol) should be used to control the heart rate. Protection of the upper airway with a cuffed tracheal tube may become necessary. Correction of fluid, electrolyte (magnesium, potassium), and metabolic (thiamine) derangements is important. Despite aggressive treatment, mortality from delirium tremens is about 10%. This mortality is often caused by hypotension, cardiac dysrhythmias, or seizures.

DISEASES OF THE BILIARY TRACT

Gallstones are reported to be present in 10% of men and 20% of women between 55 and 65 years of age. These patients usually have normal liver function test results, except for increased serum bilirubin or alkaline phosphatase concentrations because of the presence of choledocholithiasis (common bile duct stone) or chronic cholangitis.

Management of Anesthesia

Anesthesia for cholecystectomy or exploration of the common bile duct, or both, is influenced by the effect of the drugs used for anesthesia on intraluminal pressure in the biliary tract. Specifically, opioids can produce spasm of the choledochoduodenal sphincter, which increases common bile duct pressure. Such spasm may impair the passage of contrast media into the duodenum and erroneously suggest the need for sphincteroplasty or the presence of common bile duct stones. However, opioids have been used in many instances without adverse effect, which emphasizes the fact that not all patients respond to opioids with choledochoduodenal sphincter spasm.

LAPAROSCOPIC CHOLECYSTECTOMY
Anesthetic considerations for laparoscopic cholecystectomy are similar to those for other laparoscopic procedures.[14] For example, insufflation of the abdominal cavity (pneumoperitoneum) with carbon dioxide introduced through a needle placed via a supraumbilical incision results in increased intra-abdominal pressure that may interfere with ventilation of the lungs and venous return. During laparoscopic cholecystectomy, placement of the patient in the reverse Trendelenburg position favors

IV

movement of the abdominal contents away from the operative site and may facilitate mechanical ventilation of the lungs. This position, however, may further interfere with venous return. Generous fluid replacement during laparoscopic cholecystectomy may facilitate recovery from this surgery.

Monitoring end-tidal carbon dioxide concentrations during laparoscopic abdominal surgical procedures is useful because of the unpredictability of systemic absorption of the carbon dioxide used to create the pneumoperitoneum. Intraoperative decompression of the stomach with a nasogastric or orogastric tube may decrease the risk for visceral puncture at the time of needle insertion and may subsequently improve laparoscopic visualization. Administration of nitrous oxide during laparoscopic cholecystectomy is not usually recommended because of the remote possibility that it could expand bowel gas volume and thus interfere with surgical working conditions.[15] Loss of hemostasis or injury to the hepatic artery or liver may require prompt intervention via a conventional laparotomy incision.

REFERENCES

1. Norris BF, Roizen MF, Aronson S, et al. Association of preoperative risk factors with postoperative acute renal failure. Anesth Analg 1994;78: 143-149.
2. Turney JH. Acute renal failure—a dangerous condition. JAMA 1996; 275:1516-1517.
3. Kellen M, Aronson S, Roizen MF, et al. Predictive and diagnostic tests of renal failure: A review. Anesth Analg 1994;78:134-142.
4. Brater DC. Diuretic therapy. N Engl J Med 1998;339:387-402.
5. Baldwin L, Henderson A, Hickman P. Effect of postoperative low-dose dopamine on renal function after elective major vascular surgery. Ann Intern Med 1994;120:744-747.
6. Byrick RJ, Rose DK. Pathophysiology and prevention of acute renal failure:
The role of the anaesthetist. Can J Anaesth 1990;37:457-467.
7. Sladen RN. Anesthetic considerations for the patient with renal failure. Anesthesiol Clin North Am 2000; 18:863-882.
8. Eger EI. Desflurane (Suprane): A Compendium and Reference. Nutley, NJ: Anaquest, 1993, pp 1-119.
9. Njoku D, Laster MJ, Gong DH, et al. Biotransformation of halothane, enflurane, isoflurane, and desflurane to trifluoroacetylated liver proteins: Association between protein acylation and hepatic injury. Anesth Analg 1997;84:173-178.
10. Elliott RH, Strunin L. Hepatotoxicity of volatile anaesthetics. Br J Anaesth 1993;70:339-348.
11. Strunin L. Preoperative assessment of the patient with liver dysfunction.
Br J Anaesth 1978;50:25-34.
12. Ziser A, Plevak DJ, Wiesner RH, et al. Morbidity and mortality in cirrhotic patients undergoing anesthesia and surgery. Anesthesiology 1999;90:42-53.
13. Spies CD, Rommelspacher H. Alcohol withdrawal in the surgical patient: Prevention and treatment. Anesth Analg 1999;88:946-954.
14. Marco PA, Yeo CJ, Rock P. Anesthesia for the patient undergoing laparoscopic cholecystectomy. Anesthesiology 1990;73:1268-1270.
15. Taylor E, Feinstein R, White PF, et al. Anesthesia for laparoscopic cholecystectomy. Is nitrous oxide contraindicated? Anesthesiology 1992;76:541-543.

Chapter 29

ENDOCRINE AND NUTRITIONAL DISEASE

Ludwig Lin

Disorders of endocrine gland function or the presence of nutritional disease may be the primary reason for surgery or may reflect comorbidity in a preoperative patient. Coexisting endocrine and nutritional disorders can affect the patient's physiologic parameters during anesthesia.[1] The presence or absence of endocrine disease is suggested by specific observations in the preoperative evaluation (Table 29-1). In addition, the patient's nutritional status is evaluated preoperatively.

DIABETES MELLITUS

Diabetes mellitus (diabetes) is a chronic systemic disease that is characterized by an array of abnormalities, the most notable of which is disturbed glucose metabolism resulting in inappropriate hyperglycemia. In patients undergoing surgery, diabetes is the most common endocrine disease. Diabetes is classified as insulin-dependent diabetes mellitus (IDDM) and non–insulin-dependent diabetes mellitus (NIDDM) (Table 29-2). Patients with NIDDM are almost always overweight and constitute more than 90% of all diabetics. Treatment of diabetes includes diet (avoidance of obesity), oral hypoglycemic drugs, and administration of exogenous insulin.

Table 29-1 Preoperative Evaluation of Endocrine Function
Absence of glucose in urine
Systemic blood pressure and heart rate normal
Body weight unchanged
Sexual function normal
No history of relevant drug therapy

Table 29-2 Classification of Diabetes Mellitus

	Insulin-Dependent Diabetes Mellitus	Non–Insulin-Dependent Diabetes Mellitus
Alternative designations	Juvenile onset Type 1	Maturity onset Type 2
Age at onset	Child	Adult
Appearance	Abrupt	After 35 years of age
Require exogenous insulin	Always	Occasionally
Ketoacidosis prone	Yes	No
Blood glucose concentration	Wide fluctuations	Relatively stable
Body habitus	Thin	Obese

Complications

The most serious acute metabolic complication of diabetes is ketoacidosis, whereas chronic complications are manifested as macroangiopathy, microangiopathy, and disorders of the nervous system. Diabetic retinopathy occurs in 80% to 90% of those who have IDDM for at least 20 years. In young and middle-aged adults in the United States, diabetes is the leading cause of renal failure requiring hemodialysis (Table 29-3).

KETOACIDOSIS

Hyperglycemia in the presence of metabolic acidosis and a history of diabetes is sufficient to establish the diagnosis of diabetic ketoacidosis. This disorder occurs as a consequence of the absence of insulin secretion from the pancreas. Causes of diabetic ketoacidosis include poor patient compliance with insulin regimens, infection, silent myocardial infarction, and administration of a β_2-agonist to inhibit premature labor.

Treatment

Initial treatment of diabetic ketoacidosis includes aggressive repletion of intravascular fluid volume and administration of regular insulin (0.2 U/kg IV followed by a continuous low-dose infusion), potassium, and sodium bicarbonate if arterial pH is less than 7.2. Rapid shifts in the plasma potassium concentration occur as the patient's acidosis is corrected and result in the intracellular movement of potassium ions. Insulin also increases the intracellular migration of potassium. Urine output is an insensitive gauge of renal function because the osmotic diuretic effects of hyperglycemia ensure some urine output even in presence of severe hypovolemia.

AUTONOMIC NEUROPATHY

Autonomic neuropathy reflects dysfunction of the autonomic nervous system as a result of diabetes.[3] It is estimated that autonomic neuropathy will develop in 20% to 40% of patients with long-standing diabetes. The likelihood of autonomic neuropathy is increased when a patient with diabetes also manifests peripheral sensory neuropathy, renal failure, or systemic hypertension (Table 29-4). When evidence of cardiac autonomic neuropathy is clinically apparent (orthostatic hypotension, resting tachycardia, no variation in heart rate with deep breathing, prolonged QT interval on the electrocardiogram), the incidence of sudden death syndrome is increased.[3,4] Indeed, sudden and profound bradycardia unresponsive to atropine has been described during anesthesia and surgery in patients with diabetes and associated cardiac autonomic neuropathy.[5] Successful resuscitation of diabetic patients with bradycardia seems to be dependent on early intervention with epinephrine administered intravenously. The presence of autonomic neuropathy may prevent the

Table 29-3 Complications of Diabetes Mellitus

Hyperglycemia
Hypoglycemia
Ketoacidosis
Autonomic neuropathy
Coronary artery disease
Cerebral vascular disease
Peripheral vascular disease
Nephropathy
Retinopathy
Stiff joint syndrome
Sensory neuropathy

Table 29-4	Signs and Symptoms of Autonomic Neuropathy
Impotence	
Orthostatic hypotension	
Resting tachycardia	
No variation in heart rate with deep breathing	
Gastroparesis (vomiting, diarrhea, abdominal distention)	
Asymptomatic (silent) hypoglycemia	
Sudden death syndrome	

development of angina pectoris (painless myocardial infarction) and thus obscure the presence of coronary artery disease. Gastroparesis manifested as delayed gastric emptying of solids is a sign of autonomic neuropathy affecting the vagus nerves. Diabetic patients with symptoms of gastroparesis should be considered to be at increased risk for pulmonary aspiration based on the likelihood of increased residual gastric fluid volume.

PERIPHERAL NEUROPATHY

Low plasma concentrations of insulin are associated with the development of polyneuropathies regardless of the degree of blood glucose control. The incidence of peripheral neuropathy is progressive with the duration of diabetes (often present before the diagnosis of diabetes) and exceeds 50% when diabetes has been present for more than 25 years.[6] Isolated peripheral nerve lesions in patients with diabetes often occur at sites of external pressure, such as the radial nerve in the upper part of the arm or the common peroneal nerve (common fibular nerve) at the neck of the fibula, or lesions can occur at entrapment sites, such as the median nerve at the wrist (carpal tunnel syndrome) or the ulnar nerve at the elbow (cubital tunnel syndrome). It is likely that the peripheral nerves of patients with diabetes are more susceptible to compression injury. Acute hyperglycemia decreases peripheral nerve function, whereas chronic hyperglycemia is associated with loss of myelinated and unmyelinated fibers. It is conceivable that acute hyperglycemia associated with the perioperative period may unmask a previously subclinical peripheral neuropathy.

Preoperative Evaluation and Management

It is a frequent recommendation that a diabetic patient should be scheduled for surgery early in the morning. A well-controlled, diet-treated patient with NIDDM does not require special treatment (including exogenous insulin) before and during surgery. Even a patient with well-controlled IDDM undergoing a brief outpatient surgical procedure may not require any adjustment in the usual subcutaneous insulin regimen. If an oral sulfonylurea

hypoglycemic drug is being administered, it may be continued until the evening before surgery if one remembers that these drugs may produce delayed hypoglycemia in the absence of any caloric intake. The risk for hypoglycemia is less with biguanide hypoglycemic drugs, but there is a remote risk for the development of lactic acidosis intraoperatively in patients being treated with metformin.[7] If metformin cannot be discontinued for about 48 hours preoperatively, it is prudent to monitor for the development of lactic acidosis (arterial pH) in the perioperative period. Preoperative admission to the hospital may be required for an occasional patient with poorly controlled IDDM.

Preoperative evaluation and treatment of hyperglycemia, ketoacidosis, and electrolyte disturbances are important before elective surgery is performed. Measurement of the glycohemoglobin (HbA_{1c}) concentration provides information about the average blood glucose concentrations during the previous 7 to 21 days. Manifestations of coronary artery disease (electrocardiogram), cerebral vascular disease, and renal dysfunction are sought in the preoperative evaluation. The most common cause of preoperative mortality in diabetic patients is coronary artery disease. Coronary artery disease occurs more commonly and at an earlier age in diabetics than in nondiabetic controls and may be difficult to detect because of the absence of pain (silent ischemia). A careful history, including questions regarding exercise tolerance, is needed. An electrocardiogram may be indicated in the preoperative anesthetic evaluation, and perioperative β-blockade to reduce the incidence of perioperative cardiac complications should be considered. Angiotensin-converting enzyme inhibitors are commonly administered to diabetic patients for control of systemic blood pressure because this class of drugs decreases the incidence of renal insufficiency in this patient population. Excessive and persistent decreases in systemic blood pressure may occur in response to induction of anesthesia in patients being treated with angiotensin converting enzyme inhibitors.

Signs of peripheral neuropathy and autonomic nervous system insufficiency need to be noted preoperatively. The presence of peripheral neuropathy may influence the choice of anesthetic technique, such as regional anesthesia. A diabetic patient with preoperative evidence of autonomic neuropathy manifested as gastroparesis may be at increased risk for aspiration of gastric contents during induction and recovery from anesthesia. Preoperative evidence of cardiac autonomic neuropathy should alert the anesthesiologist to the possibility of intraoperative cardiovascular lability (hypotension requiring vasopressor therapy, bradycardia that is resistant to atropine).[2,5] Evaluation of a diabetic patient for evidence of limited joint mobility, including the temporomandibular joint, is important in predicting possible difficulty in performing direct laryngoscopy for tracheal intubation. The common presence of obesity in this patient population may influence the

IV

ease of tracheal intubation or performance of regional anesthetic techniques.

EXOGENOUS INSULIN

A patient with IDDM who is undergoing prolonged surgery should be treated with exogenous insulin, but there is no standardized method of administration (intravenous versus subcutaneous) (Table 29-5).[8] Regardless of the administration route selected, it is important to measure plasma glucose levels frequently. Measurement of blood glucose concentrations (every 1 to 2 hours in selected patients) is essential for adjusting the rate of intravenous infusion of glucose-containing fluids or the administration of additional regular insulin. Because the absorption of subcutaneous insulin may vary depending on regional perfusion, as well as the presence of interstitial edema, an intravenous route may be a more accurate method for delivering insulin.

Management of Anesthesia

Coronary artery disease, renal insufficiency, and poor peripheral perfusion resulting from peripheral vascular disease are the main diabetic complications to be considered when designing an anesthetic plan. The principal goal in the management of anesthesia is to maintain normal metabolism as closely as possible by avoiding hypoglycemia, hyperglycemia, ketoacidosis, dehydration,

and electrolyte disturbances.[8] Hypoglycemia is prevented by ensuring an adequate supply of exogenous glucose. Hyperglycemia and associated ketoacidosis, dehydration, and electrolyte disturbances are prevented by the exogenous administration of insulin. Perioperative monitoring of blood glucose concentrations is useful for maintaining acceptable blood glucose control. In addition to determination of blood glucose concentrations preoperatively and postoperatively, additional measurements are indicated, depending on the duration and magnitude of the surgery and the lability of the diabetes. Hourly measurements may be helpful in patients considered to be at high risk for extreme changes in their blood glucose concentrations. Maintenance of blood glucose concentrations in the range of 80 to 110 mg/dL in critically ill patients leads to improved outcomes in terms of the incidence of bacteremia and acute renal failure, as well as hospital mortality.

Induction and Maintenance of Anesthesia

The choice of drugs or techniques for induction and maintenance of anesthesia is less important than monitoring of blood glucose concentrations and treatment of the potential physiologic derangements associated with diabetes. When general anesthesia is chosen, tracheal intubation with a cuffed tube seems prudent, especially if there is preoperative evidence of gastroparesis. Although volatile anesthetics impair the release of insulin in

---

Table 29-5 Regimens for Exogenous Insulin Replacement

Subcutaneous Insulin Administration

Administer one fourth to one half the usual daily intermediate-acting dose of insulin on the morning of surgery

Initiate infusion of glucose (5-10 g/hr) with administration of insulin

Continuous Intravenous Infusion of Insulin*

Regular insulin (50 units in 500 mL normal saline at 0.5-1 U/hr)

Initiate infusion of glucose (5-10 g/hr) with initiation of insulin infusion

Measure blood glucose concentration as necessary (usually every 1 to 2 hr) and adjust insulin infusion accordingly

<80 mg/dL	Discontinue insulin infusion Administer 25 mL of 50% glucose Remeasure blood glucose concentration in 30 min
80-120 mg/dL	Decrease insulin infusion rate by 0.3 U/hr
120-180 mg/dL	No change in insulin infusion rate
180-220 mg/dL	Increase insulin infusion rate by 0.3 U/hr
>220 mg/dL	Increase insulin infusion rate by 0.5 U/hr

*Data for intravenous infusion from Hirsch IP, Magill JB, Cryer PE, et al. Perioperative management of surgical patients with diabetes mellitus. Anesthesiology 1991;74:346-359.

response to the administration of glucose, there is no evidence that maintenance of anesthesia with a specific volatile drug in a diabetic patient is advantageous. Epidural anesthesia and spinal anesthesia preserve glucose tolerance, but the high incidence of peripheral neuropathy may influence the selection of a regional anesthetic technique for fear that a diabetic sensory neuropathy could be erroneously attributed to the regional anesthetic technique. In light of the possibility of autonomic insufficiency, episodes of bradycardia and hypotension that develop suddenly and are unresponsive to atropine or ephedrine (or both) should be treated promptly with the intravenous administration of epinephrine (10 µg IV and repeated if necessary). Diabetic patients often have longstanding systemic hypertension and possible cardiac diastolic dysfunction, and they may also have chronic renal insufficiency, all of which may contribute to a possibility of intravascular fluid volume overload and resulting congestive heart failure. Therefore, invasive hemodynamic monitoring may be necessary in a patient who has a history suggestive of congestive heart failure or is undergoing a procedure associated with large intraoperative fluid shifts. In terms of dealing with the diabetic complication of peripheral neuropathy, although positioning and padding of the patient's extremities are the same regardless of whether the patient has diabetes, it may be helpful to specifically document the care taken to prevent peripheral nerve compression or stretch while the patient is sedated or unconscious because of anesthetic drugs.

HYPEROSMOLAR HYPERGLYCEMIC NONKETOTIC COMA

Hyperosmolar hyperglycemic nonketotic coma occurs most often in elderly patients with an impaired thirst mechanism (Table 29-6). Two thirds of patients in whom this syndrome develops do not have a history of diabetes, ketoacidosis does not occur, and exogenous insulin is not needed after resolution of the coma. The presence of hyperglycemia and insulin resistance in patients with NIDDM during cardiopulmonary bypass makes this patient population vulnerable to the development of hyperosmolar hyperglycemic nonketotic coma. This syndrome is treated by the intravenous administration of insulin and restoration of intravascular fluid volume with sodium-containing solutions.

HYPERTHYROIDISM

Hyperthyroidism is a generic term for all conditions in which tissues are exposed to increased circulating concentrations (5 to 15 times) of triiodothyronine (T_3), thyroxine (T_4), or both. Graves' disease (diffuse toxic goiter) is the most common form of hyperthyroidism and

Table 29-6 Signs and Symptoms of Hyperosmolar Hyperglycemic Nonketotic Coma

Plasma hyperosmolarity >330 mOsm/L
Hyperglycemia >600 mg/dL
Normal arterial pH
Osmotic diuresis (hypokalemia)
Hypovolemia
Seizures and coma (decreased intracellular brain water because of hyperosmolarity)

is typically manifested in women between 20 and 40 years of age. Hyperthyroidism occurs in about 0.2% of parturients. An autoimmune pathogenesis of Graves' disease is suggested by the presence of circulating antibodies that mimic the effects of thyroid-stimulating hormone. The diagnosis of hyperthyroidism is based on clinical signs and symptoms plus confirmation of excessive thyroid gland function as demonstrated by appropriate tests (Tables 29-7 and 29-8).

Management of Anesthesia

Elective surgery should probably be deferred until patients have been rendered euthyroid with drug therapy. Usually, medical treatment of hyperthyroidism consists of β-blockers, antithyroid medications, and iodides.[9] β-Blockers control the hyperdynamic state induced by excessive thyroid hormones, but they also inhibit the peripheral conversion of T_4 to T_3, which is the most active thyroid hormone. Selective $β_1$-antagonists such as propranolol, atenolol, or metoprolol are most often selected. The goal in hemodynamic control is to achieve a resting heart rate less than 85 beats/min. When surgery cannot be delayed, a continuous intravenous infusion of esmolol at a rate required to sustain an acceptable heart rate relative to the surgical stimulus (usually 100 to 300 µg/kg/min) is useful.[10] Antithyroid medications (propylthiouracil, methimazole) are administered to

Table 29-7 Signs and Symptoms of Hyperthyroidism

Anxiety
Fatigue
Skeletal muscle weakness
Tachycardia
Tachydysrhythmias
Exophthalmos

IV

Table 29-8   Tests for the Diagnosis of Thyroid Gland Dysfunction

	Thyroxine	Triiodothyronine	Thyroid-Stimulating Hormone
Hyperthyroidism	Increased	Increased	Normal
Primary hypothyroidism	Decreased	Decreased	Increased
Secondary hypothyroidism	Decreased	Decreased	Decreased

decrease thyroid hormone synthesis. It is important to note that these drugs block the synthesis of only new thyroid hormone and do not affect the behavior of stored thyroid hormones. Methimazole achieves a euthyroid state more rapidly than propylthiouracil does and is less likely to produce the complications of agranulocytosis, hepatitis, or vasculitis. Iodine preparations block the release of thyroid hormone from the thyroid gland, and if given 2 to 3 hours after administration of the antithyroid medications, they can further decrease circulating levels of thyroid hormones in a hyperthyroid patient.

Preoperative sedation is often produced by the oral administration of a benzodiazepine. Anticholinergic drugs are not recommended as part of the preanesthetic medication because they could interfere with heat regulation and contribute to increases in heart rate. Evaluation of the upper airway for evidence of compression by the enlarged thyroid gland is an important part of the preoperative evaluation. An enlarged thyroid gland may extend into the mediastinal space and obstruct either the great vessels or the airways. In this regard, computed tomography may be helpful in evaluating airway anatomy, especially if the patient has symptoms consistent with dynamic upper airway obstruction, such as orthopnea.

INDUCTION OF ANESTHESIA

Induction of anesthesia is acceptably achieved with a number of intravenous induction drugs. Thiopental is an attractive selection because its thiourea structure lends antithyroid activity to the drug. Nevertheless, it is unlikely that a significant antithyroid effect is produced by an induction dose of thiopental. Ketamine is not an optimal selection because it can stimulate the sympathetic nervous system. Assuming the absence of airway compression from an enlarged goiter, the administration of succinylcholine or a nondepolarizing neuromuscular blocking drug is useful to facilitate tracheal intubation. Vagolytic drugs such as pancuronium are avoided because of the potential for a drug-induced increase in heart rate.

MAINTENANCE OF ANESTHESIA

Goals during maintenance of anesthesia are to avoid the administration of drugs that stimulate the sympathetic nervous system and to provide sufficient anesthetic depression of the sympathetic nervous system to prevent an exaggerated response to surgical stimulation. The possibility of organ toxicity as a result of altered or accelerated drug metabolism in the presence of hyperthyroidism is a consideration when selecting drugs for maintenance of anesthesia. In animals rendered hyperthyroid, the administration of a volatile anesthetic was followed by evidence of hepatic centrilobular necrosis, with the greatest incidence (92%) being in animals exposed to halothane.[11] Nevertheless, liver function test results are not altered postoperatively in previously hyperthyroid patients who are rendered euthyroid before surgery and given a volatile anesthetic, including halothane, as part of the anesthesia.[12]

Despite animal evidence of hepatic necrosis after exposure to volatile anesthetics, the ability of isoflurane, desflurane, and sevoflurane to blunt exaggerated sympathetic nervous system responses to surgical stimulation and not sensitize the heart to catecholamines makes these drugs attractive selections to combine with nitrous oxide for maintenance of anesthesia in a hyperthyroid patient. Selection of desflurane may be influenced by the observation that sudden and large increases in the delivered concentration of desflurane can produce transient stimulation of the sympathetic nervous system (see Chapter 8). Nitrous oxide combined with a short-acting opioid is an alternative to the administration of a volatile anesthetic but has the disadvantage of not reliably suppressing sympathetic nervous system activity.

Anesthetic Requirements

Controlled studies in animals do not support the clinical impression that anesthetic requirements for inhaled anesthetics (minimum alveolar concentration [MAC]) are increased in the presence of hyperthyroidism.[13] In this regard, the discrepancy between clinical impression and objective data is presumed to reflect the increased cardiac output characteristic of hyperthyroidism. For example, increased cardiac output accelerates the uptake of inhaled anesthetics and thus results in the need to increase the inspired concentration of the drug to achieve a brain partial pressure similar to that achieved with a lower inspired concentration in a euthyroid patient. It should be appreciated that accelerated metabolism of the anesthetic does not alter the brain partial pressure of the drug necessary to produce the desired pharmacologic effect.

Another factor to be considered in evaluating anesthetic requirements in patients with altered thyroid gland function is body temperature. For example, increased body temperature, as could accompany thyroid storm, would be expected to increase MAC about 5% for each degree that the temperature increases above 37°C.

Neuromuscular Blocking Drugs

Selection of a neuromuscular blocking drug for production of intraoperative surgical muscle relaxation should include consideration of the theoretical advantage of drugs that lack cardiovascular effects. Conceivably, a prolonged response could occur when a traditional dose of a neuromuscular blocking drug is administered to a patient with coexisting skeletal muscle weakness. For this reason, it may be prudent to decrease the initial dose of neuromuscular blocking drug and closely monitor the effect produced at the neuromuscular junction with a peripheral nerve stimulator. Antagonism of neuromuscular blockade with an anticholinesterase drug combined with an anticholinergic drug introduces the concern for drug-induced tachycardia. Although experience is too limited to make a recommendation, it would seem unwarranted to avoid drug-enhanced antagonism of nondepolarizing neuromuscular blocking drugs in hyperthyroid patients. Perhaps glycopyrrolate, which has less of a chronotropic effect than atropine does, would be a more appropriate anticholinergic drug selection.

Monitoring

Monitoring during maintenance of anesthesia in hyperthyroid patients is directed at early recognition of increased activity of the thyroid glands suggesting the onset of thyroid storm. Constant monitoring of body temperature is particularly useful, and methods to lower body temperature, including a cooling mattress and chilled crystalloid solutions for intravenous infusion, are recommended. The electrocardiogram may reveal tachycardia or cardiac dysrhythmias and thus indicate the need for intraoperative administration of a β-antagonist (continuous infusion of esmolol) or lidocaine (or both). Patients with exophthalmos are susceptible to corneal ulceration and drying, and therefore the eyes of such patients need to be protected during the perioperative period.

Treatment of hypotension with a sympathomimetic drug must consider the possibility of the exaggerated responsiveness of hyperthyroid patients to endogenous or exogenous catecholamines. For this reason, a decreased dose of a direct-acting vasopressor, such as phenylephrine, may be more acceptable than ephedrine, which acts in part by provoking the release of catecholamines.

REGIONAL ANESTHESIA

Regional anesthesia with its associated blockade of the sympathetic nervous system is a potentially useful selection for hyperthyroid patients, assuming that there is no evidence of high-output congestive heart failure. A continuous lumbar epidural anesthetic may be preferable to a spinal anesthetic because the slower onset of sympathetic nervous system blockade makes severe hypotension less likely. If hypotension occurs, a decreased dose of phenylephrine is recommended, while keeping in mind the possible hypersensitivity of these patients to sympathomimetic drugs. Epinephrine should not be added to the local anesthetic solution because systemic absorption of this catecholamine could produce exaggerated circulatory responses. Increased anxiety and associated activation of the sympathetic nervous system can be treated in awake patients by the intravenous administration of a benzodiazepine such as midazolam.

Thyroid Storm

Thyroid storm (thyrotoxicosis) is an abrupt exacerbation of hyperthyroidism as a result of the sudden excessive release of thyroid gland hormones into the circulation. Hyperthermia, tachycardia, delirium, congestive heart failure, dehydration, and shock are likely. Thyroid storm associated with surgery can occur intraoperatively but is more likely to develop 6 to 18 hours after surgery. When thyroid storm occurs during the perioperative period, it may mimic malignant hyperthermia or pheochromocytoma. It carries a mortality rate of 10% to 75%, and supportive care should be administered in a critical setting. Thyroid storm is treated by infusion of chilled crystalloid solutions and continuous infusion of esmolol to maintain the heart rate at an acceptable level.[10]

Acetylsalicylic acid, or aspirin, should not be used as an antipyretic agent in these situations because it interferes with binding of thyroglobulin to T_4 and T_3 and can therefore increase plasma levels of free thyroid hormone. When hypotension is persistent, the administration of cortisol (100 to 200 mg IV) may be considered. Dexamethasone may inhibit the conversion of T_4 to T_3, an effect that is additive to that of propylthiouracil. It is important to also treat any suspected infection. Drugs such as propylthiouracil and sodium iodide are administered to prevent the synthesis and release of thyroid gland hormone. Ultimately, methods to enhance thyroid hormone clearance can be attempted; such methods range from the use of cholestyramine to bind and clear thyroid hormone through the gastrointestinal tract to charcoal hemoperfusion, hemodialysis, and plasmapheresis.

Complications after Total or Subtotal Thyroidectomy

Damage to the laryngeal nerves, tracheal compression, and accidental removal of the parathyroid glands are early complications that can follow thyroid surgery.

DAMAGE TO LARYNGEAL NERVES

The entire sensory and motor supply to the larynx is from the two superior and two recurrent laryngeal nerves. The superior laryngeal nerves provide the motor supply to the cricothyroid muscles and sensation above the level of the vocal cords. The recurrent laryngeal nerves supply motor innervation to all the muscles of the larynx (except the cricothyroid muscles), plus sensation below the level of the vocal cords. Function of the vocal cords after thyroid surgery can be evaluated by asking the patient to say "e." The most common nerve injury after thyroid surgery is unilateral damage to the recurrent laryngeal nerve, which is manifested as hoarseness and a paralyzed vocal cord that assumes an intermediate position. Bilateral recurrent laryngeal nerve injury results in aphonia and paralyzed vocal cords that can flap together during inspiration and produce airway obstruction. Superior laryngeal nerve paralysis is manifested as hoarseness and loss of sensation above the vocal cords, thus making patients vulnerable to the inhalation of any material present in the pharynx.

COMPRESSION OF THE TRACHEA

Compression of the trachea leading to airway obstruction may reflect a hematoma at the operative site or tracheomalacia secondary to weakening of the tracheal rings by chronic pressure from a goiter. Airway obstruction after tracheal extubation and in the presence of normal vocal cord function should suggest the diagnosis of tracheomalacia.

ACCIDENTAL REMOVAL OF THE PARATHYROID GLANDS

Hypoparathyroidism caused by accidental removal of the parathyroid glands is an uncommon, but possible complication in patients who undergo total thyroidectomy. In these patients, signs of hypocalcemia can be manifested as early as 1 to 3 hours after surgery but typically do not appear until 24 to 72 hours postoperatively. The laryngeal muscles are very sensitive to hypocalcemia, and inspiratory stridor progressing to laryngospasm may be the first suggestion that surgically induced hypoparathyroidism is present.

HYPOTHYROIDISM

Hypothyroidism is a generic term for all conditions in which tissues are exposed to decreased circulating concentrations of T_3 and T_4. Chronic thyroiditis (Hashimoto's thyroiditis), the most common cause of hypothyroidism, is manifested as an autoimmune disease characterized by progressive destruction of the thyroid gland. Medical or surgical treatment of hyperthyroidism may also become a cause of iatrogenic hypothyroidism. The incidence of hypothyroidism after radioiodine treatment of hyper-

thyroidism is at least 50% by 10 years after treatment. The diagnosis of hypothyroidism is based on clinical signs and symptoms plus confirmation of decreased thyroid gland function as demonstrated by appropriate tests (Table 29-9; also see Table 29-8). The development of hypothyroidism in adulthood is often insidious and gradual and may go unrecognized, in part because of the associated apathy that minimizes the patient's complaints. Subclinical hypothyroidism manifested only as an increased plasma thyroid-stimulating hormone concentration is present in about 5% of the American population, with a prevalence of more than 13% in otherwise healthy elderly patients, especially women.[14] There is no evidence that these asymptomatic patients are at increased risk during anesthesia or surgery.[15]

Management of Anesthesia

Elective surgery can proceed in patients with mild to moderate hypothyroidism because no clinical evidence supports a concern for increased morbidity; however, severe hypothyroidism (with manifestations of myxedema coma, pericardial effusion, or cardiac failure) necessitates surgical delay until thyroid replacement has returned the patient to normal. Thyroid replacement is initiated slowly because acute cardiac ischemia can develop in patients with coronary artery disease from the sudden increase in myocardial oxygen demand as the body's metabolism and cardiac output increase as the result of appropriate thyroid hormone presence. Although intravenous thyroid replacement therapy is available, there should be very few instances in which it is indicated, and its use should be undertaken with careful cardiac monitoring. Myxedema coma is one of the few indications for intravenous thyroid replacement. Oral thyroid medications are usually only 50% bioavailable, so conversion to an equivalent intravenous dose means reducing the amount administered by half.

No controlled data support the position that hypothyroid patients are unusually sensitive to inhaled anesthetic drugs and opioids. Nevertheless, a high index of suspicion for possible adverse effects, including exaggerated

Table 29-9 Signs and Symptoms of Hypothyroidism
Lethargy
Intolerance to cold
Bradycardia
Decreased cardiac output
Peripheral vasoconstriction
Hyponatremia
Atrophy of the adrenal cortex

effects of depressant drugs, adrenal insufficiency, hypovolemia, and prolonged gastric emptying time, would seem warranted. Furthermore, a severe nonthyroid illness may precipitate acute hypothyroidism in a vulnerable patient.[16]

When considering preoperative medication for a hypothyroid patient, the value of the preoperative visit and resultant psychological support should be emphasized. Opioid premedication has been administered safely, but there is a historical concern that the depressant effects of these drugs may be exaggerated in hypothyroid patients. It may be better to administer sedative and anticholinergic drugs intravenously after arrival in the operating room so that any unexpected effect can be promptly recognized and treated. Supplemental corticosteroids may be considered because occult adrenal insufficiency can accompany hypothyroidism.

INDUCTION OF ANESTHESIA

Induction of anesthesia is often accomplished by the intravenous administration of ketamine with the presumption that this drug's inherent support of the cardiovascular system will be beneficial. Tracheal intubation is facilitated by the administration of succinylcholine or a nondepolarizing neuromuscular blocking drug, while keeping in mind that coexisting skeletal muscle weakness could be associated with an exaggerated drug-induced response at the neuromuscular junction.

MAINTENANCE OF ANESTHESIA

Maintenance of anesthesia is often achieved by the inhalation of nitrous oxide plus supplementation, if necessary, with minimal doses of ketamine, opioids, or benzodiazepines. Volatile anesthetics are not recommended because of the exquisite sensitivity of hypothyroid patients to drug-induced myocardial depression. The failure of decreases in thyroid activity to decrease anesthetic requirements (MAC) may reflect maintenance of the cerebral metabolic requirements for oxygen that are independent of thyroid activity.[13] Decreased production of carbon dioxide associated with the decreased metabolic rate makes hypothyroid patients vulnerable to excessive decreases in $PaCO_2$ during controlled ventilation of the lungs. Pancuronium, because of its mild sympathomimetic effects, would seem to be a useful selection for production of skeletal muscle paralysis. Drug-assisted antagonism of neuromuscular blockade with an anticholinesterase drug combined with an anticholinergic drug does not pose a risk to a hypothyroid patient. Regional anesthesia is also an acceptable technique for management of anesthesia in selected hypothyroid patients.

Monitoring

Monitoring of hypothyroid patients is directed toward early recognition of congestive heart failure and detection of the onset of hypothermia. Continuous recording of systemic blood pressure and cardiac filling pressure is indicated for prolonged and complex surgical procedures. In addition to glucose, intravenous solutions should contain sodium to prevent the development of hyponatremia. The possibility of acute primary adrenal insufficiency should be entertained when hypotension persists despite intravenous infusion of fluids or the administration of sympathomimetic drugs (or both). Maintenance of body temperature is facilitated by increasing the ambient temperature of the operating room and passing intravenous fluid solutions through warming devices.

Postoperative Complications

Because recovery from the sedative effects of anesthetics may be delayed in hypothyroid patients, continued mechanical ventilation of the lungs may be necessary. Removal of the tracheal tube is logically deferred until the patient is responding appropriately and body temperature is near 37°C. The concern about possible increased sensitivity to the effects of opioids is a consideration in the management of postoperative pain, perhaps with emphasis on the use of nonopioid analgesics.

CHRONIC ADRENAL AXIS SUPPRESSION AND ADRENAL INSUFFICIENCY

Corticosteroid supplementation should be increased whenever patients who are being treated with chronic corticosteroid therapy undergo surgical procedures. In patients with known adrenal insufficiency, this recommendation is based on the concern that these patients are susceptible to cardiovascular collapse because they cannot release additional endogenous cortisol in response to the stress of surgery. More controversial is the management of patients who have possible suppression of the pituitary-adrenal axis as a result of current or previous corticosteroid administration (including epidural corticosteroids) for the treatment of diseases unrelated to abnormalities in the anterior pituitary or adrenal cortex. This category includes acute or chronic corticosteroid administration for asthma/chronic obstructive pulmonary disease, dermatologic conditions, or autoimmune disorders. The dose of corticosteroids or duration of therapy with corticosteroids that produces suppression of the pituitary-adrenal axis is not known. Suppression, however, may persist for as long as 12 months after discontinuation of therapy. Therefore, it is common practice to empirically administer supplemental corticosteroids in the perioperative period when surgery is planned in patients who are being treated with corticosteroids or who have been treated for longer than 1 month in the past 6 to 12 months.[17]

Nevertheless, it should be appreciated that cause-and-effect relationships between intraoperative hypotension and acute hypoadrenocorticism in patients previously

IV

treated with corticosteroids are very difficult to document. There is evidence supporting the administration of physiologic doses of corticosteroids when patients at risk for inhibition of the pituitary-adrenal axis undergo surgery.[18] Conversely, there is no evidence that these patients need supraphysiologic supplemental doses of corticosteroids, nor is there evidence to support the practice of increasing maintenance doses of corticosteroids preoperatively and then gradually decreasing the dose back to maintenance levels during the first few days postoperatively.

Evaluation of Adrenal Axis Responsiveness

Signs of acute adrenal insufficiency include persistent hypotension, hyponatremia, hyperkalemia, abdominal pain, nausea and emesis, and altered mental status. Diagnosis includes checking random plasma cortisol concentrations and determining preoperative and postoperative stimulation plasma levels of cortisol after the administration of adrenocorticotropic hormone (ACTH) for stimulation of the adrenal glands. Patients with a suppressed adrenal axis will fail to increase their plasma cortisol levels by at least 9 µg/dL.[1]

PHEOCHROMOCYTOMA

Pheochromocytomas are catecholamine-secreting tumors composed of chromaffin cells that originate in the adrenal medulla or along the paravertebral sympathetic chain. Although less than 0.1% of patients with systemic hypertension have a pheochromocytoma, historically, nearly 50% of deaths in patients with unsuspected pheochromocytoma have occurred during anesthesia and surgery (for reasons other than resection of the pheochromocytoma) or parturition. Pheochromocytoma can occur as part of an autosomal dominant multiglandular neoplastic syndrome (medullary thyroid carcinoma is most often present) designated multiple endocrine neoplasia (MEN). Approximately 16% of patients with pheochromocytomas have other associated disorders, such as MEN type II or neurofibromatosis type 1. It is estimated that 10% of patients with pheochromocytoma have bilateral adrenal tumors, 10% have extra-adrenal sites, and less than 10% have malignant pheochromocytomas. QT interval prolongation on the electrocardiogram is present in about 16% of patients with pheochromocytoma.

Diagnosis

The systemic hypertension and hypermetabolism associated with pheochromocytoma may mimic other diseases, including thyroid storm and malignant hyperthermia (Table 29-10). The hallmark of pheochromocytoma is paroxysmal or sustained systemic hypertension. The triad

Table 29-10 Signs and Symptoms of Pheochromocytoma

Paroxysmal hypertension
Triad of diaphoresis, tachycardia, and headache
Tremulousness
Weight loss
Decreased intravascular fluid volume 　Orthostatic hypotension 　Hematocrit >45%
Cardiomyopathy
Intracerebral hemorrhage

of diaphoresis, tachycardia/palpitations, and headache in a hypertensive patient is suggestive of the presence of pheochromocytoma. Definitive diagnosis of pheochromocytoma requires chemical confirmation of excessive catecholamine release. The most specific tests are urinary vanillylmandelic acid and urinary total metanephrines. False-positive test results may occur with caffeine ingestion, administration of tricyclic antidepressants, and treatment with phenoxybenzamine. Oral clonidine suppresses the plasma concentration of catecholamines in hypertensive patients but not in patients with pheochromocytoma. In patients with positive test results, magnetic resonance imaging and computed tomography may be useful, but small tumors may not be identified.

Treatment

Treatment of pheochromocytoma is surgical excision of the catecholamine-secreting tumor. Before surgery is scheduled, however, it is important to establish α-blockade (phenoxybenzamine, prazosin, labetalol), restore intravascular fluid volume (disappearance of orthostatic hypotension, decrease in the hematocrit), and treat cardiac dysrhythmias (β-antagonists). Preoperative normalization of intravascular fluid volume and systemic blood pressure also decreases the risk for intraoperative hypertension during manipulation of the tumor. The recommendation that β-blockade not be instituted in the absence of α-blockade is based on the concern that a heart depressed by β-blockade might not be able to maintain adequate cardiac output should unopposed α-mediated vasoconstriction from the release of catecholamines result in an abrupt increase in systemic vascular resistance. Furthermore, there is concern that any increase in α-mediated vasoconstriction without the vasodilatory effects of β-adrenoreceptors may result in severe systemic hypertension. α-Blockade will facilitate the release of insulin and decrease the likelihood of hyperglycemia. Evaluation of cardiac function with echocardiography may be useful in patients with suspected cardiomyopathy that is presumed to reflect the effects of chronic excessive concentrations of circulating catecholamines.

Medications that should be avoided in patients with pheochromocytoma include tricyclic antidepressants, metoclopramide, droperidol, and naloxone.

Management of Anesthesia

Management of anesthesia in patients requiring excision of pheochromocytoma is based on avoidance of drugs or events that might activate the sympathetic nervous system and on the use of invasive monitoring techniques (arterial and pulmonary artery catheters, transesophageal echocardiography) that permit early and appropriate interventions when changes in cardiovascular function occur.[19] Continuation of α- and β-antagonist therapy until induction of anesthesia is recommended. If bilateral adrenalectomy is anticipated, supplemental cortisol treatment may be instituted at the time of preoperative medication. Periods of significant hemodynamic instability for these patients are (1) during tracheal intubation, (2) during manipulation of the tumor, and (3) after ligation of the tumor's venous drainage.

INDUCTION OF ANESTHESIA

Placement of a catheter in a peripheral artery to provide continuous monitoring of systemic blood pressure is useful before proceeding with induction of anesthesia. Unconsciousness is produced by the administration of any intravenous anesthetic (except ketamine), followed by ventilation of the lungs with nitrous oxide plus a volatile anesthetic (most likely isoflurane, desflurane, or sevoflurane). Administration of a volatile anesthetic is intended to decrease sympathetic nervous system activity before initiation of direct laryngoscopy for tracheal intubation. These drugs do not sensitize the myocardium to catecholamines, but desflurane may produce transient stimulation of the sympathetic nervous system when its inhaled concentration is abruptly increased. Halothane is not recommended because this drug can sensitize the heart to cardiac dysrhythmias in the presence of increased plasma concentrations of catecholamines. Mechanical ventilation of the patient's lungs is facilitated by the production of skeletal muscle paralysis with a nondepolarizing neuromuscular blocking drug deemed to be devoid of vagolytic or histamine-releasing properties (vecuronium, rocuronium, cisatracurium).

TRACHEAL INTUBATION

Direct laryngoscopy for tracheal intubation is initiated only after establishment of a concentration of anesthetic drugs compatible with that judged to be appropriate for surgery (about 1.3 MAC). An adequate concentration of anesthetic drugs is necessary to minimize the increases in systemic blood pressure associated with tracheal intu-

bation. It may be helpful to administer lidocaine (1 to 2 mg/kg IV) about 1 minute before initiating laryngoscopy because this drug may attenuate the hypertensive response to tracheal intubation and decrease the likelihood of cardiac dysrhythmias. In addition, the administration of a short-acting opioid with a rapid brain-blood equilibration time (remifentanil, alfentanil) just before initiating direct laryngoscopy may attenuate the pressor and heart rate response. Nitroprusside (50 to 100 μg IV) or phentolamine (1 to 5 mg IV) should be readily available for injection should persistent systemic hypertension follow tracheal intubation.

MAINTENANCE OF ANESTHESIA

Maintenance of anesthesia is most often accomplished with nitrous oxide plus a volatile anesthetic. An opioid combined with nitrous oxide is a less likely selection because this combination does not suppress the systemic hypertensive responses caused by catecholamine release. In addition, it is not easy to decrease the concentration of anesthetic drugs should persistent hypotension occur when intravenous agents are used for maintenance of anesthesia. A continuous intravenous infusion of nitroprusside will be necessary if hypertension persists despite delivery of maximum safe concentrations of the volatile anesthetic (about 1.5 to 2 MAC). An alternative intravenous drug, fenoldopam (0.2 to 0.8 μg/kg), may be used to avoid the risk of toxic metabolites associated with the administration of nitroprusside. Fenoldopam is a dopamine$_1$ agonist drug that causes peripheral vasodilatation. The reflex tachycardia that may accompany drug-induced peripheral vasodilation is treated by continuous infusion of esmolol.

Cardiac dysrhythmias are initially treated with lidocaine administered intravenously. The decrease in systemic blood pressure that accompanies ligation of the tumor's venous drainage (reflects sudden decreases in circulating catecholamine concentrations) is treated by decreasing the delivered concentration of volatile anesthetic and rapid intravenous infusion of electrolyte-containing crystalloid solutions. Rarely, a continuous intravenous infusion of phenylephrine or norepinephrine may be required until the peripheral vasculature can adapt to a decreased level of endogenous α-adrenergic stimulation. A pulmonary artery catheter or transesophageal echocardiography is helpful in evaluating the response to therapeutic interventions. Monitoring of blood glucose concentrations is useful because hyperglycemia is common before excision of the pheochromocytoma and hypoglycemia may occur within minutes of tumor removal as α-adrenergic–induced suppression of insulin release wanes.

REGIONAL ANESTHESIA

Regional anesthesia for excision of a pheochromocytoma has the attractive features of blocking the sympathetic nervous system without sensitizing the heart to cate-

IV

cholamines. Nevertheless, postsynaptic α-receptors can still respond to the direct effects of circulating catecholamines. Furthermore, the hypotension that may accompany ligation of the veins draining the pheochromocytoma cannot be offset by sympathetic nervous system activation in the presence of epidural or spinal anesthesia. Selection of a regional anesthetic is practical only if the surgical procedure is performed in the supine position.

Postoperative Care

Invasive monitoring is continued in the postoperative period because abrupt increases or decreases in systemic blood pressure remain a possibility. An estimated 50% of patients will remain hypertensive during the early postoperative period despite removal of the pheochromocytoma. A high index of suspicion for hypoglycemia should be maintained. Relief of postoperative pain, as with neuraxial opioids, may permit early tracheal extubation in these often young and otherwise healthy patients.

MORBID OBESITY

Obesity is the most common nutritional disorder in the United States, and it affects about a third of the population as reflected by body weight more than 20% above the ideal weight.[20] Morbid obesity is present when body weight is more than 45 kg above ideal body weight. It is estimated that 3% to 5% of the U.S. population is morbidly obese. A body mass index (weight in kilograms divided by the square of height in meters) higher than 28 is associated with a risk for morbidity (stroke, coronary artery disease, diabetes mellitus) that is three to four times the risk in the general population.

Adverse Effects

The adverse effects of obesity are associated with increased morbidity and mortality and often reflect the concomitant presence of systemic hypertension, lipid abnormalities, and diabetes mellitus (Table 29-11). During anesthesia and surgery, obesity complicates airway management, positioning on a narrow operating room table, and surgical access.

CARDIOVASCULAR

There is a positive correlation between increases in systemic blood pressure, cardiomegaly, and weight gain. Increased cardiac output and blood volume are the presumed cause of systemic hypertension. It is estimated that cardiac output increases 0.1 L/min for every 1 kg of weight gain related to adipose tissue (1 kg of adipose tissue contains about 3000 m of blood vessels). When measuring systemic blood pressure in an obese patient, care should be taken to use a blood pressure cuff of the correct size. As a general rule, the width of the blood pressure cuff should be greater

Table 29-11 Adverse Effects of Obesity

Cardiovascular
   Systemic hypertension
   Cardiomegaly
   Congestive heart failure
   Coronary artery disease
   Pulmonary hypertension

Ventilation
   Decreased lung volumes and capacities
   Arterial hypoxemia
   Obesity-hypoventilation syndrome

Liver
   Abnormal liver function test results
   Fatty liver infiltration

Metabolic
   Insulin resistance (diabetes mellitus)
   Hypercholesterolemia (coronary artery disease, cholelithiasis)

than a third the circumference of the arm. When the cuff is too narrow, more pressure will be required to compress the extra tissues, and a falsely high systolic blood pressure will be recorded. Pulmonary hypertension is common in the presence of obesity and most likely reflects the effects of chronic arterial hypoxemia or increased pulmonary blood flow, or both.

VENTILATION

Obesity imposes a restrictive ventilation defect (decreased expiratory reserve, vital capacity, and functional residual capacity) because of the compressive effects on the chest and abdomen produced by the excess adipose tissue. This added weight impedes motion of the diaphragm, especially with assumption of the supine position. Fatty infiltration of the muscles of breathing further diminishes ventilation and limits exercise tolerance.

There is a predictable decrease in the PaO_2 of obese patients, presumably reflecting ventilation-to-perfusion mismatching, that is accentuated by decreases in lung volumes and capacities. Conversely, $PaCO_2$ and the ventilatory response to carbon dioxide remain normal because of the high diffusing capacity and favorable characteristics of the dissociation curve for carbon dioxide. The margin of reserve, however, is small, and the administration of ventilatory depressant drugs or assumption of the head-down position can result in hypoventilation. Furthermore, obstructive sleep apnea with accompanying sensitivity to opioids and sedatives is often associated with obesity.

Obesity-Hypoventilation Syndrome
Obesity-hypoventilation syndrome (pickwickian syndrome) occurs in about 8% of morbidly obese individuals. The

occurrence of episodic daytime somnolence and hypoventilation in a morbidly obese patient suggests the presence of this syndrome. Ultimately, hypoventilation leads to sustained pulmonary hypertension and right ventricular failure. The etiology of obesity-hypoventilation syndrome is unknown, but it may represent a disorder of central nervous system regulation of breathing or an inability of the muscles of breathing to respond to neural impulses (or both).

Management of Anesthesia

Management of anesthesia is influenced by the presence of adverse effects from the underlying obesity.

INDUCTION OF ANESTHESIA

Obese patients are likely to be at increased risk for pulmonary aspiration in view of the increased incidence of gastroesophageal reflux and hiatal hernia in this patient population. The massive amount of soft tissue about the head and upper part of the trunk can impair mandibular and cervical mobility and make maintenance of a patent upper airway and tracheal intubation difficult. For these reasons, preoperative administration of an H_2 receptor antagonist or metoclopramide, or both, may be considered in the hope of increasing gastric fluid pH and decreasing gastric fluid volume. In addition, rapid induction of anesthesia followed by prompt intubation of the trachea with a cuffed tube is often selected to minimize the risk for pulmonary aspiration. In prospectively selected patients, awake tracheal intubation, most often with the use of a fiberoptic laryngoscope, may be indicated. Despite the common belief that obesity predisposes to the presence of an increased volume of acidic gastric fluid, there is paradoxical evidence that fasted obese patients have a lower incidence of high-volume low-pH gastric fluid than lean patients do.[21]

Decreased functional residual capacity predisposes obese patients to rapid decreases in PaO_2 during any period of apnea, such as may accompany direct laryngoscopy for tracheal intubation (Fig. 29-1).[22] This risk for rapid decreases in PaO_2 emphasizes the importance of maximizing the oxygen content of the lungs before initiating direct laryngoscopy, as well as monitoring peripheral arterial hemoglobin oxygen saturation continuously with a pulse oximeter. A decrease in functional residual capacity also decreases the mixing time for any inhaled drug, thus accelerating the rate of increase in the alveolar concentration of that drug.

Predicting the behavior of intravenous drugs in an obese patient is difficult. Plasma volume is often increased in obese patients, which would tend to decrease the plasma concentrations achieved with a single rapid intravenous injection of a drug such as thiopental. Conversely, adipose tissue has low blood flow such that increased doses calculated on absolute body weight in an obese patient could

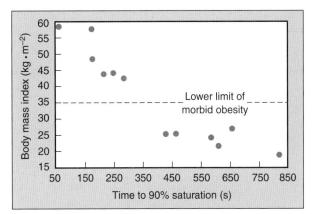

Figure 29-1 Arterial oxygen saturation decreases to 90% more rapidly in morbidly obese patients as quantitated by body mass index. (From Berthoud MC, Peacock JE, Reilly CS. Effectiveness of preoxygenation in morbidly obese patients. Br J Anaesth 1991;67:464-466.)

result in excessive plasma concentrations of drugs. The most logical approach is to use ideal body weight (reflects lean body mass) rather than actual body weight to calculate the initial drug doses. In this regard, it is rarely appropriate to base calculation of the drug dose on a weight higher than 80 kg in a female or more than 100 kg in a male.[23] Subsequent doses should be based on the patient's observed responses. On the other hand, infusions or repeated boluses of drugs can easily result in accumulation and prolonged sedation because of the storage of lipid-soluble drugs in adipose tissue and subsequent release into the circulation as the plasma concentration of the drug declines.

MAINTENANCE OF ANESTHESIA

The preferred choice of drugs or techniques for maintenance of anesthesia in obese patients is not clear. An increased incidence of fatty liver infiltration suggests caution in the selection of drugs associated with postoperative liver dysfunction. Increased defluorination of volatile anesthetics in obese patients, however, has not been shown to result in hepatic or renal dysfunction. The possibility of prolonged responses to drugs stored in adipose tissue (volatile anesthetics, opioids, barbiturates) is not supported by delayed awakening from anesthesia in obese patients.[24] To offset the increased likelihood for atelectasis as a result of increased chest wall and abdominal wall mass, controlled ventilation of the patient's lungs with large tidal volumes can act to counter the decreased functional residual capacity and PaO_2 accompanying obesity and accentuated by anesthesia. However, large tidal volumes may be detrimental because of the proinflammatory effects on the pulmonary parenchyma.[25] In this regard, an alternative approach to intraoperative

IV

recruitment of collapsed alveoli is to use positive end-expiratory pressure and standard tidal volumes.

The selection of spinal or epidural anesthesia can be technically challenging in obese patients because bony landmarks are obscured; at the same time, the level of anesthesia that will be produced by a given dose of drug is difficult to predict.

Postoperative Care

The semisitting position is often used in the postoperative care of obese patients to optimize the mechanics of breathing and to minimize the development of arterial hypoxemia. Arterial oxygenation should be closely monitored with pulse oximetry and supplemental oxygen administered if necessary, while remembering that the maximum decrease in PaO_2 typically occurs 2 to 3 days postoperatively. In addition, patients with the pickwickian syndrome may be extremely sensitive to opioids and will exhibit depressed ventilation in response to the administration of postoperative opioids. Aggressive pulmonary regimens, such as incentive spirometry or even intermittent positive-pressure breathing, may be combined with advanced analgesic techniques such as postoperative epidural infusions to optimize respiratory mechanics. The likelihood of deep vein thrombosis and the risk for pulmonary embolism are increased in obese patients, thus emphasizing the possible importance of early postoperative ambulation.

MALNUTRITION

Caloric support, in the presence of increased energy requirements, is commonly provided by enteral or total parenteral nutrition (hyperalimentation). It is often recommended that patients who have lost more than 20% of their body weight be treated nutritionally before elective surgery. Patients who are unable to eat or absorb nutrients after about 7 days postoperatively may also require parenteral nutrition.

Enteral Nutrition

The gastrointestinal tract should be used for a patient's nutritional needs as much as possible. Enteral nutrition is delivered as a continuous infusion via a nasal or oral tube. The feeding tube may be positioned in the stomach, duodenum, or jejunum. Postpyloric (duodenal and jejunal) feeding tubes will have lesser rates of regurgitation and potential aspiration; however, even gastric feeding tubes have low rates of aspiration based on radionuclide-tagged tube feeding studies.[26] Enteral nutrition is advantageous because it maintains the health of the gastrointestinal tract, thus preventing the possible complication of bacterial transfer across the gastrointestinal mucosa. Enteral

nutrition is associated with improved patient outcomes in terms of decreased infectious complications and the total number of ventilator and intensive care unit days.[27] In patients with pancreatitis, current practice is to insert a jejunal feeding tube so that feedings do not stimulate pancreatic activity. This approach has been shown to decrease the incidence of secondary infectious complications in patients with severe pancreatitis. Complications of enteral feedings are infrequent but may include hyperglycemia leading to osmotic diuresis and hypovolemia.[28] Blood glucose concentrations should be monitored and exogenous insulin administration considered when hyperglycemia (>250 mg/dL) occurs. The high osmolarity (550 to 850 mOsm/L) of elemental diets is often a cause of diarrhea; in these cases, changing the osmolarity or switching to a formula with higher fiber content will often resolve the problem.

Total Parenteral Nutrition

Total parenteral nutrition is indicated when the gastrointestinal tract is not functioning. Total parenteral nutrition with an isotonic solution delivered through a catheter placed in a large peripheral vein is acceptable when the patient requires less than 2000 calories per day and the anticipated need for nutritional support is brief. When caloric requirements are greater than 2000 calories per day or prolonged nutritional support is needed, a central venous catheter (either placed centrally or via an antecubital vein) is inserted to permit infusion of a hypertonic parenteral solution (about 1900 mOsm/L) in a daily volume of about 40 mL/kg.

ADVERSE EFFECTS

Potential adverse effects of total parenteral nutrition are numerous (Table 29-12). Blood glucose concentrations are monitored and hyperglycemia (>250 mg/dL) may require treatment with exogenous insulin. Conversely, hypoglycemia may occur if infusion of the parenteral nutrition solution is abruptly discontinued (mechanical obstruction in the delivery tubing) but increased circulating endogenous concentrations of insulin persist. A reason for considering a decrease in the infusion rate of the parenteral nutrition solution before induction of anesthesia is to avoid the possibility of plasma hyperosmolarity developing intraoperatively. Likewise, it may be appropriate to decrease the infusion rate of maintenance fluids so that the risk for fluid overload is minimized. Indeed, parenteral feeding of patients with compromised cardiac function is associated with a risk for congestive heart failure as a result of fluid overload.

Hyperchloremic metabolic acidosis may occur because of the liberation of hydrochloric acid during metabolism of the amino acids present in most parenteral nutrition solutions. Increased production of carbon dioxide resulting from the metabolism of large amounts of glucose may

Table 29-12   Adverse Effects of Total Parenteral Nutrition
Hyperglycemia
Hypoglycemia
Fluid overload
Increased carbon dioxide production
Catheter-related sepsis
Electrolyte abnormalities (hypokalemia, hypocalcemia, hypophosphatemia, hypomagnesemia)
Hepatic dysfunction
Renal dysfunction
Thrombosis of central veins

result in the need to initiate mechanical ventilation of the lungs or failure to wean a patient from long-term ventilatory support. Parenteral nutrition solutions can support the growth of bacteria and fungi, and catheter-related sepsis is a constant threat. A catheter impregnated with antimicrobials is associated with a lowered incidence of infusion site infection. In view of the risk for contamination, use of a central line port dedicated strictly to hyperalimentation is recommended, and use of that port for administration of medications, withdrawal of blood samples, or monitoring of central venous pressure as during the perioperative period is not recommended. Electrolyte abnormalities as a result of total parenteral nutrition are detected by preoperative measurement of plasma electrolyte concentrations.

ENDOCRINE AND METABOLIC CHANGES IN THE PERIOPERATIVE PERIOD

Surgical stimulation produces profound endocrine and metabolic responses that parallel the magnitude of the operative trauma.[29] Conversely, the inhaled or injected drugs used to produce anesthesia result in minimal effects on hormone secretion in the absence of surgical stimulation. An exception is etomidate, which interferes with the synthesis of cortisol in the adrenal cortex.

The initial endocrine response to surgical stimulation is an increase in the circulating concentration of cortisol and catecholamines and a decrease in the plasma concentration of insulin despite hyperglycemia. In view of the latter, excessive infusion of glucose via intravenous solutions could result in intraoperative hyperglycemia.

Surgical trauma causes protein degradation as reflected by loss of lean body weight and increased urinary excretion of nitrogen postoperatively. Sodium and water retention and excretion of potassium in the postoperative period presumably reflect release of arginine vasopressin and activation of the renin-angiotensin-aldosterone system.

Although it is difficult to quantitate the adverse effects produced by endocrine and metabolic responses to surgical stimulation, it would seem prudent to minimize the magnitude and duration of these changes whenever possible. Attenuation or prevention of the endocrine responses to surgery can be produced by afferent neuronal blockade, as with regional anesthesia (T4 sensory level), or by inhibition of hypothalamic function with large doses of opioids. It is likely, however, that regional anesthesia merely postpones the endocrine responses to surgery until the postoperative period.

IV

REFERENCES

1. Connery LE, Coursin DB. Assessment and therapy of selected endocrine disorders. Anesthesiol Clin North Am 2004;22:93-123.
2. Watkins PJ. Diabetic autonomic neuropathy. N Engl J Med 1990; 322:1078-1079.
3. Charlson ME, MacKenzie CR, Gold JP. Preoperative autonomic function abnormalities in patients with diabetes mellitus and patients with hypertension. J Am Coll Surg 1994:179:1-10.
4. Kirvela M, Yli-Hankala A, Lindgren L. QT dispersion and autonomic function in diabetic and nondiabetic patients with renal failure. Br J Anaesth 1994;73:801-804.
5. Burgos LG, Ebert TJ, Asiddao C, et al. Increased intraoperative morbidity in diabetics with autonomic neuropathy. Anesthesiology 1989;70:591-597.
6. Partanen JA, Niskanen L, Lehtinen J, et al. Natural history of peripheral neuropathy in patients with non–insulin-dependent diabetes mellitus. N Engl J Med 1995;333:89-94.
7. Mercker SK, Maier C, Doz P, et al. Lactic acidosis as a serious perioperative complication of antidiabetic biguanide medication with metformin. Anesthesiology 1997;87:1003-1005.
8. Hirsch IB, Magill JB, Cryer PE, et al. Perioperative management of surgical patients with diabetes mellitus. Anesthesiology 1991;74:346-359.
9. Cooper DS. Antithyroid drugs. N Engl J Med 2005;352:905-917.
10. Thome AC, Bedford RF. Esmolol for perioperative management of thyrotoxic goiter. Anesthesiology 1989;71:291-294.
11. Berman ML, Khunert L, Phythyon JM, et al. Isoflurane and enflurane-induced hepatic necrosis in triiodothyronine-pretreated rats. Anesthesiology 1983;58:1-5.
12. Seiuno H, Dohi S, Aiyoshi Y, et al. Postoperative hepatic dysfunction after halothane or enflurane anesthesia in patients with hyperthyroidism. Anesthesiology 1986;64:122-125.
13. Babad AA, Eger EL II. The effects of hyperthyroidism and hypothyroidism on halothane and oxygen requirements in dogs. Anesthesiology 1968;29:1087-1093.
14. Cooper DS. Subclinical hypothyroidism. JAMA 1987;258:246-247.
15. Bennett-Guerrero E, Kramer DC, Schwinn DA. Effect of chronic and acute thyroid hormone reduction on perioperative outcome. Anesth Analg 1997;85:30-36.

16. Mogensen T, Hjortso NC. Acute hypothyroidism in a severely ill surgical patient. Can J Anaesth 1988;35:74-75.

17. Symreng T, Karlberg BE, Kagedal B, et al. Physiological cortisol substitution of long-term steroid-treated patients undergoing major surgery. Br J Anaesth 1981;53:949-953.

18. Salem M, Tinsh RE, Bromberg J, et al. Perioperative glucocorticoid coverage: A reassessment 42 years after emergence of a problem. Ann Surg 1994;219:416-425.

19. Pullerits J, Ein S, Balfe JW. Anaesthesia for phaeochromocytoma. Can J Anaesth 1988;35:526-534.

20. Rosenbaum M, Leibel RL, Hirsch J. Obesity. N Engl J Med 1997;337:396-407.

21. Harter RL, Kelly WB, Kramer MG, et al. A comparison of the volume and pH of gastric contents of obese and lean surgical patients. Anesth Analg 1998;86:147-152.

22. Berthoud MC, Peacock JE, Reilly CS. Effectiveness of preoxygenation in morbidly obese patients. Br J Anaesth 1991;67:464-466.

23. Bouillon T, Shafer SL. Does size matter? Anesthesiology 1998;89:557-560.

24. Cork RC, Vaughn RW, Bentley JB. General anaesthesia for morbidly obese patients—an examination of postoperative outcomes. Anesthesiology 1981;54:310-313.

25. The Acute Respiratory Distress Syndrome Network. Ventilation with lower tidal volumes as compared with traditional tidal volumes for acute lung injury and the acute respiratory distress syndrome. N Engl J Med 2000;342:1301-1308.

26. Esparza J, Boivin MA, Hartshorne MF, et al. Equal aspiration rates in gastrically and transpylorically fed critically ill patients. Intensive Care Med 2001;27:660-664.

27. Lin L, Cohen NH. Early nutritional support for the ICU patient: Does it matter? Cont Crit Care 2005;2(9):1-10.

28. Kurian J, Kaul V. Profound postoperative hypoglycemia in a malnourished patient. Can J Anaesth 2001;28:881-883.

29. Weissman C. The metabolic response to stress: An overview and update. Anesthesiology 1990;73:308-327.

Chapter 30

CENTRAL NERVOUS SYSTEM DISEASE

Cheng Quah, Adrian W. Gelb, and Pekka Talke

Anesthesia for neurosurgery requires an understanding of the physiology of the central nervous system (CNS). The relationship between cerebral blood flow (CBF), cerebral metabolic rate for oxygen consumption ($CMRO_2$), and intracranial pressure (ICP) is influenced by physiologic and pharmacologic factors that are often under the control of the anesthesiologist. The selection of drugs, ventilation techniques, and monitors may have important implications in the care of patients with diseases involving the CNS.

NEUROPHYSIOLOGY

Cerebral Blood Flow

An understanding of neurophysiology is important for the management of patients with CNS disease. Normal CBF is 40 to 50 mL/100 g/min and represents about 15% of cardiac output. This disproportionately large CBF is due to the rapid metabolic rate of the brain and the absence of oxygen stores. Determinants of CBF include (1) $CMRO_2$, (2) $PaCO_2$, (3) cerebral perfusion pressure (CPP) and autoregulation, (4) PaO_2, and (5) anesthetic drugs (Fig. 30-1). Although cerebral blood vessels receive innervation from the autonomic nervous system, the impact on global CBF is small.

CEREBRAL METABOLIC RATE FOR OXYGEN

Changes in CBF are directly coupled with $CMRO_2$. Increases or decreases in $CMRO_2$ result in a proportional increase or decrease in CBF. Hypothermia, which reduces $CMRO_2$, also decreases CBF about 7% for every 1°C decrease in body temperature below 37°C. All intravenously administered anesthetics (thiopental, propofol, and etomidate) except for ketamine have minimal effects on or reduce $CMRO_2$ and CBF in parallel.[1] All volatile anesthetics also reduce $CMRO_2$; however, because they are cerebral vasodilators, they increase CBF.[2]

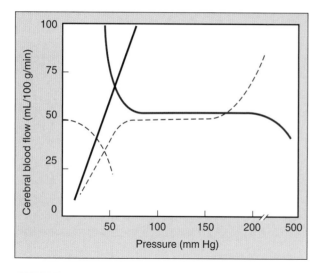

Figure 30-1 Schematic depiction of the impact of intracranial pressure (*dashed black line*), Pao$_2$ (*solid red line*), Paco$_2$ (*solid black line*), and cerebral perfusion pressure (mean arterial pressure minus intracranial pressure or central venous pressure, whichever is greater) (*dashed red line*) on cerebral blood flow. Cerebral perfusion pressure less than 50 mm Hg (mean arterial pressure of 65 mm Hg, assuming an intracranial pressure of 15 mm Hg) does not necessarily produce cerebral ischemia, but the physiologic reserve is decreased. In the presence of decreased physiologic reserve, the addition of anemia may result in cerebral ischemia.

ARTERIAL CARBON DIOXIDE PARTIAL PRESSURE

Changes in Paco$_2$ produce corresponding directional changes in CBF between a Paco$_2$ of 20 to 80 mm Hg (Fig. 30-2).[2] As a guide, CBF increases or decreases 1 mL/100 g/min for every 1–mm Hg increase or decrease in Paco$_2$ from 40 mm Hg. Such changes in CBF reflect the effect of carbon dioxide–mediated alterations in perivascular pH and lead to dilation or constriction of cerebral arterioles. These Paco$_2$-induced changes in CBF are transient because of an increase in cerebrospinal fluid (CSF) HCO$_3$ concentrations. CBF returns to normal in 6 to 8 hours, even if the altered Paco$_2$ levels are maintained.[2] The ability of decreases in Paco$_2$ (secondary to iatrogenic hyperventilation) to lower CBF and thereby cerebral blood volume and ICP is a critically important principle in neuroanesthesia.

CEREBRAL PERFUSION PRESSURE AND AUTOREGULATION

CPP is the difference between mean arterial pressure (MAP) and ICP or central venous pressure (CVP), whichever is greater. For example, assuming that ICP or CVP is 15 mm Hg, a MAP of 65 mm Hg would provide a CPP of 50 mm Hg. Autoregulation refers to the mechanism that maintains CBF constant in the presence of a changing CPP and reflects the ability of cerebral arterioles to constrict or relax in response to changes in perfusion (distending) pressure. This response normally requires 1 to 3 minutes to develop, so a rapid increase in MAP is associated with a brief period of cerebral hyperperfusion. Similarly, the

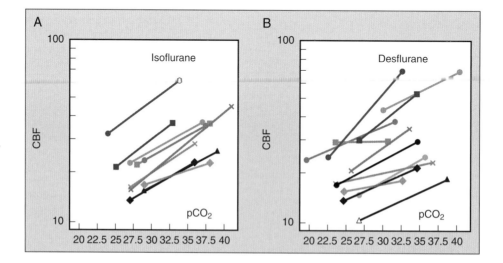

Figure 30-2 Individual cerebral blood flow (CBF) measurements (mL/100 g/min) plotted against Pco$_2$ (mm Hg) in patients receiving 1.25 MAC isoflurane or desflurane. (From Ornstein E, Young WL, Fleischer LH, et al. Desflurane and isoflurane have similar effects on cerebral blood flow in patients with intracranial mass lesions. Anesthesiology 1993;79:498-502, with permission.)

converse situation occurs with hypotension. Autoregulation maintains CBF relatively constant between a CPP of 50 and 150 mm Hg (see Fig. 30-1). With normal autoregulation and an intact blood-brain barrier, vasopressors affect CBF only when MAP is below 50 to 60 mm Hg or above 150 to 160 mm Hg.

With respect to inhaled anesthetics, autoregulation is maintained at anesthetic concentrations less than 1 minimum alveolar concentration (MAC).[3] At higher concentrations, inhaled anesthetics abolish autoregulation, and CBF becomes proportional to MAP. In contrast, intravenous anesthetics do not disrupt autoregulation. The autoregulation curve in patients with chronic hypertension is shifted to the right such that a lower MAP is less well tolerated. The anesthetic state shifts the autoregulatory response to the left, which provides for some safety from the decreases in MAP that can occur intraoperatively. Autoregulation may be impaired in patients with poorly controlled systemic hypertension and may also be impaired in the proximity of intracranial tumors.

ARTERIAL OXYGEN PARTIAL PRESSURE
Decreases in PaO_2 result in an exponential increase in CBF below a threshold value of about 50 mm Hg (see Fig. 30-1).

INHALED ANESTHETICS
Volatile anesthetics administered during normocapnia at concentrations higher than 0.5 MAC rapidly produce cerebral vasodilation and result in dose-dependent increases in CBF. CBF remains increased relative to $CMRO_2$ during administration of halothane, isoflurane, or sevoflurane (Fig. 30-3).[4] This drug-induced increase in CBF occurs despite concomitant decreases in $CMRO_2$. The largest increase in CBF occurs with halothane, with less of an effect seen with isoflurane, desflurane, and sevoflurane. Nitrous oxide also increases CBF.

INTRAVENOUS ANESTHETICS
All intravenous drugs except ketamine reduce $CMRO_2$ and CBF in a dose-dependent fashion, and this decrease is associated with a reduction in ICP. There is controversy about the effects of ketamine, which probably reflects differences in the conditions of the research study.[5] When ketamine is given on its own without control of ventilation, $PaCO_2$, CBF, and ICP all increase, whereas when given in the presence of another sedative/anesthetic drug in patients whose ventilation is controlled, these effects are not noted. Because of this controversy, however, ketamine is not usually selected for patients with known intracranial disease.

Thiopental, propofol, and etomidate are cerebral vasoconstrictors that decrease $CMRO_2$, CBF, and ICP. These drugs may be administered to patients with intracranial hypertension to decrease ICP. Large doses of propofol or thiopental may decrease systemic blood pressure sufficiently to also decrease CPP. Autoregulation of CBF is

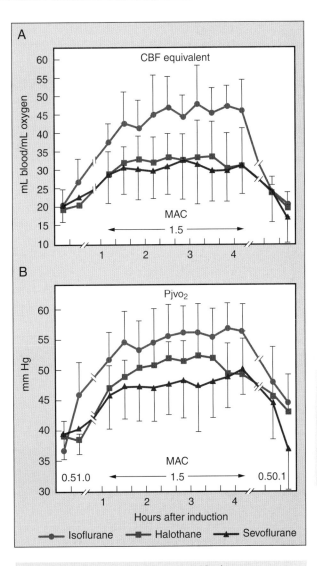

Figure 30-3 When compared at 1.5 MAC, the average increase in cerebral blood flow (CBF) in patients receiving isoflurane is greater than in those receiving halothane and sevoflurane (**A**). Likewise, the average value of the internal jugular venous oxygen tension ($Pjvo_2$) is higher in patients receiving isoflurane (**B**). The increased CBF present at 1.5 MAC was sustained over time. (From Kuroda Y, Murakanic M, Tsuruta J, et al. Preservation of the ratio of cerebral blood flow metabolic rate for oxygen during prolonged anesthesia with isoflurane, sevoflurane, and halothane in humans. Anesthesiology 1966;84:555-561, with permission.)

not altered by propofol or thiopental. Myoclonus may accompany the administration of etomidate. An increased frequency of excitatory peaks on the electroencephalogram of patients receiving etomidate, as compared with thiopental, suggests caution in the administration of etomidate to patients with a history of epilepsy. Benzodiazepines decrease $CMRO_2$ and CBF, analogous to thiopental and propofol.

Opioids decrease CBF and possibly ICP in the absence of hypoventilation. These drugs should be used with caution in patients with intracranial disease because of their (1) depressant effects on consciousness, (2) production of miosis, and (3) depression of ventilation with associated increases in ICP if $PaCO_2$ increases. Although opioids do not usually increase ICP, there is evidence that modest and transient increases in ICP may accompany administration in patients with acute head injury despite maintenance of normocapnia or even hypocapnia.[6] This is probably related to reductions in arterial blood pressure with autoregulatory-mediated cerebral vasodilation.

α_2-Agonists (clonidine and dexmedetomidine) have sedative, sympatholytic, and analgesic properties. They are unique sedatives in that they do not cause significant respiratory depression. They have no effects on ICP. Because they reduce arterial blood pressure without having an effect on ICP, they reduce CPP. α_2-Agonists reduce CBF and only slightly attenuate the cerebrovascular response to changes in $PaCO_2$. Clinically, α_2-agonists can be used intraoperatively to reduce the dose of other anesthetics and analgesics or postoperatively as sedatives and to attenuate postoperative hypertension and tachycardia.

NEUROMUSCULAR BLOCKING DRUGS
Neuromuscular blocking drugs do not usually affect ICP unless they induce release of histamine or hypotension. Histamine can cause cerebral vasodilation leading to an increase in ICP. Succinylcholine may increase ICP through stimulation of muscle spindles, which in turn either directly or indirectly results in increased $CMRO_2$.[7] Because CBF is coupled to $CMRO_2$, the increase in $CMRO_2$ is responsible for increasing CBF and thus ICP. However, the increase in ICP has not been a consistent observation.

INTRACRANIAL PRESSURE

ICP is normally less than 10 mm Hg. A sustained increase in ICP above 15 mm Hg is defined as intracranial hypertension. Marked increases in ICP can decrease CPP and thereby CBF to the point of producing regional/general ischemia. Pressure-volume elastance (change in pressure produced by a change in volume) curves reflect changes produced by expanding intracranial masses (Fig. 30-4). As the intracranial volume increases, CSF is initially translocated into the spinal canal. Once this compensation is maximized, ICP starts to rise and cerebral vessels are eventually compressed. A point is reached when even small increases in intracranial volume, as produced by drug-induced cerebral vasodilation, may result in marked increases in ICP. Ischemia will lead to cerebral edema

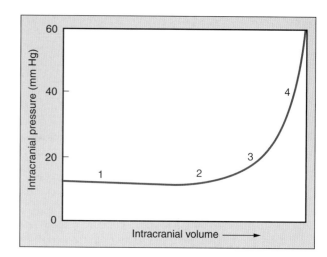

Figure 30-4 The pressure-volume compliance curve depicts the impact of increasing intracranial volume on intracranial pressure (ICP). As volume increases from point 1 to point 2 on the curve, ICP does not increase because cerebrospinal fluid is shifted from the cranium into the spinal subarachnoid space. Patients with intracranial tumors who are between point 1 and point 2 on the compliance curve are unlikely to manifest clinical symptoms of increased ICP. Patients who are on the rising portion of the pressure-volume curve (point 3) can no longer compensate for increases in intracranial volume, and ICP begins to increase. Clinical symptoms attributable to increased ICP are likely at this stage. Additional increases in volume at this point, as produced by increased CBF during anesthesia, can precipitate abrupt increases in ICP (point 4).

and further increases in ICP. It is therefore critical to prevent sustained increases in ICP (Table 30-1).

The duration of the efficacy of hyperventilation and the duration of decreased ICP are unclear. In patients, however, the effect of hyperventilation wanes with time and CBF returns to normal after about 6 hours.[2] A further concern is that hyperventilation reduces CBF and may actually produce ischemia.

Volatile anesthetics produce dose-dependent increases in ICP that parallel the increases in CBF. Patients with space-occupying intracranial lesions are most vulnerable to these drug-induced increases in ICP. Hyperventilation to decrease $PaCO_2$ to < 35 mm Hg attenuates the tendency for volatile anesthetics to increase ICP. In patients undergoing craniotomy for supratentorial tumors with evidence of a midline shift, neither isoflurane nor desflurane significantly affected lumbar CSF pressure when moderate hypocapnia ($PaCO_2$ of 30 mm Hg) was maintained.[8]

The effects of physiologic and pharmacologic interventions on ICP discussed above may be dependent on an

Table 30-1 Methods to Decrease Intracranial Pressure

Elevation of the head to improve cerebral venous outflow

Hyperventilation

Cerebrospinal fluid drainage

Osmotic and other diuretic drugs (decrease brain water content and reduce cerebrospinal fluid production)

Administration of drugs that reduce intracranial blood volume (barbiturates, propofol)

Avoidance of cerebral vasodilating drugs (volatile anesthetics)

Table 30-2 Management of Anesthesia for Patients with Intracranial Masses

Preoperative

Avoid sedatives and opioids if ICP is elevated

Standard anxiolytics if ICP is not elevated

Monitors

Supratentorial masses—standard ASA monitors (arterial line, Foley catheter)

Infratentorial masses (depending on positioning)

    Prone or park bench—standard ASA monitors (arterial line, Foley catheter)

    Sitting position associated with frequent VAE risk (standard monitors plus CVP, precordial Doppler, or TEE)

Induction

Deep anesthesia and skeletal muscle paralysis before direct laryngoscopy/tracheal intubation to avoid increasing ICP while maintaining CPP

Maintenance

Minimize ICP and maintain adequate CPP

Opioid plus propofol or a volatile anesthetic with or without nitrous oxide

Mannitol (0.25-1g/kg IV)

Maintain euvolemia

Postoperative

Avoid coughing, straining, and systemic hypertension during tracheal extubation

Rapid awakening allows early neurologic assessment

ASA, American Society of Anesthesiologists; CPP, cerebral perfusion pressure; CVP, central venous pressure; ICP, intracranial pressure; TEE, transesophageal echocardiography; VAE, venous air embolism.

intact blood-brain barrier. The blood-brain barrier, composed of capillary endothelial cells with extremely tight junctions that are almost fused, prevents extracellular passage of macromolecules (proteins), whereas lipid-soluble substances (carbon dioxide, oxygen, anesthetics) cross the blood-brain barrier easily. The blood-brain barrier may be disrupted in the event of acute systemic hypertension, trauma, infection, arterial hypoxemia, marked hypercapnia, tumors, and sustained seizure activity.

PATIENTS WITH INTRACRANIAL MASS LESIONS

Supratentorial Masses

Intracranial masses (tumors) requiring surgery occur most often in patients 40 to 60 years of age, and the initial signs and symptoms reflect increases in ICP. Seizures that appear in a previously asymptomatic adult suggest the presence of an intracranial tumor, and such tumors are usually confirmed by computed tomography (CT) or magnetic resonance imaging (MRI)

MANAGEMENT OF ANESTHESIA

Management of anesthesia for craniotomy and resection of an intracranial tumor is designed to prevent undesirable changes in CBF and ICP and result in timely awakening after surgery to allow for postoperative neurologic evaluation (Table 30-2). Preoperative evaluation of neurologic status should be carried out to determine the presence or extent of neurologic deficits. Anesthetic requirements will differ, depending on the location and type of tumor. Resection of supratentorial tumors is typically accomplished with the patient in the supine or lateral position.

Preoperative Evaluation

Evidence of increased ICP is sought during the preoperative visit. In this regard, clinical signs may be consistent with but do not reliably indicate the level of ICP (Table 30-3).

Table 30-3 Preoperative Evidence of Increased Intracranial Pressure

Nausea and vomiting

Hypertension

Bradycardia

Personality change

Altered levels of consciousness

Altered patterns of breathing

Papilledema

IV

MRI or CT may show a midline shift of more than 0.5 cm, encroachment of expanding brain on cerebral ventricles, cerebral edema, or any combination of these signs. In symptomatic patients, preoperative medications that cause sedation or depression of ventilation are usually avoided. Drug-induced depression of ventilation can lead to increased $PaCO_2$ and subsequent increases in ICP. In alert patients, small doses of benzodiazepines may provide useful relief of anxiety.

Monitors

Continuous monitoring of systemic blood pressure via a catheter in a peripheral artery is recommended because of hemodynamic perturbations occurring during induction of anesthesia, tracheal intubation, surgery, and emergence from anesthesia, all of which may compromise cerebral perfusion. Central venous catheters are used only in selected cases for estimating intravascular fluid volume. Measurement of the exhaled carbon dioxide concentration (capnography) is necessary to determine ventilation parameters. The electrocardiogram (ECG) allows prompt detection of cardiac dysrhythmias caused by surgical manipulation of cardiovascular centers. Neuromuscular blockade is monitored with a peripheral nerve stimulator. Because of the length of these surgical procedures and the use of diuretics, a bladder catheter is often necessary and helps in guiding fluid therapy. A continuous monitor of ICP is helpful but rarely used. There are two main monitors for ICP inserted by neurosurgeons. The intraventricular catheter permits direct measurement of ICP and drainage of CSF. The subarachnoid or subdural bolt is placed through a burr hole and can be inserted quickly in an emergency setting, but it does not allow for CSF drainage.

Induction of Anesthesia

The goal of induction of anesthesia is to achieve a sufficient level of anesthesia before the stimulation of direct laryngoscopy and tracheal intubation without compromising cerebral perfusion by increasing ICP or decreasing MAP. Intravenous induction with thiopental, 3 to 6 mg/kg, propofol, 1.5 to 3 mg/kg, or etomidate, 0.2 to 0.5 mg/kg, produces reliable and prompt onset of unconsciousness (anesthesia) and is unlikely to adversely increase ICP. Hemodynamic support with sympathomimetic drugs may be necessary and such drugs should be readily available, especially in cases in which CPP may already be compromised. A nondepolarizing neuromuscular blocking drug or succinylcholine is used to facilitate tracheal intubation, mechanical ventilation of the lungs, and patient positioning on the operating table. Increases in ICP may occur after the administration of succinylcholine, but the extent of the increase is quite variable and usually short-lived.[7] The patient's trachea is intubated after a peripheral nerve stimulator confirms the establishment of skeletal muscle paralysis so that coughing is avoided, which may result in marked increases in ICP. Injection of additional intravenous doses of thiopental, propofol, opioids, or lidocaine 1 to 2 minutes before beginning direct laryngoscopy may be effective in attenuating the increase in systemic blood pressure and ICP that can accompany tracheal intubation.

After tracheal intubation, ventilation of the lungs is controlled at a rate and tidal volume sufficient to maintain $PaCO_2$ between 30 and 35 mm Hg. There is no evidence of additional therapeutic benefit when $PaCO_2$ is decreased below 30 to 35 mm Hg. Positive end-expiratory pressure is not encouraged because it could impair cerebral venous drainage and increase ICP, but it can usually be counteracted by raising the head 10 to 15 cm above the level of the chest.

Maintenance of Anesthesia

After tracheal intubation, measures should be taken to optimize CPP and minimize ICP, at least until the dura is opened. Maintenance of anesthesia is often achieved with an opioid together with either a continuous infusion of propofol or inhalation of a volatile anesthetic with or without nitrous oxide. Volatile anesthetics must be used carefully because of their ability to increase ICP. Nevertheless, low concentrations of volatile anesthetics (<0.6 MAC) may be useful for decreasing the risk of awareness and blunting the increases in systemic blood pressure evoked by surgical stimulation. The minimal effects of isoflurane, desflurane, and sevoflurane on ICP, especially when used with judicious hyperventilation, make these drugs useful selections for patients undergoing intracranial operations. Direct-acting vasodilating drugs (nitroprusside, nitroglycerin, calcium channel blockers) increase CBF and ICP despite causing simultaneous decreases in systemic blood pressure; therefore, use of these drugs, particularly before the dura is open, is not encouraged.

Movement, coughing, or reacting to the presence of the tracheal tube during intracranial procedures is avoided because these responses can lead to increases in ICP, bleeding into the operative site, and a brain that bulges into the operative site and makes surgical exposure difficult. Thus, maintenance of an adequate depth of anesthesia is important. Skeletal muscle paralysis is often used to provide added insurance against movement or coughing. The choice of anesthetics is also determined in part by the use of intraoperative neurophysiologic monitoring. For example, volatile anesthetics cause dose-related decreases in the amplitude and increases in the latency of the cortical components of median nerve somatosensory evoked potentials.

Cerebral Swelling

If cerebral swelling occurs, it may be useful to administer additional doses of diuretics to decrease brain water. Mannitol (0.25 to 1 g/kg IV) acts as an osmotic diuretic and reduces cerebral water content. The onset of action is 5 to 10 minutes, maximum effects are seen in 20 to 30 minutes, and its effects last for about 2 to 4 hours. However, if administered rapidly, mannitol can also cause peripheral vasodilation (hypotension) and short-term intravascular volume expansion, which could result in increased ICP. Acute mannitol toxicity, as manifested by hyponatremia, high measured serum osmolality, and a gap between the measured and calculated serum osmolality of greater than 10 mOsm/kg, can also occur when large does of the drug (2 to 3 g/kg IV) are given. Furosemide (0.5 to 1 mg/kg IV) is effective in decreasing ICP, though less so than mannitol. Intermittent intravenous injections of thiopental or propofol may also be effective in decreasing ICP, and if surgically possible, placing the patient in a head-up position also helps. Other useful measures include hyperventilating the patient's lungs and discontinuing the administration of volatile anesthetics.

Intravenous Fluid Therapy

Maintaining euvolemia rather than fluid restriction is recommended, although the presence of cerebral edema or elevated ICP may restrict the administration of fluids. Dextrose solutions are not recommended because they are rapidly distributed throughout body water and, if blood glucose concentrations decrease more rapidly than brain glucose concentrations, water crosses the blood-brain barrier and cerebral edema results. Furthermore, hyperglycemia augments ischemic neuronal cell damage by promoting neuronal lactate production, which worsens cellular injury. Therefore, crystalloid solutions such as normal saline and lactated Ringer's solution are recommended, although normal saline is sometimes preferred because of its slightly higher osmolality. Colloids such as 5% albumin are also an acceptable replacement fluid, but no improvement in outcome has been shown.

AWAKENING

On awakening from anesthesia, coughing or straining by the patient should be avoided because these responses could increase the possibility of hemorrhage or edema formation. A prior intravenous bolus of lidocaine or an opioid, or both, may help decrease the likelihood of coughing during tracheal extubation. Postoperatively, assessing neurologic status frequently and providing adequate analgesia are important. Delayed return of consciousness postoperatively or neurologic deterioration in the postoperative period is evaluated by CT or MRI. Tension pneumocephalus as a cause of neurologic deterioration is a consideration, especially if nitrous oxide was administered during anesthesia. The postoperative stress response and resulting hyperdynamic events (hypertension, tachycardia) are attenuated with the use of hemodynamically active drugs and opioids.

Posterior Fossa Masses

Resection of posterior fossa/infratentorial tumors frequently requires placement of the patient in the sitting or prone position (see Table 30-2). The sitting position facilitates surgical exposure of posterior fossa tumors, but because the risk for venous air embolism is so high (> 25% incidence), many neurosurgeons prefer the prone position. Other risks associated with the sitting position include upper airway edema as a result of venous obstruction from excessive cervical flexion and quadriplegia from spinal cord compression and ischemia, especially in the presence of preexisting cervical stenosis. Another popular approach is the "park bench position" in which the patient is placed in a lateral position but rolled slightly forward with the head further rotated to "look" at the floor. This position allows the surgeon full access to the posterior fossa and minimizes the risk for venous air embolism.

Intraoperative management is similar to that for supratentorial masses. In addition to an arterial line, monitoring for the sitting position should include a properly positioned central venous catheter and precordial Doppler given the high incidence of venous air embolism. Operations on posterior fossa tumors can injure vital brainstem respiratory and circulatory nuclei and result in intraoperative hemodynamic fluctuations and postoperative depression of ventilation. The cranial nerves can also be affected and lead to impairment of protective airway reflexes.

Postoperatively, one needs to assess whether the patient will be able to maintain and protect the airway or whether tracheal intubation and ventilation should be continued in the intensive care unit.

VENOUS AIR EMBOLISM

Neurosurgery that requires significant elevation of the head is associated with an increased risk for venous air embolism.[9] Not only is the operative site above the level of the heart (risk increased whenever the operative field is more than 5 cm above the level of the right atrium), but the venous sinuses in the cut edge of bone or dura may not collapse when transected. Air enters the pulmonary circulation and becomes trapped in the small vessels, thereby causing an acute increase in dead space. In addition, air can enter and be trapped in the right ventricle and lead to interference with right ventricular output into the pulmonary artery. Microvascular bubbles may also cause reflex bronchoconstriction and activate the release of endothelial mediators causing pulmonary edema. Death is usually due to cardiovascular collapse and arterial hypoxemia. Air may reach the coronary and cerebral circulations (paradoxical air embolism) by crossing a patent foramen ovale (a probe-patent foramen ovale is present in 20% to 30% of adults) and result in myocardial infarction or stroke. Furthermore, transpulmonary passage of venous air is possible in the absence of a patent foramen ovale.[10]

Detection

Transesophageal echocardiography is the most sensitive method to detect air embolism, but it is invasive and cumbersome. A precordial Doppler ultrasound transducer placed over the right heart (over the second or third intercostal space to the right of the sternum to maximize audible signals from the right atrium) is the next most sensitive (detects amounts of air as small as 0.25 mL) and noninvasive indicator of the presence of intracardiac air. A sudden decrease in end-exhaled concentrations of carbon dioxide reflects increased dead space secondary to continued ventilation of alveoli no longer being perfused because of obstruction of their vascular supply by air bubbles. An increased end-tidal nitrogen concentration may reflect nitrogen from venous air embolism. Aspiration of air through a correctly positioned central venous catheter can also be used to diagnose air embolism. In this regard, a right atrial catheter with the tip positioned at the junction of the superior vena cava and the right atrium seems to provide the most rapid aspiration of air.[11] During controlled ventilation of the lungs, sudden attempts (gasps) by patients to initiate spontaneous breaths may be the first indication of the occurrence of venous air embolism. Hypotension, tachycardia, cardiac dysrhythmias, cyanosis, and a "mill wheel" murmur are late signs of venous air embolism. Insertion of a pulmonary artery catheter may provide additional evidence that venous air embolism has occurred because of increases in pulmonary artery pressure. Additional signs in awake patients include chest pain and coughing.

Treatment

The surgeon should be notified immediately whenever a venous air embolism is suspected. Venous air embolism is treated by (1) irrigation of the operative site with fluid, as well as the application of occlusive material to all bone edges so that sites of venous air entry are occluded; (2) gentle compression of the internal jugular veins; and (3) placement of the patient in a head-down position. If nitrous oxide is being administered, it should be promptly discontinued to avoid the risk of increasing the size of venous air bubbles because of diffusion of this gas into the air bubbles. Despite the logic of positive end-expiratory pressure to decrease entrainment of air, the efficacy of this maneuver has not been confirmed. Furthermore, positive end-expiratory pressure could reverse the pressure gradient between the left and right atria and predispose to passage of air across a patent foramen ovale.

INTRACRANIAL ANEURYSMS

Intracranial aneurysms are the most common cause of intracranial hemorrhage. They occur in 2% to 4% of the population, with 1% to 2% rupturing per year. Although aneurysms may be found incidentally or appear as a slowly enlarging mass, they are most frequently manifested as hemorrhage together with a sudden, severe headache, nausea, vomiting, focal neurologic signs, and depressed consciousness.

Complications

Major complications of aneurysmal rupture include death, rebleeding, and vasospasm. Early surgery is advocated for prevention of rebleeding, but it may be associated with greater technical difficulty because of a swollen inflamed brain, whereas delaying surgery increases the risk for rebleeding. Current clinical practice favors early surgery. Vasospasm of the cerebral arteries is generally manifested clinically 3 to 5 days after subarachnoid hemorrhage and is the foremost cause of morbidity and mortality. Transcranial Doppler and cerebral arteriography can detect cerebral vasospasm before clinical symptoms (worsening headache, neurologic deterioration, loss of consciousness) occur. Treatment of vasospasm includes "triple H" therapy (hypervolemia, hypertension, hemodilution), which consists of the intravenous administration of fluids or inotropic drugs, or both. The intravenous administration of a calcium entry blocker, nimodipine, decreases the morbidity and mortality from vasospasm. Other treatment modalities include selective intra-arterial injection of vasodilators and balloon dilation (angioplasty) of the affected cerebral vessels.

Other complications of subarachnoid hemorrhage include seizures (10%), acute and chronic hydrocephalus, and intracerebral hematoma. Changes on the ECG (T-wave inversions, U waves, ST depressions, prolonged QT, and rarely Q waves) are frequent but do not usually correlate with significant myocardial dysfunction or poor outcome. Hyponatremia is commonly seen after subarachnoid hemorrhage. Significant electrolyte, acid-base abnormalities or hemodynamic derangements should be corrected if present, and a cardiac workup should ensue if Q waves are seen on the ECG.

Treatment

Short-term outcomes are similar in patients treated surgically versus endovascular insertion of platinum coils (see Chapter 37). Some patients are unsuitable candidates for insertion of platinum coils because of the anatomy and location of their aneurysms and still require surgery.

Management of Anesthesia

Management of anesthesia for resection of an intracranial aneurysm is designed to (1) prevent sudden increases in systemic arterial blood pressure, which would increase the aneurysm's transmural pressure and could result in rupture, and (2) facilitate surgical exposure and access to the aneurysm (Table 30-4). Preoperative sedation may not be needed, but if used, it must be titrated to prevent hypoventilation and associated increases in ICP. Induction and maintenance of anesthesia must be designed to minimize the hypertensive responses evoked by noxious stimulation, such as direct laryngoscopy and placing the patient's head in immobilizing pins. Conversely, CPP

Table 30-4 Anesthetic Management of Patients with Intracranial Aneurysms

Preoperative

Neurologic evaluation for evidence of increased intracranial pressure and vasospasm

Electrocardiogram changes frequently present

HHH therapy if vasospasm is present

Calcium channel blockers

Induction

Avoid increases in systemic blood pressure

Maintain cerebral perfusion pressure to avoid ischemia

Maintenance

Opioid plus propofol and/or volatile anesthetic

Mannitol (0.25-1 g/kg IV)

Maintain normal to increased systemic blood pressure to avoid ischemia during temporary clipping

Postoperative

Maintain normal to increased systemic blood pressure

Early awakening to facilitate neurologic assessment

HHH therapy

HHH, hypervolemia, hypertension, hemodilution.

must be maintained to prevent ischemia during retraction or temporary vessel occlusion or as a result of vasospasm.

INDUCTION AND MAINTENANCE OF ANESTHESIA

Induction of anesthesia is most frequently achieved by the intravenous administration of propofol and an opioid plus a nondepolarizing neuromuscular blocking drug. Anesthesia is then maintained with an opioid and either an intravenous propofol infusion or inhalation of a volatile anesthetic, usually at less than 1 MAC. The exact choice may also be influenced by the use of electro-physiologic monitoring. For example, volatile anesthetics cause dose-related decreases in the amplitude and increases in the latency of the cortical components of median nerve somatosensory evoked potentials. Surgical dissection is facilitated by osmotic diuresis and moderate hyperventilation of the patient's lungs, which help decrease brain swelling.

HEMODYNAMIC CONTROL

Hemodynamic control is important during dissection of the aneurysm to prevent intraoperative rupture. In the past, deliberate hypotension was used to decrease the risk for rupture of an intracranial aneurysm and to facilitate

surgical placement of occlusive vascular clips. However, currently, temporary occlusive clips applied to the major feeding artery of the aneurysm can create regional hypotension without the need for systemic hypotension and its inherent risks on multiple organ systems. As a result, normal or even increased systemic arterial blood pressure should be instituted to facilitate perfusion through the collateral circulation. In addition to maintaining collateral cerebral circulation via systemic hypertension, drugs such as thiopental may be administered in the hope that they can provide some protection from cerebral ischemia. Occasionally, hypothermic circulatory arrest may be used for very large complex aneurysms.

The patient's trachea is generally extubated at the completion of surgery unless there is significant neurologic impairment. Measures to prevent vasospasm and seizures while maintaining adequate CPP should be continued during care of these patients postoperatively.

SPINAL CORD TRANSECTION

Spinal cord transection results in damage to the spinal cord that is manifested as paralysis of the lower extremities (paraplegia) or all the extremities (quadriplegia). Anatomically, the damaged spinal cord is not transected, but the physiologic effect is the same as though it were divided. The most common cause of spinal cord transection is trauma.

Acute Paralysis

The extent of hemodynamic instability and the difficulty in managing the patient's airway depend on the level of spinal cord injury. Further damage to the spinal cord could result from extension or flexion of the head in the presence of a cervical spine fracture. Topical anesthesia of the trachea plus intubation in an awake patient with the use of a fiberoptic bronchoscope is an alternative to rapid-sequence induction of anesthesia and subsequent endo-tracheal intubation. In both scenarios, in-line stabilization of the neck should be maintained. There is no evidence of a difference in neurologic morbidity after intubation in an anesthetized or awake patient.[12]

Succinylcholine is unlikely to provoke an excessive release of potassium in the first 24 hours after acute spinal cord transection. Nevertheless, it is common practice to avoid the use of this drug, except when rapid onset of short-duration skeletal muscle paralysis is considered necessary. Even in these situations, rocuronium may be a suitable alternative to succinylcholine (see Chapter 12). Minimal concentrations of volatile anesthetics are required because these patients are often anesthetic in the operative area. Breathing is best managed by mechanical ventilation of the lungs because abdominal and intercostal muscle paralysis as a result of spinal cord transection combined with general anesthesia makes maintenance of adequate spontaneous ventilation unlikely.

The absence of sympathetic nervous system activity below the level of spinal cord transection leaves these patients vulnerable to systemic hypotension, particularly in response to acute changes in body position, blood loss, or positive airway pressure. Hypothermia is a hazard because the patients are usually poikilothermic below the spinal cord transection.

Chronic Paralysis

The most important goal during management of anesthesia in patients with chronic transection of the spinal cord is prevention of autonomic hyperreflexia, which is manifested as abrupt systemic hypertension with an associated baroreflex-mediated compensatory bradycardia (Fig. 30-5). Spinal cord transection above T6 is frequently associated with autonomic hyperreflexia, with as many as 85% of patients manifesting this response.[13] Autonomic hyperreflexia is initiated by cutaneous or visceral stimulation below the level of the spinal cord transection. Distention of a hollow viscus, such as the bladder during cystoscopy, is a common initiating event. Stimulation elicits reflex sympathetic nervous system activity and vasoconstriction below the level of the spinal cord transection and thereby results in systemic hypertension. Vasoconstriction and hypertension persist because vasodilatory impulses from the CNS cannot traverse the spinal cord to reach the area below the level of the cord transection.

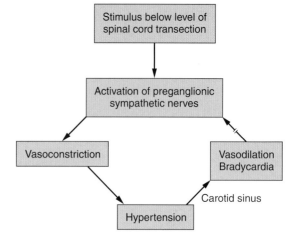

Figure 30-5 Sequence of events associated with clinical manifestations of autonomic hyperreflexia. Impulses that produce vasodilation cannot reach the neurologically isolated distal portion of the spinal cord, so vasoconstriction and hypertension persist.

Spinal anesthesia is particularly effective in preventing autonomic hyperreflexia. General anesthesia with volatile anesthetics or epidural anesthesia is also effective, but less so than spinal anesthesia. Treatment of systemic hypertension with a drug such as nitroprusside is necessary if autonomic hyperreflexia occurs despite preventive steps.

REFERENCES

1. Pinaud M, Leausquer JN, Chetanneau A, et al. Effects of propofol on cerebral hemodynamics and metabolism in patients with brain trauma. Anesthesiology 1990;73:404-409.
2. Ornstein E, Young WL, Fleischer LH, et al. Desflurane and isoflurane have similar effects on cerebral blood flow in patients with intracranial mass lesions. Anesthesiology 1993;79:498-502.
3. Cho S, Jujigake T, Uchiyama Y, et al. Effects of sevoflurane with and without nitrous oxide on human cerebral circulation. Anesthesiology 1996;85:755-760.
4. Kuroda Y, Murakami M, Tsuruta J, et al. Preservation of the ratio of cerebral blood flow/metabolic rate for oxygen during prolonged anesthesia with isoflurane, sevoflurane, and halothane in humans. Anesthesiology 1996;84:555-561.
5. Albanese J, Arnaud S, Rey M, et al. Ketamine decreases intracranial pressure and electroencephalographic activity in traumatic brain injury patients during propofol sedation. Anesthesiology 1997;87:1328-1334.
6. Sperry RJ, Bailey PL, Reichman MV, et al. Fentanyl and sufentanil increase intracranial pressure in head trauma patients. Anesthesiology 1992;77:416-420.
7. Kovarik WD, Mayberg TS, Lam AM, et al. Succinylcholine does not change intracranial pressure, cerebral blood flow velocity, or the electroencephalogram in patients with neurologic injury. Anesth Analg 1994;78:469-473.
8. Muzzi D, Losasso T, Dietz N, et al. The effect of desflurane and isoflurane on cerebrospinal fluid pressure in humans with supratentorial mass lesions. Anesthesiology 1992;76:720-724.
9. Muth CM, Shank ES. Gas embolism. N Engl J Med 2000;342:476-482.
10. Byrick RJ, Korley RE, McKee MD, et al. Prolonged coma after unreamed, locked nailing of femoral shaft fracture. Anesthesiology 2001;94:163-165.
11. Bunegin L, Albin MS, Helsel PE, et al. Positioning the right atrial catheter: A model for reappraisal. Anesthesiology 1981;55:343-348.
12. McLeod ADM, Calder I. Spinal cord injury and direct laryngoscopy—the legend lives on. Br J Anaesth 2000;84:705-709.
13. Kobayashi A, Mizobe T, Tojo H, et al. Autonomic hyperreflexia during labour. Can J Anaesth 1995;42:1134-1136.

Chapter 31

OPHTHALMOLOGY AND OTOLARYNGOLOGY

Errol Lobo, Francesca Pelegrini, and Tina Chiu

Surgical procedures involving the eyes, ears, nose, and throat require a cooperative relationship between the surgeon and the anesthesiologist. It is important for the anesthesiologist to appreciate the anatomy and physiology of the structures in the operative field. In addition, an understanding of the surgical procedure is important. Patients undergoing surgical procedures on the eye, head, and neck represent a diversity of age groups from infants to the elderly. The majority of these procedures are performed in an outpatient setting, with a significant percentage of ophthalmologic procedures performed under monitored anesthesia care.

OPHTHALMOLOGY

The majority of patients who undergo elective ophthalmologic procedures are elderly and have multiple comorbid conditions.[1] Hence an understanding of the surgical procedure, as well as a detailed preoperative evaluation, is important. Because most patients with eye problems use ophthalmic medications that may interact with the medications used in anesthesia, an understanding of drug interactions is important (Table 31-1).[2] Intraoperative management also requires that the anesthesiologist be familiar with factors and medications that influence intraocular pressure (IOP) and the hemodynamic changes associated with the oculocardiac reflex. A significant percentage of ophthalmologic procedures are performed with a retrobulbar block; hence an understanding of this technique and associated complications is useful.[3,4]

Ophthalmic Medications

Ophthalmic medications that are applied topically to the eye undergo sufficient absorption and may produce systemic effects (see Table 31-1).[2] Topically applied eye drops may be absorbed by blood vessels in the conjunctival sac and by the mucosal lining of the nasolacrimal duct. Absorption

Table 31-1 Drugs Administered to Patients Undergoing Eye Surgery

Ophthalmic Indication	Drug	Mechanism of Action	Systemic Effect
Miosis	Acetylcholine	Cholinergic agonist	Bronchospasm, bradycardia, hypotension
Glaucoma (increased intraocular pressure)	Acetazolamide	Carbonic anhydrase inhibitor	Diuresis, hypokalemic metabolic acidosis
	Echothiophate	Irreversible cholinesterase inhibitor	Prolongation of succinylcholine's effects Reduction in plasma cholinesterase activity up to 3-7 weeks after discontinuation Bradycardia, bronchospasm
	Timolol	β-Adrenergic antagonist	Atropine-resistant bradycardia, bronchospasm, exacerbation of congestive heart failure; possible exacerbation of myasthenia gravis
Mydriasis, ophthalmic capillary decongestion	Atropine	Anticholinergic	Central anticholinergic syndrome (mad as a hatter, delirium, agitation; hot as a hare, fever; red as a beet, flushing; dry as a bone, xerostomia, anhidrosis) Blurred vision (cycloplegia, photophobia)
	Cyclopentolate	Anticholinergic	Disorientation, psychosis, convulsions, dysarthria
	Epinephrine	α-, β-Adrenergic agonist	Hypertension, tachycardia, cardiac dysrhythmias; epinephrine paradoxically leads to decreased intraocular pressure and can also be used for glaucoma
	Phenylephrine	α-Adrenergic agonist, direct-acting vasopressor	Hypertension (one drop, or 0.05 mL, of a 10% solution contains 5 mg of phenylephrine)
	Scopolamine	Anticholinergic	Central anticholinergic syndrome (see atropine above)

of these topically administered drugs is prompt (more rapid than subcutaneous administration but slower than intravenous administration). Topical ophthalmic drugs (acetylcholine, anticholinesterases, cocaine, cyclopentolate, epinephrine, phenylephrine, timolol) can have profound effects on IOP and may cause adverse reactions to some medications used in the anesthetic care of these patients (see Table 31-1).[2] It is also important to note that certain ophthalmic drugs, such as glycerol, mannitol, and acetazolamide given systemically, may produce untoward side effects that influence anesthetic management.

Intraocular Pressure

It is essential that the anesthesiologist be familiar with the anatomy and physiology of the ocular system, as well as IOP and how it is influenced by medications, including anesthetics, and by disease processes. IOP is generated by the formation and drainage of aqueous humor. Most of the aqueous humor is formed in the posterior chamber by the ciliary body in an active secretory process involving both the carbonic anhydrase and cytochrome oxidase systems. The remaining aqueous humor is formed by passive filtration of fluid from the vessels on the anterior surface of the iris. Drainage of aqueous humor occurs via the trabecular network, canal of Schlemm, and the episcleral venous system. Obstruction of the drainage system or venous return at any point from the eye to the right side of the heart will elevate IOP.

In a normal eye IOP typically varies between 10 and 22 mm Hg, and it is considered abnormal when higher than 25 mm Hg. IOP varies by 1 to 2 mm Hg with each cardiac contraction. There is also a diurnal variation of 2 to 5 mm Hg, with a higher value noted on awakening. Maintenance of such a relatively high pressure in the eye is important for the integrity of the optical properties of refracting surfaces. Moreover, the corneal surface should be kept at a constant curvature, and the stroma must be under constant high pressure to maintain a uniform refractive index.

FACTORS THAT INFLUENCE INTRAOCULAR PRESSURE
IOP is primarily influenced by (1) external pressure on the eye by contraction of the orbicularis oculi muscle and an increase in tone of the extraocular muscles; (2) the development of scleral rigidity, which usually occurs with aging; and (3) hardening of semisolid intraocular contents, such as the lens and vitreous. External pressure can also

be generated by venous congestion of the orbital veins, which is accentuated during a Valsalva maneuver and during coughing and vomiting. Trauma to the eye causing engorgement with blood also elevates IOP. Hyperventilation and hypothermia decrease IOP, whereas arterial hypoxemia and hypoventilation elevate IOP.

ANESTHETIC DRUGS AND INTRAOCULAR PRESSURE

Most inhaled and injected anesthetics (with the exception of ketamine) reduce IOP. Although the mechanism of action for the reduction in IOP is unclear, it is thought that the central nervous system depression produced by these drugs contributes to the decrease in IOP. Relaxation of the extraocular muscles, a decrease in aqueous humor production, and improved drainage may also contribute to the decreased IOP. Ketamine in larger dose may increase IOP.

SUCCINYLCHOLINE AND INTRAOCULAR PRESSURE

The use of succinylcholine for eye surgery remains controversial, particularly when there is a preexisting increase in IOP.[5] Succinylcholine increases IOP about 8 mm Hg within 1 to 4 minutes after intravenous administration, followed by a return to baseline in about 7 minutes. This increase in IOP is probably due to several mechanisms, including tonic contraction of extraocular muscles, choroidal vascular dilation, and relaxation of orbital smooth muscle, as well as the cycloplegic action of succinylcholine. Pretreatment with a nondepolarizing muscle relaxant or prior intravenous administration of lidocaine, acetazolamide, or propranolol may attenuate succinylcholine-induced increases in IOP.

Oculocardiac Reflex

The oculocardiac reflex can be triggered by multiple stimuli, including (1) external pressure on the globe, (2) traction on the extraocular muscles, (3) traction on the conjunctiva, and (4) placement of a retrobulbar block. The reflex consists of a trigeminal afferent and a vagal efferent pathway. Although bradycardia is the most common clinical manifestation of the oculocardiac reflex, cardiac dysrhythmias (junctional rhythm, ectopic atrial rhythm, atrioventricular blockade, ventricular bigeminy, multifocal premature ventricular contractions, wandering pacemaker, idioventricular rhythm, ventricular tachycardia, asystole) may occur. This reflex is not suppressed by general anesthesia and may be augmented by arterial hypoxemia and hypercapnia.

PREVENTION AND TREATMENT

In children, prophylactic intravenous administration of an anticholinergic drug (atropine, glycopyrrolate) shortly before the potential evoking stimulus may be recommended. The use of intramuscular atropine for prophylactic treatment in adults scheduled for eye surgery has not been found to be effective. Treatment of the clinical manifestations of oculocardiac reflex is removal of the surgical stimulus. If the reflex persists even after removal of the surgical stimulus, the administration of atropine (10 to 20 μg/kg IV) (alternatively, glycopyrrolate) is a consideration.

Anesthesia for Eye Surgery

Patients scheduled for eye surgery range in age from infants to the elderly. In all patients scheduled for eye surgery, preoperative evaluation is very important, including knowledge of the medications used by the patient. The use of general anesthesia is necessary in infants and children because patient cooperation is essential. In adults, most eye procedures can be achieved with monitored anesthesia care, including pulse oximetry and capnography plus the use of a regional block (retrobulbar block, peribulbar block) (Table 31-2). Most anesthetic induction drugs and nondepolarizing neuromuscular blocking drugs may be used. Succinylcholine can be used if it is recognized that this drug transiently increases IOP. When general anesthesia is selected, it is desirable to avoid coughing, nausea, and vomiting on emergence and in the postoperative period.

RETROBULBAR OR PERIBULBAR BLOCK

Surgery involving the cornea, anterior chamber, and lens can be accomplished with a retrobulbar or peribulbar block, provided that the procedure does not last more than 2 hours and the patient is able to cooperate.[3,4] Communication between the anesthesiologist and the patient is important. Retrobulbar and peribulbar blocks are usually placed by the surgeon, although in some practices the anesthesiologist places such blocks.

Technique for a Retrobulbar Block

A retrobulbar block is placed with the patient supine and the nose pointing toward the ceiling. The patient is instructed to look supranasally, and the inferior orbital margin at its most lateral and inferior aspect is palpated. At this site a blunt 25-gauge needle is inserted through a

Table 31-2 Goals in Management of Anesthesia for Ophthalmic Surgery

Control of intraocular pressure
Intense analgesia
Akinesia (motionless eye)
Avoidance of the oculocardiac reflex
Awareness of possible drug interactions
Awakening without coughing, nausea, or vomiting

IV

skin wheal and directed toward the top of the orbital pyramid but remaining inferior to the globe. The needle is advanced about 35 mm to the apex of the muscle cone, at which point 2 to 5 mL of local anesthetic solution with hyaluronidase (to enhance the spread of anesthetic) is injected with frequent aspiration to minimize the risk for accidental intravascular injection. The injection site is massaged for 2 to 5 minutes to facilitate spread of the local anesthetic solution.

A retrobulbar block is relatively safe to place, although side effects may occur (Table 31-3).[6] In addition, block of the orbicularis oculi muscle should be performed to achieve adequate akinesia and analgesia of the eye (Table 31-4).

Technique for a Peribulbar Block

A peribulbar block is technically easier to place, and there is a lower risk of complications than with a retrobulbar block (Table 31-5). For example, there is a reduced risk

Table 31-3	Complications of Retrobulbar Block
Retrobulbar hemorrhage
Stimulation of the oculocardiac reflex
Puncture of the posterior of the globe
Intravenous injection of local anesthetic solution
Intraocular injection
Central retinal artery occlusion
Subdural injection
Spread of local anesthetic to the brainstem causing delayed-onset loss of consciousness because of respiratory depression (post–retrobulbar apnea syndrome)
Blindness
Penetration of the optic nerve
Staphyloma
Local anesthesia spread to the midbrain resulting in paralysis of the contralateral extraocular muscles

Table 31-4	Nerves Affected by a Retrobulbar Block
Nerves blocked are those within the cone (annulus of Zinn)
Optic
Oculomotor—superior and inferior branches
Nasociliary
Abducens

Table 31-5	Characteristics of a Peribulbar Block
Nerves Blocked
Lacrimal
Frontal
Trochlear
Oculomotor
Nasociliary
Abducens
Infraorbital
Zygomatic
Complications
Spread of local anesthetics solution to the contralateral eye
Periorbital ecchymoses
Transient blindness

for retrobulbar hemorrhage, central retinal artery occlusion, optic nerve injury, globe perforation, and intradural injection with this block. A peribulbar block is performed in the supine position with placement of a skin wheal on the lower lid just above the inferior orbital rim, 1.5 cm from the lateral canthus. Lidocaine, 4 mL of a 2% solution (alternatively, 4 mL of 0.5% bupivacaine), with hyaluronidase is injected through the wheal toward the orbit until the lower orbital septum is penetrated. The needle is then advanced toward the equator of the eye and angled in a superomedial direction. An additional 2 to 3 mL of local anesthesia solution with hyaluronidase is then injected into the upper lid, 1 to 2 mm medial and inferior to the supraorbital notch. As the needle is withdrawn, 1 mL of local anesthetic solution is injected into the orbicularis muscle. External pressure is applied to the area for 10 minutes to facilitate spread of the local anesthetic solution.

Technique for a Facial Nerve Block

A facial nerve block is often placed with a retrobulbar block to prevent squinting and to allow placement of a lid speculum. This block is achieved by injecting local anesthetic solution into the region of the outer canthus. The injection is subcutaneous and directed toward the patient's eyebrow and then again toward the infraorbital foramen. A facial nerve block can also be performed in the area of the stylomastoid as the nerve exits with the vagus and glossopharyngeal nerves. However, this technique and injection site may be accompanied by vocal cord paralysis, laryngospasm, dysphagia, and respiratory distress.

Specific Ophthalmic Procedures and Anesthetic Considerations

TRAUMATIC INJURIES TO THE EYE

Eye injuries commonly occur as a result of penetrating or blunt trauma.[7] Frequently, this means providing emergency general anesthesia for a patient with a full stomach and the associated risk of pulmonary aspiration of gastric contents. It is important to avoid any sudden increases in IOP that may cause further extrusion of the ocular contents and loss of vision. Administration of a histamine H_2 receptor antagonist such as cimetidine with metoclopramide will decrease gastric acidity and volume, respectively. Although awake tracheal intubation provides the greatest margin of safety, it is not usually feasible. Placement of a retrobulbar block is ill advised because it can lead to extrusion of the contents of the orbit. For most cases involving trauma to the eye and globe, rapid-sequence or modified rapid-sequence induction of anesthesia is recommended. Precautions that blunt the cardiovascular and IOP responses to laryngoscopy and tracheal intubation should be considered. The choice of succinylcholine (after pretreatment with a nondepolarizing neuromuscular blocking drug) may offer the advantage of rapid-sequence induction of anesthesia and tracheal intubation with minimal change in IOP. Alternatively, the use of a large ("modified rapid-sequence") dose of nondepolarizing neuromuscular blocking drug will reduce IOP and facilitate tracheal intubation (wait to initiate direct laryngoscopy until the response to a peripheral nerve stimulator confirms the onset of neuromuscular blockade).

Strabismus Surgery

Misalignment of the visual axis often requires extraocular muscle ("strabismus") surgery for realignment. Surgical intervention must occur by 4 months of age if proper stereoscopic visual development is to proceed. In older children the operation is performed for cosmetic purposes. Special considerations associated with strabismus surgery include (1) an increased risk for the development of malignant hyperthermia, (2) a high incidence of postoperative nausea and vomiting, and (3) a risk for oculocardiac reflex during surgery.

MALIGNANT HYPERTHERMIA

Strabismus is thought to reflect an underlying myopathy, which has led some to believe that malignant hyperthermia may be more likely to develop in these patients. Indeed, the incidence of isolated masseter spasm after halothane and succinylcholine administration is four times higher in these patients. This risk can be negated by avoiding drugs that are known to trigger malignant hyperthermia. For example, in most cases involving infants and children, the use of succinylcholine is avoided. Nondepolarizing neuromuscular blocking drugs that have a longer duration of action and do not trigger malignant hyperthermia

may be more useful, especially if forced duction to test extraocular muscle tone is needed.[8]

NAUSEA AND VOMITING

The incidence of nausea and vomiting in children after outpatient strabismus surgery varies from 48% to 85%. The high incidence of nausea and vomiting associated with strabismus surgery may be caused by extraocular muscle manipulation or pain that induces an oculocardiac reflex vagal response. Limiting the dose of opioids and substituting propofol for inhaled anesthetics, together with the use of a selective 5-hydroxytryptamine type 3 (5-HT$_3$) receptor antagonist, have been shown to be highly effective in reducing nausea and vomiting after strabismus surgery.

Glaucoma

Glaucoma is characterized by elevated IOP that compresses capillaries and subsequent blood flow to the optic nerve and ultimately by ischemic damage to the optic nerve and blindness.[9] Open-angle glaucoma (chronic glaucoma) and closed-angle glaucoma (acute glaucoma) are examples of glaucoma that may occur in adults.

OPEN-ANGLE GLAUCOMA

Open-angle glaucoma is the most common type of glaucoma encountered in adults. Sclerosis of trabecular tissue results in impaired aqueous filtration and drainage. The disease usually affects both eyes, and over a period of years the chronically elevated IOP slowly, but progressively damages the optic nerves. Treatment consists of lowering IOP with medications that produce miosis and trabecular stretching.

CLOSED-ANGLE GLAUCOMA

Closed-angle glaucoma may occur in individuals who were born with a narrow angle between the iris and cornea. The peripheral portion of the iris comes in direct contact with the posterior corneal surface and mechanically obstructs aqueous outflow. This type of glaucoma can also be caused by swelling of the crystalline lens or by trauma or displacement of the lens. Surgical intervention may be necessary.

GLAUCOMA IN CHILDREN

In infants and children, glaucoma may be manifested as (1) an infantile type occurring any time after birth until 3 years of age and (2) juvenile glaucoma, which can develop between the ages of 3 and 30 years. Infantile glaucoma is frequently associated with obstructed aqueous outflow, and surgical creation of a route for aqueous humor to flow into Schlemm's canal is often required.

TREATMENT

Trabeculectomy is the most common therapeutic surgical procedure to relieve high IOP in patients with glaucoma. In patients in whom surgery fails, a glaucoma seton implant (Molteno valve) is placed. Whereas trabeculectomies may

IV

be performed with monitored anesthesia care, placement of an implant is often done under general anesthesia. In children and infants, goniotomy may be performed to relieve IOP. This procedure requires general anesthesia.

MANAGEMENT OF ANESTHESIA

Special considerations for patients who are scheduled for glaucoma surgery include (1) continuation of drugs that induce miosis throughout the perioperative period; (2) avoidance of venous congestion, which could increase IOP; and (3) awareness of the interaction between antiglaucoma drugs and anesthetic drugs. As with strabismus surgery, avoidance of coughing, nausea, and vomiting is essential.

Cataract Extraction

Cataract formation, manifested as opacification of the lens of the eye, usually occurs with advancing age. Patients with this condition generally have multiple coexisting diseases.[10] Cataract extraction is usually performed under monitored anesthesia care plus a retrobulbar block.

Retinal Detachment Surgery

The retina is the neurosensory tissue that lines the posterior inside wall of the eye and functions like the film in a camera. In essence, the retina transfers the light coming into the eye into vision. The center of the retina is called the macula and is the only part capable of fine detailed vision. The rest of the retina, which makes up more than 95% of the retina, is not capable of fine detailed vision. If the retina detaches from the back wall of the eye, it loses its blood supply and source of nutrition. The lack of blood supply and nutrients causes the retina to degenerate. Retinal breaks without detachment can be treated by laser-induced scarring to seal the retina to the underlying tissue. Injection of an intravitreal bubble of gas is performed for repair of retinal detachment. The gases commonly used, sulfur hexafluoride and carbon octofluorine, are inert, very insoluble in water, and poorly diffusible. Retinal detachments can be repaired by a scleral buckle procedure, vitrectomy, and pneumatic retinopexy.

SCLERAL BUCKLE PROCEDURE

The scleral buckle procedure involves localizing the position of all retinal breaks, treating all retinal breaks with a cryoprobe, and supporting all retinal breaks with a scleral buckle, usually a piece of silicone sponge or solid silicone. The buckle is secured to the outer wall of the orbit (sclera) to create an indentation or buckle effect inside the eye.

VITRECTOMY

Vitrectomy involves making small incisions in the wall of the eye to allow the introduction of instruments for reattaching the retina to the vitreous cavity.

PNEUMATIC RETINOPEXY

Pneumatic retinopexy can be performed to repair a straightforward retinal detachment, especially if there is a single break located in the superior portion of the retina. This procedure involves injecting a gas bubble into the middle part of the eye.

MANAGEMENT OF ANESTHESIA

Anesthesia for repair of retinal detachment can be achieved by regional or general anesthesia. In most cases regional anesthesia is used. With general anesthesia, avoidance of drug-induced skeletal muscle paralysis and prevention of reaction to the tracheal tube during emergence from anesthesia are important. The use of nitrous oxide may expand a hexafluoride gas bubble because nitrous oxide is 117 times more diffusible than sulfur hexafluoride and rapidly enters the gas bubble.[11] This will significantly raise IOP and may adversely affect the outcome of surgery. Hence, if general anesthesia is used, administration of nitrous oxide should be discontinued at least 20 minutes before intravitreal injection of gas (washout of nitrous oxide from the lungs is 90% complete within 10 minutes). The gas bubble may remain in the eye for 10 to 28 days, depending on what gas is used. General anesthesia with nitrous oxide should be avoided during this period.

Injury to the Eye during Anesthesia

Eye injury is most often manifested as postoperative eye pain and is usually caused by corneal abrasion.[12]

CORNEAL ABRASION

Corneal abrasion produces the sensation of the presence of a foreign body in the eye, tearing, conjunctivitis, and photophobia. The pain is made worse by blinking. Corneal abrasions may occur because of loss of the blinking reflex and a decrease in both basal and reflex tear production during anesthesia. The exposed cornea is at high risk for abrasion. Protection against the occurrence of corneal abrasion includes applying nonionic petroleum-based ophthalmic ointment to the eye, securely taping the eyelids shut during anesthesia, and discouraging patients from rubbing their eyes on emergence. Corneal abrasions can be diagnosed by fluorescein staining, and treatment requires the application of antibiotic ophthalmic ointment and covering the eye with a patch for at least 48 hours.

ACUTE GLAUCOMA

An acute glaucoma attack caused by the use of drugs that induce mydriasis will be manifested as dull periorbital pain in the early postoperative period. Administration of mannitol and acetazolamide will reduce the acutely increased IOP and associated pain.

ISCHEMIC EYE INJURY

Ischemic eye injury can occur as a result of unrecognized external pressure on the globe while the patient is in the prone position.[13] If external pressure on the globe exceeds venous pressure, the veins may collapse, arterial inflow may continue, and arterial hemorrhage is likely. If external pressure exceeds arterial pressure, the result is ischemia of the retina.

External pressure on the globe can be prevented by the use of appropriate headrests during anesthesia and surgery. The patient's eyes should be checked throughout the operation to confirm that the position on the headrest has not changed. Confirmation of this observation with a notation on the anesthesia record may be useful.

UNEXPECTED PATIENT MOVEMENT

Unexpected patient movement during ophthalmic surgery as associated with coughing and reacting to the presence of a tracheal tube may result in ocular injury. Monitoring neuromuscular blockade with a peripheral nerve stimulator is useful for maintaining the desired level of drug-induced paralysis during ophthalmic surgery.

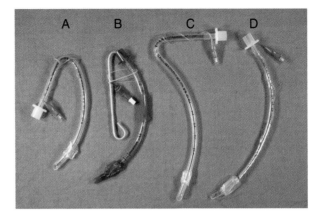

Figure 31-1 Specialized endotracheal tubes used for ear, nose, and throat procedures. Included are an oral RAE and a nasal RAE tube (**A** and **C**), used for tonsillectomies and procedures in the oral cavity, and an armored tube (**B**) and a wrapped tracheal tube (**D**), used for laser procedures. Armored tubes are also commonly used for laryngectomy.

OTOLARYNGOLOGY

Head and neck surgery requires a cooperative relationship between the surgeon and anesthesiologist, especially for surgical procedures involving the airway.[14] It is important to appreciate that manipulation of the larynx, pharynx, and neck may precipitate cardiac dysrhythmias and that blood loss can be underestimated as a result of hidden losses within the surgical drapes and blood swallowed into the stomach. The use of neuromonitoring techniques during surgery to aid the surgeon in identification of peripheral nerves in the operative area may influence the choice and dose of anesthetic and neuromuscular blocking drugs. Damage to nerves that innervate the pharynx, larynx, and especially the vocal cords (may be manifested promptly after tracheal extubation) can occur during head and neck surgery. The presence of laryngeal and pharyngeal edema should be considered before tracheal extubation.

Special Considerations for Head and Neck Surgery

Most patients scheduled for head and neck surgery will have their airway examined by the surgeon before surgery. The anesthesiologist should communicate with the surgeon about the probability of a difficult airway and whether nasal or oral tracheal intubation is indicated for optimal surgical exposure. An awake fiberoptic intubation of the trachea or a tracheostomy under local anesthesia may be indicated if difficult upper airway management is anticipated.[15] The anesthesiologist should be familiar with the variety of endotracheal tubes that are available for head and neck surgery to facilitate better surgical exposure (Fig. 31-1).

LARYNGOSPASM

Instrumentation or manipulation of the endolarynx or the presence of blood or a foreign body can induce laryngospasm. Laryngospasm is an exaggerated and prolonged response of the protective glottic closure reflex, mediated by the superior laryngeal nerve. With severe laryngospasm, the false cords and epiglottic body come together firmly. Airflow is absent, there is no vocal sound, and the true vocal cords cannot be seen. If laryngospasm persists, arterial hypoxemia and hypercapnia will decrease postsynaptic action potentials and brainstem output to the superior laryngeal nerve, and the intensity of the laryngospasm will eventually decrease. The most common method of overcoming laryngospasm is continued positive airway pressure applied by facemask or the intravenous administration of a neuromuscular blocking drug such as succinylcholine (0.25 to 1 mg/kg). Intubation of the trachea may be warranted in selected patients.

Tonsillectomy and Adenoidectomy

Patients who undergo tonsillectomy and adenoidectomy are usually young and healthy. Although recurrent upper respiratory tract infection remains a significant indication for surgery, upper airway obstruction, especially during sleep (obstructive sleep apnea [OSA]), accounts for an increasing percentage of the procedures performed, especially in children younger than 4 years.

Preoperative evaluation for tonsillectomy or adenoidectomy, or both, depends on the initial history and physical examination. In otherwise normal patients who have classic symptoms of severe upper airway obstruction and

IV

adenotonsillar hypertrophy, the preoperative evaluation rarely requires any special studies. In some patients, if severe airway obstruction is suspected, an electrocardiogram, echocardiogram, chest radiograph, and coagulation studies may be considered. Sedative premedication may be avoided in children with OSA, intermittent upper airway obstruction, or very large tonsils.

OBSTRUCTIVE SLEEP APNEA

OSA syndrome may be associated with behavior and growth disturbances. Symptoms in these patients include snoring, sleep disturbances and daytime hypersomnolence, decreased school performance and personality changes, recurrent enuresis, hyponasal speech, and growth disturbances. Patients with OSA are often obese with potentially difficult upper airway management. These individuals will probably have short, thick necks, large tongues, and redundant pharyngeal tissues such that upper airway obstruction is frequent and awake tracheal intubation will be necessary. Polysomnography to evaluate the severity of OSA requires hospitalization, is expensive, and is rarely needed.

UPPER RESPIRATORY TRACT INFECTIONS

Patients may arrive at the hospital for elective tonsillectomy and adenoidectomy with an acute upper respiratory tract infection. Surgery for these patients is usually postponed until resolution of the upper respiratory tract infection, which is typically 7 to 14 days. Laryngospasm with airway manipulation may be more likely to occur in the presence of an upper respiratory tract infection.

GASTROESOPHAGEAL REFLUX DISEASE

Gastroesophageal reflux disease (GERD) may be a significant symptom in children with chronic lung disease or upper airway obstruction (or both) secondary to increased intrathoracic negative pressure. This is particularly relevant in neurologically abnormal patients (hypotonia, developmental delay) because such patients have a high incidence of GERD even without upper airway obstruction. GERD is a consideration in young children with significant developmental delay who require tonsillectomy to treat upper airway obstruction.

MANAGEMENT OF ANESTHESIA

Management of anesthesia for patients undergoing tonsillectomy is focused on airway considerations and bleeding. Continuous positive airway pressure during induction of anesthesia may be useful for alleviating upper airway obstruction. Placement of a cuffed endotracheal tube will decrease the incidence of aspiration of blood. As with an uncuffed tube, a cuffed endotracheal tube should be appropriately sized to allow an air leak around the tube with 20 to 25 cm H_2O of peak airway pressure. The tracheal tube cuff is inflated beyond this point only if high peak airway pressure is needed to

ventilate the lungs adequately or if hemorrhage suddenly develops.[16]

When difficult tracheal intubation is anticipated, it may be helpful to have an otolaryngologist present. The use of an oral RAE tube for tracheal intubation may optimize visualization of the surgical field. The supraglottic area may be packed with petroleum gauze to minimize the likelihood of inhalation of blood from the pharynx. When gauze packing is used, it is important to maintain an appropriate leak around the tube during the application of positive airway pressure.

Surgeons are meticulous about ensuring a dry tonsillar bed at the end of surgery and often place a pack in the posterior of the pharynx to limit draining of blood into the stomach during the procedure. Inserting an orogastric tube into the stomach before extubating the trachea while being careful to not traumatize the adenoidectomy site is a frequent maneuver to remove any blood that may have drained into the stomach. Tracheal extubation is performed when the child is awake and responding. In patients with reactive airway disease, including asthma, tracheal extubation may be performed while the patient is still anesthetized to decrease the likelihood of bronchospasm and laryngospasm.

POSTOPERATIVE CARE AND COMPLICATIONS

Dexamethasone administered intravenously may be useful for decreasing postoperative pain. Adding an intraoperative dose of an antiemetic and removing blood from the stomach may combine to decrease postoperative emesis.

Hemorrhage from a bleeding tonsil in the postoperative period is a recognized complication.[17] The need for tracheal reintubation may be complicated by the presence of large amounts of swallowed blood in the stomach. In this regard, care should be taken to not oversedate these patients. If the bleeding is not controlled, the patient should be returned to the operating room for exploration and surgical hemostasis.

Acute airway obstruction such as laryngospasm can lead to negative-pressure pulmonary edema. This occurs as the patient breathes against a closed glottis and negative intrathoracic pressure is created. This pressure is transmitted to interstitial tissue, where the hydrostatic pressure gradient is increased and enhances fluid movement out of the pulmonary circulation into the alveoli. Airway obstruction in the postoperative period can also be associated with retention of a pharyngeal pack.

The practice of monitoring young children for 24 hours after surgery is based on observations of postoperative airway obstruction occurring in children younger than 4 years as late as 18 to 24 hours postoperatively. In addition to young age, risk factors associated with postoperative airway obstruction after tonsillectomy may include prematurity and recent upper respiratory infection.

Laser Surgery

Laser surgery provides precision in targeting airway lesions, minimal bleeding and edema, preservation of surrounding structures, and rapid healing. The carbon dioxide laser has particular application in the treatment of laryngeal or vocal cord papillomas, laryngeal webs, resection of redundant subglottic tissue, and coagulation of hemangiomas. In most cases laser surgery is preceded by microdirect laryngoscopy. The use of small-diameter endotracheal tubes (5.0 or 5.5 mm internal diameter) is necessary for optimum exposure. Brief skeletal muscle paralysis as provided by an infusion of succinylcholine may be useful.

MANAGEMENT OF ANESTHESIA

Anesthesia during laser surgery may be administered with or without an endotracheal tube.[18] However, appropriate laser-resistant endotracheal tubes should be available. In this regard, all polyvinyl chloride endotracheal tubes are flammable and can ignite and vaporize when in contact with the laser beam. Some surgeons may prefer using a Dedo or Marshall laryngoscope and intermittent ventilation with a Sanders jet ventilator. The Sanders jet ventilator delivers oxygen at 50 psi directly through a port in the laryngoscope. If a Dedo or Marshall laryngoscope is used, maintenance anesthesia can be accomplished with an intravenous anesthetic. Use of the Sanders jet ventilator is associated with a risk for pneumothorax and pneumomediastinum as a result of rupture of alveolar blebs or a bronchus.

Laser surgery produces a plume of smoke and particles (mean size, 0.31 μm) that can be deposited in the alveoli if aspirated (Table 31-6). This hazard can be minimized if an efficient smoke evacuator and special masks are used. A misdirected laser bean can also lead to perforation of a viscus and transection of blood vessels. Other risks include venous gas embolism and ocular injury. The patient's eyes must be protected by taping them shut, followed by the application of wet gauze pads and a metal shield to prevent laser penetration. All operating room personnel should wear special protective glasses.

AIRWAY FIRES

Airway fires are a risk with laser surgery, and thus a plan of action is necessary (Table 31-7).[19] The tracheal tube cuff may be filled with methylene blue so that appearance of the dye provides early warning of cuff rupture by the laser beam. Inspired oxygen concentrations limited to 30% (dilution with air) are often recommended because both oxygen and nitrous oxide support combustion. If a an airway fire occurs, the anesthesia delivery circuit should be immediately disconnected from the endotracheal tube (to achieve cessation of ventilation and delivery of oxygen), followed by removal of the tracheal tube from the patient's airway. If the flame persists, the field should be flooded with normal saline. Direct examination of the pharynx and larynx is indicated to evaluate the extent of the burn. The patient should be reintubated with a regular endotracheal tube after the bronchoscope is removed and monitored for at least 24 hours. Corticosteroids and antibiotics should be considered for severe burns.

Epiglottitis

Acute epiglottitis is an infectious disease caused by *Haemophilus influenzae* type B. It can progress rapidly from a sore throat, to airway obstruction, to respiratory failure and death if proper diagnosis and treatment are delayed. Patients are usually between 2 and 7 years of age, although epiglottitis has been reported in younger children and adults. Characteristic signs and symptoms of acute epiglottitis include (1) a sudden onset of fever, dysphagia, drooling, thick muffled voice, and preference for the sitting position with the head extended and leaning forward and (2) retractions, labored breathing, and cyanosis when respiratory obstruction is present.

IV

Table 31-6 *Hazards Associated with Laser Surgery*

Atmospheric contamination from vaporization of tissues (smoke and fine particles)

Misdirected laser energy (viscus perforation, transection of uncoagulable blood vessels)

Venous gas embolism

Ocular injury (cornea, retina)

Airway fire (endotracheal tube ignition)

Table 31-7 Airway Fire Protocol during Laser Surgery

Disconnect the anesthesia delivery circuit from the tracheal tube and cease ventilation of the patient's lungs (removes the enriched oxygen source)

Extubate the trachea

Extinguish the removed flaming material in water

Ventilate the patient's lungs with oxygen by facemask and reintubate the trachea

Perform rigid bronchoscopy to assess airway damage and remove debris

Assess the oropharynx and face

Obtain a chest radiograph

Consider bronchial lavage and corticosteroids

TREATMENT

Direct visualization of the epiglottis should not be attempted in an awake patient because it could lead to airway compromise and death. Interactions with the patient should be kept to a minimum. Stimulation of the patient or the onset of struggling during attempted treatment procedures may result in exacerbation of the airway obstruction. Induction of anesthesia is often accomplished with the inhalation of sevoflurane (alternatively, halothane) while maintaining spontaneous ventilation. It is important to secure the airway without stimulating the reactive airway. An emergency airway cart and tracheostomy tray should be available and open, with appropriate personnel present should an emergency surgical airway be needed.

Postoperative management takes place in the intensive care unit and consists of continued observation and radiographic confirmation of tracheal tube placement. Tracheal extubation is usually attempted 48 to 72 hours later when a significant leak around the endotracheal tube is present and visual inspection of the larynx by flexible fiberoptic bronchoscopy confirms a reduction in swelling of the epiglottis and surrounding tissue.

Foreign Body in the Airway

Aspiration of a foreign body into the trachea is an emergency, especially in the pediatric population. Clinical manifestations of this phenomenon include a sudden onset of difficulty breathing, dry cough, hoarseness, or even wheezing in young children. Treatment of foreign body aspiration into the trachea involves special cooperation between the anesthesiologist and the surgeon because care must be taken to avoid converting partial airway obstruction into total obstruction by distal displacement of the foreign body.

TREATMENT

Removal of a foreign body may include awake direct laryngoscopy or performance of a rigid bronchoscopic examination without the application of positive airway pressure.[20] During this period a surgeon should be present and prepared to perform an emergency tracheostomy or cricothyrotomy should total airway obstruction occur. When a rigid bronchoscope is used, an intravenous anesthetic may be necessary to avoid exposing the surgeon to inhaled anesthetics. All patients should be observed closely during the recovery period for airway edema and respiratory compromise. The use of humidified oxygen is suggested.

Parotid Gland Surgery

Parotid gland surgery is usually performed for tumors and occasionally for treatment of infectious disorders. Some diseases of the parotid gland may be associated with alcohol abuse, and these patients may exhibit signs and symptoms of alcohol-related diseases. Parotid gland surgery is performed under general anesthesia and often with monitoring of the facial nerve to avoid surgical damage to this important structure. Neuromuscular blocking drugs may be avoided when nerve monitoring is performed, although preservation of a twitch response with a peripheral nerve stimulator should permit identification of skeletal muscle response to direct electrical stimulation of the facial nerve.[21] When a radical parotidectomy is performed, the facial nerve may be sacrificed and reconstructed with a graft from the contralateral greater auricular nerve. Nasotracheal intubation may be preferable to orotracheal intubation if the mandible has to be dislocated during surgery.

Facial Trauma

Facial fractures are characterized by the Le Fort classification of maxilla fractures (Fig. 31-2).[22] A Le Fort I fracture extends across the lower portion of the maxilla but does not continue up into the medial canthal region. A Le Fort II fracture also extends across the maxilla, but at a more cephalad level, and it also continues upward to the medial canthal region. A Le Fort III fracture is a high-level transverse fracture above the malar bone and through the orbits. It is characterized by complete separation of the maxilla from the craniofacial skeleton. Orotracheal intubation is necessary when intranasal damage is a possibility. In cosmetic surgery, Le Fort fractures are created for cosmetic repair.

Nasal Surgery

Nasal surgery is most often performed for cosmetic purposes or for functional restoration of the upper airway. Functional restoration is usually performed for either congenital or post-traumatic deviations of the septum. Nasal surgery is typically performed in the physician's office with local anesthesia and intravenous sedation.

A special consideration in nasal surgery is drug-induced (cocaine, epinephrine) vasoconstriction of the nasal mucosa to reduce bleeding. These drugs may have a profound effect on the cardiovascular system, especially in elderly patients or those with known cardiac disease. Cardiac dysrhythmias may accompany drug-induced nasal vasoconstriction. A moderate degree of controlled hypotension combined with head elevation decreases bleeding in the surgical site. Blood may passively enter the stomach during surgery, and placement of an oropharyngeal pack or suctioning of the stomach at the conclusion of surgery may attenuate postoperative retching and vomiting.

Ear Surgery

Placement of myringotomy tubes, tympanoplasty, and placement of cochlear implants are examples of operations that may be characterized as ear surgery. These surgeries usually require general anesthesia and in some cases rely

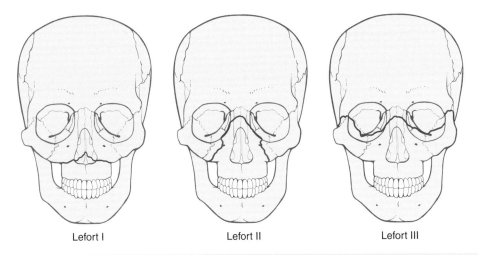

Lefort I   Lefort II   Lefort III

Figure 31-2 Facial injuries and the Le Fort fracture classification. (From Myer CM. Trauma of the larynx and craniofacial structures: Airway implications. Paediatr Anaesth 2004;14:103-106, with permission.)

on neuromonitoring. When nerve monitoring is used, neuromuscular blocking drugs are avoided or the dose is greatly decreased to preserve a skeletal muscle response with peripheral nerve stimulation.[21] Nausea and vomiting are common after ear surgery. Pretreatment with antiemetics and inclusion of propofol and sevoflurane in the management of anesthesia reduces the incidence of postoperative nausea and vomiting after ear surgery.

MYRINGOTOMY AND TUBE INSERTION

Myringotomy with tube insertion is often performed in children with disorders of the middle ear. Premedication is not recommended in these patients because most sedative drugs will outlast the duration of the surgical procedure. Anesthesia may be accomplished with a volatile drug, oxygen, and nitrous oxide administered by facemask.

MIDDLE EAR AND MASTOID

Tympanoplasty and mastoidectomy are common procedures performed on the middle ear and accessory structures. Tracheal intubation should be accomplished with an oral or nasal RAE tube to minimize intrusion into the surgical field. If nitrous oxide is included in the management of anesthesia, it is recommended that this gas be discontinued at least 30 minutes before placement of the tympanic membrane graft to avoid displacement of the graft by outward diffusion of nitrous oxide into the air-filled middle ear. Tracheal extubation is often accomplished while the patient is still anesthetized to avoid any straining that may displace the tympanic membrane graft or disrupt other repairs. Postoperative nausea and vomiting are a common problem that may be reduced by (1) decompressing the stomach after induction of anes-

thesia, (2) limiting the use of opioids, and (3) administering prophylactic antiemetics.

Neck Surgery

Neck dissection may be complete, modified, or functional. Anatomically, the structures principally involved are (1) the sternocleidomastoid muscle, (2) cranial nerve XI, and (3) the internal and external jugular veins and carotid artery. Frequently, neck dissection is performed for removal of a tumor and may also involve partial or total glossectomy. Patients with such tumors may have a history of tobacco and alcohol abuse. Pulmonary disease is likely and is an indication for a preoperative pulmonary workup.

MANAGEMENT OF ANESTHESIA

In a high percentage of cases the neck dissection may be bilateral and a tracheostomy is performed to maintain a patent airway. Upper airway management may be difficult in these patients, especially if there is a history of radiation treatment of the larynx and pharynx or if a mass is present in the oral cavity. Neuromuscular blocking drugs are avoided or the dose is greatly decreased if neuromonitoring is used. Dissection around the carotid bulb may precipitate bradycardia, which may be treated by the injection of local anesthetic solution into the bulb or by the intravenous injection of atropine or glycopyrrolate. Postoperative laryngeal edema can be a significant problem if drains are not placed in the operative area.

POSTOPERATIVE COMPLICATIONS

In the postoperative period the anesthesiologist should be aware of potential nerve injuries, including facial palsy

IV

as a result of surgical damage to branches of the facial nerve. Injury to the recurrent laryngeal nerve can cause vocal cord dysfunction and, if bilateral, results in airway obstruction. Because the phrenic nerve also traverses through the operative field, paralysis of the hemidiaphragm can occur.

Spontaneous breathing is impaired if the phrenic nerve injury is bilateral. Pneumothorax can also occur in the postoperative period. Excessive coughing or agitation can result in hematoma formation and airway compromise.

REFERENCES

1. Kubitz JC, Motsch J. Eye surgery in the elderly. Best Pract Res Clin Anaesthesiol 2003;17:245-257.
2. Koch PS. Preoperative and postoperative medications of anesthesia. Curr Opin Ophthalmol 1998;9:5-9.
3. Kallio H, Rosenberg PH. Advances in ophthalmic regional anaesthesia. Best Pract Res Clin Anaesthesiol 2005;19:215-227.
4. Ripart J, Nouvellon E, Chaumeron A. Regional anesthesia for eye surgery. Reg Anesth Pain Med 2005;30:72-82.
5. Kelly RE, Dinner M, Turner LOS, et al. Succinylcholine increases intraocular pressure in the human eye with the extraocular muscles detached. Anesthesiology 1993;79:948-952.
6. Chang J-L, Gonzales-Abola E, Larson CE. Brain stem anesthesia following retrobulbar block. Anesthesiology 1984;61:789-790.
7. Hamid RK, Newfield P. Pediatric eye emergencies. Anesthesiol Clin North Am 2001;19:257-264.
8. Geldner G, Wulf H. Muscle relaxants suitable for day case surgery. Eur J Anaesthesiol 2001;23:43-46.

9. Levin LA. Pathophysiology of the progressive optic neuropathy of glaucoma. Ophthalmol Clin North Am 2005;18:355-364.
10. Schein OD, Katz J, Bass EB, et al. The value of routine preoperative medical testing before cataract surgery. N Engl J Med 2000;342:168-175.
11. Wolf GL, Capuano C, Hartung J. Nitrous oxide increases intraocular pressure after intravitreal sulfur hexafluoride injection. Anesthesiology 1983;59:547-548.
12. Roth S, Thisted RA, Erickson JP, et al. Eye injuries after nonocular surgery. A study of 60,965 anesthetics from 1988 to 1992. Anesthesiology 1996;85:1020-1027.
13. Gild WM, Posner KL, Caplan RA, Cheney FW. Eye injuries associated with anesthesia. A closed claims analysis. Anesthesiology 1992;76:204-208.
14. Sataloff RT, Brown AC. Special equipment in the operating room for otolaryngology–head and neck surgery. Otolaryngol Clin North Am 1981;14:669-686.
15. Verghese ST, Hannallah RS. Pediatric otolaryngologic emergencies.

Anesthesiol Clin North Am 2001;19:237-256.
16. Fine GF, Borland LM. The future of the cuffed endotracheal tube. Pediatr Anesthesiol 2004;14:38-42.
17. Randall DA, Hoffer ME. Complications of tonsillectomy and adenoidectomy. Otolaryngol Head Neck Surg 1998;118:61-68.
18. Rampil IJ. Anesthetic considerations for laser surgery. Anesth Analg 1992;74:424-435.
19. Mattucci KF, Militana CJ. The prevention of fire during oropharyngeal electrosurgery. Ear Nose Throat J 2003;82:107-109.
20. Lam HC, Woo JK, van Hasselt CA. Management of ingested foreign bodies: A retrospective review of 5240 patients. J Laryngol Otol 2001;115;954-957.
21. Paloheimo M, Edmonds HL, Wirtavouri K, et al. Assessment of anaesthetic adequacy with upper facial and abdominal wall EMG. Eur J Anesthiol 1989;6:119-123.
22. Myer CM. Trauma of the larynx and craniofacial structures: Airway implications. Paediatr Anaesth 2004;14:103-106.

OBSTETRICS

Mark A. Rosen and Samuel C. Hughes

Modern-era obstetric anesthesia can be dated to January 19, 1847, when a Scottish physician, James Young Simpson, used diethyl ether to anesthetize a woman with a contracted pelvis. Fanny Longfellow, wife of Henry Wadsworth Longfellow, was the first woman in the United States to receive anesthesia for childbirth, barely 4 months after Simpson first used anesthesia in Edinburgh, and publicly proclaimed in 1847, "This is certainly the greatest blessing of this age."

Providing peripartum analgesia and anesthesia requires an understanding of the physiologic changes during pregnancy and labor, the effects of anesthetics on the fetus and neonate, and the benefits and risks associated with various techniques of analgesia and anesthesia. Furthermore, it requires an understanding of the course of labor and delivery, as well as potential obstetric emergencies and complications that demand immediate obstetric intervention and skilled anesthesia care, such as fetal distress, maternal hemorrhage, and prolapsed cord.

PHYSIOLOGIC CHANGES IN PREGNANT WOMEN

During pregnancy, labor, and delivery, women undergo fundamental changes in anatomy and physiology as a result of altered hormonal activity; biochemical changes associated with increasing metabolic demands of a growing fetus, placenta, and uterus; and mechanical displacement by an enlarging uterus.[1,2] Beyond midgestation, women are at increased risk for pulmonary aspiration of acidic gastric contents because of decreased competence of the lower esophageal sphincter, as well as delayed gastric emptying with the onset of labor or opioid administration. This has an important impact on the method of induction of general anesthesia and airway management selected by the anesthesiologist.

Cardiovascular System Changes

Changes in the cardiovascular system during pregnancy can be summarized as (1) an increase in intravascular fluid volume, (2) an increase in cardiac output, and (3) a decrease in systemic vascular resistance (Table 32-1).

INTRAVASCULAR FLUID VOLUME

Maternal intravascular fluid volume increases in the first trimester, and at term the plasma volume is increased about 45% and the erythrocyte volume about 20%. This disproportionate increase in plasma volume accounts for the relative anemia of pregnancy. The increased intravascular fluid volume offsets the 300 to 500 mL blood loss that accompanies vaginal delivery and the average 800 to 1000 mL blood loss that accompanies cesarean section. The total plasma protein concentration is decreased as a result of the dilutional effect of the increased intravascular fluid volume.

CARDIAC OUTPUT

Cardiac output increases about 10% by the 10th week of gestation and increases 40% to 50% by the third trimester. This augmentation of cardiac output is due to an increased stroke volume (25% to 30%) and heart rate (15% to 25%). The onset of labor is associated with further increases in cardiac output, with the largest increase occurring immediately after delivery, when cardiac output is increased by as much as 80%. This presents a unique postpartum risk for patients with cardiac disease, such as fixed valvular stenosis. A regional anesthetic is capable of attenuating the release of catecholamines during painful labor and the resultant maternal tachycardia and systemic hypertension. Cardiac output substantially returns toward prepregnant values by 2 weeks postpartum.

SYSTEMIC VASCULAR RESISTANCE

Systolic blood pressure decreases by as much as 15% during an uncomplicated pregnancy. Although there is an increase in cardiac output and plasma volume, systemic blood pressure does not increase because of a decrease in systemic vascular resistance (mean arterial pressure may decrease slightly). Furthermore, there is no change in central venous pressure during pregnancy despite the increased plasma volume because venous capacitance increases. Femoral venous pressure increases about 15%, presumably reflecting compression of the inferior vena cava by the gravid uterus.

AORTOCAVAL COMPRESSION (SUPINE HYPOTENSION SYNDROME)

Decreases in maternal blood pressure because of aortocaval compression by the gravid uterus are associated with the supine position. Significant aortoiliac artery compression occurs in 15% to 20% of pregnant women and vena cava compression in all such women. Vena cava compression may contribute to lower extremity venous stasis and thereby result in ankle edema and varices. Diaphoresis, nausea, vomiting, and changes in cerebration may accompany this hypotension. These symptoms are termed the "supine hypotension syndrome."

Table 32-1 Changes in the Cardiovascular System during Pregnancy	
	Value Near Term Compared with Nonpregnant Value
Intravascular fluid volume	Increased 35%
Plasma volume	Increased 45%
Erythrocyte volume	Increased 20%
Cardiac output	Increased 40%-50%
Stroke volume	Increased 30%
Heart rate	Increased 15%-25%
Peripheral circulation Mean arterial blood pressure	Decreased 15 mm Hg
Systolic blood pressure	Decreased 0-15 mm Hg
Diastolic blood pressure	Decreased 10-20 mm Hg
Systemic vascular resistance	Decreased 20%
Pulmonary vascular resistance	Decreased 35%
Central venous pressure	No change
Femoral venous pressure	Increased 15%

Mechanism and Compensatory Responses

The mechanism of supine hypotension syndrome is decreased venous return as a result of compression of the inferior vena cava by the gravid uterus when the pregnant woman assumes the supine position (Fig. 32-1). The resulting decrease in venous return leads to a decrease in cardiac output and a decline in systemic blood pressure. Fortunately, most pregnant women undergo compensatory responses on assuming the supine position that prevent hypotension despite aortocaval compression. One compensatory mechanism is increased venous pressure below the level of compression of the inferior vena cava, which serves to divert venous blood from the lower half of the body via the paravertebral venous plexuses to the azygos vein. Flow from the azygos vein enters the superior vena cava and venous return is maintained. Dilation of the epidural veins may make penetration of a vein more likely during attempted lumbar epidural anesthesia and thus could lead to accidental intravascular injection of the local anesthetic solution. This would result in a bolus delivery of local anesthetic to the heart with potentially profound consequences on the central nervous and cardiovascular systems.

Another compensatory response that prevents hypotension with aortocaval compression is a reflex increase in peripheral sympathetic nervous system activity. This results in increased systemic vascular resistance and permits systemic blood pressure to be maintained despite decreased cardiac output. It is important to recognize that compensatory increases in systemic vascular resistance are impaired by regional anesthetic techniques. Indeed, arterial hypotension is more common and profound during regional anesthesia administered to pregnant as compared with nonpregnant women.

In addition to compression of the inferior vena cava, the gravid uterus can compress the lower abdominal aorta (see Fig. 32-1). Such compression leads to arterial hypotension in the lower extremities, but maternal symptoms or decreases in systemic blood pressure as measured in the arms do not occur.

Risks

The significance of aortocaval compression is the associated decrease in uterine and placental blood flow. Even with a healthy uteroplacental unit, prolonged maternal hypotension (approximately 90 to 100 mm Hg systolic blood pressure for an average patient) for longer than 10 to 15 minutes will most likely significantly decrease uterine blood flow and lead to progressive fetal acidosis.

Venous compression by the gravid uterus diverts some blood returning from the lower extremities through the internal vertebral venous plexus to the azygos and epidural veins, thereby increasing the likelihood of epidural venous puncture with epidural or spinal techniques. Supine positioning is avoided in pregnant women during anesthetic administration in the second and third trimesters. Anesthetic techniques that interfere with increased sympathetic nervous system tone will further compromise the compensatory mechanisms for vena cava compression induced by supine positioning and potentially cause profound hypotension.

Treatment

Displacing the gravid uterus can minimize the incidence of supine hypotension syndrome, which is important for patients undergoing regional or general anesthesia because their compensatory increases in systemic vascular resistance will be impaired. Displacement of the gravid uterus can be achieved by placing the pregnant woman in the lateral position or by moving the gravid uterus to the left and off the inferior vena cava or aorta. Displacement of the uterus to the left can be accomplished manually or by elevation of the right hip 10 to 15 cm with a blanket or wedge (Fig. 32-2).

Pulmonary System Changes

The most significant changes in the pulmonary system during pregnancy include alterations in (1) the upper airway, (2) minute ventilation, (3) lung volumes, and (4) arterial oxygenation (Table 32-2).

UPPER AIRWAY

Capillary engorgement of the mucosal lining of the upper respiratory tract accompanies pregnancy, thus emphasizing the need for careful instrumentation of the upper airway during suctioning, placement of airways (avoid nasal instrumentation if possible), and direct laryngoscopy. It may be prudent to select a smaller cuffed tracheal tube (6.5 to 7.0 mm internal diameter) because the vocal cords

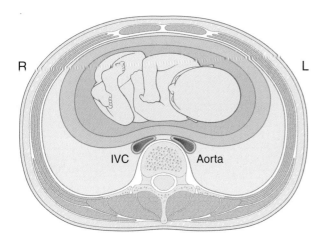

Figure 32-1 Schematic diagram showing compression of the inferior vena cava (IVC) and abdominal aorta by the gravid uterus when the parturient assumes the supine position.

IV

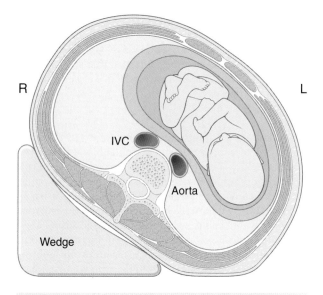

R

L

IVC

Aorta

Wedge

Figure 32-2 Schematic diagram depicting left uterine displacement by elevation of the parturient's right hip with a foam rubber wedge. This position moves the gravid uterus off the inferior vena cava (IVC) and aorta.

and arytenoids are often edematous. Weight gain associated with pregnancy, particularly in women of short stature or with coexisting obesity, can result in difficulty inserting the laryngoscope because of a short neck and large breasts.

MINUTE VENTILATION

Minute ventilation is increased about 50% above prepregnant levels during the first trimester and is maintained for the remainder of the pregnancy. This increased minute ventilation is achieved primarily by an increased tidal volume, with small increases in the respiratory rate (see Table 32-2). Increased circulating levels of progesterone are presumed to be the stimulus for increased minute ventilation.

Resting maternal $PaCO_2$ decreases from 40 to about 32 mm Hg during the first trimester as a reflection of the increased minute ventilation. Arterial pH, however, remains near normal because of increased renal excretion of bicarbonate ions. The pain associated with labor and delivery results in further hyperventilation, which can be attenuated by adequate analgesia, such as lumbar epidural analgesia.

LUNG VOLUMES

Lung volumes, in contrast to the early appearance of increased minute ventilation, do not begin to change until about the third month of pregnancy (see Table 32-2). With increasing enlargement of the uterus, the diaphragm is forced cephalad, which is primarily responsible for the 20% decrease in functional residual capacity (FRC) present at term. As a result, FRC can be less than closing capacity for many small airways and may give rise to atelectasis in the supine position. Vital capacity is not significantly changed.

The combination of increased minute ventilation and decreased FRC results in an increase in the rate at which changes in the alveolar concentration of inhaled anesthetics

Table 32-2 Changes in the Pulmonary System during Pregnancy	
	Value Near Term Compared with Nonpregnant Value
Minute ventilation	Increased 50%
Tidal volume	Increased 40%
Breathing frequency	Increased 15%
Lung volumes Expiratory reserve volume	Decreased 20%
Residual volume	Decreased 20%
Functional residual capacity	Decreased 20%
Vital capacity	No change
Total lung capacity	Decreased 0-5%
Arterial blood gases and pH PaO_2	Normal or slightly decreased
$PaCO_2$	Decreased 10 mm Hg
pH	No change
Oxygen consumption	Increased 20%

can be achieved. This affects induction of anesthesia, emergence from anesthesia, and changes in depth of anesthesia.

ARTERIAL OXYGENATION

Early in gestation, maternal PaO_2 while breathing room air is normally above 100 mm Hg because of the presence of hyperventilation. Later, PaO_2 becomes normal or even slightly decreased, most likely reflecting airway closure. During induction of general anesthesia in a pregnant patient, PaO_2 decreases more rapidly than in a nonpregnant patient because of decreased oxygen reserve (decreased FRC) and increased oxygen uptake (increased metabolic rate). For these reasons, the administration of supplemental oxygen during a regional anesthetic or "preoxygenation" (breathe oxygen for 3 minutes, four to five deep breaths, or eight maximal breaths over a 1-minute period) before any anticipated period of apnea (such as induction of general anesthesia) is recommended.[3,4]

Nervous System Changes

Anesthetic requirements (minimum alveolar concentration [MAC]) for volatile anesthetics decrease during pregnancy as demonstrated in humans and animals.[5] The sedative effects produced by progesterone may be partially responsible. The important clinical implication of decreased MAC is that alveolar concentrations of inhaled drugs that would not produce unconsciousness in nonpregnant patients may approximate anesthetizing concentrations in pregnant women. This degree of central nervous system depression can impair protective upper airway reflexes and subject pregnant women to pulmonary aspiration. Furthermore, the decreased FRC increases the rate at which potential excessive alveolar concentrations of anesthetics can be achieved.

Engorgement of epidural veins as intra-abdominal pressure increases with progressive enlargement of the uterus results in a decrease in the size of the epidural space and decreased volume of cerebrospinal fluid (CSF) in the subarachnoid space. The decreased volume of these spaces facilitates the spread of local anesthetics. The observation of increased spread of local anesthetic solutions placed in the epidural space as early as the first trimester suggests a role for biochemical as well as mechanical changes. Indeed, data from pregnant women demonstrate increased peripheral nerve sensitivity to lidocaine. These mechanical and biochemical changes are consistent with the decrease in dose requirements of local anesthetics necessary for epidural or spinal anesthesia in pregnant women at term gestation.

Renal Changes

Renal blood flow and the glomerular filtration rate are increased about 50% to 60% by the third month of pregnancy. Therefore, the normal upper limits in blood urea nitrogen and serum creatinine concentrations are decreased about 50% in pregnant women.

Hepatic Changes

Plasma protein concentrations are reduced during pregnancy because of dilution, similar to the physiologic anemia of pregnancy. Decreased serum albumin levels can result in higher free blood levels of highly protein-bound drugs. Slightly elevated liver function test results do not necessarily indicate hepatic disease. Plasma cholinesterase (pseudocholinesterase) activity is decreased about 25% from the 10th week of gestation to as long as 6 weeks postpartum. This decreased activity is unlikely to be associated with significant prolongation of the neuromuscular blocking effects of succinylcholine or mivacurium. As part of the hypercoagulable state of pregnancy, plasma concentrations of coagulation factors, including fibrinogen, are increased.

Gastrointestinal Changes

Gastrointestinal changes during pregnancy make pregnant women vulnerable to regurgitation of gastric contents and to the development of acid pneumonitis should pulmonary aspiration occur. Displacement of the pylorus cephalad by the enlarged uterus retards gastric emptying, and progesterone decreases gastrointestinal motility. As a result, gastric fluid volume tends to be increased even in the fasting state. In addition, gastrin, which is secreted by the placenta, stimulates gastric hydrogen ion secretion such that the pH of gastric fluid is predictably low in pregnant women. The enlarging uterus changes the angle of the gastroesophageal junction and thereby leads to relative incompetence of the physiologic sphincter mechanism. For this reason, gastric fluid reflux into the esophagus with subsequent esophagitis (heartburn) is common in pregnant women.

RISK OF ASPIRATION

Regardless of the time interval since the ingestion of food, women in labor must be treated as having a full stomach. Pain, anxiety, and drugs (especially opioids) administered during labor can all slow gastric emptying beyond an already prolonged transit time.

The increased risk for pulmonary aspiration of gastric contents is the reason for recommending placement of a cuffed tube in the trachea of pregnant women rendered unconscious by anesthesia. The recognition that the pH of inhaled gastric fluid is important in the production and severity of acid pneumonitis is the basis for the administration of antacids to pregnant women before induction of anesthesia. To obviate the hazards of inhalation of particulate antacids that can increase pulmonary damage, the use of a nonparticulate antacid such as sodium citrate is recommended. H_2 receptor antagonists usually increase

IV

gastric fluid pH in pregnant women without producing adverse effects and are recommended by some. H_2 receptor antagonists, unlike antacids, do not alter the pH of gastric fluid already present in the stomach. Combinations of an H_2 receptor antagonist and sodium citrate may be more useful than an antacid alone for producing a persistent increase in gastric fluid pH.

Metoclopramide can be useful for decreasing the gastric fluid volume of pregnant women in active labor who require general anesthesia and are considered to be at high risk for increased gastric fluid volume (apprehension, systemic opioid analgesia, recent solid food ingestion). The gastric hypomotility associated with opioid administration, however, may be resistant to treatment with metoclopramide.

PHYSIOLOGY OF THE UTEROPLACENTAL CIRCULATION

The placenta is a union of maternal and fetal tissue for the purpose of physiologic exchange. Maternal blood is delivered to the placenta by the uterine arteries, and fetal blood arrives via two umbilical arteries. Nutrient-rich and waste-free blood is delivered to the fetus through a single umbilical vein.

Uterine Blood Flow

Uterine blood flow increases to about 700 mL/min (about 10% of cardiac output) at term gestation, with about 80% of the uterine blood flow perfusing the intervillous space (placenta) and 20% the myometrium. The uterine vasculature is not autoregulated and remains essentially maximally dilated under normal conditions during pregnancy. Though capable of marked vasoconstriction in response to α-adrenergic drugs, pregnancy is associated with reduced uterine artery response and sensitivity to vasoconstrictors. Uterine blood flow decreases because of decreased uterine perfusion pressure as a result of systemic hypotension (shock; general, epidural, or spinal anesthesia). Uterine blood flow also decreases with aortocaval compression or increased uterine venous pressure as a result of vena cava compression (supine position) or uterine contractions (particularly uterine hyperstimulation as may occur with oxytocin administration or abruption). Epidural or spinal anesthesia does not alter uterine blood flow as long as maternal hypotension is avoided.

In an animal model, α-adrenergic stimulation produced by methoxamine and metaraminol increased uterine vascular resistance and decreased uterine blood flow, whereas administration of ephedrine was not accompanied by significant decreases in uterine blood flow despite drug-induced increases in maternal arterial blood pressure.[6] Largely based on these animal data, ephedrine has been considered the drug of choice for the treatment of hypotension caused by the administration of regional anesthesia to pregnant women. The applicability of these data to humans, however, has been questioned, and there is evidence that the use of α-adrenergic agonists to correct maternal hypotension is not associated with adverse effects on indices of fetal well-being.[7] Studies suggest that the use of ephedrine results in clinically nonsignificant increased umbilical cord blood acidemia when compared with the use of phenylephrine. Nevertheless, caution would still seem to be indicated in pregnant women with known uteroplacental insufficiency because maternal hypotension, as well as correction of the hypotension with an α-adrenergic agonist, might further compromise the fetus. Both drugs are now commonly used in practice; prompt correction of maternal hypotension will lead to the best neonatal outcome.

Increased uterine vascular resistance with decreases in uterine blood flow can also result from maternal stress or pain that stimulates the endogenous release of catecholamines (Fig. 32-3).[8] This response suggests that a

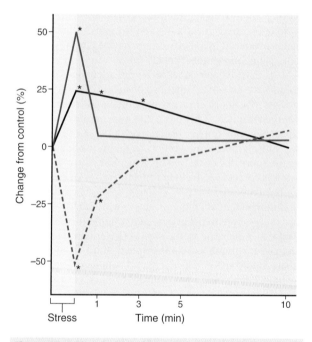

Figure 32-3 Electrically induced stress lasting 30 to 60 seconds in pregnant ewes results in increased maternal blood pressure (*solid red line*) and serum norepinephrine concentrations (*solid black line*). Uterine blood flow (*dashed red line*) is decreased about 50% at the time of the maximum increase in maternal blood pressure and catecholamines. Mean ± SEM. *Significantly different from control (*P* < .05). (From Shnider SM, Wright RG, Levinson G, et al. Uterine blood flow and plasma norepinephrine changes during maternal stress in the pregnant ewe. Anesthesiology 1979;50:524-527, with permission.)

regional or general anesthetic may be protective to the fetus in certain instances. Uterine contractions also decrease uterine blood flow secondary to increased uterine venous pressure.

Placental Exchange

Placental exchange of substances occurs principally by diffusion from the maternal circulation to the fetus and vice versa. Diffusion of a substance across the placenta to the fetus depends on maternal-to-fetal concentration gradients, maternal protein binding, molecular weight, lipid solubility, and the degree of ionization of that substance. Minimizing the maternal blood concentration of a drug is the most important method of limiting the amount that ultimately reaches the fetus.

The high molecular weight and poor lipid solubility of nondepolarizing neuromuscular blocking drugs result in limited ability of these drugs to cross the placenta. Succinylcholine has a low molecular weight but is highly ionized and therefore does not readily cross the placenta. Thus, during administration of a general anesthetic for cesarean section, the fetus/neonate is not paralyzed. Placental transfer of barbiturates, local anesthetics, and opioids is facilitated by the relatively low molecular weights of these substances. Drugs that readily cross the blood-brain barrier also cross the placenta.

FETAL UPTAKE

Fetal uptake of a substance that crosses the placenta is facilitated by the lower pH (0.1 unit) of fetal than maternal blood. The lower fetal pH means that weakly basic drugs (local anesthetics, opioids) that cross the placenta in the nonionized form will become ionized in the fetal circulation. Because an ionized drug cannot readily cross the placenta back to the maternal circulation, this drug will accumulate in the fetal blood against a concentration gradient. This phenomenon is known as ion trapping and may explain the higher concentrations of lidocaine found in the fetus when acidosis secondary to fetal distress is present (Fig. 32-4).[9] Furthermore, conversion of lidocaine to the ionized fraction maintains the concentration gradient from the mother to the fetus for continued passage of nonionized lidocaine to the fetus. Despite decreased enzyme activity in comparison to adults, neonatal enzyme systems are adequately developed to metabolize most drugs, with the possible exception of mepivacaine.

UNIQUE CHARACTERISTICS OF THE FETAL CIRCULATION

The unique characteristics of the fetal circulation influence the distribution of drugs in the fetus and protect the vital organs of the fetus from exposure to high concentrations of drugs initially present in umbilical venous blood. For example, about 75% of umbilical venous blood passes through the liver such that significant portions of drugs

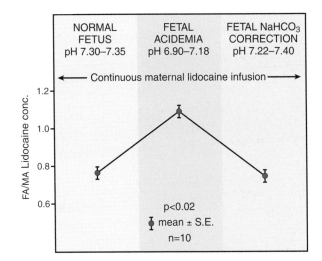

Figure 32-4 Fetal-to-maternal (FA/MA) lidocaine ratios are higher during fetal acidemia than during control (normal fetus) or during pH correction with sodium bicarbonate. This reflects ion trapping of the ionized fraction of lidocaine in the fetus in the presence of acidosis. (From Biehl D, Shnider SM, Levinson G, et al. Placental transfer of lidocaine. Effects of fetal acidosis. Anesthesiology 1978;48:409-412, with permission.)

can be metabolized before reaching the fetal arterial circulation for delivery to the heart and brain. Moreover, drugs in the portion of umbilical venous blood that enters the inferior vena cava via the ductus venosus will be diluted by drug-free blood returning from the lower extremities and pelvic viscera of the fetus.

ANATOMY OF LABOR PAIN

Pain during labor and delivery is caused by uterine contractions, dilatation of the cervix, and distention of the perineum. Somatic and visceral afferent sensory fibers from the uterus and cervix travel with sympathetic nerve fibers to the spinal cord (Fig. 32-5). These fibers pass through the paracervical tissue, with the uterine artery, and then through the inferior, middle, and superior hypogastric plexuses to the sympathetic chain. Nerve impulses from the uterus and cervix enter the spinal cord through the 10th, 11th, and 12th thoracic nerves (T10-12) and the 1st lumbar nerve (L1). Somatic perineal pain impulses travel to the 2nd, 3rd, and 4th sacral nerves primarily via the pudendal nerve (S2-4). Pain in the perineum, caused by distention of the vagina, perineum, and pelvic floor muscles, is associated with descent of the fetus into the pelvis during the second stage of labor and with delivery.

Somatic pain differs from visceral pain as reflected by different types of pain sensation. Somatic pain (incision

IV

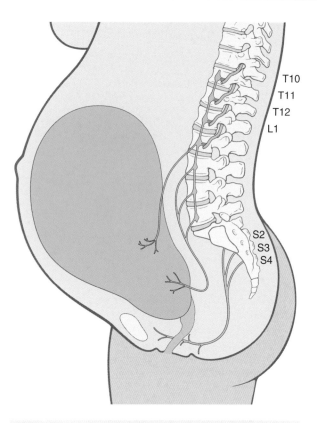

of pain (or both). Factors that may influence the perception of labor pain include the duration of labor, maternal pelvic anatomy and fetal size, use of oxytocin, parity, participation in childbirth preparation classes, fear and anxiety about childbirth, attitudes and experience of pain, and coping mechanisms. Labor analgesia may prevent reflex effects, which can be deleterious for certain high-risk patients or their fetuses (patients with severe preeclampsia, valvular heart disease, myasthenia gravis).

The choice of analgesic technique resides primarily with the pregnant woman. The medical condition of the pregnant woman, stage of labor, condition of the fetus, and availability of qualified personnel are also factors. Many different techniques are used to alleviate labor and delivery pain. Techniques for labor analgesia must be safe for the mother and fetus, be individualized to satisfy the analgesic requirement and desires of the pregnant woman, and accommodate the changing nature of labor pain and the evolving, varied course of labor and delivery (spontaneous vaginal delivery, instrumental vaginal delivery, cesarean delivery) (Table 32-3).

Nonpharmacologic Techniques: Psychological and Alternative Techniques

Psychological and alternative techniques for obstetric analgesia include hypnosis, natural childbirth, Lamaze breathing techniques, acupuncture, acupressure, transcutaneous nerve stimulation, hydrotherapy, and biofeed-

Figure 32-5 Schematic diagram of pain pathways during parturition. Visceral pain during the first stage of labor is due to uterine contraction and dilation of the cervix. Afferent pain impulses from the uterus and cervix are transmitted by nerves that accompany sympathetic nervous system fibers and enter the spinal cord at T10-L1. Somatic pain during the second stage of labor is vaginal and perineal in origin, and impulses travel via the pudendal nerves to S2-4.

pain, second-stage labor pain) is well localized and typically described as "sharp." Visceral pain (uterine contractions in the first stage of labor) is poorly localized and usually described as "dull but intense aching." Along with the subjective sensation of pain, nerve impulses of labor pain lead to stimulation of the sympathetic nervous system and result in reflex cardiovascular, respiratory, endocrine, and musculoskeletal effects, such as maternal tachycardia, hypertension, elevation in plasma concentrations of catecholamines, and reduced uterine blood flow.

METHODS OF LABOR ANALGESIA

The pain of labor is highly variable but is described by many women as severe. Analgesia for labor and childbirth reduces the psychological or subjective component

Table 32-3	Techniques for Labor Analgesia
Nonpharmacologic analgesia	
Psychological techniques	
Alternative techniques	
Systemic medications	
Sedatives and tranquilizers	
Dissociative analgesia	
Opioids	
Inhalation analgesia	
Regional analgesia	
Spinal	
Epidural	
Combined spinal-epidural	
Paracervical block	
Lumbar sympathetic block	
Pudendal block	

back.[10] These psychoanalgesic techniques require a high level of personal concentration and are not reliable or applicable to all deliveries.

Systemic Medications

Systemic medications for labor and delivery are widely used but administered in limited doses because they readily cross the placenta and can depress the fetus in a dose-dependent fashion. Opioids are the most commonly used systemic medication for relief of labor pain. However, excessive maternal sedation, maternal respiratory depression, loss of maternal protective airway reflexes, and the risk of neonatal depression limit the safe amount of opioids administered for labor analgesia. The most commonly used opioid analgesics in obstetrics are the synthetic opioids (fentanyl, butorphanol, nalbuphine, meperidine) and morphine.

Systemic administration of opioids at doses safe for the mother and newborn provides some analgesia but cannot substitute for the analgesia provided by regional anesthetic techniques. It is recommended that systemic opioids be administered in the smallest doses possible while minimizing repeated dosing to reduce the accumulation of drug and metabolites in the fetus. Opioids are most useful in *primiparas* in early labor, as adjuncts to major regional anesthetics, and in *multiparas* with relatively short, predictable labor with minimal pain.

ANXIOLYTICS

Diazepam and midazolam are used as anxiolytic drugs in obstetrics. They rapidly cross the placenta and yield approximately equal maternal and fetal blood levels within minutes of intravenous administration. Neonates have a limited ability to excrete diazepam, so the drug and its active metabolite may persist in significant amounts in neonates for a week. When used in small doses (2.5 to 10 mg IV), minimal newborn sedation and hypotonia have been observed.

KETAMINE

Intramuscular or intravenous administration of low-dose ketamine (0.25 mg/kg) produces a state called "dissociative analgesia." Profound analgesia and amnesia without loss of consciousness or protective airway reflexes characterize this state. Administered in divided doses totaling less than 1 mg/kg, ketamine can provide adequate analgesia for vaginal delivery and episiotomy repair. As the dose administered increases, airway protection cannot be guaranteed and the risk for pulmonary aspiration is a consideration. Ketamine is best reserved as a low-dose supplement to other techniques for (1) situations in which more reliable and safer drugs or techniques are contraindicated or (2) when rapid control is required because mother's pain is compromising the fetus (often in the presence of fetal heart rate deceleration).

OPIOIDS

Opioids at equipotent doses have similar effects on the fetus and newborn, and they cross the placental barrier by passive diffusion. Although systemic opioids can alleviate labor pain, the large doses necessary would introduce a risk for maternal and fetal ventilatory depression, excessive maternal sedation, loss of protective airway reflexes, impaired early breast-feeding, and neonatal neurobehavior changes. The opioid dose selected for a pregnant woman is intended to relieve pain without producing adverse effects on either the mother or baby. Nevertheless, for many pregnant women, opioids do not provide adequate analgesia during labor and delivery and their use for this purpose is declining.[11] Furthermore, all opioids readily cross the placental barrier and exert neonatal effects in normal doses, including decreased fetal heart rate variability. Routine doses also result in maternal side effects, including nausea, vomiting, pruritus, and decreased motility of the gastrointestinal tract.

Regional Analgesia

Regional analgesia (epidural, spinal, combined spinal-epidural) is the most widely used technique for labor analgesia (Fig. 32-6). Lumbar sympathetic blocks and paracervical blocks are rarely performed for labor analgesia, but pudendal blocks are used for delivery. Regional blocks generally involve the administration of local anesthetics, and some include coadministration of opioid analgesics and possibly other drugs that modulate interneuronal communication.[12]

Local Anesthetics

Clinically useful local anesthetics consist of amine moieties linked by an intermediate chain containing an ester or amide. Ester-linked local anesthetics (procaine, chloroprocaine, tetracaine) are rapidly metabolized by plasma cholinesterase, thus limiting the risk for maternal toxicity and placental drug transfer. Amide-linked local anesthetics (lidocaine, bupivacaine, ropivacaine, levobupivacaine) are slowly degraded by the liver and bind to plasma protein. Ropivacaine and levobupivacaine are (S)-enantiomer, amino amide–type local anesthetics with a chemical formula similar to that of bupivacaine, which is a racemic mixture.

OVERDOSE AND TOXICITY

Vascular absorption of local anesthetics limits the safe dose that can be administered. Toxic plasma concentrations of local anesthetics produce neurologic toxicity (seizures) or cardiovascular toxicity (myocardial depression, ventricular dysrhythmias). Accidental intravascular injection of local anesthetic solutions may result in maternal mortality. Mild overdoses of local anesthetic are exhibited by the neonate as decreases in neuromuscular tone similar to that seen with magnesium. If a direct intravascular or intrafetal injec-

IV

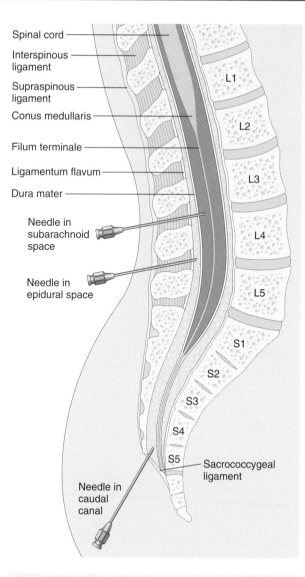

Figure 32-6 Schematic diagram of lumbosacral anatomy showing needle placement for subarachnoid, lumbar epidural, and caudal blocks.

analgesia include (1) the ability to achieve segmental bands of analgesia (T10-L1) during the first stage of labor when total anesthesia is not required, (2) the ability to extend the block to include the S2-4 segments during the second stage of labor, and (3) extension of sensory anesthesia to T4 for cesarean delivery if necessary.

TECHNIQUE

Before placing an epidural for labor analgesia, it is important to have equipment for resuscitation available (Table 32-4). The technique involves insertion of an epidural needle between vertebral spinous processes (most commonly L3-4 or L4-5) until loss of resistance with an air- or saline-filled syringe is detected by the anesthesiologist (Fig. 32-7; see Fig. 17-21).[13] Once the needle is properly placed, a catheter is inserted through the needle and left in place, and the needle is removed. Caudal anesthesia is produced by placing the local anesthetic solution in the caudal epidural space rather than the lumbar epidural space.

Table 32-4 Resuscitation Equipment for Regional Blockade
Positive-pressure breathing apparatus
Oxygen supply
Laryngoscope and blades
Endotracheal tubes: adult—6.0, 6.5, 7.0, 7.5
Stylets
Oral and nasal airways
Laryngeal mask airways
Drugs
Ephedrine, phenylephrine
Thiopental, propofol
Succinylcholine
Epinephrine, atropine
Labetalol, hydralazine
Nitroglycerin (parenteral, sublingual spray)
Calcium
Naloxone
Supplies for venous access and fluid resuscitation
Each labor room should contain an oxygen supply, suction, and a bed capable of rapid change to a Trendelenburg position
Equipment and drugs for cardiopulmonary resuscitation (including a defibrillator) should be readily available.

tion of local anesthetic occurs, significant depression can develop, as manifested by bradycardia, ventricular dysrhythmias, and severe cardiac depression with acidosis.

Epidural Analgesia

Epidural analgesia for labor and delivery is often viewed as the technique of choice for relief of labor pain. The pregnant woman remains awake and alert without sedative side effects. Maternal catecholamine concentrations are reduced, hyperventilation is avoided, and the ability of the mother to cooperate and participate actively during labor is facilitated. Further advantages of lumbar epidural

A. EPIDURAL ANALGESIA

B. COMBINED SPINAL–EPIDURAL ANALGESIA

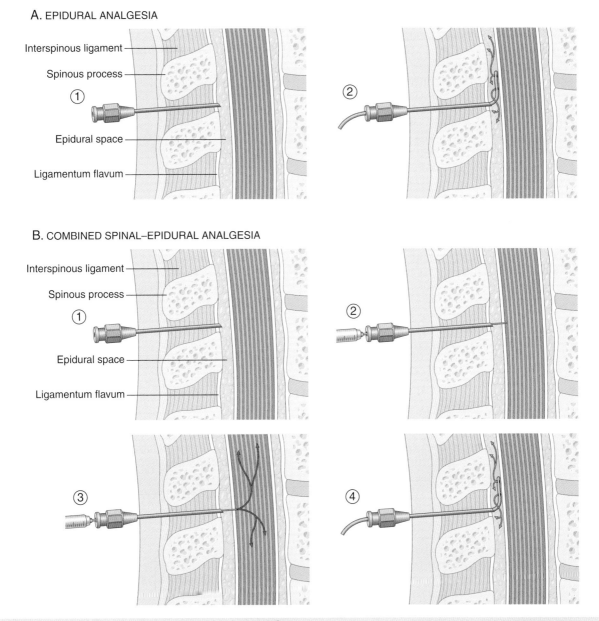

Figure 32-7 Technique of epidural analgesia and combined spinal-epidural analgesia. **A,** Epidural analgesia is achieved by placement of a catheter in the lumbar epidural space (1). After the desired intervertebral space (between L3 and L4) has been identified and infiltrated with local anesthetic, a hollow epidural needle is placed in the intervertebral ligaments. These ligaments are characterized by a high degree of resistance to penetration. A syringe connected to the epidural needle allows the anesthesiologist to confirm the resistance of these ligaments. In contrast, the epidural space has a low degree of resistance. When the anesthesiologist slowly advances the needle while feeling for resistance, the epidural space can be recognized by sudden loss of resistance as the epidural needle enters the epidural space (2). Next, an epidural catheter is advanced into the space. Solutions of a local anesthetic, opioids, or a combination of the two can now be administered through the catheter. **B,** For combined spinal-epidural analgesia, the lumbar epidural space is identified (1). Next, a very thin spinal needle is introduced through the epidural needle into the subarachnoid space (2). Correct placement can be confirmed by free flow of cerebrospinal fluid. A single bolus of solution containing local anesthetic, opioid, or a combination of the two is injected through this needle into the subarachnoid space (3). Subsequently, the needle is removed, and a catheter is advanced into the epidural space through the epidural needle (4). When the single-shot spinal analgesic wears off, the epidural catheter can be used for continuation of pain relief. (From Eltzschig HK, Lieberman ES, Camann WR. Regional anesthesia and analgesia for labor and delivery. N Engl J Med 2003;348:319-332, with permission.)

Absence of intrathecal (subarachnoid) or intravascular placement of the epidural catheter is confirmed by applying negative pressure (aspiration for blood or CSF) to the catheter, followed by administering a small test dose of local anesthetic (bupivacaine, 7.5 mg; lidocaine, 45 mg). The test dose is necessary to identify accidental intrathecal injection because aspiration of the catheter for CSF may not be diagnostic. Inclusion of epinephrine (15 µg) in the local anesthetic solution may indicate accidental intravascular injection because it causes a sudden (within 30 to 45 seconds), but transient increase in maternal systemic blood pressure and heart rate. The use of epinephrine for this purpose, however, is controversial because false-positive tests may occur as a result of similar cardiovascular changes that accompany uterine contractions and this exogenous epinephrine may decrease uteroplacental perfusion.[14] Furthermore, negative aspiration of blood through a multiorifice epidural catheter is considered by some to be sufficient evidence that the epidural catheter remains extravascular.[15] Even with negative aspiration of blood, subsequent doses of local anesthetic solution should be administered in increments to decrease the likelihood of unrecognized intravascular migration of the catheter.

MONITORING

Careful monitoring of the fetus and uterine contractions is important after the administration of regional analgesia. Fetal bradycardia from uterine hyperactivity causing decreased uteroplacental perfusion can occur and is most likely due to the rapidly decreasing maternal catecholamines after the onset of analgesia.[16] Nitroglycerin is effective in achieving uterine relaxation should the hyperactivity persist.[17]

TIMING OF PLACEMENT

An epidural block can be performed early in labor when patients request analgesia and should not be withheld simply because an arbitrary degree of cervical dilation has not yet been achieved.[18] Regional analgesia in early labor does not increase the rate of cesarean delivery, and it provides better analgesia and may lead to a shorter duration of labor than is the case with systemic analgesia.[19] During early labor, many anesthesiologists strive to provide a segmental band of analgesia (T10-L1) for the pain of uterine contractions and cervical dilation. Later, a larger volume of local anesthetic solution can be administered to provide perineal analgesia for spontaneous vaginal delivery or, if needed, an instrumental vaginal delivery. Once the catheter is placed, analgesia may be achieved and continued throughout the active phase of labor and delivery and for operative anesthesia (cesarean delivery), as well as for postoperative analgesia if necessary.

METHOD OF DELIVERY

Local anesthetics are typically infused continuously after incremental bolus doses to produce pain relief with similar or lower blood levels of local anesthetics than achieved with repetitive, intermittent boluses of these drugs. Most important, the possibility of total spinal anesthesia or intravascular injection with cardiovascular collapse secondary to large doses of local anesthetics is decreased. If an epidural catheter enters an epidural vein during continuous infusion, the analgesia merely ceases without producing neurologic or cardiovascular toxicity. If the catheter enters the subarachnoid space instead, the level of sensory and motor blockade increases slowly without the sudden onset of complete subarachnoid blockade that may occur with bolus techniques.

Patient-Controlled Epidural Analgesia

Patient-controlled epidural analgesia (PCEA) is an alternative to incremental doses or continuous infusion of the local anesthetic solution. A pump is programmed to administer a fixed continuous rate of a local anesthetic and opioid mixture through the epidural catheter, and the patient is allowed to self-administer a small additional dose at fixed intervals to reinforce the block, if desired. Use of the PCEA technique results in increased patient satisfaction and decreased workload for the anesthesiologist, with less frequent need to adjust dosing (top-ups).[20]

DRUG CHOICE AND DOSE

The choice of drugs for continuous epidural infusion includes dilute solutions of lidocaine, bupivacaine, ropivacaine, or chloroprocaine (Table 32-5).[21] The concentration and volume of the loading dose, administered before initiation of the continuous infusion, and the volume and concentration of the infusion are variable. The visceral pain of the first stage of labor can usually be relieved by injection of 6 to 10 mL of 0.125% to 0.25% bupivacaine or ropivacaine into the lumbar epidural space. These local anesthetics are often selected for labor analgesia because of their motor-sparing block and long duration of action. Higher concentrations of local anesthetics result in increased density of the motor block. With larger volumes, a greater dermatomal spread of analgesia is achieved.

Anesthesiologists often administer reduced concentrations of local anesthetics, such as 0.0625% to 0.01% bupivacaine, and coadminister an opioid such as fentanyl with both the bolus (50 to 100 µg) and infusion (2 µg/mL). Dilute solutions of local anesthetics minimize the motor block and preserve the perception of pelvic pressure with descent of the fetus. Coadministration of a local anesthetic and opioid results in an additive (perhaps synergistic) effect. Dilute concentrations of local anesthetics combined with an opioid may allow the pregnant woman to ambulate (after careful neurologic testing) (see Table 32-5).[21]

Combined Spinal-Epidural Analgesia

One variation of the lumbar epidural technique is combined spinal-epidural analgesia. After placement of the epidural

Table 32–5 Suggested Regimens for Lumbar Epidural Anesthesia for Labor and Delivery*

Initial Block (Options)

Bupivacaine, 0.125% to 0.25% (10 to 15 mL)

Bupivacaine, 0.125% (10 to 15 mL) + fentanyl, 50 to 100 μg

Fentanyl, 50 to 100 μg (or sufentanil, 10 to 15 μg) in 10 mL saline (after a 3-mL test dose of 1.5% lidocaine + epinephrine, 1:200,000)

Subsequent Analgesia (Options)

Intermittent boluses—repeat as above, as necessary, to maintain maternal comfort

Continuous infusions—10 to 15 mL/hr

Bupivacaine, 0.0625% to 0.125% + fentanyl, 1 to 2 μg/mL (or sufentanil, 0.1 to 0.3 μg/mL)

Bupivacaine, 0.1% to 0.25%, without opioid

Addition of epinephrine, 1:400,000 (2.5 μg/mL), to either of the above

Patient-Controlled Epidural Analgesia

Initial bolus

  Bupivacaine, 0.125% to 0.25% (10 to 15 mL)

  Bupivacaine, 0.125% (10 to 15 mL) + fentanyl, 50 to 100 μg

Basal infusion—8 mL/hr (bupivacaine, 0.08% + fentanyl, 1 to 2 μg/mL)

Demand bolus dose—8 mL (bupivacaine, 0.08% + fentanyl, 1 to 2 μg/mL)

Lockout interval—8 minutes

If perineal anesthesia is required, administer 10 to 15 mL local anesthetic (1% to 2% lidocaine or 2% to 3% chloroprocaine)

*Equipotent doses of local anesthetics, including bupivacaine, chloroprocaine, lidocaine, levobupivacaine, and ropivacaine, can be used interchangeably.

IV

needle, a long spinal needle is passed through the indwelling epidural needle to puncture the dura, and a small dose of local anesthetic or opioid (or both) is administered. After subarachnoid injection, the spinal needle is removed and an epidural catheter is placed. If opioid alone is administered and the epidural catheter is not activated, analgesia without motor block or sympathectomy is achieved. This allows the parturient to safely ambulate. The side effects of pruritus, nausea, and vomiting are not usually substantial with lipid-soluble opioids such as fentanyl or sufentanil, but the analgesia is limited (about 2 hours in the early active phase) and rarely effective for the second phase of labor.

If small doses of local anesthetics are administered through the spinal needle, segmental analgesia results more rapidly than with epidural administration of local anesthetics. The epidural placement of the catheter allows continuation of the segmental analgesia initiated by the spinal technique. Combined spinal-epidural analgesia is more reliable and has a faster onset of analgesia than conventional epidural analgesia for labor does. It is particularly useful when instituted in early labor with opioid alone to permit ambulation or in late, rapidly progressing labor.

Spinal Anesthesia

Spinal anesthesia administered immediately before vaginal delivery produces rapid onset of analgesia and skeletal muscle relaxation, which may be particularly important for operative delivery such as midforceps and for perineal repair. A 25- to 26-gauge "pencil-point" spinal needle is often selected to decrease the risk for post–dural puncture headache, which is the major disadvantage of spinal anesthesia for vaginal delivery. Subarachnoid placement of a dilute solution of hyperbaric lidocaine (20 to 30 mg), tetracaine (2 to 4 mg), or bupivacaine (5 to 6 mg) will reliably produce rapid and profound anesthesia of the perineum and vagina. Ropivacaine (0.5% to 0.75%) is also an effective local anesthetic for production of spinal anesthesia. Often, the pregnant woman will be maintained in the sitting position for 1 to 2 minutes in an attempt to limit the sensory block to perineal analgesia (area of the body that would be in contact with a saddle and thus the designation as "saddle block"). True saddle block anesthesia does not produce complete pain relief because afferent fibers from the uterus are not blocked.

Modified saddle block anesthesia is achieved by the subarachnoid injection of larger doses of local anesthetics (lidocaine, 30 to 50 mg; tetracaine, 6 to 8 mg), with the sitting position maintained for about 30 seconds. With this approach, sensory anesthesia typically extends to T10 or several levels higher, which prevents pain from uterine contractions.

Spinal anesthesia may also be considered for patients in advanced stages of labor. In this situation, intrathecal injection of 2.5 to 5.0 mg of isobaric bupivacaine and 10 to 25 μg of fentanyl provides satisfactory sensory analgesia for 90 to 120 minutes without profound skeletal muscle weakness.

CONTRAINDICATIONS AND COMPLICATIONS OF REGIONAL ANESTHESIA

Certain conditions such as patient refusal, infection at the needle insertion site, coagulopathy, or hypovolemic shock make regional anesthesia contraindicated. Human immunodeficiency virus (HIV) infection is not a contraindication to regional techniques in pregnant women.[22] If required to treat a post–dural puncture headache, an epidural blood patch may also be performed in an HIV-infected patient.[23]

Infrequent, but occasionally life-threatening complications can result from the administration of regional anesthesia. The most serious complications are due to accidental intravascular or subarachnoid injection of local anesthetics. Another relatively frequent complication of epidural analgesia is headache from CSF leak after accidental dural puncture.

Systemic Hypotension

Systemic hypotension secondary to sympathetic nervous system block is the most common complication of regional anesthesia for parturition.[21] Prophylactic measures include adequate hydration, avoidance of the supine position, and leftward displacement of the uterus off the abdominal aorta and vena cava. Treatment includes more uterine displacement, intravenous fluids, and administration of a vasopressor. If treated promptly, maternal hypotension does not result in fetal depression or neonatal morbidity.

Systemic Toxicity

Accidental intravascular injection of the local anesthetic solution can result in maternal seizures and possibly cardiovascular collapse. Resuscitation and support of the mother will reestablish uterine blood flow and allow adequate

fetal oxygenation and excretion of local anesthetic. Unless the mother cannot be resuscitated, delivery of the fetus should be delayed because the neonate has an extremely limited ability to excrete local anesthetics and may have prolonged convulsions. Measures that minimize the likelihood of accidental intravascular injection include careful aspiration before injection, test dosing, and administration of therapeutic doses in an incremental fashion.

Excessive Level of Neural Blockade

An excessive level of neural blockade (high or total spinal) may develop during initiation of a spinal, epidural, or caudal block or during a continuous infusion and lead to block of the motor nerves to the respiratory muscles.[24] Treatment consists of endotracheal intubation and ventilation of the pregnant woman's lungs with oxygen. The maternal circulation must be supported by avoiding aortocaval compression and, if needed, administering additional fluids and vasopressors (ephedrine). If these measures are not promptly effective in restoring and maintaining the maternal circulation, epinephrine (0.1 to 0.5 mg IV) should be administered.

MATERNAL CARDIAC ARREST

In any situation involving maternal cardiac arrest with unsuccessful resuscitation, consideration must be given to urgent delivery of the fetus. If delivered within 5 minutes of the arrest, the chance of infant survival is maximized, and evacuation of the uterus relieves the aortocaval compression and thereby improves the chance of maternal resuscitation.

Altered Progress of Labor

The progress of labor, including increasing cervical dilation, effacement, and descent over time, is unpredictable because it is influenced by many variables, including maternal pain, parity, size and presentation of the fetus, and drugs and techniques used to provide analgesia or anesthesia. Excessive sedation or premature initiation of a regional anesthetic has been proposed as a cause of prolongation of the latent phase. Some evidence, however, suggests that the need for early analgesia, either regional anesthesia or intravenous drugs, may be a characteristic of pregnant women who will experience a prolonged latent phase and dysfunctional labor, independent of the method of analgesia. Furthermore, labor can slow spontaneously during the latent phase in the absence of anesthesia. Likewise, catecholamine release in response to pain can inhibit uterine contractions such that the analgesia provided by appropriate regional anesthetic techniques might even enhance the early progress of labor. During the active phase the most likely causes of delayed progress of labor are cephalopelvic disproportion, fetal malposition, and fetal malpresentation.

The impact of anesthesia on the progress of labor is more predictable after labor has become active. For example, during the active phase a T10 sensory level produced by spinal or epidural anesthesia has no significant effect on the progress of labor, provided that fetal malpresentation is absent and hypotension is avoided. However, a regional anesthetic, by removing the reflex urge to bear down, may prolong the second stage of labor. Nevertheless, even if labor is prolonged by a regional anesthetic, there is no evidence that such prolongation is harmful to the fetus.

Increase in Core Body Temperature

The increase in core body temperature that results from epidural analgesia in labor is influenced by several factors, including the duration of labor, the ambient temperature, and possibly most important, the presence of shivering. During the first 5 hours of epidural analgesia, a significant rise in body temperature does not occur.[25] If labor is prolonged, body temperature increases at about 0.1°C/hr and may reach 38°C in some pregnant women by 12 hours. Some have suggested that epidural analgesia results in a significant increase in newborn sepsis workup rates, but others have found no association despite an increase in maternal body temperature at delivery.[26] Although the cause of the rise in maternal temperature remains uncertain, it need not affect neonatal management. The rise in temperature is not associated with a change in the leukocyte count, it is not associated with an infectious process, and treatment is not necessary.

OTHER NERVE BLOCKS FOR LABOR AND DELIVERY

Paracervical Block

A paracervical block is occasionally used by obstetricians to provide pain relief in the first stage of labor. The technique involves the submucosal administration of local anesthetic solution immediately lateral and posterior to the uterocervical junction to block transmission of pain impulses at the paracervical ganglion. Analgesia is not as profound as with an epidural or spinal regional block and the duration of analgesia is short (45 to 60 minutes), but complications and side effects of epidural analgesia such as hypotension, hypoventilation, and motor block are avoided. Convulsions, however, may occur as a result of systemic absorption of local anesthetic. When performed, the obstetrician should closely monitor the fetus and inject just beneath the vaginal mucosa after a negative aspiration for blood, and a 5-minute interval should be allowed between injection of the first and second side. Chloroprocaine is often used for this block because it undergoes rapid intravascular hydrolysis and has a very short intravascular half-time (in case of accidental intravascular or fetal injection). Lidocaine is also used, but bupivacaine is considered contraindicated.

FETAL BRADYCARDIA

A paracervical block is associated with a relatively high incidence of fetal bradycardia after the block. The cause of this phenomenon is unclear but probably involves decreased uterine blood flow secondary to the vasoconstrictive properties of local anesthetics. The bradycardia is usually limited to less than 15 minutes, and treatment is supportive and includes lateral positioning and administration of oxygen. Because fetal bradycardia is associated with increased neonatal morbidity and mortality, this block is rarely performed and should be avoided in patients with evidence of uteroplacental insufficiency or nonreassuring fetal heart rate patterns.

Pudendal Nerve Block

A pudendal block is performed by obstetricians via a transvaginal technique in which a sheathed needle is guided to the vaginal mucosa and sacrospinous ligament just medial and posterior to the ischial spine. Although the technique provides analgesia for vaginal delivery or uncomplicated instrumental vaginal delivery, the rate of failure is high, and the block achieved is often inadequate for midforceps application, examination of the cervix and upper vagina, or manual exploration of the uterus after delivery. This block may be used when epidural or spinal blocks are unavailable. Complications, besides failure, include vaginal lacerations, systemic local anesthetic toxicity, ischiorectal or vaginal hematoma, and rarely, fetal injection of the local anesthetic solution.

Perineal Infiltration

Infiltration of the perineum is commonly performed by obstetricians to provide anesthesia for episiotomy and its repair. Care is taken to avoid injection into the fetal scalp and the administration of excessive (total) doses of local anesthetic drugs. This is a common and useful technique alone or in conjunction with other regional blocks.

INHALATION ANALGESIA FOR VAGINAL DELIVERY

Some birthing centers use nitrous oxide, usually administered by a device that delivers 50% nitrous oxide in oxygen. This concentration of nitrous oxide without coadministration of opioids provides safe and satisfactory analgesia in some pregnant women and is insufficient to result in unconsciousness or loss of protective airway reflexes.[21] Maternal cardiovascular and respiratory depression is minimal, uterine contractility is not affected, and neonatal depression does not occur regardless of the duration of nitrous oxide administration. Appropriate equipment and fully trained personnel are essential to ensure safety when delivering this gas mixture. Overall, however, 50% nitrous oxide is a weak analgesic.

ANESTHESIA FOR CESAREAN DELIVERY

Although the majority of cesarean deliveries are performed with regional anesthesia, sometimes the severity of the fetal condition (severe fetal heart rate deceleration) necessitates the use of general anesthesia for its rapidity, and at other times it is required when regional anesthesia is contraindicated. Regardless, in preparation for cesarean delivery, all pregnant women should receive an oral antacid (nonparticulate such as sodium citrate) to reduce gastric fluid pH. In addition, some anesthesiologists routinely administer a drug to accelerate gastric emptying (metoclopramide) or an H_2 receptor antagonist (ranitidine), or both, to reduce gastric acid production.

Spinal Anesthesia

For a pregnant woman without an epidural catheter, spinal anesthesia is the most common regional anesthetic technique used for cesarean delivery (Table 32-6). The block is technically easier than an epidural anesthetic, more rapid in onset, and more reliable in providing surgical anesthesia from the midthoracic level to the sacrum.[27] The incidence of post–dural puncture headache has become low with the introduction of noncutting, "pencil-point" spinal needles. However, maternal hypotension is more likely and more profound with spinal anesthesia than with epidural anesthesia because the onset of sympathectomy is more rapid. Prehydration, avoidance of aortocaval compression, and aggressive use of ephedrine (even as a prophylactic) may minimize the risk for hypotension. Spinal anesthesia can be safely used in patients with preeclampsia.[20]

Lumbar Epidural Anesthesia

Epidural anesthesia is an excellent choice for surgical anesthesia when an indwelling, functioning epidural catheter has been placed for labor analgesia. It is also ideal for patients who cannot tolerate the sudden onset of sympathectomy or in some patients with cardiac disease. The volume and concentration of local anesthetic drugs used for surgical anesthesia are larger than those used for labor analgesia; however, the technique of catheter placement, test dosing, and potential complications are similar. Typically, the anesthesiologist attempts to provide sensory anesthesia from the T4 level to the sacrum. This level of anesthesia may not always alleviate the visceral pain associated with peritoneal manipulation, and adjuvant drugs may be necessary (see Table 32-5).

Local Anesthesia

Although cesarean delivery can be performed by local infiltration, it is accompanied by considerable discomfort and risks the possibility of local anesthetic overdose; moreover, most obstetricians have not been trained to do this. However, in rare circumstances of acute fetal distress, when a regional block is inadequate, and when induction of general anesthesia is considered dangerous (morbid obesity), local infiltration can be helpful to at least deliver the baby. General anesthesia can then be induced after securing the patient's airway with appropriate techniques, which may include awake fiberoptic tracheal intubation.

General Anesthesia

General anesthesia is used in obstetric practice for cesarean section, typically when regional anesthesia is contraindicated (coagulopathy, certain cardiac lesions, hemorrhage) or for emergencies (placental abruption, uterine rupture, fetal bradycardia, prolapsed umbilical cord) because of its rapid and predictable action (Table 32-7).

After rapid-sequence induction of anesthesia and placement of a cuffed tracheal tube facilitated by the administration of succinylcholine or a nondepolarizing neuromuscular blocking drug, anesthesia is maintained by inhalation of nitrous oxide and a volatile anesthetic, often in combination with sedative-hypnotics or opioids (or both). Nondepolarizing neuromuscular blocking drugs are subsequently administered to facilitate surgery.

INDUCTION DRUGS

A number of different drugs are used by anesthesiologists to rapidly induce unconsciousness.

Thiopental

Thiopental (4 to 6 mg/kg IV) is the most commonly used drug for induction of general anesthesia in obstetrics because it renders the patient unconscious within 30 seconds of administration. This dose of thiopental has no significant clinical impact on neonatal well-being. Neonatal depression may, however, occur with higher doses of thiopental, and cardiorespiratory supportive techniques are necessary until the neonate can excrete the drug (may take up to 48 hours).

Ketamine

Ketamine produces a rapid onset of anesthesia and, unlike thiopental, increases systemic blood pressure, heart rate, and cardiac output by central stimulation of the sympathetic nervous system. Increased uterine tone and decreased uterine blood flow can accompany excessively large doses of ketamine. In contrast to thiopental, low doses of ketamine (0.25 mg/kg IV) have profound analgesic effects. The undesirable psychotomimetic side effects (hallucinations, bad dreams) associated with ketamine administrations can be lessened by coadministration of benzodiazepines.

Table 32-6 Regional Anesthesia for Cesarean Section: Suggested Technique

Spinal Anesthesia (use a small-gauge, pencil-point [noncutting] spinal needle, 24 gauge or smaller)

Local Anesthetic Options
Bupivacaine, 12 to 15 mg (1.6 to 2 mL 0.75% bupivacaine in 8.25% glucose; most common choice)

Lidocaine, 60 to 75 mg (1.2 to 1.5 mL 5% lidocaine in 7.5% glucose diluted with equal volumes of cerebrospinal fluid)

Tetracaine, 8 to 10 mg hyperbaric tetracaine (0.8 to 1 mL 1% tetracaine with equal volumes of 10% glucose in water)

Intrathecal Opioid Options (added to local anesthetic solutions)
Fentanyl, 10 to 25 µg (0.1 to 0.5 mL fentanyl, 50-µg/mL solution)

Morphine, 0.1 to 0.25 mg (0.2 to 0.5 mL preservative-free morphine, 5 mg/10 mL)

Fentanyl plus morphine in above doses

Epinephrine
0.1 to 0.2 mg added to the local anesthetic solution may prolong and/or improve the quality of the block

Epidural Anesthesia

Local Anesthetic Options*
Lidocaine, 1.5% to 2%, plus epinephrine, 1:200,000

Bupivacaine, 0.5%

Chloroprocaine, 3%

Test Dose (administered through the epidural catheter to detect intrathecal or intravascular injection)
Lidocaine, 45 mg (spinal block within 3 to 5 minutes)

Epinephrine, 15 µg (heart rate increase within 60 seconds if intravascular)

Negative Test Dose
Administer up to 20 mL of local anesthetic solution in fractional increments of no more than 5 mL every 30 seconds

Inject additional local anesthetic solution as required through the catheter to obtain a sensory block up to T4

If the local anesthetic solution is initially injected through the needle, an additional test dose should be administered through the catheter before its use

pH Adjustment Options
Add 1 mL (1 mEq) sodium bicarbonate (8.4%) to 10 mL lidocaine

Epidural Opioid Options
Fentanyl, 50 to 100 µg, or sufentanil, 10 to 20 µg, may be added to the local anesthetics to potentiate intraoperative analgesia

Morphine, 4 to 5 mg, may be administered through the epidural catheter after delivery

Patient Position
Left uterine displacement

Slight (10 degree) Trendelenburg tilt may improve venous return

Monitor
Blood pressure every minute for the first 20 minutes and then every 5 minutes for the duration of surgery

Electrocardiogram and oxygen saturation

*Equipotent doses of other local anesthetics to include levobupivacaine and ropivacaine may be used.

IV

Table 32-7 General Anesthesia for Cesarean Section: A Suggested Technique

Administer a nonparticulate oral antacid (sodium citrate) within 15 minutes of induction of anesthesia

Maintain left uterine displacement

Start an infusion of crystalloid solution through a large-bore intravenous catheter

Preoxygenate for 3 minutes

When the surgeon is ready to begin, an assistant should apply cricoid pressure (and maintain until the position of the endotracheal tube is verified and the trachea is sealed by an inflated cuff)*

Administer thiopental, 4 to 5 mg/kg, and succinylcholine, 1 to 1.5 mg/kg, wait 30 to 60 seconds, and then initiate direct laryngoscopy for tracheal intubation

Administer 50% nitrous oxide in oxygen plus 0.5 MAC of a volatile anesthetic

Begin deliberate hyperventilation of the patient's lungs

After delivery, anesthesia may be deepened by increasing the nitrous oxide concentration and/or administering opioids, barbiturates, or propofol while continuing the volatile anesthetic

Extubate the trachea when the patient is fully awake

*Not all agree that cricoid pressure is efficacious or required in every patient.
MAC, minimal alveolar concentration.

Many anesthesiologists consider ketamine the appropriate drug for induction of anesthesia in a pregnant woman who is actively hemorrhaging, has uncertain blood volume, and is at risk for profound hypotension in response to intravenous thiopental.

Etomidate

Etomidate, like thiopental, has a rapid onset of action because of its high lipid solubility, and redistribution results in a relatively short duration of action. Although etomidate has minimal effects on the cardiovascular system, unlike thiopental and ketamine, it is painful on injection, induces extrapyramidal motor activity, and thus is rarely used in obstetrics.

Propofol

The need to have syringes of induction drugs ready to administer for rapid response to urgent situations requiring induction of general anesthesia (fetal distress) detracts from the value of preservative-free propofol in the obstetric suite. For an elective cesarean section, this highly lipid-soluble drug results in rapid onset of action similar to

thiopental and rapid and complete recovery with less residual sedative effect than is the case with thiopental. Nevertheless, propofol has not been demonstrated to be superior to thiopental in maternal or neonatal outcome. Furthermore, propofol has been associated with maternal bradycardia when administered with succinylcholine for induction of general anesthesia for cesarean section.

MAINTENANCE OF ANESTHESIA

Maintenance of anesthesia for cesarean section often includes the inhalation of 50% nitrous oxide in combination with a low concentration of volatile anesthetic. A volatile anesthetic is an important component of general anesthesia for cesarean section because the incidence of maternal recall of intraoperative events without these drugs is unacceptably high. During a typical general anesthetic for cesarean delivery, opioids are administered after the baby is delivered to avoid the concern of placental transfer to the neonate.

Placental transfer of volatile anesthetics is rapid because they are nonionized, highly lipid-soluble substances of low molecular weight. Fetal concentrations depend on the concentration and duration of anesthetic administered to the mother. If excessive concentrations of volatile anesthetics are administered for prolonged periods, neonatal effects of these drugs, as evidenced by flaccidity, cardiorespiratory depression, and decreased tone, may be anticipated. It is important to recognize that if neonatal depression is due to transfer of anesthetic drugs, the infant is merely lightly anesthetized and should respond easily to simple treatment measures such as assisted ventilation of the lungs to facilitate excretion of the inhalation anesthetic. Rapid improvement of the infant should be expected, and if it does not occur, it is important to search for other causes of depression.

There may be confusion regarding the presence of fetal distress, the use of general anesthesia, and subsequent delivery of a depressed neonate. A depressed fetus is likely to be associated with a depressed neonate, and general anesthesia is selected because it is the most rapidly acting anesthetic technique to allow cesarean delivery. For a healthy fetus, the interval from induction to delivery is not as important to neonatal outcome as the interval from uterine incision to delivery, when uterine blood flow may be compromised and fetal asphyxia may occur. A long time from induction to delivery may result in a lightly anesthetized neonate, but not an asphyxiated neonate.

NEUROMUSCULAR BLOCKING DRUGS

Succinylcholine remains the neuromuscular blocking drug of choice for obstetric anesthesia because of its rapid onset and short duration of action. This depolarizing neuromuscular blocking drug is normally hydrolyzed in maternal blood by the enzyme pseudocholinesterase and does not generally interfere with fetal neuromuscular activity. If the hydrolytic enzyme is present either in low concentration or in a genetically determined atypical form, prolonged maternal or neonatal respiratory depression secondary to muscular paralysis can occur.

Nondepolarizing neuromuscular blocking drugs are titrated to response with the use of a peripheral nerve stimulator. Under normal circumstances, the poorly lipid-soluble, highly ionized, nondepolarizing neuromuscular blocking drugs do not cross the placenta in amounts significant enough to cause neonatal skeletal muscle weakness. This placental impermeability is only relative, however, and when large doses are given over long periods, as for the treatment of maternal tetanus or status epilepticus, neonatal neuromuscular blockade can occur.

The diagnosis of neonatal depression secondary to drug-induced neuromuscular blockade may be made on the basis of the maternal history (prolonged administration of neuromuscular blocking drugs, history of atypical pseudocholinesterase), the response of the mother to neuromuscular blocking drugs, and physical examination of the newborn. A paralyzed neonate will have normal cardiovascular function and good color, but no spontaneous ventilatory movements or reflex responses, and skeletal muscle flaccidity is present. The anesthesiologist can test the neonate with a peripheral nerve stimulator and demonstrate the classic signs of neuromuscular blockade. Treatment consists of respiratory support until the neonate excretes the drug (may take up to 48 hours). Antagonism of nondepolarizing neuromuscular blocking drugs with cholinesterase inhibitors (neostigmine, edrophonium) may be attempted, but adequate respiratory support is the mainstay of treatment.

ADJUVANT MEDICATIONS

In addition to opioids, anesthesiologists may administer additional drugs such as benzodiazepines and antiemetics, but typically after the baby is delivered and the cord is clamped. Rarely are these drugs administered before delivery in doses large enough that placental transfer results in a clinically important neonatal effect.

ABNORMAL PRESENTATIONS AND MULTIPLE BIRTHS

Description of fetal position is based on the relationship of the fetal occiput, chin, or sacrum to the left or right side of the pregnant woman. Approximately 90% of all deliveries are cephalic presentations in either the occiput transverse or occiput anterior position. All other presentations and positions are considered abnormal.

Persistent Occiput Posterior

During active labor, the occiput undergoes internal rotation to the occiput anterior position. If this rotation does not occur, the persistent occiput posterior position can result in prolonged and painful labor with back pain, probably reflecting pressure on the posterior sacral nerves by the fetal occiput.

Breech Presentation

Breech deliveries are associated with increased maternal (cervical lacerations, retained placenta, hemorrhage) and neonatal (intracranial hemorrhage, prolapse of the umbilical cord) morbidity. Most breech presentations are delivered by elective cesarean section.[29] If cesarean section is planned, either a regional or general anesthetic may be selected. It should be recognized that during regional anesthesia there can be difficulty in extracting the infant through the uterine incision. If uterine hypertonus is the cause, administration of nitroglycerin (50 to 150 μg) may be effective in relaxing the hypertonic uterus. Alternatively, metered-dose sublingual nitroglycerin (400 μg per spray) can be used. It may be necessary to rapidly induce general anesthesia, intubate the trachea, and administer a volatile anesthetic to relax the uterus.

When vaginal delivery is planned for a breech presentation, a common approach is the use of a continuous lumbar epidural anesthetic. For example, a lumbar epidural anesthetic provides analgesia and maximal perineal relaxation for delivery of the fetal head. The ability of the pregnant woman to bear down ("push") during delivery can be preserved by using low concentrations of local anesthetics (0.125% bupivacaine) and providing constant maternal encouragement. More concentrated epidural local anesthetic solutions (2% chloroprocaine, 2% lidocaine) can be administered in the late second stage of labor to provide perineal anesthesia and relaxation to facilitate delivery of the fetal head.

In the absence of a regional anesthetic, administration of nitroglycerin or even rapid induction of general anesthesia and tracheal intubation facilitated by a neuromuscular blocking drug may be necessary to permit administration of a volatile anesthetic should perineal muscle relaxation be inadequate for delivery of the after-coming fetal head or if the lower uterine segment contracts and traps the fetal head.

Multiple Gestations

The use of a continuous lumbar epidural anesthetic for vaginal delivery is a method of anesthesia that provides flexibility, particularly for the birth of the second twin. When selecting anesthesia in the presence of multiple gestations, the frequent occurrence of prematurity and breech presentation and the potential for emergency cesarean delivery for the second twin must be considered. These pregnant women should give birth in a room in which an emergency cesarean section can be performed and adequate help for neonatal resuscitation is also available. Multiple gestations with more than two fetuses always involve cesarean delivery.

IV

PREGNANCY-ASSOCIATED HYPERTENSION

Pregnancy-associated hypertension encompasses a range of disorders (gestational proteinuric hypertension, preeclampsia, eclampsia) formerly designated toxemia of pregnancy. Occurring in 5% to 15% of all pregnancies, hypertension is a major cause of obstetric and perinatal morbidity and mortality. The pathophysiology of preeclampsia involves nearly every organ system (Table 32-8).

Preeclampsia is a syndrome manifested after the 20th week of gestation that is characterized by systemic hypertension (>140/90 mm Hg), proteinuria (>0.5 g/day), general-ized edema, and complaints of headache. Hemolysis (H), elevated liver enzymes (EL), and a low platelet count (LP) are elements of the HELLP syndrome, which represents a severe form of preeclampsia. The manifestations of preeclampsia usually abate within 48 hours after delivery. Eclampsia is present when seizures are superimposed on preeclampsia, and it is potentially life threatening. Causes of maternal mortality in women with preeclampsia include congestive heart failure, myocardial infarction, coagulopathy, and cerebral hemorrhage.

Treatment

Definitive treatment of preeclampsia/eclampsia is delivery of the fetus and placenta. In the interim, magnesium and antihypertensive drugs may be required. A general or regional anesthetic should not be used in attempts to lower maternal blood pressure. If these anesthetic approaches are used, the dose of antihypertensive drugs may need to be reduced.

MAGNESIUM

Magnesium is effective in pregnant women with preeclampsia and acts by decreasing the irritability of the central nervous system, which decreases the likelihood of seizures. Magnesium also decreases hyperactivity at the neuromuscular junction, presumably by decreasing the presynaptic release of acetylcholine, as well as by decreasing the sensitivity of postjunctional membranes to acetyl-choline. In addition, magnesium relaxes uterine and vascular smooth muscle, which contributes to an increase in uterine blood flow.

Clinically, the therapeutic effects of magnesium therapy are estimated by the responsiveness of deep tendon reflexes. Marked depression of these reflexes is an indication of impending magnesium toxicity. Periodic determination of serum magnesium concentrations is also helpful in adjusting supplemental doses of magnesium so that the level is kept in the therapeutic range of 4 to 6 mEq/L. Serum magnesium levels in excess of this range can lead to severe skeletal muscle weakness, hypoventilation, and cardiac arrest. Intravenous administration of calcium is the antidote for toxic effects of magnesium. Magnesium is excreted by the kidneys, so intravenous administration of this electrolyte must be carefully titrated when renal function is impaired, as in pregnant women in whom preeclampsia has developed.

Magnesium inhibits the release of acetylcholine from motor nerve terminals, thus enhancing the effects of nondepolarizing neuromuscular blocking drugs at the neuromuscular junction. Furthermore, preeclampsia may be associated with decreases in plasma cholinesterase activity that are greater than those normally associated with pregnancy, thereby resulting in potentiation of the effects of succinylcholine and mivacurium independent of magnesium therapy. This introduces the need for

Table 32-8 Pathophysiology of Pregnancy-Associated Hypertension
Cardiovascular system
Generalized vasoconstriction
Increased vascular responsiveness to sympathetic nervous system stimulation
Decreased uteroplacental perfusion
Hepatorenal system
Decreased hepatic blood flow
Decreased glomerular filtration rate
Decreased renal blood flow
Retention of sodium and water
Pulmonary system
Interstitial accumulation of fluid
Decreased arterial oxygenation
Exaggerated edema of the upper airway and larynx
Central nervous system
Hyperreflexia
Cerebral edema
Seizure activity
Intravascular fluid volume
Hypovolemia
Coagulation
Decreased platelet count
Increased fibrin split products
Uterus
Hyperactivity
Premature labor

careful titration of the doses of neuromuscular blocking drugs and monitoring their effects at the neuromuscular junction. Likewise, doses of sedatives and opioids should be decreased because magnesium can also enhance the effects of these drugs. Magnesium readily crosses the placenta, so neonatal skeletal muscle tone could be decreased at birth.

ANTIHYPERTENSIVES

Antihypertensive drugs are likely to be administered when maternal diastolic blood pressure is higher than 110 mm Hg. Hydralazine and labetalol are the most commonly administered antihypertensives. Hydralazine has the advantage of being a vasodilator, and therefore it increases uteroplacental and renal blood flow. The presence of tachycardia may dictate the simultaneous administration of an adrenergic blocking drug such as labetalol, which also has the advantage of rapid onset of action. The goal is to decrease maternal diastolic blood pressure to about 100 mm Hg. The peak effect of hydralazine does not occur until about 30 minutes after initial administration, thus emphasizing the need to delay subsequent doses for this period. The fetal heart rate should be monitored continuously during drug-induced decreases in maternal blood pressure to ensure an early warning should the uteroplacental circulation be jeopardized by decreased perfusion pressure.

Management of Anesthesia

Continuous lumbar epidural analgesia is acceptable for vaginal delivery by a preeclamptic pregnant woman in good medical control. Epidural analgesia negates the need for administration of parenteral opioids and the possible adverse effects of these drugs on a premature fetus. The presence of analgesia decreases the likelihood that maternal blood pressure will increase in response to painful uterine contractions. Before epidural analgesia is instituted, the pregnant woman is often prehydrated as guided by clinical examination, urine output, oxygenation, and occasionally, central venous pressure monitoring. Aggressive fluid administration may precipitate pulmonary edema, especially in the postpartum period. For severely preeclamptic women, coagulation studies are performed before placement of the epidural catheter because both a quantitative and a qualitative platelet defect can occur. For women with mild preeclampsia, platelet count or coagulation studies are not necessary before regional anesthesia. If maternal hypotension occurs, a decreased dose of ephedrine (2.5 mg IV) or phenylephrine (25 µg IV) is initially selected because of the presumed hypersensitivity of the maternal vasculature to catecholamines.

For cesarean delivery, either spinal or epidural anesthesia can be used safely.[30] Treatment of hypotension should be prompt, with decreased doses of vasopressors. Continuous monitoring of intra-arterial blood pressure, cardiac filling pressure, and urine output can be useful for severely preeclamptic women.

When emergency cesarean delivery is required and general anesthesia is used, it is important to recognize that the incidence of difficult tracheal intubation is increased in pregnant women in whom preeclampsia develops. Exaggerated edema of the upper airway structures may require the use of smaller tracheal tubes than anticipated. Induction of anesthesia is often performed with thiopental (4 to 6 mg/kg IV) or propofol (2 to 4 mg/kg IV) followed immediately by succinylcholine (1 to 1.5 mg/kg IV) to facilitate tracheal intubation. The systemic blood pressure increases elicited by direct laryngoscopy and tracheal intubation are predictably exaggerated in these pregnant women. A short duration of direct laryngoscopy is helpful for minimizing the magnitude and duration of the increase in systolic blood pressure. Nitroglycerin (1 to 2 µg/kg IV) administered just before initiating direct laryngoscopy has been used to attenuate this blood pressure response. Alternatively, fentanyl (1 µg/kg IV), lidocaine (1.5 mg/kg IV), or esmolol (1 mg/kg IV) may be selected. Remifentanil as a continuous intravenous infusion may be useful in such circumstances.

A volatile anesthetic can be administered to control intraoperative hypertension. Enhancement of the effects of all neuromuscular blocking drugs by magnesium must be remembered and a peripheral nerve stimulator used to monitor the effect of decreased doses of these drugs at the neuromuscular junction. Magnesium will also decrease uterine tone, thus increasing the risk for bleeding after delivery. Although pitocin and prostaglandin $F_{2\alpha}$ are safe for administration to preeclamptic pregnant women with uterine atony, methylergonovine (Methergine) should be used with caution because it can precipitate a hypertensive crisis.

HEMORRHAGE IN PREGNANT WOMEN

Hemorrhage in pregnant women is one of the leading causes of maternal mortality (Table 32-9). Placenta previa and abruptio placentae are the major causes of bleeding during the third trimester. Uterine rupture can be responsible for uncontrolled hemorrhage during labor. Postpartum hemorrhage occurs in 3% to 5% of all vaginal deliveries and is typically due to uterine atony, retained placenta, placenta accreta, or lacerations involving the cervix or vagina (or both).

Placenta Previa

Placenta previa is abnormally low implantation of the placenta in the uterus. The cardinal symptom of placenta previa is painless vaginal bleeding that typically occurs around the 32nd week of gestation, when the lower uterine segment is beginning to form. When this diagnosis is

IV

Table 32-9 Hemorrhage in a Pregnant Woman

Placenta Previa

Painless vaginal bleeding associated with advanced age and/or multiple parity

Abruptio Placentae

Abdominal pain is a poor sign

Bleeding partially or entirely concealed

Hemorrhagic shock

Disseminated intravascular coagulation

Acute renal failure

Fetal distress

Uterine Rupture

Abdominal pain

Hypotension

Disappearance of fetal heart tones

Associated with excessive uterine stimulation and/or rapid spontaneous delivery, as well as previous cesarean section (incidence, 0.4%-1.0%)

Retained Placenta

Necessitates manual exploration of the uterus; nitroglycerin may be useful

May require general anesthesia with a volatile anesthetic or, if hemodynamically stable, intravenous sedation or a regional anesthetic

Uterine Atony

Occurs in 2%-5% of all deliveries

Associated with increased multiparity, multiple births, polyhydramnios, large infants

Retained placenta and chorioamnionitis

Pharmacologic interventions include pitocin, ergot alkaloids, and prostaglandin $F_{2\alpha}$

suspected, the position of the placenta should be confirmed by ultrasonography. Regional anesthesia is appropriate for elective cesarean delivery in a woman with known placenta previa. The use of two large-bore intravenous lines is suggested to allow rapid infusion of fluids or blood, if needed. For emergency situations with active hemorrhage, general anesthesia may be required, and ketamine (1 to 1.5 mg/kg IV) is a useful drug for induction of anesthesia. Neonates delivered from pregnant women in hemorrhagic shock are likely to be acidotic and hypovolemic.

Abruptio Placentae

Abruptio placentae is separation of a normally implanted placenta after 20 weeks of gestation. When the separation involves only the placental margin, the escaping blood can appear as vaginal bleeding. Alternatively, large volumes of blood loss can remain entirely concealed in the uterus. Chronic bleeding and clotting between the uterus and placenta can cause maternal disseminated intravascular coagulation. Definitive treatment of abruptio placentae is to empty the uterus. If there are no signs of maternal hypovolemia, clotting abnormalities, or fetal distress, continuous lumbar epidural anesthesia can be used to provide analgesia for labor and vaginal delivery. However, severe hemorrhage necessitates emergency cesarean section and the use of a general anesthetic similar to that described for placenta previa. It is predictable that neonates born under these circumstances will be acidotic and hypovolemic.

Uterine Rupture

Uterine rupture can be associated with separation of a previous cesarean section and healed incision (scar) in the uterus, rapid spontaneous delivery, or excessive oxytocin stimulation. Overall, however, more than 80% of uterine ruptures are spontaneous and without an obvious explanation. After previous cesarean section, vaginal birth is associated with a 0.4% to 1% incidence of uterine rupture.[31] When vaginal birth is planned after a previous cesarean section, it is required that a surgical team, including an obstetrician, anesthesiologist, and nursing staff, be available so that emergency cesarean section can be initiated without delay should uterine rupture occur.

Retained Placenta

Retained placenta occurs in about 1% of all vaginal deliveries and usually necessitates manual exploration of the uterus. If a lumbar epidural or spinal anesthetic was not used for vaginal delivery, manual removal of the placenta may be initially attempted with analgesia provided by the intravenous administration of opioids or the inhalation of nitrous oxide. If uterine relaxation is necessary, nitroglycerin (50 to 150 µg IV) may be effective in relaxing the uterus. Rarely, induction of general anesthesia with tracheal intubation and administration of a volatile drug to provide uterine relaxation will be necessary if the uterus remains firmly contracted around the placenta.

Uterine Atony

Uterine atony as a cause of postpartum hemorrhage can occur immediately after delivery or be manifested several hours later. Retained placenta is a common accompaniment of uterine atony. Uterine atony is treated with synthetic oxytocins, which do not contain vasopressin. Dilute solutions of synthetic oxytocins exert no cardiovascular effects, but rapid intravenous injections may be associated with tachycardia, vasodilation, and hypotension.[32] These cardiovascular effects are avoided by infusion of 10 to 15 units of synthetic oxytocin in 500 mL of balanced salt solution until uterine contraction is adequate. Other drugs can be used if oxytocin alone is not effective, including methylergonovine (0.2 mg IM), prostaglandin $F_{2\alpha}$ (0.25 mg IM), and misoprostol, a prostaglandin E_1 analog.

Placenta Accreta

Placental implantation beyond the endometrium gives rise to (1) placenta accreta, which is implantation onto the myometrium; (2) placenta increta, which is implantation into the myometrium; and (3) placenta percreta, which is penetration through the full thickness of the myometrium (Fig. 32-8).[33] With placenta percreta, implantations may occur onto bowel, bladder, or other pelvic organs and vessels. Any of these placental implantations can produce a markedly adherent placenta that cannot be removed without tearing the myometrium.

These abnormal placental implantations occur more frequently in association with placenta previa. In the general obstetric population, placenta accreta occurs in approximately 1 in 2500 and cannot be reliably diagnosed by ultrasonography. In patients with placenta previa and no previous cesarean sections, the incidence is 5% to 7%. However, the risk of placenta accreta associated with placenta previa in women who have had a previous cesarean delivery is much greater. With one previous uterine incision, the incidence of placenta accreta has been reported to be between 24% and 31%, and with two or more previous uterine incisions, the incidence rises to about 50%.

In patients with placenta previa and accreta, massive intraoperative blood loss is common. Reported average blood loss has ranged from 2000 to 5000 mL, with some patients requiring more than 30 units of blood. Coagulopathies develop in approximately 20% of these patients. Between 30% and 72% have required cesarean hysterectomies. Placenta accreta is not reliably diagnosed until the uterus is open. The anesthesiologist must keep in mind this possibility and be prepared to treat sudden massive blood loss. Although anesthetic care must be individualized, it is believed that regional anesthesia does not contribute to increased maternal morbidity and may be appropriate in many cases of placenta accreta.

AMNIOTIC FLUID EMBOLISM

Amniotic fluid embolism is signaled by the sudden onset of respiratory distress, systemic hypotension, and arterial hypoxemia as a reflection of the cardiopulmonary effects of the entrance of amniotic fluid into the circulation. The precise pathophysiology of amniotic fluid embolism remains unclear, partially because there are no animal models that reproduce the syndrome. It is presumed that some pregnant women experience an anaphylactoid reaction to their amniotic fluid that results in pulmonary hypertension, right heart failure, and subsequently, biventricular cardiac failure, probably from the ensuing arterial hypoxemia. Multiparous pregnant women who experience a tumultuous labor are more likely to experience amniotic fluid embolism.

Treatment

Treatment of amniotic fluid embolism is supportive and directed toward cardiopulmonary resuscitation with inotropic support and correction of arterial hypoxemia. Tracheal intubation and mechanical support of ventilation are almost always required. Rapid onset of coagulopathy may occur and result in life-threatening hemorrhage. Conditions that mimic amniotic fluid embolism include venous air embolism, pulmonary embolism, and inhalation of gastric contents. Definitive diagnosis is extremely difficult or impossible, even postmortem, should amniotic fluid embolism result in death.

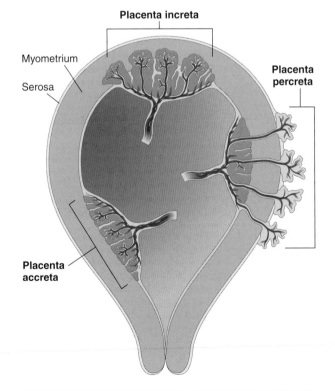

Figure 32-8 Classification of placenta accreta based on the degree of penetration of myometrium. (From Kamani AAS, Gambling DR, Chritilaw J, et al. Anesthetic management of patients with placenta accreta. Can J Anaesth 1987;34:613-617, with permission.)

IV

ANESTHESIA FOR NONOBSTETRIC SURGERY DURING PREGNANCY

The unique anesthesia management objectives for pregnant women undergoing nonobstetric surgery, such as excision of an ovarian cyst or appendectomy, include avoidance of teratogenic drugs, avoidance of intrauterine fetal hypoxia and acidosis, and prevention of spontaneous abortion early in pregnancy and premature labor later in pregnancy.[34] There is always the possibility that anesthesia will be unknowingly administered to women with early undiagnosed pregnancy. For this reason, routine pregnancy testing may be recommended before elective surgery for women of childbearing age.

Avoidance of Teratogenic Drugs

Most drugs, including anesthetics, have been demonstrated to be teratogenic in at least one animal species. In humans, the critical period of organogenesis is between 15 and 56 days of gestation. Nevertheless, there is no evidence that any of the currently used anesthetics administered during pregnancy are teratogenic. The available evidence in pregnant women suggests that exposure to nitrous oxide during clinical anesthesia does not alter reproductive outcome beyond the effects of the medical condition and surgery.[34] The use of nitrous oxide for in vitro fertilization and fallopian transfer procedures is controversial but has not been proved to be harmful.[34] There is no evidence in humans that drugs administered to produce analgesia during labor and vaginal delivery adversely affect later mental and neurologic development of the newborn.

Avoidance of Intrauterine Fetal Hypoxia and Acidosis

The development of intrauterine fetal hypoxia and acidosis is minimized by avoiding maternal hypotension with left uterine displacement after the 20th week of gestation, as well as by preventing arterial hypoxemia and excessive changes in $PaCO_2$. High inspired concentrations of oxygen do not increase the risk for in utero retrolental fibroplasia (retinopathy) because the high oxygen consumption of the placenta plus the uneven distribution of maternal and fetal blood flow in the placenta prevent fetal PaO_2 from exceeding about 60 mm Hg, even if maternal PaO_2 exceeds 500 mm Hg. The normal fetal umbilical vein (arterialized) blood has a pH of 7.35, PCO_2 of 38 mm Hg, and PO_2 of 30 mm Hg.

Prevention of Preterm Labor

The underlying pathology requiring surgery, and not the anesthetic technique, has been associated with an increased risk for preterm labor and delivery; intra-abdominal procedures have more risk than peripheral, minor procedures

do. After successful completion of surgery, it is advisable to monitor the fetal heart rate and maternal uterine activity. Preterm labor can be treated with β_2-agonists (terbutaline), magnesium, indomethacin, or calcium channel blockers such as nifedipine. These drugs relax uterine smooth muscle and thereby result in inhibition of uterine contractions and improved uteroplacental blood flow. Side effects of β_2-agonist therapy include maternal hypokalemia and cardiac dysrhythmias and fetal tachycardia and hypoglycemia. Prolonged use of indomethacin is contraindicated because of its vasoconstrictive effect on the fetal ductus arteriosus.

Management of Anesthesia

Elective surgery for pregnant women should be deferred until after delivery. When surgery is necessary, it is best to delay the operation until the second or third trimester. Emergency surgery in the first trimester is often performed with lumbar epidural anesthesia or spinal anesthesia. Spinal anesthesia seems uniquely advantageous because it limits fetal drug exposure to a minimum. Continuous intraoperative monitoring of the fetal heart rate after about the 16th week of gestation is helpful in providing early warning of fetal distress as a result of impaired uteroplacental perfusion (see the next section). When a general anesthetic is chosen, it should be appreciated that volatile anesthetics are not associated with significant decreases in uterine blood flow if maternal systemic blood pressure is maintained in the normal range. Regardless of the technique of anesthesia selected, it is recommended that inhaled concentrations of oxygen be at least 50%.

DIAGNOSIS AND MANAGEMENT OF FETAL DISTRESS

Fetal well-being is often determined by evaluation of the fetal electrocardiogram, including beat-to-beat variability in fetal heart rate as computed from R-wave intervals and fetal heart rate changes in association with uterine contractions (periodic changes). The fetal electrocardiogram is obtained by placing an electrode on the presenting fetal part, or the fetal heart rate can be determined indirectly by ultrasound with a sensor placed on the maternal abdomen. Fetal heart rate decelerations are most often classified as late or variable and typically signify compromise in uteroplacental function or cord compression, respectively (Figs. 32-9 and 32-10).[35] Fetal scalp blood sampling for determination of pH, which is not commonly performed, is a consideration when abnormal fetal heart rate patterns occur. It has been observed that the fetus is usually depressed when one or more fetal scalp pH values are near 7.0, whereas values higher than 7.2 to 7.25 most often indicate a vigorous infant at birth. Fetal pulse oximetry (normal values exceed 30%) may also be used.

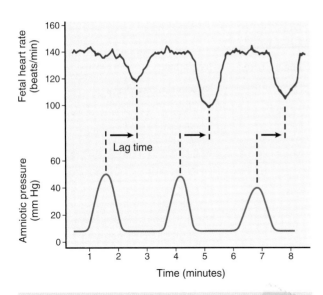

Figure 32-9 Late decelerations of the fetal heart rate are characterized by a delay between the onset of uterine contraction and the beginning of fetal heart rate slowing. The fetal heart rate does not return to normal until after the contraction has ceased. Late decelerations often indicate uteroplacental insufficiency. (From Shnider SM. Diagnosis of fetal distress: Fetal heart rate. *In* Shnider SM [ed]: Obstetrical Anesthesia: Current Concepts and Practice. Baltimore: Williams & Wilkins, 1970, pp 197-203, with permission.)

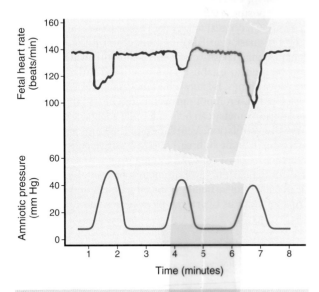

Figure 32-10 Variable decelerations of the fetal heart rate are characterized by varying magnitudes and times of onset of heart rate slowing. This pattern is usually benign but, if persistent, may reflect compression of the umbilical cord. (From Shnider SM. Diagnosis of fetal distress: Fetal heart rate. *In* Shnider SM [ed]: Obstetrical Anesthesia: Current Concepts and Practice. Baltimore: Williams & Wilkins, 1970, pp 197-203, with permission.)

Beat-to-Beat Variability

The normal fetal heart rate ranges between 110 and 160 beats/min with a beat-to-beat fluctuation of about 5 to 20 beats/min. This normal variability reflects the integrity of the neural pathway from the fetal cerebral cortex through the medulla, vagus nerves, and cardiac conduction system. Fetal well-being is ensured when beat-to-beat variability is present. Conversely, fetal distress secondary to arterial hypoxemia, acidosis, or central nervous system damage is associated with minimal to absent variability of the fetal heart rate. Opioids and anticholinergics administered to pregnant women may eliminate fetal heart rate variability, even in the absence of fetal distress, as does general anesthesia. This drug-induced effect does not appear to be deleterious but may cause difficulty in the interpretation of fetal heart rate monitoring.

Late Decelerations

Late decelerations are characterized by slowing of the fetal heart rate beginning 10 to 30 seconds after onset of the uterine contraction, probably mediated by chemoreceptors triggered by hypoxia (see Fig. 32-9).[35] This deceleration pattern consists of a gradual decrease and return to baseline, with the time from onset of the deceleration to its nadir being greater than 30 seconds. It is associated with fetal compromise (hypoxia and acidosis), most likely reflecting myocardial hypoxia secondary to uteroplacental insufficiency, which can be produced by maternal hypotension, partial placental abruption, preeclampsia, or other conditions of reduced placental reserve. Interventions may include a change in maternal position or administration of oxygen or tocolytic agents. If maternal blood pressure has decreased as a result of epidural anesthesia, it must be promptly treated with fluids and vasopressors.

Variable Decelerations

As the designation indicates, these deceleration patterns are variable in magnitude, duration, and time of onset, although they are generally characterized by a steep descent of the fetal heart rate (see Fig. 32-10).[35] Variable decelerations are thought to be caused by umbilical cord compression. Unless prolonged beyond 30 seconds or associated with fetal bradycardia (<70 beats/min), they are usually benign. Changing the maternal position often lessens or abolishes this pattern.

EVALUATION OF THE NEONATE AND NEONATAL RESUSCITATION

The transition from fetal to neonatal life involves major physiologic changes in the pulmonary and circulatory systems. Although these changes most often occur spontaneously, some infants require assistance to safely and

IV

successfully make the complex transition from a dependent fetus to an independent neonate. Assessment of neonates immediately after birth is important to promptly identify depressed infants who require active resuscitation. The Apgar score, described by Dr. Virginia Apgar in 1953,[36] assigns a numerical value to five vital signs measured or observed 1 and 5 minutes after delivery and has not been surpassed as a method of facilitating recognition and guiding management of a newborn who requires active resuscitation (Tables 32-10 and 32-11).

Apgar Scores of 8 and 9

Most newborns fall into this category, which requires little treatment other than suctioning the nose and mouth, tactile stimulation to promote breathing, and avoiding hypothermia. A neonate has a large surface area–to–volume ratio and therefore will cool quickly. The neonate's skin should be wiped dry and the baby placed in a radiantly heated bed, covered with warm blankets, or placed in skin-to-skin contact with the mother and covered. Apgar scores of 10 are very rare because acrocyanosis persists in a normal newborn well past 5 minutes of life.

Apgar Score of 5 to 7

These newborns may have experienced mild asphyxia before birth. Depressed Apgar scores can also result from maternally administered central nervous system depressants, birth trauma, or reflex bradycardia from suctioning of the airway. These newborns usually respond to tactile stimulation and delivery of supplemental oxygen over the face. If they do not respond in 1 to 2 minutes and the heart rate is less than 100 beats/min, ventilation of the newborn's lungs with oxygen should be instituted via a bag and facemask.

Apgar Score of 0 to 4

These newborns are often severely to moderately depressed and cyanotic and have poor breathing effort. If ventilation is inadequate and unresponsive to tactile stimulation or the heart rate remains less than 100 beats/min after about 30 seconds, positive-pressure ventilation with 100%

Table 32–11 Apgar Score as a Guide to Newborn Resuscitation

Apgar Score	Treatment
>8	Suction the pharynx Place in a warm environment
5-7	External stimulation Oxygen by mask Mechanical ventilation by facemask if no response
3-6	Initiate mechanical ventilation by facemask Tracheal intubation if spontaneous ventilation does not occur promptly Analysis of arterial blood gases from a doubly clamped segment of the umbilical cord
<2	Tracheal intubation and mechanical ventilation of the lungs with oxygen External cardiac compression if the heart rate is <60 beats/min

oxygen should be initiated with a bag and properly fitted facemask (avoiding excessive inspiratory pressure). Proper neonatal head positioning for airway management is a neutral position with the neck slightly extended. Alternatively, a laryngeal mask airway or tracheal intubation (if bag-and-mask ventilation is ineffective or it is anticipated that prolonged positive-pressure ventilation will be needed) can be used to establish an airway for ventilation of the newborn's lungs. Bilateral chest movement, air exchange on auscultation, prompt improvement in heart rate and color, and pulse oximetry can help assess the adequacy of positive-pressure ventilation. Ventilation of the lungs is controlled at a rate of about 40 breaths/min. Positive end-expiratory pressure to 3 to 5 cm H_2O is often useful. Airway pressure greater than 30 cm H_2O should not be used. Blood should be obtained from a doubly clamped segment of the umbilical cord for analysis of arterial blood gases and pH.

Table 32–10 Evaluation of a Neonate with the Apgar Score

	Two	One	Zero
Heart rate (beats/min)	>100	<100	Absent
Breathing	Irregular, crying	Slow	Absent
Reflex irritability	Cry	Grimace	No response
Muscle tone	Active	Flexion of the extremities	Limp
Color	Pink	Body pink, extremities cyanotic	Cyanotic

CARDIOPULMONARY RESUSCITATION

After about 30 seconds of effective ventilation, if the heart rate remains below 60 beats/min, external cardiac compressions are instituted.[37] External cardiac massage increases intrathoracic pressure to circulate blood to vital organs. The recommended technique is compression of the sternum, one fingerbreadth below an imaginary line drawn between the nipples, by the resuscitator's thumbs with hands encircling the neonate's thorax or by using the middle and ring fingertips. Firm support for the newborn's back is necessary and can be provided by the other hand (if it is not provided by the surface on which the baby lies). The sternum is depressed 1 to 2 cm at a rate of 120 times per minute. This should be accompanied by positive-pressure ventilation at a rate of 40 to 60 breaths per minute, preferably through an endotracheal tube. Evaluation by assessing peripheral pulses, stopping to assess spontaneous cardiac rhythm, and ideally monitoring the electrocardiogram and systemic blood pressure with an indwelling catheter are helpful. Improper resuscitation techniques introduce a risk for pneumothorax and liver injury.

Epinephrine

Epinephrine is indicated for heart rates remaining below 80 beats/min after 30 seconds of adequate ventilation and chest compression or immediately if asystole is present. The dose is 0.1 to 0.3 mL/kg of a 1:10,000 solution given rapidly intravenously into the trachea or into the aorta through an umbilical artery catheter. The dose may be repeated every 3 to 5 minutes if necessary, but if the heart rate remains lower than 100 beats/min, the resuscitator should consider plasma volume expansion if hypovolemia is suspected or sodium bicarbonate if metabolic acidosis is documented. If repetitive doses of epinephrine are required to maintain a heart rate higher than 100 to 120 beats/min, an infusion of isoproterenol may be considered. Intracardiac administration of epinephrine is not recommended because this route of administration does not show increased efficacy over intravenous or endotracheal administration and may be associated with major complications.

Sodium Bicarbonate

Administration of sodium bicarbonate for correction of neonatal acidosis has the objectives of reversing both the cardiac failure and the pulmonary vasoconstriction associated with asphyxia. Additionally, there may be benefits to sodium bicarbonate administration for partial volume expansion. A 4.2% solution of sodium bicarbonate is administered intravenously at a dose of 2 mEq/kg given slowly at a rate of 1 mEq/kg/min for documented severe metabolic acidosis (base deficit >15 mEq). If blood gas analysis is not immediately available, sodium bicarbonate is given to neonates who remain severely depressed despite adequate ventilation. Effective ventilation must precede and accompany bicarbonate administration to minimize the risk for intracranial hemorrhage, which can result from rapid bicarbonate administration and accompanying increases in cerebral blood flow. Another potential problem of sodium bicarbonate administration is unmasking the presence of hypovolemia when correction of the acidosis and hyperventilation results in dilation of peripheral blood vessels that had previously been intensely vasoconstricted.

An alternative to the use of sodium bicarbonate is tromethamine (THAM) solution, which has the advantage of reducing $PaCO_2$. It is particularly useful in the presence of combined respiratory and metabolic acidosis.

Volume Expanders

Volume expanders are indicated for evidence of acute bleeding or signs of hypovolemia, such as hypotension, pallor, poor capillary refill, tachycardia with faint pulses, and tachypnea. Hypovolemia is suspected in asphyxiated newborns or neonates born with cord compression, abruptio placentae, or placenta previa. Volume expanders may include blood, fresh frozen plasma, 5% albumin solutions, or isotonic crystalloid solutions. The appropriate volume is 10 mL/kg intravenously (or into the aorta via an umbilical artery catheter) over a period of 5 to 10 minutes and repeated if signs of hypovolemia (shock) persist. If there is little or no improvement, consideration should be given to the possibility of persistent metabolic acidosis.

Vascular Access

Vascular access can be established by umbilical venous catheterization. A 3.5- to 5.0-gauge catheter is advanced into the umbilical vein under sterile conditions. Technically more difficult to place, an umbilical arterial catheter permits analysis of arterial blood gases, pH, and systemic blood pressure and allows the administration of volume expanders and drugs. Before anything is injected into the umbilical artery, blood must be withdrawn to clear air from the catheter.

Naloxone

Naloxone is indicated only for neonatal respiratory depression associated with maternal opioid administration. It is contraindicated in newborns of opioid-addicted mothers. Naloxone can be given to the neonate at a dose of 0.1 mg/kg intravenously, intramuscularly, or into the trachea. Commonly, neonates born in the presence of opioids will be vigorous at birth but subsequently become lethargic and even apneic within a few minutes after the stimulation of the birth experience subsides.

Glucose

Glucose (dextrose) is indicated for hypoglycemia during resuscitation. Hypoglycemia should be suspected in neonates with intrauterine growth restriction, those born with severe asphyxia, and neonates born to diabetic mothers. Glucose can be measured by heel stick during resuscitation of a depressed neonate.

IV

MECONIUM ASPIRATION

Meconium aspiration is a common neonatal outcome of intrauterine asphyxia and requires expert and prompt management to avoid the risks associated with meconium aspiration pneumonitis. Immediate endotracheal intubation and tracheal/bronchial suctioning, with the tracheal tube used as a suction catheter, should be performed in all depressed newborns born through meconium staining. This procedure will remove particulate material that is impossible to dislodge with smaller suction catheters and should be repeated until suctioning through the endotracheal tube retrieves no meconium.

POSTPARTUM TUBAL LIGATION

Postpartum tubal ligation is the most common type of surgery performed in the early postpartum period. Residual epidural anesthesia from the preceding delivery may be used to perform the intra-abdominal procedure, which necessitates a T5 sensory level to ensure patient comfort. When epidural or spinal anesthesia is not used for delivery, it is common to wait 6 to 8 hours postpartum before tubal ligation in the hope of improving the likelihood of gastric emptying. Evaluation of the patient for postpartum tubal ligation should include assessment of hemodynamic status (blood loss) and consideration of anesthetic risk. Both the timing of the procedure and the decision to use a particular anesthetic technique (regional versus general) should be individualized. A spinal anesthetic is often the preferred choice. The timing of postpartum tubal ligation should not compromise other aspects of patient care in the labor and delivery area.[38]

REFERENCES

1. Parer JT, Rosen MA, Levinson G. Uteroplacental circulation and respiratory gas exchange. *In* Hughes SC, Levinson G, Rosen MA (eds): Shnider and Levinson's Anesthesia for Obstetrics, 4th ed. Philadelphia: Lippincott, Williams & Wilkins, 2002, pp 19-40.
2. Cheek TG, Gutsche BB. Pulmonary aspiration of gastric content. *In* Hughes SC, Levinson G, Rosen MA (eds): Shnider and Levinson's Anesthesia for Obstetrics, 4th ed. Philadelphia: Lippincott, Williams & Wilkins, 2002, pp 391-407.
3. Hughes SC, Levinson G, Rosen MA. Anesthesia for cesarean section. *In* Hughes SC, Levinson G, Rosen MA (eds): Shnider and Levinson's Anesthesia for Obstetrics, 4th ed. Philadelphia: Lippincott, Williams & Wilkins, 2002, pp 216-217.
4. Baraka AA, Taha SK, Aouad MT, et al. Preoxygenation, comparison of maximal breathing and tidal volume breathing techniques. Anesthesiology 1999;91:612-616.
5. Palahniuk RJ, Shnider SM, Eger EI II. Pregnancy decreases the requirement of inhaled anesthetic agents. Anesthesiology 1974;41:82-83.
6. Ralston DH, Shnider SM, deLorimier AA. Effects of equipotent ephedrine, metaraminol, mephentermine, and methoxamine on uterine blood flow in the pregnant ewe. Anesthesiology 1974;40:354-370.
7. Lee A, Ngan Kee WD, Gin T. A quantitative, systematic review of randomized controlled trials of ephedrine versus phenylephrine for the management of hypotension during spinal anesthesia for cesarean delivery. Anesth Analg 2002;94:920-926.
8. Shnider SM, Wright RG, Levinson G, et al. Uterine blood flow and plasma norepinephrine changes during maternal stress in the pregnant ewe. Anesthesiology 1979;50:524-527.
9. Biehl D, Shnider SM, Levinson G, et al. Placental transfer of lidocaine. Effects of fetal acidosis. Anesthesiology 1978;48:409-412.
10. Anderson DL, Hughes SC. Nonpharmacologic methods of pain relief during labor. *In* Hughes SC, Levinson G, Rosen MA (eds): Shnider and Levinson's Anesthesia for Obstetrics, 4th ed. Philadelphia: Lippincott, Williams & Wilkins, 2002, pp 95-104.
11. Douglas MJ, Levinson G. Systemic medication for labor and delivery. *In* Hughes SC, Levinson G, Rosen MA (eds): Shnider and Levinson's Anesthesia for Obstetrics, 4th ed. Philadelphia: Lippincott, Williams & Wilkins, 2002, pp 105-121.
12. Eisenach JC. Intraspinal analgesia in obstetrics: Part I. Opioids and other non-local anesthetics. *In* Hughes SC, Levinson G, Rosen MA (eds): Shnider and Levinson's Anesthesia for Obstetrics, 4th ed. Philadelphia: Lippincott, Williams & Wilkins, 2002, pp 149-154.
13. Eltzschig HK, Lieberman ES, Camann WR. Regional anesthesia and analgesia for labor and delivery. N Engl J Med 2003;348:319-332.
14. Mulroy M, Glosten B. The epinephrine test dose in obstetrics: Note the limitations. Anesth Analg 1998;86:923-925.
15. Norris MC, Ferrenbach D, Dalman H, et al. Does epinephrine improve the diagnostic accuracy of aspiration during labor epidural analgesia? Anesth Analg 1999;88:1073-1076.
16. Friedlander JD, Fox HE, Cain CF, et al. Fetal bradycardia and uterine hyperactivity following subarachnoid administration of fentanyl during labor. Reg Anesth 1997;22:378-381.
17. Segal S, Csavoy AN, Datta S. Placental tissue enhances uterine relaxation by nitroglycerin. Anesth Analg 1998;86:304-309.
18. Camann W. Pain relief during labor. N Engl J Med 2005;352:718-720.
19. Wong CA, Scavone BM, Peaceman AM, et al. The risk of cesarean delivery with neuraxial analgesia given early versus late in labor. N Engl J Med 2005;352:655-665.
20. van der Vyver M, Halpern S, Joseph G. Patient-controlled epidural analgesia versus continuous infusion for labour analgesia: A meta-analysis. Br J Anaesth 2002;89:459-465.
21. Rosen MA, Hughes SC, Levinson G. Regional anesthesia for labor and delivery. *In* Hughes SC, Levinson G, Rosen MA (eds): Shnider and Levinson's Anesthesia for Obstetrics, 4th ed. Philadelphia: Lippincott, Williams & Wilkins, 2002, pp 123-148.
22. Hughes SC, Dailey PA, Landers D, et al. Parturients infected with human immunodeficiency virus and regional anesthesia: Clinical and immunologic response. Anesthesiology 1995;82:32-37.

23. Hughes SC. HIV and anesthesia. Anesthesiol Clin North Am 2004;22:379-404.

24. Yentis S. High regional block—the failed intubation of the new millennium? Int J Obstet Anesth 2001;10:159-161.

25. Mercier FJ, Benhamou D. Hyperthermia related to epidural analgesia during labor. Int J Obstet Anesth 1997;7:19-24.

26. Kaul B, Vallejo M, Ramanathan S, Mandell G. Epidural labor analgesia and neonatal sepsis evaluation rate: A quality improvement study. Anesth Analg 2001;93:986-990.

27. Riley ET, Cohen SE, Macario A, et al. Spinal versus epidural anesthesia for caesarean section: A comparison of time efficiency, costs, charges, and complications. Anesth Analg 1995;80:709-712.

28. Aya AG, Mangin R, Vialles N, et al. Patients with severe preeclampsia experience less hypotension during spinal anesthesia for elective cesarean delivery than healthy parturients: A prospective cohort comparison. Anesth Analg 2003;97:867-872.

29. Su M, Hannah WJ, Willan A, et al. Term Breech Trial collaborative group. Planned caesarean section decreases the risk of adverse perinatal outcome due to both labour and delivery complications in the Term Breech Trial. Br J Obstet Gynaecol 2004;111:1065-1074.

30. Gaiser RR, Gutsche BB, Cheek TG. Anesthetic considerations for the hypertensive disorders of pregnancy. *In* Hughes SC, Levinson G, Rosen MA (eds): Shnider and Levinson's Anesthesia for Obstetrics, 4th ed. Philadelphia: Lippincott, Williams & Wilkins, 2002, pp 297-321.

31. Lydon-Rochelle M, Holt VL, Easterling TR, Martin DP. Risk of uterine rupture during labor among women with a prior cesarean delivery. N Engl J Med 2001;345:3-8.

32. Pinder AJ, Dresner M, Calow C, et al. Haemodynamic changes caused by oxytocin during caesarean section under spinal anaesthesia. Int J Obstet Anesth 2002;11:156-159.

33. Kamani AAS, Gambling DR, Chritilaw J, et al. Anesthetic management of patients with placenta accreta. Can J Anaesth 1987;34:613-617.

34. Rosen MA. Management of anesthesia for the pregnant surgical patient. Anesthesiology 1999;91:1159-1163.

35. Shnider SM (ed): Obstetrical Anesthesia: Current Concepts and Practice. Baltimore: Williams & Wilkins, 1970, pp 197-203.

36. Apgar V. A proposal for a new method of evaluation of the newborn infant. Anesth Analg 1953;32:260-267.

37. Davis PG, Tan A, O'Donnell CP, Schulze A. Resuscitation of newborn infants with 100% oxygen or air: A systematic review and meta-analysis. Lancet 2004;364:1329-1333.

38. American Society of Anesthesiologists (ASA) Taskforce on Obstetrical Anesthesia. Practice guidelines for obstetrical anesthesia. Anesthesiology 1999;90:600-611.

IV

PEDIATRICS

Claire Brett

Age-related mortality and morbidity have been measured with a wide variety of markers over the last 50 years. Although the risks associated with anesthesia (cardiac arrest, critical events) have decreased dramatically over the past 40 to 50 years, the incidence of anesthesia-related mortality and morbidity remains higher in infants than in adults and higher in younger than older children.[1-3] In the postanesthesia care unit, problems primarily or secondarily related to airway complications are more likely to develop in the youngest infants. The incidence of critical events (most often respiratory) is higher in infants younger than 1 year than in children older than 1 year, especially in infants weighing less than 2 kg.[4]

Credentialing policies for the practice of pediatric anesthesia remain controversial. The logical argument supporting subspecialization in many areas of medicine revolves around the concept that outcome is optimized by concentrating high-risk procedures in the hands of physicians who provide care for large numbers of such patients. Indeed, the frequency of anesthetic cardiac arrest in infants is less when care is delivered by pediatric-trained/experienced practitioners.[5]

FLUIDS AND ELECTROLYTES

Managing fluids and electrolytes during anesthesia for young infants, especially neonates, is challenging (Tables 33-1 and 33-2). Considerations that influence fluid homeostasis include (1) anatomic factors related to the distribution of body fluids, (2) physiologic factors such as basal requirements and abnormal metabolic rate, (3) functional immaturity of the kidneys and liver, and (4) pathologic factors secondary to the special setting of illness, anesthesia, and surgery.

Normal Distribution of Water

Total-body water consists of extracellular fluid (ECF) and intracellular fluid (ICF) (Fig. 33-1).[6] ECF includes plasma

Table 33–1 Fluid Replacement in Children

Maintenance Requirements		
Weight (kg)	**Hourly Fluid Requirements**	**24-hr Fluid Requirements**
<10	4 mL/kg	100 mL/kg
11-20	40 mL + 2 mL/kg >10 kg	1000 mL + 50 mL/kg >10 kg
>20	60 mL + 1 mL/kg >20 kg	1500 mL + 20 mL/kg >20 kg
Replacement of Ongoing Losses		
Type of Surgery	**Specific Example**	**Hourly Fluid**
Noninvasive	Inguinal hernia repair, clubfoot repair	0-2 mL/kg/hr
Mildly invasive	Ureteral reimplantation	2-4 mL/kg/hr
Moderately invasive	Elective bowel reanastomosis	4-8 mL/kg/hr
Significantly invasive	Bowel resection for necrotizing enterocolitis	≥10 mL/kg/hr

Replacement for ongoing losses with crystalloid must always be integrated with the current cardiorespiratory status, constant evaluation of the status of the surgical procedure, estimate of blood loss and plans for blood product replacement, and baseline medical problems.

Table 33–2 Clinically Important Formulas for Perioperative Management of Children

Volume of Packed Red Blood Cells (PRBCs)

PRBCs (mL) = EBV × Desired Hct × (Actual Hct/Hct of PRBCs)

EBV, estimated blood volume; Hct, hematocrit

Intraoperative Fluid Administration (Consider Four Factors)

1. "Catch up" (maintenance rate × hours NPO)

2. Maintenance fluid

3. Ongoing losses (blood loss, third spacing)

4. Special considerations (calcium, glucose, coagulation factors)

Intraoperative Glucose

Maintenance requirement of glucose for newborn (4 mg/kg/min = 240 mg/kg/hr)

Maintenance fluid (D_5 = 50 mg glucose/mL) (4 mL/kg/min = 200 mg/kg/hr)

Delivery of a D_5 solution at a rate greater than 4 mL/kg/hr may lead to hyperglycemia; preoperative evaluation includes noting the blood glucose concentration (Chemstrip/Dextrostix) level at a specific infusion (mg/kg/min) of glucose

volume and interstitial fluid volume. In the early stages of fetal development, water constitutes approximately 94% of body weight. As gestation continues, total-body water decreases so that at 32 weeks' gestation, 80% of body weight is water and, at term, total-body water is 78% of

IV

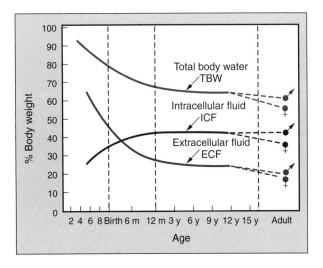

Figure 33-1 Total-body water, intracellular fluid, and extracellular fluid as a percentage of body weight and a function of age. (From Winters RW. Water and electrolyte regulation. *In* Winters RW [ed]: The Body Fluids in Pediatrics. Boston: Little, Brown, 1973, with permission.)

body weight. Adult proportions of fluid to body weight are reached between the age of 9 months and 2 years. Adult females have approximately 55% of their body weight as total-body water, with males averaging 60%.

RELATIONSHIP OF BODY FLUID COMPARTMENTS

The relationship of ECF and ICF also changes during fetal growth. ECF decreases from 60% of body weight at the fifth month to approximately 45% at term. ICF increases from 25% in the fifth month of fetal life to 33% at birth. In adult males, the ICF and ECF compartments approximate 40% and 20% of body weight, respectively. The plasma volume component of ECF remains constant at about 5% of body weight throughout life. Thus, interstitial water is greater in infants (40%) and declines to 15% and 10% of body weight in men and women, respectively (see Fig. 33-1).

ELECTROLYTE COMPOSITION OF BODY FLUIDS

The electrolyte composition of the body fluids of infants is also different from that in adults. Higher plasma chloride and lower bicarbonate and pH imply a mild metabolic acidosis with reduced buffering power (Tables 33-3 and 33-4).[7] In the first 10 days of postnatal life (term infants), serum potassium levels may be as high as 6.0 to 6.5 mEq/L. In term infants, serum potassium ranges from 3.5 to 5.5 mEq/L after the first 2 to 3 weeks of life. Another unique feature of newborns is the reduced protein concentration, which results in lower intravascular oncotic pressure.

Over the first week of life, water exchange is often negative because of ongoing losses through the skin, lungs, and urine in the setting of limited intake. A 7-kg infant with a 2100-mL ECF volume takes in and excretes approximately 700 to 1000 mL of fluid daily, which represents a 33% turnover in ECF. By comparison, a 70-kg adult with a 14,000-mL ECF volume excretes approximately 2000 mL of fluid daily for a 14% turnover. This high rate of fluid exchange may expose infants to more rapid development of both dehydration and overhydration.

PEDIATRIC AIRWAY

Preoperatively, the anesthesiologist must meticulously assess all aspects of the airway to develop detailed and flexible plans for (1) intubating the trachea, (2) intraoperative airway management, and (3) postoperative recovery (Table 33-5). The anesthetic plan for management of the child's airway may be influenced by the site of surgery. Maintaining upper airway patency is an active process that is depressed during general anesthesia.[8]

During spontaneous ventilation, the upper airway is exposed to potentially collapsing negative pressure during inspiration, but the pharynx is kept open by the upper airway muscles. The pharynx is prone to collapse because negative pressure pulls the tongue against the pharynx. The genioglossus is the principal muscle that dilates the pharynx, and it serves to keep the upper airway patent. This muscle receives feedback from the central nervous system via the hypoglossal nerve and from the lower airway via the vagus nerve.

General anesthesia depresses activity of the upper airway and thereby predisposes to oropharyngeal obstruction, especially in newborns and young infants, whose upper airways and chest wall are easily compressible. The contribution of the tongue to airway obstruction is exaggerated in infants because the tongue is large relative to the total volume of the mouth. Infants or children with small upper airways secondary to craniofacial anomalies, weakness as a result of neuromuscular or central nervous system disorders, impingement on the airway secondary to tumors or hemangiomas, or dysfunction of the tracheobronchial tree because of an upper respiratory infection (URI) are especially prone to pharyngeal obstruction by the tongue.

Head position is important in maintaining upper airway patency during anesthesia. Flexing an infant's head may cause the upper airway to collapse more readily. This is particularly important during induction of anesthesia in children with abnormal upper airways. In addition, the

Table 33–3 Laboratory Values in Children				
	Newborn	**1 Week Old**	**1 Month Old**	**1 Year Old**
Glucose (mg/dL)	40-60	50-80	60-100	60-100
Total CO$_2$ (mEq/L)	13-22	15-22	20-28	22-28
Chloride (mEq/L)	98-113	98-113	98-107	98-107
Potassium (mEq/L)	3.9-5.9	4.1-5.5	3.4-4.7	3.4-4.7
Total calcium (mg/dL)	7.6-10.4	9.0-11.0	9.0-11.0	8.8-10.8
Ionized calcium (mmol/L)	1.05-1.37	1.10-1.42	1.20-1.38	1.20-1.38
Total protein (g/dL) Albumin (g/dL)	4.4-7.6 2.2-4.0	4.4-7.6 2.5-5.5	3.6-7.4 2.1-4.8	3.7-7.5 1.9-5.0

Data from The Harriet Lane Handbook: A Manual for Pediatric House Officers, 16th ed. St Louis: CV Mosby, 2002.

Table 33-4 Developmental Changes in Blood Gas Values in Children

Age	pH	Pao$_2$	Paco$_2$
1 hour	7.26-7.29	60	55
24 hours	7.37	70	33-35
1 week	7.40	70-80	35
1-10 months	7.40	85-90	35
4-8 years	7.39-7.40	90-95	37
12-18 years	7.35-7.45	95-100	35-45

Data from The Harriet Lane Handbook: A Manual for Pediatric House Officers, 16th ed. St Louis: CV Mosby, 2002.

Table 33-5 Endotracheal Tube Sizes

Age	Size: ID (mm)	Depth (cm)
Preterm	2.5	6-8
Term	3.0	9-10
6 months	3.0-3.5	10
1-2 years	4.0	10-11
3-4 years	4.5	12-13
5-6 years	5.0	14-15
10 years	6.0	16-17

To maintain the same external diameter, the size of a cuffed endotracheal tube (ETT) is generally about 0.5 mm smaller than the uncuffed device. For example, a 4-year-old who requires a 4.5-mm uncuffed ETT should probably be intubated with a 4.0-mm cuffed ETT. Because of the need to decrease the size when substituting a cuffed for an uncuffed ETT, the benefit of the cuff must be balanced against the decrease in cross-sectional area of the smaller tube. That is, replacing a 5.5-mm uncuffed with a 5.0-mm cuffed ETT is less of an "insult" in the percent decrease in cross sectional area than when a 3.0-mm cuffed ETT replaces an uncuffed 3.5-mm tube.

small, soft airways of neonates (especially premature neonates) are more compressible if the neck is flexed. Extending or keeping the neck in a neutral position while applying positive airway pressure during ventilation with a bag and facemask is important, particularly during induction of general anesthesia.

Unique Anatomic Features

The larynx of infants is higher in the neck (C3-4) than in adults (C4-5). An infant's epiglottis is large, but it is narrow and short. Because of these anatomic features, a straight laryngoscope blade may allow the larynx of a normal infant to be visualized more easily. When laryngeal anatomy is distorted by craniofacial anomalies (micrognathia or midface hypoplasia), direct visualization of the larynx may be impossible, and alternative methods of securing the airway should be available.

An infant's vocal cords are slanted such that the posterior commissure is more cephalad than the anterior commissure. This arrangement may predispose the anterior sublaryngeal airway to trauma from an endotracheal tube. The subglottic area is prone to traumatic injury from an endotracheal tube because the narrowest portion of an infant's larynx is at the cricoid cartilage. In adults, the narrowest portion is the glottic rim. Thus, an endotracheal tube that easily passes through the vocal cords of an infant or child may fit snugly in the subglottis and cause subglottic edema and symptoms of increased airway resistance after tracheal extubation. This increased resistance is usually reversible, but subglottic stenosis may develop after prolonged tracheal intubation with an oversized endotracheal tube.

Airway Assessment

Difficult tracheal intubation generally occurs when facial or oral pathology prevents visualization of the larynx or when the larynx is easily visualized by direct laryngoscopy but a lesion in the supraglottic, glottic, or subglottic region interferes with insertion of the endotracheal tube. Circumstances that may result in difficult intubation may also be categorized by anatomic location or by etiology (congenital, inflammatory, traumatic, metabolic, or neoplastic).

When the past medical history documents previous difficult airway management and tracheal intubation, it is recommended that a physician experienced in performing pediatric bronchoscopy be present during initial airway management. Fiberoptic airway endoscopy with or without the aid of a laryngeal mask airway (LMA) may be indicated for securing a difficult airway. In some circumstances, it may be prudent to have available a surgeon skilled in performing cricothyrotomy or tracheostomy (or both). Preoperatively, the patient's parents should be informed of the risks and the potential need for a tracheostomy. In some situations, performing a controlled tracheostomy may be less traumatic than persisting with multiple attempts at direct laryngoscopy.

DEVELOPMENTAL PHYSIOLOGY

Respiratory System (Table 33-6)

LUNG DEVELOPMENT

Alveoli develop mainly after birth and increase from 20 million terminal air sacs in a newborn to approximately 300 million alveoli at 18 months of age. In general, extrauterine viability is first likely after 26 weeks when the respiratory saccules have developed and vascularization

Table 33-6 Comparison of Pulmonary Variables

	Neonate	Infant	5 Years of Age	Adult
Weight (kg)	3	4-10	18	70
Breathing frequency (breaths/min)	35	24-30	20	15
Tidal volume (mL/kg)	6	6	6	6
Vital capacity (mL/kg)	35			70
Alveolar ventilation (mL/kg/min)	130			60
Carbon dioxide production (mL/kg/min)	6			3
Functional residual capacity (mL/kg)	25	25	35	40

by capillaries has occurred. Supportive care of a premature infant commonly includes oxygen and positive-pressure ventilation, and infections are inevitable.

RIB CAGE

The compliant rib cage of a newborn produces a mechanical disadvantage to effective ventilation. The negative intrapleural pressure produced by normal inspiratory effort tends to collapse the cartilaginous, compliant chest of an infant (especially a premature newborn), which causes paradoxical chest wall motion and limits airflow during inspiration. The circular configuration of the rib cage (ellipsoid in adults) and the horizontal angle of insertion of the diaphragm (oblique in adults) cause distortion of a newborn's rib cage and inefficient diaphragmatic contraction.

DIAPHRAGM

An adult diaphragm contains 55% type I fibers (fatigue-resistant, slow-twitching, highly oxidative fibers), whereas the diaphragm of a full-term infant has 25% and that of a preterm infant has 10%. A lower proportion of type I fibers predisposes these primary respiratory muscles to fatigue. The intercostal muscles show a similar developmental pattern.

PULMONARY SURFACTANT

Pulmonary surfactant effects dramatic changes in lung mechanics, including distensibility and end-expiratory volume stability. The development of respiratory distress syndrome of the newborn correlates with insufficient (premature infants) or delayed (infants of diabetic mothers) synthesis of surfactant. The most significant decrease in infant mortality observed in 20 years in the United States occurred in 1990, the year that surfactant was released commercially. However, chronic lung disease persists as a common problem in approximately 20% of premature infants as a result of the complex interplay of many factors in addition to surfactant during normal growth and development of the lungs.

Circulatory System (Table 33-7)

FETAL CIRCULATION

The fetal circulation is characterized by (1) increased pulmonary vascular resistance, (2) decreased pulmonary blood flow, (3) decreased systemic vascular resistance, and (4) right-to-left blood flow through the patent ductus arteriosus and foramen ovale. At birth, the onset of spontaneous ventilation and elimination of the placental circulation decrease pulmonary vascular resistance and increase pulmonary blood flow. Simultaneously, systemic vascular resistance increases, left atrial pressure increases, the foramen ovale closes functionally, and the right-to-left shunting ceases. When anatomic closure is achieved and cardiac anatomy is normal, shunting through the ductus arteriosus is eliminated. Arterial hypoxemia or acidosis in a newborn can precipitate return to a fetal pattern of circulation (pulmonary arterial vasoconstriction, pulmonary hypertension, reduced pulmonary blood flow). This combination leads to right atrial pressure increasing above left atrial pressure and thereby results in right-to-left shunting through the foramen ovale and ductus arteriosus. This return to a fetal circulatory pattern, termed persistent fetal circulation or persistent pulmonary hypertension of the newborn, further exacerbates the arterial hypoxemia and acidosis.

MYOCARDIAL FUNCTION

The ability of fetal and adult myocardium to contract and relax depends on the same basic processes. However, the membranes in the myocardium that control calcium flux and the contractile system that responds to calcium undergo qualitative and quantitative age-related changes (postnatal myocardial development).

The major differences in myocardial function between the neonatal and adult heart translate to important principles of clinical care. The relative noncompliance of the neonatal heart implies a limited capacity to handle a volume load or to increase stroke volume for augmentation of cardiac output (or both). Thus, the "Frank-Starling" response

Table 33-7 Comparison of Cardiovascular Variables

	Neonate	Infant	5 Years of Age	Adult
Weight	3	4-10	18	70
Oxygen consumption (mg/kg/min)	6	5	4	3
Systolic blood pressure (mm Hg)	65	90-95	95	120
Heart rate (beats/min)	130	120	90	80

is considered to play a limited role, whereas the heart rate is critical for maintaining cardiac output in a newborn. Over the first months of life, myocardial contractility gradually increases, which allows cardiac output to be maintained over a wide range of preload and afterload.

EVALUATION OF CARDIOPULMONARY FUNCTION

The initial step in evaluating the cardiopulmonary system of a newborn begins with the physical examination. Skin color, capillary filling time, trends in blood pressure, heart rate, intensity of peripheral pulses, presence of a murmur or S_3 or S_4 heart sounds, respiratory rate, effort, and breath sounds, as well as decreased urine output or metabolic acidosis, should be assessed. Murmurs, abnormal heart sounds, cardiac dysrhythmias, and cardiomegaly are rarely innocuous findings in a newborn. Interpretation of the electrocardiogram, chest radiograph, and echocardiogram will allow rational planning for intraoperative monitoring, selection of anesthetic drugs, delivery of intravenous fluids, postoperative recovery, and the extent of the proposed surgical procedure (total correction or staged procedure).

Renal Function

The fetal kidneys are a passive organ that undergoes transition to an active organ at birth. Urine production increases from about 5 mL/hr at 20 weeks, to about 18 mL/hr at 30 weeks, to about 50 mL/hr at 40 weeks of gestation. Although the kidneys are not essential for maintaining normal fluid and electrolyte balance in a fetus, urine production contributes to normal amniotic fluid volume and is critical for normal pulmonary and urinary tract development.

GLOMERULAR FILTRATION RATE

The renal function of a newborn versus an adult is characterized by a decreased glomerular filtration rate (GFR), decreased excretion of solid materials, and decreased urine concentrating ability. The GFR increases with gestational age, and by 34 to 36 weeks of gestation, values are similar to those reported for full-term infants. Over the first 3 months of life, the GFR increases twofold to threefold.

Thereafter, a slower rise is noted until adult values are reached by 12 to 24 months of life.

RENAL TUBULAR FUNCTION

Limited renal tubular reabsorptive function is the basis for the loss of bicarbonate and the "normal" acidosis that occur in a newborn, particularly premature newborns (sometimes called renal tubular acidosis type 4). Similarly, proximal renal tubular reabsorption of sodium increases with gestational age. Of note, arterial hypoxemia, respiratory distress, and hyperbilirubinemia can increase fractional sodium excretion. The limited distal renal tubular function also impairs the ability of the kidneys to excrete a sodium load. In addition, tubular immaturity affects the conservation of amino acids, nucleosides, glucose, and other essential substrates.

Hematology

At birth, a full-term newborn normally has a hemoglobin concentration of 18 to 20 g/dL; a preterm infant usually has a lower hemoglobin concentration ranging between 13 and 15 g/dL (Tables 33-8 and 33-9).[7] Approximately 70% to 80% of the hemoglobin at birth is fetal hemoglobin (HgF), but the concentration of HgF decreases to physiologically insignificant levels by 3 to 6 months of age. The high affinity of HgF for oxygen shifts the oxyhemoglobin dissociation curve to the left so that P_{50} (normally 18 to 20 mm Hg) is less than the adult value (27 mm Hg). Although high oxygen affinity improves the fetus's ability to uptake oxygen from the mother at the placental interface, after birth this same high affinity decreases the amount of oxygen released at tissue levels. In a normal newborn, higher hemoglobin levels, greater blood volume, and increased cardiac output (per unit weight) compensate adequately for HgF. Such normal, term infants tolerate the gradual decrease in hematocrit (and HgF) over the first few months of life, with the nadir reaching values as low as 9 to 10 g/dL. By comparison, the concentration of hemoglobin in a very-low-birth-weight (VLBW, <1500 g) or extremely-low-birth-weight (ELBW, <1000 g) infant at birth normally ranges between 13 and 15 g/dL. Of note, the nadir of a premature (<30 weeks' gestation) infant's

IV

Table 33-8 Hematologic Values in Children

Age	Hemoglobin (g/100 mL) (Mean)	Platelets (/mm³)
26-27 weeks	13.4	254,000
28 weeks	14.5	275,000
32 weeks	15.0	290,000
Term (cord)	16.5	290,000
1-3 days	18.5	192,000
2 weeks	16.6	252,000
1 month	13.9	250,000
2 months	11.2	200,000-250,000
6 months	12.6	150,000-350,000
6-24 months	12.0	150,000-350,000
2-6 years	12.5	150,000-350,000
6-12 years	13.5	150,000-350,000
12-18 years (male)	14.5	150,000-350,000
12-18 years (female)	14.0	150,000-350,000
Adult male	15.5	150,000-350,000
Adult female	14.0	150,000-350,000

Data from The Harriet Lane Handbook: A Manual for Pediatric House Officers, 16th ed. St Louis: CV Mosby, 2002.

Table 33-9 Developmental Changes in Blood Volume

Age	Blood Volume (ml/kg)
Preterm infant	90-105
Term infant	78-86
1-12 months	73-78
1-3 years	74-82
4-6 years	80-86
7-18 years	83-90
Adults	68-88

hemoglobin may be as low as 6 to 7 g/dL by 3 to 4 months of age. However, erythropoietin is now routinely administered to infants in the neonatal intensive care unit, thereby avoiding such profound anemia.

Newborns with cardiovascular or respiratory instability often benefit from a hematocrit higher than 40% to 45% to facilitate adequate oxygen delivery. Blood loss exceeding 10% to 15% of blood volume (or even less in some patients) may not be tolerated by newborns, especially VLBW infants. Cross-matched blood should be available for surgery in a newborn, especially when blood loss is anticipated.

Assessment of clotting function should be considered before major surgery in a newborn because the synthesis of prothrombin and factors II, VII, and X is limited in an immature liver. Perinatal asphyxia and septicemia affect the function and concentration of both clotting factors and platelet count and thereby result in coagulopathies. Before surgical intervention, the availability of fresh frozen plasma, fibrinogen, and platelets must be considered.

MEDICAL AND SURGICAL DISEASES THAT AFFECT THE NEWBORN

Necrotizing Enterocolitis

Necrotizing enterocolitis (NEC) is a gastrointestinal emergency that primarily affects premature infants younger than 32 weeks' gestational age. Though centered in the gastrointestinal tract, NEC is a systemic process primarily related to the sepsis that accompanies intestinal necrosis and increased mucosal permeability.

NEC is frequently linked to intestinal mucosal injury from ischemia caused by reduced mesenteric blood flow.

The most common anatomic site is the ileocolic region, but NEC is frequently discontinuous and involves both the small and large intestine (Fig 33-2). The primary pathologic finding in NEC is coagulative or ischemic necrosis, but inflammation is also prominent. The combination of ischemia and bacteria (no specific organism) seems to be essential. The formation of gas bubbles (pneumatosis intestinalis) reflects fermentation of intraluminal substrate by bacteria.

CLINICAL MANIFESTATIONS

Typically, a preterm baby in whom NEC develops has a history of perinatal asphyxia or postnatal cardiorespiratory instability and manifests gastrointestinal signs between the 1st and 10th days of life (abdominal distention, retained gastric secretions that may be bile tinged, vomiting, bloody or mucoid diarrhea, and occult blood loss in stools). Bowel necrosis and perforation may develop and be accompanied by sepsis with thermal instability, lethargy, metabolic acidosis, hypotension, hypoxia, jaundice, disseminated intravascular coagulation, and generalized bleeding. Most infants with NEC have a decreased platelet count (50,000 to 75,000/mm^3) and prolonged prothrombin and partial thromboplastin times. Abdominal radiographs may reveal dilated, fixed (adynamic ileus) loops of bowel, gas in the portal venous system, and pneumoperitoneum.

TREATMENT

Unless there is evidence of intestinal necrosis or perforation, the initial treatment of NEC is nonoperative and includes decompression of the stomach, cessation of feeding, broad-spectrum antibiotics, fluid and electrolyte therapy, parenteral nutrition, and correction of hematologic abnormalities. Inotropic drugs may be needed to maintain hemodynamic stability. Bowel perforation is the most important indication for surgery. Other events that increase the likelihood for surgical intervention include peritonitis, air in the portal system, bowel wall edema, ascites, and progressively deteriorating hemodynamic status.

MANAGEMENT OF ANESTHESIA

The preoperative assessment of infants with NEC should focus on evaluating and correcting the respiratory, circulatory, metabolic, and hematologic disorders. During fluid resuscitation these infants must be monitored carefully for signs of patent ductus arteriosus or congestive heart failure. Most require mechanical ventilatory support because of metabolic acidosis and respiratory complications of fluid administration and sepsis.

Depending on the hemodynamic status of the infant, intraoperative monitoring may include continuous monitoring of intra-arterial and central venous pressure and blood gas analysis. At a minimum, intravenous access should be adequate to allow vigorous crystalloid and colloid administration. Fresh frozen plasma, platelets, and red blood cells may be administered early in surgery in response to blood loss, hemodynamic instability, or coagulopathy. In preterm infants, inspired oxygen concentrations should be adjusted to produce a PaO$_2$ of 50 to 70 mm Hg (SpO$_2$ of 90% to 95%). Nitrous oxide should be avoided, especially in the presence of free air in the gastrointestinal and portal venous systems.

Volatile anesthetics are often poorly tolerated and should be introduced only in low concentrations to supplement intravenous drugs (opioids, ketamine). Fentanyl or remifentanil combined with low doses of volatile anesthetics can provide analgesia and amnesia and allow cardiovascular stability. Neuromuscular blocking drugs facilitate surgical exposure. Inotropes are occasionally needed to support the cardiovascular system when fluid therapy alone fails to maintain adequate perfusion. Observing bowel perfusion during surgery may provide a useful guide to the effectiveness of fluid and inotropic support. Postoperatively, mechanical ventilation and cardiovascular support are usually required in the neonatal intensive care unit. Parenteral nutrition is essential after sepsis is controlled and metabolic stability is established.

Abdominal Wall Defects

Omphalocele and gastroschisis are distinct lesions despite a similar physical appearance (Figs. 33-3 and 33-4). Omphalocele is a central defect of the umbilical ring, and the abdominal contents are within a sac, unless the sac ruptures in utero. Gastroschisis is an abdominal wall defect, usually to the right of the umbilical cord. This defect is

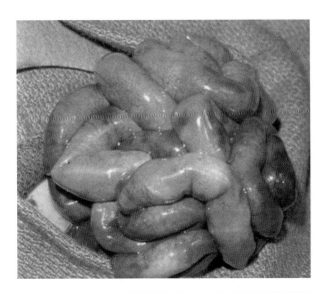

Figure 33-2 Necrotizing enterocolitis is characterized by patchy areas of involvement in the small bowel. Areas of dark, underperfused bowel are scattered among normal-appearing, well-perfused, "pink" bowel.

IV

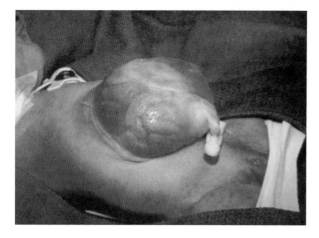

Figure 33-3 An omphalocele is a central defect of the umbilical ring, and the abdominal contents are within a sac. Note that the umbilical cord is inserted into the sac.

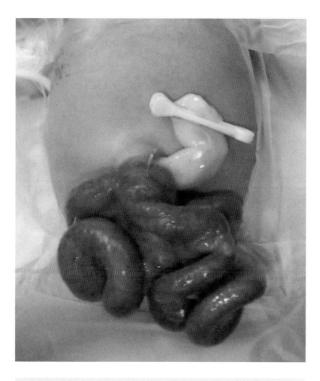

Figure 33-4 Gastroschisis is an abdominal wall defect, usually to the right of the umbilical cord. Note that the bowel loops are matted, thick, and without a sac. The umbilical cord is separate from the abdominal wall defect.

matted, thickened, and often covered with an inflammatory coating or peel. This anatomic defect can be diagnosed in utero with fetal ultrasound.

TREATMENT
Preoperative management of abdominal wall defects is directed primarily toward fluid resuscitation and minimizing heat loss, treating sepsis, avoiding direct trauma to the herniated organs, and identifying other anomalies. A bowel bag may be used to minimize fluid and heat loss. Decompression of the stomach with an orogastric or nasogastric tube is important to prevent regurgitation, aspiration pneumonia, and further bowel distention.

Fluid Therapy
Intravenous fluid therapy (as much as two to four times [150 to 300 mL/kg/day] the usual maintenance infusion rate [80 to 100 mL/kg/day]) is infused to ensure adequate hydration and to compensate for peritonitis, bowel ischemia, and significant third-space loss. Initially, a balanced salt solution is used, and urine output is monitored. Urine output of 1 to 2 mL/kg/hr suggests adequate hydration. Because of the large fluid requirements, acid-base status and electrolyte levels should be monitored. Rarely, colloid is required to maintain hemodynamic stability preoperatively.

Surgical Treatment
Surgical management is aimed at repairing the abdominal wall defect and reducing the protruded viscera. Forcing the viscera into an underdeveloped abdominal cavity that cannot easily accommodate the herniated bowel can have dramatic effects on ventilation and oxygenation, as well as on cardiac output and systemic blood pressure (secondary to impaired venous return from the inferior vena cava). Excessive compression of the intestine can produce ischemia. Thus, during abdominal closure, the anesthesiologist must anticipate the potential effects of decreased pulmonary compliance (increased airway pressure, decreased oxygen saturation, hypercapnia) and inadequate cardiac output. If primary closure is not possible, a Silastic mesh prosthesis ("silo") is sutured to the fascia of the defect. After the silo is in place, the extra-abdominal organs are then gradually returned to the peritoneal cavity over a period of 3 to 10 days.

Management of Anesthesia
Depending on the size of the defect, the anticipated difficulty with closure, and the preoperative status of the infant, continuous invasive monitoring of arterial and central venous pressure may be indicated. Vigorous fluid therapy (10 to 100 mL/kg/hr) is often critical to maintain perfusion and hemodynamic stability, but glucose should be delivered at maintenance rates (3 to 4 mg/kg/min). Heat loss should be minimized and a warm environment maintained.

Neuromuscular blockade is essential to maximize efforts for primary closure of the abdomen. The inspired oxygen

generally larger than 5 cm in diameter and typically contains only large and small bowel (rarely the liver may exit through the defect). The bowel is exposed to the intrauterine environment with no sac, so the loops are

concentration must be adjusted to maintain oxygen saturation between 95% and 97% while recognizing that the physiologic range of PaO₂ in newborns is 50 to 70 mm Hg. Nitrous oxide may increase bowel distention and is therefore avoided. A variety of combinations of intravenous drugs and volatile anesthetics can provide adequate surgical conditions. High doses of opioids are acceptable because except in infants with a small defect, mechanical ventilation of the lungs must be maintained postoperatively. Prolonged postoperative total parenteral nutrition is generally required, especially in infants with a large omphalocele or gastroschisis, so appropriate intravenous access should be established in the operating room to facilitate early postoperative nutritional support.

Tracheoesophageal Fistula

Different anatomic variations of tracheoesophageal fistula (TEF) occur, and in most cases (type B, C, E), TEF and esophageal atresia occur together (Fig. 33-5).[9] The most common lesion (>90%) is type C, in which a fistula exists between the trachea and the lower esophageal segment at a point slightly above the carina, whereas the upper esophageal segment ends blindly in the mediastinum at the level of the second or third thoracic vertebra. Approximately 20% to 25% of these infants also have a congenital heart defect (ventricular septal defect, atrial septal defect, tetralogy of Fallot, atrioventricular canal, coarctation of the aorta), and about 20% to 30% are born prematurely.

The acronym VATER refers to a group of anomalies including V, vertebral defects; A, anal defects; TE, tracheoesophageal atresia; and R, renal anomalies.[10] Another acronym includes a C and L because cardiac and limb anomalies are also common. As many as 20% to 25% of

infants with esophageal atresia will have at least three of the defects included in VACTERL. Between 50% and 65% of infants with esophageal atresia with or without TEF will have at least one additional anomaly.

TREATMENT

Surgical ligation of a TEF is performed promptly. Preoperatively, several interventions are undertaken to protect the lungs from aspiration of gastric fluids (Table 33-10). Optimally, the surgical repair can be accomplished as a one-stage procedure in which the fistula is ligated and the esophagus is primarily anastomosed. In infants with significant associated anomalies or sepsis, a thoracotomy may be considered too risky, and instead, a palliative procedure (gastrostomy) is performed under local or general anesthesia and the definitive repair performed within 24 to 72 hours, when the extent of other anomalies is defined, cardiovascular stability is established, and a clear surgical plan has been defined. Often, the gastrostomy tube is kept patent to decompress the stomach and minimize regurgitation into the lungs.

MANAGEMENT OF ANESTHESIA

Awake tracheal intubation is likely to be considered the safest approach to secure the airway in infants with TEF. It allows appropriate positioning of the endotracheal tube without positive-pressure ventilation, as well as minimizes the risk for gastric distention from inspired gases passing through the fistula during positive-pressure ventilation of the newborn's lungs. Titrating small doses of fentanyl (0.2 to 0.5 µg/kg IV) or morphine (0.02 to 0.05 mg/kg IV) before tracheal intubation may be helpful, but this must be considered from the perspective of the infant's clinical status at the time of the procedure.

IV

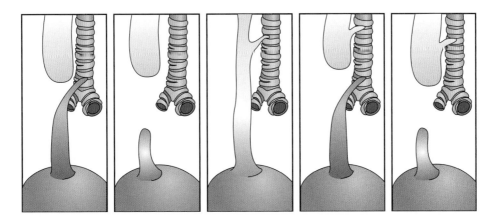

Figure 33-5 Classification of tracheoesophageal anomalies in descending order of incidence. Type C (86%) is esophageal atresia with a distal tracheoesophageal fistula. Type A (8%) is esophageal atresia without a tracheoesophageal fistula. Type E (4%) is an H-type fistula without esophageal atresia. Type D (1%) is esophageal atresia with both proximal and distal tracheoesophageal fistulas. Type B (1%) is esophageal atresia with a proximal tracheoesophageal fistula. (From Gross RE. The Surgery of Infancy and Childhood. Philadelphia: WB Saunders, 1953.)

Table 33-10 Interventions to Protect the Lungs from Aspiration in the Presence of a Tracheoesophageal Fistula

Avoidance of feedings

Upright positioning of the infant to decrease the likelihood of gastroesophageal reflux

Intermittent suctioning of the upper blind esophageal pouch

Antibiotic therapy and physiotherapy if pneumonia is diagnosed

An alternative to awake tracheal intubation is inhalation induction of anesthesia (after pharyngeal suctioning), with or without a neuromuscular blocking drug, plus gentle positive-pressure ventilation of the infants' lungs.

After the endotracheal tube is in place, end-tidal carbon dioxide and oxygen saturation are monitored and the stomach and chest auscultated to ensure that the lungs are adequately ventilated and the stomach is not being inflated with inspired gas. Blood clots or secretions may block the endotracheal tube, and thus frequent suctioning is usually required.

After the TEF is ligated, a catheter passed through the nose or mouth by the anesthesiologist into the blind upper pouch identifies the upper esophageal structure. The surgeon passes a catheter into the lower part of the esophagus, and the anastomosis is fashioned over the catheter. When the anastomosis is complete, the catheter is withdrawn to just above the suture line, and the proximal end of the catheter is marked at the mouth. The distance from the mouth to the distal tip is noted. Only catheters of this length or shorter should be used to suction postoperatively.

Some term infants can be extubated after simple ligation of a TEF, but more often postoperative ventilation is maintained for at least 24 to 40 hours. Tracheomalacia or a defective tracheal wall at the site of the fistula is common and can predispose to collapse of the airway during spontaneous ventilation. Most surgeons recommend that ventilation with a mask and bag be avoided for at least several days after an esophageal anastomosis.

PERSISTENT EFFECTS AFTER SURGICAL REPAIR

TEF cannot be considered a simple anatomic problem cured by a surgical intervention. Many patients have anatomic narrowing of the esophagus at the site of anastomosis or ligation of the fistula, and this narrowing may progress to a severe stricture. Esophageal dysmotility and reflux are common and may also lead to esophageal stricture. Recurrent upper and lower respiratory infections occur in 35% to 75% of patients. Pulmonary function studies 7 to 18 years after repair show a high incidence of obstructive and restrictive forms of lung disease.

Congenital Diaphragmatic Hernia

Congenital diaphragmatic hernia (CDH) is a defect in the diaphragm that develops early in gestation and is accompanied by extrusion of intra-abdominal organs into the thoracic cavity and other associated abnormalities (Table 33-11) (Fig. 33-6). In many infants with CDH, the herniated abdominal viscera that occupy the thoracic cage interfere with development of the lungs. Typically, some degree of pulmonary hypoplasia is present on the ipsilateral side, but often also on the contralateral side.

CLINICAL MANIFESTATIONS

The classic triad of CDH consists of cyanosis, dyspnea, and apparent dextrocardia. Physical examination reveals a

Table 33-11 Abnormalities That May Be Associated with Congenital Diaphragmatic Hernia

Bilateral lung hypoplasia (varying degrees)

Pulmonary hypertension

Pulmonary arteriolar hyperreactivity and arteriolar reactivity

Congenital anomalies

Cardiac

Chromosomal

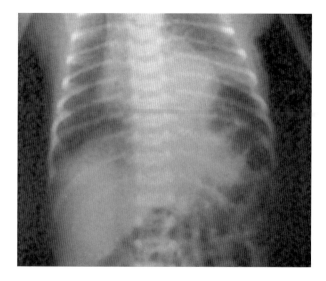

Figure 33-6 Chest radiograph of a newborn with a congenital diaphragmatic hernia. Note the bowel gas pattern in the left hemithorax with absence of lung tissue in the left costophrenic sulcus, deviation of the mediastinum, and cardiac silhouette to the right.

scaphoid abdomen, bulging chest, decreased breath sounds, distant or right-displaced heart sounds, and bowel sounds in the chest. Radiographs may show a bowel gas pattern in the chest, mediastinal shift, and minimal lung tissue at the left costophrenic sulcus.

TREATMENT

The goal of initial management of CDH is to avoid a surgical intervention when the infant is hypoxic and acidotic. Instead, medical management is directed to stabilizing the infant's cardiorespiratory status by improving oxygenation, correcting metabolic acidosis, reducing the right-to-left shunting, and increasing pulmonary perfusion.

Positive-pressure ventilation with a facemask is particularly risky for infants with CDH because attempting to expand the noncompliant lungs may distend the stomach and intestines, which are in the left thoracic cavity, and thereby further decrease chest compliance. Early tracheal intubation and decompression of the stomach are important initial steps to prevent further compression of the infant's lungs by the displaced abdominal viscera.

In the early neonatal period, some infants exhibit a honeymoon period characterized by adequate oxygenation and ventilation with minimal ventilatory support. However, this period is often followed by a sudden and often unexplained return to a state of persistent pulmonary hypertension (persistent fetal circulation) and clinical deterioration (acidosis, arterial hypoxemia, hypercapnia, pulmonary hypertension, and right-to-left shunting through the foramen ovale and ductus arteriosus). Efforts at manipulating pulmonary vascular resistance (pharmacologic means or hyperventilation, or both) are not predictably successful. If conventional mechanical ventilation of the infant's lungs is not effective, a trial of high-frequency oscillatory support may be considered. Other therapeutic interventions to consider include the administration of inhaled nitric oxide and extracorporeal membrane oxygenation (ECMO) to achieve cardiorespiratory stability before surgery. If an infant does require either nitric oxide or ECMO, surgery is likely to be performed in the neonatal intensive care unit so that these therapies can be maintained.

MANAGEMENT OF ANESTHESIA

Usually, surgical repair is approached through an abdominal incision, but a transthoracic or thoracoabdominal approach is also possible. With rare exception, infants with a moderate or large CDH require ventilatory support preoperatively, and most receive neuromuscular blockade. The goals of ventilation in the operating room (optimize pH and pulmonary blood flow with minimal barotrauma) are the same as preoperatively. Hyperventilation of the infant's lungs is reserved to treat acute episodes of pulmonary hypertension. If sudden deterioration in ventilation or hemodynamic status (or both) occurs, pulmonary hypertension must be quickly differentiated from a contralateral pneumothorax because treatment of pneumothorax is needle thoracostomy and chest tube placement rather than hyperventilation.

The selection of specific anesthetic drugs is logically based on cardiorespiratory status, the site of surgical repair (neonatal intensive care nursery or operating room), and the plans for intraoperative ventilatory support. Nitrous oxide is avoided in infants with CDH because most require high inspired oxygen concentrations and nitrous oxide can diffuse inside the viscera and exaggerate lung compression. If an anesthesia machine is available, a low concentration of a volatile anesthetic can be administered and the dose increased if the newborn is hemodynamically stable. In most cases, opioids (usually intravenous fentanyl) are administered and an opioid infusion is continued into the postoperative period.

Myelomeningocele

The primary defect in a myelomeningocele is localized failure of the neural tube to close. The lesion appears most often in the lumbar area as a sac on the back of the infant. In addition, because the vertebral arches in the area fail to fuse or are totally absent, the spinal canal is widened.

CLINICAL MANIFESTATIONS

The clinical manifestations of myelomeningocele relate to the level of neural tube involvement, the existence of any other neurologic anomalies, and the development of hydrocephalus (develops in about 90% of infants with thoracolumbar, lumbar, or lumbosacral lesions). In addition, the Arnold-Chiari malformation is identified in most infants with this lesion.

TREATMENT

Treatment of myelomeningocele is based on the predicted prognosis. In some infants, supportive care is an appropriate level of conservative intervention. In many infants, prenatal diagnosis introduces the consideration of fetal treatment or cesarean section, or both, to avoid trauma during spontaneous vaginal delivery.

In most cases of thoracolumbar, lumbar, and lumbosacral lesions, surgical intervention is initiated in the first 24 hours of life. Early surgical treatment decreases the incidence of infection and further neurologic injury. The main anesthetic considerations are related to avoiding injury during induction and tracheal intubation and meticulous attention to ventilation in the prone position. The infant can be supported on "bolsters" while supine during induction and again when positioned prone for surgical treatment. Placement of a ventriculoperitoneal shunt is generally performed in a separate surgery. The need for frequent surgical interventions is the basis for initiating latex precautions from the neonatal period in the hope of minimizing the risk for development of latex allergy.

IV

Pyloric Stenosis

The abnormal anatomy leading to pyloric stenosis is thickened circular smooth muscle of the pylorus. The gastric outlet gradually becomes obstructed over the first days to weeks of life and leads to projectile, nonbilious vomiting and failure to thrive, with body weight less than birth weight at 2 to 3 weeks of age. The pathognomonic physical finding is an olive-sized mass in the upper left to midportion of the abdomen. The condition is more common in white, first-born males.

The most significant preoperative considerations are fluid and electrolyte imbalance and a full stomach. Because of recurrent vomiting of acidic gastric fluid, hypokalemic hypochloremic metabolic alkalosis and dehydration may develop. Administration of intravenous fluids allows rehydration and correction of the metabolic abnormalities within 6 to 12 hours in most infants. At that point, surgical treatment is indicated.

MANAGEMENT OF ANESTHESIA

Some anesthesiologist prefer to consider an infant as having a full stomach and recommend a rapid-sequence induction of anesthesia after emptying the stomach with a nasogastric tube. Others suggest that the stomach empties spontaneously and believe that a inhalational or intravenous (not necessarily rapid-sequence) induction of anesthesia is acceptable. A history of a barium swallow may affect the decision regarding the technique for induction of anesthesia. However, sonography and not a barium swallow is the most frequent technique for confirming the diagnosis of pyloric stenosis.

Although the surgical procedure is a simple pyloromyotomy that takes only about 15 minutes, the current trend is to perform a laparoscopic procedure to minimize recovery time and the likelihood of ileus. The infant may be able to eat within several hours of surgery, and discharge is often possible within about 12 hours.

COMPLICATING ISSUES IN THE CLINICAL MANAGEMENT OF PEDIATRIC PATIENTS

Upper Respiratory Infection

URI has diffuse effects on the respiratory epithelium, mucociliary function, and airway reactivity. These effects combine to provide the potential for an increased risk for anesthesia in specific clinical settings. If the planned surgical procedure is short and airway support is restricted to the use of a facemask, the risk for an adverse respiratory event is minimal. If an endotracheal tube is required, the risk for an adverse respiratory event is increased (up to 10-fold) over that in an infant without a URI whose trachea is not intubated. An LMA seems to be associated with risks midway between those associated with a facemask and those with an endotracheal tube. Younger age plus a URI seems to be associated with an increased risk from anesthesia. URIs develop recurrently in 1- to 6-year-olds, and if reactive airways accompany the infection, the effect on the airway persists for 2 to 6 weeks.

The decision to cancel surgery on a child with an uncomplicated URI always requires assessment from the viewpoint of a specific patient and family, a specific procedure, and a specific surgeon. A strict protocol for when to cancel surgery is impractical. The patient's age, medical and anesthetic history, current physical examination, planned surgery (placement of tympanostomy tubes versus surgery for craniofacial repair), and anticipated postoperative care (need for mechanical ventilatory support) must be analyzed. Ultimately, the preoperative evaluation must weigh the inconvenience of rescheduling against ignoring possible risks. If the decision is to proceed with elective surgery, the infant should be considered to have reactive airways.

OUTPATIENT SURGERY

Inguinal herniorrhaphy, hypospadias repair, and various orthopedic procedures are commonly performed in young children as outpatient surgery (Table 33-12). The use of an LMA plus a caudal block (1 mg/kg of 0.125% to 0.25% bupivacaine or ropivacaine) provides excellent postoperative pain control while decreasing intraoperative anesthetic requirements. The more dilute local anesthetic solution may be of benefit to ambulatory children by avoiding significant motor blockade. Laparoscopic inguinal hernia repair, unlike an open repair, generally requires endotracheal intubation, and caudal anesthesia is not needed.

EX-PREMATURE INFANT

Despite many studies dealing with postoperative apnea in ex-premature infants, a precise protocol defining the need for postoperative monitoring cannot be developed.[11] This may reflect the difficulty in defining an ex-premature infant. For example, a 36-week-gestation infant who had an unremarkable 3-day stay in the intensive care nursery is distinct from a 28-week-gestation infant who had NEC, respiratory insufficiency, and chronic lung disease and is continuing oxygen therapy and diuretics at home. Furthermore, although apnea is rare after about 48 weeks' postconceptual age, the incidence is not zero. Even the definition of apnea varies from study to study. Thus, the decision to admit an ex-premature infant after surgery requires individual assessment of the patient, consideration of the surgical procedure, and the time when the surgery is completed (early morning, late afternoon). The most conservative approach is to admit every ex-premature infant who is younger than 60 weeks' postconceptual age, but this is impractical in many cases.

Table 33-12 Preoperative Medication in Children

	Oral	Nasal	Intravenous
Midazolam (mg/kg)	0.5-1.0		0.05-0.1
Fentanyl (μg/kg)			1-3
Morphine (mg/kg)			0.05-01
Sufentanil (μg/kg)		0.25-0.5	

In addition to the potential risk for postoperative apnea, ex-premature infants commonly have chronic lung conditions characterized by reactive airways disease and abnormal pulmonary function for the first decade of life, if not longer. Developmental delay may affect plans for premedication and may contribute to unexpected responses to sedatives and anesthetics. Hepatic and renal dysfunction is not uncommon.

REFERENCES

1. Morray JP, Geiduschek JM, Ramamoorthy C, et al. Anesthesia-related cardiac arrest in children. Anesthesiology 2000;93:6-14.
2. Cohen MM, Cameron CB, Duncan PG. Pediatric anesthesia morbidity and mortality in the perioperative period. Anesth Analg 1990;70:160-167.
3. Murat I, Constant I, Maud'Huy H. Perioperative anaesthetic morbidity in children: A database of 24,165 anaesthetics over a 30-month period. Paediatr Anaesth 2004;14:158-166.
4. Tay CLM, Tan GM, Ng SBA. Critical incidents in paediatric anaesthesia: An audit of 10,000 anaesthetics in Singapore. Paediatr Anaesth 2001;11:711-718.
5. Keenen RL, Shapiro JH, Dawson K. Frequency of anesthetic cardiac arrests in infants: Effect of pediatric anesthesiologists. J Clin Anesth 1991;3:433-437.
6. Winters RW. Water and electrolyte regulation. *In* Winters RW (ed): The Body Fluids in Pediatrics. Boston: Little, Brown, 1973.
7. The Harriet Lane Handbook: A Manual for Pediatric House Officers, 16th ed. St Louis: CV Mosby, 2002.
8. Mathew OP: Maintenance of upper airway patency. J Pediatr 1985;106:863-869.
9. Gross RE: The Surgery of Infancy and Childhood. Philadelphia: WB Saunders, 1953.
10. Quan L, Smith DW. The VATER association: Vertebral defects, anal atresia, T-E fistula with esophageal atresia, radial and renal dysplasia; a spectrum of associated defects. J Pediatr 1973;82:104-107.
11. Coté CJ, Zaslavsky A, Downes JJ, et al. Postoperative apnea in former preterm infants after inguinal herniorrhaphy: A combined analysis. Anesthesiology 1995;82:809-822.

IV

ELDERLY PATIENTS

Jacqueline M. Leung

The changing demography in the United States has a direct impact on the practice of anesthesia. It is estimated that 12% of the U.S. population (35 million people) is 65 years or older, and they represent the fasting growing age group in the United States. If aging of the U.S. population continues at the same rate, it is projected that by 2030, 20% of the U.S. population (>70 million people) will be 65 years or older.

The use of health care resources, including surgical services, is disproportionately higher in the elderly than in their younger counterparts. Many elderly patients who were denied surgical treatment in the past because of their age now routinely undergo operative procedures as a result of improvement in anesthetic, surgical, and medical care. Approximately 35% of all surgical procedures are performed in elderly patients.[1]

NORMAL PHYSIOLOGIC CHANGES WITH AGING

Functional and structural changes occur in most of the organ systems with aging (Table 34-1). The decline in each organ system has been described to occur independently of changes in other organ systems. The rate of aging varies in these organ systems and is influenced by genetic factors, environment, and diet.

Cardiovascular System

Aging in healthy individuals affects the peripheral vasculature through increases in wall thickness and the diameter and vascular stiffness of the aorta and large arteries. Systolic and mean arterial blood pressure increases with widening of the pulse pressure. Aortic impedance and systemic vascular resistance increase, and there is a decrease in β-adrenergic–mediated vasodilatation of the systemic vasculature. Aging also affects the heart through increases in left ventricular wall thickness secondary to enlargement

Table 34–1 Age-Related Changes in Selected Organ Systems

Organ System	Structural Changes	Functional Changes
Body composition	Decreased skeletal muscle mass Increased percentage of body fat Decreased total body water	Increased storage size for lipid-soluble drugs Decreased O_2 consumption and heat production
Central nervous system	Loss of neural tissue Decreased number of serotonin, acetylcholine, and dopamine receptors	Reduction in cerebral blood flow Decline in memory, reasoning, perception Disturbed sleep/wake cycle
Cardiovascular system	LV hypertrophy and decreased compliance Increase in vascular rigidity Decreased compliance of venous vessels	Decreased parasympathetic nervous system tone Increased sympathetic neuronal activity Desensitization of β-adrenergic receptors Increase in SVR and SBP Decrease in stroke volume and cardiac output Diastolic LV dysfunction Decreased maximally attainable HR
Pulmonary system	Increase in central airway size Decrease in small-airway diameter Decrease in elastic tissue, reorientation of elastic fibers, increased amount of collagen Decrease in respiratory muscle strength Increased chest wall stiffness Decrease in chest wall height and increase in AP diameter	Decreased respiratory center sensitivity Decreased effectiveness of coughing and swallowing Increase in lung compliance and decrease in chest wall compliance Decreased function alveolar surface area Decrease in D_{LCO_2} Decrease in P_{Imax} and P_{Emax} Decrease in ERV and VC Increase in RV and FRC with no change in TLC Increase in RV/TLC and FRC/TLC ratios Increase in closing volume and closing capacity Decrease in FVC, FEV_1, FEV_1/VC, and FEF at low lung volumes Increased A-a gradient and decrease in Pa_{O_2}
Renal system	Loss of tissue mass Decreased perfusion	Decreased GFR Reduced ability to dilute and concentrate urine and conserve sodium Decreased drug clearance
Hepatic system	Decrease in tissue mass Decrease in blood flow	Possible decrease in affinity for substrate Possible decrease in intrinsic activity Decreased first-pass metabolism of some drugs

A-a, alveolar-arterial; AP, anteroposterior; D_{LCO}, single-breath carbon monoxide diffusion capacity; ERV, expiratory reserve volume; FEF, peak expiratory flow rate—the peak flow rate during expiration; FEV_1, the amount that can be forcefully exhaled in the first second from a full inspiration, FRC, functional residual capacity; FVC, forced vital capacity; GFR, glomerular filtration rate; HR, heart rate; LV, left ventricle; RV, residual volume; SBP, systolic blood pressure; SVR, systemic vascular resistance; TLC, total lung capacity; VC, vital capacity.

of cardiac myocytes. Myocardial compliance is decreased, with a reduction in the early diastolic filling rate and compensatory augmentation of the contribution of atrial contraction to late left ventricular filling. Ventricular diastolic dysfunction, with prolonged relaxation, should be considered in any elderly patient who has a history of decreased exercise tolerance. Despite the common belief that systolic cardiac function decreases with age, it is

recognized that in the absence of coexisting cardiovascular disease, resting systolic cardiac function is well preserved, even at very advanced ages.

Other cardiovascular-related changes in aging include sclerosis and calcification of the cardiac conduction system and thickening of the aortic valve cusps. Turbulent blood flow caused by thickening of the aortic valve cusps results in the midsystolic ejection murmur that is commonly present in elderly individuals. In addition, the incidence of aortic stenosis increases with aging secondary to cusp calcification because of mechanical wear and tear on the collagenous core of the valve cusp.

Pulmonary System

With aging, the central airways increase in size with a resultant increase in the anatomic and physiologic dead spaces. Small airways decrease in diameter secondary to loss of connective tissue support. However, total airway resistance is unchanged, possibly because of opposite changes in the distal and proximal airways. There is a progressive loss in elastic tissue and an increase in the amount of collagen within the lung parenchyma. Lung elastic recoil and tethering support of the small airways are both reduced with consequent dilatation of respiratory bronchioles and alveolar ducts. This results in an approximately 15% reduction in the functional alveolar surface area available for gas exchange by the age of 70 years.[2]

Chest wall compliance decreases with aging. Decreased intervertebral space and age-associated kyphoscoliosis lead to decreased chest height and increased anteroposterior diameter, which may alter respiratory mechanics. Respiratory muscle strength decreases with aging secondary to multiple factors such as selective denervation of skeletal muscle fibers and atrophy and degeneration of motor nerves and muscle fibers.

Static and dynamic lung volumes also undergo age-related changes. The loss of elastic elements results in increased lung compliance and residual volume. As a result, functional residual capacity (FRC) is increased, though to the lesser degree than residual volume, because the decrease in chest wall compliance in part counteracts the decrease in lung recoil. In contrast, total lung capacity decreases minimally, mainly secondary to a decrease in inspiratory muscle strength and a loss of height. Vital capacity declines progressively with aging because of decreases in chest wall compliance, loss of lung elastic recoil, and decreases in respiratory muscle strength.

As a result of loss of tethering support of the small airways, closing volume and closing capacity increase. Closing capacity approaches or exceeds FRC, and the decreased ability of elderly individuals to keep the airways open during expiration and to reopen collapsed alveoli during inspiration results in an increase in ventilation-to-perfusion mismatching.

Although closing capacity and closing volume increase during general anesthesia, the deterioration in arterial oxygenation during general anesthesia is more related to the development of atelectasis in the dependent lung areas with the formation of a shunt, changes that have not been reported to be influenced by aging.[3]

Airway reflexes are more sluggish in elderly patients secondary to diminished laryngeal and pharyngeal responses. The cough reflex is less efficient, and the risk for pulmonary aspiration is increased.

Gastrointestinal System

The swallowing and motility function of the esophagus and the gastric emptying time are usually unchanged with aging. Liver size decreases progressively with aging, and it is estimated that by the age of 80 years, liver mass is decreased by 40% with a parallel decline in hepatic blood flow. However, the content of both microsomal and nonmicrosomal liver enzymes is unchanged with aging. Liver function test results are generally normal.

Renal System

The kidneys lose approximately 50% of their functional glomeruli with similar decreases in renal blood flow by 80 years of age. The decline in both renal mass and renal blood flow occurs primarily in the cortex with compensatory changes in the juxtamedullary region. The glomerular filtration rate is decreased by 30% at 60 years of age and by 50% at 80 years of age. In addition, elderly individuals have a decreased ability to dilute and concentrate urine and to conserve sodium. The decrease in renal function with aging may affect the pharmacokinetics (prolonged elimination half-times) of certain drugs used in anesthesia.

The overall decline in renal functional reserve usually has no effect on an elderly individual's ability to maintain extracellular fluid volume and electrolyte concentrations. Similarly, serum creatinine remains relatively stable because of a parallel decrease in overall skeletal muscle mass. However, in situations in which renal blood flow is compromised, the decreased renal functional reserve characteristic of elderly individuals may increase the risk for perioperative renal insufficiency or failure.

Central Nervous System

Aging is associated with a progressive loss of neural tissue and a parallel reduction in cerebral blood flow and cerebral oxygen consumption. On average, 30% of total brain mass is lost by 80 years of age. In addition, the number of neuroreceptors generally declines with aging in various regions of the central nervous system. For example, a reduction is seen in the number of serotonin receptors in the cortex, acetylcholine receptors in multiple brain regions, and dopamine receptors in the neostriatum. Levels of dopamine in the neostriatum and substantia nigra are also decreased. These structural changes are not necessarily associated with a decline in cognitive function. However, the incidence of postoperative delirium and cognitive dysfunction is higher in elderly individuals. Patients with a history of cognitive impairment are at even higher risk for further impairment postoperatively.

Pharmacokinetic and Pharmacodynamic Changes

The pharmacokinetics of drugs is influenced by changes in plasma protein binding, the percentage of body content that is fat or skeletal muscle (lean mass), circulating blood volume, and metabolism and excretion of drugs.

PROTEIN BINDING

With aging, protein binding sites are reduced secondary to both quantitative (decreased level of circulating protein) and qualitative changes. In addition, elderly individuals frequently take multiple medications that might interfere with the binding of drugs to protein active sites (Table 34-2). These changes may increase the level of free, unbound drug in plasma with a resulting enhanced pharmacologic effect.

LEAN AND FAT BODY MASS

Older individuals have decreased skeletal muscle mass and an increased percentage of body fat. These changes result in an increased ability to store lipid-soluble drugs, which may lead to a more gradual and prolonged release of the drugs used during anesthesia from lipid storage sites and, consequently, an increased elimination time and prolonged effect.

CIRCULATING BLOOD VOLUME

Circulating blood volume generally decreases with aging and results in a higher than expected initial plasma drug concentration for the same amount of drug administered. Gradual declines in hepatic and renal function may lead to decreased metabolism and prolonged elimination of drugs and their metabolites and thus may contribute to a more gradual decline in plasma drug concentrations and a prolonged effect of anesthetic drugs.

Basal Metabolic Rate

The basal metabolic rate declines with aging, and elderly surgical patients may have difficulty maintaining normothermia during general anesthesia. The development of hypothermia may lead to slower metabolism and excretion of drugs in elderly patients. Furthermore, hypothermia may lead to shivering, which will increase the basal metabolic rate and oxygen consumption and result in arterial hypoxemia or myocardial ischemia, or both.

Endocrine Changes

Endocrine changes occur with aging. The response of arginine vasopressin (formerly known as antidiuretic hormone) to hypovolemia and hypotension is reduced, but it remains sensitive to changes in serum osmolarity. The renal tubules are less sensitive to this hormone and atrial natriuretic peptide. During hyperglycemia, insulin release is impaired. However, because of increased peripheral tissue resistance and decreased clearance, plasma insulin levels are elevated, which results in an enlarging fat depot. Serum levels of renin and aldosterone decline, and the response of both hormones to sodium restriction and postural changes is blunted, with a decreased ability to

Table 34-2 Drugs Often Taken by Elderly Patients That May Contribute to Adverse Effects or Drug Interactions

Drug	Response
Diuretics	Hypokalemia Hypovolemia
Centrally acting antihypertensives	Decreased autonomic nervous system activity
β-Adrenergic antagonists	Decreased autonomic nervous system activity Decreased anesthetic requirements Bronchospasm Bradycardia
Cardiac antidysrhythmics	Potentiation of neuromuscular blocking drugs
Digitalis	Cardiac dysrhythmias Cardiac conduction disturbances
Tricyclic antidepressants	Anticholinergic effects
Antibiotics	Potentiation of neuromuscular blocking drugs
Oral hypoglycemics	Hypoglycemia
Alcohol	Increased anesthetic requirements Delirium tremens

IV

conserve sodium and excrete potassium. In contrast, adreno-corticotropic hormone, cortisol, catecholamine production by the adrenal medulla, and thyroid-stimulating hormone and thyroxine levels are unchanged with aging.

PREOPERATIVE EVALUATION AND ANESTHETIC CONSIDERATIONS

The prevalence of coexisting diseases increases with aging (Table 34-3). In older individuals undergoing surgery, the most common coexisting diseases are systemic hypertension, diabetes mellitus, cardiovascular disease, pulmonary disease, neurologic disease, and renal disease.[4] Optimizing the patient's medical condition before surgery is essential because baseline health status is an important predictor of postoperative complications. However, for elderly patients, delaying surgery to optimize a medical condition must be weighed against the risk of delaying surgery because emergency surgical treatment is associated with higher morbidity and mortality. Furthermore, delaying certain surgical procedures, such as cancer surgery, may substantially alter the patient's prognosis. In this regard, communication among the anesthesiologist, surgeon, and primary care physician is critical to developing an optimal plan regarding the timing of each elderly patient's surgery.

Laboratory Testing

Data suggest that routine laboratory testing should not be performed simply on the basis of age alone but, rather, it should be based on a thorough preoperative evaluation to determine coexisting medical conditions and on the

Table 34-3 Age-Related Concomitant Diseases in Elderly Patients
Systemic hypertension
Coronary artery disease
Congestive heart failure
Peripheral vascular disease (stroke, claudication)
Chronic obstructive pulmonary disease
Anemia
Renal disease
Liver disease
Diabetes mellitus
Subclinical hypothyroidism
Arthritis
Dementia

type of planned surgical procedures.[5] This approach is likely to be more cost-effective than routine testing in all elderly patients.

ELECTROCARDIOGRAM

Elderly patients with a history of coronary artery disease may benefit from a preoperative 12-lead electrocardiogram (ECG) to determine the presence and location of any previous myocardial infarction, left ventricular hypertrophy, conduction abnormalities, and ST-T wave changes indicative of ischemia. If an abnormality is present, comparison with a previous ECG is needed to determine the timing of the occurrence. However, in elderly patients, abnormalities on the preoperative ECG are common and of limited value in predicting postoperative cardiac complications in noncardiac surgery.[6] The low specificity of the preoperative ECG in predicting postoperative cardiac complications also suggests that a normal ECG does not rule out occult cardiac disease.

CHEST RADIOGRAPH

In patients undergoing high-risk surgery, a chest radiograph may be useful in providing noninvasive information regarding ventricular function (cardiomegaly may indicate an ejection fraction <40%). The pulmonary vasculature should also be examined to rule out preoperative congestive heart failure. However, the cost-effectiveness of routine preoperative chest radiographs in elderly patients undergoing surgery has not been defined.

EVALUATION OF CARDIAC STATUS

Because the prevalence of cardiovascular disease increases with aging, evaluation of cardiac status is an integral part of the preoperative evaluation of elderly patients. Poor functional status in elderly patients may reflect cardiac causes or be secondary to chronic pain, physical deconditioning, or obesity (or any combination of these causes).

Blood Pressure Control

Systemic hypertension (systolic blood pressure ≥180 mm Hg, diastolic blood pressure ≥110 mm Hg) increases the risk for cardiac and cerebrovascular disease.[7] Adverse intraoperative events in hypertensive patients include perioperative myocardial ischemia, cardiac dysrhythmias, and cardiovascular lability. Although data are limited, there is little evidence of increased perioperative cardiac risk if systolic blood pressure is less than 180 mm Hg or diastolic blood pressure is less than 110 mm Hg.

Even though there is no evidence that deferring anesthesia and surgery reduces perioperative risk, careful determination of the baseline blood pressure range for each patient is critical and requires more than one measurement preoperatively. If systemic blood pressure is consistently elevated, optimization with appropriate anti-hypertensive drugs preoperatively is often recommended for elective surgery. Checking compliance with blood pressure medication is important because elderly patients frequently take multiple medications, and therefore preoperative instructions on which medications to discontinue need to be carefully conveyed (see Table 34-2). In patients scheduled for urgent or emergency surgery with a preinduction systolic blood pressure higher than 180 mm Hg or diastolic blood pressure higher than 110 mm Hg, induction of anesthesia may proceed carefully, often with invasive monitoring. In these patients, administration of a small dose of an anxiolytic drug before induction of anesthesia may result in more gradual lowering of systemic blood pressure.

In elderly patients with uncontrolled systemic hypertension who are about to undergo emergency surgery, the use of continuous invasive blood pressure monitoring and postoperative surveillance in the intensive care unit may be indicated.

Protection from Perioperative Myocardial Ischemia

Postoperative myocardial ischemia is the strongest clinical predictor of adverse postoperative cardiac events in high-risk surgical patients, with most ischemic events occurring within the first 24 hours after surgery.[8,9] Therefore, reducing the number and duration of perioperative ischemic events by improving the myocardial oxygen supply-demand balance during surgery may potentially improve postoperative cardiac outcomes. Reduction of myocardial metabolic oxygen demand can be achieved by perioperative administration of β-blockers to decrease myocardial contractility and heart rate.

Elderly patients (≥65 years of age) who have one or more risk factors (systemic hypertension, current smoking, hypercholesterolemia, diabetes mellitus) may benefit from prophylactic perioperative β-blockade as evidenced by decreased circulating levels of troponin I.[10] However, in elderly patients at low risk for ischemic heart disease, this prophylactic therapy may be potentially costly and unnecessary.[11] Because sympathetic nervous system tone is increased with aging, administration of β-blockers during the perioperative period may result in hypotension, especially in the presence of relative hypovolemia secondary to preoperative fasting. Furthermore, autonomic control of hemodynamics in the elderly may be compromised as a result of the decrease in baroreceptor reflex activity with aging. Because perioperative tachycardia is one of the most important hemodynamic abnormalities that has been shown to be associated with myocardial ischemia, the adequacy of the heart rate response to β-blockers is critical to guide therapy. Individualized dosing of β-blockers for control of postoperative myocardial ischemia rather than a fixed-dose regimen may be more beneficial because patients with coronary artery disease have different coronary anatomy and therefore different ischemic thresholds.

Physical Examination

Elderly individuals are more likely to be edentulous, and although removal of dentures preoperatively may facilitate direct laryngoscopy and tracheal intubation, positive-pressure ventilation by facemask may be difficult. Range of neck motion should be evaluated because older individuals may have limitations as a result of degenerative spine disease. Auscultation of the carotid arteries over the neck bilaterally is helpful to rule out carotid artery disease but requires confirmation by carotid ultrasound if loud carotid bruits are present. Auscultation of the heart may reveal additional heart sounds such as S_3 or S_4, which are commonly associated with decreased left ventricular compliance. A midsystolic ejection murmur is often present in elderly patients secondary to thickening of the aortic cusps or calcification, or both. A laterally displaced point of maximal impulse together with increased heart size on the chest radiograph suggests cardiomegaly. Auscultation of the lungs is performed to evaluate the presence of rales or wheezes, which may be associated with congestive heart failure or lung disease (or both). Examination of the extremities should be performed to rule out the presence of peripheral edema, which may be indicative of congestive heart failure.

Risk Assessment

Although elderly patients are at increased risk for perioperative morbidity and mortality, advanced age by itself is not a contraindication to surgery. General factors that should be evaluated when performing a preoperative risk assessment include age, functional status, cognition, nutrition, and comorbid conditions (cardiac, pulmonary, renal, and endocrine disease) (see Table 34-3). When both age and comorbidity are considered, the latter is a better predictor of adverse postoperative outcomes. Functional limitation increases perioperative risk, and preoperative evaluation of functional status with common measures such as activities of daily living and instrumental activities of daily living is informative (Table 34-4). Preoperative cognitive status has been shown to be associated with adverse postoperative outcome and functional recovery, thus emphasizing that assessment of preoperative baseline cognitive status may be useful. Depression is also common in elderly patients and may increase perioperative morbidity, including postoperative delirium.

Management of Preoperative Medication

Elderly patients are typically taking multiple prescription and over-the-counter medications (see Table 34-2). In general, all antihypertensive and cardiac medications should be continued until surgery, with the exception of diuretics, which are preferably withheld on the day of surgery because the patient will be fasting before surgery. For those taking aspirin or warfarin for treatment of

Table 34–4 Activities of Daily Living and Instrumental Activities of Daily Living*

Activities of Daily Living
Bathing
Dressing
Toileting
Transferring
Eating

Instrumental Activities of Daily Living
Use of telephone
Use of public transportation
Shopping
Preparation of meals
Housekeeping
Taking medications properly
Managing personal finances

*The ability of the patient to perform the above tasks independently, partially independently, or with complete assistance required is recorded.

cerebral vascular or coronary artery disease, atrial fibrillation, or deep vein thrombosis, the risks associated with discontinuing anticoagulation should be weighed against the benefits of reduced bleeding from discontinuation of such drugs. Warfarin is typically withheld (often four doses) to allow normalization of the international normalized ratio. In case of emergency surgery, fresh frozen plasma or vitamin K can be administered to reverse warfarin's effects. For patients at high risk for thromboembolism, such as those with a prosthetic heart valve, a history of pulmonary embolism, or a recent history of deep vein thrombosis, a transition using low-molecular-weight heparin or intravenous heparin is indicated when oral anticoagulation is discontinued. Antibiotic prophylaxis is indicated for patients with valvular heart disease and mitral valve prolapse.

INTRAOPERATIVE MANAGEMENT

No single anesthetic drug or technique has been demonstrated to be superior for elderly surgical patients (Table 34-5). However, familiarity with the pharmacokinetics of anesthetic drugs and how age-related changes may affect drug dosing is important.

Inhaled Anesthetics

The minimum alveolar concentration (MAC) for various inhaled anesthetics is reduced by approximately 6% per year after the age of 40 years.[12] The onset of action of volatile anesthetics may be more rapid if cardiac output is reduced, particularly for more lipid-soluble drugs, but decreased lung function secondary to an increased shunt fraction has an opposite effect. Recovery from the depressant effects of volatile anesthetics may be more prolonged because of an increased volume of distribution

Table 34–5 Adjustments of Anesthetic and Adjuvant Drugs in Elderly Patients

Drug	Adjustment
Volatile anesthetics	Decrease inspired concentration
Intravenous induction drugs (thiopental, propofol)	Small to moderate decreases in initial dose Decreased maintenance infusion
Opioids	Decrease initial dose* Increased incidence of skeletal muscle rigidity Increased duration of systemic and neuraxial effects Increased incidence of depression of ventilation
Local anesthetics (spinal and epidural)	Small to moderate decrease in segmental dose requirements Anticipate prolonged effects
Benzodiazepines	Modest decrease in initial dose Anticipate marked increase in duration of action
Atropine	Increased dose needed for comparable heart rate response Anticipate possible central anticholinergic syndrome
Isoproterenol	Increased dose needed for comparable heart rate response

*Supportive data not available.

secondary to increased body fat and decreased pulmonary gas exchange.

Intravenous Anesthetics and Neuromuscular Blocking Drugs

Dose requirements for barbiturates, opioids, and benzodiazepines are likely to be decreased in elderly patients.

OPIOIDS

The elimination half-time of fentanyl is longer in elderly patients than younger patients because of the larger volume of distribution. As a result, depression of ventilation and prolonged analgesia may ensue with the same dose administered to younger patients. Decreased hepatic clearance may contribute to prolonged opioid effects, especially when high does of these drugs are administered to elderly patients.

PROPOFOL

Propofol is highly lipid soluble and produces rapid loss of consciousness when administered intravenously. A decreased induction dose or slow titration is recommended for elderly patients. A decrease in age-related clearance of propofol may result in reduced anesthetic requirements with aging. Propofol, because of its negative inotropic and vasodilatory effects, may give rise to exaggerated decreases in systemic blood pressure when used for induction of anesthesia in elderly patients. Despite these characteristics, propofol may be superior to thiopental for recovery of mental function.

ETOMIDATE

Etomidate produces rapid loss of consciousness and has been frequently chosen for induction of anesthesia in elderly patients with cardiovascular instability. The initial volume of distribution of etomidate is decreased such that an 80-year-old patient requires less than half the dose of etomidate to produce the same magnitude of depression on the electroencephalogram as in younger patients.

MIDAZOLAM

Midazolam has increased potency and decreased clearance in elderly individuals. Context-sensitive half-times are prolonged. Accordingly, doses of midazolam should be decreased and a longer duration of action is expected.

NEUROMUSCULAR BLOCKING DRUGS

Despite age-related changes in the neuromuscular junction, the effects of depolarizing and nondepolarizing neuromuscular blocking drugs are not altered in elderly patients. Rather, the altered pharmacokinetics of these drugs in older individuals is secondary to decreases in renal and hepatic function and the altered volume of distribution that accompanies aging. Clearance is decreased for nondepolarizing neuromuscular blocking drugs (vecuronium, rocuronium) that are dependent on either the kidneys or the liver for elimination from plasma. The duration of action of atracurium and cisatracurium is not prolonged because these drugs are eliminated by Hofmann degradation, which is independent of renal and hepatic clearance mechanisms. Monitoring of neuromuscular function and recovery is important in elderly patients because incomplete recovery of neuromuscular function may lead to a higher incidence of postoperative pulmonary complications.

Regional Anesthesia

Cardiovascular responses to either spinal or epidural anesthesia may be exaggerated in older individuals. The decrease in cardiac output is thought to primarily be due to a decrease in stroke volume.[13] Treatment of the resultant hypotension typically consists of the administration of crystalloid solutions or vasopressors such as phenylephrine.

Surgical procedures that are amenable to regional anesthesia include transurethral resection of the prostate, orthopedic procedures such as hip or knee replacement, inguinal herniorrhaphy, and minor gynecologic procedures. Technical difficulties in performing regional anesthesia probably reflect age-related decreases in the intervertebral spaces and scoliosis. A thorough examination of the targeted spinal segment must be performed before initiating regional anesthesia.

Intraoperative Monitoring

Because of the prevalence of coexisting disease involving the cardiac and pulmonary systems, consideration should be given to using invasive monitoring such as arterial and central venous catheterization in elderly patients undergoing major surgical procedures, which are likely to be prolonged and include large body fluid shifts.

Postoperative Pain Therapy

The concept that pain perception decreases with aging and that elderly individuals have a low tolerance of opioids is unsubstantiated. Elderly individuals are commonly afflicted with osteoarthritic disease that results in chronic pain, which may influence requirements for postoperative pain medications. In addition, because elderly surgical patients have an increased likelihood of postoperative delirium or cognitive dysfunction, or both, assessment of the adequacy of postoperative pain control may be difficult.

STRATEGIES TO IMPROVE PERIOPERATIVE MANAGEMENT AND POSTOPERATIVE OUTCOME

Decreasing Cardiovascular Complications

Cardiovascular complications (cardiac dysrhythmias, myocardial ischemia, congestive heart failure) may influence

IV

postoperative outcomes in elderly patients.[14] Perioperative planning includes (1) identifying elderly patients who are at higher risk for postoperative cardiovascular complications, (2) optimizing preoperative medical therapies, (3) modifying known risk factors preoperatively (pharmacologic therapy), and (4) planning of postoperative care (pain control, admission to intensive care units).

Assessment of Cardiac Function

Congestive heart failure is a common problem in the elderly population. It is estimated that congestive heart failure will develop in 10% of persons 80 years and older and will lead to increased mortality within 2 years.[15] Because clinical signs or a history of congestive heart failure is associated with postoperative cardiac complications, special attention should be directed to preoperative optimization of heart function in elderly surgical patients.[4,14]

DIAGNOSIS OF CONGESTIVE HEART FAILURE

Clinical diagnosis of congestive heart failure can be particularly challenging in elderly patients because of the lack of typical symptoms and physical findings.[15] When present, symptoms of congestive heart failure are often nonspecific and frequently misdiagnosed as symptoms of concomitant disease (chronic pulmonary disease) or interpreted as changes associated with aging.

DIASTOLIC CONGESTIVE HEART FAILURE

Despite the common preservation of left ventricular systolic function, congestive heart failure may result from left ventricular diastolic dysfunction.[16] Patients with diastolic congestive heart failure have a leftward shift in the pressure-volume relationship such that their hearts operate on the steep portion of the curve (Fig. 34-1). Small changes in volume may result in substantial increases in diastolic pressure to the extent that pulmonary congestion may occur, even at relatively normal left ventricular volume. Such changes may be accentuated by exercise, and many elderly individuals with diastolic dysfunction exhibit exercise intolerance as one of their major symptoms. Other symptoms may include dyspnea, cough, edema, or fatigue. Preoperatively, noninvasive approaches to diagnosing diastolic dysfunction include Doppler echocardiography and radionuclide ventriculography.[17] With Doppler echocardiography, measurement of the ratio between the peak early filling wave (E wave) and the atrial filling wave (A wave) is a useful screening tool for detecting abnormal left ventricular relaxation (Fig. 34-2).

Disorders associated with diastolic dysfunction include systemic hypertension, coronary artery disease, cardiomyopathies, diabetes, chronic renal disease, aortic stenosis, and atrial fibrillation.[18] Potentially reversible causes of diastolic congestive heart failure in elderly patients include myocardial ischemia and accelerated hypertension.

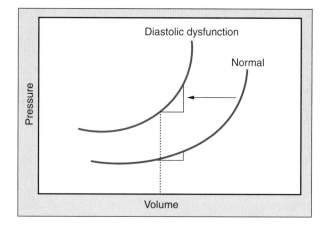

Figure 34-1 Depiction of the diastolic function pressure-volume relationship. In diastolic dysfunction, there is a leftward shift of the pressure-volume curve. As a result, small volume changes result in exaggerated increases in atrial and ventricular filling pressure, which may lead to pulmonary congestion. In addition, reduced left ventricular filling may result in decreased stroke volume and symptoms of low cardiac output.

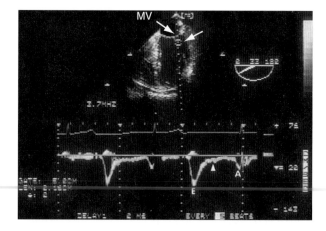

Figure 34-2 Interrogation of the mitral valve (MV) by pulsed-wave Doppler imaging. The E wave represents early diastolic filling and the A wave represents late filling secondary to atrial contraction. Measurement of the ratio between these two waveforms is a useful screening tool for determining the presence of abnormal left ventricular relaxation. The normal E/A range is 1 to 2.

Perioperative goals in elderly patients with diastolic dysfunction include (1) maintenance of normal sinus rhythm and a slow heart rate, (2) control of systemic blood pressure, (3) optimization of blood volume, and (4) detection and treatment of myocardial ischemia. The use of invasive monitoring such as central venous pressure or pulmonary artery catheterization may be indicated in managing patients with a history of congestive heart failure secondary to diastolic dysfunction. Treatment of diastolic congestive heart failure may include pharmacologic interventions (Table 34-6).[18]

Impact of Anesthetic Technique on Cardiovascular Complications

The view that regional anesthesia is better than general anesthesia in reducing adverse cardiac outcomes has not been consistently demonstrated.[19] There is no difference in 30-day mortality in patients undergoing major abdominal surgery with epidural or spinal anesthesia versus general anesthesia.[20]

Decreasing Perioperative Pulmonary Complications

Advanced age is not considered to be an independent risk factor for perioperative pulmonary dysfunction. In contrast, other factors that have been shown to be associated with postoperative pulmonary complications include (1) emergency surgery, (2) anatomic site of surgery (upper abdominal and thoracic procedures), (3) duration of anesthesia, (4) general anesthesia, (5) hypercapnia, (6) history of smoking, (7) obesity, and (8) preexisting pulmonary disease (chronic obstructive pulmonary disease [COPD] and asthma).

CIGARETTE SMOKING

Cessation of cigarette smoking and the use of oxygen therapy may improve outcomes in patients with COPD. Preoperative cessation of smoking immediately before surgery serves only to decrease carboxyhemoglobin levels (half-time of about 6 hours). Prolonged cessation of smoking (8 weeks) is necessary to result in a decrease in postoperative pulmonary complications because of the period necessary for improvement in mucociliary action and a decrease in mucus secretion.[21] Differentiation of reversible and irreversible airflow obstruction is important to guide the use of anti-inflammatory medications, β_2-agonists, and anticholinergic agents.

ASTHMA

Asthma is often underdiagnosed and not optimally treated in elderly individuals. There is a tendency to label elderly patients with symptoms of airflow obstruction as having COPD. Differentiation between asthma and COPD is important because the therapeutic strategies may be different. A postbronchodilator increase in forced exhaled volume in 1 second (FEV_1) of 200 mL or 15% is considered a sign of reversibility of airflow obstruction and suggests a diagnosis of asthma rather than COPD. However, an overlap between asthma and COPD may be more common in elderly patients because older asthmatics may have a propensity for irreversible airway obstruction and some patients with smoking-related COPD may have some response to bronchodilator therapy. Although pulmonary function tests assess the presence and severity of the disease, they do not have great predictive value for postoperative pulmonary complications.

Treatment

Administration of β-agonists is relatively safe in elderly patients, although systemic absorption of inhaled β-agonists may result in tachycardia, systemic hypertension, and skeletal muscle tremors. Patients with asthma may be

IV

Table 34–6 Pharmacologic Management of Diastolic Dysfunction

Drugs	Goals of Acute Perioperative Therapy	Considerations
Diuretics	Decrease central blood volume and left ventricular filling pressure	Acute reduction in blood volume may decrease cardiac output and cause hypotension
Calcium channel blockers	Decrease afterload Relieve myocardial ischemia Slow the heart rate Enhance ventricular relaxation	Acute reduction in afterload may decrease cardiac output and cause hypotension Exercise caution when used in conjunction with β-adrenergic blockers
β-Adrenergic blockers	Decrease afterload Relieve myocardial ischemia Slow the heart rate Enhance ventricular relaxation	Exercise caution when used in conjunction with calcium channel blockers
Angiotensin-converting enzyme inhibitors	Decrease afterload Enhance ventricular relaxation	Acute reduction in afterload may decrease cardiac output and cause hypotension

Data from Tresch D, McGough M: Heart failure with normal systolic function: A common disorder in old people. J Am Geriatr Soc 1995;43:1035-1042.

receiving corticosteroid therapy, which may result in adverse effects such as osteoporosis, psychiatric disturbances, and exacerbation of chronic conditions such as systemic hypertension and diabetes mellitus. Patients being treated with corticosteroids should receive supplemental corticosteroid before induction of anesthesia. Medication such as β-blockers may exacerbate asthma. The use of selective β-blockers such as metoprolol or atenolol is preferable for the treatment of systemic hypertension or congestive heart failure.

Intraoperative Management

INITIATION OF POSTOPERATIVE PAIN MANAGEMENT

Epidural analgesia with local anesthetics and opioids provides considerable benefit in terms of pulmonary outcomes after surgery, including (1) a decrease in the incidence of atelectasis, pulmonary infections, and complications; (2) better postoperative pain relief than with parenteral opioids; (3) shorter time to tracheal extubation; and (4) less time in the intensive care unit.[22] Indeed, the quality and possibly the modality of postoperative pain relief may be more important than the choice of intraoperative anesthetic.

INTERVENTIONS TO IMPROVE POSTOPERATIVE PULMONARY FUNCTION

Certain intraoperative strategies may improve pulmonary function. Measures such as adding positive end-expiratory pressure (5 to 10 cm H_2O) can increase FRC and restore the closing capacity–to–FRC ratio. The use of higher inspired oxygen concentrations (FIO_2) may provide (1) a better proinflammatory and antimicrobial response of alveolar macrophages than that associated with 30% oxygen, (2) a lower incidence of postoperative nausea and vomiting, and (3) a reduced incidence of surgical wound infections.[23,24] A high FIO_2 does not influence postoperative pulmonary mechanical dysfunction or alter the incidence of postoperative complications such as pulmonary atelectasis.

Reducing Postoperative Delirium

Delirium, an acute disorder of attention and cognition, occurs in 14% to 50% of hospitalized medical patients (especially elderly patients) and is accompanied by a mortality rate ranging from 10% to 65%.[25] In general, delirium is the manifestation or symptom of an underlying medical illness for which multiple causes exist. Delirium can be superimposed on dementia or other neurologic disorders associated with global cognitive impairment. As a result, the course of delirium can vary considerably and depends on resolution of the causative factors.

PREDISPOSING FACTORS

Factors that predispose elderly patients to delirium include aging processes in the brain, structural brain disease, a reduced capacity for homeostatic regulation and therefore resistance to stress, visual and hearing impairment, a high prevalence of chronic disease, reduced resistance to acute diseases, and age-related changes in the pharmacokinetics and pharmacodynamics of drugs.[25] Sleeping disorders, sensory deprivation or overload, and psychological stress resulting from bereavement or relocation to an unfamiliar environment are common precipitants of delirium.

Certain drugs administered during anesthesia may be associated with postoperative delirium, but it is not possible to determine whether elimination of these drugs will actually lead to a lower incidence of delirium postoperatively. Controversy persists regarding whether any anesthetic technique (regional versus general) has an impact on postoperative delirium. Earlier studies suggested an association between general anesthesia and a higher incidence of cognitive dysfunction relative to epidural anesthesia.[26] However, recent studies have concluded that there was no relationship between anesthetic technique and the magnitude or pattern of postoperative cognitive dysfunction.[27] Intraoperative hypotension does not appear to influence the occurrence of postoperative cognitive dysfunction.[28]

Until more definitive clinical studies become available, minimizing the number of medications used, avoiding arterial hypoxemia and extremes of hypocapnia or hypercapnia, and providing adequate postoperative pain control appear to be the best approach to minimizing the occurrence of postoperative delirium in elderly surgical patients.[29]

REFERENCES

1. Anderson R. United States Life Tables, 1998. Washington, DC: Department of Health and Human Services, Center for Disease Control and Prevention, National Center for Health Statistics, 2001, pp 1-39.
2. Niederman MS. Respiratory Infections in the Elderly. New York: Raven Press, 1991.
3. Gunnarsson L, Tokics L, Gustavsson H, Hedenstierna G. Influence of age on atelectasis formation and gas exchange impairment during general anaesthesia. Br J Anaesth 1991;66:423-432.
4. Leung J, Dzankic S. Relative importance of preoperative health status versus intraoperative factors in predicting postoperative adverse outcomes in geriatric surgical patients. J Am Geriatr Soc 2001;49:1080-1085.
5. Dzankic S, Pastor D, Gonzalez C, Leung J. Prevalence and predictive value of abnormal preoperative laboratory tests in elderly surgical patients. Anesth Analg 2001;93:301-308.

6. Liu LL, Dzankic S, Leung JM. Preoperative electrocardiogram abnormalities do not predict postoperative cardiac complications in geriatric surgical patients. J Am Geriatr Soc 2002;50:1186-1191.

7. Howell SJ, Sear JW, Foex P. Hypertension, hypertensive heart disease and perioperative cardiac risk. Br J Anaesth 2004;92:570-583.

8. Mangano D, Browner W, Hollenberg M, et al. SPI Research Group: Association of perioperative myocardial ischemia with cardiac morbidity and mortality in men undergoing noncardiac surgery. N Engl J Med 1990;323:1781-1788.

9. Von Arnim T, TIBBS Investigators. Medical treatment to reduce total ischemia burden: Total Ischemic Burden Bisoprolol Study (TIBBS), a multicenter trial comparing bisoprolol and nifedipine. J Am Coll Cardiol 1996;28:20-24.

10. Auerbach AD, Goldman L. Beta-blockers and reduction of cardiac events in noncardiac surgery: Scientific review. JAMA 2002;287:1435-1444.

11. Zaugg M, Tagliente T, Lucchinetti E, et al. Beneficial effects from beta-adrenergic blockade in elderly patients undergoing noncardiac surgery. Anesthesiology 1999;91:1674-1686.

12. Mapleson WW. Effect of age on MAC in humans: A meta-analysis. Br J Anaesth 1996;76:179-185.

13. Rooke G, Freund P, Jacobson A. Hemodynamic response and change in organ blood volume during spinal anesthesia in elderly men with cardiac disease. Anesth Analg 1997;85:99-105.

14. Liu L, Leung J. Predicting adverse postoperative outcomes in patients aged 80 years or older. J Am Geriatr Soc 2000;48:405-412.

15. Tresch D. The clinical diagnosis of heart failure in older patients. J Am Geriatr Soc 1997;45:1128-1133.

16. Vasan R, Benjamin E, Levy D. Prevalence, clinical features and prognosis of diastolic heart failure: An epidemiologic perspective. J Am Coll Cardiol 1995;26:1565-1574.

17. Hurrell D, Nishimura R, Ilstrup D, Appleton C. Utility of preload alteration in assessment of left ventricular filling pressure by Doppler echocardiography: A simultaneous catheterization and Doppler echocardiographic study. J Am Coll Cardiol 1997;30:459-467.

18. Tresch D, McGough M. Heart failure with normal systolic function: A common disorder in old people. J Am Geriatr Soc 1995;43:1035-1042.

19. Bode R, Lewis K, Zarich S, et al. Cardiac outcome after peripheral vascular surgery. Anesthesiology 1996;84:3-13.

20. Rodgers A, Walker N, Schug S, et al. Reduction of postoperative mortality and morbidity with epidural or spinal anaesthesia: Results from overview of randomized trials. BMJ 2000;321:1493-1501.

21. Warner MA, Offord KP, Warner ME, et al. Role of preoperative cessation of smoking and other factors in postoperative pulmonary complications: A blinded prospective study of coronary artery bypass patients. Mayo Clin Proc 1989;64:609-616.

22. Rigg JR, Jamrozik K, Myles PS, et al. Epidural anaesthesia and analgesia and outcome of major surgery: A randomized trial. Lancet 2002;359:1276-1282.

23. Greif R, Akça O, Horn EP, et al. Supplemental perioperative oxygen to reduce the incidence of surgical-wound infection. Outcomes Research Group. N Engl J Med 2000;342:161-167.

24. Kotani N, Hashimoto H, Sessler DI, et al. Supplemental intraoperative oxygen augments antimicrobial and proinflammatory responses of alveolar macrophages. Anesthesiology 2000;93:15-25.

25. Lipowski Z. Delirium in the elderly patient. N Engl J Med 1989;320:578-582.

26. Berggren D, Gustafson Y, Eriksson B, et al. Postoperative confusion after anesthesia in elderly patients with femoral neck fractures. Anesth Analg 1987;66:497-504.

27. O'Hara D, Duff A, Berlin J, et al. The effect of anesthetic technique on postoperative outcomes in hip fracture repair. Anesthesiology 2000;92:947-957.

28. Williams-Russo P, Sharrock N, Mattis S, et al. Randomized trial of hypotensive epidural anesthesia in older adults. Anesthesiology 1999;91:926-935.

29. Inouye S, Charpentier P. Precipitating factors for delirium in hospitalized elderly persons. A predictive model and interrelationship with baseline vulnerability. JAMA 1996;275:852-857.

IV

Chapter 35

ORGAN TRANSPLANTATION

Claus U. Niemann and C. S. Yost

Solid organ transplantation has become a well-accepted treatment modality for patients with end-stage organ disease.[1,2] The role of the anesthesiologist in organ transplantation may involve caring for organ donors, prospective recipients, or patients who have already received transplants but require further surgery. Organs that are most frequently transplanted are the kidneys and the liver. An extensive preoperative workup with an emphasis on the cardiopulmonary system and conditions related to the failing organ is required for all potential transplant candidates.

UNIQUE CONSIDERATIONS FOR ORGAN TRANSPLANTATION

Organ transplantation unavoidably exposes the anesthesiologist to issues related to biomedical ethics, the diagnosis of death, and transplantation immunology (Tables 35-1 and 35-2). Death is always certified before the donor procedure. Anesthetic care for organ procurement requires a focus on maintenance of donor organ perfusion and oxygenation and recognition of common physiologic derangements associated with brain death (see Table 35-2). Organ preservation after removal from the donor includes hypothermia to decrease metabolism with preservative solutions of specific additives to maintain cellular integrity and decrease hypothermia-mediated injury.

Refinement of perioperative care plus improved management of patients after transplantation has resulted in a dramatic improvement in both 1- and 5-year graft survival. Postoperative organ function after transplantation depends on multiple factors, including donor demographics, organ ischemia time, mechanism of death of the donor, and medical condition of the recipient. Improvement in immunosuppressive regimens and better tissue typing have contributed to the increasing success of organ transplantation. Infection (bacterial, fungal, viral) attributable to chronic immunosuppression is the most common cause of death in transplant recipients, thus

Table 35-1 Criteria for the Diagnosis of Brain Death

Loss of Cerebral Cortical Function

No spontaneous movement

Unresponsive to external stimuli

Loss of Brainstem Function

Apnea

Absent cranial nerve reflexes (papillary, corneal, oculocephalic, oculovestibular)

Supporting Documentation

Electroencephalogram

Cerebral blood flow studies (angiography, transcranial Doppler, xenon scan)

Table 35-2 Common Physiologic Derangements after Brain Death

Derangement	Mechanism
Hypotension	Hypovolemia (diabetes insipidus, hemorrhage) Neurogenic shock
Arterial hypoxemia	Neurogenic pulmonary edema Aspiration Pneumonia
Hypothermia	Hypothalamic infarction
Cardiac dysrhythmias	Hypothermia Arterial hypoxemia Electrolyte abnormality Myocardial ischemia

emphasizing the importance of strict asepsis during the management of anesthesia. The frequency of cancer (especially skin and lymphoproliferative) is increased in transplant patients, perhaps reflecting loss of the protective effects of an active immune system.

CONTRAINDICATIONS TO SOLID ORGAN TRANSPLANTATION

Absolute and relative contraindications to solid organ transplantation have diminished over recent years. For instance, candidates for kidney transplantation are increasingly older and have more complex medical problems. Evidence of malignancy is not a contraindication per se. For example, hepatocellular carcinoma with underlying cirrhosis is considered to be an indication for liver trans-

plantation as long as the tumor has not reached a certain size. Active infection is an absolute contraindication until it has been treated and the infection has resolved. Severe irreversible pulmonary hypertension is a contraindication to heart transplantation, but these patients may be candidates for combined heart-lung transplantation.

KIDNEY TRANSPLANTATION

Approximately 16,500 kidney transplants are performed in the United States annually (Table 35-3).[3] The number of kidneys available for transplantation from deceased donors is around 7000 to 8000 annually, with living donors making up the difference. More than 75,000 patients are registered and await kidney transplantation. A small subset of diabetic patients undergo combined kidney/pancreas transplantation.

The graft survival rate of kidney transplants from deceased donors is approximately 65% at 5 years, whereas it is 80% in recipients who receive a kidney from a living donor. Although transplants involving deceased donor organs are often scheduled as urgent or emergency operations, prolonged cold preservation of the donor kidney is generally well tolerated and provides enough time for transplant candidates to be well prepared for surgery. This time allows for normalization of electrolyte imbalance, volume status, and if necessary, renal dialysis before surgery. Donor kidneys, whether from a living or a deceased donor, are usually implanted in the iliac fossa. Either side of the abdomen can be used. Although vascular anastomoses can be performed to a variety of recipient vessels, the external iliac artery and vein are most frequently used (Fig. 35-1).[4] The ureter is anastomosed directly to the bladder.

Management of Anesthesia

The majority of patients with end stage renal disease have significant comorbid conditions that may influence the anesthetic approach that is chosen for these patients (Table 35-4).[4] Management of anesthesia for renal transplantation follows the same principles as described for patients with chronic renal failure, including possible renal dialysis before surgery to optimize fluid, electrolyte, and acid-base status (see Chapter 28).

Table 35-3 Major Indications for Kidney Transplantation

Diabetes mellitus

Hypertension–induced nephropathy

Glomerulonephritis

Polycystic kidney disease

IV

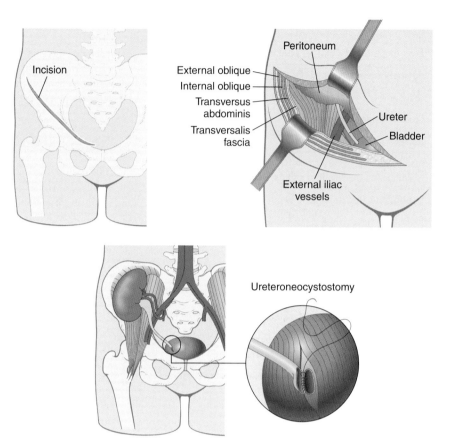

Figure 35-1 Kidney transplantation. The recipient operation is performed through a retroperitoneal incision, and the iliac vessels are used to revascularize the kidney and a ureteroneocystostomy is used to establish urinary continuity. (From Markmann JF, Brayman KL, Naji A, et al. Transplantation of abdominal organs. *In* Townsend CM Jr, Beauchamp RD, Evers MB, Mattox KL [eds]: Sabiston Textbook of Surgery: The Biological Basis of Modern Surgical Practice, 17th ed. Philadelphia: WB Saunders, 2004, p 709.)

Table 35–4 Physiologic Disturbances Often Present before Renal Transplantation

Peripheral neuropathy
Lethargy
Anemia
Platelet dysfunction
Pericarditis
Systemic hypertension
Depressed ejection fraction
Pleural effusions
Skeletal muscle weakness
Ileus
Glucose intolerance

A variety of anesthetic techniques (most often general anesthesia) have been used successfully for renal transplantation.[3] Selection of monitors may be influenced by the patient's comorbid conditions. For example, patients with long-standing diabetes mellitus may require more extensive monitoring (continuous arterial or central venous pressure [CVP] monitoring, or both) than a young patient with glomerulonephritis and well-controlled systemic hypertension. When CVP monitoring is used, the goal is to maintain CVP in the 10– to 15–mm Hg range to optimize fluid status and renal perfusion. Surgical stimulation after dissection of the fascia for placement of the donor kidney is minimal, and systemic hypotension may ensue as a result of the effects of anesthetic drugs.

Effort should be made to avoid episodes of hypotension after reperfusion because renal graft function is critically dependent on perfusion pressure. Excessive opioid administration coupled with minimal surgical stimulation may contribute to hypotension. Intravenous administration of α-adrenergic drugs such as phenylephrine may be avoided inasmuch as animal models have demonstrated that vessels in the transplanted kidney are sensitive to sympathomimetics, which can compromise blood flow to the transplanted organ. Of note, convincing scientific data in humans are not available. Mannitol, loop diuretics, and dopamine may be used intraoperatively to improve renal perfusion pressure and enhance urine production. Low-dose mannitol (12.5 to 25 g IV) and loop diuretics are usually administered before unclamping the vascular supply to the transplanted kidney. The role of dopamine in kidney transplantation remains controversial.

Prompt urine production is seen in more than 90% of living donor kidney transplants and in 40% to 70% of deceased donor transplants. During the latter stages of closure of the surgical wound, a decrease in urine output suggests mechanical impingement of the graft, vessel, or ureter. If impingement occurs, the Foley catheter should be irrigated and checked for patency. If intraoperative ultrasound is immediately available, it can be used to examine flow through the arterial and venous anastomoses.

Moderate to severe systemic hypertension can accompany emergence from anesthesia after renal transplantation. Antihypertensive therapy may be initiated in the operating room and continued during the recovery period. Postoperative pain is generally mild to moderate and can be well controlled with intravenous opioids. Epidural catheters are not usually placed in this patient population.

LIVER TRANSPLANTATION

Approximately 6400 liver transplantations are performed in the United States annually, including a small number with living liver donors.[5] Roughly 17,500 patients are on the waiting list for liver transplantation in the United States. The 3-year survival rate after transplantation in the United States is greater than 75%. The most common causes of end-stage liver disease requiring liver transplantation are chronic viral hepatitis C or B and alcoholic and cholestatic cirrhosis (primary sclerosing cholangitis). Patients are categorized by either the Child-Pugh classification (see Chapter 28) or the Model for End-stage Liver Disease (MELD). The MELD risk score is a mathematical formula that uses creatinine, bilirubin, and INR (international normalized ratio for prothrombin time). MELD calculates a single numerical value (0.40) using a formula that gives each value specific weight. Of note, for adult patients on dialysis within the last week, the creatinine value will be automatically set to 4 mg/dL.

Candidates for liver transplantation have various symptoms ranging from chronic fatigue with mild jaundice to coma with multiple organ failure (Table 35-5). The severity of hepatic dysfunction and the urgent nature of the operation often limit the time available to optimize preoperative disturbances before proceeding with liver transplantation surgery.

IV

Table 35-5 Comorbid Conditions Associated with Liver Failure	
Central nervous system	Hepatic encephalopathy Increased intracranial pressure (acute liver failure)
Cardiac system	Hyperdynamic circulation Cirrhotic cardiomyopathy
Respiratory system	Hepatopulmonary syndrome (arterial hypoxemia) Portopulmonary hypertension
Gastrointestinal system	Portal hypertension Upper gastrointestinal bleeding Ascites
Hematologic system	Anemia Thrombocytopenia Prolonged prothrombin time and plasma thromboplastin time Decreased plasma fibrinogen concentration Disseminated intravascular coagulation Protein C and S deficiency
Renal system	Hepatorenal syndrome Acute tubular necrosis
Miscellaneous	Electrolyte disturbances (hypokalemia, hypocalcemia) Malnutrition Hypoglycemia Metabolic acidosis

Phases of Liver Transplantation

Liver transplant surgery can be divided into three phases (Fig. 35-2).[4] The dissection phase includes lysis of adhesions and mobilization of the liver. The anhepatic phase consists of removal of the native liver and implantation of the donor liver. The reperfusion or neohepatic phase involves surgical completion of the remaining anastomoses, hemostasis, and closure. Intraoperative complications arise from medical conditions of the recipient that may be aggravated by intraoperative hemodynamic instability (see Table 35-5).

Management of Anesthesia

Management of anesthesia during liver transplantation includes invasive monitoring of arterial blood pressure and CVP. The decision to place a pulmonary artery catheter or transesophageal echocardiography (TEE) probe varies between institutions and often depends on the medical condition of the patient. Large-bore intravenous access is mandatory because of the significant blood loss that may be encountered during surgery.

Before induction of anesthesia it is important to consider the impact of ascites and its effect on gastric emptying and pulmonary function. Several different anesthetic drugs can be used for induction and maintenance of anesthesia. Although a significant number of anesthetic drugs rely

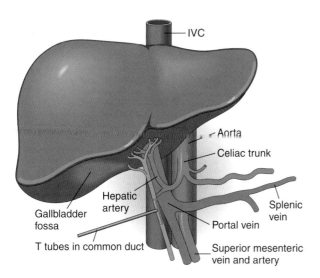

Figure 35-2 Liver transplantation: the recipient procedure. IVC, inferior vena cava. (Modified from Markmann JF, Brayman KL, Naji A, et al. Transplantation of abdominal organs. *In* Townsend CM Jr, Beauchamp RD, Evers MB, Mattox KL [eds]: Sabiston Textbook of Surgery: The Biological Basis of Modern Surgical Practice, 17th ed. Philadelphia: WB Saunders, 2004, p 728.)

on hepatic metabolism and excretion, titration of their use is generally safe because of the subsequent implantation of a functioning liver. Nitrous oxide, however, is generally avoided.

DISSECTION PHASE

During the dissection phase, cardiovascular instability from hemorrhage, venous pooling as a result of sudden decreases in intra-abdominal pressure, and impaired venous return secondary to surgical retraction may occur. Hypocalcemia, hyperkalemia, and metabolic acidosis may also be encountered.

ANHEPATIC PHASE

The anhepatic phase begins when the native liver is removed after transection and clamping of the suprahepatic and infrahepatic portions of the inferior vena cava and portal vein. The hepatic artery is usually ligated before the anhepatic phase. A venovenous bypass system is used in some cases to minimize decreases in preload and cardiac output and to prevent splanchnic congestion. Cardiac output and systemic blood pressure may need to be supported with inotropes and vasoconstrictors during this phase. Citrate intoxication from rapid blood transfusion is more likely during the anhepatic phase because of the complete absence of any liver metabolic function. Calcium may need to be administered rapidly to prevent hypocalcemia.

REPERFUSION PHASE

The reperfusion phase begins with release of the clamps on the major vascular structures. The sequence of reperfusion depends on surgical preference. Severe hemodynamic instability may occur during unclamping of the portal vein (reperfusion syndrome); this effect appears to be multifactorial in origin and may require pharmacologic intervention with potent vasopressors such as epinephrine or norepinephrine, or both.[6] Once the allograft begins to function, hemodynamic and metabolic stability is gradually restored, and the need for inotropic support decreases. Indirect signs of a functioning graft include intraoperative bile production, correction of the negative base excess, and improvement in coagulation.

Postoperative Care

Continued intubation of the patient's trachea may not be required in the postoperative period, especially in patients with active protective airway reflexes and no preexisting respiratory compromise.[7] Blood loss per se should not be considered an indication for postoperative intubation. Most often patients are admitted directly to the intensive care unit for monitoring. Ultrasound is warranted if there is any doubt about hepatic artery or portal vein patency. Thrombosis of the hepatic artery usually requires retransplantation.

LUNG TRANSPLANTATION

Approximately 1000 to 1200 lung transplants are performed annually in the United States, whereas fewer than 40 heart-lung transplants are performed annually.[8] Lung transplantation for adults generally refers to (1) single-lung transplantation (SLT), (2) bilateral sequential lung transplantation (BSLT), and (3) heart-lung transplantation (HLT). Patients with primary lung pathology typically undergo SLT or BSLT (Table 35-6). When significant left ventricular dysfunction is present as a result of underlying coronary artery disease or dilated cardiomyopathy, patients may instead undergo HLT.

Management of Anesthesia

The derangement in pulmonary mechanics assumes central importance in the intraoperative management of patients with end-stage lung disease.[9] Lung transplant patients have varying degrees of impaired gas exchange, altered pulmonary mechanics, and impaired right ventricular function that are largely determined by the underlying cause of the pulmonary failure.

Lung transplantation begins with a pneumonectomy performed through either a standard posterolateral thoracotomy incision or a bilateral thoracosternotomy incision. With the assistance of one-lung ventilation, the lung is dissected and the hilar structures are identified, clamped, and divided. After the native lung is removed, the lung graft is placed in the patient's hemithorax, and anastomosis of the hilar structures is performed (bronchial and arterial anastomoses). Cardiopulmonary bypass (CBP) may or may not be used, depending on the exact surgical procedure performed and the patient's medical condition. In select cases (severe pulmonary hypertension), cannulation of the femoral vessels may be indicated before induction of anesthesia in preparation for emergency institution of CPB.

If postoperative neuraxial analgesia is planned, the best time for injection of subarachnoid opioids or placement of an epidural catheter is before induction of anesthesia,

Table 35–6 Most Frequent Indications for Lung Transplantation

Chronic obstructive pulmonary disease
Idiopathic pulmonary fibrosis
Cystic fibrosis
α_1-Antitrypsin deficiency
Sarcoidosis
Congenital heart disease (Eisenmenger's syndrome with concomitant cardiac repair)

although some have preferred to postpone this until the postoperative period. In addition to standard monitors and intravenous access, appropriate adjuncts include arterial, central, and pulmonary arterial pressure monitoring. The decision whether to place invasive monitors before or immediately after induction of anesthesia is made after considering the individual patient's degree of cardiovascular impairment or instability. TEE assists in the intraoperative assessment of right ventricular function, pulmonary hypertension, intracardiac air, and unexplained hypotension.

INDUCTION OF ANESTHESIA

The anesthetic induction technique should preserve ventricular contractility and avoid elevation of pulmonary vascular resistance. Consideration should be given to temporary placement of a single-lumen endotracheal tube to facilitate fiberoptic bronchoscopic assessment of the tracheobronchial tree and allow thorough suctioning, especially in patients with cystic fibrosis. Ultimately, however, provision will need to be made for single-lung ventilation.

MAINTENANCE OF ANESTHESIA

Volatile anesthetics are generally well tolerated, especially when combined with intravenous drugs to lower dose requirements for the inhaled drugs. Nitrous oxide is not recommended because of its potential to increase pulmonary vascular resistance, aggravate intravascular air by expansion, and substantially limit FIO_2 when administered at clinically relevant doses. Occasionally, positive-pressure ventilation to maintain normocapnia during one-lung ventilation results in unacceptably high airway pressure, breath stacking, or both in patients with chronic obstructive pulmonary disease. Consequently, many anesthesiologists adopt a ventilation strategy that allows permissive hypercapnia. Patients with predominantly restrictive pulmonary physiology, such as those with idiopathic pulmonary fibrosis, are not generally subject to gas trapping or breath stacking but instead have decreased parenchymal compliance. Unplanned CPB is most characteristically prompted by a deterioration in gas exchange during one-lung ventilation or by hemodynamic decompensation (right heart failure) at the time of pulmonary artery clamping.

Allograft reperfusion begins when the pulmonary artery is unclamped. It is usually accompanied by a reduction in mean pulmonary artery pressure and pulmonary vascular resistance. The concomitant resumption of bilateral lung ventilation generally results in improvement in both pulmonary gas exchange and overall pulmonary mechanics. When a second contralateral transplant is planned, dissection of the remaining native lung begins. This procedure is facilitated by single-lung ventilation of the newly implanted lung. Hypotension can be encountered at the time of reperfusion, and the newly transplanted lungs may exhibit features of the pulmonary reimplantation response, which is characterized by low-pressure pulmonary edema leading to deterioration in compliance and oxygenation and increased pulmonary vascular resistance.

After implantation of the graft or grafts, ventilation is reestablished to both lungs. F_{IO_2} is titrated to maintain acceptable systemic oxygen saturation while keeping in mind the concern for pulmonary toxicity with sustained administration of high concentrations of oxygen. The use of positive end-expiratory pressure (5 cm H_2O) and inhaled nitric oxide may facilitate this goal. Bronchoscopy is useful for the evaluation of anastomosis integrity, whereas TEE may reveal pulmonary venous obstruction.

Before leaving the operating room, the double-lumen tube is removed from the patient's trachea and replaced with a single-lumen tube. The single-lumen tube is necessary to facilitate bronchoscopic inspection of the anastomoses, allow tracheobronchial suctioning, and assist in postoperative ventilatory care.

Mechanical ventilation is typically provided for 1 or more days in the absence of complications. It may be prolonged in the presence of early graft dysfunction, acute rejection episodes, bronchial anastomosis stricture or failure, pneumonia, and complications related to bleeding.

HEART TRANSPLANTATION

Between 2000 and 2200 heart transplantation procedures are performed each year in the United States.[10] A significant number of patients who undergo heart transplantation have end-stage cardiac failure as a result of ischemic or idiopathic dilated cardiomyopathy. Most of the remainder suffer from congenital defects, valvular heart disease, or increasingly, dysfunction of a previously placed cardiac graft (retransplantation). In a small minority of patients without heart failure per se, a heart transplant is indicated to treat uncontrolled ventricular dysrhythmias, idiopathic hypertrophic cardiomyopathy, intracardiac tumors, or life-threatening myocardial ischemia that is not amenable to revascularization.

Significant comorbid conditions (renal and hepatic dysfunction) are common sequelae of severe cardiac disease. Transplantation is generally considered appropriate in patients with mild organ system dysfunction that is deemed likely to normalize with the improved cardiac output after transplantation. Many patients awaiting transplantation are stabilized with intravenous inotropes, intra-aortic balloon pumps, ventricular assist devices, or mechanical ventilation (or any combination of these measures).

Preoperative measurement of pulmonary vascular resistance is of major importance because engraftment of a normal donor heart into a patient with high, fixed pulmonary vascular resistance may cause acute right ventricular failure. In these patients, pulmonary vascular resistance may be normalized by treating with intravenous or inhaled pulmonary vasodilators. Those who show significant improvement with this treatment may safely undergo cardiac transplantation.

Management of Anesthesia

During the operation the patient is placed on CPB, and the operative technique consists of anastomosis of the aorta, pulmonary artery, and left and right atria. Anesthetic induction should be conducted by following principles similar to those for any patient with end-stage cardiac failure.[10] Standard anesthetic monitoring is supplemented by invasive hemodynamic monitoring, including peripheral arterial, central venous TEE, and pulmonary artery pressure lines (RV assist device support may preclude pulmonary artery catheterization until weaning from CPB). It will be necessary to withdraw a central venous catheter or pulmonary artery catheter back into the internal jugular vein when the recipient's heart is removed. The catheter can then be repositioned when the donor heart is in place.

Vasopressors or inotropes may be instituted in the operating room before induction of anesthesia. For patients who are at the limit of their hemodynamic compensatory mechanisms, subsequent institution of extracorporeal membrane oxygenation or CPB support may be necessary.

Anesthetic induction drugs that do not cause significant myocardial depression are a consideration. Many variations of anesthetic technique have been used with success. Balanced anesthesia with continuous infusion or intermittent bolus administration of opioids, benzodiazepines, and neuromuscular blocking drugs is typical and may be supplemented with low doses of volatile anesthetics. However, the required dose of any drug may vary significantly and should be titrated according to the patient's hemodynamics. Hypotension may ensue regardless of the specific drugs used because of a reduction in preload or afterload secondary to a decrease in sympathetic nervous system tone induced by the onset of anesthesia.

Surgical preparations that occur before the initiation of CPB create few problems for hemodynamic stability, provided that intravascular fluid volume is carefully maintained along with myocardial contractility and systemic vascular resistance.

Separation from Cardiopulmonary Bypass

Once all anastomoses are completed, anesthetic goals include the provision of optimal conditions for separation from CPB and the anticipation of probable hemodynamic derangements.[10] In patients with bradycardia or atrioventricular conduction heart block, an adequate heart rate and cardiac rhythm may be achieved by the intravenous infusion of a chronotropic drug (isoproterenol or dobutamine) or the use of a temporary artificial cardiac pacemaker. An appropriate target heart rate for weaning from CPB is in the range of 90 to 110 beats/min. Because of the absence of autonomic nervous system innervation to the transplanted heart, only direct-acting sympathomimetics such as catecholamines or phosphodiesterase inhibitors are effective for inotropic or chronotropic effect. Drugs that increase the heart rate with a vagolytic effect (atropine) are ineffective.

Separation from CPB may also be complicated by myocardial dysfunction, which is often attributable to incomplete or prolonged cardiac preservation (cold ischemia time) or circumstances of the critical illness of the donor. Although left ventricular function is generally adequate, right ventricular function is also important after heart transplantation for adequate cardiac output, hemodynamic stability, and end-organ perfusion. The persistence of significant pulmonary hypertension or right ventricular failure despite pharmacologic interventions may warrant the administration of other drugs with pulmonary vasodilating properties. Nonpharmacologic measures to minimize pulmonary vascular resistance include the avoidance of hypercapnia, delivery of high F_{IO_2} concentrations, and maintenance of normothermia. Refractory right ventricular failure may be treated with a right ventricular assist device in an attempt to restore acceptable hemodynamics and systemic perfusion during the postoperative period. Cardiac dysrhythmias, hypovolemia, left ventricular dysfunction, and even anastomotic obstruction can contribute to hemodynamic compromise during reperfusion.

Postoperative Management

Tracheal extubation most often occurs in an intensive care unit setting in the absence of significant hemodynamic instability or other complications. Although normal or near-normal biventricular function is expected in most cases, right ventricular dysfunction may develop postoperatively and persist because of increased pulmonary vascular resistance.

REFERENCES

1. Baker J, Yost CS, Niemann CU. Organ transplantation. *In* Miller RD (ed): Miller's Anesthesia, 6th ed. Philadelphia: Elsevier, 2005, pp 2231-2283.
2. Csete M, Glas K. Anesthesia for organ transplantation. *In* Barash PG, Cullen BF, Stoelting RK (eds): Clinical Anesthesia, 5th ed. Philadelphia: Lippincott, Williams & Wilkins, 2006, pp 1358-1376.
3. Lemmens HJ. Kidney transplantation: Recent developments and recommendations for anesthetic management. Anesthesiol Clin North Am 2004;22:651-652.
4. Markmann JF, Brayman KL, Naji A, et al. Transplantation of abdominal organs. *In* Townsend CM Jr, Beauchamp RD, Evers MB, Mattox K (eds): Sabiston Textbook of Surgery: The Biological Basis of Modern Surgical Practice, 17th ed. Philadelphia: WB Saunders, 2004.
5. Steadman RH. Anesthesia for liver transplant surgery. Anesthesiol Clin North Am 2004;22:687-711.
6. Vater Y, Levy A, Martay K, et al. Adjuvant drugs for end-stage liver failure and transplantation. Med Sci Monit 2004;10:77-88.
7. Catron EG, Rettke SR, Plevak DJ, et al. Perioperative care of the liver transplant patient. Anesth Analg 1994;78:382-399.
8. Bracken CA, Gurkowski MA, Naples JJ. Lung transplantation: Historical perspective, current concepts, and anesthetic considerations. J Cardiothorac Vasc Anesth 1997;11:220-241.
9. Rosenberg AL, Rao M, Benedict PE. Anesthetic implications for lung transplantation. Anesthesiol Clin North Am 2004;22:767-788.
10. Shanewise J. Cardiac transplantation. Anesthesiol Clin North Am 2004;22:753-765.

IV

OUTPATIENT SURGERY

Martin S. Bogetz

Outpatient (ambulatory, day-case, same-day, come-and-go) surgery and anesthesia continue to evolve in scope and complexity throughout the world. The development of surgical techniques based on new technology, along with refinement in anesthetic techniques, has promoted the continuing transition of traditionally inpatient and more complex procedures (knee and shoulder reconstruction, laparoscopic cholecystectomy, splenectomy, adrenalectomy, vaginal hysterectomy) to the outpatient venue.[1] Multimodal regimens for the management of postoperative pain, nausea, and vomiting promote more timely discharge, a better quality of recovery, and greater patient satisfaction.[2,3] These advances allow patients at the extremes of age and infirmity to safely undergo surgery on an outpatient basis. The elements of care that provide for safe and uncomplicated anesthesia in the outpatient venue are no less important when the patient is to be discharged after an overnight hospital stay.

Outpatient surgery and diagnostic and therapeutic procedures occur in a variety of settings designed to eliminate the need for prior or subsequent hospitalization. Sites for outpatient surgery include main operating room complex or separate operating rooms within a hospital, a separate facility physically attached to a hospital or on hospital grounds, or a hospital-independent facility (freestanding "surgicenter.")

Diagnostic or therapeutic procedures that are associated with some discomfort or require immobility (or both) are usually performed on an outpatient basis in other venues (see Chapter 37). Such procedures commonly involve children and include radiation therapy, interventional radiologic procedures, neuroradiologic interventions, computed tomography/magnetic resonance imaging, endoscopy, examination under anesthesia, auditory evoked potentials, electroretinography, bone marrow biopsy, and intrathecal drug therapy.

ADVANTAGES OF OUTPATIENT SURGERY

When compared with inpatient surgery, advantages of performing the same operation on an outpatient basis theoretically include (1) decreased medical costs, (2) increased availability of beds for patients who require hospitalization, (3) protection of immunocompromised patients from hospital-acquired infections, and (4) avoidance of disruption of the family unit by hospitalization. The ability to rehabilitate soon after outpatient surgery decreases surgical and anesthetic complications and reduces mental and physical disability.[1] Cost savings may extend beyond actual medical expenses inasmuch as patients can often return to daily activity or work sooner. On the other hand, offloading the patient's recovery to the patient or other individuals may require additional absence from work and financial expense. The short separation time from one's usual environment provided by outpatient surgery is especially important for children and the elderly because it decreases the order and magnitude of postoperative psychological and behavioral problems caused by separation-induced anxiety, unfamiliar surroundings, and unfamiliar routines.

An alternative to the same-day surgical concept is a planned overnight admission to the hospital after surgery. This approach (AM admit, 23 hour, short stay, come and stay) is often classified as outpatient surgery and preserves many of its advantages. Physician, patient, or family concerns regarding the ability to manage potential anesthetic or operative complications in the early postoperative period are mitigated.

OFFICE-BASED ANESTHESIA

Physicians' offices and their operatories are increasingly becoming the site for elective outpatient surgical procedures (office-based surgery and office-based anesthesia). Patient preference, convenience, and privacy, along with theoretically reduced expenses, are the public's push behind this trend. Surgeons enjoy convenience and control over a lower overhead. Third-party payers leverage procedures to the office setting to reduce their costs. Traditionally, office-based care was limited to disciplines such as aesthetic surgery, dermatology, and oral surgery. Today, virtually every medical and surgical discipline has its office-based procedures, many of which still require only local anesthesia and minimal sedation. However, the escalating scope and complexity of office-based procedures make provision of monitored anesthesia care (MAC), regional anesthesia, or general anesthesia an increasingly common requirement. Lessons learned over years in the transition from inpatient to outpatient surgery have been applied promptly in the transition to the office venue.

Patient Safety Considerations

Rapid expansion in the context of financial incentives and entrepreneurship raises concern about procedure selection, patient selection, and patient safety. The public deserves and expects a single safety and quality standard of anesthetic and surgical care regardless of venue. An increasing number of states have instituted regulations that attempt to maintain standards through accreditation of facilities, credentialing of individuals, requirement for an on-site anesthesiologist or nurse anesthetist, reporting of adverse outcomes, and limitations on the nature and scope of procedures. Accreditation requirements deal with physical resources, credentialing, policies, and procedures. The American Society of Anesthesiologists (ASA) has promulgated guidelines on the delivery of high-quality anesthesia care in the office setting.[4] When outpatient surgery is performed in a freestanding facility or the physician's office, a transfer and admission agreement with a nearby affiliated hospital must be in place should unexpected hospitalization be required in the immediate perioperative period.

The need to deliver a safe anesthetic with minimal undesirable side effects and rapid recovery is critically important for office-based surgery. Short-acting, fast emergence (SAFE) anesthetics such as propofol, remifentanil, desflurane, and sevoflurane facilitate timely achievement of discharge criteria. More sophisticated regimens for MAC have also been developed.[5] Regional anesthesia with longer-acting local anesthetics can provide excellent analgesia during surgery and effective postoperative pain relief for complex surgical procedures.

FACILITIES

A basic tenet of outpatient surgery is that the operating rooms, anesthetic equipment, and recovery facilities used for outpatient surgery not differ in quality from those used for inpatient surgery.[4] Policies and procedures should be consistent and staff should possess equivalent skills and be equally competent. The postanesthesia care unit (PACU) and its staff must be capable of permitting patients to remain for several hours after surgery if needed. Some facilities are capable of caring for patients overnight.

Outpatient surgical facilities have a medical director, often an anesthesiologist, who is responsible for the medical care delivered in the facility. Physician behavior, adherence to medical staff bylaws, and the propriety of a patient or a procedure fall under the director's purview. Administrative responsibility may be the medical director's or be under the purview of an individual with administrative expertise. Some facilities employ staff with specific expertise in marketing and financial operations.

PATIENT SELECTION

Selection of individuals appropriate for outpatient surgery was once solely determined by the characteristics of the patient and the type of operation. A healthy patient could

IV

undergo a more sophisticated procedure—a more infirm patient, a lesser one. Today, other elements must be considered, including the psychosocial aspects of the patient, human and physical resources for preoperative and postoperative care, proximity to emergency care, resources of the facility and the skill set of both the surgeon and the anesthesiologist.

Characteristics of the Patient

Reimbursement agencies (third-party payers, governmental agencies) usually dictate the venue for elective surgical procedures independent of the patient's wishes. Nevertheless, the patient and caregivers must accept performance of surgery on an outpatient basis. Many patients are in good general health or have systemic diseases (non–insulin-dependent diabetes mellitus, essential hypertension, seizure disorder, asthma) that are controlled and medically stable. The development and application of less invasive surgical techniques and better anesthetic regimens have promoted the performance of more complex procedures in those more infirm. As outpatient surgery continues to expand in scope, more patients will have severe conditions (poorly controlled hypertension, morbid obesity, sleep apnea, chronic renal failure, insulin-dependent diabetes, difficult airway, history of organ transplantation).

The patient or a responsible adult must be reliable and mentally and physically competent to ensure compliance with preoperative and postoperative instructions. Ideally, the venue the night after surgery (home, stay with a relative, motel/hotel, postoperative care facility) will have proximity to emergency care should postoperative complications occur. Patient or caretaker competence and proximity to emergency care may permit discharge in one case and prohibit it in another.

PEDIATRIC PATIENTS

Age is usually not a factor in the selection of patients for outpatient surgery. It has been noted that many operations and diagnostic/therapeutic procedures in children are amenable to being performed on an outpatient basis. The American Academy of Pediatrics Section on Anesthesiology has published guidelines that detail the essential components needed to create an environment of care that promotes the safety and well-being of infants and children.[6]

Postoperative Apnea

The age at which premature or full-term infants can safely undergo surgery and return home remains controversial.[7] A combined analysis of eight studies concluded that in nonanemic infants free of apnea in the PACU, the subsequent incidence of apnea after inguinal herniorrhaphy was not less than 5% until postconceptual age was 48 weeks and gestational age was 35 weeks. The risk for subsequent apnea was not less than 1%, for the same subset of infants,

until postconceptual age was 56 weeks with a gestational age of 32 weeks or postconceptual age was 54 weeks with a gestational age of 35 weeks. Any infant with apnea in the PACU or anemia, regardless of age, should be admitted to the hospital.[8]

ELDERLY PATIENTS

Advanced age alone is not a reason to avoid outpatient surgery.[9] More important than advanced age is the medical control of diseases often associated with aging, as well as provision for social and physical support of the elderly patient both before and after surgery and anesthesia. An elderly patient often depends on another elderly individual for support and postoperative care.

TYPES OF PROCEDURES

Practically speaking, the question to answer when considering the propriety of a certain procedure is simply, "Can the patient return home afterward?" Procedural factors may predict prolonged PACU stay or unplanned admission to the hospital.[10] Such factors include intraoperative blood loss and duration of the procedure. Patient or caregiver (parent/guardian) sophistication and competence may facilitate discharge in one case and prevent it in another. Appropriate procedures for outpatient surgery include those associated with postoperative care that can first be managed in the facility and then managed relatively easily outside the surgical facility. Postoperative complications that might require intensive physician or nursing management should be very rare. Pain should be manageable with the use of local anesthetics and enteral (oral or rectal) analgesics. Postoperative nausea and vomiting (PONV) should be minimal to absent.

Operations that require major intervention into the cranium and thorax remain unacceptable for outpatient surgery, but new and minimally invasive surgical techniques will certainly change this limitation in the future. Infected patients and emergency surgery are "disruptive" and not usually welcome in an outpatient facility. However, some facilities may be able to accommodate such cases.

PREOPERATIVE PREPARATION AND INSTRUCTIONS TO THE PATIENT

Evaluation and preparation of the patient have both medical and practical importance (see Chapter 13). The ASA has produced a "Practice Advisory for Preanesthesia Evaluation."[11] Coexisting medical conditions must be evaluated to determine whether the patient's health is acceptable, in need of further evaluation, or in need of intervention. Instructions need to be understood, the patient's support network assessed, and preoperative teaching accomplished.

Patient safety and quality of care are the ultimate goals, but maintaining an efficient operating room schedule is the practical goal. How the evaluation is accomplished depends on the nature of the patient and procedure, whether the patient lives locally, the resources of the facility, and the nature of the evaluation supplied by the surgeon or referring physician.

Psychosocial issues can be even more important than medical issues. Examples include third-party authorization for the procedure, transportation to and from the facility, local lodgings before and after surgery, access to a telephone, the ability to understand and follow instructions, the availability of translation services, proximity to emergency care, and the competence of the patient's supportive network. Children often need additional effort to help prepare them and their parents or guardians.

Timing of Preoperative Evaluation

Most evaluation systems triage patients into those who need to be seen, or at least contacted before the day of surgery, and those who can be seen on the day of surgery.[12] Sick patients or those with psychosocial issues are best identified early in the process (days before) so that additional information can be gathered, evaluations performed, arrangements made, and interventions accomplished. Some systems rely on the surgeon to identify such patients. Others ask that at least the patient's history be made available beforehand so that the anesthesiologist can make a determination.

Historical Information

Historical information (medical history, medications, previous anesthetic history) is often obtained through an oral (over the telephone or in person), written, or electronic questionnaire. The questionnaire can be self-administered or administered by trained staff, a registered nurse, a nurse practitioner, a nurse anesthetist or an anesthesiologist. Screening then reveals issues that may have an impact on the perioperative experience. Web- and e-mail–based systems for preoperative evaluation are in their infancy. Security of confidential information is one of the major concerns.

Medical conditions may require active intervention and management or just awareness. Examples commonly include poorly controlled systemic hypertension, diabetes, anticoagulation, and chronic pain.

Medications

Most medications should be continued and administered at their usual time. Most patients undergoing outpatient surgery can be expected to be able to take oral medications soon after surgery and anesthesia. Insulin, oral hyperglycemic agents, diuretics, aspirin, nonsteroidal anti-inflammatory drugs (NSAIDs), and some psychiatric medications are examples of drugs that might require

adjustment. Taking an oral drug with a sip of water is clearly acceptable. Patients who require food along with their medication present an issue that must be dealt with on an individual basis. Preoperative interventions now common to inpatient care, such as perioperative β-blockade to reduce the incidence of myocardial ischemia, medications or compression devices to reduce venous thrombosis, and aggressive glucose control, may be applicable to surgical outpatients, depending on the patient or the procedure.

Orientation to the Facility

Some facilities provide information through a tour, video, or web-based material. Play therapy, introduction to the facemask, or behavioral rehearsal can be used along with the services of a child life specialist. If parents are allowed to be present for induction of anesthesia, they should be educated so that they have realistic expectations of the experience.

Laboratory Data Required Preoperatively

Laboratory data required preoperatively depend on the patient's age, medical history, physical examination, and current drug therapy. Routine laboratory tests in the absence of positive findings on the history or physical examination are not usually warranted.[11]

Patient Instructions

Preoperative instructions should be provided in writing or at least by telephone in the relevant language (Table 36-1). It is best to contact the patient or caretaker personally because telephone messages can be misunderstood, if they are listened to at all. Translation services may be needed. The threat of cancellation or postponement of one's procedure is generally all that can be done to force compliance with preoperative instructions.

Patients are usually asked to arrive 1 to 2 hours before the expected time of surgery. When one surgeon performs a series of relatively short cases, patients may be asked to arrive earlier and as a single group. Patient groups associated with a higher cancellation rate (children and the mentally challenged) may also be asked to arrive earlier. Convenience for the facility often outweighs convenience for the patient.

FASTING

The historical practice of prohibiting the ingestion of solids and liquids after midnight (*NPO after midnight*) is no longer appropriate. The ASA has issued a practice guideline for preoperative fasting in healthy patients undergoing elective surgery.[13] Clear fluids (water, black coffee, clear tea, pulp-free juice, carbonated beverage) in reasonable volumes are permissible up to 2 hours before induction

IV

Table 36-1 Information Often Provided on the Written Instruction Sheet Given to Patients When Outpatient Surgery Is Scheduled

Verify that the requested laboratory tests are completed
Fasting for solids for 6 hours or longer
Clear fluids are permissible up to 2 hours before induction of anesthesia as approved by the anesthesiologist
What medications to take (or not take)
Bring inhalers and sleep apnea devices
Wear minimal to no cosmetics or jewelry
Where and when to report for surgery and estimate of discharge time
Must be accompanied by a responsible adult to provide transportation home
Notify the surgeon if there is a change in the patient's medical condition before surgery
After surgery, resume eating when hungry, starting with clear liquids and progressing to soups and then a regular diet
Do not drive an automobile (or other mechanized equipment), make important decisions, or ingest alcohol or depressant drugs for 24 to 48 hours
Telephone number to contact a nurse or physician regarding postoperative complications

of anesthesia. Adults and children can now be spared the discomfort of thirst. Adults can avoid hypoglycemia and caffeine withdrawal.[1] Some facilities find it difficult to accurately predict the time of induction, so times for fasting can be referenced to arrival time. Breast milk is permissible up to 4 hours before induction, and infant formula, up to 6 hours. It may be acceptable to permit a "light meal" (dry toast, milk) up to 6 hours before induction of anesthesia. Both the amount and type of food need to be taken into account. Consideration must also be made for conditions (gastroparesis) that slow the transport of food through the gastrointestinal tract.

In practice, misunderstanding or failure to follow fasting instructions is a very common reason for cancellation or postponement of surgery. Such instructions can be complicated and inconsistent, particularly when multiple staff members contact the patient before surgery. Most facilities do contact the patient the day before surgery to reiterate the instructions and detect anything that might delay or cancel the patient's arrival. Confidentiality can be an issue when a telephone message is left. When patients live far away from the surgical facility, local contact information must be obtained and confirmed.

ARRIVAL ON THE DAY OF SURGERY

The greeting and initial contact that a patient receives on arrival at the facility can set the tone for the entire experience. Compliance with preoperative instructions is verified, particularly with respect to the ingestion of solid

food and clear liquids. The individual designated as the responsible escort needs to be verified in person or by telephone, and third-party authorization needs to be confirmed. Ideally, the preoperative database has been collated—it now must be rechecked for completeness, including the patient's health history and physical examination, indicated laboratory or study results, and surgical consent.

Check-in Procedure

State requirements for timeliness of the history and physical examination vary and may be different from requirements of the Joint Commission on the Accreditation of Healthcare Organizations (JCAHO). Some states require that the history and physical examination be performed within 7 days of the procedure. At the time of surgery or within 24 hours of surgery, an interval update is often performed and any changes documented. A check-in procedure confirms the identification of the patient, the nature of the procedure, and the surgical site. Patients change into a gown if indicated, NPO times are confirmed, vital signs are obtained, and if indicated, an intravenous catheter is inserted. At this time blood glucose can be checked along with any indicated laboratory tests.

ROLE OF THE ANESTHESIOLOGIST
At some point before the procedure, the anesthesiologist reviews the patient's medical record, laboratory data, and surgical consent and verifies the site of surgery. Some facilities have a separate consent for anesthesia. Vital signs are noted and current medications and medication allergies reviewed. Often, this is the start of the anesthesiologist-

patient relationship, the tone and quality of which are set by this initial interaction. It is important to elicit any change in the patient's medical condition that may have developed since the preanesthetic evaluation was performed. For example, pediatric patients must be thoroughly evaluated for the recent onset of an upper respiratory tract infection.

PEDIATRIC PATIENTS AND RHINORRHEA

Rhinorrhea can be an enigma in pediatric patients scheduled for outpatient surgery. Benign rhinorrhea is usually an allergic rhinitis that does not contraindicate elective surgery. If there is any doubt, rhinorrhea should be assumed to be an acute upper respiratory infection, and consideration should be given to delaying elective surgery. In this regard, an ill appearance and a body temperature higher than 38°C are suggestive of an infectious rather than a noninfectious process.

Preoperative Medication

As with inpatients, preoperative medication may be useful for ameliorating anxiety and addressing preoperative discomfort. Additional medication may be given acutely to treat systemic hypertension, institute β-blockade, treat bronchoconstriction, prevent infection (prophylactic antibiotics), control blood glucose concentrations, and provide corticosteroid coverage. Unlike an inpatient, an outpatient is going home on the day of surgery, so drugs administered for preoperative medication should neither delay recovery from anesthesia nor produce excessive amnesia. Most drugs used for preoperative medication do not prolong recovery when administered in appropriate doses for appropriate indications.[14] For example, fentanyl (1.0 μg/kg IV) and midazolam (0.04 mg/kg IV) administered before induction of anesthesia tend to decrease anesthetic requirements and airway irritability and do not delay recovery. Communication with and reassurance by the anesthesiologist and surgeon are potent antidotes to preoperative anxiety.

PEDIATRIC PATIENTS

Children are most likely to experience the highest level of anxiety at the time of separation from parents. The need for pharmacologic premedication may be less if the parents are calm and can participate in the induction of general anesthesia or physical transfer of the child to the nurse or anesthesiologist. Preoperative administration of midazolam (0.5 to 1.0 mg/kg orally or rectally) is effective in promoting separation from the parents within 20 to 30 minutes and is not associated with delayed recovery.

MENTALLY CHALLENGED PATIENT

Uncooperative, mentally challenged adults pose unique issues because they cannot be physically manipulated as easily as children. Some will cooperate and accept insertion of an intravenous catheter; others may cooperate with inhalation induction of anesthesia. The most uncooperative patients require pharmacologic premedication. Regimens include midazolam, up to 20 mg orally, ketamine, 2 to 3 mg/kg intramuscularly, or a combination of midazolam (0.3 mg/kg) and ketamine (2 mg/kg) intramuscularly.

GOALS

Preoperative medication intended to decrease preoperative anxiety in adults is most often provided by the administration of small doses of midazolam (1 to 2 mg IV).[14] When the patient does not have an intravenous catheter in place, sedation can be produced by the oral administration of a benzodiazepine such as diazepam. Orally administered diazepam (2 to 5 mg) is well absorbed from the gastrointestinal tract, with the plasma level reaching a peak about 60 minutes after ingestion. Unmedicated patients may walk to the operating room, whereas others may be transported by gurney or wheelchair.

Prophylaxis against Postoperative Nausea and Vomiting

A prophylactic antiemetic (serotonin antagonists, corticosteroid) may be useful for patients who (1) have a history of PONV, (2) are subject to motion sickness, or (3) are undergoing operations associated with a high incidence of PONV. Nausea with or without vomiting is an important factor contributing to a delay in discharge of patients and unanticipated admission of both children and adults after outpatient surgery.[15] Nevertheless, the routine use of prophylactic antiemetics remains controversial because a large percentage of patients do not experience nausea and vomiting.[3,16] The association of opioids with PONV may be a reason to limit the use of these drugs. Patients who undergo outpatient surgery are at no greater risk for aspiration than inpatients are. As with inpatients, outpatients considered to be at risk for pulmonary aspiration may receive preoperative pharmacologic therapy intended to speed gastric emptying, increase gastric fluid pH, or decrease gastric fluid volume (or any combination of these effects). Any antacid administered orally should be clear, not particulate.[13]

Use of Anticholinergics

Routine use of anticholinergic drugs is not needed, although an antisialagogue effect may be useful before procedures involving the oropharynx, where excessive secretions could interfere with the production of topical anesthesia. Otherwise, the discomfort of a dry mouth and throat and the possibility of residual mydriasis are undesirable in adult outpatients.

TECHNIQUES OF ANESTHESIA

All techniques of anesthesia (general anesthesia, regional anesthesia, local anesthesia with or without sedation, and

MAC) and most drugs available to inpatients are also appropriate for outpatients. The use of techniques or drugs that permit prompt and nearly complete recovery with minimal side effects (residual sedation, PONV, orthostatic hypotension, pain) is important for optimal patient safety and satisfaction. In practice, anesthetic regimens are a combination of evidence-based and experience-based care. In some facilities, expense may be a factor in the choice of anesthetics, and in this regard it should be kept in mind that the cost of sedation is usually less than the cost of a general anesthetic. The incidence of PONV tends to be less after local anesthesia and MAC than after general anesthesia. Likewise, awakening is usually more rapid after local anesthesia and MAC than after general anesthesia. Overall, the safety of modern ambulatory anesthesia is impressive, and the complications that occur in these patients are generally easily managed and self-limited.[15]

General Anesthesia

General anesthesia is frequently selected for outpatient surgery. Its onset is fast and it can be controlled easily. Administration of so-called SAFE drugs for general anesthesia is uniquely important for promoting timely recovery and minimal side effects. Propofol has become the induction drug of choice for patients undergoing outpatient surgery despite the availability of alternative drugs (thiopental, etomidate). Psychomotor recovery is more rapid after induction of anesthesia with propofol than with thiopental.[17] Postoperatively, patients have less nausea and vomiting after induction of anesthesia with propofol, and this effect is even more apparent when propofol is also used for maintenance of anesthesia.[16] Furthermore, patients may experience euphoria on emergence from propofol anesthesia, especially when combined with the ultrashort-acting opioid remifentanil. Etomidate is associated with rapid awakening, but the increased incidence of myoclonic movements and PONV detracts from its use for outpatients.

INDUCTION OF ANESTHESIA IN PEDIATRIC PATIENTS

Local custom often determines whether pediatric patients are given an inhalation induction of anesthesia or the needlestick required for placement of an intravenous catheter for intravenous induction of anesthesia. Introduction to the facemask, choice of "flavored medicine," parental presence, involvement of the child in a game or story, and premedication all facilitate cooperation for inhalation induction of anesthesia. With skill, a small-gauge intravenous catheter can be placed with minimal discomfort, particularly if a topical local anesthetic preparation (EMLA cream) is used. When inhalation induction of anesthesia is planned, the most frequently selected drug is sevoflurane. Sevoflurane does not cause airway irritation,

and its poor solubility in blood permits more rapid achievement of an anesthetizing concentration than is possible with halothane (use is decreasing). Desflurane's solubility characteristics resemble those of sevoflurane, but its airway irritant effects make it a poor choice for inhalation induction of anesthesia. Postoperative delirium in children may result from the rapid offset of drugs such as sevoflurane.

AIRWAY ADJUVANTS

Facemasks and oral airways may be used during anesthesia for brief and superficial surgical procedures. Many patients and outpatient procedures do not require tracheal intubation. The laryngeal mask airway (LMA) and other supraglottic airway devices have completely changed airway management for such patients. Successful placement of an LMA does not require the same constellation of factors associated with successful direct laryngoscopy and tracheal intubation. Such factors include neck mobility, mouth opening, pharyngeal space, and submandibular compliance. When compared with tracheal intubation, use of an LMA does not require neuromuscular blocking drugs nor their antagonism. An LMA tends to be less irritating, and placement is associated with a smaller hemodynamic response and a smaller rise in intraocular pressure. The original LMA Classic™ does not protect the airway from aspiration, and the use of positive-pressure ventilation may be questionable. The LMA ProSeal™ attempts to address both issues.

TRACHEAL INTUBATION

Some patients and procedures require tracheal intubation. Facilitation of tracheal intubation is provided by the intravenous administration of succinylcholine or a nondepolarizing neuromuscular blocking drug. A disadvantage of succinylcholine in outpatients is the occasional occurrence of myalgia. This problem does not occur with nondepolarizing neuromuscular blocking drugs. Spontaneous recovery from the effects of mivacurium is prompt. Atracurium, cisatracurium, vecuronium, and rocuronium are somewhat longer-acting alternatives. Some believe that any nondepolarizing neuromuscular blockade should be antagonized by an anticholinesterase drug such as neostigmine. Others feel comfortable if the blockade has fully resolved spontaneously as reflected by neuromuscular blockade monitoring or clinical criteria.

MAINTENANCE OF ANESTHESIA

Maintenance of anesthesia is often achieved with the combination of nitrous oxide and a volatile anesthetic (desflurane or sevoflurane) because of the desire for prompt awakening after inhaled drugs are discontinued. Nitrous oxide may be avoided based on the concern that this gas promotes PONV.[16] The low blood and tissue solubility of these inhaled drugs results in rapid recovery. The utility of brain function monitoring to minimize the dose of anesthetics and still prevent intraoperative awareness is controversial and has been addressed by an ASA practice advisory on such devices.[18,19]

An alternative to volatile anesthetics for maintenance of anesthesia is the continuous intravenous infusion of propofol, usually with an adjunct such as fentanyl, remifentanil, or ketamine. Total intravenous anesthesia (TIVA) techniques avoid all inhaled anesthetics and may include a neuromuscular blocking drug. Inhaled and intravenous anesthetics are not mutually exclusive, and many use them in combination.

ANALGESIA

Analgesia during and after the procedure is best provided by the use of a local anesthetic administered by infiltration, nerve block, plexus block, or intra-articular, intracavitary, or topical delivery. The benefit of administering a local anesthetic solution before the surgical incision (preemptive analgesia) remains controversial.[2] Opioids such as fentanyl and meperidine have traditionally been used to provide perioperative analgesia. Unfortunately, such drugs are associated with side effects, including respiratory depression, drowsiness, PONV, pruritus, and urinary retention—each of which can delay discharge and produce dissatisfaction. Other analgesic modalities include NSAIDs, acetaminophen, ketamine, and α_2-agonists such as clonidine and dexmedetomidine. The initial promise of cyclooxygenase inhibitors has been tempered by the potential for adverse cardiovascular effects and concern for deleterious effects on bone growth and healing.

Severe postoperative pain in adults may require acute treatment by the intravenous administration of an opioid such as fentanyl, meperidine, or hydromorphone. PONV and sedation may accompany the administration of an opioid for this purpose. Conversely, PONV often accompanies pain and can be relieved when analgesia is provided by the intravenous administration of an opioid. Severe, protracted pain remains a common reason for unanticipated hospital admission after planned outpatient surgery.

POSTOPERATIVE NAUSEA AND VOMITING

Treatment of severe postoperative vomiting may include the rescue administration of ondansetron, dexamethasone, promethazine, or dimenhydrinate.[20] The use of droperidol, a popular and effective antiemetic, has been curtailed by the Food and Drug Administration's "black box" warning concerning rare, but possible deleterious electrophysiologic effects (prolongation of the QT interval on the electrocardiogram).[21] For motion-related PONV, some find intramuscular hydroxyzine or ephedrine (or both) efficacious. Protracted PONV is a common reason for prolonged time in the PACU or unanticipated hospital admission after planned outpatient surgery.[15,22,23]

Regional Anesthesia

Regional anesthetic techniques, including peripheral nerve blocks (femoral, median, sciatic nerve), a combination of peripheral nerve blocks (ankle, hand block), brachial or lumbar plexus blocks, and neuraxial blocks (spinal and epidural), are increasing in popularity for outpatient surgery. Performing a regional anesthetic may take longer than inducing general anesthesia, and the possibility of failure exists. Logistics and competence play important roles in the success of regional anesthesia.

TECHNIQUE

Regional anesthesia may be used in combination with intravenous sedation or general anesthesia. Except in children, the administration of a neuraxial block is not recommended when the patient is unconscious. Still controversial, except in children, is the performance of a peripheral nerve or plexus block when the patient is unconscious. An unconscious patient cannot report pain or severe paresthesia. Adjuncts to improve the success and reduce the complications associated with regional anesthesia include the use of an electrical stimulator with an insulated needle and ultrasound guidance to localize the nerve. Because the duration of effect of certain injected and inhaled anesthetic drugs is very brief, recovery from the effects of a regional anesthetic (sensory, motor, and sympathetic nervous system blockade) can take longer and delay ambulation when compared with recovery from a general anesthetic.[24] The use of slings, crutches, and wheelchairs along with special education for PACU nurses and patients mitigates the impact of delayed recovery from the effects of regional anesthesia.

SPINAL ANESTHESIA

Spinal anesthesia does not need to be avoided in outpatients. The use of very thin ($\geq$25-gauge), rounded- or pencil-point needles (Sprotte, Whitacre, Pencan) reduces the incidence of post–dural puncture headache (PDPH), and the headaches that do occur are usually mild and self-limited. Many believe that early ambulation does not increase the incidence of PDPH. In younger patients or those in whom the potential for PDPH is considered an unacceptable risk, epidural anesthesia may become a suitable alternative to spinal anesthesia. Prolonged spinal block can delay discharge and lead to patient frustration and urinary retention in susceptible males.[24] Epinephrine should not be added to the local anesthetic solution. Traditionally, lidocaine has been used for spinal anesthesia in the outpatient setting because of its short duration of action. Concern about painful transient radicular symptoms after spinal anesthesia with lidocaine has reduced its popularity substantially.[25] Procaine, mepivacaine, bupivacaine, ropivacaine, and levobupivacaine may provide alternatives to lidocaine. The concomitant administration of intrathecal fentanyl can also be useful. For patients who are given a spinal anesthetic, it is imperative that follow-up telephone

IV

contact confirm the absence of PDPH or transient radicular symptoms.

POSTOPERATIVE ANALGESIA

Postoperative use of patient-controlled analgesia or epidural local anesthetic/opioid infusions has not proved practical for analgesia after outpatient surgery. Indwelling peripheral nerve and plexus catheters that allow continuous instillation of low doses of local anesthetic solution may be used for postoperative analgesia after more complex procedures involving the extremities. Such techniques give the patient a reusable or disposable reservoir and pump to use at home. Patient and caretaker education about its proper use and potential complications is mandatory. The quest to prolong the action of local anesthetics includes mixing α_2-adrenergic agonists (clonidine) with the local anesthetic and the development of local anesthetic suspensions using liposomes or microspheres.[2]

Sedation and Analgesia

Anesthesia for many outpatient surgical procedures, invasive medical procedures, and diagnostic tests can be accomplished simply and effectively by the use of intravenous sedative-hypnotics and analgesics. MAC entails the administration of these drugs and monitoring of the patient's vital signs by an anesthesiologist.[5] A practice guideline for sedation and analgesia by nonanesthesiologists has been developed by the ASA.[26] The combination of a regional anesthetic or local infiltration anesthesia with the intravenous injection of drugs to produce sedation or analgesia (or both) is particularly well suited for outpatient surgery.[27] However, there can be marked variation in individual patient responses to given doses of sedative-hypnotic and analgesic drugs.

Drugs commonly administered to adults to produce sedation and amnesia include midazolam or propofol.[2] Propofol is particularly well suited and extremely versatile in producing varying degrees of sedation.[27] For example, a continuous low-dose intravenous infusion of propofol (25 to 100 μg/kg/min) is particularly useful for producing sedation that can be adjusted precisely. For more painful procedures or when a peripheral nerve block requires supplementation, an opioid such as fentanyl (25 to 50 μg IV) or an infusion of remifentanil (0.075 to 0.15 μg/kg/min) or ketamine (5 to 20 μg/kg/min) may be useful.

DISCHARGE FROM THE OUTPATIENT FACILITY

Discharge from the outpatient PACU is based on specific criteria and documentation that the residual effects of anesthesia have dissipated.[15,28] Nursing policies that dictate a mandatory minimal stay in the labor-intensive PACU

are obsolete given today's anesthetic techniques. More important is the use of criterion-based milestones to determine the propriety of discharge.

Variability between nursing personnel remains the largest, single variable in determining discharge from an outpatient surgical facility.[22] Hospital-based outpatient facilities may admit postoperative outpatients to a PACU more suited for inpatient care (first stage or phase I). When defined criteria are met, patients then transfer to a less intensive and acute care area where they may still recover on a gurney or flattened recliner (second stage or phase II). Patients who meet these criteria in the operating room or very soon after leaving the operating room may be admitted directly to this phase II area (Table 36-2).[15] Admitting a postoperative patient directly to a less acute PACU environment from the operating room is called "fast tracking."[28] A light snack may be offered and the family allowed to visit. Slightly different criteria apply for determining "home readiness" (Table 36-3).[15] Eating or drinking successfully is seldom a criterion for discharge unless the patient has diabetes mellitus, has a long trip home, or is at risk for dehydration. Forcing food often leads to PONV.

Postoperative Instructions

Before discharge, postoperative instructions for wound care, medications, and return to activities and telephone contact information for questions and emergencies are reviewed with the patient or the caregiver (or both). Expected postoperative symptoms (incisional pain, drowsiness) should be distinguished from more important complications (bleeding, fever). All instructions are given in writing, and translated versions should be available for non–English-speaking patients. Instruction sheets specific to a surgeon or a surgical procedure add detail. Ensuring the availability of a competent (adult) escort to listen to the postoperative instructions and accompany the patient after discharge is essential to making sure that the discharge time is not delayed despite recovery from the effects of the anesthetic.[22] Most facilities ask that surgeons give patients prescriptions for postoperative medications before the time of surgery so that such medications can be obtained before the trip home. Some facilities give a patient a "starter pack" containing enough oral analgesics for the first night.

Common Postoperative Problems

Managing common problems in the postoperative period is as important as appropriate patient selection and the choice of anesthetic technique if the patient is to return home on the day of surgery.[22] In this regard, PONV, pain, and drowsiness are the most common reasons for protracted stay in the PACU. Urinary retention in those at risk may also delay discharge.[29] Traditionally, the unanticipated postoperative admission rate to the hospital is less than 1%. A greater incidence calls for review of patient selection

Table 36-2 Fast-Track Criteria for Direct Transfer from the Operating Room to the Phase II Unit after General Anesthesia*

	Score
Level of Consciousness	
Aware and oriented	2
Arousable with minimal stimulation	1
Responsive only to tactile stimulation	0
Physical Activity	
Able to move all extremities on command	2
Some weakness in movement of extremities	1
Unable to voluntarily move extremities	0
Hemodynamic Stability	
Systemic blood pressure <15% of baseline MAP value	2
Systemic blood pressure 15% to 30% of baseline MAP value	1
Systemic blood pressure >30% below baseline MAP value	0
Respiratory Stability	
Able to breathe deeply	2
Tachypnea with good cough	1
Dyspnea with cough	0
Oxygen Saturation Status	
Maintains value >90% on room air	2
Requires supplemental oxygen (nasal prongs)	1
Saturation <90% with supplemental oxygen	0
Postoperative Pain Assessment	
No or mild discomfort	2
Moderate to severe pain controlled with IV analgesics	1
Persistent severe pain	0
Postoperative Emetic Symptoms	
No or mild nausea with no active vomiting	2
Transient vomiting or retching	1
Persistent moderate to severe nausea and vomiting	0
TOTAL SCORE	**14**

*A minimal score of 12 (with no score less than 1 in any individual category) is required for a patient to bypass the postanesthesia care unit ("fast-tracked") after general anesthesia.

IV, intravenous; MAP, mean arterial pressure.

Data from White PF, Song D. New criteria for fast-tracking after outpatient anesthesia: A comparison with the modified Aldrete's scoring system. Anesth Analg 1999;88:1069-1072.

IV

Table 36–3 Criteria for Determination of a Discharge Score for Release Home to a Responsible Adult

Variable Evaluated	Score*
Vital signs (stable and consistent with age and preanesthetic baseline	
Systemic blood pressure and heart rate within 20% of preanesthetic level	2
Systemic blood pressure and heart rate within 20% to 40% of preanesthetic level	1
Systemic blood pressure and heart rate >40% of preanesthetic level	0
Activity level	
Steady gait without dizziness or meets preanesthetic level	2
Requires assistance	1
Unable to ambulate	0
Nausea and vomiting	
None to minimal	2
Moderate	1
Severe (continues for repeated treatment)	0
Pain (minimal to no pain, controllable with oral analgesics)	
Yes	2
No	1
Surgical bleeding (consistent with that expected for the surgical procedure)	
Minimal (does not require dressing change)	2
Moderate (up to two dressing changes required)	1
Severe (more than two dressing changes required)	0

*Patients achieving a score of at least 9 are acceptable for discharge.
Data from Marshall SI, Chung F. Discharge criteria and complications after ambulatory surgery. Anesth Analg 1999;88:508-517.

and procedure selection and an analysis of the care given by individual anesthesiologists and surgeons.[15]

Patient Expectations

A patient's expectations of the postoperative period should be realistic. Too often, pain, malaise, and recovery time are minimized in preoperative discussions. Staff members should be encouraging and the patient reassured that efforts to control pain and PONV will not stop after discharge. Patients should be reminded that mental clarity and dexterity may remain impaired for as long as 24 to 48 hours despite an overall feeling of well-being. Therefore, important decisions, driving an automobile, or operation of complex equipment should not be attempted during this period. Ingestion of alcohol or depressant drugs should be discouraged because additive responses with residual anesthetic effects are possible. The diet should initially consist of clear liquids and progress to easily digested food (soups, cereal) and then a regular diet as tolerated.

Quality improvement and accreditation require that the patient be contacted the next day, usually by telephone, to ensure that recovery is progressing without complications. Patient satisfaction may be assessed at this time or through a mail-in questionnaire. Complications need to be addressed immediately and dissatisfaction addressed in a timely and appropriate manner.

REFERENCES

1. White PF. Ambulatory anesthesia advances into the new millennium. Anesth Analg 2000;90:1234-1235.

2. White PF. The changing role of non-opioid analgesic techniques in the management of postoperative pain. Anesth Analg 2005;101:S5-S22.

3. Eubanks S, Kovac A, Philip B, et al. Consensus guidelines for managing postoperative nausea and vomiting. Anesth Analg 2003;97:62-71.

4. American Society of Anesthesiologists Committee on Ambulatory Surgical Care and the American Society of Anesthesiologists Task Force on Office-Based Anesthesia. Considerations for anesthesiologists in setting up and maintaining a safe office anesthesia environment. Available at http://www.asahq.org/ Accessed 2000.

5. Sá Rêgo MM, Watcha MF, White PF. The changing role of monitored anesthesia care in the ambulatory setting. Anesth Analg 1997;85:1020-1036.

6. American Academy of Pediatrics, Section on Anesthesiology. Guidelines for the pediatric perioperative anesthesia environment. Pediatrics 1999;103:512-515.

7. Fisher DM. When is the ex-premature infant no longer at risk for apnea? Anesthesiology 1995;82:807-808.

8. Cote CJ, Zaslavsky A, Downs JJ, et al. Postoperative apnea in former preterm infants after inguinal herniorrhaphy: A combined analysis. Anesthesiology 1995;82:809-822.

9. Fleisher LA, Pasternal LR, Herbert R, et al. Inpatient hospital admission and death after outpatient surgery in elderly patients: Importance of patient and system characteristics and location of care. Arch Surg 2004;139:67-72.

10. Junger A, Klasen J, Benson M, et al. Factors determining length of stay of surgical day-case patients. Eur J Anaesthesiol 2001;18:314-321.

11. American Society of Anesthesiologists. Practice Advisory for Preanesthesia Evaluation. Available at http://www.asahq.org/ Accessed 2003.

12. Parker BM, Tetzlaff JE, Litaker DL. Redefining the preoperative evaluation process and the role of the anesthesiologist. J Clin Anesth 2000;12:350-356.

13. American Society of Anesthesiologists Task Force on Preoperative Fasting. Practice guidelines for preoperative fasting and the use of pharmacologic agents to reduce the risk of pulmonary aspiration: Application to healthy patients undergoing elective procedures. Anesthesiology 1999;90:896-905.

14. Van Vlymen JM, Sá Rêgo MM, White PF. Benzodiazepine premedication: Can it improve outcome in patients undergoing breast biopsy? Anesthesiology 1999;90:740-747.

15. Marshall SI, Chung F. Discharge criteria and complications after ambulatory surgery. Anesth Analg 1999;88:508-517.

16. Apfel CC, Korttila K, Abdalla M, et al. A factorial trial of six interventions for the prevention of postoperative nausea and vomiting. N Engl J Med 2004;350:2441-2451.

17. Korttila K, Nuotto EJ, Lichtor JL, et al. Clinical recovery and psychomotor function after brief anesthesia with propofol or thiopental. Anesthesiology 1992;76:676-681.

18. Gan TJ, Glass PS, Windsor A, et al. Bispectral index monitoring allows faster emergence and improved recovery from propofol, alfentanil, and nitrous oxide anesthesia. Anesthesiology 1997;87:808-815.

19. American Society of Anesthesiologists. Practice advisory for intraoperative awareness and brain function monitoring. Available at http://www.asahq.org/ Accessed 2005.

20. Habib AS, Gan TJ. The effectiveness of rescue antiemetics after failure of prophylaxis with ondansetron or droperidol: A preliminary report. J Clin Anesth 2005;17:62-65.

21. Gan TJ. "Black box" warning on droperidol: Report of the FDA convened expert panel. Anesth Analg 2004;98:1809.

22. Pavlin DJ, Rapp SE, Polissar NL, et al. Factors affecting discharge time in adult outpatients. Anesth Analg 1998;87:816-826.

23. Chung F, Mezei G. Factors contributing to a prolonged stay after ambulatory surgery. Anesth Analg 1999;89:1352-1359.

24. Watcha MF, Chiu JW, Li H, et al. Comparison of the costs and recovery profiles of three anesthetic techniques for ambulatory anorectal surgery. Anesthesiology 2000;93:1225-1230.

25. Pollock JE, Neal JM, Stephenson CA et al. Prospective study of the incidence of transient radicular irritation in patients undergoing spinal anesthesia. Anesthesiology 1996:84:1361-1367.

26. American Society of Anesthesiologists Task Force on Sedation and Analgesia by Non-Anesthesiologists. Practice guidelines for sedation and analgesia by non-anesthesiologists. An updated report. Anesthesiology 2002;96:1004-1017.

27. Smith I, Monk TG, White PF, Ding Y. Propofol infusion during regional anesthesia: Sedative, amnesic, and anxiolytic properties. Anesth Analg 1994;79:313-318.

28. White PF, Song D. New criteria for fast-tracking after outpatient anesthesia: A comparison with the modified Aldrete's scoring system. Anesth Analg 1999;88:1069-1072.

29. Pavlin DJ, Pavlin EG, Fitzgibbon DR, et al. Management of bladder function after outpatient surgery. Anesthesiology 1999;91:42-50.

IV

Chapter 37

PROCEDURES PERFORMED OUTSIDE THE OPERATING ROOM

Lawrence Litt and William L. Young

The number of diagnostic and therapeutic medical procedures that require specialized environments such that they must be performed away from traditional hospital and outpatient operating room suites is increasing (Table 37-1). In addition to "remote locations" in medical centers are off-site medical offices established by surgeons who choose to perform outpatient surgery in private settings that they find more convenient and economical. Office-based anesthesia has become a primary mode of practice for many anesthesiologists.

CHARACTERISTICS OF REMOTE LOCATIONS

Remote locations are much different from self-contained operating rooms. The anesthesiologist should have a basic understanding of logistic arrangements between the anesthesia department and the various medical and nursing departments that host the remote location. Within the anesthesia department detailed arrangements must be in place regarding immediate contacts that can be established between remote locations and centrally located anesthesia colleagues and technicians, especially when help is required or vital information needs to be transmitted. There should also be clear policies for dealing with remote equipment problems and unexpected escalations of medical problems.

It is important for an anesthesiologist working in an unfamiliar remote location to keep track of the identity and role of personnel who participate in the surgical procedure or patient care. During times when the anesthesiologist may need experienced medical assistance (tracheal intubation, placement of a central venous catheter), it can be important to know which of the available staff members are qualified to render assistance. Readily available preoperative documents for all patients in remote locations must include the attending surgeon's history and physical examination. Arrangements for patient arrival and check-in should be similar to those for outpatients and inpatients undergoing procedures in a traditional operating room setting.

Table 37-1 Remote Locations That Commonly Require Anesthesia Services

Radiology and Nuclear Medicine

Diagnostic radiology and nuclear medicine

　Computed tomography

　Fluoroscopy

Therapeutic radiology

　Interventional body angiography (can involve embolization or stent placement)

　Interventional neuroangiography (can involve embolization or stent placement)

Magnetic resonance imaging

Ultrasound imaging

Radiation Therapy

Standard x-ray therapy with collimated beams

GammaKnife x-ray surgery for brain tumors and A-V malformations

CyberKnife x-ray surgery for central nervous system, body tumors, and A-V malformations

Electron beam radiation therapy (usually intraoperative)

Cardiology

Cardiac catheterization with or without electrophysiologic studies

Cardioversion

Gastroenterology

Endoscopy

Colonoscopy

Endoscopic retrograde cholangiopancreatography

Pulmonary Medicine

Tracheal and bronchial stent placement

Bronchoscopy

Pulmonary lavage

Psychiatry

Electroconvulsive therapy

Urology

Extracorporeal shock wave lithotripsy

General Dentistry and Oral and Maxillofacial Surgery

Dental surgery

Remote locations must provide for the same basic anesthesia care that is possible in any operating room. There must be adequate monitoring capabilities, the means to deliver supplemental oxygen by facemask with positive pressure, the availability of suction, equipment for providing controlled mechanical ventilation, an adequate supply of anesthetic drugs and ancillary equipment, and supplemental lighting for procedures that involve darkness. Although new, portable anesthesia machines (Fig. 37-1) can sometimes be placed very close to the patient to facilitate gas connections, it is often not possible to have an anesthesia machine as close to the patient as in the operating room (Fig. 37-2). The use of sedation, as for placement of a nerve block, should take place in an area (block room) where adequate equipment, drugs, and support personnel are available for immediate intervention.

If anesthetic gases are to be used, scavenging must be sufficient to ensure that trace amounts are below the upper limits set by the Occupational Safety and Health Administration (OSHA). Remote locations frequently involve additional hazards, such as exposure to radiation, high sound levels, and heavy mechanical equipment. Advance preparation should be made to have all needed equipment available, such as lead aprons, portable lead-glass shields, and earplugs. At the end of the procedure one must often travel distances that are typically greater than the usual distance to the postanesthesia care unit or other patient units. So that patients can be safely and

IV

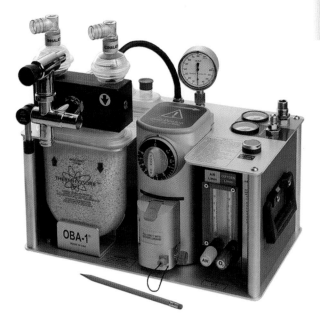

Figure 37-1 The OBA-1, a 14-kg, MRI compatible, portable anesthesia machine that may also be taken to a physician's office, a hospital block room, a bedside, or a field location. (Shown courtesy of OBAMED, Inc. Louisville, KY.)

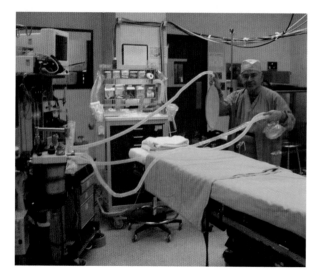

Figure 37-2 Example of an operating room setup for use when it is not possible to locate equipment in close proximity to the patient.

expeditiously taken to a recovery area, remote locations should always have available sufficient supplies of supplemental oxygen, appropriate transport monitoring equipment, and elevator and passageway keys. The anesthesiologist should always know the location of the nearest defibrillator, fire extinguisher, gas shutoff valves, and exits.

RADIATION SAFETY

Ionizing radiation and radiation safety issues may be present in remote locations.[1,2] Radiation intensity and exposure decrease with the inverse square of the distance from the emitting source. It is often possible for the anesthesiologist to be immediately behind a movable lead-glass screen. Regardless of whether this is possible, the anesthesiologist should wear a lead apron and a lead thyroid shield and remain at least 1 to 2 m from the radiation source. Clear communication between the radiology and anesthesia teams is crucial for limiting radiation exposure.

Monitoring the Radiation Dose

Anesthesiologists, like all other health care workers who are at risk for radiation exposure, can monitor their monthly dosage by wearing radiation exposure badges. The physics unit of measurement for a biologic radiation dose is the sievert; 100 rem = 1 Sv. Because some types of ionizing radiation are more injurious than others, the biologic radiation dose is obtained by multiplying together a "quality factor" and the ionizing energy absorbed per gram of tissue. Radiation exposure can be monitored with

one or more film badges. In the United States, the average annual dose from cosmic rays and naturally occurring radioactive materials is about 3 mSv (300 mrem). Patients undergoing a chest radiograph receive a dose of 0.04 mSv, whereas those undergoing a computed tomography (CT) scan of the head receive 2.00 mSv. Federal guidelines give a limit of 50 mSv for the maximum annual occupational dose.

ALLERGIC REACTIONS

Contrast agents are used in more than 10 million diagnostic radiology procedures performed each year. In 1990, fatal adverse reactions after the intravenous administration of contrast media were estimated to occur approximately once for every 100,000 procedures, whereas serious adverse reactions were estimated to occur 0.2% of the time with ionic agents and 0.4% of the time with low osmolarity agents. Radiocontrast agents can produce anaphylactoid reactions in sensitive patients, and such reactions necessitate aggressive intervention, including the administration of oxygen, intravenous fluids, and epinephrine, with epinephrine being the essential component of therapy.[3]

Adverse drug reactions are more common after the injection of iodinated contrast agents (used for x-ray examinations such as CT) than after gadolinium contrast agents (used for magnetic resonance imaging [MRI]).[4] The signs and symptoms of anaphylactoid reactions can be mild (nausea, pruritus, diaphoresis), moderate (faintness, emesis, urticaria, laryngeal edema, bronchospasm), or severe (seizures, hypotensive shock, laryngeal edema, respiratory distress, cardiac arrest). Prophylaxis against anaphylactoid reactions is directed against the massive vasodilatation that results from mast cell and basophil release of inflammatory cytokines such as histamine, serotonin, and bradykinin. The main approach to prophylaxis is steroid and antihistamine administration on the night before and the morning of the procedure. A typical regimen for a 70-kg adult is 40 mg prednisone, 20 mg famotidine, and 50 mg diphenhydramine. Patients undergoing contrast procedures usually have an induced diuresis from the osmotic load presented by the contrast agent. In this regard, adequate hydration of these patients is important to prevent aggravation of coexisting hypovolemia or azotemia. Chemotoxic reactions to contrast media are typically dose dependent (unlike anaphylactoid and anaphylactic reactions) and related to osmolarity and ionic strength.

NONINVASIVE X-RAY PROCEDURES

Sedation and General Anesthesia

Radiology departments commonly use remote locations where anesthesia services are required for patient immobility, maintenance of adequate oxygenation and perfusion, and minimization of pain and anxiety. Most adult patients, when provided with adequate instructions and preparation, do not need sedation or general anesthesia for noninvasive radiologic procedures. For many other adults, conscious sedation can be provided by qualified nurses. In contrast, sedation or general anesthesia is often required to enable children to cooperate.

PHYSIOLOGIC MONITORING

Normal physiologic monitoring is essential, as is supplemental oxygen, which is usually supplied by nasal cannula attached to a capnograph. Capnography provides the respiratory rate and pattern, as well as the end-tidal CO_2 concentration. Anesthesiologists commonly use specially constructed nasal cannulas that have a sample line for a capnograph. If capnography is not possible, ventilation must be assessed by continuous visual inspection or auscultation, or both.

SUPPLEMENTAL OXYGEN

It is preferable to have nasal cannula oxygen come from a separate flowmeter instead of from the common gas outlet of the anesthesia machine to permit more rapid deployment of the anesthesia machine's breathing circuit for delivering facemask oxygen. For long procedures it is best to administer humidified oxygen through the nasal cannula to avoid leaving the patient with an uncomfortably dry mouth and throat. Certain patients, including infants and small children, will not tolerate a nasal cannula but will do well with an oxygen "blow-by" technique.

PHARMACOLOGICALLY INDUCED SEDATION

Conscious sedation can usually be managed successfully with a continuous propofol infusion, with or without supplemental intravenous opioids or benzodiazepines (or both). A low dose of a rapid-onset, short-acting opioid such as remifentanil or alfentanil is also an appropriate selection. Dexmedetomidine is another useful drug, primarily in procedures lasting more than an hour.[5] This drug is especially useful for patients who cannot tolerate CO_2 retention, such as those with severe pulmonary hypertension, or those who require frequent assessment of mental status. Dexmedetomidine should be used cautiously in patients who require strict blood pressure maintenance at or above their baseline levels.[5] Because dexmedetomidine tends to lower systemic arterial pressure, its use might require pressure support or even be inappropriate in patients at risk for cardiac or cerebrovascular insufficiency.

COMPUTED TOMOGRAPHY

CT is most often used for intracranial imaging and for studies of the thorax and abdomen. Because CT is painless and noninvasive, adult patients undergoing elective scans rarely require more than emotional support. CT scanning is a crucial diagnostic tool in several acute settings, including traumatic injury (head and abdominal) and stroke (hemorrhagic and nonhemorrhagic). It is also used for rapid assessment of expanding intracranial masses when an increase in intracranial pressure may be a concern. Sedation or general anesthesia is often essential for such patients, as well as for children and adults who have difficulty remaining motionless.

Airway management and adequate oxygenation are the anesthesiologist's primary concerns when providing sedation or general anesthesia to patients undergoing CT. During CT scanning the anesthesiologist steps behind radiation shielding as a controlled, mechanized table moves the patient. Airway hoses, intravenous delivery tubing, and monitors can become kinked or disconnected when the table moves the patient.

MAGNETIC RESONANCE IMAGING

MRI is a standard diagnostic tool and is likely to supplant or replace conventional x-ray techniques. Patient immobility is the primary indication for sedation or general anesthesia, which is routinely needed for children, adults who are claustrophobic or in pain, and critical care patients. Although ionizing radiation is not a safety issue because no x-rays or radioactive substances are involved, other important safety issues pertain to the magnet suite. For example, missile injuries can occur if ferromagnetic objects are brought near the magnet. In addition, hearing loss may occur from high sound levels during a scan, as can electrical burns if incompatible monitoring equipment is attached to the patient. Patients with implanted devices or ferromagnetic material should never be inside a large magnetic field.

Safety Considerations

Objects in the magnet room need to be both MRI safe and MRI compatible. Before an MRI scan is started, the anesthesiologist should be sure that the patient has been screened and cleared by MRI technicians responsible for knowing that the patient's body does not contain susceptible metal objects, such as incompatible orthopedic hardware, cardiac pacemakers, wire-reinforced epidural catheters, or a pulmonary artery catheter with a temperature wire. Pulse oximetry is essential during MRI scans, and only an MRI-compatible fiberoptic pulse oximeter should be used. (Patient burns can result at the point of attachment if one uses a standard pulse oximeter.) Similar concerns pertain to any other monitoring or management devices that make actual or potential patient contact.

MISSILE INJURY

Missile injury in an MRI suite is a serious and life-threatening risk. The superconducting electrical currents that generate an MRI scanner's large magnetic field are always "on." Therefore, MRI scanners are also always

IV

surrounded by large magnetic field gradients (up to 6 m away). Magnetic field gradients can pull magnetic objects into the magnet with alarming speed and force.[6]

Whereas certain metals (nickel, cobalt) are dangerous because they are magnetic, other metals (aluminum, titanium, copper, silver) do not pose a missile danger. These metals are used to make MRI-compatible intravenous poles, fixation devices, and nonmagnetic anesthesia machines. MRI-compatible intravenous infusion pumps are clinically available. If one must bring susceptible metal items such as infusion pumps into the MRI magnet room, they should be safely located and fixed, preferably bolted to a wall or floor, with everything being done and checked before the patient enters the MRI scanner. Anesthesiologists should know that if a missile does fly into the magnet and cause injury while pinning the patient to the inside of the scanner, there is a way that the superconducting magnet can be turned off immediately. However, this is something that should be done only by MRI technicians, and while it is being done, the anesthesiologist should initiate removal of the patient from the scanner because it can become extremely cold during magnet shutdown.

Monitoring Issues

Many anesthesiologists prefer to be outside the magnet room during the scan. This would seem to be acceptable if in addition to having monitor displays of vital signs, sufficient simultaneous vigilance can also take place via video cameras and windows.

INVASIVE BLOOD PRESSURE MONITORING

Critically ill patients undergoing MRI may require invasive systemic blood pressure monitoring. Long lengths of pressure tubing are added so that pressure transducers and their electrical cables can be far from the magnet, preferably outside the magnet room. All arterial catheter stopcocks should be capped so that hemorrhage is impossible in the event of accidental perturbations in the stopcock setting. Radiofrequency pulsing can sometimes cause the pressure transducer to generate artifactual spikes, which in turn cause the monitoring equipment to falsely calculate an erroneously high blood pressure and possibly mislead the anesthesiologist. Visual inspection of the waveform can lead to rapid detection of this type of artifact.

Compatible Equipment

The MRI-compatible equipment that goes into the magnet room is really a second anesthesia station.[7] Although suction, physiologic monitoring, and mechanical ventilation must be possible inside the magnet room, it is nevertheless crucial that a primary anesthesia station be located just outside the magnet room. If a potentially life-threatening problem arises, it must be possible to promptly remove the patient from the scanner for transfer to the primary anesthesia station so that optimum care and additional help can be provided more efficiently.

Management of Anesthesia

Inhalation induction with sevoflurane plus subsequent establishment of intravenous access for infusion of propofol is a useful technique for pediatric patients requiring anesthesia for MRI.[8] Mechanical ventilation via an endotracheal tube may be needed (concern about aspiration risk, presence of increased intracranial pressure); alternatively, a laryngeal mask airway may be placed after sevoflurane induction for continued maintenance of anesthesia. General anesthesia for adults undergoing MRI brain scans usually requires an endotracheal tube, although a laryngeal mask airway will sometimes suffice. Upper airway obstruction during an MRI brain scan results in motion artifact that is unacceptable. Because hyperoxia can increase signal intensity in brain cerebrospinal fluid, the radiologist must consider this possibility when interpreting the MRI scan.[9]

INVASIVE X-RAY PROCEDURES

Interventional Radiology—Neuroangiography and Body Angiography

Interventional neuroradiology (endovascular neurosurgery) mixes traditional neurosurgery with neuroradiology while also including certain aspects of head and neck surgery. Body angiography mixes general surgery with general radiology. In angiographic procedures the relevant blood vessel trees are imaged, after which a decision is made to continue by providing one or more therapeutic interventions via drugs or devices (or both).

MANAGEMENT OF ANESTHESIA

Anesthesia-related concerns include (1) maintenance of patient immobility and physiologic stability, (2) perioperative management of anticoagulation, (3) readiness for sudden unexpected complications during the procedure, (4) provision of smooth and rapid emergence from anesthesia and sedation at appropriate times (may be required during the procedure), and (5) appropriate monitoring and management during transport after completion of the procedure, particularly for critically ill patients, who may require continuous evaluation of breathing and systemic blood pressure.[10]

Physiologic Stability

Maintenance of blood pressure is particularly important in patients with cerebrovascular disease. Blood pressure targets should always be discussed preoperatively with the surgical team. Maintaining a higher than normal blood pressure is important in cases in which the patient has occlusive cerebrovascular disease. Such cases include patients undergoing emergency thrombolysis and patients with aneurysmal subarachnoid hemorrhage in whom vasospasm has developed. Conversely, prevention of blood pressure increases may be critical in certain groups. Examples include patients with recently ruptured intracranial aneurysms or recently obliterated intracranial A-V malformation and patients who have undergone cerebrovascular angioplasty and stent placement in extracranial conductance vessels such as the carotid artery. These patients are also susceptible to post-treatment cerebral hyperperfusion injury and require careful control of systemic blood pressure after the procedure.

Anticoagulation

Anticoagulation is often needed during intracranial catheter navigation to prevent thromboembolic complications. Heparin (70 U/kg) is commonly used to prolong the baseline activated clotting time (ACT) by a factor of 2 to 3. Hourly monitoring of the ACT is performed to assess the need for additional heparin, which can be given continuously or as intermittent boluses. Hemorrhagic complications during the procedure may necessitate emergency reversal of anticoagulation. If heparin has been administered, a full reversal dose of protamine (1 mg for each 100 units of heparin activity) should always be available for immediate injection. At the completion of uneventful procedures, heparin can be reversed with protamine, if deemed appropriate.

Antiplatelet agents (aspirin, ticlopidine, and antagonists to glycoprotein IIb/IIIa receptors) are often used together with heparin, particularly when placing intra-arterial stents. Although antiplatelet drugs decrease the incidence of serious thromboembolic complications, emergency reversal of their anticoagulant effects is difficult. The only practical approach to antagonism of these drugs is empirical provision of exogenous platelets.

Patient Transport

During transport from the imaging suite, airway management equipment, including a facemask and an Ambu bag or a Jackson-Rees circuit, should be immediately available for providing positive-pressure ventilation. It is not unusual to maintain an intravenous sedation regimen (propofol infusion) during transport or to have given additional medications just before transport.

RADIATION THERAPY

Patient immobility during radiation therapy is the primary goal of sedation or general anesthesia so that the delivered radiation can be precisely targeted. Radiation therapy may involve daily treatments for several weeks. Treatments frequently take very little time, and patients want to quickly resume normal daily activities. In such instances, sedation or general anesthesia should be achieved with fast-onset, short-acting drugs appropriate for brief duration and rapid emergence while keeping in mind that sedation or anesthesia will be repeated daily. Anesthesia may also be required for lengthy or complex cases.

Devices to Deliver Large Targeted Doses of Radiation

Radiation therapy for cancer delivers large radiation doses to target tissues. In some patients, radiation is used to kill vulnerable cancer cells while only minimally injuring noncancer cells. In others, radiation is used to kill all cells in the target region (reason that the radiation device may be referred to as a "knife"). Such radiation therapy is known as stereotactic because three-dimensional MRI and CT images are used by the radiation instrument to target specific tissue volumes. For example, the GammaKnife simultaneously directs multiple carefully aligned, pencil-thin gamma ray beams into the targeted area. The CyberKnife is also characterized by delivery of a large number of ovelapping pencil-thin gamma-ray beams to provide lethal radiation. In contrast to the GammaKnife, which exposes the patient to the gamma rays as a simultaneous single dose, the CyberKnife exposes the patient to a sequence of several hundred gamma-ray beams, each being delivered from a computer-controlled robot arm that moves around the patient and shoots the beams at cancer regions from different directions.

ANESTHESIA REQUIREMENTS

Anesthesia for GammaKnife procedures can involve general anesthesia or sedation for placement of a head frame, subsequent MRI or CT (or both), transport to the recovery room where anesthesia or sedation is maintained as one waits for generation of the computer data needed by the GammaKnife, and finally transport of the anesthetized or sedated patient to the GammaKnife room for the treatment. CyberKnife procedures require prior surgical implantation of radiopaque markers. The anesthesiologist must keep the anesthesia machine, the drug cart, and all tubes and hoses away from all locations that will be occupied by the robot arm. Robot motions can be monitored closely by a remote video connection to verify that one's setup is appropriate. Scattered gamma radiation during therapy reaches high enough levels in the treatment room to require that all health care personnel be outside. Treatments occur in a heavily shielded room with health care personnel typically waiting on the other side of a large lead or iron door that takes 30 to 60 seconds to open. Physiologic monitoring is accomplished via two or more remote video connections.

Alternative Radiation Therapy Delivery Devices

Other external beam radiation therapy modalities for cancer include electron beam radiation and heavy particle ion beam radiation. The "heavy particles" are nuclei from atoms

IV

larger than helium. This treatment mode has limited availability, but it has significant advantages because the energy deposition of a heavy ion beam is very concentrated and it can be targeted with millimeter precision. Intraoperative use of particle beams has become popular in cancer surgery. During intraoperative radiation therapy (IORT), a giant linear accelerator is placed in the operating room, and the depth and width of the electron beam are adjusted according to the patient's needs. Adjacent organs and tissues are shielded with lead. All personnel must leave the room during the radiation treatment, but thick shielding walls are not necessary. A single IORT session will typically provide as much therapy as 10 to 20 daily gamma-ray treatments.

In some instances the patient cannot receive IORT in the operating room when an intraoperative gamma-ray treatment is needed. In such cases, the anesthesiologist must transport the anesthetized patient to the alternative treatment area.

ELECTROCONVULSIVE THERAPY

Electroconvulsive therapy (ECT) is used primarily after failure of pharmacotherapy for affective disorders, most notably severe depression, but also bipolar syndrome and schizophrenia. Because the ECT effect is evident within only a few treatments, it has been proposed for the treatment of psychiatric disorders of high acuity, such as suicidal patients or those unable to take food. There is little doubt about the short-term effectiveness of ECT for depression, but controversies remain regarding its place in long-term management, as well as the definition of failed pharmacotherapy. ECT's therapeutic effects are thought to result from the release of neurotransmitters during the electrically induced grand mal seizure or, perhaps, from the reestablishment of neurotransmitter levels that occurs after seizure activity.

Characteristics of Electrically Induced Seizures

It is important that an electrically induced seizure be of sufficient duration (>20 seconds) for optimal therapeutic effect. In this regard, the anesthesiologist must consider the impact of selected anesthetic drugs on the duration of seizure activity. Electrically induced seizures are characterized by an initial tonic phase (lasts 10 to 15 seconds), followed by a second myoclonic phase (lasts 30 to 60 seconds). Seizure duration is monitored by motor activity and usually a single-channel electroencephalogram. Needs for adjustments in seizure length should be discussed with the anesthesiologist before ECT.

Management of Anesthesia

The two goals of anesthetic management are to (1) provide partial neuromuscular blockade because unmitigated motor activity can result in long bone fractures and skeletal muscle injury and (2) render the patient briefly unconscious for application of the electrical stimulus.[11] The seizure is associated with a profound amnestic response and is not painful if motor activity is blocked. In the past, anesthetics most often used for ECT were the short-acting barbiturates methohexital (0.5 to 1.0 mg/kg IV) and thiopental (1.0-2.0 mg/kg IV). More recently, propofol (1 mg/kg IV) and etomidate (0.3 mg/kg IV) have become popular.[12]

PROPOFOL

Although studies have found that systemic hemodynamics during ECT is more stable under propofol anesthesia than under barbiturate anesthesia, it appears that propofol tends to shorten seizure duration.[12] In this regard, reducing the propofol dose while adding a short-acting opioid (alfentanil or remifentanil) increases seizure duration by about 50% without causing significant differences in hemodynamics or recovery time.[13]

ETOMIDATE

Etomidate may be preferred over propofol because of its association with longer electrically induced seizures and minimal cardiovascular and respiratory depression. However, a 50% to 80% incidence of myoclonus has been reported with etomidate. Although myoclonus is quickly terminated by the succinylcholine dose that immediately follows the etomidate injection, it and the skeletal muscle response to succinylcholine (fasciculations) can produce myalgias. Large doses of etomidate are known to cause adrenocortical suppression, and after a single dose some suppression has been found at 6 hours, with responses being normal at 24 hours. The adrenocortical effects of daily doses of etomidate as administered for ECT are not known.

Psychotropic Medications

In many instances, patients selected for ECT will have had their psychotropic medications tapered for 1 or 2 weeks before a series of 10 to 20 ECT treatments delivered over a period of several weeks. However, it is also not unusual for ECT patients to be taking one or more psychotropic drugs when they arrive for treatment. Such drugs include monoamine oxidase inhibitors, serotonin uptake inhibitors, tricyclic antidepressants, lithium, and benzodiazepines. Hypothyroidism is known to occur in patients who have been taking lithium for a long time (15 years or more).

Delivery of Electroconvulsive Therapy

ECT treatments are usually performed as morning cases in a procedure room that is fully equipped for general anesthesia, typically in or close to the postanesthesia care unit. Patients should be NPO during the preceding night. Preoperative evaluation of ECT patients should follow the guidelines for other surgical patients, including a current medical history and physical examination.

On the morning of the procedure the anesthesiologist should document any interval change in the patient's medical condition. Such changes can occur during a course of several ECT treatments, with anesthesia having been provided by multiple personnel. Generally, ECT should not be performed on patients with intracranial mass lesions. If a pregnant patient undergoes ECT, close monitoring of the fetus is recommended. Although the overall risk of aspiration in ECT cases is very small (less than 1 per 2000 cases), esophageal reflux and hiatal hernia are common findings in ECT patients. Some centers use drugs before the procedure to increase gastric fluid pH or decrease gastric fluid volume, or both. However, there are no data to support this practice. External cardiac pacemaker function should not be affected by ECT because the current path is far from the heart. Patients with a history of coronary artery disease, congestive heart failure, and valvular heart disease may benefit from invasive monitoring to assess myocardial function and permit aggressive hemodynamic control.

PREPARATION FOR ANESTHESIA
Anesthesia for ECT begins with attachment of all monitors, administration of 100% oxygen by facemask, and acquisition of vital signs. Supplemental oxygen is continued during and after ECT. A second blood pressure cuff is placed on the lower part of the leg or forearm. This cuff is inflated before administration of the neuromuscular blocking drug to allow monitoring of motor activity during the seizure. Standard neuromuscular blockade monitoring may be carried out distal to the cuff, if desired.

INDUCTION OF ANESTHESIA
After preoxygenation, anesthesia is induced by the administration of propofol (1 to 1.5 mg/kg IV) or etomidate (0.15 to 0.30 mg/kg IV), alone or in combination with esmolol and/or a rapidly acting opioid such as remifentanil or alfentanil. After the patient loses consciousness, the blood pressure cuff on the leg or arm is inflated above arterial pressure so that it functions as a tourniquet to prevent distal perfusion. During this time, ECT electrodes are applied by the psychiatrist to one or both sides of the head, and an oral airway, if placed previously, is removed and replaced with a bite block to protect the tongue. Because hypercapnia can increase a patient's seizure threshold, the anesthesiologist often provides ventilatory support via the mask just before the therapist energizes the electrodes. Indeed, ECT therapists often prefer that the anesthesiologist hyperventilate the patient's lungs to generate hypocapnia and a lower seizure threshold.

PREVENTION OF EXCESS SKELETAL MUSCLE ACTIVITY
Succinylcholine (0.5 to 1 mg/kg IV) is injected just before application of the electrical current. Full relaxation is not required to prevent seizure-induced skeletal muscle and bone injury. When succinylcholine is contraindicated, a short-acting nondepolarizing neuromuscular blocking drug such as mivacurium is selected. Succinylcholine is known to increase intragastric pressure, and suction must be available to treat regurgitation.

AIRWAY MANAGEMENT AND MONITORING
Endotracheal intubation is rarely required, but it is important to have available all necessary equipment should unexpected airway problems arise. Monitoring with pulse oximetry is used to guide the need for continued administration of supplemental oxygen. The use of a second peripheral nerve stimulator, placed anywhere proximal to the leg tourniquet, will confirm the degree of neuromuscular blockade produced by the neuromuscular blocking drug and will also identify unexpected prolonged neuromuscular blockade, which will occur in patients with previously unrecognized cholinesterase deficiency. The electrocardiogram (ECG) is a necessary monitor because cardiac dysrhythmias can occur during ECT.

PRODUCTION OF THE SEIZURE
Visual monitoring of the seizure is possible by observing the tonic contractions and myoclonus distal to the previously inflated tourniquet (blood pressure cuff) that has been placed on an extremity (serves to isolate this portion of the body from the circulation and the effects of the neuromuscular blocking drug). The electrodes are energized by the psychiatrist once it is clear from fasciculations or the neural blockade monitor that succinylcholine has acted throughout the body (except below the inflated blood pressure cuff). Just before the ECT shock one can give the patient a few breaths of supplemental oxygen via the anesthesia mask, which serves to reduce end-tidal CO_2, denitrogenate the functional residual capacity (FRC), and help prevent airway collapse during apnea. During the ECT shock it is safe for the anesthesiologist to be using gloved hands to gently displace the mandible forward to ensure that the tonic phase of the seizure does not displace the bite block.

PHYSIOLOGIC RESPONSES TO THE SEIZURE
The two phases of the electrically induced seizure (tonic and clonic) have characteristic and highly predictable effects on the vital signs. The initial tonic phase is characterized by profound stimulation of the parasympathetic nervous system that results in a consistent brief period of bradycardia. Blood pressure may decrease as well. This phase quickly converts to a state of sympathetic nervous system stimulation as the seizure enters the clonic phase. Systemic hypertension and tachycardia are often observed but usually abate at or soon after the conclusion of the seizure. During this time cardiac dysrhythmias may be visible on the ECG, as well as changes indicative of myocardial ischemia. Because the maximum blood pressure and heart

IV

rate occur and end so quickly, medications to reduce these self-limited changes must be used with great caution. If used, they are most effective when given before the seizure is induced. In appropriate patients, esmolol (0.15 to 1.50 mg/kg IV) or labetalol (0.13 mg/kg IV) may be administered 30 to 60 seconds before the seizure is induced.[14] Similarly, remifentanil or alfentanil may also be administered just before seizure induction. However, routine blunting of sympathetic nervous system responses by β-adrenergic antagonists is not recommended because severe bradycardia has been observed.

ANALYSIS OF RESPONSES TO SEIZURES

Because patients undergo a series of ECT sessions, after the first treatment one can evaluate previous cardiovascular responses to the electrical shocks and revise whatever decision one made before about esmolol and other drugs. One can similarly assess the dose used to produce neuromuscular blockade. On rare occasion a seizure will not abate. Seizures that last longer than 90 seconds should generally be terminated with a repeat dose of propofol or equivalent drug.

CARDIAC CATHETERIZATION— ANGIOGRAPHY, INTERVENTION, ELECTROPHYSIOLOGY

Pediatric cardiac catheterization is usually performed for the diagnosis and evaluation of congenital heart disease. However, septal defects can sometimes be repaired. Intravenous sedation or general anesthesia must be adequate to prevent stress-induced changes in heart rate and systemic blood pressure without interfering with existing intracardiac shunts as reflected by arterial blood gas measurements. Excess myocardial depression or changes in preload as a result of fluid imbalance must be avoided. Normocapnia is a goal of ventilation during anesthesia for cardiac catheterization. A high hematocrit may be associated with an increased risk for thrombosis, whereas lowering the hematocrit may jeopardize tissue oxygen delivery. Cardiac dysrhythmias and heart block are important causes of morbidity, thus emphasizing the need for prompt access to a defibrillator and resuscitation drugs.

Premedication and sedation (often combinations of midazolam and a short-acting opioid) may be sufficient to allay the anxiety that could exacerbate coexisting cardiopulmonary problems. Atropine premedication is sometimes useful, particularly if cyanotic congenital heart disease is present. The onset of action of injected or inhaled drugs (or both) may be influenced by the presence of a left-to-right or right-to-left intracardiac shunt, as well as by coexisting congestive heart failure and associated low cardiac output. Patient monitoring during cardiac catheterization may include arterial blood gas data. Access to the patient can be limited by fluoroscopy and the presence of surgical equipment on all sides of the patient during the procedure.

Adult cases can be extremely challenging, particularly in patients with advanced myocardial disease, who routinely have an ejection fraction (EF) below 20% and who come for installation of programmable pacemaker that is also an implanted cardioverter/defibrillator (ICD). It is not uncommon for such pacemakers to provide right and left dual-chamber pacing. Timing parameters are adjusted during the electrophysiology session, and the session is concluded with repeated defibrillator tests during which the cardiologist induces fibrillation and the device automatically delivers a rescue shock. Conscious sedation with spontaneous respiration is best in such cases. Before starting the procedure the anesthesiologist should be sure to check the filter setting on the ECG monitoring setup. Many ECG monitors routinely filter out sharp pulses, thus making pacemaker spikes invisible unless "HIDE" is changed to "SHOW" under the setting for pacemakers. Using a minidrip intravenous set can be very helpful in avoiding inadvertent administration of intravenous fluids. A primary element in the anesthesia plan is avoidance of positive-pressure ventilation whenever possible because it will increase pulmonary vascular resistance, decrease left ventricular filling, and decrease arterial pressure. Systemic blood pressure in cardiomyopathy patients with a low EF should be monitored continuously via an arterial catheter; if necessary, the pressure can often be raised with low-dose boluses of phenylephrine (e.g., 25 to 50 µg per bolus), but response is slower than in patients with normal cardiac output. In rare cases phenylephrine can cause an increase in systemic vascular resistance that is not tolerated by a cardiomyopathic heart. If such is the case when blood pressure is dangerously low, gentle inotrope administration is needed, as sometimes occurs when inducing anesthesia for cardiac transplantation. Although patients with ICDs have many indwelling catheters and lie on a narrow table, brief neuromuscular blockade is rarely needed to avoid adverse sudden muscle movements at the time of ICD testing. At that time a small dose of propofol after voluntary preoxygenation and hyperventilation is usually sufficient for patients undergoing conscious sedation with spontaneous ventilation. Once ICD testing is complete, gentle hand ventilation via a mask can be used if needed to maintain oxygenation until spontaneous respirations return. Cases will occur in which general anesthesia, endotracheal intubation, and mechanical ventilation are all unavoidable. Low-dose etomidate is a useful induction agent in such instances. Supplementation with midazolam is helpful in minimizing the likelihood of awareness. However, spontaneous ventilation will be reduced by midazolam, and it is important later on to not have serious interference from this adverse secondary effect. During general anesthesia, maintenance typically consists of 50% or more nitrous oxide and a small amount of vapor. Blood pressure is often improved when dual-chamber cardiac pacing is initiated by the cardiologist.

CARDIOVERSION

Elective cardioversion requires a brief period of sedation and amnesia for the discomfort produced by the electric shock. After monitors are attached and emergency drugs and equipment have been checked, including the availability of suction, the patient is preoxygenated and the desired level of sedation is typically produced by the intravenous administration of a short-acting drug such as propofol. After loss of consciousness, the electrical charge is delivered to the patient, and gentle assisted ventilation of the patient's lungs with 100% oxygen is provided as needed, with a bag and mask used until consciousness has returned. Decreases in systemic blood pressure, especially after the administration of propofol, can be minimized by the use of a low dose at a reduced rate of injection. Etomidate is an unlikely selection despite its reduced cardiac depression because the myoclonus that it often induces can make airway management and ECG analysis difficult. Because of slower onset, a less profound degree of central nervous system depression, and duration of action, benzodiazepines are not as useful for cardioversion.

EXTRACORPOREAL SHOCK WAVE LITHOTRIPSY

Extracorporeal shock wave lithotripsy (ESWL) uses focused shock waves (high-intensity pressure waves of short duration) to pulverize renal and ureteral calculi into very small fragments, which are then washed out by normal urine flow. Modern lithotripters deliver several precisely focused, simultaneous shock waves that have been generated in water-filled cushions at the surface of a special table on which the patient lies. Pain at the skin is usually tolerable or amenable to short-acting drugs. Patient immobility during lithotripsy is very important.

Ureteroscopic Lithotripsy

Ureteroscopic lithotripsy (also referred to as "endoscopic lithotripsy") is needed for the disintegration of complex upper urinary tract calculi. A powerful yttrium-aluminum-garnet (YAG) laser is aimed directly at the stones. ESWL and ureteroscopic lithotripsy are routinely performed on an outpatient basis.

Immersion Lithotripsy

ESWL was initially possible only by immersing the patient from the neck down in a water bath. Modern ESWL has eliminated numerous concerns unique to patient immersion, which produces effects similar to those of a G-suit. For example, immersion causes peripheral venous compression, thereby increasing central intravascular volume and central venous pressure—typically by 8 to 11 mm Hg.

Immersion lithotripsy also increases the work of breathing, and breathing in awake patients often becomes shallow and rapid. Extrinsic pressure on the abdomen and chest results in a decrease in vital capacity and FRC. Patients with preexisting pulmonary disease may experience impaired ventilation and oxygenation during water immersion. Despite the increased central venous pressure, some patients will exhibit hypotension secondary to vasodilatation as a result of the effects of warm water. Hypotension may also occur during removal from the water bath. During immersion or emersion, cardiac dysrhythmias can occur, presumably reflecting abrupt changes in right atrial pressure and rapid changes in central venous return. Because placement in a water bath puts patients with marginal cardiovascular reserve at greater risk for congestive heart failure or myocardial ischemia, such patients should undergo lithotripsy only in modern units that do not involve immersion.

Risk for Cardiac Dysrhythmias

To minimize the risk of initiating cardiac dysrhythmias (especially ventricular tachycardia), shock waves are triggered from the ECG to occur 20 msec after the R wave, which corresponds to the absolute refractory period of the heart. The concern that shock waves could interfere with functioning of external cardiac pacemakers has not been validated, and the presence of such a device is not considered a contraindication to ESWL, assuming that the external cardiac pacemaker is not positioned in the path of the shock waves.

Side Effects

Hematuria occurs in nearly all patients, presumably from renal parenchymal damage or dislodgement of calculi. In very rare instances, calcifications in blood vessels near the kidney can unintentionally be disintegrated by shock waves aimed at renal stones. Thus, vigilance must always be maintained for bleeding, hematoma formation, or emboli. Other very rare side effects of shock wave damage include pulmonary contusions and pancreatitis. Flank pain may persist for several days after ESWL, and petechiae and soft tissue swelling are common at the shock wave entry site.

Management of Anesthesia

Shock waves cause cutaneous pain as they traverse the water-skin interface. With modern lithotripters the pain is minimal, and intravenous sedation and analgesia are usually sufficient. Supplemental oxygen should be administered during the procedure. It is often possible to avoid endotracheal intubation and use a laryngeal mask, an ordinary facemask, or simply nasal prongs. The pain is greater with immersion lithotripsy, and general or regional

IV

anesthesia is needed. If an epidural technique is used, air should never be injected because it can create a significant density difference just outside the dura. It is not uncommon for midline back pain to develop postoperatively in patients who have had air injected into their epidural space during immersion lithotripsy. Adequate intravenous fluid administration is essential during lithotripsy to facilitate the passage of disintegrated stones and maintenance of systemic blood pressure.

DENTAL SURGERY

Anesthesia for dental surgery is commonly needed for patients who are very young, as well as for mentally handicapped patients. Special considerations must often be incorporated into the anesthetic plan for a patient with developmental delay as associated with congenital heart disease. Because the teeth and gums are highly innervated, the ECG may reveal cardiac dysrhythmias during periods of intense stimulation.

Management of Anesthesia

Management goals include rapid induction and prompt emergence from anesthesia. Ketamine injected intramus-cularly is commonly used for induction of anesthesia. After onset of the effects of ketamine, it is convenient to establish intravenous access and administer short-acting drugs (thiopental, etomidate, propofol). Inhalation induction of anesthesia with sevoflurane is also commonly used. Tracheal intubation, often via a nasal route, is recommended for lengthy or unusually bloody procedures. Because tracheal suction through a nasal tube can sometimes be difficult, consideration should be given to the preoperative or intraoperative use of atropine to reduce secretions. A cuffed endotracheal tube is preferred. If an esophageal stethoscope cannot be used, a precordial stethoscope can be placed to monitor breath and heart sounds. The choice of maintenance anesthesia drugs depends on the probable duration of the planned dental surgery. It is not unusual to use combinations of inhaled and intravenous agents. The antiemetic properties of propofol may be useful in this setting. Short-acting opioids such as remifentanil and alfentanil may also be considered. Bleeding and the use of oropharyngeal packing during dental procedures emphasize the need for close observation and maintenance of airway patency during emergence, as well as the immediate availability of appropriate personnel and equipment (airways, drugs, suction).

REFERENCES

1. Brateman L. Radiation safety considerations for diagnostic radiology personnel. Radiographics 1999;19:1037-1055.
2. Miller KL. Operational health physics. Health Phys 2005;88:1-15.
3. Robertson PS, Rhoney DH. Prophylaxis for anaphylactoid reactions in high risk patients receiving radiopaque contrast media. Surg Neurol 1997;48:292-293.
4. Ketkar M, Shrier D. An allergic reaction to intraarterial nonionic contrast material. AJNR Am J Neuroradiol 2003;24:292.
5. Nichols DP, Berkenbosch JW, Tobias JD. Rescue sedation with dexmedetomidine for diagnostic imaging: A preliminary report. Paediatr Anaesth 2005;15:199-203.
6. Litt L, Cauldwell C. Being extra safe when providing anesthesia for MRI examinations. ASA Newsletter 2002;66.
7. Miyasaka K, Kondo Y, Tamura T, Sakai H. Anesthesia-compatible magnetic resonance imaging. Anesthesiology 2005;102:235, author reply 235-236, discussion 236.
8. Gooden CK, Dilos B. Anesthesia for magnetic resonance imaging. Int Anesthesiol Clin 2003;41:29-37.
9. Frigon C, Shaw DW, Heckbert SR, et al. Supplemental oxygen causes increased signal intensity in subarachnoid cerebrospinal fluid on brain FLAIR MR images obtained in children during general anesthesia. Radiology 2004;233:51-55.
10. Hashimoto T, Gupta DK, Young WL. Interventional neuroradiology—anesthetic considerations. Anesthesiol Clin North Am 2002;20:347-359.
11. Ding Z, White PF. Anesthesia for electroconvulsive therapy. Anesth Analg 2002;94:1351-1364.
12. Avramov MN, Husain MM, White PF. The comparative effects of methohexital, propofol, and etomidate for electroconvulsive therapy. Anesth Analg 1995;81:596-602.
13. Recart A, Rawal S, White PF, et al. The effect of remifentanil on seizure duration and acute hemodynamic responses to electroconvulsive therapy. Anesth Analg 2003;96:1047-1050.
14. Castelli I, Steiner LA, Kaufmann MA, et al. Comparative effects of esmolol and labetalol to attenuate hyperdynamic states after electroconvulsive therapy. Anesth Analg 1995;80:557-561.

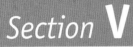

Section **V**

RECOVERY PERIOD

POSTANESTHESIA RECOVERY

Dorre Nicholau

The postanesthesia care unit (PACU) is the area designated for the monitoring and care of patients who are recovering from the immediate physiologic derangements produced by anesthesia and surgery. The PACU is staffed by specially trained nurses skilled in prompt recognition of postoperative complications. Location of the PACU in close proximity to the operating rooms facilitates rapid access to physician consultation and assistance.

Care of patients in the PACU is a vital part of anesthesia practice. This care spans the transition from delivery of anesthesia care in the operating room to less acute monitoring on the hospital ward and, in some cases, independent function of the patient at home. To serve this unique transition period, the PACU must be equipped to monitor and resuscitate unstable patients while simultaneously providing a tranquil environment for the "recovery" and comfort of stable patients. Standards for postanesthesia care have been adopted by the American Society of Anesthesiologists (see Appendix).[1]

ADMISSION TO THE POSTANESTHESIA CARE UNIT

On arrival in the PACU, the anesthesiologist provides the PACU nurse with pertinent details of the patient's history, medical condition, anesthesia, and surgery (Table 38-1). Particular attention is directed to monitoring oxygenation (pulse oximetry), ventilation (breathing frequency, airway patency, capnography), and circulation (systemic blood pressure, heart rate, electrocardiogram [ECG]). Most patients receive supplemental oxygen during transfer from the operating room to the PACU and during initial recovery in the PACU. Vital signs are recorded as often as necessary but at least every 15 minutes while the patient is in the PACU. The vital signs and other pertinent information are recorded on a document that becomes part of the patient's medical record.

Table 38-1 Information Often Given to the Nurse at the Time of Admission to the Postanesthesia Care Unit

Patient's name and age
Surgical procedure and type of anesthesia (drugs used)
Other intraoperative drugs (antagonists, antibiotics, diuretics, vasopressors, cardiac antidysrhythmics)
Preoperative vital signs
Coexisting medical diseases
Preoperative drug therapy, including preoperative medication
Allergies
Intraoperative estimated blood loss and measured urine output
Intraoperative fluid and blood replacement
Anesthetic and surgical complications (if any)
Special medications or procedures that will be necessary in the postanesthesia care unit (pain management, arterial blood gases, radiographs)

Table 38-2 Physiologic Disorders That May Be Manifested in the Postanesthesia Care Unit

Upper airway obstruction
Arterial hypoxemia
Hypoventilation
Hypotension
Hypertension
Cardiac dysrhythmias
Oliguria
Bleeding
Decreased body temperature
Agitation (emergence delirium)
Delayed awakening
Nausea and vomiting
Pain

EARLY POSTOPERATIVE PHYSIOLOGIC DISORDERS

A variety of physiologic disorders affecting multiple organ systems must be diagnosed and treated in the PACU during emergence from the effects of anesthesia and surgery (Table 38-2).[2-4] Nausea and vomiting, the need for upper airway support, and systemic hypertension requiring treatment have been observed to be the most frequently encountered PACU complications (Fig. 38-1).[2]

UPPER AIRWAY OBSTRUCTION

Loss of Pharyngeal Muscle Tone

Airway obstruction is a common and potentially devastating complication in the postoperative period. The most frequent cause of airway obstruction in the PACU is the loss of pharyngeal muscle tone in a sedated or obtunded patient. Residual depressant effects of inhaled and injected anesthetics and persistent effects of neuromuscular blocking drugs contribute to the loss of pharyngeal tone in the immediate postoperative period.

In an awake patient, the pharyngeal muscles contract synchronously with the diaphragm to pull the tongue forward and tent the airway open against the negative inspiratory pressure generated by the diaphragm. This pharyngeal muscle activity is depressed during sleep, and the resulting decrease in tone promotes airway obstruction.

With the collapse of compliant pharyngeal tissue during inspiration, a viscous cycle may ensue in which a reflex compensatory increase in respiratory effort and negative inspiratory pressure promotes further airway obstruction. This effort to breathe against an obstructed airway is characterized by a paradoxical breathing pattern consisting of retraction of the sternal notch and exaggerated abdominal muscle activity. Collapse of the chest wall plus protrusion of the abdomen with inspiratory effort produces a rocking motion that becomes more prominent with increasing airway obstruction.

TREATMENT

Obstruction secondary to loss of pharyngeal tone can be relieved by simply opening the airway with the "jaw thrust maneuver" or continuous positive airway pressure (CPAP) applied via a facemask (or both). Support of the airway is needed until the patient has adequately recovered from the effects of drugs administered during anesthesia. In selected patients, placement of an oral or nasal airway, laryngeal mask airway, or endotracheal tube may be required.

IMPLICATIONS OF OBSTRUCTIVE SLEEP APNEA

Patients with obstructive sleep apnea (OSA) are particularly prone to airway obstruction and should not be extubated until they are fully awake and following commands.[5] Any redundant compliant pharyngeal tissue in these patients not only increases the incidence of airway obstruction but also often makes intubation by direct laryngoscopy difficult or impossible. Once in the PACU, an extubated patient with OSA is exquisitely sensitive to opioids, and when

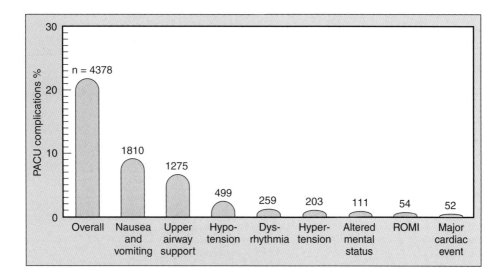

Figure 38-1 The overall complication rate in 18,473 consecutive patients entering a postanesthesia care unit (PACU) was 23.7%. Nausea and vomiting, the need for upper airway support, and hypotension were the most frequent individual complications. (From Hines HR, Barash PG, Watrous G, et al. Complications occurring in the postanesthesia care unit: A survey. Anesth Analg 1992;74:503-509, with permission.)

possible, continuous regional anesthesia techniques should be used to provide postoperative analgesia. Interestingly, benzodiazepines can have a greater effect on pharyngeal muscle tone than opioids, and the use of benzodiazepines in the preoperative setting can contribute to airway obstruction in the PACU.

When caring for a patient with OSA, plans should be made preoperatively to provide CPAP in the immediate postoperative period. Patients are often asked to bring their CPAP machines with them on the day of surgery so that the equipment can be set up before the patient's arrival in the PACU. Patients who do not routinely use CPAP at home or who do not have their machines with them may require additional attention from the respiratory therapist to ensure proper fit of the CPAP delivery device (mask or nasal airways) and determine the amount of positive pressure needed to prevent upper airway obstruction.

Residual Neuromuscular Blockade

When evaluating upper airway obstruction in the PACU, the possibility of residual neuromuscular blockade must be considered in any patient who received neuromuscular blocking drugs during anesthesia. Residual neuromuscular blockade may not be evident on arrival in the PACU because the diaphragm recovers from neuromuscular blockade before the pharyngeal muscles do. With an endotracheal tube in place, end-tidal carbon dioxide concentrations and tidal volumes may indicate adequate ventilation while the ability to maintain a patent upper airway and clear upper airway secretions remain compromised. The stimulation

associated with tracheal extubation, followed by the activity of patient transfer to the gurney and subsequent mask airway support, may keep the airway open during transport to the PACU. Only after the patient is calmly resting in the PACU does upper airway obstruction become evident. Even patients treated with intermediate- and short-acting neuromuscular blocking drugs may manifest residual paralysis in the PACU despite what was deemed clinically adequate pharmacologic reversal in the operating room.

CLINICAL ASSESSMENT OF RESIDUAL NEUROMUSCULAR BLOCKADE

Measurement of the train-of-four (TOF) ratio is a subjective assessment, and a decline in the TOF ratio may not be appreciated until it reaches a value less than 0.4 to 0.5, whereas significant clinical weakness may persist to a ratio of 0.7. Five seconds of sustained tetanus to 100-Hz stimulation is probably the most reliable indicator of adequate reversal of drug-induced neuromuscular blockade.

When patients with residual neuromuscular blockade are awake in the PACU, an inability to breathe adequately can result in agitation. In an awake patient, clinical assessment of reversal of neuromuscular blockade is preferred to the application of painful TOF or tetanic stimulation. Clinical evaluation includes grip strength, tongue protrusion, the ability to lift the legs off the bed, and the ability to lift the head off the bed for a full 5 seconds. Of these maneuvers, the 5-second sustained head lift is considered the gold standard because it reflects not only generalized motor strength but, more importantly, the patient's ability to maintain and protect the airway.

V

FACTORS THAT CONTRIBUTE TO PROLONGED NEUROMUSCULAR BLOCKADE

Persistence or return of neuromuscular weakness in the PACU should prompt a review of possible etiologic factors (Table 38-3). Common etiologic factors include respiratory acidosis and hypothermia, alone or in combination. Upper airway obstruction as a result of the residual depressant effects of volatile anesthetics or opioids (or both) may result in progressive respiratory acidosis only after the patient is admitted to the PACU and external stimulation is minimized. Similarly, a patient who becomes hypothermic during anesthesia and surgery may show signs of weakness in the PACU that were not noted on extubation in the operating room. Simple measures such as warming the patient, airway support, and correction of electrolyte abnormalities can facilitate recovery from neuromuscular blockade.

Laryngospasm

Laryngospasm refers to a sudden spasm of the vocal cords that completely occludes the laryngeal opening. It typically occurs in the transitional period when the extubated patient is emerging from general anesthesia. Although it is most likely to occur in the operating room at the time of tracheal extubation, patients who arrive in the PACU asleep after general anesthesia are also at risk for laryngospasm on awakening.

TREATMENT

Jaw thrust with CPAP (up to 40 cm H_2O) is often sufficient stimulation to "break" the laryngospasm. If jaw thrust and CPAP maneuvers fail, immediate skeletal muscle relaxation can be achieved with succinylcholine (0.1 to 1.0 mg/kg IV or 4 mg/kg IM). It is not acceptable to attempt to forcibly pass a tracheal tube through a glottis that is closed because of laryngospasm.

Airway Edema

Airway edema is a possible operative complication in patients undergoing prolonged procedures in the prone or Trendelenburg position. It can be particularly significant in procedures that involve a large amount of blood loss requiring aggressive fluid resuscitation. Surgical procedures on the tongue, pharynx, and neck, including thyroidectomy, carotid endarterectomy, and cervical spinal procedures, can result in upper airway obstruction because of tissue edema or hematoma, or both. Although facial and scleral edema is an important physical sign that can alert the clinician to the presence of airway edema, significant edema of pharyngeal tissue is often not accompanied by visible external signs. If tracheal extubation is to be attempted in these patients in the PACU, evaluation of airway patency must precede removal of the endotracheal tube. The patient's ability to breathe around the endotracheal tube can be evaluated by suctioning the oral pharynx and deflating the endotracheal tube cuff. With occlusion of the proximal end of the endotracheal tube, the patient is then asked to breathe around the tube. Good air movement suggests that the patent's airway will remain patent after tracheal extubation.

Table 38–3 Factors Contributing to Prolonged Nondepolarizing Neuromuscular Blockade

Drugs
Inhaled anesthetic drugs
Local anesthetics (lidocaine)
Cardiac antidysrhythmics (procainamide)
Antibiotics (polymyxins, aminoglycosides, lincosamines [clindamycin], metronidazole [Flagyl], tetracyclines)
Corticosteroids
Calcium channel blockers
Dantrolene
Furosemide
Metabolic and Physiologic States
Hypermagnesemia
Hypocalcemia
Hypothermia
Respiratory acidosis
Hepatic/renal failure
Myasthenia syndromes
Factors Contributing to Prolonged Depolarizing Blockade
I. Excessive dose of succinylcholine
II. Reduced plasma cholinesterase activity
Decreased levels
Extremes of age (newborn, old age)
Disease states (hepatic disease, uremia, malnutrition, plasmapheresis)
Hormonal changes
Pregnancy
Contraceptives
Glucocorticoids
III. Inhibited activity
Irreversible (echothiophate)
Reversible (edrophonium, neostigmine, pyridostigmine)
IV. Genetic variant (atypical plasma cholinesterase)

Management of Upper Airway Obstruction

An obstructed upper airway requires immediate attention. Efforts to open the airway by noninvasive measures should be attempted before reintubation of the trachea. Jaw thrust with CPAP (5 to 15 cm H_2O) is often enough to tent the upper airway open in patients with decreased pharyngeal muscle tone. If CPAP is not effective, an oral, nasal, or laryngeal mask airway can be inserted rapidly. After successfully opening the upper airway and ensuring adequate ventilation, the cause of the upper airway obstruction should be identified and treated. The sedating effects of opioids and benzodiazepines can be reversed with persistent stimulation or small titrated doses of naloxone (0.3 to 0.5 µg/kg IV) or flumazenil, respectively. Residual effects of neuromuscular blocking drugs can be reversed pharmacologically or by correcting contributing factors such as hypothermia.

TREATMENT OF UPPER AIRWAY OBSTRUCTION CAUSED BY EDEMA OR HEMATOMA

It may not be possible to mask-ventilate a patient with severe upper airway obstruction as a result of edema or hematoma. In the case of hematoma after thyroid or carotid surgery, an attempt can be made to decompress the airway by releasing the clips or sutures on the wound and evacuating the hematoma. This maneuver is recommended as a temporizing measure, but it will not effectively decompress the airway if a significant amount of fluid or blood (or both) has infiltrated the tissue planes of the pharyngeal wall. If emergency tracheal intubation is required, it is important to have ready access to difficult airway equipment and, if possible, surgical backup for performance of an emergency tracheostomy. If the patient is able to move air by spontaneous ventilation, an awake technique is preferred because visualization of the cords by direct laryngoscopy may not be possible.

MONITORING AIRWAY PATENCY DURING TRANSPORT

It is imperative to monitor upper airway patency and the effectiveness of the patient's respiratory efforts during transportation from the operating room to the PACU. Hypoventilation in a patient receiving supplemental oxygen will not be reliably detected by monitoring with pulse oximetry during transport. Adequate ventilation must be confirmed by watching for the appropriate rise and fall of the chest wall with inspiration, listening for breath sounds, or simply feeling for exhaled breath with the palm of one's hand over the patient's nose and mouth.

ARTERIAL HYPOXEMIA

Atelectasis and alveolar hypoventilation are the most common causes of transient postoperative arterial hypoxemia in the immediate postoperative period (Fig. 38-2; Table 38-4).[6] Filling the patient's lungs with oxygen at the

$$PAO_2 = FIO_2(PB - PH_2O) - \frac{PCO_2}{RQ}$$

$PaCO_2 = 40$ mm Hg
$$PAO_2 = .21(760 - 47) - \frac{40}{0.8} = 150 - 50 = 100 \text{ mm Hg}$$

$PaCO_2 = 80$ mm Hg
$$PAO_2 = .21(760 - 47) - \frac{80}{0.8} = 150 - 100 = 50 \text{ mm Hg}$$

PAO_2	= alveolar oxygen pressure
FIO_2	= fraction of inspired oxygen concentration
PB	= barometric pressure
PH_2O	= vapor pressure of water
RQ	= respiratory quotient

Figure 38-2 Hypoventilation as a cause of arterial hypoxemia.

conclusion of anesthesia, as well as the administration of supplemental oxygen, should blunt any effect of diffusion hypoxia as a contributor to arterial hypoxemia. Clinical correlation should guide the workup of a postoperative patient who remains persistently hypoxic. Review of the patient's history, operative course, and clinical signs and symptoms will direct the workup to rule in possible causes.

Postoperative ventilatory failure can result from a depressed drive to breathe or generalized weakness from either residual neuromuscular blockade or underlying neuromuscular disease. Restrictive pulmonary conditions such as preexisting chest wall deformity, postoperative abdominal binding, or abdominal distention can also contribute to inadequate ventilation.

Alveolar Hypoventilation (Table 38-5)

Review of the alveolar gas equation demonstrates that hypoventilation alone is sufficient to cause arterial hypoxemia in a patient breathing room air (see Fig. 38-2). At sea level, a normocapnic patient breathing room air will have an alveolar oxygen pressure of 100 mm Hg. Thus, a healthy patient without a significant alveolar-arterial (A-a) gradient will have a PaO_2 near 100 mm Hg. In the same patient, a rise in $PaCO_2$ from 40 to 80 mm Hg (alveolar hypoventilation) results in an alveolar oxygen pressure (PAO_2) of 50 mm Hg. This exercise demonstrates that even a patient with normal lungs will become hypoxic if allowed to significantly hypoventilate while breathing room air.

Normally, minute ventilation increases by approximately 2 L/min for every 1–mm Hg increase in arterial PCO_2. This linear ventilatory response to carbon dioxide can be significantly depressed in the immediate post-

Table 38–4 Factors Leading to Postoperative Arterial Hypoxemia

Right-to-left intrapulmonary shunt (atelectasis)
Mismatching of ventilation to perfusion (decreased functional residual capacity)
Congestive heart failure
Pulmonary edema (fluid overload, postobstructive)
Alveolar hypoventilation (residual effects of anesthetics and/or neuromuscular blocking drugs)
Diffusion hypoxia (unlikely if receiving supplemental oxygen)
Inhalation of gastric contents (aspiration)
Pulmonary embolus
Pneumothorax
Posthyperventilation hypoxia
Increased oxygen consumption (shivering)
Sepsis
Transfusion-related lung injury
Adult respiratory distress syndrome
Advanced age
Obesity

Table 38–5 Factors Leading to Postoperative Hypoventilation

Drug-induced central nervous system depression (volatile anesthetics, opioids)
Residual effects of neuromuscular blocking drugs
Suboptimal ventilatory muscle mechanics
Increased production of carbon dioxide
Coexisting chronic obstructive pulmonary disease

operative period by the residual effects of drugs (inhaled anesthetics, opioids, sedative-hypnotics) administered during anesthesia.

TREATMENT

Arterial hypoxemia secondary to hypercapnia alone can be reversed by the administration of supplemental oxygen or by normalizing the $PaCO_2$ (or both) (Fig. 38-3).[7] In the PACU, $PaCO_2$ can be normalized by external stimulation of the patient to wakefulness, pharmacologic

reversal of opioid or benzodiazepine effect, or controlled mechanical ventilation of the patient's lungs. Figure 38-3 demonstrates why pulse oximetry is an unreliable marker of hypoventilation in a patient receiving supplemental oxygen.

Decreased Alveolar Partial Pressure of Oxygen

Diffusion hypoxia refers to the rapid diffusion of nitrous oxide into alveoli at the end of a nitrous oxide anesthetic. Nitrous oxide dilutes the alveolar gas and produces a transient decrease in PaO_2 and $PaCO_2$. In a patient breathing room air, the resulting decrease in PaO_2 can produce arterial hypoxemia. In the absence of supplemental oxygen administration, diffusion hypoxia can persist for 5 to 10 minutes after a nitrous oxide anesthetic and thus contribute to arterial hypoxemia in the initial moments as the patient is admitted to the PACU.

When providing supplemental oxygen to a patient during transport to the PACU, care should be taken to avoid the relative decrease in FiO_2 that can result from an unrecognized disconnection of the oxygen source or empty oxygen tank.

Ventilation-to-Perfusion Mismatch and Shunt

Hypoxic pulmonary vasoconstriction (HPV) is an attempt of normal lungs to optimally match ventilation and perfusion. This response constricts vessels in poorly ventilated regions of the lung and directs pulmonary blood flow to well-ventilated alveoli. The HPV response is inhibited by

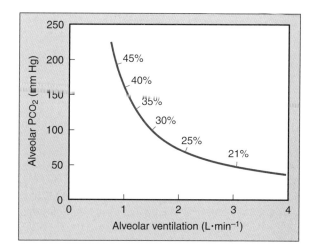

Figure 38-3 Alveolar PCO_2 as a function of alveolar ventilation at rest. The percentages indicate the inspired oxygen concentration required to restore alveolar PO_2 to normal. (Adapted from Nunn JF. Nunn's Applied Respiratory Physiology, 6th ed. Butterworth-Heinemann, with permission.)

a number of conditions and medications, including pneumonia, sepsis, and vasodilators. In the PACU, the residual effects of inhaled anesthetics and vasodilators such as nitroprusside and dobutamine used to treat systemic hypertension or improve hemodynamics will blunt HPV and contribute to arterial hypoxemia.

Unlike a ventilation-to-perfusion mismatch, a true shunt will not respond to supplemental oxygen. Causes of postoperative pulmonary shunt include atelectasis, pulmonary edema, gastric aspiration, pulmonary emboli, and pneumonia. Of these, atelectasis is probably the most common cause of pulmonary shunting in the immediate postoperative period. Mobilization of the patient to the sitting position, incentive spirometry, and positive airway pressure by facemask can be effective in treating atelectasis.

Increased Venous Admixture

Increased venous admixture typically refers to low–cardiac output states. It is due to mixing of desaturated venous blood with oxygenated arterial blood. Normally, only 2% to 5% of cardiac output is shunted through the lungs, and this shunted blood with a normal mixed venous saturation has a minimal effect on PaO_2. In low–cardiac output states, blood returns to the heart severely desaturated. Additionally, the shunt fraction increases significantly in conditions that impede alveolar oxygenation, such as pulmonary edema and atelectasis. Under these conditions, mixing of desaturated shunted blood with saturated arterialized blood decreases PaO_2.

Decreased Diffusion Capacity

A decreased diffusion capacity suggests the presence of underlying lung disease such as emphysema, interstitial lung disease, pulmonary fibrosis, or primary pulmonary hypertension. In this regard, the differential diagnosis of arterial hypoxemia in the PACU must include the contribution of any preexisting pulmonary condition.

PULMONARY EDEMA

Pulmonary edema in the PACU may be due to intravascular fluid volume overload, congestive heart failure, and causes of noncardiogenic edema such as sepsis. Occasional causes of pulmonary edema in the immediate postoperative period may include postobstructive pulmonary edema and transfusion-related pulmonary edema.

Postobstructive Pulmonary Edema

Postobstructive pulmonary edema and the resulting arterial hypoxemia are rare, but significant consequences of upper airway obstruction, as may follow tracheal extubation at the conclusion of anesthesia and surgery. It is a transudative edema produced by the exaggerated negative pressure generated by inspiration against a closed glottis. This exaggerated negative intrathoracic pressure increases venous return, which further promotes the transudation of fluid. Muscular healthy patients are at increased risk because of their ability to generate significant inspiratory force.

Laryngospasm is the most common cause of upper airway obstruction leading to postobstructive pulmonary edema, but it may result from any condition that occludes the upper airway. Arterial hypoxemia is usually manifested within 90 minutes of the upper airway obstruction and is accompanied by bilateral fluffy infiltrates on the chest radiograph. The diagnosis depends on clinical suspicion once other causes of pulmonary edema are ruled out. Treatment is supportive and includes supplemental oxygen, diuresis, and in severe cases, positive-pressure ventilation of the patient's lungs.

Transfusion-related Lung Injury

The differential diagnosis of pulmonary edema in the PACU should include transfusion-related lung injury in any patient who received blood, coagulation factor, or platelet transfusions intraoperatively. Transfusion-related lung injury is typically manifested within 1 to 2 hours after the transfusion of plasma-containing blood products, including packed red blood cells, whole blood, fresh frozen plasma, or platelets. Because reactions can occur up to 6 hours after transfusion, the syndrome may develop during the patient's stay in the PACU after a transfusion in the operating room. The resulting noncardiogenic pulmonary edema is often associated with fever and systemic hypotension. If a complete blood count is obtained with the onset of symptoms, it is possible to document an acute drop in the white blood cell count (leukopenia) reflecting the sequestration of granulocytes within the lung and exudative fluid. The diagnosis is made clinically with the appearance of bilateral pulmonary infiltrates and an increased alveolar-to-arterial oxygen difference that is temporally related to the transfusion. Treatment is supportive and includes supplemental oxygen and drug-induced diuresis.

HEMODYNAMIC INSTABILITY

Patients arriving in the PACU may demonstrate systemic hypertension, systemic hypotension, tachycardia, or bradycardia. It is not surprising that hemodynamic instability in the PACU has a negative impact on long-term outcome. Somewhat surprising, however, is the fact that postoperative systemic hypertension and tachycardia are more predictive of an adverse outcome than are hypotension and bradycardia.

Systemic Hypertension

Patients with a history of essential hypertension are at greatest risk for significant systemic hypertension in the PACU. Other patient characteristics that may increase the incidence of systemic hypertension during recovery in the PACU include postoperative pain, hypoventilation and associated hypercapnia, emergence excitement, advanced age, a history of cigarette smoking, and pre-existing renal disease (Table 38-6).[8,9] Patients undergoing intracranial operations seem to be at increased risk for postoperative hypertension. Postoperative nausea and vomiting (PONV) may be associated with systemic hypertension, which resolves when the nausea and vomiting are treated. A significant number of patients, especially those with a known history of hypertension, will require pharmacologic blood pressure control in the PACU.

Systemic Hypotension

Systemic hypotension that is present in the PACU may be characterized as (1) hypovolemic (decreased preload), (2) cardiogenic (intrinsic pump failure), and (3) distributive (decreased afterload) (Table 38-7).

HYPOVOLEMIC (DECREASED PRELOAD)

Systemic hypotension in the PACU is usually due to decreased intravascular fluid volume and preload, and as such it responds favorably to intravenous fluid administration. The most common causes of decreased intravascular fluid volume in the immediate postoperative period include ongoing third-space translocation of fluid, inadequate intraoperative fluid replacement (especially in patients who undergo major intra-abdominal procedures or preoperative bowel preparation), and loss of sympathetic nervous system tone as a result of neuraxial (spinal or epidural) blockade.

Table 38–6 Factors Leading to Postoperative Hypertension

Arterial hypoxemia
Preoperative essential hypertension
Enhanced sympathetic nervous system activity (hypercapnia from hypoventilation, pain, gastric distention, bladder distention)
Hypervolemia
Emergence excitement
Shivering
Drug rebound
Increased intracranial pressure

Table 38–7 Causes of Hypotension in the Postanesthesia Care Unit

Intravascular Fluid Volume Depletion
Ongoing fluid losses (bowel preparation, gastrointestinal losses, surgical bleeding)
Increased capillary permeability (sepsis, burns, transfusion-related lung injury)
Decreased Cardiac Output
Myocardial ischemia/infarction
Cardiomyopathy
Valvular disease
Pericardial disease
Cardiac tamponade
Cardiac dysrhythmias
Pulmonary embolus
Tension pneumothorax
Drug induced (β-blockers, calcium channel blockers)
Decreased Vascular Tone
Sepsis
Allergic reactions (anaphylactic, anaphylactoid)
Spinal shock (cord injury, iatrogenic high spinal)
Adrenal insufficiency

Ongoing bleeding should be ruled out in hypotensive patients who have undergone a surgical procedure in which significant blood loss is possible. This is true regardless of the estimated intraoperative blood loss because the measured blood loss may be inaccurate. Blood loss is often underestimated in procedures in which blood is not readily suctioned into canisters. If the patient is unstable, hemoglobin can be measured at the bedside to eliminate laboratory turnover time. It is also important to remember that tachycardia may not be a reliable indicator of hypovolemia or anemia (or both) if the patient is taking β-blockers or calcium channel blockers.

CARDIOGENIC (INTRINSIC PUMP FAILURE)

Significant cardiogenic causes of postoperative systemic hypotension include myocardial ischemia and infarction, cardiomyopathy, and cardiac dysrhythmias. The differential diagnosis depends on the surgical procedure and patient's preoperative medical condition. To determine the cause of the hypotension, central venous pressure monitoring, echocardiography, and rarely, pulmonary artery catheter monitoring may be required.

DISTRIBUTIVE (DECREASED AFTERLOAD)

Iatrogenic Sympathectomy

Iatrogenic sympathectomy secondary to regional anesthetic techniques is an important cause of hypotension in the perioperative period. A high sympathetic block (to T4) will decrease vascular tone and block the cardioaccelerator fibers. If not treated promptly, the resulting bradycardia in the presence of severe hypotension can lead to cardiac arrest, even in young healthy patients. Vasopressors, including phenylephrine and ephedrine, are pharmacologic treatments of hypotension caused by residual sympathetic nervous system blockade.

Critically Ill Patients

Critically ill patients may rely on exaggerated sympathetic nervous system tone to maintain systemic blood pressure and heart rate. In these patients even minimal doses of inhaled anesthetics, opioids, or sedative-hypnotics can decrease sympathetic nervous system tone and produce marked systemic hypotension.

Allergic Reactions

Allergic (anaphylactic or anaphylactoid) reactions may be the cause of hypotension in the PACU as a reflection of decreased afterload. Epinephrine is the drug of choice to treat hypotension secondary to an allergic reaction. Increased serum tryptase concentrations confirm the occurrence of an allergic reaction, but this change does not differentiate anaphylactic from anaphylactoid reactions. The blood specimen for tryptase determination must be obtained within 30 to 120 minutes after the allergic reaction, but the results may not be available for several days. Neuromuscular blocking drugs are the most common cause of anaphylactic reactions in the operative setting.

Sepsis

If sepsis is suspected as the cause of hypotension in PACU, blood should be obtained for culture and empirical antibiotic therapy initiated before transfer of the patient to the ward. Urinary tract manipulations and biliary tract procedures are examples of interventions that can result in a sudden onset of severe systemic hypotension secondary to sepsis. Neo-Synephrine and Levophed are the first-line pressors for the treatment of sepsis and neurogenic shock.

Myocardial Ischemia

Interpretation of changes on the ECG in the PACU is influenced by the patient's cardiac history and risk index.[10]

LOW-RISK PATIENTS

In low-risk patients (<45 years of age, no known cardiac disease, only one risk factor), postoperative ST changes on the ECG do not usually indicate myocardial ischemia. Relatively benign causes of ST changes in these low-risk patients include anxiety, esophageal reflux, hyperventilation, and hypokalemia. In general, low-risk patients require only routine PACU observation unless associated signs and symptoms warrant further clinical evaluation. A more aggressive evaluation is indicated if the changes are accompanied by cardiac rhythm disturbances, hemodynamic instability, or both.

HIGH-RISK PATIENTS

In contrast to low-risk patients, ST and T-wave changes on the ECG in high-risk patients can be significant even in the absence of typical signs or symptoms. In this patient population, any ST or T-wave changes that are compatible with myocardial ischemia should prompt further evaluation to rule out myocardial ischemia. Determination of serum troponin levels is indicated when myocardial ischemia or infarction is suspected in the PACU. Once blood samples for measurement of troponin and the MB fraction of creatine phosphokinase are obtained and a 12-lead ECG is completed, arrangements must be made for the appropriate cardiology follow-up.

CARDIAC MONITORING

In the immediate postoperative period, myocardial ischemia is rarely accompanied by chest pain, and confirming myocardial ischemia in a PACU patient is dependent on the sensitivity of the cardiac monitoring. Although a combination of leads II and V_5 will reflect 80% of the ischemic events detected on a 12-lead ECG, visual interpretation of the cardiac monitor is often inaccurate. Because of human error, the American College of Cardiology guidelines recommend that computerized ST-segment analysis be used (if available) to monitor high-risk patients in the immediate postoperative period.[11] A routine postoperative 12-lead ECG is recommended only for patients with known or suspected coronary artery disease who have undergone high- or intermediate-risk surgery. However, a postoperative 12-lead ECG may also be a valuable tool to adjust risk stratification in low-risk patients older than 50 years.

Cardiac Dysrhythmias

Perioperative cardiac dysrhythmias are frequently transient and multifactorial in cause (Table 38-8). Reversible causes of cardiac dysrhythmias in the perioperative period include hypoxemia, hypoventilation and associated hypercapnia, endogenous or exogenous catecholamines, electrolyte abnormalities, acidemia, fluid overload, anemia, and substance withdrawal.

TACHYDYSRHYTHMIAS

Common causes of sinus tachycardia in the PACU include postoperative pain, agitation (rule out arterial hypoxemia), hypoventilation with associated hypercapnia, hypovolemia (continued postoperative bleeding), shivering, and the

Table 38–8 Factors Leading to Postoperative Cardiac Dysrhythmias

Hypoxemia

Hypercarbia

Volume shifts

Pain, agitation

Hypothermia

Hyperthermia

Anticholinesterases

Anticholinergics

Myocardial ischemia

Electrolyte abnormalities

Respiratory acidosis

Hypertension

Digitalis intoxication

Preoperative cardiac dysrhythmias

presence of a tracheal tube.[8,12] Additional causes include cardiogenic or septic shock, pulmonary embolism, thyroid storm, and malignant hyperthermia.

ATRIAL DYSRHYTHMIAS

The incidence of new postoperative atrial dysrhythmias may be as high as 10% after major noncardiothoracic surgery. The incidence is even higher after cardiac and thoracic procedures, and the cardiac dysrhythmia is often attributed to atrial irritation. These new-onset atrial dysrhythmias are not benign because they are often associated with a longer hospital stay and increased mortality.

Atrial Fibrillation

Control of the ventricular response rate is the immediate goal in the treatment of new-onset atrial fibrillation. Hemodynamically unstable patients may require prompt electrical cardioversion, but most patients can be treated pharmacologically with intravenous β-blocker or calcium channel blocker. Diltiazem is the calcium channel blocker of choice for patients in whom β-blockers are contraindicated. If hemodynamic instability is a concern, the short-acting β-blocker esmolol is an option. Rate control with these agents is often enough to chemically cardiovert the postoperative patient whose arythythmia may be catecholamine driven. If the goal of therapy is chemical cardioversion, an amiodarone load can be initiated in the PACU, as long as one recognizes that bradycardia and hypotension may accompany the intravenous infusion of this drug.

VENTRICULAR DYSRHYTHMIAS

Ventricular tachycardia is uncommon, whereas premature ventricular contractions (PVCs) and ventricular bigeminy are common. PVCs most often reflect increased sympathetic nervous system stimulation, as may accompany tracheal intubation and transient hypercapnia. True ventricular tachycardia is indicative of underlying cardiac pathology, and in the case of torsades de pointes, QT prolongation on the ECG may be intrinsic or drug related (amiodarone, procainamide, or droperidol).

BRADYDYSRHYTHMIAS

Bradycardia in the PACU is often iatrogenic. Drug-related causes include β-blocker therapy, anticholinesterase reversal of neuromuscular blockade, opioid administration, and treatment with dexmedetomidine. Procedure- and patient-related causes include bowel distention, increased intracranial or intraocular pressure, and spinal anesthesia. A high spinal that blocks the cardioaccelerator fibers originating from T1 through T4 can produce severe bradycardia. The resulting sympathectomy, bradycardia, and possible intravascular fluid volume depletion and associated decreased venous return can produce sudden bradycardia and cardiac arrest, even in young healthy patients.

TREATMENT

The urgency of treatment of a cardiac dysrhythmia depends on the physiologic consequences (principally systemic hypotension) of the dysrhythmia. Tachydysrhythmia decreases diastolic and coronary perfusion time and increases myocardial oxygen consumption. Its impact depends on the patient's underlying cardiac function, and it is most harmful in patients with coronary artery disease. Bradycardia has a more deleterious effect in patients with a fixed stroke volume, such as infants and patients with restrictive pericardial disease or cardiac tamponade. The possible role of myocardial ischemia or the occurrence of pulmonary embolism must be considered when contemplating treatment options.

DELIRIUM

The American Psychiatric Association defines delirium as an acute change in cognition or disturbance of consciousness that cannot be attributed to a preexisting medical condition, substance intoxication, or medication. Approximately 10% of adult patients older than 50 years who undergo elective surgery will experience some degree of postoperative delirium within the first 5 postoperative days. The incidence is much higher (>30%) for certain procedures, such as repair of a hip fracture and bilateral knee replacement. The incidence of delirium in the PACU is not well known because many studies of acute postoperative delirium do not include the PACU stay (Table 38-9).

Table 38–9   Differential Diagnosis of Postoperative Delirium

Arterial hypoxemia
Preexisting cognitive disorder (dementia, Parkinson's disease)
Hypoventilation with associated hypercapnia
Metabolic derangements (renal dysfunction, hepatic insufficiency)
Drugs (anticholinergics, benzodiazepines, opioids, β-blockers)
Electrolyte abnormalities
Seizures
Acute central nervous system event (ischemic stroke, hemorrhage)
Infection
Emergence excitement

Risk Factors

Persistent postoperative delirium is generally a condition of elderly patients. It is a costly complication in both human and monetary terms because it increases the length of hospital stay, pharmacy costs, and mortality. In adults, patients at risk for postoperative delirium can be identified before surgery. The most significant preoperative risk factors include (1) advancing age, (2) preoperative cognitive impairment, (3) decreased functional status, (4) alcohol abuse, and (5) a previous history of delirium.

In addition to iatrogenic factors, including inadequate hydration and medications, the workup for postoperative delirium must exclude arterial hypoxemia, hypercapnia, pain, sepsis, and electrolyte abnormalities. Intraoperative factors that are predictive of postoperative delirium include surgical blood loss, hematocrit less than 30%, and the number of intraoperative blood transfusions.[13] Intraoperative hemodynamic derangements and the anesthetic technique do not seem to be predictors of postoperative delirium. Clinical evaluation of a delirious patient in the PACU includes a thorough evaluation of any underlying disease and metabolic derangements, such as hepatic- and renal-related encephalopathy.

Management

It is useful to identify a high-risk patient before admission to the PACU.[14] Severely agitated patients may require restraints and additional personnel to control their behavior and avoid self-inflicted injury or dislodgment of intravascular catheters and the endotracheal tube. Early identification of patients at risk for delirium can also guide pharmacologic therapy postoperatively. Patients who are tolerant to alcohol or opioids will probably require increased opioid doses to treat pain and anxiety and avoid the onset of alcohol withdrawal. Conversely, in the elderly population it is best to decrease drug therapy and doses as much as possible to minimize the probable onset of delirium.

Emergence Excitement

Persistent delirium may mimic a transient confusional state ("emergence excitement") that is associated with emergence from general anesthesia. Emergence excitement is common in children, with more than 30% experiencing agitation or delirium at some period during their PACU stay.[15] The peak age of emergence excitement in children is between 2 and 4 years.

Unlike delirium, emergence excitement typically resolves quickly and is followed by uneventful recovery. Emergence excitement is more frequent with rapid "wake up" from inhalational anesthesia. In children, preoperative medication with midazolam has been associated with an increase in the incidence and duration of postoperative delirium, but whether midazolam is an independent factor or merely a reflection of other preoperative variables remains unclear.

RENAL DYSFUNCTION

The differential diagnosis of postoperative renal dysfunction includes preoperative, intraoperative, and postoperative causes (see Chapter 28). Frequently, the cause is multifactorial, with a preexisting renal insufficiency that is exacerbated by an intraoperative insult. In the PACU, diagnostic efforts should focus on identification and treatment of the readily reversible causes of oliguria (urine output <0.5 mL/kg/hr). For example, urinary catheter obstruction or dislodgment is easily remedied and often overlooked (Table 38-10). Preoperative or intraoperative angiography can result in ischemic injury secondary to renal vasoconstriction and direct renal tubular injury. Intravascular fluid volume depletion can exacerbate hepatorenal syndrome or acute tubular necrosis caused by sepsis.

Oliguria Secondary to Depletion of Intravascular Fluid Volume

The most common cause of oliguria in the immediate postoperative period is depletion of intravascular fluid volume. In this regard, fluid challenge (500 to 1000 mL of crystalloid) is usually effective in restoring urine output. A hematocrit measurement is indicated when surgical blood loss is suspected and repeated volume boluses are

Table 38–10 Postoperative Oliguria
Prerenal
Hypovolemia (bleeding, sepsis, third-space fluid loss, inadequate volume resuscitation)
Hepatorenal syndrome
Low cardiac output
Renal vascular obstruction or disruption
Intra-abdominal hypertension
Renal
Ischemia (acute tubular necrosis)
Radiographic contrast dyes
Rhabdomyolysis
Tumor lysis
Hemolysis
Postrenal
Surgical injury to the ureters
Obstruction of the ureters with clots or stones
Mechanical (urinary catheter obstruction or malposition)

required to maintain urine output. Volume resuscitation to maximize renal perfusion is particularly important in order to prevent ongoing ischemic injury and the development of acute tubular necrosis.

If a fluid challenge is contraindicated or oliguria persists, assessment of intravascular fluid volume status and cardiac function is indicated to differentiate hypovolemia from sepsis and low–cardiac output states. Fractional excretion of sodium can be useful in determining the adequacy of renal perfusion (assuming that diuretics have not been given), but the diagnosis of prerenal azotemia will not differentiate between hypovolemia, congestive heart failure, or hepatorenal syndrome. Further evaluation with central venous monitoring or echocardiography, or both, may facilitate the differential diagnosis.

Intra-abdominal Hypertension

Major abdominal surgery and increased intra-abdominal pressure (intra-abdominal hypertension) can impair renal perfusion and should be considered in any oliguric patient with a tense abdomen after surgery. An intra-abdominal pressure higher than 30 cm H_2O can impede renal perfusion and lead to renal ischemia and postoperative renal dysfunction.[16] Bladder pressure should be measured in patients in whom intra-abdominal hypertension is suspected so that prompt intervention can be initiated to relieve intra-abdominal pressure and restore renal perfusion.

Rhabdomyolysis

Rhabdomyolysis is a possible cause of postoperative renal insufficiency in patients who have suffered major crush or thermal injury. The incidence of rhabdomyolysis may be increased in morbidly obese patients who undergo gastric bypass procedures. Patient history and the operative course guide the decision for measuring creatine phosphokinase in the PACU. Volume loading, mannitol, and alkalinization of urine to flush the renal tubules can prevent ongoing renal tubular damage and subsequent acute renal failure. Loop diuretics can be used to maintain urine output and avoid fluid overload, thus simplifying management in the immediate postoperative setting. The role of renal-dose dopamine remains controversial because there is no evidence that it affords renal protection in this setting.

BODY TEMPERATURE AND SHIVERING

Postoperative shivering is a dramatic consequence of general and epidural anesthesia. The incidence of postoperative shivering may be as high as 65% (range, 5% to 65%) after general anesthesia and 33% after epidural anesthesia.[17] Identified risk factors include male gender and the choice of drug (propofol more likely than thiopental) for induction of anesthesia.

Mechanism

Postoperative shivering is usually, but not always associated with a decrease in the patient's body temperature. Although thermoregulatory mechanisms can explain shivering in a hypothermic patient, a separate mechanism has been proposed to explain shivering in normothermic patients. The proposed mechanism is based on the observation that the brain and spinal cord do not recover simultaneously from general anesthesia. The more rapid recovery of spinal cord function is thought to result in uninhibited spinal reflexes manifested as clonic activity. This theory is supported by the fact that doxapram, a central nervous system stimulant, is somewhat effective in abolishing postoperative shivering.

Treatment

Intervention includes the identification and treatment of hypothermia if present. Accurate core body temperatures can be most easily obtained at the tympanic membrane. Axillary, rectal, and nasopharyngeal temperature measurements are less accurate and may underestimate core temperature. Forced air warmers are used to actively warm the hypothermic patient. A number of opioids and clonidine are effective in abolishing shivering once it starts, but meperidine (12.5 to 25 mg IV) is the most effective treatment.

Clinical Effects

In addition to significant patient discomfort, postoperative shivering increases oxygen consumption and carbon dioxide production. Cardiac output, heart rate, and systemic blood pressure are increased during shivering. Patients who are hypothermic on arrival in the PACU should be actively warmed. Mild to moderate hypothermia (33°C to 35°C) inhibits platelet function, coagulation factor activity, and drug metabolism. It exacerbates postoperative bleeding, prolongs neuromuscular blockade, and may delay awakening. Whereas these immediate consequences are associated with a prolonged PACU stay, long-term deleterious effects include an increased incidence of myocardial ischemia and myocardial infarction, delayed wound healing, and increased perioperative mortality.

POSTOPERATIVE NAUSEA AND VOMITING

Without prophylactic intervention, PONV will develop in an estimated one third of patients (range, 10% to 80%) who undergo inhalational anesthesia.[18-20] The consequences of PONV include delayed discharge from the PACU, unanticipated hospital admission, increased incidence of pulmonary aspiration, and significant postoperative discomfort. The ability to identify high-risk patients for prophylactic intervention can significantly improve the quality of patient care and satisfaction in the PACU. From a patient's perspective, PONV may be more uncomfortable than postoperative pain.

High-Risk Patients

Specific risk factors for PONV include (1) female gender, (2) history of motion sickness or PONV, (3) nonsmoking, and (4) the use of postoperative opioids (Table 38-11). The incidence of PONV correlates with the number of factors present: zero, one, two, three, or four factors correspond to an incidence of 10%, 21%, 39%, 61%, and 79%, respectively.[18-20]

The efficacy of prophylactic treatment is dependent on the patient's preoperative risk. A single intervention in a patient with four risk factors will result in an absolute risk reduction of 21% (59% to 80%) compared with a 3% risk reduction in a patient with an initial risk of only 10%.[18-20] These numbers correlate to a number needed to treat of 5 and 40, respectively. Hence cost-effective management of PONV takes into consideration the patient's underlying risk.

Table 38-11 Factors Associated with an Increased Incidence of Postoperative Nausea and Vomiting

History of postoperative vomiting with previous anesthesia and surgery
Female gender
Obesity
Postoperative pain
Type of surgery (eye muscle surgery, middle ear surgery, laparoscopic surgery)
Anesthetic drugs (opioids, nitrous oxide[?])
Gastric distention (swallowed blood)

Prevention and Treatment

Prophylactic measures against PONV include modification of the anesthetic technique and pharmacologic intervention. The use of propofol decreases the incidence of PONV by 19%, whereas the administration of an antiemetic (ondansetron, dexamethasone, or droperidol) decreases the risk by 26%.[18] Although prophylactic measures to prevent PONV are clearly more effective than rescue, a subset of patients will require treatment in the PACU even after appropriate prophylactic treatment. When choosing an antiemetic for these patients, both the class of drug and the timing of administration are factors (Table 38-12). For instance, dexamethasone has been shown to be effective when given prophylactically at the start of surgery, whereas serotonin receptor antagonists are effective when given 30 minutes before the end of anesthesia.[18] Furthermore, there is no evidence that any of the serotonin receptor antagonists commonly precribed at this time are more effective than any others. Table 38-12 lists the different classes of antiemetic medications commonly prescribed in the PACU. Droperidol, a favorite cost-effective antiemetic in the past, has recently fallen out of favor because of a Food and Drug. Administration warning regarding its use. The warning is based on case reports of torsades de pointes, a rare complication of its use. If an adequate dose of antiemetic given at the appropriate time is ineffective, simply giving more of the same class of drug in the PACU is unlikely to be of significant benefit.

BLEEDING ABNORMALITIES

Bleeding in the postoperative period is most often due to inadequate surgical hemostasis. Alternatively, postoperative bleeding may be due to a coagulopathy, which can be diagnosed with specific laboratory tests (Table 38-13). A platelet count is useful for evaluation of bleeding after massive transfusions of blood. A qualitative platelet defect

Table 38-12 Commonly Used Antiemetics (Adult Doses)

Anticholinergics

Scopolamine (0.3-0.65 mg IV, IM)

Scopolamine (2.5 cm²) transdermal patch to a hairless area behind the ear before surgery (remove 24 hours postoperatively)

Antihistamines

Hydroxyzine (12.5-25 mg IM)

Phenothiazines

Promethazine (12.5-25 mg IV or IM)

Butyrophenones

Droperidol (0.625-1.25 mg IV); monitor the ECG for prolongation of the QT interval for 2-3 hours after administration—preoperative 12-lead ECG recommended

Prokinetic

Metoclopramide (10-20 mg IV; avoid if any possibility of gastrointestinal obstruction)

Serotonin Receptor Antagonists

Ondansetron (4 mg IV 30 minutes before the conclusion of surgery)

Anzemet (12.5 mg IV 15-30 minutes before the end of surgery)

Vasopressors

Ephedrine (25 mg IM with hydroxyzine, 25 mg)

Corticosteroids

Dexamethasone (4-8 mg IV with induction of anesthesia)

Table 38-13 Laboratory Tests for Evaluation of Postoperative Bleeding Abnormalities

Test	Normal Value	Abnormality Detected
Platelet count	>150,000 cells/mm³	Dilutional thrombocytopenia Disseminated intravascular coagulation
Bleeding time	3-10 minutes	Platelet-inhibiting (acetylsalicylic acid–containing) drug
Prothrombin time	12-14 seconds	Disseminated intravascular coagulation Vitamin K deficiency Liver disease Warfarin
Partial thromboplastin time	25-35 seconds	Factor V and VIII deficiencies Heparin Hemophilia
Fibrinogen	200-400 mg/dL	Disseminated intravascular coagulation
Fibrin split products	<4 µg/mL	Disseminated intravascular coagulation
Thromboelastography		Platelet and clotting factor deficiencies

may be due to drugs ingested preoperatively, such as aspirin. In these situations, administration of platelets will reverse the thrombocytopenia and also return bleeding times to normal. Disseminated intravascular coagulation is suggested by thrombocytopenia, a prolonged prothrombin time, decreased serum concentrations of fibrinogen, and increased circulating levels of fibrin split products. Dilution of factors V and VIII by massive transfusions of whole blood or inadequate reversal of heparin will be manifested as prolonged plasma thromboplastin times. Fresh frozen plasma will reverse prolongation of the prothrombin time and plasma thromboplastin time when these abnormalities are due to liver disease or factor V or VIII deficiency. Protamine reverses heparin-induced prolongation of the partial thromboplastin time.

DELAYED AWAKENING

Even after prolonged surgery and anesthesia, it is reasonable to expect a response to stimulation in 60 to 90 minutes.[21] When delayed awakening occurs, it is important to evaluate the vital signs (systemic blood pressure, arterial oxygenation, ECG, body temperature) and perform a neurologic examination (patients may be hyperreflexic in the early postoperative period (Table 38-14). Monitoring with pulse oximetry and analysis of arterial blood gases and pH can be used to detect problems of oxygenation and ventilation. Additional blood studies may be indicated to evaluate possible electrolyte derangements and metabolic disturbances (blood glucose concentration). Radiographic procedures may be needed for evaluation of possible intracranial or intrathoracic abnormalities.

Treatment

Residual sedation from drugs used during anesthesia is the most frequent cause of delayed awakening in the PACU.

Table 38–14 Possible Explanations for Delayed Awakening in the Postanesthesia Care Unit

Residual drug effects (opioids, benzodiazepines, anticholinergics)
Hypothermia
Hypoglycemia
Electrolyte abnormalities
Arterial hypoxemia
Increased intracranial pressure (cerebral hemorrhage)
Air embolism
Hysteria

If residual effects of opioids are a possible cause of delayed awakening, it is appropriate to administer carefully titrated doses of IV naloxone (20-40 µg increments in adults), while keeping in mind that this treatment will also antagonize opioid-induced analgesia. Physostigmine may be effective in reversing the central nervous system sedative effects of anticholinergic drugs (especially scopolamine). Flumazenil is a specific antagonist for the residual depressant effects of benzodiazepines. In the absence of pharmacologic effects to explain delayed awakening, it is important to consider other causes, such as hypothermia (especially <33°C), hypoglycemia, and increased intracranial pressure. Computed tomography may be indicated in patients in

Table 38–15 Criteria for Determination of Discharge Score for Release from the Postanesthesia Care Unit

Variable Evaluated	Score
Activity	
Able to move four extremities on command	2
Able to move two extremities on command	1
Able to move no extremities on command	0
Breathing	
Able to breathe deeply and cough freely	2
Dyspnea	1
Apnea	0
Circulation	
Systemic blood pressure ≠20% of the preanesthetic level	2
Systemic blood pressure is 20% to 49% of the preanesthetic level	1
Systemic blood pressure +50% of the preanesthetic level	0
Consciousness	
Fully awake	2
Arousable	1
Not responding	0
Oxygen Saturation (Pulse Oximetry)	
>92% while breathing room air	2
Needs supplemental oxygen to maintain saturation >90%	1
<90% even with supplemental oxygen	0

Adapted from Aldrete JA. The post anaesthesia recovery score revisited. J Clin Anesth 1995;7:89-91.

V

whom a central nervous system cause of delayed awakening is a consideration. A stat glucoscan measurement of serum glucose is indicated if hypoglycemia is a possibility, as in patients with known insulin-dependent diabetes mellitus.

DISCHARGE CRITERIA

Specific PACU discharge criteria may vary, but certain general principles are universally applicable (Tables 38-15

Table 38-16 Criteria for Determination of Discharge Score for Release Home to a Responsible Adult

Variable Evaluated	Score*
Vital signs (stable and consistent with age and preanesthetic baseline)	
Systemic blood pressure and heart rate within 20% of the preanesthetic level	2
Systemic blood pressure and heart rate 20% to 40% of the preanesthetic level	1
Systemic blood pressure and heart rate >40% of the preanesthetic level	0
Activity level	
Steady gait without dizziness or meets the preanesthetic level	2
Requires assistance	1
Unable to ambulate	0
Nausea and vomiting	
None to minimal	2
Moderate	1
Severe (continues after repeated treatment)	0
Pain (minimal to no pain, controllable with oral analgesics)	
Yes	2
No	1
Surgical bleeding (consistent with that expected for the surgical procedure)	
Minimal (does not require dressing change)	2
Moderate (up to two dressing changes required)	1
Severe (more than three dressing changes required)	0

*Patients achieving a score of at least 9 are acceptable for discharge.
Modified from Marshall SI, Chung F. Discharge criteria and complications after ambulatory surgery. Anesth Analg 1999;88:508-517.

to 38-17) (see Appendix).[22-23] For example, a mandatory minimum stay in the PACU is not required (see Table 38-17). Patients must be observed until they are no longer at risk for ventilatory depression and their mental status is clear or has returned to baseline. Hemodynamic criteria are based on the patient's baseline hemodynamics without specific systemic blood pressure and heart rate requirements. An assessment and written documentation of the patient's peripheral nerve function on discharge from the PACU may become useful information should a new peripheral neuropathy develop in the later postoperative period (Table 38-18).

Table 38-17 General Principles for Discharge from the Postanesthesia Care Unit

Patients should be routinely required to have a responsible individual accompany them home

Requiring patients to urinate before discharge should not be part of a routine discharge protocol and may be necessary only in selected patients

The demonstrated ability to drink and retain clear fluids should not be part of a routine discharge protocol but may be appropriate for selected patients

A minimum mandatory stay in the unit should not be required

Patients should be observed until they are no longer at increased risk for cardiorespiratory depression

Table 38-18 Neurologic Examination before Discharge from the Postanesthesia Care Unit

Ulnar nerve	Normal sensation on the palmar surface of the fifth finger
Medial nerve	Normal sensation on the palmar surface of the second finger
Radial nerve	Ability to abduct the thumb
Sciatic nerve	Ability to flex the leg at the knee
Peroneal nerve	Ability to dorsiflex the first toe
Tibial nerve	Ability to plantar-flex the first toe

REFERENCES

1. American Society of Anesthesiologists Task Force on Post Anesthetic Care. Practice guidelines for postanesthetic care: A report by the American Society of Anesthesiologists Task Force on Post Anesthetic Care. Anesthesiology 2002;96:742-752.

2. Hines HR, Barash PG, Watrous G, et al. Complications occurring in the postanesthesia care unit: A survey. Anesth Analg 1992;74:503-509.

3. Rose DK, Cohen M, DeBoer DP. Cardiovascular events in the postanesthesia care unit: Contribution of risk factors. Anesthesiology 1996;84:772-781.

4. Rose DK, Cohen MM, Wigglesworth DF, et al. Critical respiratory events in the postanesthesia care unit: Patient, surgical and anesthetic factors. Anesthesiology 1994;81:410-418.

5. Benumof JL. Obstructive sleep apnea in the adult obese patient: Implications for airway management. J Clin Anesth 2001;13:144-156.

6. Daley MD, Norman PH, Colmenares ME, et al. Hypoxaemia in adults in the post-anesthetic unit. Can J Anaesth 1992;38:740-746.

7. Lumb AB. Nunn's Applied Respiratory Physiology, 6th ed. Philadelphia: Butterworth-Heinemann, 2005.

8. Zelcer J, Wells DG. Anaesthetic-related recovery room complications. Anaesth Intensive Care 1996;15:168-176.

9. Gal TJ, Cooperman LH. Hypertension in the immediate postoperative period. Br J Anaesth 1975;47:70-74.

10. Rinfret S, Goldman L, Polanczyk CA, et al. Value of immediate postoperative electrocardiogram to update risk stratification after major noncardiac surgery. Am J Cardiol 2004;94:1017-1022.

11. Eagle KA, Berger PB, Calkins H, et al. ACC/AHA Guideline Update for Perioperative Cardiovascular Evaluation for Noncardiac Surgery— Executive Summary. A report of the American College of Cardiology/American Heart Association Task Force on Practice Guidelines (Committee to Update the 1996 Guidelines on Perioperative Cardiovascular Evaluation for Noncardiac Surgery. Anesth Analg 2002;94:1052-1064.

12. Brathwaite D, Weissman D. The new onset of atrial arrhythmias following major noncardiothoracic surgery is associated with increased mortality. Chest 1998;114:462-468.

13. Mercantonio E, Goldman L, Orav EJ, et al. The association of intraoperative factors with the development of postoperative delirium. Am J Med 1998;105:380-384.

14. Litaker D, Locala J, Franco K, et al. Preoperative risk factors for postoperative delirium. Gen Hosp Psychiatry 2001;23:84-89.

15. Cole J, Murray D, McAllister D, Hershberg GE. Emergence behavior in children: Defining the incidence of excitement and agitation following anaesthesia. Paediatr Anaesth 2002;12:442-447.

16. Sugrue M, Jones F, Deane SA, et al. Intra-abdominal hypertension is an independent cause of postoperative renal impairment. Arch Surg 1999;134:1082-1085.

17. Buggy DJ, Crossley AWA. Thermoregulation, mild perioperative hypothermia and post-anaesthetic shivering. Br J Anaesth 2000;84:615-628.

18. Habib AS, Tong JG. Pharmacotherapy of postoperative nausea and vomiting. Exp Opin Pharmacother 2003;4:457-473.

19. Apfel C, Korttila K, Abdalla M, et al. A factorial trial of six interventions for the prevention of postoperative nausea and vomiting. N Engl J Med 2004;350:2441-2451.

20. Apfel C, Laara E, Koivuranta M, et al. A simplified risk score for predicting postoperative nausea and vomiting. Anesthesiology 1999;91:693-700.

21. Pavlin DJ, Rapp SE, Polissar NL, et al. Factors affecting discharge time in adult patients. Anesth Analg 1998;87:816-821.

22. Aldrete JA. The post anaesthesia recovery score revisited. J Clin Anesth 1995;7:89-91.

23. Marshall SI, Chung F. Discharge criteria and complications after ambulatory surgery. Anesth Analg 1999;88:508-517.

V

Chapter 39

ACUTE POSTOPERATIVE PAIN MANAGEMENT

Robert K. Stoelting

NEUROPHYSIOLOGY OF PAIN
  Nociception
  Modulation of Nociception

ANALGESIC DELIVERY SYSTEMS
  Oral Administration
  Intramuscular Administration
  Intravenous Administration
  Patient-Controlled Analgesia
  Neuraxial Analgesia

ALTERNATIVE APPROACHES TO MANAGEMENT OF ACUTE POSTOPERATIVE PAIN
  Peripheral Nerve Blocks
  Intrapleural Regional Analgesia
  Transcutaneous Electrical Nerve Stimulation

Acute postoperative pain is a complex physiologic reaction to tissue injury, visceral distention, or disease. Patients often consider "postoperative pain" the most frightening aspect of undergoing a surgical procedure. Postoperative pain produces adverse physiologic effects with manifestations on multiple organ systems (Table 39-1).[1] For example, pain after upper abdominal or thoracic surgery often leads to hypoventilation from splinting. This change promotes atelectasis, which impairs ventilation-to-perfusion relationships and increases the likelihood of arterial hypoxemia and pneumonia. Pain that limits postoperative ambulation combined with a stress-induced hypercoagulable state may contribute to an increased incidence of deep vein thrombosis.[2] Catecholamines released in response to pain may result in tachycardia and systemic hypertension, which may induce myocardial ischemia in susceptible patients.

Improved understanding of the epidemiology and pathophysiology of pain has translated into the polymodal management of pain in an effort to improve patient comfort, decrease perioperative morbidity, and reduce cost by shortening the time spent in postanesthesia care units, intensive care units, and hospitals. The natural progression of the expanding awareness of the adverse physiologic effects of postoperative pain has been the formation of acute pain management services, most often directed by an anesthesiologist.[3] In this regard, the continuity of acute postoperative pain management is enhanced because the anesthesiologist is routinely involved in preoperative assessment, intraoperative management, and postoperative follow-up of surgical patients.

The complexity of new analgesic techniques (patient-controlled analgesia [PCA], central neuraxial analgesia, peripheral nerve blocks, oral and parenteral analgesics) for the management of acute postoperative pain requires the adoption of written policies and procedures (medication protocols, algorithms, preprinted postoperative orders) to maximize efficacy while minimizing adverse effects (Tables 39-2 and 39-3).[1] Ultimately, the goals of

Table 39-1 Adverse Physiologic Effects of Postoperative Pain

Pulmonary system (decreased lung volumes)
Atelectasis
Ventilation-to-perfusion mismatching
Arterial hypoxemia
Hypercapnia
Pneumonia
Cardiovascular system (sympathetic nervous system stimulation)
Systemic hypertension
Tachycardia
Myocardial ischemia
Cardiac dysrhythmias
Endocrine system
Hyperglycemia
Sodium and water retention
Protein catabolism
Immune system
Decreased immune function
Coagulation system
Increased platelet adhesiveness
Decreased fibrinolysis
Hypercoagulation
Deep vein thrombosis
Gastrointestinal system
Ileus
Genitourinary system
Urinary retention

Table 39-2 Important Elements of Intravenous Patient-Controlled Analgesia Preprinted Orders

1. Drug(s), concentration(s)
2. Pump settings
   Incremental dose
   Lockout interval
   Other limits
3. Mode of use
   Patient-controlled analgesia only
   Continuous infusion
4. Initial drug-loading instructions
5. Instructions for treating breakthrough pain
6. Statement to prevent the ordering of central nervous system depressants by others
7. Monitoring instructions
8. Availability of drugs to treat side effects
9. Instructions for treatment of side effects
   Depression of ventilation
   Nausea and/or vomiting
   Pruritus
   Urinary retention
10. Instructions about concurrent use of other central nervous system depressants
11. Instructions for whom to contact if problems occur
12. Date, time, signature

Modified from Ready LB, Ashburn M, Caplan RA, et al. Practice guidelines for acute pain management in the perioperative setting. Anesthesiology 1995;82:1071-1081, with permission.

NEUROPHYSIOLOGY OF PAIN

Understanding the mechanisms of pain and its pharmacologic modification is essential to optimal treatment of acute postoperative pain.[4]

Nociception

Nociception involves the recognition and transmission of painful stimuli. Stimuli generated from thermal, mechanical, or chemical tissue damage may activate nociceptors, which are free afferent nerve endings of myelinated A-delta and unmyelinated C fibers (Fig. 39-1).[5] These peripheral afferent nerve endings send axonal projections into the dorsal horn of the spinal cord, where they synapse with second-order afferent neurons. Axonal projections of second-order neurons cross to the contralateral hemisphere of the spinal cord and ascend as afferent sensory pathways (spinotha-

the acute pain management service are (1) evaluation and treatment of postoperative pain and (2) identification and management of undesirable side effects related to postoperative analgesic techniques. This is a 24-hour-a-day commitment to postoperative patients by the anesthesiologist responsible for the acute pain management service. In addition, there must be cooperation between anesthesiology, nursing, pharmacy, and surgery personnel.

Table 39–3 Important Elements of Epidural Analgesia Preprinted Orders

1. Drug(s), concentration(s)

2. Instructions for administration
   If boluses—drug dose and interval between injections
   If infusion—loading dose and infusion rate

3. Instructions for treating breakthrough pain

4. Maintain intravenous access for immediate infusion of necessary drugs (naloxone)

5. Statement to prevent ordering of central nervous system depressants by others

6. Monitoring instructions
   For effects of opioids—consider pulse oximetry and capnography, respiratory rate every hour for 24 hours, availability of naloxone
   For effects of local anesthetics—sensory and motor block, hypotension, bradycardia

7. Observations and vital signs that should be communicated to the anesthesiologist

8. Instructions for treatment of side effects
   Depression of ventilation
   Nausea and vomiting
   Pruritus
   Urinary retention

9. Instructions about concurrent use of other central nervous system depressants

10. Instructions for whom to contact if problems occur

11. Date, time, signature

Modified from Ready LB, Ashburn M, Caplan RA, et al. Practice guidelines for acute pain management in the perioperative setting. Anesthesiology 1995;82:1071-1081, with permission.

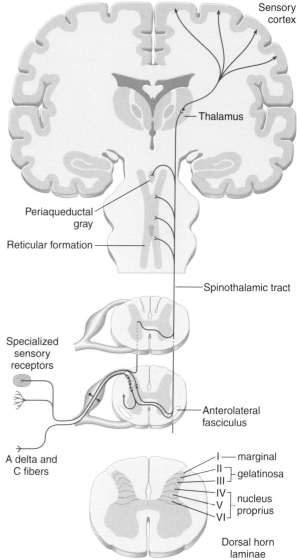

Figure 39-1 Afferent sensory pathways for recognition and transmission of painful stimuli. (From Lubenow TH, Ivankovich AD, Barkin RL. Management of acute postoperative pain. *In* Barash PG, Cullen BF, Stoelting RK [eds]: Clinical Anesthesia. Philadelphia: Lippincott Williams & Wilkins, 2006, pp 1405-1440, with permission.)

lamic tract) to the level of the thalamus (see Fig. 39-1).[5] Along the way, these neurons divide and send axonal branches to the reticular formation and periaqueductal gray matter. In the thalamus, second-order neurons synapse with third-order neurons, which send axonal projections into the sensory cortex.

Modulation of Nociception

Modulation of nociception can occur at several levels of the afferent sensory pathway before perception of pain at the sensory cortex. For example, modulation of a painful impulse may occur at the origin of the stimulus (nociceptor) and at any point in the ascending sensory afferent pathways where synaptic transmission occurs (see Fig. 39-1).[5] Furthermore, modulation of nociception may occur through descending efferent inhibitory pathways that originate at the level of the brainstem (Fig. 39-2).[5]

PERIPHERAL
Peripheral modulation of nociception occurs by either the liberation or elimination of endogenous mediators of inflammation in the vicinity of the nociceptor (Table 39-4).

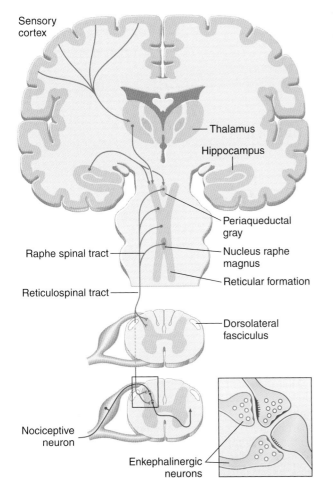

Sensory cortex

— Thalamus

Hippocampus

— Periaqueductal gray

Raphe spinal tract —

— Nucleus raphe magnus

— Reticular formation

Reticulospinal tract —

— Dorsolateral fasciculus

Nociceptive neuron

Enkephalinergic neurons

Figure 39-2 Descending efferent inhibitory (modulating) pathways involved in nociceptive regulation. (From Lubenow TR, Ivankovich AD, Barkin RL. Management of acute postoperative pain. *In* Barash PG, Cullen BF, Stoelting RK [eds]: Clinical Anesthesia. Philadelphia: Lippincott Williams & Wilkins, 2006, pp 1405-1440, with permission.)

These mediators sensitize (hyperalgesic effect) and excite nociceptors, especially in tissues that have been subjected to trauma and inflammation. Aspirin and other nonsteroidal anti-inflammatory drugs (NSAIDs), including nonspecific cyclooxygenase (COX-1) and specific cyclooxygenase (COX-2) inhibitors, exert an analgesic effect by inhibiting the action of the enzyme COX, which is necessary for the conversion of arachidonic acid into prostaglandins. By decreasing prostaglandin synthesis, these NSAIDs also modulate (block) nociception (sensitization) at peripheral sites.

SPINAL CORD

Modulation of nociception in the spinal cord results from the effects of excitatory or inhibitory neurotransmitters in the dorsal horn or by spinal reflexes that transmit efferent impulses back to peripheral nociceptors (Table 39-5) (see Fig. 39-2).[5]

SUPRASPINAL

Modulation of nociception may occur through descending efferent inhibitory pathways that originate at the level of the brainstem and synapse in the substantia gelatinosa region of the dorsal horn (see Fig. 39-2).[5] An opioid descending inhibitory pathway releases endorphins and enkephalins, which act presynaptically to hyperpolarize nerve fibers; this action serves to negate the current (action potential) to the next synapse and subsequent release of neurotransmitter. Morphine and other exogenous opioids act as agonists at stereoselective membrane-bound receptors that are distributed throughout the central nervous system

Table 39–4 Endogenous Mediators of Inflammation
Prostaglandins ($PGE_1 > PGE_2$)
Histamine
Bradykinin
Serotonin
Acetylcholine
Lactic acid
Hydrogen ions
Potassium ions

Table 39–5 Examples of Pain-Modulating Neurotransmitters
Excitatory
Glutamate
Aspartate
Vasoactive intestinal polypeptide
Cholecystokinin
Gastrin-releasing peptide
Angiotensin
Substance P
Inhibitory
Enkephalins
Endorphins
Substance P
Somatostatin

V

(see Table 10-2). In addition to the opioid descending inhibitory pathway, there is an α-adrenergic descending inhibitory pathway that terminates in the substantia gelatinosa region of the dorsal horn. Norepinephrine is released from these nerve terminals and produces hyperpolarization of nerve fibers, which serves to negate the current to the next synapse and subsequent release of neurotransmitter. The analgesic effects of clonidine most likely reflect its actions through this α-adrenergic inhibitory pathway.

DYNAMIC MODULATION OF NEURAL IMPULSES

The dynamic nature of the nociceptive response to injury is described by neural activity–dependent plasticity. As peripheral nociceptors are sensitized by local tissue mediators of injury (bradykinin, prostaglandins, potassium ions), the excitability and frequency of neural discharge increase. The primary hyperalgesia permits previously subnoxious stimuli to generate action potentials that are transmitted in the spinal cord. As peripheral nerve firing increases, changes in the excitability of spinal cord neurons take place and alter their response to afferent impulses. This central sensitization to afferent impulses results from functional changes in spinal cord processing known as neuroplasticity. Action potentials may persist after discontinuation of the stimulus and result in changes in spinal cord processing that can last for 1 to 3 hours. Spinal cord plasticity involves binding of glutamate to N-methyl-D-aspartate receptors, as well as binding of substance P and neurokinins. These changes in spinal cord processing occur after even a minor surgical incision and result in hyperalgesic responses to noxious stimuli that persist for days in the area of the incision.[6]

ANALGESIC DELIVERY SYSTEMS

Traditional delivery systems for the management of acute postoperative pain as represented by oral and parenteral on-demand administration of analgesics are being replaced by more efficacious techniques such as neuraxial analgesia or PCA (Table 39-6). New drug delivery techniques are based on improved understanding of the neurophysiology of pain and the potential deleterious effects of postoperative pain. The formation of acute pain management services directed by anesthesiologists with expertise in regional anesthesia and the pharmacology of analgesics has facilitated the widespread application of these new analgesic delivery systems.

Oral Administration

Oral administration of analgesics is not considered optimal for the management of moderate to severe acute postoperative pain, principally because of the lack of titratability and a prolonged time to peak effect (Table 39-7).[7,8] Traditionally, postoperative patients are switched to oral

Table 39–6 Routes of Delivery for Analgesic Drugs
Oral
Transmucosal
Transdermal
Intramuscular
Intravenous
Intermittent
Continuous
Patient controlled
Neuraxial
Epidural
Intrathecal
Peripheral nerve block
Intrapleural regional analgesia

analgesics (aspirin, acetaminophen, COX-1/COX-2 inhibitors) when pain has diminished to the extent that the need for rapid adjustments in the level of analgesia is unlikely. COX-2 inhibitors exhibit a postoperative opioid-sparing effect. Perioperative administration of NSAIDs is an integral component of polymodal analgesic treatment plans. Ketorolac is an NSAID that exhibits potent analgesic effects (30 mg IM has analgesic effects equivalent to 10 mg morphine) but has only moderate anti-inflammatory effects. Unlike opioids, ketorolac has little or no effect on biliary tract dynamics. NSAIDs have a dose ceiling effect beyond which no additional therapeutic benefit occurs. The increased complexity of outpatient surgical procedures has introduced the need for oral opioid analgesics that are efficacious in the treatment of moderate to severe acute postoperative pain (see Table 39-7).[7,8] Transmucosal delivery of analgesics such as fentanyl may serve as an alternative to the oral administration of NSAIDs and opioids, especially when a prompt drug effect is desirable.[9]

Intramuscular Administration

Intramuscular administration of analgesics is the traditional method for treating moderate to severe postoperative pain because it provides a more rapid onset and time to peak effect than oral analgesics do. Nevertheless, plasma concentrations of opioids achieved after intramuscular administration may vary as much as threefold to fivefold.[10] Plasma concentrations of opioids after intramuscular administration at a fixed time interval (typically every 3 to 4 hours) result in a cyclic period of sedation, analgesia, and finally, inadequate analgesia (Fig. 39-3).[11] It is estimated

Table 39–7 Oral and Parenteral Analgesics for Treatment of Acute Postoperative Pain

| | | | | Analgesic Action (hr) | | |
	Route of Administration	Dose (mg)	Half-Life (hr)	Onset	Peak	Duration
Naturally Occurring Alkaloids						
Morphine	Intravenous	2.5-15	2-3.5		0.125	
	Intramuscular	10-15	3	0.3	0.5-1.5	3-4
	Oral	30-60		0.5-1	1-2	4
Codeine	Intramuscular	15-60		0.25-0.5	1-5	4-6
	Oral	15-60		0.25-1	0.5-2	3-4
Synthetic Derivatives of Morphine						
Hydromorphone	Intramuscular	1-4	2-3	0.3-0.5	1	2-3
	Oral	1-4	2-3	0.5-1	1	3-4
Oxymorphone	Intramuscular	1.0-1.5	3.3-4.5	0.5	1	2-4
Hydrocodone	Oral	5-7.5	2-3			3-8
Oxycodone	Oral	5		0.5	1-2	3-6
Synthetic Compounds						
Methadone	Oral	2.5-10	3-4	0.5-1	1.5-2	4-8
Propoxyphene	Oral	32-65	12-16	0.25-1	1-2	3-6
Nonsteroidal Anti-inflammatory Drugs						
Ketorolac	Intramuscular	30	5		0.75-1	3-6

Adapted from Lubenow TR, Ivankovich AD, Barkin RL. Management of acute postoperative pain. *In* Barash PG, Cullen BF, Stoelting RK (eds): Clinical Anesthesia. Philadelphia: Lippincott Williams & Wilkins, 2006, pp 1405-1440.

Figure 39-3 Relationship between serum drug concentrations, pharmacologic effects, and route of administration. IM, intramuscular; IV, intravenous; PCA, patient-controlled analgesia. (From Tuman KJ, McCarthy RJ, Ivankovich AD. Pain control in the postoperative cardiac surgery patient. Hosp Formul 1988;23:580-595, with permission.)

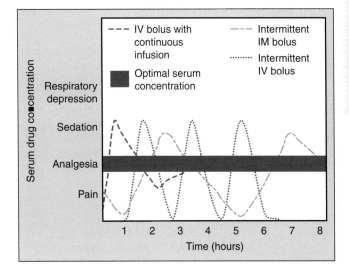

that plasma concentrations will exceed or equal analgesic concentrations only 35% of the time during such a fixed dosing interval. As a result, an estimated 75% of patients receiving intermittent intramuscular opioids postoperatively remain in moderate to severe pain. Delivery of opioids by PCA circumvents many of the problems of intramuscular opioid administration and is predicted to provide more effective analgesia with fewer side effects by maintaining plasma concentrations in a more narrow, but analgesic range (see the section "Patient-Controlled Analgesia"). An alternative to intramuscular administration of opioids is the injection of ketorolac, an NSAID with efficacy equal to that of moderate doses of opioids but lacking depressant effects on ventilation.

Intravenous Administration

Intermittent intravenous administration of small doses of opioids (morphine, 0.5 to 3 mg; fentanyl, 15 to 50 µg; sufentanil, 3 to 15 µg) is commonly used to treat acute and severe pain in the postanesthesia or intensive care unit, where continuous nursing surveillance and monitoring (pulse oximetry, capnography) are available. With a small intravenous dose of an opioid, the time delay for analgesia and the variability in plasma concentrations characteristic of intramuscular injections are minimized. Rapid redistribution of the opioid results in a shorter duration of analgesia after a single intravenous administration than after an intramuscular injection.

Patient-Controlled Analgesia

PCA is dependent on the use of drug delivery systems that allow the patient to titrate analgesic needs by activating a switch that results in the intravenous delivery of a solution containing a small dose of an opioid. Limits are placed on the number of doses per unit of time that will be administered to the patient on activation of the delivery system, and there is also a minimum time interval that must elapse between activations (lockout interval) (Tables 39-8 and 39-9).[12] It is also possible for these delivery devices to record a profile of the drug administration, including the number and time of bolus delivery, number of activations that did not result in drug delivery, and total amount of drug that was administered per unit time. Further refinement of these delivery systems permits the physician to administer a continuous background intravenous infusion of opioid superimposed on patient-controlled boluses. Most patients tend to determine a level of pain that they view as acceptable and taper their dosage requirements as they convalesce. Patient acceptance of PCA is high because patients feel that they have significant

control of their therapy. When compared with traditional methods of intermittent intramuscular injections of opioids to manage acute postoperative pain, PCA provides better analgesia with less total drug use, less sedation, fewer nocturnal sleep disturbances, and more rapid return to physical activity.[13]

Neuraxial Analgesia

Placement of an opioid in the intrathecal or epidural space (neuraxial placement) to manage acute postoperative pain is based on the knowledge that opioid receptors are present in the substantia gelatinosa of the spinal cord.[14] Presumably, opioids placed in the epidural space diffuse across the dura to gain access to opioid receptors on the spinal cord. The analgesia produced by neuraxial opioids, in contrast to intravenous administration of opioids or regional anesthesia with local anesthetics, is not associated with sympathetic nervous system denervation, skeletal muscle weakness, or loss of proprioception. As a result, it is possible to render postoperative patients pain free without interfering with their ability to ambulate. There is evidence that neuraxial analgesia improves postoperative pulmonary function, decreases cardiovascular and infectious complications, and decreases total hospital costs.[2]

Table 39–8 Postoperative Patient-Controlled Analgesia Order Sheet

Morphine, 30 mg per 30 mL prefilled syringe

Loading dose, 2 mg IV (range, 1 to 4 mg)

Maintenance dose, 1 mg IV

Lockout interval, 8 minutes (range, 6 to 10 minutes)

Limit dose to 20 mg over 4 hours (may be increased to 30 mg if analgesia is inadequate)

Monitor vital signs as ordered

Assess pain level and effectiveness of patient-controlled analgesia as ordered

Record drug administered every 8 hours

Table 39–9 Guidelines for Delivery Systems Used in Patient-Controlled Analgesia

	Bolus Dose (mg)	Lockout Interval (min)	Continuous Infusion (mg/hr)	4-Hour Limit (mg)
Morphine	0.5-3	5-20	1-10	20-30
Meperidine	5-15	5-15	5-40	200-300
Fentanyl	0.015-0.05	3-10	0.02-0.1	0.2-0.4
Sufentanil	0.003-0.015	3-10	0.004-0.03	

SIDE EFFECTS

Side effects of neuraxial opioids are due to the presence of drug in cerebrospinal fluid or the systemic circulation, or both (see Table 10-4).[15] Early depression of ventilation (within 2 hours of neuraxial administration) reflects systemic absorption of opioid from its epidural placement site, whereas delayed depression of ventilation (6 to 12 hours after neuraxial administration) is due to cephalad spread of the opioid in cerebrospinal fluid and interaction with opioid receptors located in the medullary centers in the area of the fourth cerebral ventricle.

Factors that increase the risk for delayed depression of ventilation, especially concomitant use of any intravenous opioids or sedatives, must be considered when determining the total dose of neuraxial opioid (see Table 10-4).[15] Detection of depression of ventilation induced by neuraxial opioids may be difficult. Pulse oximetry reliably detects opioid-induced arterial hypoxemia, and supplemental oxygen is an effective treatment.[16] Monitoring of end-tidal carbon dioxide concentrations is a consideration inasmuch as opioid-induced hypoventilation may be masked by supplemental oxygenation. A depressed level of consciousness in a patient being treated with neuraxial opioids should arouse suspicion of opioid-induced depression of ventilation. Opioids with high lipid solubility, such as fentanyl or sufentanil, attach to lipid components in the spinal cord; as a result, less drug is available to diffuse cephalad, thus making delayed depression of ventilation less likely than after the injection of poorly lipid-soluble morphine.

INTRATHECAL ADMINISTRATION

Intrathecal administration of an opioid provides long-lasting postoperative analgesia after a single injection. The intrathecal route offers the advantage of precise and reliable placement of low concentrations of drug near its site of action.[17] The onset of analgesic effects after the intrathecal administration of an opioid is directly proportional to the lipid solubility of the drug, whereas the duration of effect is longer with more hydrophilic compounds. Morphine, for example, has been shown to produce peak analgesic effects in 20 to 60 minutes and postoperative analgesia for 12 to 36 hours. The onset of analgesic effect may be enhanced by adding a small dose of fentanyl to the morphine-containing opioid solution. For example, intrathecal placement of morphine (0.6 to 0.8 mg) plus fentanyl (25 µg) at the conclusion of a thoracotomy is likely to permit an early onset of analgesia. As a result, the patient is able to breathe deeply without pain and the trachea can often be extubated at the conclusion of surgery. This analgesia may also be supplemented by the intraoperative performance of intercostal nerve blocks by the surgeon. For lower abdominal procedures performed with spinal anesthesia (cesarean section, transurethral resection of the prostate), morphine (0.2 to 0.4 mg) may be added to the local anesthetic solution at the time that anesthesia is induced to ensure analgesia at the conclusion of surgery.

A clinical impression that the incidence of side effects, particularly delayed depression of ventilation, is higher after intrathecal than after epidural opioid injection is most likely the result of excessive intrathecal opioid doses.[17] For example, the analgesic effect of neuraxial opioids exerted through receptors in the substantia gelatinosa should be the same regardless of whether the drug is placed in the epidural space and diffuses across the dura or is placed directly in cerebrospinal fluid. On the basis of this logic, equally potent doses of opioids placed in the epidural or intrathecal space (dose about $\frac{1}{10}$ the epidural dose) should produce similar effects at opioid receptors in the substantia gelatinosa and hence a comparable degree of analgesia and a similar incidence of side effects because of effects of the opioid in cerebrospinal fluid.

The principal disadvantage of an intrathecal opioid injection is its lack of titratability and the need to either repeat the injection or consider other options when the analgesic effect of the initial dose wanes. Nevertheless, it is common clinical experience that after the analgesic effect of the initial intrathecal dose wanes, the intensity of postoperative pain is greatly diminished and can be satisfactorily managed with oral analgesics or PCA. The practical aspects of leaving a catheter in the intrathecal space for either continuous or repeated intermittent opioid injections is controversial, especially in view of reports of cauda equina syndrome after continuous spinal anesthesia with hyperbaric local anesthetic solutions injected through a small-diameter catheter.[18]

EPIDURAL ADMINISTRATION

Epidural administration of an opioid as either an intermittent injection or a continuous epidural infusion through an epidural catheter is a common method of providing postoperative analgesia (Tables 39-10 to 39-12).[12] A low dose of local anesthetic may be added to the opioid-containing solution for injection into the epidural space. When an opioid is placed in the epidural space, it must cross the dura to reach opioid receptors in the substantia gelatinosa of the spinal cord. Besides the physical barrier presented by the dura, opioid is deposited in the fat and connective tissues present in the epidural space. The impact of these factors on the pharmacokinetics of drugs placed in the epidural space is evidenced by the estimated 10-fold increase in dose requirements for epidural opioids versus intrathecal opioids to produce a similar analgesic effect. Furthermore, the epidural space is highly vascularized, and there is significant absorption of drug in the systemic circulation. In fact, plasma concentrations of fentanyl are similar after placement of this opioid in the epidural space and intravenous injection (Fig. 39-4).[19] Clearly, part of the analgesic effect, as well as side effects (early depression of ventilation), reflects systemic absorption of the opioid from the epidural space.

It may take as long as 3 to 4 hours to provide effective analgesia when epidural opioids are administered by inter-

Table 39-10 Guidelines for Epidural Analgesia

	Bolus Dose (mg)	Onset (min)	Analgesic Peak Effect (min)	Duration (hr)	Continuous Infusion Concentration (%)	Infusion Rate (mL/hr)
Morphine	5	20	30-60	12-24	0.01	1-6
Meperidine	30-100	5-10	12-30	4-6		
Fentanyl	0.1	4-10	20	2-4*	0.001	4-12
Sufentanil	0.03-0.05	7	25	3*	0.0001	10
Bupivacaine†		2.5-5			0.1	4-6

*Estimates.
†Combined with an opioid.

Table 39-11 Postoperative Epidural (Lumbar or Thoracic) Analgesia Infusion Order Sheet (<70 Years Old, >50 kg)

Select epidural infusion contents (morphine [30 mg] or fentanyl plus bupivacaine [300 mg])

Maximum continuous infusion rate, 6 mL/hr

Supplemental oxygen

Monitor arterial oxygen saturation with pulse oximetry

Consider monitoring end-tidal carbon dioxide concentration with capnography

Observe level of consciousness and breathing rate at periodic intervals (every 1 hour may be recommended)

Record pain score at periodic intervals

Naloxone at bedside (administer if slow respiratory rate and/or sudden decrease in level of consciousness; contact anesthesiologist)

Morphine, ? mg IV, for breakthrough pain (alternatively, ketorolac, 30 mg IM)

mittent injection or continuous infusion. This delayed onset of effective analgesia can readily be overcome by adjusting the infusion rate to provide the equivalent of a small bolus (5 to 10 mL) before beginning the maintenance infusion. Alternatively, a short-action opioid such as fentanyl may be added to the morphine-containing solution, or the drug-containing analgesic solution can be injected preoperatively to ensure the presence of analgesia when the patient awakens at the conclusion of surgery. Bupivacaine (1 mg/mL) may also be added to the opioid-containing solution. The synergy between the analgesic effects of opioids and local anesthetics may be the result of blockade of afferent impulses at two different sites in the spinal cord. Opioids produce analgesia by binding to opioid receptors in the substantia gelatinosa, whereas local anesthetics block transmission of afferent impulses at the nerve roots and dorsal root ganglia. α_2-Agonists (clonidine, dexmedetomidine) may be used in combination with opioids and local anesthetics to potentiate analgesia.[20] A possible benefit of these combinations is a decrease in the dosage of individual drugs with a concomitant reduction in the incidence of side effects.

Table 39-12 Comparison of Epidural Administration Techniques

Intermittent Epidural Injection	Continuous Epidural Injection
No need for infusion devices	Need sophisticated infusion devices
Requires personnel to inject catheter periodically	Removes need for personnel to inject catheter periodically
Limited number of suitable opioids	Allows administration of short-acting opioids such as fentanyl or sufentanil
Difficult to titrate dose	Provides continuous analgesia, thereby avoiding peaks and valleys in plasma opioid concentration
Higher incidence of side effects	Less rostral spread, so side effects are minimized

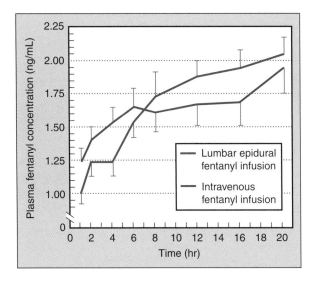

Figure 39-4 Plasma fentanyl concentrations postoperatively were similar in patients receiving a lumbar epidural fentanyl infusion (*blue line*) or intravenous fentanyl infusion (*red line*). (From Sandler AN, Stringer D, Panos L, et al. A randomized, double-blind comparison of lumbar epidural and intravenous fentanyl infusions for postthoracotomy pain relief. Analgesic, pharmacokinetic, and respiratory effects. Anesthesiology 1992;77:626-634, with permission.)

Intermittent intravenous injections of an opioid may be necessary to treat "breakthrough" pain until epidural analgesia is adequate. Ketorolac administered parenterally may also be a useful nonopioid analgesic in these situations. An advantage of continuous epidural infusion versus intermittent epidural injection is the ability to titrate the infusion rate to the desired level of analgesia. It is even possible to combine a continuous epidural infusion regimen with patient-activated intermittent boluses (patient-assisted epidural analgesia). Patient-assisted epidural analgesia is particularly useful for the management of dynamic changes in pain related to patient activity (coughing, chest physiotherapy). Complications that can occur with a continuous epidural technique include accidental intrathecal administration of the drug, infection, and depression of breathing.

Hydrophilic opioids such as morphine, when injected into the epidural space, result in cerebrospinal fluid concentrations of the opioid that allow the drug to follow the rostral spread of cerebrospinal fluid and saturate the entire length of the spinal cord.[21] Because of this property, epidural morphine may be infused at a lower lumbar level and still provide analgesia for surgical procedures performed on the upper abdominal region and thorax. Lipophilic opioids such as fentanyl and sufentanil tend to provide more of a segmental analgesic effect, perhaps reflecting more intense drug binding to opioid receptors. The segmental nature of analgesia produced by these lipophilic opioids is the basis for the recommendation by some anesthesiologists that the epidural catheter be placed in a position to cover the dermatomes included in the surgical field (thoracic epidural for analgesia after thoracotomy) when a lipophilic opioid (fentanyl, sufentanil) is selected.

Achievement of optimal results with continuous epidural analgesia techniques requires appropriate perioperative planning and assessment, including identification of patients who may benefit from epidural analgesia and scheduling placement of the epidural catheter as part of the anesthetic plan. This may include placement of the epidural catheter in the holding area before the patient is brought to the operating room so that the anesthesiologist can administer a test dose of the local anesthetic (usually bupivacaine) while the patient is still awake. This practice facilitates the diagnosis of intrathecal or intravascular placement and allows confirmation of epidural catheter placement by virtue of segmental epidural analgesia when the test dose of local anesthetic is administered. It also allows initiation of the continuous epidural infusion intraoperatively (morphine or fentanyl with bupivacaine at 4 to 6 mL/hr), thereby augmenting the general anesthetic and providing sufficient time to achieve analgesia at the time of emergence from anesthesia. If the surgical procedure is expected to exceed 3 to 4 hours, sufficient solution can be infused into the epidural space to achieve analgesia on awakening of the patient. If the surgical procedure is to be less than 2 hours in duration, a 5- to 10-mL dose of the epidural solution may be administered as a rapid infusion to hasten the onset of analgesia. Alternatively, a rapid epidural infusion of 0.5% bupivacaine combined with either fentanyl (50 to 100 μg) or morphine (2 to 5 mg) may be administered.

Venous Thromboembolism Prophylaxis

Prophylaxis against the occurrence of postoperative thromboembolic complications often involves the perioperative administration of low doses of subcutaneous heparin ("minidose heparin," 5000 units of unfractionated heparin every 12 hours). Knowledge that this prophylaxis will be used may influence the anesthesiologist's decision to place an epidural catheter for postoperative pain management inasmuch as the risk for epidural hematoma formation may be increased in the presence of abnormal coagulation (Table 39-13).[22] Several large studies have confirmed the safety of instituting heparin therapy in patients in whom the epidural catheter was placed without clinically detectable bleeding at least 1 hour previously.[23,24] Postponement of surgery for 24 hours may be recommended if placement of the epidural catheter is associated with a bloody tap. Timing of removal of the epidural catheter is also considered to be critical because epidural bleeding could be initiated at this time. In this regard, it is often recommended that the epidural catheter be removed 10 to 12 hours after the last dose of heparin and subsequent

Table 39-13 Recommendations for Performance of Neuraxial Analgesia/Anesthesia in the Presence of Anticoagulants Administered for Thromboembolism Prophylaxis or Intraoperative Coagulation

Unfractionated (standard) minidose subcutaneous heparin

  No contraindication to neuraxial block

  May consider delaying initiation of heparin therapy until after neuraxial block

Unfractionated (standard) intravenous heparin for intraoperative coagulation

  Delay initiating heparin administration for 1 hour after needle placement for the neuraxial block

  Remove the epidural catheter 1 hour before any subsequent intravenous dose of heparin (assumes a 12-hour dosing interval) or 2 to 4 hours after the last previous dose of heparin

  Consider the use of minimal concentrations of local anesthetic to permit early clinical detection of neurologic changes

  Bloody or difficult neuraxial needle and/or catheter placement does not mandate cancellation of the surgical procedure, but if it proceeds, frequent postoperative monitoring of neurologic status must be performed

Low-molecular-weight heparin

  Decision to perform a neuraxial block is made on an individual patient basis

  Bloody or difficult neuraxial and/or catheter placement does not mandate cancellation of the surgical procedure, but if it proceeds, initiation of low-molecular-weight heparin administration should be delayed for 24 hours

  Delay epidural catheter removal for 10 to 12 hours after the last dose of low-molecular-weight heparin and do not administer any subsequent doses of heparin for 2 hours

  Consider single-dose spinal anesthesia if regional anesthesia is required in patients receiving low-molecular-weight heparin preoperatively

  Perform frequent postoperative monitoring of neurologic status

Oral anticoagulants

  Stop anticoagulant and allow normalization of prothrombin time before performance of neuraxial block

Antiplatelet drugs

  Use does not interfere with performance of a neuraxial block

Fibrinolytic and thrombolytic drugs

  Neuraxial block not recommended within 10 days of receiving these drugs

Modified from Neuraxial Anesthesia and Anticoagulation, Consensus Statements. American Society of Regional Anesthesia, 1998.

dosing with heparin be delayed for at least 1 hour after removal of the catheter (see Table 39-13).[22] Patients must be monitored closely in the perioperative period, including the time following catheter removal, for early signs of cord compression (back pain, progression of numbness or weakness, bowel or bladder dysfunction) from a developing epidural hematoma. Prompt recognition of an epidural hematoma (confirmed by computed tomography or magnetic resonance imaging) is followed by decompressive laminectomy. Recovery of spinal cord function is unlikely if surgery is delayed more than 8 hours.[25]

In contrast to unfractionated heparin, low-molecular-weight heparin was hoped to provide the potential for separating the antithrombotic from the bleeding effects of heparin. However, reports of epidural hematoma occurring spontaneously and in association with regional anesthesia have created concern regarding the safety of spinal or epidural anesthesia in patients receiving low-molecular-weight heparin (see Table 39-13).[22] These same concerns would also seem to apply to these regional techniques as used for neuraxial analgesia.

Management of Inadequate Analgesia

In the event of inadequate analgesia provided by the epidural infusion, it is important to verify proper placement of the catheter. The initial step is rapid epidural infusion of 5 to 7 mL of the opioid and local anesthetic solutions. If analgesia remains inadequate after 15 to 30 minutes, a test dose of a local anesthetic solution, such as 2% lidocaine with 1:200,000 epinephrine, can be administered to further evaluate catheter location. If this test dose produces a bilateral sensory block in a few segmental dermatomes, epidural catheter location is confirmed. Based on this observation, it is presumed that the rate of epidural infusion was insufficient for adequate analgesia and increasing the rate of infusion may produce acceptable analgesia. If the test dose of local anesthetic solution produces a unilateral sensory block, it is likely that the catheter is placed laterally and withdrawal of the catheter 1 to 2 cm is indicated. A lack of sensory block in response to the local anesthetic solution test dose confirms that the catheter is not in the epidural space. In this situation, the catheter is removed and the patient is given the option of having another epidural catheter placed or switching to PCA.

ALTERNATIVE APPROACHES TO MANAGEMENT OF ACUTE POSTOPERATIVE PAIN

Alternative approaches to analgesia delivery systems for the treatment of acute postoperative pain include peripheral nerve blocks, intrapleural regional analgesia, and transcutaneous electrical nerve stimulation (TENS).

Peripheral Nerve Blocks

Peripheral nerve blocks may provide effective postoperative analgesia, but their relatively short duration of analgesia and their selective nature preclude their general application to all patient populations. Nevertheless, the pain relief afforded by a regional nerve block may be superior to that achievable with systemic opioids. For example, intercostal nerve blocks may be useful for providing postoperative analgesia after abdominal or thoracic operations (see Chapter 18).

Intrapleural Regional Analgesia

Intrapleural regional analgesia is produced by the injection of a local anesthetic solution through a catheter inserted percutaneously into the intrapleural space. The local anesthetic diffuses across the parietal pleura to the intercostal neurovascular bundle and produces a unilateral intercostal nerve block at multiple levels. Effective postoperative pain relief requires intermittent intrapleural injections approximately every 6 hours with approximately 20 mL of 0.25% to 0.5% bupivacaine. Pleural drainage tubes as placed after a thoracotomy may result in loss of the local anesthetic solution and inadequate analgesia.

Transcutaneous Electrical Nerve Stimulation

TENS is a simple conservative technique that uses electrical stimulation of the skin to provide pain relief (see Chapter 43). The mechanism by which TENS produces pain relief is presumed to involve the release of endogenous endorphins by the electrical stimulation of afferent cutaneous nerves. Endorphins exert an inhibitory effect on the dorsal horn and augment the descending inhibitory modulating pathways. The degree of acute pain relief provided by TENS is variable and less effective than that produced by neuraxial opioids or PCA.

REFERENCES

1. Ready LB, Ashburn M, Caplan RA, et al. Practice guidelines for acute pain management in the perioperative setting. Anesthesiology 1995;82:1071-1081.
2. Tuman KJ, McCarthy RJ, March R et al. Effects of epidural anesthesia and analgesia on coagulation and outcome after major vascular surgery. Anesth Analg 1991;73:696-704.
3. Lubenow TR, Ivankovich AD. Organization of an acute pain management service. In Stoelting RK, Barash PG, Gallagher TJ (eds): Advances in Anesthesia, vol 8. St Louis: Mosby–Year Book, 1991, pp 1-28.
4. Sorkin L, Wallace MS. Acute pain mechanisms. Surg Clin North Am 1999;79:213-231.
5. Lubenow TR, Ivankovich AD, Barkin RL. Management of acute postoperative pain. In Barash PG, Cullen BF, Stoelting RK (eds): Clinical Anesthesia. Philadelphia: Lippincott Williams & Wilkins, 2006, pp 1405-1440.
6. Zahn PK, Brennan TJ. Primary and secondary hyperalgesia in a rat model for human postoperative pain Anesthesiology 1999;91:863-869.
7. Buvanderan A, Kroin JS, Tuman KJ, et al. Effects of perioperative administration of a selective cyclooxygenase 2 inhibitor on pain management and recovery of function after knee replacement. JAMA 2003;290:2411-2416.
8. Ginsberg B, Sinatra RS, Adler LJ, et al. Conversion to oral controlled-release oxycodone from intravenous opioid analgesic in the postoperative setting. Pain Med 2003;4:31-36.
9. Macaluso AD, Connelly AM, Hayes B, et al. Oral transmucosal fentanyl citrate for premedication in adults. Anes Analg 1996; 84:1513-1515.
10. Rigy JR, Browne RA, Davis C, et al. Variation in the disposition of morphine after administration in surgical patients. Br J Anaesth 1978;50:1125-1130.
11. Tuman KJ, McCarthy RJ, Ivankovich AD. Pain control in the postoperative cardiac surgery patient. Hosp Formul 1988;23:580-595.
12. Ready LB, Oden R, Chadwick HS, et al. Development of an anesthesiology-based postoperative pain management service. Anesthesiology 1988;68:100-106.
13. Egbert AM, Parks LH, Short LM, et al. Randomized trial of postoperative patient-controlled analgesia vs. intramuscular narcotics in frail elderly men. Arch Intern Med 1990;150:1897-1903.
14. Cousins MJ, Mather LE. Intrathecal and epidural administration of opioids. Anesthesiology 1984;61:276-310.
15. Chaney MA. Side effects of intrathecal and epidural opioids. Can J Anaesth 1995;42:891-903.

16. Bailey PL, Rhondeau S, Schafer PG, et al. Dose-response pharmacology of intrathecal morphine in human volunteers. Anesthesiology 1990;73:566-568.

17. Stoelting RK. Intrathecal morphine—an underused combination for postoperative pain management. Anesth Analg 1989;68:707-709.

18. Rigler ML, Drasner K, Krejcie TC, et al. Cauda equina syndrome after spinal anesthesia. Anesth Analg 1991;72:275-281.

19. Sandler AN, Stringer D, Panos L, et al. A randomized, double-blind comparison of lumbar epidural and intravenous fentanyl infusions for postthoracotomy pain relief. Analgesic, pharmacokinetic, and respiratory effects. Anesthesiology 1992;77:626-634.

20. Curatolo M, Schnider TW, Petersen-Felix S, et al. A direct search procedure to optimize combinations of epidural bupivacaine, fentanyl, and clonidine for postoperative pain. Anesthesiology 2000;92:325-331.

21. Angst MS, Ramaswamy B, Riley ET, et al. Lumbar epidural morphine in humans and supraspinal analgesia to experimental heat pain. Anesthesiology 2000;92:312-318.

22. Horlocker TT, Heit JA. Low molecular weight heparin: Biochemistry, pharmacology, perioperative prophylaxis regimens, and guidelines for regional anesthetic management. Anesth Analg 1997;85:874-885.

23. Rao TLK, El-Etr AA. Anticoagulation following placement of epidural and subarachnoid catheters: An evaluation of neurologic sequelae. Anesthesiology 1981;55:618-620.

24. Neuraxial Anesthesia and Anticoagulation, Consensus Statements. American Society of Regional Anesthesia, 1998.

25. Vandermeulen EP, VanAken H, Vermylen J. Anticoagulants and spinal-epidural anesthesia. Anesth Analg 1994;79:1165-1177.

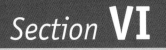

Section VI

CONSULTANT ANESTHETIC PRACTICE

Chapter 40

CRITICAL CARE MEDICINE

Lundy Campbell and Michael Gropper

The practice of critical care medicine, which originated in the 1940s with anesthesiologists providing life support to patients with poliomyelitis, has undergone revolutionary change. The development of equipment, procedures, and medications has enabled intensivists to treat critically ill patients and support them through increasingly invasive procedures. In the past decade another revolution has taken place with the introduction of evidence-based medicine into the practice of critical care medicine.

Ironically, anesthesiologists, who founded critical care medicine, represent a shrinking percentage of these specialists. Anesthesiologists are particularly well trained to manage critically ill patients in the intensive care unit (ICU) and do so on a regular basis in the operating room. Anesthesiologists may be required to care for patients in the operating room who either have been or will be admitted to the ICU, and familiarity with the unique challenges that these patients present may dramatically improve their care.

MECHANICAL VENTILATION

ICUs were developed to support patients in respiratory failure, and this function remains a major feature of modern units. The availability of modern mechanical ventilators has made ventilatory support routine.

Indications

Mechanical ventilatory support is typically initiated for the treatment of respiratory failure (impaired oxygenation), ventilatory failure (impaired carbon dioxide excretion), and airway protection. Causes of respiratory failure include trauma, acute respiratory distress syndrome (ARDS), sepsis, pneumonia, and pulmonary edema (both cardiogenic and noncardiogenic). Ventilatory failure may be due to chronic obstructive pulmonary disease (COPD), asthma, and drug intoxication. Intubation plus mechanical ventilation for airway protection is usually limited to disorders such as acute airway edema, altered mental status, and significant neuromuscular disorders. Patients receive mechanical ventilatory support to (1) reduce the work of breathing, (2) reverse progressive respiratory acidosis or hypoxemia, (3) reduce the risk for aspiration, or (4) ensure a patent airway with severe neck and facial swelling or trauma.

Modes of Mechanical Ventilation

The goal of the several different modes of mechanical ventilation is to provide adequate oxygenation and removal of carbon dioxide.

CONTINUOUS MANDATORY VENTILATION

Continuous mandatory ventilation (CMV) is present when the ventilator is programmed to deliver a set tidal volume at a set respiratory rate, thereby resulting in the delivery of a predictable minute ventilation. Regardless of patient effort, the ventilator will deliver its preset tidal volume at its preset time. If the patient makes additional efforts between delivered breaths, these breaths are unsupported. To regulate the amount of time that the ventilator spends cycling in inspiration and expiration, the inspiratory flow rate is set. By increasing inspiratory flow, the set tidal volume is delivered in a shorter time, which allows more time for exhalation.

A related mode of CMV is assist-control ventilation. Like intermittent mandatory ventilation (IMV), set tidal volume breaths are delivered at a set rate; however, additional breaths are detected by the ventilator and supported to full tidal volume. CMV is the most commonly used mode of mechanical ventilation in ICUs.

SYNCHRONIZED INTERMITTENT MANDATORY VENTILATION

In synchronized intermittent mandatory ventilation (SIMV), the tidal volume and respiratory rate are set as in IMV, but the ventilator attempts to synchronize the mandatory breaths that it delivers with the patient's own spontaneous breaths. If the patient does not initiate a breath within a set time, the ventilator delivers the set tidal volume machine breath as in the CMV mode. In this way, the ventilator ensures that the patient maintains the desired minimum ventilation. If a patient initiates additional breaths beyond those that are set in the SIMV mode to maintain the set minute ventilation, the ventilator can be programmed to deliver a pressure-supported breath. This combined mode of ventilation is known as SIMV with pressure support.

PRESSURE SUPPORT VENTILATION

In pressure support ventilation, the ventilator does not deliver a preset tidal volume but, instead, relies on the patient's intrinsic respiratory drive. When the machine senses the patient initiating a breath, the ventilator delivers a preset positive pressure to assist the patient in obtaining an adequate breath. Typically, the amount of pressure support is set between 5 and 20 cm H_2O to ensure adequate tidal volume and minute ventilation. In this mode, the ventilator stops its delivery of positive pressure when it senses that the patient's airflow has dropped below a preset level. Therefore, tidal volume will vary with patient effort. To use pressure support ventilation, the patient must possess an intact respiratory drive, and no residual skeletal muscle paralysis can be present. However, as an added safety precaution, all modern ventilators with this mode also have a backup mode of emergency assist-control ventilation in the event that a patient's minute ventilation falls below a set threshold.

POSITIVE END-EXPIRATORY PRESSURE

Positive end-expiratory pressure (PEEP) is constant positive airway pressure that is applied throughout the respiratory cycle. PEEP functions to increase mean airway pressure and thereby prevent atelectasis. It increases the functional residual capacity of the lungs and, in patients with lung injury, results in improved pulmonary compliance. The process of inflating collapsed alveoli is known as recruitment, and when properly applied, PEEP can improve oxygenation in a mechanically ventilated patient.

The typical PEEP range is between 5 and 20 cm H_2O. High levels of PEEP can overdistend and damage alveoli and may cause hemodynamic collapse by reducing preload to both the right and the left ventricles with a resultant fall in cardiac output. If sufficient time for exhalation of the delivered tidal breath is not allowed, a phenomenon known as intrinsic PEEP or auto-PEEP may occur. It results in a buildup of end-expiratory pressure, and when excessive, hemodynamic collapse may occur. Treatment of auto-PEEP entails disconnecting the patient from the ventilator to release the PEEP and increasing expiratory time to prevent recurrence.

Weaning from Mechanical Ventilation

To decrease the risks associated with continued mechanical ventilation, such as ventilator-associated pneumonia, patients are weaned from the ventilator as soon as possible. To consider weaning, a patient must have recovered from the process that originally required mechanical ventilatory support. In addition, the patient should be hemodynamically stable and receiving minimal vasopressor support because weaning may increase the work of breathing and thereby cause cardiovascular strain.

Postsurgical cardiac patients may be an exception to this rule. Although these patients still need to be hemodynamically stable to consider weaning, they may remain on relatively high-dose vasopressors during the weaning and tracheal extubation period. This select group is treated differently because patients who have undergone cardiopulmonary bypass often have myocardial dysfunction and peripheral vasodilatation that will quickly resolve.

TRIAL OF WEANING

Generally, patients are not considered candidates for a trial of weaning and tracheal extubation until certain criteria are met.

Inspired Oxygen Needed to Maintain Oxygenation

The patient's required inspired oxygen concentration to maintain adequate oxygenation saturation should be less than 40% to 50%. This amount of oxygen is chosen because this level can be reasonably and reliably delivered in the absence of a tracheal tube via facemask or nasal cannula. An oxygen requirement greater than this denotes that the patient still has a large shunt fraction through the lung and the underlying pulmonary process has not adequately resolved.

Tidal Volume

Patients must be strong enough to generate an adequate tidal volume. This can be ascertained by having the patient inhale as forcefully as possible. The negative inspiratory force of this breath (maximum negative inspiratory force) or the absolute size of the inhaled breath (vital capacity) can then be measured. For weaning, a negative inspiratory force of at least –20 cm H_2O pressure or a vial capacity of at least 10 mL/kg is required. In normal tidal breathing, a tidal volume of at least 5 mL/kg and a minute ventilation of no more than 10 L/min may also be used.

Protect the Airway against Aspiration

Patients must be able to protect their airway against aspiration, and they must be able to adequately clear their own pulmonary secretions. The ability to protect an airway usually requires an intact mental status and gag reflex. The ability to clear pulmonary secretions requires a strong cough. However, if a patient continues to have a large amount of pulmonary secretions, weaning may be delayed despite the presence of an adequate cough because these patients may fatigue under the work of clearing copious thick secretions.

EVIDENCE-BASED WEANING STRATEGIES

A randomized controlled clinical trial comparing four modes of weaning (IMV, pressure support ventilation, intermittent trials of spontaneous breathing with continuous positive airway pressure [CPAP] or a T-piece, and once-daily trials of spontaneous breathing) found that patients weaned an average of 1 to 2 days sooner with spontaneous breathing trials versus IMV or pressure support weaning.[1] In addition, it was shown that once-daily weaning trials were just as effective as intermittent (more than one trial per day) weaning trials.

In another trial, physician-directed weaning was compared with protocol-driven weaning managed by nurses and respiratory therapists.[2] When a patient met the criteria for extubation, a physician was notified and the patient's trachea was subsequently extubated if the physician agreed. The patients in the protocol arm weaned an average of 1.5 days sooner than the control (physician-directed) group did. From these trials, it is now recommended that the fastest and most cost-effective weaning method is once-daily CPAP or T-piece weaning trials that are protocol driven by nurses and respiratory therapists.

NONINVASIVE POSITIVE-PRESSURE VENTILATION

Noninvasive positive-pressure ventilation (NIPPV) is frequently used in the ICU to provide support for both oxygenation and ventilatory failure. NIPPV is positive-pressure ventilation delivered without the use of an endotracheal tube. Positive airway pressure is delivered by a facemask that covers either the nose and mouth or the nose only or by "nasal pillows," which are similar to a large nasal cannula that fits into the nares. All NIPPV masks are held firmly in place by a tight-fitting strap.

Modes of Delivery

Noninvasive ventilation is typically administered as (1) CPAP or (2) bilevel positive airway pressure (BiPAP).

CONTINUOUS POSITIVE AIRWAY PRESSURE

CPAP is constant positive airway pressure that is applied throughout both the inspiratory and expiratory phases of ventilation. CPAP improves oxygenation and ventilation by recruitment of collapsed alveoli in acute lung injury, helps maintain a patent airway in the setting of airway obstruction such as sleep apnea, and increases mean airway pressure with respect to ambient atmospheric pressure in patients with COPD.

BILEVEL POSITIVE AIRWAY PRESSURE

BiPAP is similar to pressure support with PEEP ventilation because the ventilator cycles between two sets of positive-pressure settings. Positive pressure is delivered throughout the respiratory cycle, and higher positive pressure is applied during inspiration only. The ventilator is set by adjusting the level of both the inspiratory high pressure and the expiratory low pressure values.

Advantages

NIPPV has the advantage of being less invasive than traditional endotracheal intubation and ventilation. Patients can be rapidly supported with NIPPV by simply fitting a proper facemask and can be removed from ventilatory support just as easily. NIPPV allows for ventilation during short periods only, such as while sleeping or immediately after discontinuation of traditional mechanical ventilation.

VI

Indications

NIPPV is indicated in a patient who has a potentially rapidly reversible pulmonary process that requires ventilatory support. NIPPV reduces the morbidity associated with endotracheal intubation and allows the patient to remain awake and interactive during the period of ventilatory support.

In patients with acute exacerbations of COPD, there is evidence that NIPPV is an effective treatment that can reduce the need for subsequent endotracheal intubation and reduce mortality.[3] NIPPV has been used successfully to treat other forms of acute respiratory failure such as pneumonia, congestive heart failure, and postsurgical respiratory failure. NIPPV may be just as effective as conventional ventilation with respect to oxygenation and removal of carbon dioxide in these patients, and it is associated with fewer serious complications and shorter ICU stay.[4]

A multicenter study comparing the use of NIPPV with standard treatment (oxygen, bronchodilator therapy, reintubation when necessary) in postlaparotomy patients who had recently been extubated and subsequently suffered postextubation respiratory failure concluded that both groups had the same reintubation rate but the NIPPV group had a significantly longer time to reintubation.[5] However, the NIPPV group also had significantly higher mortality than did the standard medical treatment group (25% versus 14%).

Disadvantages

There are certain unique disadvantages to the use of NIPPV. The most frequently encountered problem is lack of patient compliance. Because NIPPV requires a tight-fitting mask for effective ventilation, many patients find it uncomfortable and it is poorly tolerated by those who are claustrophobic. Additionally, because NIPPV provides no airway protection, patients must be awake and able to follow commands and must possess an adequate cough and gag reflex such that it is certain that they will be able to protect their own airway against aspiration. Other problems associated with NIPPV include gastric distention from swallowing air when using high inspiratory pressure and difficulty delivering adequate enteral nutrition to patients while they are being ventilated.

ACUTE RESPIRATORY DISTRESS SYNDROME

ARDS and acute lung injury (ALI) encompass a broad array of causes of respiratory failure and result in a similar clinical picture (Table 40-1).[6] ARDS may arise from an infectious insult such as pneumonia or sepsis, or it can develop from a noninfectious process such as trauma, pulmonary aspiration, burns, or transfusion-related acute lung injury (TRALI) (Table 40-2).[7] Typically, ARDS arising

Table 40-1 Acute Respiratory Distress Syndrome and Acute Lung Injury Definitions from the American-European Consensus Conference

Acute onset
Gas exchange
Acute lung injury: $Pa_{O_2}/F_{IO_2} \leq 300$
Acute respiratory distress syndrome: $Pa_{O_2}/F_{IO_2} \leq 200$
Bilateral infiltrates on the chest radiograph
Pulmonary artery occlusion pressure ≤18 mm Hg or clinical absence of left atrial hypertension

Data from Bernard GR, Artigas A, Brigham KL, et al. The American-European Consensus Conference on ARDS: Definitions, mechanisms, relevant outcomes, and clinical trial coordination. Am J Respir Crit Care Med 1994;149:818-824.

Table 40-2 Causes of Acute Respiratory Distress Syndrome

Causes of Direct Lung Injury	Causes of Indirect Lung Injury
Pneumonia	Sepsis
Aspiration of stomach contents	Severe trauma
Pulmonary contusion	Cardiopulmonary bypass
Reperfusion pulmonary edema	Drug overdose
Amniotic fluid embolus	Acute pancreatitis
Inhalational injury	Near drowning Transfusion-related acute lung injury

Data from Ware LB, Matthay MA. The acute respiratory distress syndrome. N Engl J Med 2000;342:1334-1349.

from causes such as trauma and TRALI has better outcomes and lower mortality than does ARDS resulting from sepsis, pneumonia, and burns. Sepsis is associated with an unusually high incidence of ALI or ARDS approximating 40%.[8]

Treatment

Treatment of ARDS remains supportive. There have been multiple clinical trials of pharmacotherapies targeting specific inflammatory mediators that are thought to be involved in the pathogenesis of ALI and ARDS, but thus far these treatments have been unsuccessful.

VENTILATOR MANAGEMENT

The ARDSnet trial of low–tidal volume ventilation in patients with ALI or ARDS showed decreased mortality in those receiving low tidal volumes (6 mL/kg) versus standard tidal volumes (12 mL/kg).[9] The hypothesis of the ARDSnet trial was that lower tidal volumes would "protect" the lung by preventing overdistention of normal regions of the lung. As a result of this study, it has become the standard of care in critical care medicine to ventilate all patients who have known or suspected lung injury with a low–tidal volume ventilation strategy.

When patients are ventilated with lower tidal volumes, they tend to have lower arterial oxygen tension and higher arterial carbon dioxide tension. This is termed permissive hypercapnia in recognition of the fact that to normalize arterial blood gas, significantly more harmful mechanical ventilation may be required. Although higher tidal volumes may improve oxygenation, they ultimately increase mortality. This is thought to be due to "biotrauma," in which excessive stretching of the lung releases injurious cytokines into the circulation.

SEDATION AND ANALGESIA IN THE INTENSIVE CARE UNIT

Sedation is used in the ICU to provide analgesia, anxiolysis, and amnesia and to protect the patient from dislodging or removing any indwelling lines, catheters, drains, or tubes. In certain instances, sedation is used to control or prevent seizures, reduce elevated intracranial pressure (ICP), and provide treatment for withdrawal from substances such as ethanol, benzodiazepines, and opioids. If patients are paralyzed with neuromuscular blocking drugs either as a result of a recent surgical procedure or for severe respiratory distress, effective and adequate sedation is essential.

Because of the risks associated with excessive sedation (prolonged mechanical ventilation, ventilator-associated pneumonia, pressure ulceration), sedation should be continuously evaluated with a sedation score and weaned as soon as possible (Table 40-3).[10] To achieve appropriate sedation, a variety of classes of sedative drugs (opioids, benzodiazepines, propofol, barbiturates, N-methyl-D-aspartate [NMDA] antagonists such as ketamine, and α_2-receptor agonists) are used (Table 40-4). The choice of the specific drug used depends on the clinical situation and the drug effects that are desired. For example, an opioid is used to treat pain, whereas a benzodiazepine or propofol may be chosen to treat anxiety, withdrawal symptoms, seizures, or elevated ICP.

Opioids

Opioids (fentanyl, morphine, methadone, hydromorphone) are used primarily for analgesia and usually in combination with a sedative drug. As a class, opioids have

Table 40–3 The Ramsay Sedation Scoring System

Score	Response
1	Anxious and agitated or restless, or both
2	Cooperative, oriented, and tranquil
3	Responding to commands only
4	Brisk response to a light glabellar tap
5	Sluggish response to a light glabellar tap
6	No response to a light glabellar tap

Data from Ramsay MAE, Savege TM, Simpson BRJ, et al. Controlled sedation with alphaxalone-alphadolone. BMJ 1974;2:656-659.

very little effect on anxiolysis or amnesia, unless the cause of anxiety is pain. Pain in the ICU may arise from a number of sources, including indwelling lines, catheters, and tubes; procedures performed in the ICU; recent surgeries; and simply lying in bed for an extended period. Fentanyl is most often used for its ease of administration, rapid pharmacokinetics, and lack of active or toxic metabolites.

Opioids are typically administered intravenously in the ICU, although certain drugs such as methadone have excellent bioavailability when given orally. When used intravenously, opioids may be administered by either repeated bolus injections or continuous infusion. Either method works satisfactorily to ensure adequate pain relief, provided that the bolus dosing interval is based on the drug's pharmacokinetics and pharmacodynamics and is titrated appropriately. If a continuous infusion is used, it must be done with caution because the infused drug may accumulate.

SIDE EFFECTS

The most dangerous side effects of opioids include respiratory and central nervous system (CNS) depression. Other side effects include constipation, urinary retention, and tolerance (manifested as escalating doses of drug to achieve the desired effect). It is important to note that a patient never becomes tolerant to the constipating effects of opioids, and as the dose escalates, this effect becomes even more pronounced. As a class, opioids are well tolerated with minimal effects on hemodynamics and organ perfusion and very little impact on the metabolism of other drugs. However, when opioids are used in conjunction with other CNS depressants such as benzodiazepines or barbiturates, drug-induced CNS and respiratory depression may be amplified synergistically.

Benzodiazepines

Benzodiazepines (midazolam, lorazepam) are administered to decrease anxiety and promote amnesia. In addition,

VI

Table 40–4   Commonly Used Sedatives and Analgesics

Drug	Elimination Half-Time	Peak Effect (IV)	Suggested Dose
Morphine	2 to 4 hours	30 minutes	1- to 4-mg bolus 1 to 10 mg/hr
Fentanyl	2 to 5 hours	4 minutes	25- to 100-μg bolus 25 to 200 μg/hr
Hydromorphone	2 to 4 hours	20 minutes	0.2- to 1-mg bolus 0.2 to 5 mg/hr
Ketamine	2 to 3 hours	30 to 60 seconds	1 to 20 mg/hr
Midazolam	3 to 5 hours	2 to 5 minutes	1- to 2-mg bolus 0.5 to 10 mg/hr
Lorazepam	10 to 20 hours	2 to 20 minutes	1- to 2-mg bolus 0.5 to 10 mg/hr
Propofol	20 to 30 hours	90 seconds	25 to 100 μg/kg/min
Dexmedetomidine	2 hours	1 to 2 minutes	0.2 to 0.7 μg/kg/hr

they are often used to prevent or treat both seizures and alcohol withdrawal symptoms. Like opioids, benzodiazepines can be given either enterally or parenterally, but in the ICU they are most often given parenterally. Similar to opioids, a continuous infusion results in more stable and reliable plasma concentrations; however, the effects of the drug may accumulate. The effects become even more intensified when this class of drug is used in the elderly or patients with hepatic or renal failure. Weaning from mechanical ventilation after prolonged administration of these drugs must be done slowly because benzodiazepine withdrawal (as with ethanol withdrawal) can be life threatening.

Propofol

Propofol is a hypnotic anesthetic with extremely rapid pharmacokinetics and pharmacodynamics, even when given by prolonged continuous infusion. It is this property that makes propofol so useful in the ICU. Propofol provides excellent amnesia and anxiolysis, but it has no significant analgesic effects. Therefore, an opioid is usually administered concomitantly with propofol. Propofol is especially useful in patients who require frequent neurologic examination. Because of its short elimination half-time and minimal accumulation, a patient can "wake up" a few minutes after discontinuation of a continuous propofol infusion and a reliable neurologic examination can be performed. It is also useful in preventing and treating seizures and in lowering ICP.

SIDE EFFECTS

Hemodynamically, propofol has significant effects on decreasing myocardial contractility and reducing systemic

vascular resistance. In hemodynamically unstable patients with low cardiac output or low afterload (or both), propofol must be used with caution. This property limits its usefulness in many unstable patients, such as postsurgical cardiac patients and those in profound shock.

Propofol is a profound respiratory depressant. Although most patients who receive propofol in the ICU are intubated and maintained on mechanical ventilation, occasionally propofol may be used in nonintubated patients. An example is its use for procedural sedation. In this specific instance, extreme caution must be exercised to prevent severe respiratory depression with profound respiratory acidosis.

Propofol is formulated in a lecithin (egg white) solution, and as such, it is an excellent bacterial growth medium. Consequently, when a bottle is opened, it must be used relatively quickly to avoid contamination. Propofol also has a high fat content because of its lecithin base. Patients who are receiving long-term infusions of this drug must be periodically checked for hypertriglyceridemia. Because of this high fat content, if a patient is receiving total parenteral nutrition (TPN) and then propofol is started, the Intralipid portion of the TPN needs to be reduced or eliminated altogether.

Ketamine

Ketamine is a dissociative anesthetic with profound analgesic effects even at low doses. Ketamine acts as an antagonist at NMDA receptors in the CNS. It produces potent psychomimetic effects with vivid hallucinations, similar to phencyclidine. As such, ketamine is usually prescribed along with a benzodiazepine or propofol, which will decrease its hallucinogenic effects. When given at low doses by continuous infusion (1 to 5 µg/kg/min), these adverse effects tend to be minimal.

Ketamine has proved to be useful in the ICU because of its ability to produce profound analgesia without significant respiratory depression. This makes ketamine an excellent choice for patients with chronic pain who may require excessively large doses of opioids for pain relief. Ketamine is also useful for patients who need to undergo brief, painful procedures (burn dressing changes) in the ICU.

Ketamine has intrinsic sympathomimetic properties that increase systemic blood pressure and heart rate during infusion. This may be useful when sedation and analgesia are required for a hemodynamically unstable patient. Ketamine is often combined with propofol in such patients to counteract the reduced blood pressure associated with propofol while providing adjuvant analgesia. Ketamine raises ICP, increases the cerebral metabolic consumption of oxygen ($CMRO_2$), and decreases the seizure threshold. For these reasons, ketamine is infrequently used in neurosurgical patients or in any patients with an increased risk for seizures.

Barbiturates

Barbiturates are used primarily to place patients in a "barbiturate coma" to suppress seizures in the setting of status epilepticus or to reduce ICP or $CMRO_2$ in the setting of brain injury. However, barbiturates also decrease systemic blood pressure and may therefore significantly decrease cerebral perfusion pressure. Because of its rapid metabolism, propofol has supplanted the use of barbiturates in the setting of pharmacologic neuroprotection. Recently, there has been less enthusiasm for placing patients in a pharmacologic coma to reduce $CMRO_2$ because many well-designed trials have failed to show significant benefit from this practice.

α_2-Receptor Agonists

Examples of α_2-receptor agonists are clonidine and dexmedetomidine. These drugs act by binding to α_2-receptors both centrally and peripherally. Central α_2-binding at presynaptic neurons inhibits the release of norepinephrine. The central effects of these drugs produce analgesia, sedation, anxiolysis, and hypotension. At high doses, these drugs are anesthetics and induce a state that is very much like regular sleep. Patients will arouse when stimulated but rapidly fall back to sleep once the stimulation decreases. These properties make α_2-receptor agonists very effective drugs when patient cooperation is occasionally required, such as for frequent neurologic examinations.

At the level of the spinal cord, α_2-activation is thought to modulate pain pathways, and this is the probable site of action for the analgesic effects of these drugs. Peripheral activation of the presynaptic α_2-receptor also decreases the release of norepinephrine; however, these drugs possess weak α_1-receptor activity, and binding of these receptors on vascular smooth muscle cells induces vasoconstriction. Overall, in the recommended dosage range, their effect is to decrease systemic blood pressure by means of a decrease in both systemic vascular resistance and heart rate. Within the usual dose range, these drugs do not cause respiratory depression. However, because patients tend to fall asleep at higher dosages, these drugs can still cause upper airway obstruction and resultant hypoventilation.

CLONIDINE

Clonidine can be administered by the oral, intravenous, intramuscular, transdermal, intrathecal, and epidural routes. It has a broad therapeutic index and as such is quite safe when given over a wide range of doses. Hypotension tends to be the limiting factor when administering this drug. At excessively high doses, essentially all α_2-receptors are saturated with agonist, and the less potent α_1-effects tend to predominate.

DEXMEDETOMIDINE

Dexmedetomidine is an α_2-receptor agonist that is formulated for intravenous use only. It has a relatively short elimination half-time and is given by continuous infusion. Like clonidine, it has the same sedating and hemodynamic effects at lower doses, with increasing systemic vascular resistance secondary to α_1-effects at higher dosage ranges. However, dexmedetomidine has a much higher affinity for α_2-receptors than clonidine does, and as such it has an even broader therapeutic index. The usual dosage range for dexmedetomidine is 0.2 to 0.7 µg/kg/min.

Sedative Titration and Weaning

As patients recover from their illness, they need to be weaned from mechanical ventilatory support and from sedation. Continuous sedative infusion is an independent risk factor for prolongation of mechanical ventilation. Patients who receive a continuous infusion have significantly longer periods of mechanical ventilation with correspondingly longer stays in both the ICU and hospital than do those who receive sedation by bolus administration or no sedation.[11] Nevertheless, continuous sedation is widely used because it is believed to provide improved patient comfort and hemodynamic control.

The preferred method for weaning from sedation is protocol driven.[12] Patients treated by daily interruption of their sedatives with retitration versus weaning only at the discretion of the ICU physician are successfully weaned from mechanical ventilation earlier and have shorter ICU lengths of stay. Rapid weaning of sedation does not increase complications such as inadvertent tracheal extubation. Protocolized weaning also decreases the length of ICU and hospital stay, which is not only cost-effective but also likely to reduce time-dependent complications such as infection.

VI

SHOCK

Shock is a common clinical condition in the ICU. Shock in any form results in inadequate tissue perfusion to end organs such as the brain, heart, liver, kidneys, and abdominal viscera. Shock represents an imbalance between oxygen demand and delivery. As such, when faced with inadequate oxygen delivery, organs begin to fail and multisystem organ dysfunction and death result. Early in its course, shock may be reversible with proper diagnosis and effective treatment. However, if shock remains untreated, irreversible shock develops and death becomes inevitable.

Categories of Shock

The major categories of shock include hypovolemic, cardiogenic, septic, and other forms of vasodilatory shock (Table 40-5). Although all forms of shock are characterized by low systemic blood pressure and inadequate tissue perfusion, the root cause of this hypotension is different in each case. In hypovolemic shock, hypotension is due to inadequate preload, whereas in cardiogenic shock, hypotension results from poor pump function and, in septic or vasodilatory shock, from low afterload.

HYPOVOLEMIC SHOCK

Hypovolemic shock is caused by decreased effective circulating blood volume and therefore inadequate ventricular preload. The most common cause of hypovolemic shock is major blood loss, such as occurs with trauma, surgery, or massive gastrointestinal hemorrhage.

Clinical Manifestations

With decreased preload, left ventricular end-diastolic volume falls and cardiac output decreases. In response to baroreceptor stimulation, the heart rate increases to maintain cardiac output. There is increased sympathetic nervous system outflow that constricts blood vessels, increases systemic vascular resistance, and diverts blood away from the skin and skeletal muscle beds to the brain and heart. As a result, the patient appears cool and clammy and has pale mucosa. Activation of the renin-angiotensin system ensues to increase sodium reabsorption and restore circulating blood volume. In addition, the release of cate-cholamines from the adrenal glands acts to inhibit insulin secretion and induce gluconeogenesis. The result is dramatically increased plasma glucose levels that help restore circulating blood volume by increasing the osmotic gradient for fluid reabsorption into the intravascular space.

Treatment

Treatment of hypovolemic shock involves restoration of circulating blood volume and treatment of the underlying cause of the hypovolemia. Treatment of the underlying cause of hypovolemic shock can be undertaken only when adequate intravenous access and aggressive fluid therapy are achieved. Vasopressor therapy may be used to increase systemic blood pressure, but it will probably be unsuccessful until intravascular volume is restored. Resuscitation can be guided with the use of data from central venous pressure or pulmonary artery catheters in concert with physical examination and measurement of metabolic parameters.

CARDIOGENIC SHOCK

Cardiogenic shock is characterized by failure of either or both ventricles. When the ventricle fails, preload increases and the ventricle cannot adequately eject the end-diastolic volume. This serves to further increase ventricular end-diastolic pressure, and eventually the ventricle becomes overdistended, which hastens the ventricular failure.

Clinical Manifestations

If the right ventricle is the initial site of failure, the increased right-sided preload will be noted as increased central venous pressure, detected clinically as distended neck veins, peripheral edema, or hepatic congestion. If the left ventricle fails, the increased preload can be detected as increased pulmonary capillary wedge pressure, which causes cardiogenic pulmonary edema and rales on physical examination. In this case, the right ventricle eventually fails under the increased pulmonary artery pressure afterload, and biventricular failure results.

In either scenario, cardiac output is low, and systemic blood pressure is therefore reduced. To counteract the hypotension, there is increased sympathetic outflow with resultant tachycardia and increased systemic vascular resistance. This compensatory mechanism initially works

Table 40-5 Characteristics of Various Shock States

Shock Type	Cardiac Output	Systemic Vascular Resistance	Central Venous Pressure	Pulmonary Capillary Wedge Pressure*	Mixed Venous Oxygen Saturation
Hypovolemic	↓	↑	↓	↓	↓
Cardiogenic	↓	↑	↑	↑*	↓
Vasodilatory	↑ or ⇔	↓	↓	↓	↑ or ⇔

*Pulmonary capillary wedge pressure is normal to low in right ventricular failure.

to increase blood flow to the brain and failing ventricle, but it simultaneously increases myocardial oxygen demand. Increased myocardial oxygen demand ultimately leads to worsening cardiac failure. On physical examination, a patient in cardiogenic shock appears cool and pale secondary to the high systemic vascular resistance and shunting of blood away from the skin and skeletal muscle beds.

Treatment

The goals in treatment of cardiogenic shock are to improve cardiac output and decrease afterload. These interventions allow the ventricle to eject more efficiently, decrease myocardial work, lower myocardial oxygen consumption, and reverse the dangerous spiral of cardiac failure. To oversee treatment, adequate monitoring is required, including the use of direct arterial and central venous pressure monitoring. In addition, echocardiographic and possibly pulmonary artery catheter measurements may be required to adequately treat these patients.

Depending on the type of cardiac failure and ventricular filling conditions, diuretics are generally indicated but must be used judiciously to avoid worsening the hypotension. Afterload and preload can be reduced with vasodilators and venodilators such as nicardipine, nitroglycerin, or nitroprusside. For inotropy, dobutamine is preferred because it improves cardiac output and reduces afterload with a minimal increase in myocardial oxygen demand. Additional interventions for left-sided cardiogenic shock include the use of intra-aortic balloon counterpulsation and ventricular assist devices.

For right-sided failure, the goal of treatment is to reduce afterload with pulmonary vasodilators such as nitroglycerin, dobutamine, and even inhaled nitric oxide.

VASODILATORY SHOCK

Sepsis is the most common cause of vasodilatory shock, which is characterized by a low afterload state in which organ perfusion is impaired. Other major causes of this form of shock include anaphylaxis and neurologic dysfunction, such as stroke or spinal shock from a high spinal cord injury. Vasodilatory shock is often the final common pathway for the prolonged and severe hypotension resulting from late-stage shock of other causes, such as cardiogenic or hypovolemic shock. In all these conditions there is markedly reduced afterload with a redistribution of blood away from normally highly perfused organs (brain, heart, liver, and kidney) to large capacitance areas such as the skin and skeletal muscles.

Clinical Manifestations

Compensation for vasodilatory shock includes an increase in cardiac output mediated by increasing stroke volume and heart rate. Initially, increased cardiac output may provide adequate compensation. If left untreated, systemic vascular resistance continues to decrease with worsening metabolic acidosis. Myocardial perfusion becomes impaired, and

the patient eventually progresses to cardiac failure as well. On physical examination, a patient in vasodilatory shock initially appears warm and vasodilated with increased peripheral blood flow secondary to vasodilatation in the skin and skeletal muscle beds. However, with progression to late, irreversible shock, the extremities become increasingly cold and poorly perfused.

Treatment

Treatment of vasodilatory shock involves initial intravenous fluid therapy until adequate preload is established, typically at a central venous pressure of approximately 8 to 12 cm H_2O. Vasopressors (phenylephrine, dopamine, epinephrine [especially for anaphylaxis], norepinephrine) are added if the patient remains hypotensive in an effort to increase systemic vascular resistance and cardiac output. The choice of drug depends on the specific clinical situation. As with all other forms of shock, the underlying cause of the disorder should be treated as soon as possible.

SEPSIS AND SEPTIC SHOCK

Septic shock is the final pathway of disseminated infection and, after respiratory failure, is the most common cause for admission to the ICU. The diagnosis of severe sepsis and septic shock is based on identifying the probable source of infection, the systemic inflammatory response to infection, and concomitant organ failure (Table 40-6).[13]

Morbidity and mortality in patients with septic shock result from an overwhelming systemic inflammatory response, with the final common pathway being multiple organ dysfunction and death. Essential for successful treatment of sepsis is early recognition, rapid resuscitation, early administration of broad-spectrum antibiotics, and efforts to identify and treat the source of infection.

INOTROPES AND VASOPRESSORS

In the ICU patient population, shock is a common clinical disorder. As a result, inotropes and vasopressors are often required to support cardiac output and systemic blood pressure. Many choices of vasopressors are available to the clinician, but there is little evidence regarding which vasopressor is preferred in a given clinical scenario.

Dopamine

Dopamine has both direct and indirect agonist activity at the dopamine$_1$ (DA$_1$), β_1-, and α_1-receptors. Its pharmacologic action varies with dose and within individuals as well. At low doses (0 to 5 µg/kg/min), dopamine has predominantly DA$_1$-receptor agonist activity. This causes dilatation of the renal arterioles and promotes diuresis. Low-dose dopamine may help convert oliguric renal failure to nonoliguric renal failure, which makes fluid management easier, but it does not protect the kidneys from failure.

VI

Table 40-6 American College of Chest Physicians/Society of Critical Care Medicine (ACCP/SCCM) Consensus Conference Definitions for Sepsis

Definition	Criteria
Infection	Inflammatory response to microorganisms or invasion of normally sterile tissues SIRS (systemic inflammatory response syndrome)
	Clinical response to infection manifested by two of the following:
	Temperature >38°C or <36°C
	HR >90 bpm
	Respirations >20 breaths/min or $Paco_2$ <32 mm Hg
	WBC count >12,000 cells/L or <4000 cells/L or 10% immature neutrophils
Sepsis	Confirmed or suspected infection plus two SIRS criteria
Severe sepsis	Sepsis and one organ dysfunction
Septic shock	Sepsis plus hypotension (<90 mm Hg) despite fluid resuscitation

HR, heart rate; WBC, white blood cell.
Data from Bone RC, Balk RA, Cerra FB, et al. Definitions for sepsis and organ failure and guidelines for the use of innovative therapies in sepsis: The ACCP/SCCM Consensus Conference Committee–American College of Chest Physicians/Society of Critical Care Medicine. Chest 1992;101:1644–1655.

At moderate doses (5 to 10 μg/kg/min), the β_1-effects of dopamine begin to dominate. These β_1-effects cause an increase in myocardial contractility, heart rate, and cardiac output. As a result, myocardial oxygen demand increases as well. In fact, oxygen demand can increase more than myocardial oxygen delivery, with resultant myocardial ischemia.

At high doses (10 to 20 μg/kg/min), the α_1-agonist effects predominate and dopamine acts to increase vascular smooth muscle tone, which increases systemic vascular resistance. This causes a decrease in splanchnic and renal blood flow similar to the effects of high-dose phenylephrine. At all doses, dopamine mediates the indirect release of norepinephrine, which may be responsible for the tachycardia seen in some patients when dopamine is used at any dosage range.

Clinically, dopamine is regarded as a relatively weak vasopressor and is useful in mild hypotensive states. In patients who are in profound shock, dopamine is generally regarded as a second-line drug, and other more potent, direct-acting adrenergic agonists are preferred.

Epinephrine

Epinephrine causes direct stimulation of α_1-, β_1-, and β_2-receptors. At lower doses, epinephrine acts primarily as a β-receptor agonist, whereas at higher doses, it has increasing α_1-receptor effects. Increases in heart rate, myocardial activity, and cardiac output reflect β_1-receptor effects. The principal β_2-effects are bronchial and vascular smooth muscle relaxation. At higher doses, the α_1-effects of epinephrine act to increase systemic vascular resistance and reduce splanchnic and renal blood flow

while maintaining both cerebral and myocardial perfusion pressure.

Epinephrine also has anti-inflammatory effects by blocking the release of inflammatory mediators from mast cells and basophils. β-Activation in liver and skeletal muscle cells leads to increased gluconeogenesis via the adenylate cyclase signaling pathway. Both these actions function to increase blood glucose levels.

The main indications for epinephrine are in the management of cardiac arrest, severe cardiogenic shock, and anaphylactic and anaphylactoid reactions. When given as a continuous infusion, the usual range of epinephrine is between 1 and 20 μg/min. However, in patients with refractory, life-threatening shock, it may be necessary to administer epinephrine at even higher doses.

Norepinephrine

Norepinephrine is a direct-acting adrenergic agonist with activity at both the α_1- and β_1-receptors. It is similar to epinephrine except that norepinephrine lacks the β_2-effect of epinephrine and has much stronger α_1-activity. As a result, norepinephrine increases blood pressure through its α_1-effects on increasing systemic vascular resistance. The β_1-effects of norepinephrine also contribute to increased myocardial contractility and cardiac output.

There has recently been renewed interest in norepinephrine for the treatment of septic shock. It is thought that the β_1-activity may help offset the myocardial dysfunction associated with severe sepsis and septic shock. Both preclinical and limited clinical data suggest that norepinephrine is the pressor of choice for patients in septic shock.

Norepinephrine must be given by continuous infusion, and the typical dose range is between 1 and 20 µg/min. At the lower end of this range there are more β_1-effects, whereas α_1-activity dominates at the higher dosages.

Phenylephrine

Phenylephrine is a direct-acting, highly selective α_1-receptor agonist. As such, it acts to increase systemic vascular resistance and thereby raises systemic blood pressure. Phenylephrine has no direct effect on myocardial function, but it can cause reflex bradycardia, which may decrease cardiac output. Phenylephrine is frequently used for the treatment of septic and other forms of vasodilatory shock to increase systemic blood pressure. However, it can also cause splanchnic ischemia, especially when used chronically at high doses.

Phenylephrine is often administered to brain-injured patients to improve cerebral perfusion pressure. Because it does not cross the blood-brain barrier, phenylephrine has no effect on the cerebral vasculature, but its ability to increase systemic blood pressure leads to increased cerebral blood flow. The typical dosage range for phenylephrine is up to 200 µg/min. Higher doses have little therapeutic effect, with only worsening of splanchnic ischemia.

Dobutamine

Dobutamine is a mixed β_1- and β_2-receptor agonist. As a result, the primary effect of dobutamine is to increase both heart rate and myocardial contractility. Dobutamine also relaxes vascular smooth muscle via binding at β_2-receptors. This combination acts to increase cardiac output by improving ventricular function (β_1-effect) and decreasing systemic vascular resistance (β_2-effect). Dobutamine is typically indicated for the treatment of patients in cardiogenic shock with high afterload and low cardiac output. It is one of the few drugs available to the clinician that will reduce pulmonary vascular resistance and possibly improve right heart function.

Because of its β_2-effects, some patients may become hypotensive, particularly those with decreased intravascular volume. However, because dobutamine has a relatively short elimination half-time, its effects rapidly disappear once the infusion is discontinued. Dobutamine is given by continuous infusion only, and the usual dosage range is between 1 and 20 µg/kg/min.

Vasopressin

Vasopressin is a potent vasoconstrictor that does not work via the adrenergic receptor system as do most other vasopressors. Rather, vasopressin binds to peripheral vasopressin receptors to induce potent vasoconstriction.

Vasopressin provides a useful alternative to catecholamines, which do not function well in the setting of profound acidemia. Vasopressin remains efficacious as a vasoconstrictor even in the setting of severe acidosis.

Patients with severe sepsis and septic shock have a relative deficiency of vasopressin. This group of patients is remarkably sensitive to the effects of vasopressin, and the usual dose ranges for vasopressin need to be reduced. For septic shock, the recommendation is to infuse vasopressin at 0.04 U/min. If the patient improves, the vasopressin infusion is discontinued, not weaned.

Vasopressin has been successfully used for cardiogenic shock. Patients who have recently been weaned from cardiopulmonary bypass may remain hypotensive secondary to a low afterload state. There is evidence that these patients also have a relative vasopressin deficiency, and vasopressin may be used to treat this form of vasodilatory shock. In these patients, the dose of vasopressin (0.1 U/min) is significantly higher than that used for septic shock.

ACUTE RENAL FAILURE

Acute renal failure (ARF) is a commonly encountered complication in the ICU. The consequences of ARF are devastating, and it has higher attributable mortality than does acute respiratory failure. The definition of ARF varies, but it is often described as an abrupt decrease in renal function, which is defined as urine output less than 0.5 mL/kg/hr or a 50% increase in serum creatinine over a 24-hour period.[14] Renal failure is normally categorized as prerenal (inadequate renal perfusion pressure), intrarenal (vascular, glomerular, or interstitial dysfunction), or postrenal (usually obstructive). In the management of ARF, it is essential to recognize and treat prerenal failure by ensuring adequate fluid resuscitation and systemic blood pressure, as well as identify any postrenal obstruction through the use of ultrasound or other imaging techniques.

If the ARF has been determined to be intrarenal, it probably represents acute tubular necrosis. In addition to the history, which may include exposure to nephrotoxic drugs or prolonged hypotension, examination of urinary sediment may show renal tubular epithelial cells or granular casts. Management of ARF is supportive, with many patients ultimately requiring hemodialysis for the complications of ARF. Indications for acute hemodialysis include volume overload, hyperkalemia, acidemia, uremia, or other electrolyte abnormalities. Hemodialysis may be intermittent or continuous (continuous renal replacement therapy), with no definitive data to support the use of continuous hemodialysis. Hypotensive patients often require continuous hemodialysis because of their inability to tolerate the volume shifts associated with intermittent hemodialysis.

VI

NUTRITIONAL SUPPORT

Critically ill patients require optimal nutrition for wound healing, maintenance of skeletal muscle mass, and prevention of infection. The nutritional status of most patients declines throughout the length of their ICU stay. Malnourished patients become increasingly catabolic and may have significant skeletal muscle wasting. Loss of skeletal muscle causes weakness, which may prolong ventilator weaning and decreases the ability to tolerate rehabilitation. Optimal nutrition may directly reduce infectious complications by maintaining immunocompetence, enhancing wound healing, and preventing bacterial translocation across gut mucosal cells.

Enteral versus Parenteral Feeding

Patients may be fed either enterally (usually by a naso-jejunal feeding tube) or parenterally (intravenously). If possible, it is always preferable to feed enterally. Advantages of enteral feeding include decreased cost, ease of administration, maintenance of normal gastrointestinal physiology, and less risk for infection. For example, parenteral nutrition formulas are easily infected, which greatly increases the risk for catheter sepsis. Additionally, without enteral feeding, the normal gastrointestinal tract begins to atrophy. Such atrophy causes loss of mucosal thickness, alteration of pH, and loss of gastrointestinal tract–associated lymphoid tissue. These changes can result in replacement of normal gastrointestinal tract flora with more pathologic organisms and increased translocation of these organisms across the increasingly atrophic gastrointestinal tissue.

Candidates for Enteral Feeding

Enteral feeding is often selected for patients with pancreatitis, enteric fistulas, inflammatory bowel disease, short-bowel syndrome, acute pancreatitis, hyperemesis gravidarum, and bone marrow transplants. Parenteral feeding is selected only for patients who cannot tolerate sufficient enteral feeding.

INTENSIVE INSULIN THERAPY

Critically ill patients often display hyperglycemia that appears to be associated with insulin resistance. Hyperglycemia appears to be a risk factor for adverse outcomes in critically ill and other stressed patients. Strict glucose control improves outcomes in critically ill patients. For example, patients who had blood glucose levels maintained between 80 and 110 mg/dL had lower ICU mortality (4.6%) than did those who had blood glucose levels maintained between 180 and 200 mg/dL (8.0% mortality).[15] It is common practice in critical care medicine to tightly control the blood glucose levels of critically ill patients, and it seems logical to extend this practice to the operating room. The most effective means of achieving such control is through the use of protocol-driven insulin infusion orders.

END-OF-LIFE ISSUES

Despite delivering the best care possible, a large number of ICU patients will ultimately succumb to their illness. It is estimated that approximately one in five Americans will die in the ICU.[16] Because of this fact, ICU physicians needs to be as skilled in end-of-life care as they are in caring for critically ill patients. It is important for ICU physicians to regard death not as failure but as a normal part of life. Patients deserve the right to die with dignity and, if at all possible, in the manner that they see fit. Families deserve the right to assist in making decisions regarding their loved ones and to be treated with respect.

Occasionally, when a patient is suffering from a critical illness, the patient (or the family in accordance with the patient's wishes) may elect to stop treatment. Sometimes only specific treatments are discontinued, and in other instances, all support (including mechanical ventilation, vasopressor support, and dialysis) is withdrawn. This is usually a difficult decision for patients and their families to make, and frequently the ICU physician is called on to help with this decision-making process.

Patients can be removed from mechanical ventilatory support and placed on T-piece ventilation or extubated, depending on family and physician preference. This can be accomplished in a peaceful and dignified manner. The patient is usually sedated during this process to relieve any discomfort that may be present. Patients should be given adequate sedation during the dying process, but the goal of sedation is always the relief of patient discomfort. Sedation is never given to hasten a patient's demise. Sedation that is given to relieve suffering may have the "double effect" of hastening death, but it is important that the intent of sedative or analgesic administration be the relief of discomfort. The ICU physician must convey to patients and their families that death is an inevitable part of life and can be approached with dignity.

REFERENCES

1. Esteban A, Frutos F, Tobin MJ, et al. A comparison of four methods of weaning patients from mechanical ventilation. N Engl J Med 1995;332:345-350.

2. Ely EW, Baker AM, Dunagan DP, et al. Effect on the duration of mechanical ventilation of identifying patients capable of breathing spontaneously. N Engl J Med 1996;335:1864-1869.

3. Brochard L, Mancebo J, Wysocki M, et al. Noninvasive ventilation for

acute exacerbations of chronic obstructive pulmonary disease. N Engl J Med 1995;333:817-822.

4. Antonelli M, Conti G, Rocco M, et al. A comparison of noninvasive positive-pressure ventilation and conventional mechanical ventilation in patients with acute respiratory failure. N Engl J Med 1998;339:429-435.

5. Esteban A, Frutos-Vivar F, Ferguson ND, et al. Noninvasive positive-pressure ventilation for respiratory failure after extubation. N Engl J Med 2004;350:2452-2460.

6. Bernard GR, Artigas A, Brigham KL, et al. The American-European Consensus Conference on ARDS: Definitions, mechanisms, relevant outcomes, and clinical trial coordination. Am J Respir Crit Care Med 1994;149:818-824.

7. Ware LB, Matthay MA. The acute respiratory distress syndrome. N Engl J Med 2000;342:1334-1349.

8. Pepe PE, Potkin RT, Reus DH, et al. Clinical predictors of the adult respiratory distress syndrome. Am J Surg 1982;144:124-130.

9. The Acute Respiratory Distress Syndrome Network. Ventilation with lower tidal volumes as compared with traditional tidal volumes for acute lung injury and the acute respiratory distress syndrome. N Engl J Med 2000;342:1301-1308.

10. Ramsay MAE, Savege TM, Simpson BRJ, et al. Controlled sedation with alphaxalone-alphadolone. BMJ 1974;2:656-659.

11. Kollef MH, Levy NT, Ahrens TS, et al. The use of continuous IV sedation is associated with prolongation of mechanical ventilation. Chest 1998;114:541-548.

12. Kress JP, Pohlman AS, O'Connor MF, Hall JB. Daily interruption of sedative infusions in critically ill patients undergoing mechanical ventilation. N Engl J Med 2000;342:1471-1477.

13. Bone RC, Balk RA, Cerra FB, et al. Definitions for sepsis and organ failure and guidelines for the use of innovative therapies in sepsis: The ACCP/SCCM Consensus Conference Committee–American College of Chest Physicians/Society of Critical Care Medicine. Chest 1992;101:1644-1655.

14. Lameire N, Van Biesen W, Vanholder R. Acute renal failure. Lancet 2005;365:417-430.

15. Van den Berghe G, Wouters P, Weekers F, et al. Intensive insulin therapy in critically ill patients. N Engl J Med 2001;345:1359-1367.

16. Angus DC, Barnato AE, Linde-Zwirble WT, et al. Robert Wood Johnson Foundation ICU End-Of-Life Peer Group. Use of intensive care at the end of life in the United States: An epidemiologic study. Crit Care Med 2004;32:638-643.

VI

TRAUMA

J. F. Tang and J. F. Pittet

Trauma and associated life-threatening injuries account for 10% to 15% of all patients hospitalized. Rapid transport of a trauma victim to a trauma center rather than to the nearest hospital has resulted in improved outcome for the victim. A level I trauma center is characterized by the immediate availability of medical and nursing personnel (emergency medicine physician, trauma surgeon, neurosurgeon, orthopedic surgeon, plastic surgeon, anesthesiologist, critical care specialist, radiologist, and nurses), as well as the facilities needed to treat trauma patients (emergency room, operating rooms, radiology suite, intensive care unit [ICU], central laboratory, and blood bank). The anesthesiologist is a critical member of the trauma team and must be available 24 hours a day to take care of severely traumatized patients from the moment that the patient arrives at the emergency department of the trauma center.

INITIAL EVALUATION

On arrival at the hospital, the patient's airway, breathing, circulation, and neurologic status (Glasgow Coma Scale, computed tomography [CT], magnetic resonance imaging) must be rapidly evaluated with the advanced trauma life support (ATLS) protocol. The first priority is establishment of an airway and administration of oxygen. Occasionally, the trauma victim's trachea has been intubated by the paramedic before arrival at the hospital. Confirmation of tube placement as reflected by a sustained end-tidal CO_2 waveform needs to be established and documented immediately on arrival at the hospital.

Early tracheal intubation in selected patients has been a major factor in decreasing mortality from trauma. Nasotracheal intubation should not be attempted if there is the possibility of a basal skull fracture. If airway obstruction exists and tracheal intubation cannot be accomplished, emergency cricothyrotomy or tracheostomy is indicated. All trauma victims are assumed to be at risk for pulmonary aspiration of gastric contents (Table 41-1).

Table 41-1 Airway Management in the Emergency Room

Indications for tracheal intubation or confirmation of existing tube placement

Universal precautions (eye goggles, masks, gloves)

Airway equipment (laryngoscopes, endotracheal tubes, laryngeal mask airways, cricothyrotomy kit, fiberoptic scopes)

Oxygen source, suction device, capnography device

Vital sign monitoring device, pulse oximeter

Cervical spine, full stomach, and tension pneumothorax precautions

Establish intravenous access

Medications (hypnotics, neuromuscular blocking drugs, vasopressors)

Tracheotomy tray, electrical defibrillator

Additional experienced assistant

Follow American Society of Anesthesiologists difficult airway algorithm

Cervical Spine Injury

In patients with a possible cervical spine injury (present in 1.5% to 3% of all major trauma victims), orotracheal intubation should be attempted only with the patient's head stabilized in a neutral position (a rigid collar decreases flexion and extension to about 30% of normal and rotation and lateral movement to about 50% of normal).[1] CT is the best way to diagnose cervical spine injury, although two thirds of all trauma victims have multiple injuries that may interfere with the ability or safety of performing routine CT.

Thoracic Trauma

Thoracic trauma may involve the lungs or cardiovascular system, or both. An upright inspiratory chest radiograph is preferred for visualization of a pneumothorax (high index of suspicion if rib fractures are present), although the more likely radiograph will be an anteroposterior supine film. Pneumothorax or hemothorax is treated with a tube thoracostomy (tube placed in the fourth or fifth interspace in the midaxillary line and directed posteriorly and attached to suction). Intrathoracic vascular injury is suggested by a widening mediastinum, whereas lung contusion is predictable when a flail chest is present.

Abdominal Trauma

Abdominal injuries after blunt trauma are most often splenic rupture or laceration of the liver, with both resulting in profound hemorrhage. Intra-abdominal hemorrhage is diagnosed by diagnostic peritoneal lavage (DPL), abdominal ultrasound, or CT. Continued hematuria after placement of a bladder catheter indicates a possible bladder injury and the need for a cystogram or intravenous pyelogram.

Orthopedic Trauma

If suspicion of a pelvic fracture is entertained, the patient should be placed in a pelvic binder and transferred to interventional radiology for an emergency angiogram and possible intravascular embolization instead of rushing the patient to the operating room. Evaluation of the extremities includes palpation of distal pulses and visual inspection for symmetry of the extremities to detect evidence of bleeding, especially in the thighs after femur fractures. Early immobilization of fractures is indicated.

INITIAL STABILIZATION OF TRAUMA PATIENTS

Care for trauma patients is initiated in the emergency department and continued in the operating room.

Management of Anesthesia

General anesthesia is necessary for most trauma patients who require surgical intervention. A "trauma operating room" should be designated and appropriately equipped (Table 41-2). There is no ideal anesthetic drug or technique for a trauma patient. If the patient's trachea has not already been intubated, rapid-sequence induction of anesthesia is indicated. In the presence of hypovolemia, etomidate (0.1 to 0.3 mg/kg IV) or ketamine (1.0 to 3.0 mg/kg IV) is often selected for induction of anesthesia because these drugs are usually able to maintain stable hemodynamics. In patients with suspected or known cervical spine injury, avoidance of excessive head movement during direct laryngoscopy is necessary.[1]

Frequently, the dose of anesthetic tolerated by the patient is too small to prevent movement, thus necessitating skeletal muscle paralysis with a neuromuscular blocking drug. In this regard, some patients may experience recall of intraoperative events. Hemodynamic stability results from control of surgical bleeding and restoration of the patient's blood volume. Arterial blood gases, pH, and hematocrit are measured at frequent intervals during anesthesia and surgery. On a less frequent basis, it may be useful to analyze blood for electrolytes, glucose, and coagulation factors.

Fluid Resuscitation

Hypotension plus cellular hypoxia as a result of massive hemorrhage is the reason for anaerobic metabolism and

Table 41–2 Devices and Equipment Needed in a Trauma Operating Room

Well-equipped anesthesia machine and carts
Ventilator able to deliver assist-control and pressure-control modes
Level 1 rapid infusion devices and fluid warmer devices
Cell saver machine
Bair hugger and warm ambient environment
Eye goggles, masks, gloves, gowns
Anesthesia records, laboratory slips
Optional bronchoscopes
Echocardiography machine
Direct telephone lines to the clinical laboratory/blood bank
Emergency resuscitation cart
Electrical defibrillator, external pacer device
Arterial blood gas machine, hemoglobin machine, glucometer
Crystalloid solutions and colloid solutions
Emergency type O-negative blood (preferred)

Table 41–3 Stages of Hypovolemic Shock

Nonprogressive Stage
Compensating mechanisms (baroreceptor reflexes, systemic sympathetic stimulation, arginine vasopressin hormone, tachycardia, peripheral vasoconstriction, renal conservation of fluid)
Progressive Stage
Extensive tissue hypoxia (anaerobic glycolysis, increased lactic acidosis, decreased tissue pH, blunted vasomotor response)
Disseminated intravascular coagulation
Altered mental status
Decreased urinary output
Irreversible Stage
Extensive tissue injury (lysosomal enzyme leakage, myocardial depression, complete renal shutdown, acute tubular necrosis)

the production of lactic acid (Table 41-3). Goal-directed fluid resuscitation should be initiated immediately after the establishment of venous access because it serves to improve poorly perfused organs, including the liver and skeletal muscles. Initially, administration of a crystalloid solution such as lactated Ringer's or Plasma-Lyte solution restores intravascular fluid volume to help maintain venous return and cardiac output.

SELECTION OF INTRAVENOUS FLUIDS

There is no advantage in using colloid for initial resuscitation. When hemorrhage is extreme, it will be necessary to eventually administer blood products. Dilutional thrombocytopenia may accompany the massive blood transfusion necessary to reestablish intravascular fluid volume, whereas disseminated intravascular coagulation may accompany persistent hypotension. Rarely, transfusion-related acute lung injury can also occur in trauma victims receiving blood transfusions. A fluid warmer device should be used for all intravenous fluids to minimize the likelihood of hypothermia. The ambient operating room temperature should be kept warm. A massive transfusion protocol should be established. Invasive monitoring, including an intra-arterial and central venous pressure catheter, is recommended. A

pressurized infusion device is helpful in selected patients. Unfortunately, assessment of blood loss and adequacy of replacement can be very difficult in a trauma victim.

Transport from the Operating Room

Severely injured patients often require continued postoperative support of major organ function in an ICU, especially mechanical ventilation of the lungs. Patients usually remain intubated, sedated, and paralyzed during transport to the ICU. Appropriate and necessary drugs and equipment should accompany the patient to the ICU. A transport ventilator is preferred if the patient's oxygenation or ventilation (or both) needs to be continuously supported.

TRAUMATIC BRAIN (HEAD) INJURY

Traumatic brain injury (TBI) reflects an insult to the brain from an external mechanical force (high-energy acceleration or deceleration) that might cause a temporary or permanent impairment of physical and cognitive functions along with changes in mental status. TBI resulting from head injury is the leading cause of death in individuals younger than 45 years and accounts for approximately 40% of all deaths from acute injuries in the United States.

Recognition

The hallmark of closed head injury is loss of consciousness. CT should be performed early because it is the most important diagnostic test (evidence of increased intracranial pressure [ICP], types of hematoma, and hemorrhage), and the level of consciousness should be classified according to the Glasgow Coma Scale (Table 41-4). Patient age, imaging studies, pupillary response, mean arterial pressure, and initial Glasgow Coma Scale score have been used to predict the overall outcome in TBI patients.

Hypotension, hyperthermia, hypoxia, and elevated ICP are strong predictors of a poor outcome. Patients with a Glasgow Coma Scale score of less than 8 by definition have severe TBI, and the mortality rate is about 33% to 55%. In contrast, the mortality rate is lower (around 2.5%) in patients with mild to moderate TBI (Glasgow Coma Scale score of 8 or greater).

Critical Care

Critical care of a head-injured patient is based on recognition and treatment of hazardous increases in ICP. Interventions designed to provide cerebral protection and resuscitation have been successful in patients who experience TBI. Invasive monitoring, including intra-arterial and central venous catheter, is recommended. Fluid resuscitation to maintain adequate hemodynamics is important. Low-volume resuscitation with hypertonic saline, dextran, or a hemoglobin-based oxygen carrier may be favored over conventional crystalloid therapy. Jugular venous oxygen saturation (SjO_2), potentially representing cerebral tissue oxygenation, may be used to guide therapy. Administration of barbiturates is recommended when ICP remains increased despite traditional therapy.

MANAGEMENT OF INTRACRANIAL PRESSURE

A catheter placed through a burr hole in a cerebral ventricle or a transducer placed on the surface of the brain is used to monitor ICP. Normally, ICP is around 15 mm Hg. Cerebral perfusion pressure is the difference between mean arterial pressure and ICP. Patients with a Glasgow Coma Scale score less than 8 should probably have their ICP monitored in a neurosurgery ICU. An abrupt increase in ICP during continuous monitoring is known as a plateau wave (Fig. 41-1). Painful stimulation in an otherwise unresponsive patient can initiate a plateau wave. Hence, the liberal use of analgesics to avoid pain is indicated even in unresponsive patients. Efforts to minimize the secondary injury from hypoxia or decreased cerebral perfusion will ultimately be the main goal for the care of TBI patients.

TREATMENT

Early tracheal intubation plus mechanical ventilation of the patient's lungs to avoid arterial hypoxemia has been shown to improve outcome in the presence of TBI. Hyperventilation may be deleterious because of cerebral vasoconstriction. Methods to decrease ICP include posture; administration of osmotic diuretics, hypertonic

Table 41-4 Glasgow Coma Scale	
Eye Opening (E4)	
Spontaneous	4
To speech	3
To painful stimulation	2
No response	1
Verbal Response (V5)	
Oriented to person, place, and date	5
Converses but is disoriented	4
Says inappropriate words	3
Says incomprehensible sounds	2
No response	1
Motor Response (M6)	
Follows commands	6
Makes localizing movements to pain	5
Makes withdrawal movements to pain	4
Flexor (decorticate) posturing to pain	3
Extensor (decerebrate) posturing to pain	2
No response	1

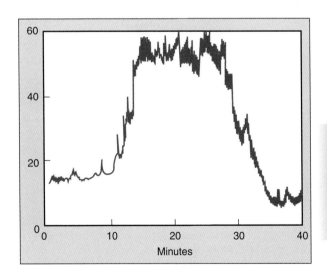

Figure 41-1 Schematic diagram of a plateau wave characterized by an abrupt and sustained (10 to 20 minutes) increase in intracranial pressure followed by a rapid decrease in intracranial pressure, often to a level lower than that present before the onset of the plateau wave.

VI

saline, or barbiturates; institution of cerebrospinal fluid drainage; and craniectomy, lobectomy, and craniotomy. A frequent recommendation is to treat sustained increases in ICP greater than 20 mm Hg. Treatment may be indicated when ICP is less than 20 mm Hg if the appearance of an occasional plateau wave suggests low intracranial compliance.

Posture

Elevation of the head to about 30 degrees is useful in the care of head-injured patients to encourage venous outflow from the brain and thus lower ICP. It should also be appreciated that extreme flexion or rotation of the head can obstruct the jugular veins and restrict venous outflow from the brain. Placement of a central catheter via the subclavian or the internal jugular vein should be guided by the ultrasonic technique. If central venous pressure monitoring is needed, the patient's neck should be prepared and draped before the patient is placed in the Trendelenburg position. The procedure should be terminated if ICP increases during placement.

Hyperventilation

In the past, deliberate hyperventilation of an adult patient's lungs to a $PaCO_2$ between 25 and 30 mm Hg to decrease ICP has been recommended. It was presumed that the beneficial effects of hyperventilation of the lungs on ICP reflect decreased cerebral blood flow and resulting decreases in intracranial blood volume. However, deliberate hyperventilation as a treatment to lower ICP has been questioned because of data showing an increase in mediators, lactate, and glutamate, even with a short period of hyperventilation.[2] Hyperventilation of a head-injured patient's lungs as a technique to reduce ICP is recommended only in the presence of a mass lesion and impending herniation before definitive surgical intervention.

Osmotic Diuretics

Administration of hyperosmotic drugs, such as mannitol (0.25 to 1 g/kg IV over a period of 15 to 30 minutes), decreases ICP by producing a transient increase in the osmolarity of plasma, which acts to draw water from tissues, including the brain. However, if the blood-brain barrier is disrupted, mannitol may pass into the brain and cause cerebral edema by drawing water into the brain. The duration of the hyperosmotic effect of mannitol is about 6 hours. The brain eventually adapts to sustained increases in plasma osmolarity such that chronic use of hyperosmotic drugs is likely to become less effective. The diuresis induced by mannitol may result in acute hypovolemia and adverse electrolyte changes (hypokalemia, hyponatremia), thus emphasizing the need to replace intravascular fluid volume with infusions of crystalloid and colloid solutions. A rule of thumb is to replace urine output with an equivalent volume of crystalloids, most often lactated Ringer's solution. Glucose and water solutions are not recommended because they are rapidly distributed in total-body water, including the brain. If the blood glucose concentration decreases more rapidly than the brain glucose concentration, the brain water becomes relatively hyperosmolar, and water enters the central nervous system and exaggerates the existing cerebral edema.

Hypertonic Saline

Hypertonic saline decreases ICP, improves cerebral perfusion pressure, and enhances hemodynamic function in TBI patients. In addition to its osmotic effect on edematous brain tissue, hypertonic saline also has vasoregulatory, neurochemical, and immunologic effects. Nevertheless, there is no significant outcome difference in patients who receive either 7.5% hypertonic solution or 20% mannitol.[3]

Corticosteroids

Corticosteroids such as dexamethasone or methylprednisolone have been used to decrease ICP for more than 30 years. The mechanism for the beneficial effect of corticosteroids is not known, but it may involve stabilization of capillary membranes or a decrease in the production of cerebrospinal fluid, or both. Nevertheless, there is no reduction in mortality in patients treated with methylprednisolone in the first 2 weeks after TBI, thus suggesting that steroids should no longer be routinely administered to these patients.[4,5]

Decompression Craniectomy

Emergency decompression craniectomy is a surgical procedure performed to resolve the elevated ICP and prevent herniation after head insults, especially severe TBI.

Barbiturates

Administration of barbiturates may be recommended when ICP remains increased despite deliberate controlled hyperventilation of the lungs and drug-induced diuresis. This recommendation is based on the predictable ability of these drugs to decrease ICP, presumably by decreasing cerebral blood volume secondary to cerebral vasoconstriction and decreased cerebral blood flow. The goal of barbiturate therapy is to maintain ICP at less than 20 mm Hg without the occurrence of plateau waves. Discontinuation of the barbiturate infusion can be considered when ICP has remained in a normal range for 48 hours. Failure of barbiturates to decrease ICP is a grave prognostic sign. Even when barbiturates are effective, overall morbidity and mortality in TBI patients have not been shown to be improved by the use of these drugs when compared with aggressive treatment consisting of deliberate hyperventilation of the lungs and drug-induced diuresis.[6] A hazard of barbiturate therapy to lower ICP is hypotension, which can jeopardize the maintenance of adequate cerebral perfusion pressure.

Such hypotension is particularly likely in the presence of decreased intravascular fluid volume. Dopamine or dobutamine may be necessary in the event of barbiturate-induced hypotension secondary to myocardial depression. Transthoracic echocardiography can be useful for evaluating cardiac function in head-injured patients.

CHEST INJURIES

Chest injuries are a significant cause of mortality in injured patients and account for 20% of trauma-related deaths in the United States. Both blunt and penetrating chest injuries are treated with similar principles of management. The initial evaluation of patients with chest injuries should emphasize the presence of an adequate airway and ventilation. The chest radiograph is analyzed for the presence of pneumothorax, hemothorax, pulmonary contusion, deviation of the tracheobronchial tree, widening of the mediastinum, and abnormal mediastinal shadows. These findings determine the need for additional diagnostic or therapeutic interventions.

Tension Pneumothorax

Tension pneumothorax is a relatively common cause of respiratory distress in a patient with chest trauma. Placement of a chest tube without waiting for a chest radiograph is warranted in patients with penetrating chest trauma who are in significant respiratory distress or have systemic hypotension. Patients with chest trauma may also have significant hemorrhage that requires prompt administration of crystalloid solutions and blood.

Urgent Thoracotomy

The need for urgent thoracotomy because of chest trauma is rare. In fact, because lobectomy and pneumonectomy are associated with high mortality in trauma patients, treatment techniques have been developed that emphasize rapid and minimal lung resection.[7] Guidelines for the need for emergency thoracotomy include an initial blood loss of 1500 mL on placement of the chest tube and continued bleeding of 200 to 300 mL/hr. Additional indications for thoracotomy consist of injuries to the heart or great vessels and tracheal, bronchial, or esophageal injuries. Diaphragmatic repair is usually performed via an abdominal approach.

MANAGEMENT OF ANESTHESIA

Before induction of general anesthesia for trauma patients undergoing emergency thoracotomy, it is critical to exclude the presence of a pneumothorax that could become a tension pneumothorax with the institution of mechanical ventilation of the patient's lungs.

Management of these patients often includes an intra-arterial and central venous pressure catheter, as well as peripheral large-bore intravenous catheters placed above the diaphragm. Because of the presence of lung injury, these patients' lungs need to be ventilated with low–tidal volume ventilation (6 mL/kg ideal body weight) and a small amount of positive end-expiratory pressure. Placement of a double-lumen endotracheal tube to perform one-lung ventilation may be warranted for lung resection or repair of the esophagus or large intrathoracic vessels. These patients are usually transferred to the ICU with the trachea intubated and the lungs mechanically ventilated.

ABDOMINAL INJURY

Abdominal injury accounts for a small, but significant number of trauma-related deaths, especially when the abdominal injury is not recognized. One of the major reasons for a fatal outcome is that the peritoneal cavity and retroperitoneal space are potential reservoirs for large and occult blood loss. During initial evaluation of the trauma victim, peritoneal signs of abdominal trauma are often subtle and difficult to diagnose because of the intense pain associated with extra-abdominal injuries or because of the presence of TBI and altered mental status. Thus, during the initial evaluation of a severely traumatized patient, the first step is to diagnose the presence of abdominal trauma.

Classification

Traumatic abdominal injuries are classified as penetrating or blunt injuries. Penetrating injuries associated with overt signs of peritoneal irritation or acute blood loss (or both) are clear indications for surgery. If there is no violation of the peritoneum, local exploration is usually sufficient. Blunt trauma is generally caused by collisions or falls. The severity of the injury is determined by the acceleration-deceleration process sustained by the victim. The organs most commonly injured are the liver, spleen, and kidneys.

Diagnosis

Ultrasound performed in the emergency department is an important diagnostic tool for detecting the presence of an abdominal injury, including the presence of blood in the abdomen. Diagnostic peritoneal lavage (DPL) is a sensitive method for detecting the presence of serious intra-abdominal bleeding. The classic indication for DPL is suspicion of intra-abdominal bleeding associated with arterial hypotension. In stable patients, an abdominal CT scan with radiocontrast is often performed instead of DPL. A CT scan allows the clinician to detect the location

VI

and magnitude of intra-abdominal injuries in hemodynamically stable patients. CT may also be important for investigating genitourinary injuries when intravenous radiocontrast is used.

Management of Anesthesia

Severe abdominal injuries require general anesthesia and often placement of an intra-arterial and central venous pressure catheter. In many institutions, a large-bore catheter is placed in a femoral vein on arrival at the emergency department. It is important to recognize that the femoral venous catheter should not be used for rapid blood transfusions when abdominal venous injuries are suspected. It is good practice to place an additional large-bore catheter above the diaphragm for rapid intravenous administration of volume to these patients.

PELVIC FRACTURES

Pelvic fractures are the third most frequent injury in victims of motor vehicle accidents and are often associated with other abdominal injuries. The overall mortality from pelvic fractures is between 15% and 50%, depending on the extent of the injuries. The combination of pelvic fracture and severe TBI has high mortality. The initial treatment of pelvic fractures associated with bleeding is nonoperative, and they are managed by angiographic embolization.[8] In addition to this treatment, patients may require external fixation of the fractures to allow mobilization. Alternatively, stabilization of the pelvis can be achieved with the use of military antishock trousers (MAST). The anesthesiologist has a critical role to play during the initial resuscitation of patients with severe pelvic fractures. These patients frequently require the administration of large volumes of blood, thus necessitating activation of the massive transfusion protocol. As with other abdominal injuries, it is also imperative to place large-bore intravenous catheters above the diaphragm.

BLUNT SPLENIC AND LIVER INJURIES

There has been a change in the management of blunt splenic and liver injuries toward a more conservative approach. Patients without signs of hemodynamic instability or intra-abdominal bleeding can be monitored closely in the ICU after the initial evaluation and placement of large-bore intravenous catheters. Usually, it is mandatory to obtain sequential hematocrit measurements during the first 24 hours and to frequently examine these patients for detection of any signs of new intra-abdominal bleeding. Furthermore, these patients are at risk for abdominal compartment syndrome because of the increased vascular permeability associated with severe trauma.

THERMAL (BURN) INJURY

Continuous improvement in the care of burned patients for the last 30 years has resulted in an increase in survival after the initial insult. It is not uncommon to see patients with burns affecting 70% to 80% of the total body surface area to survive this injury. Critical factors that affect mortality in these patients include age older than 60 years, third-degree burns over more than 40% of the total body surface area, and smoke inhalation. Mortality increases in proportion to the number of risk factors present.[9] In addition, the mortality rate of burned patients is also affected by the presence of significant coexisting diseases and delays in treatment.

Initial Evaluation

The initial clinical evaluation of an acutely burned patient includes a careful analysis of the burned body surface area, the depth of the burns, the mechanisms of injury (electrical, smoke inhalation), and the presence of associated traumatic injuries (Table 41-5). Furthermore, information should be obtained as soon as possible about the presence of significant comorbid conditions that may affect the survival of a severely burned patient.

Initial Fluid Resuscitation

The initial treatment of burned patients includes an assessment of the fluid resuscitation requirements for the first 24 hours. The most commonly used guideline for calculation of fluid replacement needs is the Parkland formula (4 mL/kg/% burn); the replacement fluid is given as lactated Ringer's solution. Half the volume should be given during the first 8 hours and the other half during the following 16 hours. After the first 24 hours, protein repletion is frequently needed and is typically provided by 5% albumin (0.3 to 0.5 mL/kg/total body surface area of burned tissue). In addition to colloid replacement, a burned patient should receive maintenance fluid, which can be estimated as basal maintenance (1500 mL/m² +

Table 41–5 Evaluation of an Acutely Burned Patient
Age
Burned body surface area
Depth of burns
Mechanism of injury
Presence of inhalation injury
Associated traumatic injuries
Significant comorbid conditions

evaporative water loss [(25 + % burn) × m² × 24]). Clinical evidence of adequate fluid resuscitation includes normalization of systemic blood pressure, urine output (>1 mL/kg/hr), and values for blood lactate, base deficit, plasma sodium concentration, and central venous pressure. Urine output is not a reliable guide to the adequacy of resuscitation after the first 24 to 48 hours following a burn injury because of the presence of osmotic diuresis associated with glucose intolerance and high caloric feeding. Furthermore, a non–anion gap arterial base deficit may reflect the excessive intravenous administration of 0.9% sodium chloride solution. In elderly patients or those with significant preexisting cardiac disease, hemodynamic parameters should be monitored carefully, possibly with placement of a pulmonary artery catheter, to prevent the development of acute congestive heart failure as a result of vigorous fluid resuscitation. Rapid fluid resuscitation can be associated with the development of severe tissue edema compromising limb perfusion or an abdominal compartment syndrome.

Management of Anesthesia

Burned patients will require general anesthesia, initially for escharotomy of the limbs, thorax, and/or abdomen and later for excision of the burned skin and grafting. If the injuries do not preclude conventional airway management, standard anesthesia induction and tracheal intubation procedures are appropriate. However, succinylcholine should not be administered when the burn injury is older than 24 hours because drug-induced hyperkalemia may result in cardiac arrest. The trachea of a severely burned patient should remain intubated after the initial escharotomies because the aggressive fluid management that occurs during the following 24 to 48 hours to compensate for the burn shock often causes airway edema and compromise. The patient's lungs should be ventilated with low–tidal volume ventilation (6 mL/kg ideal body weight) if smoke inhalation injury or acute lung injury from another origin is present. Placement of an intra-arterial and central venous catheter should be done under sterile conditions. Particular attention should be paid to the impaired temperature regulation associated with severe burns. Excision of burned skin is accompanied by substantial blood loss, which can be estimated at 0.5 mL/cm² of burned area. At the conclusion of surgery, transport of severely burned patients to the ICU should be planned carefully because accidental extubation during the transport of these patients may result in an inability to ventilate the patient's lungs by mask because of face and neck burns.

REFERENCES

1. Hastings RH, Marks JD. Airway management for trauma patients with potential cervical spine injuries. Anesth Analg 1991;73:471-482.
2. Marion DW, Puccio A, Wisniewski SR, et al. Effect of hyperventilation on extracellular concentrations of glutamate, lactate, pyruvate, and local cerebral blood flow in patients with severe traumatic brain injury. Crit Care Med 2002;30:2619-2625.
3. Bhardwaj A, Ulatowski JA. Hypertonic solutions in brain injury. Curr Opin Crit Care 2004;10:126-131.
4. Roberts I, Yates D, Sandercock P, et al. CRASH collaborators. Effect of intravenous corticosteroids on death within 14 days in 10,008 adults with clinically significant head injury (MRC CRASH trial): Randomized placebo-controlled trial. Lancet 2004;364:1321-1328.
5. Alderson P, Roberts I. Corticosteroids for acute traumatic brain injury. Cochrane Database Syst Rev 2005;Jan 25:CD000196.
6. Miller JD, Barbiturates and raised intracranial pressure. Ann Neurol 1979;6:189-193.
7. Wall MJ, Soltero E. Damage control for thoracic injuries. Surg Clin North Am 1997;77:863-878.
8. Hak DJ. The role of pelvic angiography in evaluation and management of pelvic trauma. Orthop Clin North Am 2004;35:445-449.
9. Ryan CM, Schoenfeld DA, Thorpe WP, et al. Objective estimates of the probability of death from burn injuries. N Engl J Med 1998;338:362-366.

VI

Chapter 42

BIOTERRORISM AND NATURAL DISASTERS

Robert K. Stoelting and Ronald D. Miller

Although natural (e.g., earthquakes, floods) and accidental (e.g., industrial, plane) disasters have occurred for years, terrorist attacks had been limited in the United States. *Salmonella* being introduced into food in Oregon is an example. The 1993 attack on the World Trade Center and the sarin attack in Japan proved to be hints of the future.

The September 11, 2001, airplane attack on the World Trade Center in New York was a sentinel event in establishing an era characterized by the concept that conventional, nuclear, biologic, and chemical attack can occur at any time.[1-3] Anesthesiologists must now be prepared at any time to care for victims of such assaults and to protect their own welfare so that they do not become casualties and an additional burden on the health care system. Terrorist attacks will also probably be associated with widespread public fear and panic. Although natural disasters require different responses and resources, they share some common needs, especially the organization to provide emergency care to large numbers of patients.[1-4]

COMMUNITY-WIDE EMERGENCY PREPAREDNESS

The Joint Commission on Accreditation of Healthcare Organizations (JCAHO) has published guidelines to help hospitals develop systems to create and sustain community-wide emergency preparedness.[4] These guidelines acknowledge that a system of preparedness across communities must be in place on a daily basis. Despite decreasing health care resources, a "surge capacity" is needed within health care systems to handle the potentially thousands of patients who might be victims of catastrophic events. The JCAHO guidelines focus on three major areas, including a community preparedness coordination response and a local approach to take care of patients and protect the medical staff.[5] Anesthesia teams *must* be familiar with what their hospital has done to comply with the JCAHO guidelines in anticipation of what their roles may be should the need occur.

Enlisting the Community

Emergency management standards for disaster preparedness as promulgated by the JCAHO recognize that the initial response to terrorist attacks or natural disasters needs to be a local response in which community hospitals and citizens may have to manage the events that they are confronted with in the first 24 to 72 hours (Table 42-1).[1-3] Investigation of responses after the 2001 terrorist attacks and natural disasters (floods) has called attention to the fact that law enforcement agencies, fire and rescue services, and health care provider organizations need to communicate more efficiently with one another. Furthermore, the attacks or disasters may be so extensive that outside help may be delayed (e.g., Katrina hurricane and floods).

Focusing on Key Aspects of the System

To respond to a mass casualty event, an emergency medical system must be able to assess and expand its surge capacity (ability to provide care for and transport countless numbers of patients to facilities with appropriate capacity, resources, and staff). To preserve the functionality of the system, the staff must also protect themselves (decontaminate patients before rendering care). After having established the basics, the most important aspect of managing a mass casualty event (natural, unintentional, intentional) is having a command and control structure that is familiar to everyone (Table 42-2).[1-3]

Establishing a Community Preparedness System

At the community level, most of the responsibility for preparedness is with the local, state, and federal governments in conjunction with hospitals and hospital organizations. Physicians need to be familiar with the clinical competencies needed for emergency preparedness in the event of bioterrorism (Table 42-3).[1-4]

DISASTER PREPAREDNESS

Being prepared to deal with terrorist attacks and the possible use of weapons of mass destruction is critically important, but the reality is that management of patients who are victims of natural and unintentional disasters is more likely (see Table 42-3).[1] Hurricanes, tsunamis, tropical storms, earthquakes, and tornadoes are the most likely to create chaos and mass casualties. Hospital facilities are often damaged or destroyed in affected areas. When hospitals are compromised, the government may need to establish field hospitals or, if near a body of water, bring in U.S. naval hospital ships.[6] Based on previous experience, it has been concluded that victims of entrapment from earthquakes can survive up to 5 days.[7]

Table 42–1 Emergency Management Standards (JCAHO)

Develop a management plan that addresses emergency management

Mitigation

Preparedness

Response

Recovery

Perform a hazard vulnerability analysis

Establish emergency procedures in response to a hazard vulnerability analysis

Define the organization's role with that of other community agencies

Notify external authorities of emergencies

Notify hospital personnel when emergency procedures are initiated

Assign available personnel to cover necessary positions

Manage the following activities

Patient/resident activities

Staff activities

Staff/family support

Logistics of critical supplies

Security

Evacuation of the facility if necessary

Establish internal/external communication systems

Establish an orientation/education program

Monitor ongoing drills and real emergencies

Determine how an annual evaluation will occur

Provide alternative means of meeting essential building and utility needs

Identify radioactive and biologic isolation and decontamination sites

Clarify alternative responsibility of personnel

Involve the community in the response

Reestablish and continue operations after a disaster

Adapted from Murray MJ. Disaster preparedness and weapons of mass destruction. *In* Barash PG, Cullen BF, Stoelting RK (eds): Clinical Anesthesia, 5th ed. Philadelphia: Lippincott Williams and Wilkins, 2006, pp 1521-1537.

VI

Table 42-2 Disasters That Result in Mass Casualties
Natural
Hurricanes
Tornados
Floods
Earthquakes
Fires
Unintentional
Public transportation accident
Boat accident
Nuclear accident
Industrial accident
Building collapse/sports stadium disaster
Intentional
Bombing
Nuclear
Biologic
Chemical

Adapted from Murray MJ. Disaster preparedness and weapons of mass destruction. *In* Barash PG, Cullen BF, Stoelting RK (eds): Clinical Anesthesia, 5th ed. Philadelphia: Lippincott Williams and Wilkins, 2006, pp 1521-1537.

Table 42-3 Clinical Competencies for Clinicians and Emergency Preparedness
Clinicians Should Be Able To:
Describe their role in the emergency response
Respond to an emergency event within the emergency management system
Recognize an illness or injury as potentially resulting from exposure to weapons of mass destruction
Report identified cases or events through the public health care system
Recognize that your institution may be a target
Be prepared to diagnose and treat victims of bioterrorism
Be familiar with the characteristics of (investigational) vaccines (efficacy, side effects/benefits) that you may be offered as a potential first responder
Identify and manage expected stress and anxiety
Participate in postevent feedback (afteraction report)

Role of Government

The initial response to any disaster (natural, unintentional, intentional) begins at the local level and involves law enforcement agencies, firefighters, and paramedics. Fire departments are trained to deal with toxic chemicals, whereas first responders who have not had appropriate training are at risk of becoming secondary victims. If the incident is more than local agencies can handle, state emergency management systems, including the National Guard, are activated by the governor of the state.

If the event supersedes the state's ability to respond, the federal government becomes involved. The Federal Bureau of Investigation has the responsibility for domestic terrorism and crisis management. The Federal Emergency Management Agency (FEMA) is responsible for providing assistance to local and state governments, providing emergency relief to affected individuals and businesses, and helping to ensure public safety. In addition to FEMA, the Department of Health and Human Services is the lead agency for providing health-related and medical services. The Department of Defense is also capable of assisting with incidents of biologic or chemical terrorism, bomb disposal, and decontamination. The Centers for Disease Control and Prevention has established a national pharmaceutical stockpile program as a national repository of antibiotics, chemical antidotes, life support medications, intravenous administration systems, airway management supplies, and medical/surgical items.[1] These materials are prepackaged and deployed throughout the United States for prompt delivery to disaster sites.

Triage of Victims

Though ideal, triage at the scene is rarely accomplished and most often occurs on arrival at the emergency department of the hospital. Triage is designed to identify individuals who are most critically wounded and who will most likely benefit from emergency intervention and surgery. There may be critically injured patients who are expected to die of their injuries (classified as "expectant"). These patients should be separated from the main patient flow and kept in a quiet, reassuring environment with attention to providing analgesia and comfort. Surgeons must prioritize injuries by focusing on patients and surgical interventions that are most likely to have the greatest benefit. Burn, crush, and blast injuries are common, but one must also be prepared to treat chemical, biologic, or radiation injuries while decontaminating the patient and protecting oneself.[2,3]

Role of the Anesthesiologist in Managing Mass Casualties

The anesthesia team needs to know that a number of local, state, and federal agencies are mobilizing to provide assistance during the initial phases of management after a disaster. It is difficult to predict the role that anesthesiologists may be required to fulfill in managing victims of terrorist attacks or natural disasters. Although anesthesiologists are most likely to be used in the operating room, it is also possible that participation in the triage area, emergency department, and intensive care unit may be needed (Table 42-4).[1-3,5] Familiarity with the hospital's disaster plan is imperative. Ensuring the safety of health care personnel through the appropriate use of protective devices to serve as barriers against radiologic, biologic, and chemical weapons must be considered.

The anesthesia team must understand physiology and pharmacology, possess airway management skills and fluid resuscitation expertise, and have the ability to manage ventilators and provide anesthesia at multiple sites (disaster site, emergency department, operating room, intensive care unit). The anesthesia team must focus on interventions that provide the most benefit for the largest number of victims.[1-3,5]

Prehospital Care

In mass casualty situations, patients are likely to have burns, fractures, lacerations, soft tissue trauma, and amputations that require initial stabilization and subsequent definitive treatment in the operating room or intensive care unit. Patients with large burn areas will require establishment of intravenous access. If chemical weapons are involved, tracheal intubation and ventilator management may be needed in addition to the administration of appropriate antidotes.

Table 42–4   Role of the Anesthesiologist at the Command and Control Center
Decontamination
Triage
Dead
Expectant (not expected to survive)
Operating room
Intensive care unit (to the operating room later)
Stabilize—floor
Minor
Operating room—intervention
Intensive care unit (burns, flail chest, traumatic amputations)

Adapted from Murray MJ. Disaster preparedness and weapons of mass destruction. *In* Barash PG, Cullen BF, Stoelting RK (eds): Clinical Anesthesia, 5th ed. Philadelphia: Lippincott Williams and Wilkins, 2006, pp 1521-1537.

From an anesthesia perspective, the situation most frequently encountered at the disaster site includes airway management and ensuring adequate ventilation and oxygenation. Ketamine, with or without a benzodiazepine or upload, is the anesthetic of choice for the care of patients who are entrapped at the injury site and may require amputations to facilitate extraction. Inclusion of benzodiazepines or uploads (or both) is limited by the possible presence of hypovolemia in these individuals.

Patients who have already been extracted from buildings or vehicles may need more invasive support of ventilation.[3] Tracheal intubation in this setting may be difficult, and the administration of drugs to facilitate the process is based on the expertise of the health care provider and the availability of drugs.[8] An awake, blind nasotracheal intubation may be the preferred technique, especially since these victims are likely to be at increased risk for pulmonary aspiration of gastric contents.

Hospital Care

Although anesthesiologists may be deployed in the emergency department, their expertise will most often be used in the operating rooms, where the majority of surgical procedures may be limited to lifesaving and limb salvage operations.[2] Frequently, there is no time for preoperative evaluation, and intravascular volume resuscitation may be limited because supplies are scarce.[5]

ANESTHETIC TECHNIQUES

Ketamine is an appropriate anesthetic, with or without a benzodiazepine. Alternatively, a peripheral nerve block may be appropriate, but a central neuraxial block should probably be avoided because many of these patients are hypovolemic and may be more prone to severe hypotension. Depending on the conditions at the time, an inhaled anesthetic may be used. In addition to being hypovolemic, it must be assumed that these patients may also have a full stomach or anemia (or both). Extensive burns may limit intravenous access. Chest and head injuries may complicate management, and unrecognized injuries must be considered. If tracheal intubation cannot be accomplished, a laryngeal mask airway or surgical airway may be needed (see Chapter 16).

POSTOPERATIVE CARE

As with the management of any trauma victim, these patients may require continued intravascular fluid volume resuscitation, mechanical ventilation, and frequent assessment.[5] Invasive monitoring is continued, and provision of additional sedation and analgesia may be required. The postoperative period may also be the first time available to document the patient's name and injuries and complete the anesthetic record.

VI

NUCLEAR ACCIDENTS

Exposure of large populations to ionizing radiation is most likely to result from (1) nuclear power plant or reactor accidents, (2) terrorist actions, or (3) detonation of nuclear bombs. Predictable injuries from nuclear accidents include radiation burns, bone marrow suppression, destruction of the gastrointestinal tract mucosa and bleeding with translocation of bacteria, and septic shock.[9] Although the effects of a blast, crush, or thermal injury are readily apparent, the effects of ionizing radiation are not usually evident.

Radiation Exposure

Radiation exposure may result from external sources (beta particles, gamma rays), contaminated debris, or inhaled gases. Tissues with the most frequent turnover rate (lymphoid tissues, bone marrow) are most susceptible to radiation injury. Thrombocytopenia, granulocytopenia, and gastrointestinal injury lead to sepsis and bleeding, which are the hallmarks of acute radiation syndrome. Patients with nausea, vomiting, diarrhea, and fever are likely to have severe acute radiation syndrome. Hypotension and central nervous system dysfunction typically develop later. Hematopoietic syndrome from lymphoid and bone marrow suppression may lead to death in 8 to 50 days.[9]

Response to Ionizing Radiation Exposure

If possible, patients should be decontaminated at the site of exposure rather than risk bringing material emitting ionizing radiation to the hospital. Removal of clothing is important to eliminate any residual beta and gamma rays and neutrons. Subsequently, the patient's skin should be rinsed with warm soapy water. As with clothing, biologic materials (saliva, blood, urine, stool) must be isolated because they may be contaminated with radioisotopes. Potassium iodide (Lugol's solution) can prevent radiation-induced thyroid effects, but it must be given within 24 hours to be effective.[10] Granulocyte colony-stimulating factor may be helpful for the management of postirradiation sepsis.[9] Other treatments may include oral and gastrointestinal decontamination via nasopharyngeal lavage, early stomach lavage, or the administration of emetics and osmotic laxatives. Ammonium chloride, calcium gluconate, and diuretics may be administered to facilitate renal excretion. Chelation therapy may include calcium and zinc diethylenetriamine pentaacetic acid.[11]

Initial Evaluation

For all patients with confirmed or suspected radiation exposure, a complete blood count should be obtained on initial contact and after 24 hours to determine the absolute lymphocyte count.[9] At 24 hours, an absolute lymphocyte count less than 1000 cells/mm^3 suggests moderate exposure and less than 500 cells/mm^3 suggests severe exposure. All body orifices (nostrils, ears, mouth, rectum) should be swabbed and a 24-hour stool and urine collection performed if internal contamination is considered.

Initial Treatment

The initial care of radiation-exposed victims includes measures to decrease infection, including food with a low microbial content, clean water supplies, frequent hand washing, and air filtration. When possible, oral feeding is preferred over intravenous feeding to maintain the immunologic and physiologic integrity of the gastrointestinal tract.

The mainstay of therapy during the neutropenic phase of acute radiation syndrome is prevention and management of infection.[12] In addition to institution of empirical antibiotic regimens, hematopoietic growth factors may shorten the duration of neutropenia. Administered blood products should be irradiated and cytomegalovirus negative.

Surgery in Patients Exposed to Radiation

Surgical treatment of life-threatening injuries must precede any treatment of associated radiation injury.[9] Because radiologic contamination poses little risk to health care providers, these patients are prioritized by standard trauma protocols. In the presence of traumatic injury, hypotension must be considered to be due to hypovolemia and not radiologic injury. The skin is impermeable to most radionuclides, but particles can be absorbed through open wounds. In this regard, contaminated wounds should be decontaminated with copious irrigation.

BIOLOGIC DISASTERS

In addition to biologic terrorism, anesthesiologists need to be familiar with contagious diseases (influenza, severe acute respiratory syndrome, West Nile virus). Influenza has killed more people in the 20th century than any other infectious disease has. Only subtypes of influenza A virus normally infect people. Typically, birds do not get sick when they are infected, but avian viruses can transform and infect humans, with subsequent human-to-human transmission and a resulting pandemic. The airway and ventilator management skills possessed by anesthesiologists may become essential for the care of these patients. Health care workers may be at risk for infection when asked to mange these patients in the operating rooms and intensive care units.

CHEMICAL-BIOLOGIC TERRORISM

Special requirements exist for the diagnosis and treatment of patients who are victims of biologic terrorism

(Table 42-5). Several infectious agents possess characteristics considered important for biologic weapons (Table 42-6).[13,14] The main difference between chemical-biologic and conventional mass disaster is that medical responders may be at risk themselves. An effective chemical-biologic agent needs to be toxic, have a specific latency, and be persistent and transmissible. Such agents include viruses, bacteria, toxins, neuropeptides, nerve agents, vesicants (mustard gas), cyanogens, and lung-damaging agents (phosgene). Three categories of biologic weapons are recognized (Table 42-7).[2,3] Category A consists of weapons that are highly contagious and for which there is currently no natural immunity. Health care providers must remain alert to illness patterns and diagnostic clues that might signal an unusual infection process secondary to a bioterrorist attack (Tables 42-8 and 42-9).[13] Immediate access to vital treatment information is available from the web sites of agencies such as the Centers for Disease Control and Prevention, public health organizations, and the Department of Defense.

Table 42–6 Characteristics of Effective Biologic Weapons

Easy to produce in large quantities
Inexpensive
Readily transported and disseminated (inhalational more effective than oral ingestion)
Odorless and tasteless
Survives drying and aerosolization
Highly infectious and contagious
Results in widespread morbidity and mortality
Lacks natural immunity
Places significant demands on public health and governmental resources
Results in panic and social disruption

Adapted from Coursin DB, Ketzler JT, Kumar A, et al. Bioterrorism may overwhelm medical resources. Anesthesia Patient Safety Foundation Newsletter. Spring 2002, pp 4-8. Available at http://www.apsf.org.

Table 42–5 Information Needed for Each Toxic Hazard to Provide a Safe and Effective Response

Physical, pharmacologic, and immunologic methods of individual protection
Immediate measures for life support
Specific antidote therapy
Measures to limit the effects of toxicity and latency of action

From Baker DJ. Chemical and biologic warfare agents: The role of the anesthesiologist. *In* Miller RD (ed): Anesthesia, 6th ed. Philadelphia: Churchill Livingstone, 2005, pp 2497-2526.

Role of the Anesthesiologist in Bioterrorism

Although the anesthesia team may not be at the point of origin of a biologic attack or be involved in the initial assessment of patients with suspected biologic toxicity, they may be involved in the care of acutely ill patients in the emergency department, operating rooms, and intensive care unit.[1-3,13] It is likely that the anesthesia team will be responsible for provision of life-sustaining interventions such as airway management, ventilatory support, hemodynamic monitoring, and initiation of definitive

Table 42–7 Biologic Agents Used for Warfare

Category A	Category B	Category C
Bacillus anthracis (anthrax)	*Coxiella burnetii* (Q fever)	Various equine encephalitic viruses
Variola major (smallpox)	*Vibrio cholerae* (cholera)	
Yersinia pestis (plague)	*Burkholderia mallei* (glanders)	
Clostridium botulinum (botulism)	Enteric pathogens (*Escherichia coli, Salmonella, Shigella*)	
Francisella tularensis (tularemia)	Water safety threats (*Vibrio cholerae, Cryptosporidium*)	
Viral hemorrhagic fever (Ebola, Lassa, Marburg, Argentine)	Various encephalitic viruses Various biologic toxins	

Adapted from Coursin DB, Ketzler JT, Kumar A, et al. Bioterrorism may overwhelm medical resources. Anesthesia Patient Safety Foundation Newsletter. Spring 2002, pp 4-8. Available at http://www.apsf.org.

VI

Table 42–8 Features Suggesting Exposure or Infection with Biologic Weapons

Unusually high incidence or mortality from a disease cluster

Single case of an unusual pathogen (inhaled anthrax, smallpox)

Cluster of patients with a suspicious clinical illness

  Flulike illness leading to acute respiratory distress syndrome, shock, meningitis (anthrax)

  Acute febrile illness with pustular lesions (smallpox)

Occurrence of a disease outside its natural geographic boundaries (hemorrhagic fever, tularemia, plague)

Cluster of patients with acute flaccid paralysis (botulism)

Clustering of diseases that affect animals as well as humans

Adapted from Coursin DB, Ketzler JT, Kumar A, et al. Bioterrorism may overwhelm medical resources. Anesthesia Patient Safety Foundation Newsletter. Spring 2002, pp 4-8. Available at http://www.apsf.org.

Table 42–9 Initial Management of Suspected Victims of Bioterrorism

High index of suspicion based on clustering of unusual illnesses

Protection of health care workers (gowns, gloves, masks)

Notify hospital, public health, and governmental officials

Decontaminate sick and exposed individuals

Triage (some require isolation)

  Designate a hospital ward and selected health care workers to care for patients with suspected infectious diseases

  Stable and noninfectious patients should be discharged to reduce the risk of exposure to contagious diseases

Label all materials from affected patients with bioterrorist/biohazard tags

Supportive therapy (fluids, ventilation, circulatory support)

Anti-infectives (see Tables 42-12 to 42-16)

Adapted from Coursin DB, Ketzler JT, Kumar A, et al. Bioterrorism may overwhelm medical resources. Anesthesia Patient Safety Foundation Newsletter. Spring 2002, pp 4-8. Available at http://www.apsf.org.

antimicrobial therapy. In this regard, anesthesiologists are at increased risk for inhaled exposure, direct contact with pathogens, or spread of blood-borne infection. It is important for those involved in this care to be familiar with basic isolation and decontamination techniques. When patients arrive in the emergency department, it is essential to triage them outside normal patient care areas in a designated decontamination area to prevent secondary exposure.

Anthrax

Anthrax is a gram-positive, spore-forming bacillus that is transmitted to humans from contaminated animals or their by-products (Table 42-10).[13,15] The three primary types of anthrax are cutaneous, inhalational, and gastrointestinal. Weaponized anthrax is intended to infect by inhalation. It causes influenza-like symptoms (fever, malaise, myalgia, nonproductive cough), followed by a period of seeming recovery (Table 42-11).[13] After a few days the patient suddenly appears critically ill with dyspnea, cyanosis, hemoptysis, stridor, and chest pain. The most notable radiographic finding is a widened mediastinum (Fig. 42-1).[13] Usually, when profound dyspnea develops, death ensues within 1 to 2 days. Weaponized anthrax has been engineered to be resistant to penicillin G. Ciprofloxacin or doxycycline is effective treatment of anthrax.

Smallpox

Routine vaccination for smallpox was discontinued in 1972 in the United States, and in 1980 the World Health Organization announced that the world was free of the variola virus.[16] Smallpox is highly infective, with only 10 to 100 organisms required to infect an individual.

CLINICAL MANIFESTATIONS AND TREATMENT

The clinical manifestations of smallpox in an unvaccinated individual include a prodrome of malaise, headache, and fever as high as 40°C (Table 42-12).[13] The fever decreases over the next 72 to 96 hours, at which time the rash appears. This pattern contrasts with chickenpox, in which the rash and fever develop simultaneously. All cutaneous lesions of smallpox are at the same stage, whereas chickenpox lesions are at multiple stages (papules, vesicles, pustules, scabs). Most cases of smallpox are transmitted through aerosolized droplets that are inhaled, but clothes and blankets that have come in contact with pustules are infectious. Strict isolation of patients with smallpox is critically important. Vaccination of contacts is effective in the first 3 to 7 days after exposure.

Plague

Rodents and fleas are the natural hosts for the gram-positive bacillus that causes plague (Table 42-13).[13] Humans are accidental hosts and most commonly acquire the disease

Table 42–10   Pathophysiology of Anthrax (*Pasturella anthracis*)

Infectivity	Airborne
Incubation period	1-7 days
Features	Inhalational: flulike illness followed by respiratory distress, shock, meningitis Gastrointestinal: abdominal pain, peritonitis, shock Contact or cutaneous: painless ulcers progressing to a black eschar
Mortality	80%-95% in 3-5 days (inhalational or gastrointestinal) 25% (contact or cutaneous)
Chance of secondary infection or spread	Little or none from a victim with an established infection Bleach environmental surfaces For human contamination, wash clothes and shower
Diagnosis	Gram-positive bacilli on Gram stain and blood culture Widened mediastinum on chest radiograph or computed tomography
Precautions	Avoid contact
Treatment	Ciprofloxacin Penicillin Doxycycline
Prophylaxis for exposed patients	Ciprofloxacin for 60 days Vaccination?

Adapted from Coursin DB, Ketzler JT, Kumar A, et al. Bioterrorism may overwhelm medical resources. Anesthesia Patient Safety Foundation Newsletter. Spring 2002, pp 4-8. Available at http://www.apsf.org.

Table 42–11   Differentiation of Viral Flulike Illness from Inhalational Anthrax

	Viral Flu	Inhalational Anthrax
Fever, chills, myalgia	Yes	Yes
Nasal coryza	Yes	No
Pharyngitis	Common	Occasional
Cough	Yes	Yes
Substernal chest pain	Rare	Common
Dyspnea	Rare	Common
Abdominal pain	Rare	Common
Leukocytosis	No	Yes
Arterial hypoxemia	Rare	Common
Sepsis syndrome	Rare	Common
Mediastinal adenopathy on chest radiograph	No	Yes

Adapted from Coursin DB, Ketzler JT, Kumar A, et al. Bioterrorism may overwhelm medical resources. Anesthesia Patient Safety Foundation Newsletter. Spring 2002, pp 4-8. Available at http://www.apsf.org.

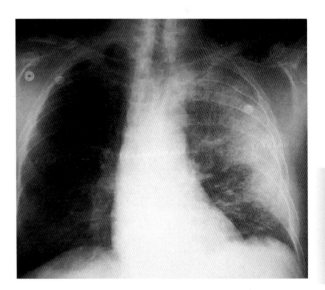

Figure 42-1 Chest radiograph showing a widened mediastinum in a patient with inhalational anthrax. (From Coursin DB, Ketzler JT, Kumar A, et al. Bioterrorism may overwhelm medical resources: New and different patient safety challenges must be anticipated. Anesthesia Patient Safety Foundation Newsletter. Spring 2002, pp 4-8. Available at http://www.apsf.org, with permission.)

VI

Table 42–12 Pathophysiology of Smallpox (Variola Major)

Infectivity	High
Incubation period	7-14 days
Features	Fever Headache Cough Centripetal pustular rash involving the palms and soles
Mortality	Overall, 35% No previous vaccination, >50% Vaccination >20 years before exposure, 11.1% Vaccination within 10 years of exposure, 1.4%
Chance of secondary infection or spread	Very high
Diagnosis	Electron microscopic evaluation of pustular material Culture
Precautions	Strict isolation (negative-pressure room)
Treatment	Supportive Cidofovir or ribavirin (?) Antibiotics for secondary bacterial infections
Prophylaxis for exposed patients and health care workers	Vaccination within 4 days of exposure (may prevent or significantly ameliorate infection)

Adapted from Coursin DB, Ketzler JT, Kumar A, et al. Bioterrorism may overwhelm medical resources. Anesthesia Patient Safety Foundation Newsletter. Spring 2002, pp 4-8. Available at http://www.apsf.org.

from a flea bite. As an aerosolized weapon the bacillus is viable for approximately 60 minutes. The two types of plague are bubonic and pneumonic. With bubonic plague, there is a 2- to 6-day incubation period after a flea bite, followed by a sudden onset of fever, chills, weakness, and headache. Intense painful swelling occurs in the lymph nodes, and this swelling ("buboes") is typically oval (1 to 10 cm in diameter) and extremely tender. Without treatment (streptomycin), patients become septic, and septic shock with cyanosis and gangrene in peripheral tissues ("black death") ensues. Pneumonic plague is highly contagious. The diagnosis is made by Gram stain or culture of organisms from blood, sputum, or buboes.

Tularemia

Tularemia as a result of bioterrorism is caused by aerosolization of the gram-negative coccobacillus *Francisella tularensis*, and a plague-like respiratory illness develops (Table 42-14).[13,17] Transmission of tularemia from person to person has not been documented.

Botulism

Botulism is a neuroparalytic disease caused by toxin from *Clostridium botulinum*. Unlike all the other bioterrorist agents, botulism is not caused by a live organism and is not contagious (Table 42-15).[13,18] Ingestion or inhalation of *C. botulinum* is followed by distribution of the toxin to cholinergic receptors, where it blocks the release of acetylcholine by inhibiting the intracellular fusion of acetylcholine vesicles to the membranes for release. *C. botulinum* toxin is the most potent known poison.

CLINICAL MANIFESTATIONS AND TREATMENT
Skeletal muscle weakness (diplopia, dysphagia, dyspnea, paralysis) occurs between 12 and 36 hours after ingestion or inhalation of the toxin.[19] There is decreased salivation, ileus, and urinary retention. The toxin can be removed by gastric lavage and the use of cathartics. Tracheal intubation and mechanical ventilation of the patient's lungs may be required. Administration of trivalent antitoxin is indicated.

Viral Hemorrhagic Fever Syndrome

Viral hemorrhagic fever syndrome describes a viral process that is spread in nature by arthropod vectors but becomes highly infectious when weaponized as an aerosol (Table 42-16).[20] There is an abrupt onset of a febrile illness that may evolve to shock and generalized mucous membrane hemorrhage.

Table 42–13 Pathophysiology of Plague (*Yersinia pestis*)

Infectivity	Moderate to high for the pneumonic form
Incubation period	2-8 days

Features	Pneumonic form:
	    Fever
	    Mucopurulent sputum
	    Chest pain
	    Hemoptysis
	    Bronchopneumonia on chest radiograph
	    Severe toxicity (shock common)

Mortality	Nonpneumonic form, 50% Pneumonic form, 100% if treatment is delayed
Chance of secondary infection or spread	High with the pneumonic form
Diagnosis	Sputum Blood culture
Precautions	Respiratory and contact isolation for 48 hours after initiation of antibiotics or negative sputum culture
Treatment	Streptomycin Gentamicin Tetracycline
Prophylaxis for exposed patients and health care workers	Postexposure prophylaxis for 7 days with tetracycline, doxycycline, sulfonamides, or chloramphenicol

Adapted from Coursin DB, Ketzler JT, Kumar A, et al. Bioterrorism may overwhelm medical resources. Anesthesia Patient Safety Foundation Newsletter. Spring 2002, pp 4-8. Available at http://www.apsf.org.

Table 42–14 Pathophysiology of Tularemia (*Francisella tularensis*)

Infectivity	High
Incubation period	3-5 days
Features	Acute onset of nonspecific febrile illness (dry cough, pleuritic chest pain) Atypical pneumonia on chest radiograph
Mortality	Undiagnosed, 30%
Chance of secondary infection or spread	None
Diagnosis	High index of suspicion Blood and sputum cultures Serology
Precautions	No isolation required
Treatment	Streptomycin
Prophylaxis for exposed victims	Streptomycin

Adapted from Coursin DB, Ketzler JT, Kumar A, et al. Bioterrorism may overwhelm medical resources. Anesthesia Patient Safety Foundation Newsletter. Spring 2002, pp 4-8. Available at http://www.apsf.org.

VI

Table 42–15   Pathophysiology of Botulism (*Clostridium botulinum*)

Infectivity	Moderate to high with intentional inhalational or gastrointestinal exposure
Incubation period	12-36 hours after inhalation or ingestion
Features	Acute onset of bilateral neuropathy with symmetric descending weakness No sensory deficit No fever No hemodynamic instability
Mortality	Appropriate supportive care, <5%
Chance of secondary infection or spread	None
Diagnosis	Toxin detection in blood or stool
Precautions	Toxin is not contagious
Treatment	Trivalent equine antitoxin
Prophylaxis for exposed victims	Trivalent equine antitoxin if signs or symptoms are present

Adapted from Coursin DB, Ketzler JT, Kumar A, et al. Bioterrorism may overwhelm medical resources. Anesthesia Patient Safety Foundation Newsletter. Spring 2002, pp 4-8. Available at http://www.apsf.org.

Table 42–16   Pathophysiology of Hemorrhagic Fever Viruses (Ebola, Marburg, Lassa, Machupo Viruses)

Infectivity	Modest (inhalational)
Incubation period	5-10 days
Features	Typical—acute onset of fever, myalgia, and headache Common—chest pain, cough, pharyngitis, nausea, vomiting, diarrhea Maculopapular rash on trunk after about 5 days of illness Hemorrhagic complications (petechiae, ecchymoses)
Mortality	25% to 90%
Chance of secondary infection or spread	Modest
Diagnosis	High index of suspicion Enzyme-linked immunosorbent assay
Precautions	Respiratory and contact isolation
Treatment	Ribavirin Immune serum (?)
Prophylaxis for exposed victims or health care workers	Ribavirin Immune serum (?)

Adapted from Coursin DB, Ketzler JT, Kumar A, et al. Bioterrorism may overwhelm medical resources. Anesthesia Patient Safety Foundation Newsletter. Spring 2002, pp 4-8. Available at http://www.apsf.org.

CHEMICAL AGENTS

Emergency management teams in the United States have traditionally been prepared to respond to chemical spills (chlorine spills) and industrial accidents.[1-3] The use of chemical agents in warfare was introduced during World War I and has recurred during isolated conflicts since that time. Chemical weapons are inexpensive in comparison to conventional and nuclear weapons and, when used against populations, create fear and panic combined with overwhelming demands on the health care system (see Table 42-17).[1-3,20-22]

Most chemical agents are liquid at room temperature, and when vaporized, all are heavier than air (hydrogen cyanide is an exception) and concentrate in low areas (trenches, basements). If exposed, individuals should ascend to higher levels, and even standing provides some protection as opposed to lying down. Paramedics and emergency medical personnel are at risk for exposure when participating in rescue attempts. Onset latency is greatest with phosgene and chlorine, whereas nerve and blood agents have the shortest latency times, usually seconds to minutes.

Treatment Principles

In the presence of a chemical exposure it is critical to (1) clearly demarcate the contaminated zone, (2) establish entry and exit points, and (3) institute existing procedures to provide self-protection and decontaminate victims.[20] Antidotes to specific chemicals are readily available from national pharmaceutical stockpiles and would be rushed to the site, although treatment of nerve agent and cyanide toxicity requires the administration of antidote within minutes rather than hours to be effective.

SELF-PROTECTION

The type of self-protection is dictated by the chemical agent involved. If the chemical is a pulmonary agent, the health care provider must wear a gas mask. A chemical protective suit is required if the chemical agent is a nerve agent or a vesicant. The protective garment should be impermeable to all classes of chemical agents because unprotected exposure to any of these compounds can result in cutaneous absorption and the rescuer becoming a casualty.

DECONTAMINATION

Hospitals should have decontamination facilities as part of their disaster preparedness plan.[20] Contaminated clothing is removed and the skin decontaminated at the scene before transportation. Soap and water are effective decontaminants, and if available, a dilute solution (0.5% to 2%) of hypochlorite (household bleach) can be used to decontaminate the skin.[20]

Nerve Agents

Nerve agents are chemicals (anticholinesterases) that affect nerve transmission by inhibiting acetylcholinesterase so that acetylcholine accumulates at peripheral muscarinic and nicotinic acetylcholine receptors and in the central nervous system. Physostigmine, neostigmine, and pyridostigmine are examples of "carbamate nerve agents" used clinically by anesthesiologists to antagonize the effects of nondepolarizing neuromuscular blocking drugs. Savin is a carbamate compound that is used as an insecticide. The remaining nerve agents are classified as organophosphates. Nerve agents are clear, colorless liquids that vaporize at room temperature and can penetrate clothing, skin, and the epithelium of the lungs and gastrointestinal tract (Table 42-17).[1-3,20,21]

Table 42-17 Examples of Chemical Weapons

Common Name	U.S. Military Code
Nerve Agents	
Tabun	GA
Sarin	GB
Soman	GD
	GF
	VX
Pulmonary Agents	
Chlorine	CL
Phosgene	CG
Skin (Vesicants)	
Sulfur mustard	HD
Nitrogen mustard	HN1
Lewisite	L
Phosgene oxime	CX
Blood Agents	
Hydrogen cyanide	AC
Cyanogen chloride	CK
Arsine	

Adapted from Murray MJ. Chemical weapons compromise provider safety. Anesthesia Patient Safety Foundation Newsletter. Spring 2002, pp 12-14. Available at http://www.apsf.org.

CLINICAL MANIFESTATIONS

Binding of nerve agents to acetylcholinesterase results in clinical manifestations that reflect excess concentrations of acetylcholine at muscarinic (miosis, gastrointestinal contraction, bradycardia, salivation, bronchoconstriction) and nicotinic (tachycardia, systemic hypertension, fasciculations, skeletal muscle paralysis) receptors. The net effect of this mixed receptor stimulation is difficult to predict because the victim's heart rate may be normal, low, or elevated. Unopposed parasympathetic nervous system activity leads to diarrhea, urination, miosis, bronchorrhea, bronchoconstriction, emesis, lacrimation, and salivation.

TREATMENT

Atropine, 2 to 6 mg IV, is administered every 5 to 10 minutes (in extreme cases, doses of atropine may exceed 100 mg) until secretions begin to decrease and ventilation is improved. Pralidoxime is a longer-acting anticholinergic drug that may be administered in doses up to 8 mg. The U.S. military travels with automatic injectors containing 2 mg of atropine and 600 mg of pyridostigmine or pralidoxime. Pyridostigmine administered 30 minutes before exposure is effective protection against subsequent nerve agent exposure. The use of pyridostigmine to treat exposure to nerve agents will have implications if these patients require surgery and anesthesia that may include the administration of nondepolarizing neuromuscular blocking drugs.

Pulmonary Agents

Phosgene is a colorless gas with an odor of recently cut hay and is the most deadly of the pulmonary agents. Because of a vapor density of 3.4, it stays in the air for prolonged periods and accumulates in low-lying areas. It is highly soluble in lipids and can easily penetrate pulmonary epithelium and cells lining the alveoli. Phosgene reacts with water to form hydrochloric acid and carbon dioxide. Hydrochloric acid is irritating to tissues and causes capillary leak and the development of acute lung injury. Coughing, nausea, vomiting, choking, and chest tightness occur. After initial exposure there may be a brief symptom-free period (1 to 24 hours), but lung injury is occurring and pulmonary edema follows.

TREATMENT

Gas masks provide the best protection against the effects of phosgene and chlorine gas. When sufficient quantities of phosgene are inhaled to cause acute lung injury, management is similar to that for patients with noncardiogenic pulmonary edema (acute respiratory distress syndrome). Anesthesiologists possess the expertise to manage the patient's airway and ventilation, as well as monitor hemodynamics and oxygenation.

Blood Agents

Blood agents are cyanogens and, when inhaled, release hydrogen cyanide, which impairs cytochrome oxidase and aerobic metabolism at the level of the mitochondria. The resulting metabolic acidosis and the sequelae of cellular hypoxemia are lethal. Hydrogen cyanide is a colorless liquid that is absorbed through the skin. Symptoms depend on the exposure dose and range from dyspnea and restlessness to convulsions, coma, and cardiac arrest. The high volatility of hydrogen cyanide would make it difficult to use as a biologic weapon.

TREATMENT

Treatment of nitroprusside toxicity by anesthesiologists is the basis for the treatment of hydrogen cyanide toxicity. Cyanide ions are normally metabolized by the enzyme rhodanese in the liver, which is a sulfur-requiring step that leads to the formation of methemoglobin. Administration of thiosulfate provides sulfur substrate for the rhodanese system. Supportive care includes tracheal intubation, administration of supplemental oxygen, and support of hemodynamics with vasopressors and inotropes.

Vesicants

These compounds produce burns and blisters on contact with the skin and eyes and, when inhaled, cause damage to the lungs and multiple organ dysfunction syndrome. Mild poisoning (tearing, erythema, cough, hoarseness) does not require treatment other than supportive care. More severe poisoning may result in blindness, nausea, vomiting, diarrhea, leukopenia, anemia, and severe respiratory difficulty.

TREATMENT

A nuclear-biologic-chemical protective suit and gas mask provide the best protection against vesicants such as sulfur mustard. Exposed individuals should be decontaminated as though they were exposed to a nerve agent (remove clothing and wash with warm soapy water with or without 0.5% to 2% hypochlorite). Tracheal intubation and mechanical ventilation of the patient's lungs may be required. There are no specific antidotes for sulfur mustard. Dimercaprol is a specific antidote for lewisite.[20]

REFERENCES

1. Murray MJ. Disaster preparedness and weapons of mass destruction. *In* Barash PG, Cullen BF, Stoelting RK (eds): Clinical Anesthesia, 5th ed. Philadelphia: Lippincott Williams and Wilkins, 2006, pp 1521-1537.
2. Baker DJ. Chemical and biologic warfare agents: The role of anesthesiologists. *In* Miller RD (ed): Anesthesia, 6th ed. Philadelphia: Churchill Livingstone, 2005, pp 2497-2526.
3. Murray MJ, Merridwe CG. Anesthesiologists must now prepare for biologic, nuclear, or chemical terrorism. Anesthesia Patient Safety Foundation Newsletter. Spring 2002, pp 1-3. Available at http://www.apsf.org.
4. Joint Commission on Accreditation of Healthcare Organizations: Healthcare at the Crossroads: Strategies for Creating and Sustaining Community Wide Emergency Preparedness Systems. Available at http://www.jcaho.org.
5. Dutton RP, McCunn M: Anesthesia for trauma. *In* Miller RD (ed): Miller's Anesthesia, 6th ed. Philadelphia: Churchill Livingstone, 2005, pp 2451-2496.
6. Halpern P, Rosen B, Carasso S, et al. Intensive care in a field hospital in an urban disaster area: Lessons from the August 1999 earthquake in Turkey. Crit Care Med 2003;31:1410-1415.
7. Sever MS, Erek E, Vanholder R, et al. Lessons learned from the Marmara disaster: Time period under the rubble. Crit Care Med 2002;30:2443-2447.
8. Lockey D, Davies G, Coats T. Survival of trauma patients who have prehospital tracheal intubation without anaesthesia or muscle relaxants: Observational study. BMJ 2001;323:141-146.
9. Mongan PD, Shields C, Via D. Threat of radiologic terrorism increases. Anesthesia Patient

Safety Foundation Newsletter. Spring 2002, pp 9-11. Available at http://www.apsf.org.

10. American Academy of Pediatrics Committee on Environmental Health. Radiation disasters and children. Pediatrics 2003;111:1455-1461.

11. Reves GI. Radiation injuries. Crit Care Clin 1999;15:457-462.

12. Klastersky J. Empirical treatment of sepsis in neutropenic patients. Hosp Med 2001;62:101-103.

13. Coursin DB, Ketzler JT, Kumar A, et al. Bioterrorism may overwhelm medical resources: New and different patient safety challenges must be anticipated. Anesthesia Patient Safety Foundation Newsletter. Spring 2002, pp 4-8. Available at http://www.apsf.org.

14. Lane HC, Fauci A. Bioterrorism on the home front: A new challenge for American medicine. JAMA 2001;286:2595-2597.

15. Swartz MN. Recognition and management of anthrax—an update. N Engl J Med 2001;345:1621-1626.

16. Breman JG, Henderson DA. Diagnosis and management of smallpox. N Engl J Med 2002;346:1300-1306.

17. Dennis DT, Inglesby TV, Henderson DA, et al. Tularemia as a biological weapon: Medical and public health management. JAMA 2001;285:2763-2773.

18. Arnon SS, Schechter R, Inglesby TV, et al. Botulinum toxin as a biological weapon: Medical and public health management. JAMA 2001;285:1059-1070.

19. Bhalla KD, Warheit DB. Biological agents with potential for misuse: A historical perspective and defensive measures. Toxicol Appl Pharmacol 2004;199:71-77.

20. Murray MJ. Chemical weapons compromise provider safety. Anesthesia Patient Safety Foundation Newsletter. Spring 2002, pp 12-14. Available at http://www.apsf.org.

21. Evison D, Hinsley D, Rice P. Chemical weapons. BMJ 2002;324:332-337.

22. Wetter DC, Daniell WD, Treser CD. Hospital preparedness for victims of chemical or biological terrorism. Am J Public Health 2001;91:710-716.

VI

Chapter 43

CHRONIC PAIN MANAGEMENT

David J. Lee

INTRODUCTION

Pain is the most frequent cause of suffering and disability and is the most common reason that people seek medical attention. Pain is defined as an unpleasant sensory and emotional experience associated with actual or potential tissue damage. Acute pain is a symptom of disease or injury, whereas chronic pain is the disease itself. Chronic pain seriously impairs the quality of life of millions of people throughout the world. Education of health care professionals and the general public remains fundamental to the proper management of patients with pain.

Pain Management

Pain management seeks to relieve pain, restore function, and prevent or eliminate disability. Prevention, diagnosis, and treatment of pain remain one of the most important and pressing issues of society. Pain relief does not necessarily improve function, functional restoration does not necessarily reduce disability, and behavioral and cognitive therapy improves disability but does not eliminate pain. Hence, the inherent complexity of pain management requires a multidisciplinary approach, one that incorporates a variety of diagnostic tools and therapeutic modalities in evaluating and treating patients with chronic pain.

Evaluation of Chronic Pain

With respect to the evaluation of chronic pain, a systematic approach in obtaining a detailed history and physical examination, establishing a differential diagnosis, and assessing the patient's psychosocial behavior and beliefs is essential. Treatment of chronic pain encompasses medications, physical therapy, behavioral and cognitive therapy, and minimally invasive procedures. Medications commonly prescribed are analgesics, nonsteroidal anti-inflammatory drugs (NSAIDs), centrally acting muscle relaxants, opioids, tricyclic antidepressants, and anticonvulsants. Minimally invasive procedures provide diagnosis and treatment options.

COMMON PAIN SYNDROMES

The most common pain syndromes that cause a patient to seek medical care include chronic low back pain, headache, neuropathic pain, complex regional pain syndrome, cancer pain, and fibromyalgia. Specific diagnostic criteria and treatment modalities, including minimally invasive pain management techniques, are useful in the management of these pain syndromes.

Chronic Low Back Pain

Low back pain originates in the lumbosacral spinal region. Chronic low back pain is characterized by pain that has been present for longer than 3 months and includes the reactions and responses to the persistence of pain. The natural history of low back pain is important in counseling a patient and planning treatment. Most patients with acute low back pain recover within 2 months.

CLINICAL MANIFESTATIONS

Clinical manifestations associated with chronic low back pain include avoidance of physical activity for fear of injury, high scores on the Minnesota Multiphasic Personality Inventory, mental depression, poor coping skills, sickness impact, duration and past history of low back pain, lower extremity pain, and job dissatisfaction. Fever and postsurgical procedures may be associated with spinal infections. A past history of cancer, age older than 50 years, prolonged illness despite treatment, and unexplained weight loss may reflect the presence of unrecognized cancer. The hallmarks of ankylosing spondylitis are morning stiffness, age younger than 30 years, and improvement with exercise. Lumbar disk herniation and radiculopathy, spinal stenosis, cauda equina syndrome, and failed back surgery syndrome often accompany chronic low back pain.

AXIAL JOINT PAIN

The most common causes of chronic low back pain are internal disk disruption, facet joint pain, and sacroiliac joint pain. Magnetic resonance imaging (MRI) is the best available imaging modality for patients with chronic low back pain. The high-intensity zone seen on T2-weighted MRI is a bright signal of edema surrounded by the dark signal of the annulus fibrosus in the posterior annulus of the lumbar intervertebral disk. It predicts internal disk disruption and strongly correlates with the patient's pain. The prevalence of discogenic pain as a result of internal disk disruption is 39% in patients with chronic back pain.[1] Provocative diskography is the only established means of diagnosing discogenic pain. The prevalence of facet joint

pain is 40% in older patients and 15% in injured workers.[2-4] Facet joint medial branch blocks and facet joint blocks provide a valid diagnosis, and radiofrequency ablation provides pain relief for an average of 12 months. The prevalence of sacroiliac joint pain is about 15%.[5,6] Sacroiliac joint blocks provide a valid diagnosis. A multidisciplinary approach encompassing medications, physical therapies that strengthen the abdominal and multifidus muscles, pool therapy, behavioral and cognitive therapy, diagnostic and therapeutic injection, intradiskal electrothermal therapy, annuloplasty, and intrathecal infusion is essential.

RADICULAR PAIN

Radicular pain is caused by stimulation of the nerve roots or dorsal root ganglion of a spinal nerve. Sixty percent of patients with lumbar disk herniation and radiculopathy improve in the first 2 months, and 20% to 30% of patients have persistent back or leg pain (or both) at 1 year.[7] Patients typically have unilateral lumbar radiculopathy. Sitting, flexion, and increased abdominal pressure tend to exacerbate the pain, whereas standing alleviates it. Physical examination is generally positive for straight leg raise, decreased sensation to pinprick and temperature, and decreased or absent deep tendon reflex. A multidisciplinary approach encompassing medications, physical therapy, transcutaneous electrical nerve stimulation (TENS), functional restoration, behavioral and cognitive therapy, epidural steroid injection, selective nerve root block, spinal cord stimulation, nucleoplasty, and percutaneous decompression is essential.

SPINAL STENOSIS AND CAUDA EQUINA SYNDROME

Degenerative lumbar spinal stenosis is three to five times more common in women than men, and it most commonly affects the L4-5 segment, followed by the L3-4 segment; in approximately 5% of cases it is associated with cervical stenosis.[8-10] Lumbar spinal stenosis is not necessarily progressive. Patients typically have an insidious onset of chronic low back pain that progresses to bilateral lumbar radiculopathy. Walking and extension exacerbate the pain, and sitting and flexion alleviate the pain. Patients can often increase walking tolerance when leaning forward over a shopping cart. Because degenerative lumbar spinal stenosis typically occurs in older patients, vascular claudication from peripheral vascular disease needs to be ruled out. Physical examination is generally negative for straight leg raise and focal neurologic deficit.

The classic clinical manifestation of cauda equina syndrome is low back pain, bilateral lower extremity radiculopathy, weakness, saddle anesthesia, and bowel and bladder dysfunction. MRI is the initial imaging modality of choice. Computed tomography (CT) or myelography is the imaging modality of choice if the patient has had previous surgery with instrumentation. A multidisciplinary approach encompassing medications, physical therapy, TENS, functional restoration, behavioral and cognitive

VI

therapy, epidural steroid injection, and intrathecal infusion is essential.

FAILED BACK SURGERY (POSTLAMINECTOMY SYNDROME)

Failed back surgery syndrome is characterized by persistent or recurring back pain, with or without sciatica, after one or more back surgeries. It may be due to incorrect diagnosis, poor patient selection, inadequate surgical decompression or fusion, infection, epidural fibrosis, or repeat surgical intervention. With a second intervention, the rate of epidural fibrosis and instability is greater than 60%.[11] MRI with gadolinium is the gold standard for detecting epidural fibrosis. A multidisciplinary approach encompassing medications, physical therapy, behavioral and cognitive therapy, and minimally invasive procedures based on the diagnosis of treatable sources of chronic low back pain is essential.

Headache

Primary headaches—migraine, tension, and cluster headaches—are those without a clear organic cause. Secondary headaches occur as a symptom of another disease. Organic causes such as trauma, vascular disorder, intracranial disorder, substance abuse or withdrawal, infection, and metabolic disorder, as well as psychosocial behavior and beliefs that compound the patient's disability, should be explored. CT and MRI may be indicated in patients with atypical headache patterns, a history of seizures, or focal neurologic signs and symptoms. Lumbar puncture should be performed after CT or MRI.

MIGRAINE HEADACHE

Migraine headache is bilateral in 40% of patients and unilateral in the remaining patients.[12] Nausea, vomiting, photophobia, and phonophobia often accompany the headache. Migraine headache has a female-to-male ratio of 3:1. Hormonal factors, excessive sleep, missed meals, alcohol, and weather changes are the most reliable factors that provoke migraine. The most predictable time for migraine is around the menstrual period. A multidisciplinary approach encompassing medications, physical therapy, and behavioral and cognitive therapy is essential. Symptomatic medications include triptans, NSAIDs, Midrin, and dihydroergotamine. When attacks occur more than two times per week, preventive medications are provided, including β-blockers, calcium channel blockers, tricyclic antidepressants, anticonvulsants, and NSAIDs. Children with migraine often respond to biofeedback and behavioral and cognitive therapy.

TENSION HEADACHE

Tension headache is not clearly distinguished from migraine, and it may represent a different point on a continuum. Tension headache is bilateral, usually mild, and associated with stress, anxiety, and depression. The same multidisciplinary approach for migraine headache is taken for tension headache.

CLUSTER HEADACHE

Cluster headache is a periodic onset of severe pain that frequently occurs during sleep, and it is primarily localized to the face and usually accompanied by ipsilateral Horner's syndrome. Cluster headache affects predominantly males. Alcohol typically provokes an attack. A multidisciplinary approach encompassing medications, physical therapy, and behavioral and cognitive therapy is essential. Preventive medications include calcium channel blockers, steroids, and anticonvulsants. Symptomatic medications include oxygen, triptans, NSAIDs, and intranasal lidocaine.

Neuropathic Pain

Neuropathic pain is defined as pain initiated or caused by injury or dysfunction of the nervous system. Peripheral neuropathic pain is chronic distal burning or deep aching pain accompanied by signs of sensory loss with or without skeletal muscle weakness, atrophy, and reflex loss; it is due to generalized or focal disease of peripheral nerves. Appropriate laboratory studies, MRI, and electrophysiologic studies may be indicated.

DIABETES MELLITUS

Diabetes mellitus is the most common cause of painful peripheral neuropathy. Peripheral neuropathic pain symptoms tend to predominate in the distal end of limbs, typically involving the feet to a greater degree than the hands. Sensory neuropathy appears to be the most common cause of a painful or burning foot.

POSTHERPETIC NEURALGIA

Postherpetic neuralgia is defined as the presence of pain more than a month after the onset of herpes zoster eruption. The incidence of herpes zoster increases with age and decreased immunity. The risk for postherpetic neuralgia increases with age. Sensory function is often altered in patients with postherpetic neuralgia. Acyclovir is recommended within 72 hours after appearance of the rash.

TRIGEMINAL NEURALGIA (TIC DOULOUREUX)

Trigeminal neuralgia is a clinical syndrome characterized by paroxysmal, unilateral lancinating facial pain. It is confined to the trigeminal distribution, with the second and third divisions affected most often, but sensory or reflex deficit does not occur. It can be triggered by tactile stimuli. The precise cause of trigeminal neuralgia has not been established.

TREATMENT

A multidisciplinary approach encompassing medications, physical therapy, and behavioral and cognitive therapy is essential for the treatment and management of neuropathic pain. Duloxetine (Cymbalta) is approved for diabetic peripheral neuralgia, gabapentin and lidocaine patches are approved for postherpetic neuralgia, and carbamazepine is approved for trigeminal neuralgia. "Off-label" antidepressants, such as tricyclic antidepressants, bupropion, and venlafaxine, and anticonvulsants, such as oxcarbazepine, lamotrigine, baclofen, tramadol, and opioids, are recommended for neuropathic pain. When medications for trigeminal neuralgia are ineffective or associated with significant side effects, creation of selective percutaneous lesions of the gasserian ganglion, such as by radiofrequency ablation, glycerol neurolysis, balloon compression, and gamma knife stereotactic radiosurgery, and microvascular decompression via a posterior fossa craniotomy can be considered.

Complex Regional Pain Syndrome

Complex regional pain syndrome is characterized by continuing pain, allodynia, or hyperalgesia disproportionate to the inciting event; it is not limited to the distribution of a single peripheral nerve and is associated with evidence of edema and changes in vasomotor and sudomotor activity. The precise cause of complex regional pain syndrome has not been established. The same multidisciplinary approach for neuropathic pain is taken for complex regional pain syndrome. Minimally invasive procedures include sympathetic ganglion blocks such as stellate ganglion block and lumbar sympathetic block, spinal cord stimulation, and intrathecal infusion.

Cancer Pain

Treatable sources of cancer-related pain, a patient's cognitive dimension, and detection of delirium and psychosocial behavior and beliefs that compound the patient's disability should be explored. A multidisciplinary approach encompassing medications, physical therapy, behavioral and cognitive therapy, and minimally invasive procedures is essential for management of a patient with cancer pain. Aspirin, indomethacin, and naproxen rectal suppositories, fentanyl lozenges, sustained-release morphine pellets, liquid hydrocodone, oxycodone, morphine and methadone, and fentanyl transdermal patches (for patients who have dysphagia) are available. Subcutaneous, intravenous, epidural, and intrathecal infusion of medications is available for patients whose pain is uncontrolled. Constipation is the most common and recalcitrant side effect of opioid therapy. Preventive stool softeners and symptomatic laxatives need to be provided. External beam radiation, radioactive strontium chloride 89, and the bisphosphonate pamidronate are effective treatments of bone pain. Neurolytic block of the gasserian ganglion, splanchnic nerves and celiac plexus, and hypogastric plexus is indicated for patients with cancer of the head and neck, abdomen, and pelvis, respectively. Early hospice referral and consultation are crucial.

The philosophy of hospice care is to provide the best possible quality of life for patients with terminal illnesses who are expected to live for 6 months or less and to assist the family through bereavement.

Fibromyalgia

Patients with fibromyalgia have diffuse musculoskeletal aching and pain with multiple predictable tender points. The precise cause of fibromyalgia has not been established. A multidisciplinary approach encompassing medications, physical therapy, and behavioral and cognitive therapy is essential to improve coping and stress management.

MINIMALLY INVASIVE PROCEDURES

Zygapophyseal Joint Block

The lumbar facet joint is formed by the articulation of the superior and inferior articular processes of adjacent vertebrae. Each joint is innervated by the medial branch from the same level as the vertebra, as well as the medial branch of the vertebra above. A facet joint block is produced by the intra-articular technique or the medial branch technique with the patient in the prone position (Fig. 43-1A and B).[13]

INTRA-ARTICULAR TECHNIQUE
In the intra-articular technique, the facet joint is visualized with medial lateral rotation under an anteroposterior (AP) fluoroscopic view. After sterile preparation and draping and administration of a local anesthetic, a 22-gauge, 7.5-cm-long needle is used to access the facet joint. Needle placement is confirmed by contrast and negative aspiration for blood or cerebrospinal fluid, and 0.5 to 1 mL of local anesthetic solution, with or without steroid, is injected through the needle.

MEDIAL BRANCH TECHNIQUE
In the medial branch technique, the junction of the superior articular process and the transverse process is visualized with an AP fluoroscopic view. After sterile preparation and draping and administration of a local anesthetic, a 22-gauge, 7.5-cm-long needle is used to access the junction in a lateral-to-medial approach. Needle placement is confirmed by AP and lateral fluoroscopic views and negative aspiration for blood or cerebrospinal fluid, and 0.75 mL of local anesthetic solution is injected through the needle.

RADIOFREQUENCY ABLATION
Radiofrequency ablation of the lumbar medial branches is indicated if the facet joint block provides significant, but transient pain relief. The same approach as for the medial branch technique is used. A 20-gauge, 10-cm-long radiofrequency ablation needle with a 10-mm active tip is used to access the junction of the superior articular

VI

Figure 43-1 A, Facet joint intra-articular block. **B,** Facet joint medial branch block. (From Waldman SD. Atlas of Interventional Pain Management, 2nd ed. Philadelphia: WB Saunders, 2004.)

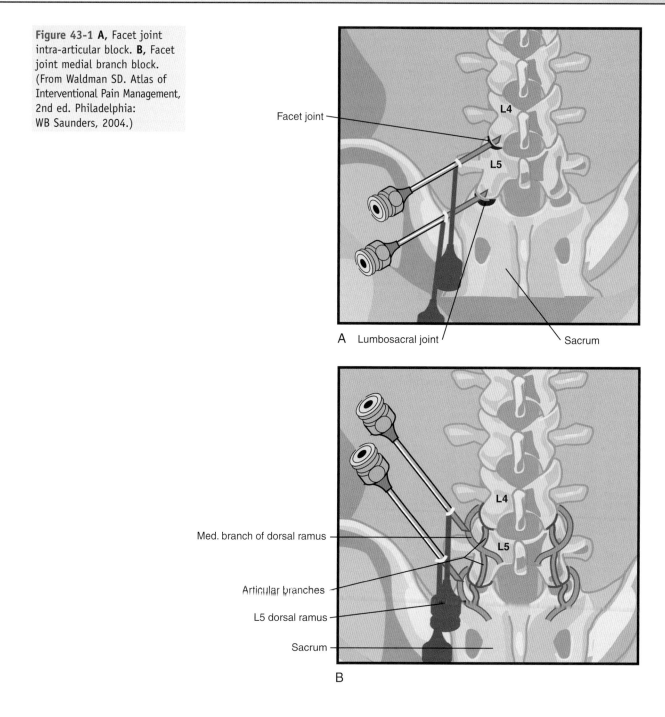

Facet joint

L4

L5

A Lumbosacral joint Sacrum

Med. branch of dorsal ramus

L4

L5

Articular branches

L5 dorsal ramus

Sacrum

B

process and the transverse process. Needle placement is confirmed by AP and lateral fluoroscopic views, and sensory and motor stimulation is performed. After obtaining appropriate stimulation and negative aspiration for blood or cerebrospinal fluid, 0.75 mL of local anesthetic solution is injected through the needle, followed by radiofrequency ablation at 80°C for 90 seconds.

Sacroiliac Joint Injection

The sacroiliac joint is formed by the articular surfaces of the sacrum and ilium. With the patient in the prone position, the sacroiliac joint is visualized with medial lateral rotation under an AP fluoroscopic view. After sterile preparation and draping and administration of a local anesthetic, a 22-gauge, 7.5-cm-long needle is used to access the sacroiliac joint. Needle placement is confirmed by contrast and negative aspiration for blood, and 5 mL of local anesthetic solution, with or without steroid, is injected through the needle (Fig. 43-2).[13]

Diskography

The intervertebral disk is innervated by the sinuvertebral nerve posteriorly and the nerves along the sympathetic nervous system anteriorly and laterally. Preoperative antibiotic is given intravenously and the patient is placed prone. The intervertebral disk is visualized after aligning the inferior end plate and rotating the fluoroscope to place the superior articular process at the midpoint of the inferior end plate. After sterile preparation and draping and administration of a local anesthetic, a 20-gauge, 7.5-cm-long needle is placed adjacent and anterolateral to the midpoint of the superior articular process. A 25-gauge, 15-cm-long needle is passed through the 20-gauge needle to access the intervertebral disk. Midline needle placement in the nucleus is confirmed by AP and lateral fluoroscopic views, and incremental infusion of 0.5 mL of a solution containing contrast and cefazolin (10 mg/mL) is delivered via an in-line pressure transducer monitor such as the Intellisystem (Fig. 43-3).[13] Based on pain concordance and spread of contrast, an intervertebral disk is determined to be positive or negative. Within 2 hours, the patient is sent for CT to confirm spread of contrast.

Intradiskal Electrothermal Therapy

The same approach as for standard lumbar diskography is used. After sterile preparation and draping and administration of a local anesthetic, a 17-gauge, 15-cm-long introducer needle is placed adjacent and anterolateral to the midpoint of the superior articular process to access the intervertebral disk. Needle placement in the nucleus is confirmed by AP and lateral fluoroscopic views, and the SpineCATH catheter is passed through the introducer needle into the nucleus and navigated well across the midline of the posterior interface of the nucleus and the annular wall. After confirmation of SpineCATH position by AP and lateral fluoroscopic views and verification of impedance, thermal energy is delivered at 80°C and 90°C for 6 and 4 minutes, respectively, as the patient tolerates (Fig. 43-4).[13]

Annuloplasty

The same approach as for standard lumbar diskography is used. After sterile preparation and draping and administration of a local anesthetic, a 17-gauge, 15-cm-long discTRODE introducer needle is placed adjacent and anterolateral to the midpoint of the superior articular process to access the intervertebral disk. Following confirmation of needle placement in the annulus by AP and lateral fluoroscopic views and verification of impedance, the discTRODE RF catheter is passed through the introducer needle into the contralateral annulus. After confirmation of discTRODE RF catheter position by AP

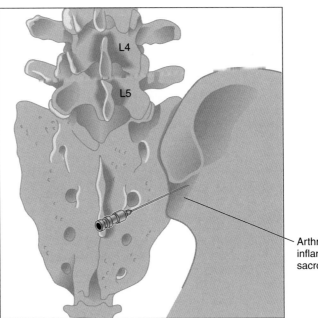

Figure 43-2 Sacroiliac joint block. (From Waldman SD. Atlas of Interventional Pain Management, 2nd ed. Philadelphia: WB Saunders, 2004.)

L4

L5

Arthritic and inflamed sacroiliac joint

VI

Figure 43-3 Diskography. (From Waldman SD. Atlas of Interventional Pain Management, 2nd ed. Philadelphia: WB Saunders, 2004.)

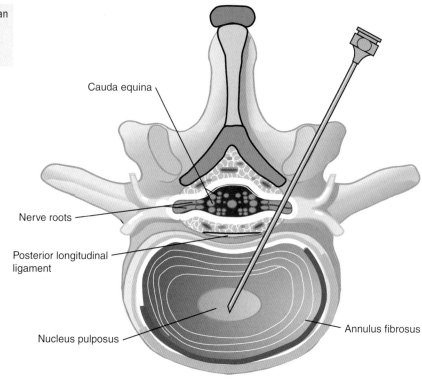

Cauda equina

Nerve roots

Posterior longitudinal ligament

Nucleus pulposus

Annulus fibrosus

and lateral fluoroscopic views and verification of impedance, radiofrequency energy is delivered at 65°C for 4 minutes, as the patient tolerates (Fig. 43-5).[14]

Nucleoplasty

The same approach as for standard lumbar diskography is used. After sterile preparation and draping and administration of a local anesthetic, a 17-gauge, 15-cm-long introducer needle is placed adjacent and anterolateral to the midpoint of the superior articular process to access the disk annulus. Needle placement in the annulus is confirmed by AP and lateral fluoroscopic views, and the spine wand is passed through the introducer needle into the nucleus. After confirmation of the depth of the nucleus by AP and lateral fluoroscopic views, six channels covering 360 degrees are created to perform coblation at 125 V on entry and coagulation at 65 V on exit, as the patient tolerates (Fig. 43-6).[15]

Percutaneous Decompression

The same approach as for standard lumbar diskography is used. After sterile preparation and draping and administration of a local anesthetic, a 17-gauge, 15-cm-long Dekompressor introducer needle is placed adjacent and anterolateral to the midpoint of the superior articular process to access the disk annulus. The dimension of the

nucleus is confirmed by the spread of a mixture of contrast and cefazolin (10 mg/mL) under AP and lateral fluoroscopic views, and the Dekompressor device is passed through the introducer needle into the nucleus. After confirmation of the position of the Dekompressor device by AP and lateral fluoroscopic views, an average of 1 mL of nucleus is decompressed, as the patient tolerates (Fig. 43-7).[16]

Spinal Cord Stimulation

Spinal cord stimulation is based on the Melzack-Wall gate control theory of pain. The exact mechanism remains unknown. Before implantation, a spinal cord stimulation trial is indicated. Because the patient's feedback in matching the stimulation pattern to the pain pattern is key, the trial is generally performed under local anesthesia. A preoperative antibiotic is given intravenously, and the patient is placed prone. After sterile preparation and draping and administration of a local anesthetic, a 15-gauge epidural needle is used to access the selected epidural space via a paramedian approach. Needle placement in the epidural space is confirmed by the loss-of-resistance technique and AP and lateral fluoroscopic views, and a spinal cord stimulation lead is passed through the needle into the epidural space and threaded to the desired vertebral level (Fig. 43-8).[17] With the patient awake and alert, proper placement of the spinal cord stimulation lead is established by matching the stimulation pattern to the pain

Anterior

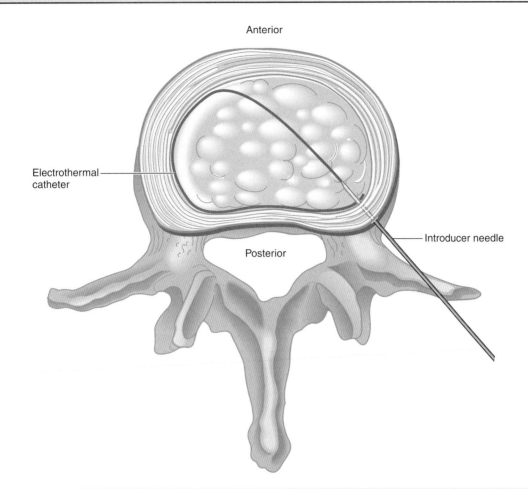

Electrothermal catheter

Introducer needle

Posterior

Figure 43-4 Intradiskal electrothermal therapy. (From Waldman SD. Atlas of Interventional Pain Management, 2nd ed. Philadelphia: WB Saunders, 2004.)

pattern. The epidural needle is removed and the lead is secured and connected to an external programmer. The patient then undergoes a spinal cord stimulation trial to evaluate its efficacy and tolerability. If the patient derives significant pain relief with minimal side effects, patient consent is obtained for spinal cord stimulation implantation.

GENERATOR (RECEIVER) AND LEAD IMPLANTATION

The generator or receiver is implanted subcutaneously, usually in the upper gluteal region. The implantation is generally performed under local anesthesia plus intravenous sedation (monitored anesthesia care [MAC]). Using the same approach as for the spinal cord stimulation trial, proper lead placement is established. The lead is then secured to the supraspinous ligament or the paraspinous fascia. The lead is tunneled subcutaneously to the pocket and connected to the generator or receiver. After confirmation of proper lead placement and system function by

matching the stimulation pattern to the pain pattern and AP and lateral fluoroscopic views, both the back incision and pocket incision are closed after hemostasis and antibiotic irrigation.

Intrathecal Infusion

Before implantation, an intrathecal infusion trial is indicated. A preoperative antibiotic is given intravenously, and the patient is placed prone. After sterile preparation and draping and administration of a local anesthetic, an 18-gauge Tuohy needle is used to access the intrathecal space via a paramedian approach. Needle placement in the intrathecal space is confirmed by the return of clear cerebrospinal fluid and AP and lateral fluoroscopic views, and a 20-gauge catheter is passed through the 18-gauge needle into the intrathecal space and threaded to the desired vertebral level (Fig. 43-9).[18] After confirmation of correct catheter placement by return of clear cere-

VI

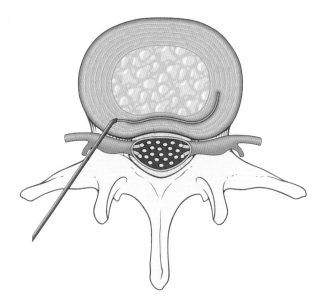

Figure 43-5 Annuloplasty. (Modified from discTRODE RF Catheter Electrode System, 2002 Radionics, 945612005, 12/02, with permission.)

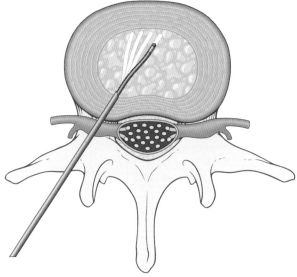

Figure 43-6 Nucleoplasty. (From DISC Nucleoplasty Perc-DLE SpineWand Technique Guide, P/N07452 Rev B, 2002 ArthroCare Corporation, with permission.)

Figure 43-7 Percutaneous decompression. (From Dekompressor Product Guide, Percutaneous Discectomy Probe, 1000-906-001 Rev. A, with permission.)

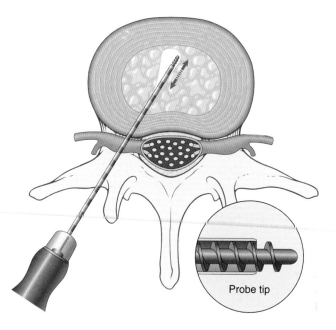

Probe tip

brospinal fluid and the pattern of contrast spread under AP and lateral fluoroscopic views, the 18-gauge needle is removed and the catheter is secured and connected to an external infusion pump. The patient then undergoes an intrathecal infusion trial with combinations of medications to evaluate the efficacy and tolerability. If the patient derives significant pain relief with minimal side effects,

consent is obtained for implantation of the intrathecal infusion pump.

PUMP IMPLANTATION

The pump is implanted subcutaneously, usually in the lower part of the abdomen. The implantation is generally performed under MAC and regional anesthesia. The

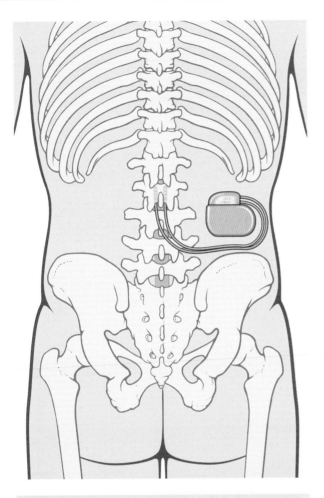

Figure 43-8 Spinal cord stimulation. (From Medtronic Pain Neurostimulation, Patient Information, page 3, UC199400762b EN N12056b, Medtronic, Inc., 2002, with permission.)

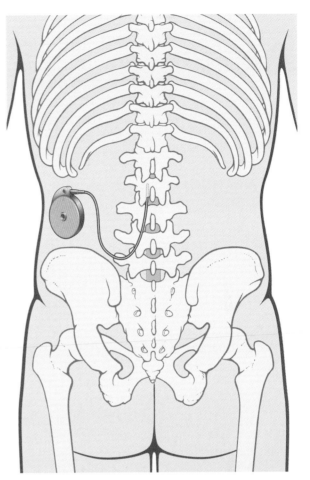

Figure 43-9 Intrathecal infusion. (From Medtronic Pain Therapies Intrathecal Drug Delivery, Patient Information for the SynchroMed and IsoMed Infusion Systems, Figure 8: Pump and catheter placement for intrathecal drug delivery, page 14, UC199603123a EN NP2686a, Medtronic, Inc., 2001, with permission.)

patient is placed in the lateral decubitus position with the implanted side up. Using the same approach as for the intrathecal infusion trial, the catheter is passed into the intrathecal space to the desired vertebral level. At this time, local anesthetic solution can be injected through the intrathecal catheter to produce regional anesthesia. The catheter is secured to the supraspinous ligament or paraspinous fascia and tunneled subcutaneously to the pump pocket. After confirmation of catheter patency by flow of cerebrospinal fluid, the catheter is connected to the pump. Both the back incision and the pocket incision are closed after hemostasis and antibiotic irrigation.

Gasserian Ganglion Block

The trigeminal nerve transmits sensory information from the face and head. A gasserian ganglion block is indicated for trigeminal neuralgia and facial pain refractory to conventional medical management. The patient is placed supine. The foramen ovale is visualized with medial lateral rotation under the submental AP fluoroscopic view. After sterile preparation and draping and administration of a local anesthetic, a 22-gauge, 7.5-cm-long needle is placed 2 cm lateral to the corner of the mouth to access the gasserian ganglion through the foramen ovale (Fig. 43-10).[13] Needle placement is confirmed by contrast and negative aspiration for blood or cerebrospinal fluid, and increments of local anesthetic solution to a total of 1 mL are injected through the needle to evaluate clinical response.

A glycerol neurolytic block and pulse radiofrequency ablation are indicated if the gasserian ganglion block provides significant, but transient pain relief.

VI

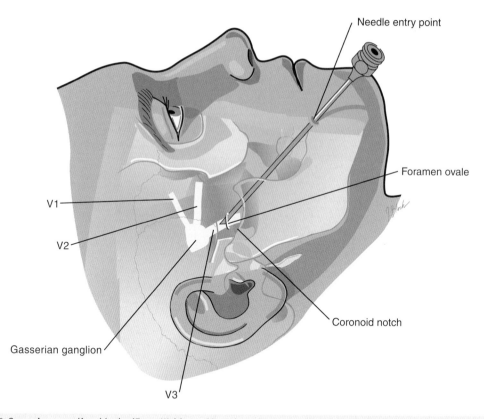

Needle entry point

Foramen ovale

V1

V2

Coronoid notch

Gasserian ganglion

V3

Figure 43-10 Gasserian ganglion block. (From Waldman SD. Atlas of Interventional Pain Management, 2nd ed. Philadelphia: WB Saunders, 2004.)

GLYCEROL NEUROLYTIC BLOCK

For a glycerol neurolytic block, the same approach as for a gasserian ganglion block is used. After confirmation of needle placement by AP and lateral fluoroscopic views and positive aspiration for cerebrospinal fluid, the patient is placed in the semisitting position with the neck flexed. Needle placement is confirmed by return of clear cerebrospinal fluid and contrast, and increments of glycerol solution to a total of 0.5 mL are injected through the needle. The needle is flushed with sterile saline.

PULSE RADIOFREQUENCY ABLATION

For pulse radiofrequency ablation, the same approach as for a gasserian ganglion block is used. A 22-gauge, 10-cm-long radiofrequency ablation needle with a 5-mm active tip is used to access the gasserian ganglion through the foramen ovale. Needle placement is confirmed by AP and lateral fluoroscopic views, and sensory and motor stimulation is performed. After appropriate stimulation and negative aspiration for blood or cerebrospinal fluid, increments of local anesthetic solution to a total of 0.5 mL are injected through the needle, followed by pulse radiofrequency ablation at 42°C for 3 minutes.

Stellate Ganglion Block

The stellate ganglia provide sympathetic innervation of the head, neck, and upper extremities. The stellate ganglion usually lies anterior to the transverse process of C7 and the neck of the first (T1) rib. Even though a stellate ganglion block can be performed without imaging, it is generally performed under fluoroscopic guidance. With the patient in the supine position, the ventrolateral aspect of the C7 vertebral body at the junction of the C7 vertebral body and the transverse process is visualized with an AP fluoroscopic view. After sterile preparation and draping and administration of a local anesthetic, a 22-gauge, 7.5-cm-long needle is used to access the ventrolateral aspect of the C7 vertebral body (Fig. 43-11).[13] Needle placement is confirmed with contrast, and increments of local anesthetic solution to a total of 10 mL are injected through the needle to evaluate clinical response.

Pulse radiofrequency ablation and an alcohol or phenol neurolytic block are indicated if the stellate ganglion block provides significant, but transient pain relief.

PULSE RADIOFREQUENCY ABLATION

For pulse radiofrequency ablation, the same approach as for a stellate ganglion block is used. A curved 20-gauge,

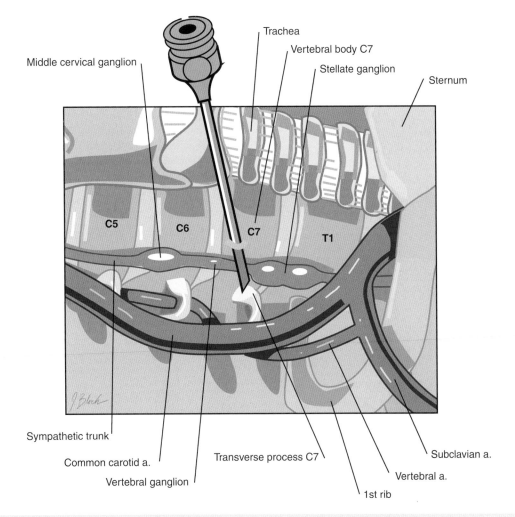

Middle cervical ganglion

Trachea

Vertebral body C7

Stellate ganglion

Sternum

C5 C6 C7 T1

Sympathetic trunk

Common carotid a.

Vertebral ganglion

Transverse process C7

1st rib

Subclavian a.

Vertebral a.

Figure 43-11 Stellate ganglion block. (From Waldman SD. Atlas of Interventional Pain Management, 2nd ed. Philadelphia: WB Saunders, 2004.)

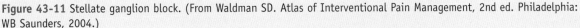

10-cm-long radiofrequency ablation needle with a blunt 5-mm active tip is used to access the ventrolateral aspect of the C7 vertebral body. Needle placement is confirmed by AP and lateral fluoroscopic views, and sensory and motor stimulation is performed. After appropriate stimulation is obtained and negative aspiration for blood or cerebrospinal fluid, 1 mL of local anesthetic solution is injected through the needle, followed by radiofrequency ablation at 80°C for 90 seconds and repeat radiofrequency ablation after turning the needle 180 degrees.

NEUROLYTIC BLOCK
For a neurolytic block, the same approach as for a stellate ganglion block is used. After appropriate response is obtained and negative aspiration for blood, increments of absolute alcohol solution to a total of 5 mL are injected through the needle. The needle is flushed with sterile saline.

Lumbar Sympathetic Block
The lumbar sympathetic ganglia provide sympathetic innervation of the lower extremities. These ganglia usually lie in the space between the anterolateral aspect of the L2 to L5 vertebral bodies and the origin of the psoas muscles. The patient is placed prone. The anterolateral border of the L3 vertebral body is visualized after aligning the inferior end plate and rotating the fluoroscope to place the superior articular process at one third of the inferior end plate. After sterile preparation and draping and administration of a local anesthetic, a 22-gauge, 15-cm-long needle is advanced to the anterolateral aspect of the L3 vertebral body (Fig. 43-12).[13] Needle placement is confirmed with contrast and negative aspiration for blood, and increments of local anesthetic solution to a total of 20 mL are injected through the needle to evaluate clinical response.

VI

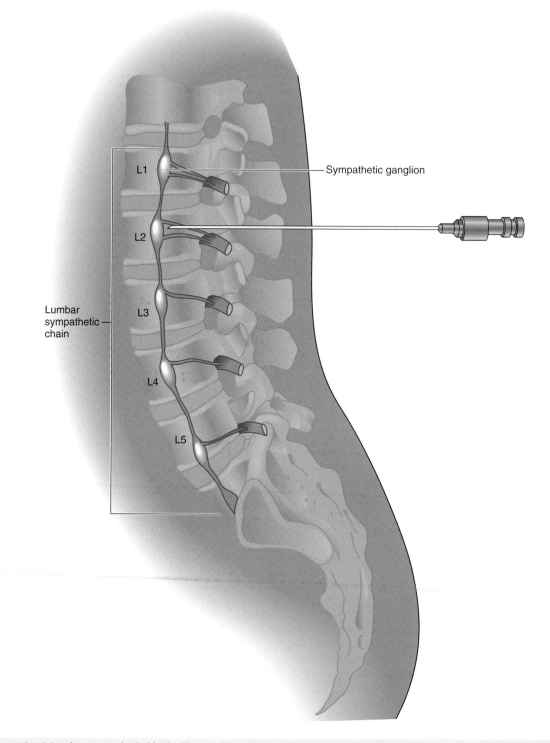

Figure 43-12 Lumbar sympathetic block. (From Waldman SD. Atlas of Interventional Pain Management, 2nd ed. Philadelphia: WB Saunders, 2004.)

Pulse radiofrequency ablation at the L2 to L4 vertebral levels and an alcohol or phenol neurolytic block are indicated if the lumbar sympathetic block provides significant, but transient pain relief.

PULSE RADIOFREQUENCY ABLATION

For pulse radiofrequency ablation, the same approach as for a lumbar sympathetic block is used. A curved 20-gauge, 15-cm-long radiofrequency ablation needle with a blunt 10-mm active tip is advanced to the anterolateral aspect at the inferior third of L2, upper third of L3, and middle third of L4. Needle placement is confirmed by AP and lateral fluoroscopic views, and sensory and motor stimulation is performed. After appropriate stimulation is obtained and negative aspiration for blood, 1 mL of local anesthetic is injected through the needle, followed by radiofrequency ablation at 80°C for 90 seconds and repeat radiofrequency ablation after turning the needle 180 degrees.

NEUROLYTIC BLOCK

For a neurolytic block, the same approach as for a lumbar sympathetic block is used. After an appropriate response is obtained and negative aspiration for blood, increments of absolute alcohol solution to a total of 5 to 10 mL are injected through the needle. The needle is flushed with sterile saline.

Splanchnic Nerve Block

The splanchnic nerves transmit sensory information from the abdominal viscera. A splanchnic nerve block is indi-

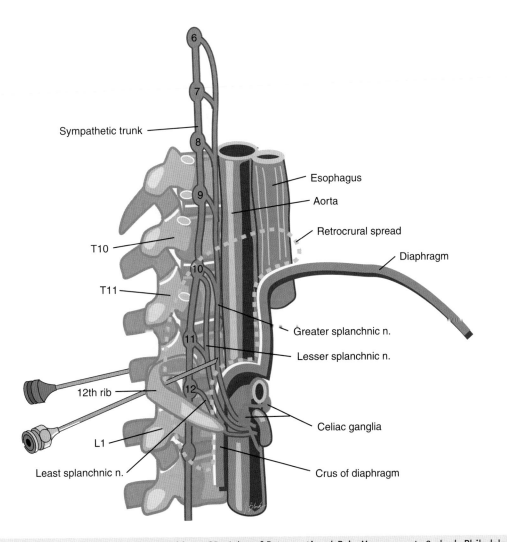

Figure 43-13 Splanchnic nerve block. (From Waldman SD. Atlas of Interventional Pain Management, 2nd ed. Philadelphia: WB Saunders, 2004.)

cated for chronic nonmalignant and malignant abdominal pain. A bolus of intravenous fluid is given preoperatively to attenuate the hypotension associated with a splanchnic nerve block. The patient is placed prone. The junction of the rib and the T12 vertebral body is visualized after aligning the inferior end plate and rotating the fluoroscope to place the superior articular process at one third of the inferior end plate. After sterile preparation and draping and administration of a local anesthetic, a 20-gauge, 15-cm-long needle is advanced to the junction of the anterior third and posterior two thirds of the T12 vertebral body (Fig. 43-13).[13] Needle placement is confirmed with contrast and negative aspiration for blood, and increments of local anesthetic solution to a total of 10 mL are injected through the needle to evaluate clinical response.

Pulse radiofrequency ablation and an alcohol or phenol neurolytic block are indicated if the splanchnic nerve block provides significant, but transient pain relief.

PULSE RADIOFREQUENCY ABLATION

For pulse radiofrequency ablation, the same approach as for a splanchnic nerve block is used. A curved 20-gauge, 15-cm-long radiofrequency ablation needle with a blunt 15-mm active tip is used to access the junction of the anterior third and posterior two thirds of the T12 vertebral body while hugging the middle third of the T12 vertebral body. Needle placement is confirmed by AP and lateral fluoroscopic views, and sensory and motor stimulation is performed. After appropriate stimulation is obtained and negative aspiration for blood, 2 mL of local anesthetic

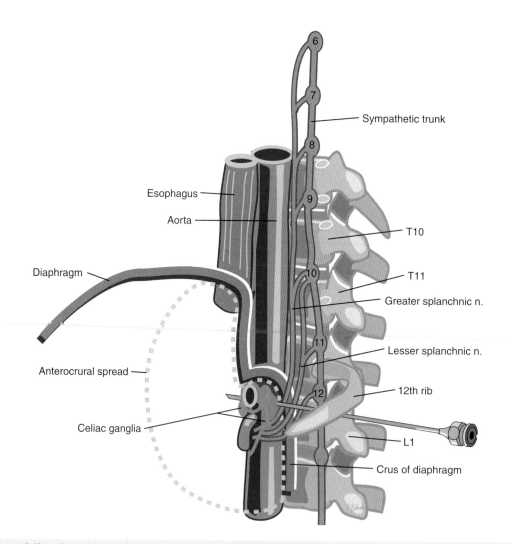

Figure 43-14 Celiac plexus block. (Modified from Waldman SD. Atlas of Interventional Pain Management, 2nd ed. Philadelphia: WB Saunders, 2004.)

solution is injected through the needle, followed by radiofrequency ablation at 80°C for 90 seconds and repeat pulse radiofrequency ablation after turning the needle 180 degrees.

NEUROLYTIC BLOCK

For a neurolytic block, the same approach as for a splanchnic nerve block is used. After appropriate response is obtained and negative aspiration for blood, increments of absolute alcohol solution to a total of 5 to 10 mL are injected through the needle. The needle is flushed with sterile saline.

Celiac Plexus Block

The celiac plexus lies anterior to the aorta at the origin of the celiac artery and is the major postsynaptic ganglia of the splanchnic nerves. The celiac plexus transmits sensory information from the abdominal viscera. A celiac plexus neurolytic block is indicated for malignant abdominal pain. A bolus of intravenous fluid is given preoperatively to attenuate the hypotension associated with a celiac plexus block. The patient is placed prone. The left anterolateral border of the L1 vertebral body is visualized after aligning the inferior end plate and rotating the fluoroscope to place the superior articular process at one third of the inferior end plate. After sterile prepara-

tion and draping and administration of a local anesthetic, a 20-gauge, 15-cm-long needle is advanced to the left anterolateral border of the L1 vertebral body. The needle is advanced to the celiac plexus via either a periaortic or transaortic approach (Fig. 43-14).[13] Needle placement is confirmed with contrast and negative aspiration for blood, and increments of local anesthetic solution to a total of 10 mL are injected through the needle to evaluate clinical response.

An alcohol or phenol neurolytic block is indicated if the celiac plexus block provides significant, but transient pain relief.

NEUROLYTIC BLOCK

For a neurolytic block, the same approach as for a celiac plexus block is used. After an appropriate response is obtained and negative aspiration for blood, increments of absolute alcohol solution to a total of 10 to 20 mL are injected through the needle. The needle is flushed with sterile saline.

Hypogastric Plexus Block

The hypogastric plexus lies anterior to the L5 and S1 vertebral bodies and transmits sensory information from the pelvic viscera. A hypogastric plexus neurolytic block

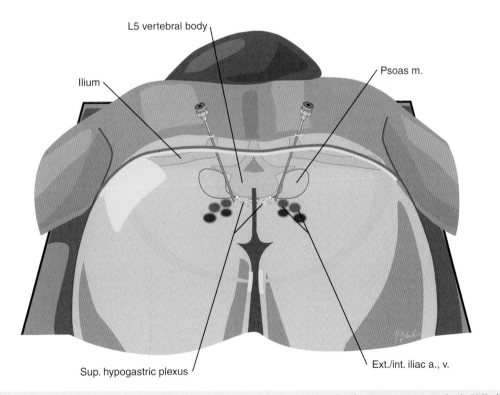

L5 vertebral body

Ilium

Psoas m.

Sup. hypogastric plexus

Ext./int. iliac a., v.

Figure 43-15 Hypogastric plexus block. (From Waldman SD. Atlas of Interventional Pain Management, 2nd ed. Philadelphia: WB Saunders, 2004.)

VI

is indicated for malignant and nonmalignant pelvic pain. The patient is placed prone. The anterolateral border of the L5 vertebral body is visualized after aligning the inferior end plate and rotating the fluoroscope to place the superior articular process at one third of the inferior end plate. After sterile preparation and draping and administration of a local anesthetic, a 20-gauge, 15-cm-long needle is advanced to the anterolateral border of the L5 vertebral body (Fig. 43-15).[13] Needle placement is confirmed with contrast and negative aspiration for blood, and increments of local anesthetic solution to a total of 10 mL are injected through the needle to evaluate clinical response. An alcohol or phenol neurolytic block is indicated if the hypogastric plexus block provides significant, but transient pain relief.

NEUROLYTIC BLOCK

For a neurolytic block, the same approach as for a hypogastric plexus block is used. After appropriate response is obtained and negative aspiration for blood, increments of absolute alcohol to a total of 10 mL are injected through the needle. The needle is flushed with sterile saline.

REFERENCES

1. Schwarzer AC, Aprill CN, Derby R, et al. The prevalence and clinical features of internal disc disruption in patients with chronic low back pain. Spine 1995;20:1878-1883.
2. Schwarzer AC, Aprill CN, Derby R, et al. Clinical features of patients with pain stemming from the lumbar zygapophyseal joints: Is the lumbar facet syndrome a clinical entity? Spine 1994;19:1132-1137.
3. Schwarzer AC, Wang S, Bogduk N, et al. Prevalence and clinical features of lumbar zygapophyseal joint pain: A study in an Australian population with chronic low back pain. Ann Rheum Dis 1995;54:100-106.
4. Manchikanti L, Pampati V, Fellows B, et al. Prevalence of lumbar facet joint pain in chronic low back pain. Pain Phys 1999;2:59-64.
5. Schwarzer AC, Aprill CN, Bogduk N. The sacroiliac joint in chronic low back pain. Spine 1995;20:31-37.
6. Maigne JY, Aivaliklis A, Pfefer F. Results of sacroiliac joint double block and value of sacroiliac pain provocation tests in 54 patients with low back pain. Spine 1996;21:1889-1892.
7. Benoist M. The natural history of lumbar disc herniation and radiculopathy. Joint Bone Spine 2002;69:155-160.
8. Grabias S. Current concepts review: The treatment of spinal stenosis. J Bone Joint Surg Am 1980;62:308-313.
9. Hall S, Bartleson JD, Onofrio BM, et al. Lumbar spinal stenosis: Clinical features, diagnostic procedures, and results of surgical treatment in 68 patients. Ann Intern Med 1985;103:271-275.
10. Tile M, McNeil SR, Zarins RK, et al. Spinal stenosis: Results of treatment. Clin Orthop 1976;115:104-108.
11. Fritsch WE, Heisel J, Rupp S. The failed back surgery syndrome—reasons, intraoperative findings, and long-term results: A report of 182 operative treatments. Spine 1996;21:626-633.
12. Saper JR, Silberstein S, Gordon CD, et al. Handbook of Headache Management: A Practical Guide to Diagnosis and Treatment of Head, Neck, and Facial Pain, 2nd ed. Baltimore: Lippincott, Williams & Wilkins, 1999.
13. Waldman SD. Atlas of Interventional Pain Management, 2nd ed. Philadelphia: WB Saunders, 2004.
14. discTRODE RF Catheter Electrode System, 2002 Radionics, 945612005, 12/02.
15. DISC Nucleoplasty Perc-DLE SpineWand Technique Guide, P/N07452 Rev B, 2002, ArthroCare Corporation.
16. Dekompressor Product Guide, Percutaneous Discectomy Probe, 1000-906-001 Rev. A.
17. Medtronic Pain Therapies Neurostimulation, Patient Information, page 3, UC199400762b EN N12056b, Medtronic, Inc., 2002.
18. Medtronic Pain Therapies Intrathecal Drug Delivery, Patient Information for the SynchroMed and IsoMed Infusion Systems, Figure 8: Pump and catheter placement for intrathecal drug delivery, page 14, UC199603123a EN NP2686a, Medtronic, Inc., 2001.

Chapter 44

CARDIOPULMONARY RESUSCITATION

David Shimabukuro and Linda Liu

Cardiopulmonary resuscitation (CPR) is a term that was first used in the early 1960s by Safar and Kouvenhowen to describe a combined technique of mouth-to-mouth ventilation and closed cardiac chest compressions in a pulseless patient. Since then, significant advances in CPR and life support have been made. Today, the early descriptions of CPR would be considered basic life support (BLS), whereas adult advanced cardiovascular life support (ACLS) and pediatric advanced cardiovascular life support (PALS) include the more sophisticated use of pharmacotherapy and other definitive techniques.

In 1986 the American Heart Association published the first ACLS algorithms in its emergency cardiovascular care (ECC) and CPR guidelines. In 2000, the International Liaison Committee on Resuscitation assembled the first international conference to produce worldwide guidelines for ECC and CPR. Guidelines and algorithms for CPR continue to be revised and updated.[1-3]

THE ABCDs

Interventions described by the letters "ABCD" are vital for successful CPR. For any patient in cardiac arrest, the most important steps are to (1) provide a patent upper airway, (2) maintain the rate of external chest compression near 100 compressions per minute, (3) minimize interruptions in external chest compressions, and (4) provide prompt electrical defibrillation.

Airway

"*A*" represents assessment and opening of the airway, which can be achieved by a simple head tilt–chin lift technique (Fig. 44-1). A jaw thrust maneuver can be used in patients with suspected cervical spine injury. Simple airway devices, such as nasal or oral airways, can be inserted as well to displace the tongue from the posterior oropharynx.

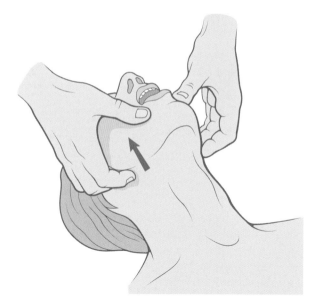

Figure 44-1 The head tilt–jaw thrust maneuver provides a patent upper airway by tensing the muscles attached to the tongue, thus pulling the tongue away from the posterior pharynx. Forward displacement of the mandible is accomplished by grasping the angles of the mandible and lifting with both hands, which serves to displace the mandible forward while tilting the head backward.

Breathing

"*B*" represents assessment and aid, if necessary, of breathing. It includes looking for normal or adequate breathing. If the patient is not breathing effectively or has agonal gasps, the provider should assist the patient's ventilation by using either mouth-to-mouth, mask-to-mouth, or bag-mask ventilation. Two rescue breaths should be given. Each breath should be delivered over a 1-second period and should produce visible chest expansion. Although a recent study showed that effective closed-chest compressions can lead to a small movement of air and ventilation with changing intrathoracic pressure, it is recommended that assisted ventilation be performed by all health care providers, even outside the hospital setting.[4] Care should be taken to avoid rapid or forceful breaths. A normal minute ventilation should be strived for because hyperventilation has proved to be detrimental.

Circulation

"*C*" is for circulation. Because a pulse can be very difficult to assess, it may be necessary to use other clues, such as whether the patient is breathing on his own or moving. The health care provider should take no more than 10 seconds to check for a pulse (most often a carotid pulse).

If the patient has no pulse or no signs of life, chest compressions should be started immediately. The heel of the hand should be placed longitudinally on the lower half of the sternum, between the nipples (Fig. 44-2).[5] The sternum should be depressed 3.75 to 5 cm at a rate of 100 compressions per minute. Complete chest recoil is necessary to allow for venous return and is important for effective CPR. The pattern should be 30 compressions to 2 breaths (30:2 = 1 cycle of CPR) until the airway is secured, regardless of whether one or two rescuers are present. Once the airway is secure, synchronous CPR is no longer necessary. Instead, the compressing rescuer should continue with chest compressions at 100 per minute, and the ventilating rescuer should continue with ventilations at 8 to 10 breaths per minute without pausing for each other.

Defibrillation

"*D*" stands for electrical defibrillation. A defibrillator, preferably an automatic external defibrillator (AED), should be attached immediately to the patient as soon as it becomes available. In unwitnessed arrests, rescuers may give five cycles of CPR before checking the rhythm and attempting defibrillation. In most cases (witnessed arrests, in-hospital setting, or immediately available defibrillator), a defibrillator should be used as soon as it is available. Proper electrode pad placement on the chest wall should be to the right of the upper sternal border below the clavicle and to the left of the nipple with the center in the midaxillary line (Fig. 44-3). Most electrode pads are now clearly labeled and accompanied by diagrams for correct positioning.

ENERGY USED FOR DEFIBRILLATION

The amount of energy (joules) delivered is dependent on the type of defibrillator used. Two major waveform types (monophasic and biphasic) are available. Monophasic waveform defibrillators deliver a unidirectional energy charge, whereas biphasic waveform defibrillators deliver an in-series bidirectional energy charge. Evidence from implantable defibrillators has suggested that bidirectional energy delivery is more successful in the termination of ventricular tachycardia (VT) and ventricular fibrillation (VF). In addition, biphasic waveform shocks require less energy than traditional monophasic waveform shocks do (120 to 200 J with biphasic versus 360 J with monophasic) to terminate cardiac dysrhythmias and may therefore cause less myocardial damage.

TIME TO DEFIBRILLATION

The time until defibrillation is critical to survival, especially since the most frequent initial cardiac rhythm in adult patients is VT/VF. Survival rates after VF cardiac arrest have been shown to decrease by 7% to 10% with every passing minute. If adequate chest compressions are provided,

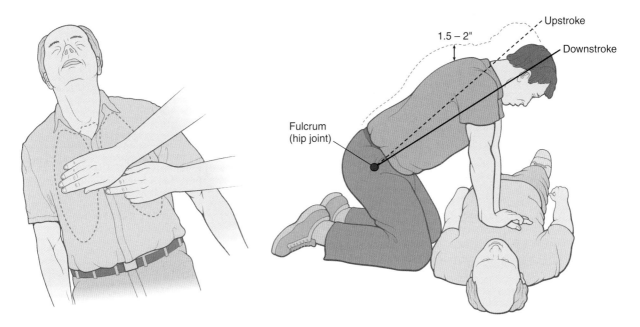

Figure 44-2 Proper hand and body position for performance of closed-chest (external) cardiac compressions in an adult. (From Guidelines for cardiopulmonary resuscitation and emergency cardiac care. JAMA 1999;268:2171-2295, with permission.)

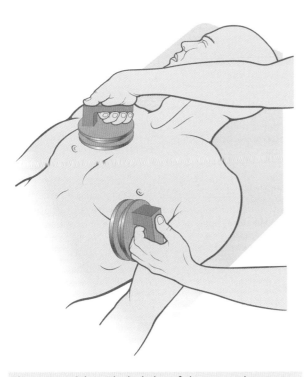

Figure 44-3 Schematic depiction of the proper placement of paddle electrodes in an adult.

this decrease in survival improves to 3% to 4% with every minute of delay until defibrillation.[6]

ALGORITHMS

Three CPR algorithms relevant to the anesthesiologist in the operating room are (1) pulseless cardiac arrest, (2) symptomatic bradycardia, and (3) symptomatic tachycardia (Figs. 44-4 to 44-6).[2,3]

Pulseless Cardiac Arrest

Cardiac dysrhythmias that produce pulseless cardiac arrest are (1) VF, (2) rapid VT, (3) pulseless electrical activity (PEA), and (4) asystole (see Fig. 44-4).[2]

TREATMENT
During pulseless cardiac arrest, the primary goals are to provide effective chest compressions and early defibrillation if the rhythm is VF or VT. Drug administration is of secondary importance because the efficacy of pharmacologic intervention is difficult to document. After initiating CPR and defibrillation, rescuers can then establish intravenous access, obtain a more definitive airway, and consider drug therapy, all while providing continued chest compressions and ventilation. Establishing intravenous

VI

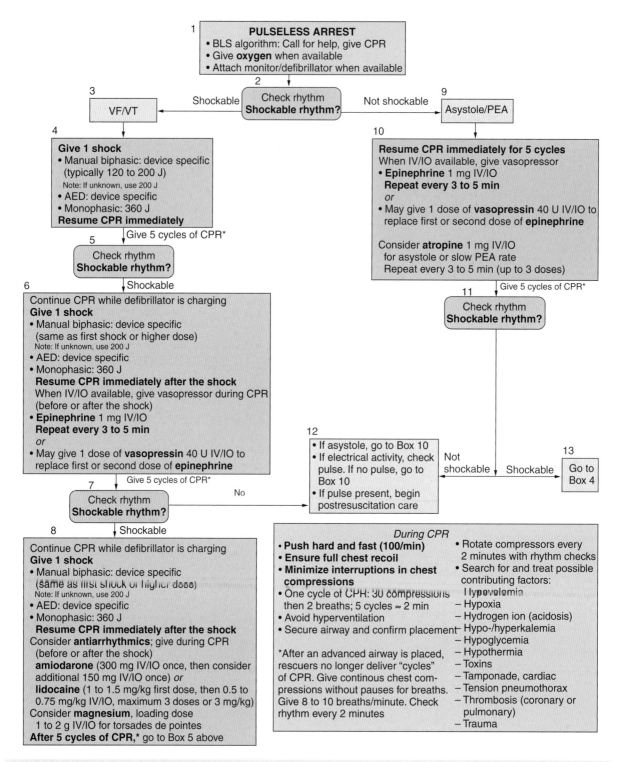

Figure 44-4 Resuscitation algorithm for pulseless arrest. AED, automatic external defibrillator; BLS, basic life support; CPR, cardiopulmonary resuscitation; IO, intraosseous; IV, intravenous; PEA, pulseless electrical activity; VF, ventricular fibrillation; VT, ventricular tachycardia. (From 2005 American Heart Association Guidelines for Cardiopulmonary Resuscitation and Emergency Cardiovascular Care, Part 7.2: Management of cardiac arrest. Circulation 2005;112(Suppl IV):IV-58, ©2005, American Heart Association, with permission.)

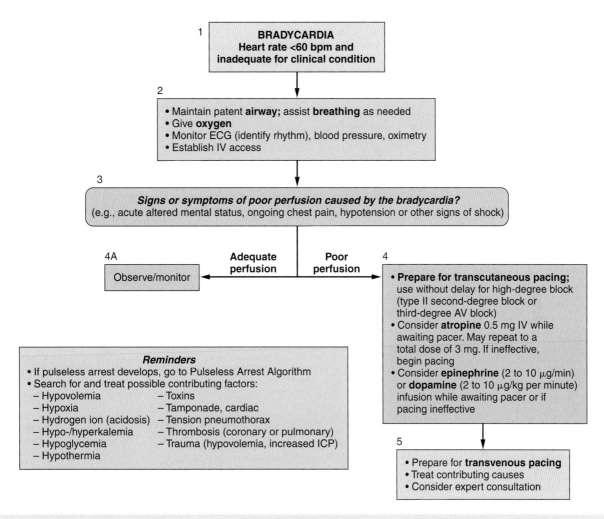

Figure 44-5 Resuscitation algorithm for symptomatic bradycardia. AV, atrioventricular; ECG, electrocardiogram; ICP, intracranial pressure; IV, intravenous. (From 2005 American Heart Association Guidelines for Cardiopulmonary Resuscitation and Emergency Cardiovascular Care, Part 7.3: Management of symptomatic bradycardia and tachycardia. Circulation 2005;112(Suppl IV):IV-68, ©2005, American Heart Association, with permission.)

access is important, but it should not interfere with CPR and defibrillation. A large peripheral venous catheter is sufficient in most resuscitations.

Drugs

Drugs should be administered by bolus injection and followed with a 20-mL fluid bolus if given peripherally. If intravenous access cannot be obtained, certain drugs (epinephrine, lidocaine, vasopressin, atropine, naloxone) can be given via the endotracheal tube. The endotracheal tube dose is 2 to 2.5 times the recommended intravenous dose, and the drug should be diluted in 5 to 10 mL of water or saline before instillation down the endotracheal tube.

Airway Management

Bag-mask ventilation and ventilation through an advanced airway (endotracheal tube, Combitube, or laryngeal mask airway) are acceptable methods of ventilation during CPR. Because chest compressions are not performed during tracheal intubation, the rescuer has to weigh the need for compressions against the need for definitive airway management. It is not unreasonable to defer insertion of an advanced airway until after the patient fails to respond to CPR and defibrillation.

If a more definitive airway has been established, the adequacy of ventilation should be evaluated again. The chest should rise bilaterally and breath sounds should be auscultated. In addition, proper positioning of the endo-

VI

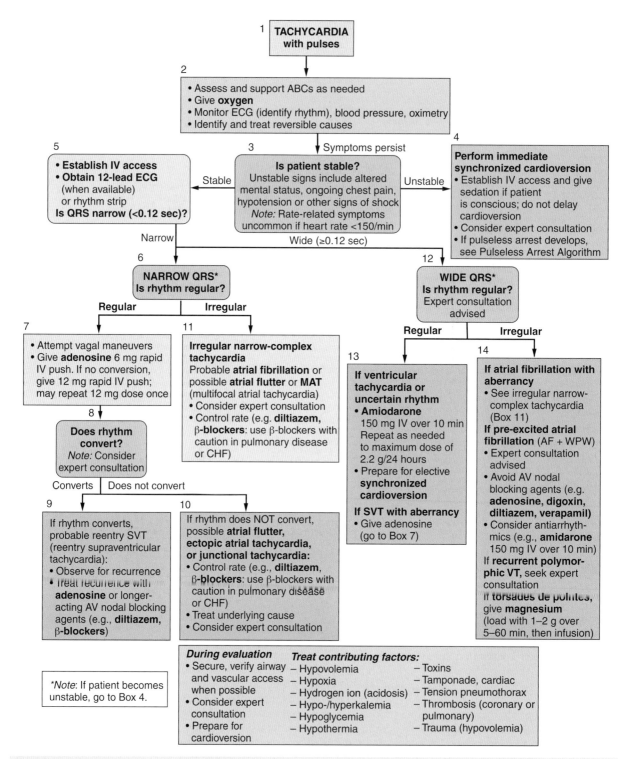

Figure 44-6 Resuscitation algorithm for symptomatic tachycardia. AF, atrial fibrillation; AV, atrioventricular; CHF, congestive heart failure; ECG, electrocardiogram; IV, intravenous; SVT, supraventricular tachycardia; VT, ventricular tachycardia; WPW, Wolff-Parkinson-White. (From 2005 American Heart Association Guidelines for Cardiopulmonary Resuscitation and Emergency Cardiovascular Care, Part 7.3: Management of symptomatic bradycardia and tachycardia. Circulation 2005;112(Suppl IV):IV-70, ©2005, American Heart Association, with permission.)

tracheal tube should be confirmed with a second test to decrease false positives and false negatives. Capnography to measure end-tidal carbon dioxide is the most ideal test. However, outside the operating room and emergency department, this can be difficult. Small portable capnographs may not be readily available. Alternative tests include pH paper (color change) and an esophageal detector device (EDD). An EDD involves using a bulb suction that is attached to the end of the endotracheal tube once the bulb is compressed. If the endotracheal tube is in the trachea, the bulb quickly inflates from the air in the lungs because the tracheal rings are stiff and do not collapse around the tube. If the endotracheal tube is in the esophagus, the esophageal walls, which are pliable, oppose around the end of the endotracheal tube, and the bulb remains in the compressed state.

Once the endotracheal tube is confirmed to be in the trachea, it should be secured in place. Specific devices are commercially available for this task, but tape can work just as well. Failed resuscitation may reflect migration of the endotracheal tube out of the trachea during chest compressions or transport of the patient (or both). If continuous end-tidal carbon dioxide monitoring is not available, tube placement should be checked periodically, especially during prolonged resuscitation.

Ventricular Fibrillation/Ventricular Tachycardia

If the pulseless cardiac arrest was witnessed, the health care provider should immediately place the defibrillator pads on the patient's chest, determine the rhythm, and deliver a shock if VF or VT is present (see Fig. 44-4).[2] If the arrest was not witnessed, the provider may give five cycles of CPR before defibrillation. CPR should be resumed immediately after delivery of the shock and continued for five cycles or about 2 minutes. Cardiac rhythm should then be re-evaluated. If the patient remains in VF/VT, the defibrillator should be charged to the appropriate energy level (360 J for monophasic or 120 to 200 J for biphasic) while CPR is still being performed.

DRUGS

If VF or VT persists after one to two sets of CPR-defibrillation-CPR-defibrillation, a vasopressor should be given (Table 44-1). Epinephrine, 1 mg IV, may be administered every 3 to 5 minutes. One dose of vasopressin, 40 units IV, may replace either the first or second dose of epinephrine. Drug administration should be timed to minimize interruptions in chest compressions. If VF/VT persists after another set of CPR-defibrillation and vasopressor administration, an antidysrhythmic medication should be given. Amiodarone and lidocaine are recommended for VF/VT, whereas magnesium should be considered for torsades de pointes.

Asystole and Pulseless Electrical Activity

Asystole is usually an agonal rhythm, whereas PEA is often caused by a reversible condition and can be treated if the inciting cause is identified (Table 44-2). These two cardiac rhythms have been combined as the second part of the Pulseless Arrest algorithm because of similarities in their management (see Fig. 44-4).[2] Neither will benefit from defibrillation, so the focus should be on performing effective CPR with minimal interruptions, identifying reversible causes, and establishing an advanced airway (see Table 44-1).

A vasopressor may be administered after initiation of CPR. Epinephrine, 1 mg IV, may be given every 3 to 5 minutes. Alternatively, a single dose of vasopressin, 40 units IV, may replace either the first or second dose of epinephrine. Atropine, 1 mg IV, may be given to patients with asystole or slow PEA. Cardiac rhythm checks should be performed after every five cycles or 2 minutes of CPR. If an organized cardiac rhythm is present, the rescuer should check for a pulse. If there is no pulse, CPR should be continued. If a pulse is present, the rescuer should identify the rhythm and treat accordingly. Given the poor survival and neurologic recovery of patients in asystole, the length and effort of resuscitation should be carefully considered.

Bradycardia

Bradycardia is defined as a heart rate lower than 60 beats/min (see Fig. 44-5).[3] Some patients, especially young athletes, may have a resting heart rate lower than 60 beats/min yet continue to exhibit signs of adequate perfusion. Asymptomatic patients do not require treatment. Intervention by pharmacologic treatment or electrical pacing should be based on signs and symptoms of inadequate perfusion. Symptoms cannot be obtained under anesthesia, so the anesthesiologist should use discretion in determining whether end-organ perfusion is compromised by the slow heart rate.

TREATMENT

Initial treatment of symptomatic bradycardia should focus on support of airway, breathing, and circulation. Supplemental oxygen should be delivered, and continuous cardiac rhythm, systemic blood pressure, and pulse oximetry should be monitored. Further therapies include transcutaneous pacing (especially if a type II second-degree heart block or third-degree atrioventricular [AV] heart block is present), atropine (0.5 mg IV every 3 to 5 minutes), or infusion of epinephrine or dopamine.

Tachycardia with Pulse

Regardless of the underlying origin of the tachycardia, unstable or symptomatic patients should be immediately shocked via synchronized cardioversion (see Fig. 44-6).[3]

VI

Table 44–1   Drugs Used During Adult Cardiopulmonary Resuscitation

Drug Name	Dose	Indication
Adenosine	6 mg by IV push May repeat 12 mg by IV push	For stable narrow QRS tachycardia (contraindicated with pre-excitation syndrome)
Amiodarone	300 mg IV Additional 150 mg IV if necessary 150 mg IV over a 10-minute period Repeat as needed until a maximum dose of 2.2 g/24 hr	For pulseless VT/VF For stable VT or uncertain wide QRS tachycardia and narrow QRS tachycardias
Atropine*	1 mg IV Repeat every 3 to 5 minutes (up to 3 doses) 0.5 mg IV May repeat to a total dose of 3 mg	For asystole or slow PEA For bradycardia
Diltiazem	15 to 20 mg (0.25 mg/kg) IV over a 2-minute period May repeat in 15 minutes at 20-25 mg/kg (0.35 mg/kg) Maintenance infusion of 5-15 mg/hr, titrate to heart rate	For stable narrow QRS tachycardia (contraindicated with pre-excitation syndrome)
Dopamine	2 to 10 µg/kg/min by infusion	For bradycardia while awaiting a pacer or if a pacer is ineffective
Epinephrine*	1 mg IV Repeat every 3 to 5 minutes 2 to 10 µg/min by infusion	For pulseless cardiac arrest For bradycardia while awaiting a pacer or if a pacer is ineffective
Esmolol	0.5 mg/kg IV load, followed by an infusion at 0.05 mg/kg/min Repeat the 0.5-mg/kg bolus and increase the infusion to 0.1 mg/kg/min Max infusion, 0.3 mg/kg/min	For stable narrow QRS tachycardias (contraindicated with pre-excitation syndrome)
Lidocaine*	1 to 1.5 mg/kg IV Then 0.5 mg to 0.75 mg/kg IV/IO Maximum, 3 doses or 3 mg/kg	For pulseless VT/VF
Magnesium	1 to 2 g IV	For torsades de pointes
Metoprolol	5 mg IV Repeat every 5 minutes Maximum dose, 15 mg	For stable narrow QRS tachycardias (contraindicated with pre-excitation syndrome)
Vasopressin*	40 U IV	To replace the first or second dose of epinephrine in pulseless VT/VF, asystole, or PEA
Verapamil	2.5 to 5 mg IV over a 2-minute period Repeat 5 to 10 mg over a 15- to 30-minute period Maximum dose, 20 mg	For stable narrow QRS tachycardia (contraindicated with pre-excitation syndrome)

*Also effective by tracheal mucosal absorption when administered through an endotracheal tube.
IV, intravenous; IO, intra-osseous; PEA, pulseless electrical activity; VF, ventricular fibrillation; VT, ventricular tachycardia.

In stable patients with fast ventricular rates, determining whether the underlying rhythm has a narrow or wide QRS complex (>0.12 second) on the electrocardiogram is important. Patients with symptomatic tachycardias, especially those with wide-complex tachycardias, should be evaluated by a consultant to help determine whether the rhythm is ventricular in origin or atrial in origin with aberrant conduction. Treatment should be guided by the consultant's opinion but includes the use of antidysrhythmic medication or AV nodal blocking drugs.

Table 44–2	Causes of Pulseless Electrical Activity
Five "H's"	
Hypovolemia	
Hypoxia	
Hydrogen (acidosis)	
Hyperkalemia/hypoglycemia/hypokalemia	
Hypothermia	
"T's"	
Tablets/toxins	
Tamponade	
Tension pneumothorax	
Thrombosis (coronary or pulmonary)	
Trauma (hypovolemia)	

NARROW-COMPLEX TACHYCARDIA

If the rhythm is an irregular narrow-complex tachycardia, the underlying rhythm is probably atrial fibrillation, and heart rate control should be attempted with AV nodal blocking drugs. If the rhythm is a regular narrow-complex tachycardia, conversion should be attempted by vagal maneuvers or the administration of adenosine, or both. Cardiac rhythm conversion signifies probable reentry supraventricular tachycardia, and recurrence can be treated with adenosine or longer-acting AV nodal blocking drugs. If cardiac rhythm conversion does not occur, the underlying rhythm is possibly atrial flutter or junctional tachycardia. Effort should be made to achieve rate control with the use of AV nodal blocking drugs.

DRUG THERAPY

Epinephrine, vasopressin, and amiodarone are the most commonly used drugs in ACLS algorithms (see Table 44-1).

Epinephrine

Epinephrine is a combined direct α- and β-receptor agonist. It is dysrhythmogenic and known to increase myocardial oxygen consumption by increasing heart rate and cardiac afterload. Although it has never been proved to be effective in a randomized double-blinded placebo-controlled trial, in multiple animal studies epinephrine has shown to be of benefit in establishing return of spontaneous circulation. Epinephrine can increase diastolic pressure and thereby restore coronary perfusion pressure and blood flow back to the myocardium. High-dose epinephrine results in a higher rate of return of spontaneous circulation, but there is no improvement in the rate of hospital discharge after cardiac arrest.[7]

Vasopressin

Vasopressin is a naturally occurring antidiuretic hormone with a half-time of 10 to 20 minutes. It is a nonadrenergic peripheral vasoconstrictor that acts by direct stimulation of smooth muscle vasopressin-1 receptors and thus leads to intense vasoconstriction of the vasculature in the skin, skeletal muscles, intestine, and fat. Vasopressin has also been found in animals to selectively vasodilate the cerebral, coronary, and pulmonary vascular beds. Like epinephrine, vasopressin is believed to increase diastolic pressure and therefore increase coronary perfusion pressure with restoration of blood flow to the myocardium. Given its relatively long half-time, it is recommended that vasopressin be given only once during resuscitation for VF and VT.

There are no significant differences in rates of hospital admission or survival between patients with out-of-hospital VF/VT or PEA who receive vasopressin or epinephrine. When compared with epinephrine in patients with asystole, vasopressin is associated with higher rates of hospital admission and hospital discharge, but neurologically intact survival is not different between treatment groups.[8] Because the effects of vasopressin and epinephrine in patients with cardiac arrest have not been shown to be significantly different, one dose of vasopressin may substitute for either the first or second dose of epinephrine in the treatment of pulseless cardiac arrest.

Amiodarone

Amiodarone was initially developed as an antianginal drug in the 1950s but was abandoned because of its side effects. Because it has effects on cardiac sodium and potassium channels, as well as α- and β-receptors, amiodarone has been reinvestigated for its antidysrhythmic effects. In this regard, amiodarone prolongs repolarization and refractoriness in the sinoatrial node, the atrial and ventricular myocardium, the AV node, and the His-Purkinje cardiac conduction system. Amiodarone can exacerbate or induce dysrhythmias, especially torsades de pointes. This drug may also interact with volatile anesthetics to produce heart block, profound vasodilation, myocardial depression, and severe hypotension. Increases in the effects of oral anticoagulants, phenytoin, digoxin, and diltiazem may occur.

Despite its multiple disadvantages, amiodarone has been shown in adults with out-of-hospital VF/VT arrest to improve survival to hospital admission when compared with placebo and lidocaine.[9,10] The recommended dose of amiodarone for VF/VT is 300 mg IV, with an additional dose of 150 mg IV for persistent VF/VT.

PEDIATRIC ADVANCED LIFE SUPPORT

Resuscitation of infants and children follows the same basic principles as those for adults. It is important to remember that most pediatric cardiac events are a result of arterial hypoxemia and respiratory compromise. Thus, airway management and breathing are critical to successful pediatric resuscitation. In contrast, adults tend to experience cardiac arrest as a result of VT or VF secondary to myocardial ischemia, and defibrillation is the more important early intervention.

BLS has many differences between adult and pediatric patients because of the smaller size of the latter. For the health care provider, infants are considered to be younger than 1 year, whereas children are considered to be between 1 year old and adolescence. Adult resuscitation guidelines can be used for adolescent children (Table 44-3).

Airway

The airway of pediatric patients is slightly different than that of an adult, but head tilt–chin lift is still the technique of choice to open the airway. Children tend to have a larger tongue and epiglottis in relation to their mouth and larynx. In addition, they have a larger head in relation to their body. Overextension or excessive flexion of the head can lead to difficulty visualizing the glottic opening during direct laryngoscopy. Straight laryngo-

Table 44-3 Comparative Resuscitation Techniques between Adults, Children, and Infants

	Adult	Child (1 Year to Adolescence)	Infant (<1 year)*
Airway Management		Head tilt–chin lift Jaw thrust if trauma suspected	
Check breathing		Adequate breathing within 10 seconds	
Rescue breaths		Two breaths, each over 1 second Enough volume to produce visible chest rise	
Rescue breathing rate		10 to 12 breaths/min 12 to 20 breaths/min	
Pulse check		Carotid or femoral	Brachial or femoral
Chest compression method	Two hands Lower half of the sternum, in the center	One or two hands Compress at the nipple line	Two fingers on the sternum Just below the nipple line
Chest compression depth	3.75 to 5 cm Allow complete chest recoil	About 1/3 to 1/2 the depth of the chest	
Chest compression rate		100 compressions/min	
Compression-ventilation ratio	30:2	30:2 (one rescuer) 15:2 (two rescuers)	
Automatic external defibrillator	Recommended with adult pads	Recommended with a pediatric dose attenuator system (if not available, a standard external defibrillator is acceptable)	No recommendations
Sequence for lone rescuer and unwitnessed arrest	Call for help Obtain an external defibrillator Provide CPR Use the external defibrillator	CPR first Call for help after 5 cycles or 2 minutes of CPR	

*Excludes newborns.
CPR, cardiopulmonary resuscitation.

scope blades may be preferred over curved blades to lift the epiglottis anteriorly and away from the glottic opening in young children.

Circulation

Pulse checks and closed chest compressions are performed slightly differently than in an adult. In adults and children, the pulse is palpated at the carotid or femoral artery, whereas in infants, the pulse is checked at the brachial or femoral artery.

External Compressions

In a child, the heel of one or both hands should be placed on the lower half of the sternum, between the nipples, while keeping the fingers off the rib cage and staying above the xiphoid process. In an infant, chest compressions are delivered via the two-finger or two-thumb–encircling hands technique. Two fingers of one hand are placed over the lower half of the sternum approximately one finger's width below the intermammary line while keeping above the xiphoid process. For both infants and children, the sternum should be depressed one third to one half the anterior-posterior diameter of the chest at a rate of at least 100 compressions per minute. The pattern should be 30 compressions to 2 breaths (30:2) if there is a single rescuer and 15 compressions to 2 breaths (15:2) if there are at least two rescuers.

Defibrillation

In children, defibrillation should be performed when a pulseless rhythm (VT, VF) is present. An initial energy of 2 J/kg should be attempted, regardless of the waveform type. Subsequent defibrillations should be delivered at 4 J/kg. Biphasic external defibrillators can be used in children older than 1 year outside the hospital setting. American Heart Association guidelines recommend the use of a pediatric dose attenuator system that will decrease the amount of delivered energy. If one is not available, a standard external defibrillator can be substituted.

Drugs

Most drug dosages are calculated by using current known weight or ideal body weight based on height. Most pediatric units have resuscitation carts divided by weight to facilitate drug administration in an emergency so that calculations do not need to be performed and valuable time wasted.

POSTRESUSCITATION CARE

After successful resuscitation with return of spontaneous circulation and a stable cardiac rhythm, patients should be admitted to the intensive care unit for further definitive treatment or close hemodynamic monitoring, or both. It is not uncommon for vasopressors and inotropes to be administered during the immediate postresuscitation period because of the presence of myocardial stunning and hemodynamic instability. Central venous access for drug administration may be necessary, along with an intra-arterial catheter to facilitate hemodynamic monitoring.

Mild Hypothermia

Temperature should be monitored closely, and hyperthermia should be avoided. Mild hypothermia for the first 24 hours may be beneficial to the neurologic recovery of patients after out-of-hospital VF/VT arrest.[11,12] It is recommended that patients successfully resuscitated from out-of-hospital VF/VT arrest who are comatose be cooled to 32°C to 34°C for the first 12 to 24 hours. Hypothermia has not been well studied in patients with an initial rhythm of asystole or PEA.

Glucose Levels

Elevated blood glucose concentrations after resuscitation from cardiac arrest have been associated with poor neurologic outcome, but studies have not shown that control of serum glucose levels alters outcome. Glucose levels after resuscitation should be monitored closely to avoid hypoglycemia and hyperglycemia, but additional studies are needed before recommendations can be made for the precise glucose levels that require insulin therapy in patients after cardiac arrest.

Normocapnia

Hyperventilation has not been shown to protect the brain or other vital organs after resuscitation from cardiac arrest. There is evidence that iatrogenic hyperventilation of the resuscitated patient's lungs can lead to increased airway pressure, intrinsic positive end-expiratory pressure ("auto-PEEP"), increased intrathoracic pressure, and increased intracranial pressure. In patients with brain injury, hyperventilation may worsen the neurologic outcome. Because no data support targeting a specific $PaCO_2$ after resuscitation, ventilation to normocapnic levels is recommended.

VI

REFERENCES

1. American Heart Association Guidelines for Cardiopulmonary Resuscitation and Emergency Cardiovascular Care, Part 4: Adult basic life support. Circulation 2005;112(Suppl IV):IV-18-IV-34.

2. American Heart Association Guidelines for Cardiopulmonary Resuscitation and Emergency

Cardiovascular Care, Part 7.2: Management of cardiac arrest. Circulation 2005;112(Suppl IV): IV-57-IV-66.

3. American Heart Association Guidelines for Cardiopulmonary Resuscitation and Emergency Cardiovascular Care, Part 7.3: Management of symptomatic bradycardia and tachycardia. Circulation 2005;112(Suppl IV): IV-67-IV-77.

4. Berg RA, Kern KB, Hilwig RW, et al. Assisted ventilation during "bystander" CPR in a swine acute myocardial infarction model does not improve outcome. Circulation 1997;96:1364-1371.

5. Guidelines for cardiopulmonary resuscitation and emergency cardiac care. JAMA 1999;268:2171-2295.

6. Valenzuela TD, Roe DJ, Cretin S, et al. Estimating effectiveness of cardiac arrest interventions: A logistic regression survival model. Circulation 1997;96:3308-3313.

7. Gueugniaud PY, Mols P, Goldstein P, et al. A comparison of repeated high doses and repeated standard doses of epinephrine for cardiac arrest outside the hospital. European Epinephrine Study Group. N Engl J Med 1998;339:1595-1601.

8. Wenzel V, Krismer AC, Arntz HR, et al. A comparison of vasopressin and epinephrine for out-of-hospital cardiopulmonary resuscitation. N Engl J Med 2004;350:105-113.

9. Kudenchuk PJ, Cobb LA, Copass MK, et al. Amiodarone for resuscitation after out-of-hospital cardiac arrest due to ventricular fibrillation. N Engl J Med 1999;341:871-878.

10. Dorian P, Cass D, Schwartz B, et al. Amiodarone as compared with lidocaine for shock-resistant ventricular fibrillation. N Engl J Med 2002;346:884-890.

11. Mild therapeutic hypothermia to improve the neurologic outcome after cardiac arrest. N Engl J Med 2002;346:549-556.

12. Bernard SA, Gray TW, Buist MD, et al. Treatment of comatose survivors of out-of-hospital cardiac arrest with induced hypothermia. N Engl J Med 2002;346:557-563.

Chapter 45

MEDICAL DIRECTION IN THE OPERATING ROOM

Jeffrey A. Katz, Eric Huczko, and J. Renee Navarro

The operating room (OR) is a unique and dynamic environment that is responsible for a substantial and significant source of revenue for hospitals.[1] However, ORs are resource intensive and incur significant costs in staffing and materials. Hospital administrations have focused their attention on the contribution margin or profitability that emanates from the OR service, and this emphasis has led to rapid growth and the need for structured management in the OR. Because medical needs and regulatory requirements are constantly changing, the concept of appointing a medical director in the OR has gained acceptance. This chapter will review the OR management structure and the complexities involved in OR function and the process involved in improving OR efficiency. Prior to delving into these OR management issues, we review some practical considerations facing the anesthesiologist.

ANESTHESIA PRACTICE

Modern-day anesthesia practice requires that the anesthesiologist fulfill and meet the expectations of patients, health care facilities, payers, and regulatory agencies.

Credentialing Process and Clinical Privileges

The process of credentialing health care professionals involves verifying the appropriate education, training, and experience of the candidate and identifying providers who fail to disclose adverse past experiences. The intense scrutiny at the time of appointment is a result of public and political pressure by various regulatory and licensing agencies requiring health care institutions to discover and remove fraudulent and incompetent health care providers whose histories show repeated poor patient outcomes.

Privileges to administer anesthesia must be formally granted and delineated in writing. Examples of such privileges are available from the American Society of Anesthesiologists (ASA).[2] An important question in procedure-oriented specialties such as anesthesiology is whether it is reasonable to grant "blanket" privileges, in effect authorizing the practitioner to provide any treatment or procedure normally considered within the purview of the applicant's medical specialty. In this regard, many institutions are moving toward granting procedure-specific privileges. Examples in anesthesia practice include intraoperative transesophageal echocardiography, performance of neurolytic celiac plexus blocks, and surgical implantation of pain management devices.

Each department or institution should develop methods to determine whether the skills of the provider are appropriate for the privileges requested and that patient safety is ensured. Regular review of these skills should be performed and all morbidity and mortality carefully assessed. Anesthesiologists must periodically (biannually) renew their clinical privileges. Renewal of clinical privileges is no longer automatic; careful checking of the renewal application and awareness of relevant peer review information are mandatory.

Policy and Procedure Manual

Each department or institution is required to have a policy and procedure manual that contains organizational and procedural elements. The organizational component of this manual includes a clear explanation of who is responsible for specific functions along with attendant detail such as expectations for the practitioner's clinical and administrative responsibilities. Also included in this section are details concerning orientation and proctoring of new providers, introducing new equipment, and continuing medical education requirements.

The procedural component of the manual provides helpful practice guides (anesthesia machine checkout as suggested by the Food and Drug Administration) and other specific information for particular circumstances (policy on blood transfusion for Jehovah's Witnesses), Standards, guidelines, and statements developed by the ASA and the Joint Commission on Accreditation of Healthcare Organizations (JCAHO) are often included in a policy and procedure manual (Table 45-1).[2,3]

Typically, policy and procedure manuals are reviewed and updated as needed, with a particularly thorough review preceding each JCAHO inspection. Ideally, each member of the department of anesthesia should review the manual on appointment and after major updates to be familiar with the ever-changing practices in the organization.

INFORMED CONSENT

Informed consent is a clinical and legal expectation and an important aspect of risk management. Most institutions require that patients sign an operative consent

Table 45-1 Examples of Statements Included in a Policy and Procedure Manual

Preanesthesia evaluation
Immediate preinduction reevaluation
Safety of the patient during the anesthetic period
Recording of all pertinent events during anesthesia
Release of the patient from the postanesthesia care unit
Recording of postanesthesia visits
Guidelines defining the role of anesthesia services in hospital infection control

form, but few mandate the use of a separate document for anesthesia consent. Although the consent form has value, informed consent should be viewed as a process rather than merely a signature on the form.

The elements of informed consent include discussions with the patient (and family/guardian if applicable), review of the risks and benefits of the proposed anesthesia plan of care, review of the alternatives, and the reason that the proposed plan is recommended. The standard for disclosing risk now centers on the concept of "material risk," or a risk that a physician knows or ought to know would be significant to a reasonable person in the patient's position on deciding whether to submit to the proposed medical treatment or procedure. There are no firm guidelines for anesthesia informed consent, although it is wise to state that all anesthesia procedures have some risk, including a risk for injury and death, just as crossing the street or riding in a car does. Statistics regarding the incidence of rare complications can be cited. Patients can identify with these analogies. Any special risk dependent on the patient's medical or surgical condition should be discussed in more detail. The patient should have an opportunity to ask questions and raise concerns. Finally, these elements of the discussion and the proposed plan should be documented in the medical record.

When a patient is unable to consent, the anesthesiologist should determine whether there is a conservator or whether the patient has completed a durable power of attorney for health care; the person who has the durable power of attorney serves to represent the patient's wishes and has the authority to provide consent.

Do Not Resuscitate

A special challenge with respect to informed consent is perioperative management of a patient with a "do-not-resuscitate" (DNR) order. Typically, a DNR order is rescinded when the patient is scheduled for surgery. Because of patient autonomy, the surgeon and anesthesiologist should discuss with the patient whether the DNR order will be removed or remain active during the procedure. If there is agreement to maintain the DNR order, it is essential that all providers agree and clarify with the patient (and family) in writing exactly what care will be provided should an untoward event occur.

OPERATING ROOM MANAGEMENT DECISIONS

Guiding principles in OR management decisions should be sufficiently clear and consistent to produce an environment that is safe, effective, and efficient. In order of priority, these principles include (1) ensuring patient safety and the highest quality of care; (2) providing surgeons with access to the OR; (3) maximizing the efficiency of OR utilization, staff, and materials to reduce costs; (4) decreasing patient delays; and (5) enhancing satisfaction among patients, staff, and physicians (Table 45-2).[4] These ordered priorities are sufficient to specify how cases are scheduled and sequenced in each OR, how staff members are assigned on the day of surgery, how OR time is allocated/released, and how urgent cases are completed on the day of surgery.

MEDICAL DIRECTOR

Historically, nurses have been in charge of ORs, but because of the frequent need to base decisions on medical judgment, it may be more effective to have a physician as the medical director. This individual provides leadership and organizational skills within the OR environment and brings nurses, anesthesiologists, surgeons, and hospital administrators together, often through the OR committee, to provide for safe and efficient patient care (Fig. 45-1).[5]

Qualifications

The medical director should be a senior-level physician with excellent clinical skills who can command the respect of peers. This individual must have intimate knowledge of the OR environment, experience in administration, knowledge of information systems, and preferably some training in business management. An effective medical director will display flexibility and receptiveness to new ideas and possess excellent interpersonal skills for defining priorities and negotiating conflict.

An anesthesiologist may be uniquely qualified to function as medical director of the ORs because of the inherent clinical relationship with nursing and the various surgical specialties, as well as an understanding of the overall needs of ORs. Anesthesiologists are present for and have the most complete understanding of the perioperative process (preoperative, intraoperative, and postoperative care) and can make these processes function as a single unit. Typically, anesthesiologists are readily available to the ORs during the day and can intervene when an urgent situation arises.

Responsibilities

The medical director in collaboration with the OR nursing manager ensures that nursing staff levels are sufficient and service-specific training is addressed. Management of access to the OR is critical. Ongoing evaluation of the total number of rooms (including off-site anesthetizing locations), hours of operation, and their assignment to various services represents a significant responsibility for the medical director. The director must work collaboratively to define OR demands based on the scope of services offered and the needs for emergency access to the ORs. Ongoing analysis of OR utilization, backlog of elective surgical cases, and ease of scheduling hospitalized patients for surgery will help guide changes in the assignment of scheduling time to individual surgical services.

The medical director must provide leadership through participation and implementation of regulations governing the safe functioning of the ORs. The director should facilitate a supportive work environment that encourages active participation in the evaluation and improvement of processes to enhance patient safety, patient flow, and satisfaction of the entire OR department.

SCHEDULING OF SURGICAL PROCEDURES

Proper scheduling of cases, including the needed level of staffing and the availability of equipment and instruments, is perhaps the most important part of running an efficient surgical enterprise. An inaccurate schedule that is revised with substitutions on the day of surgery may decrease the efficiency of the system and increase costs.

Most ORs have evolved from handwritten schedules to a computerized scheduling system. Such systems verify the availability of specialized equipment or other resource needs to prevent overbooking of items such as micro-

Table 45-2	Guiding Principles for Operating Room Management
Promote patient safety and provide the highest quality of care
Provide surgeons with access to operating room time
Maximize the efficiency of operating room utilization (staff and materials)
Decrease patient delays
Enhance professional satisfaction

VI

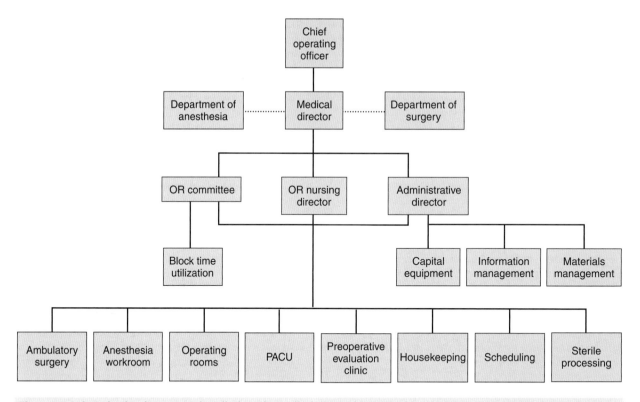

Figure 45-1 Organizational structure that displays the medical director's relationship within the perioperative arena. The *solid vertical lines* indicate direct reporting relationships; the *dashed horizontal lines* imply a collaborative relationship. OR, operating room; PACU, postanesthesia care unit.

scopes, C-arm machines, or neuromonitoring personnel. Surgical case duration is also important because it has a great impact on the predicted start of subsequent procedures in the same operating room. Most systems provide an ongoing average of surgical case duration that is surgeon specific. Anesthesia services are also needed outside the OR (see Chapter 37). To properly apportion and prioritize anesthesia resources, virtual ORs are designated in the computerized scheduling system to permit scheduling of these "out of OR cases."

Open-Block System

Historically, scheduling of surgical cases was under an open-block system in which surgeons were granted OR time on a first-come basis. This approach works when competition for OR time is minimal and all operations could be performed in any OR. However, today, specialty-specific surgical care often has its own equipment needs that are not readily interchangeable. Moving complex equipment from one OR to another is inefficient. In addition, regardless of specialty, it is more convenient for surgeons to schedule several cases sequentially in the same OR. Such sequential scheduling is extremely difficult in a completely open scheduling system, especially as competition for OR time increases. Furthermore, the open-block system often results in high cancellation rates, long waiting lines, and disparity between OR utilization rates in the various surgical subspecialities.[6]

Block Schedule

A system of guaranteed ORs, or block scheduling, is commonly used to negate the inefficiencies inherent with open-block scheduling. The distribution of blocks is often based on the number of surgical hours performed per week. Block schedules work best when allocated to a specific surgical service rather than individual surgeons and when granted for the entire day rather than half days.[7]

Rules governing the block schedule must be developed and strictly followed.[8] These rules encompass advance scheduling and release times, as well as thresholds for decreasing or increasing block time allocation. Release time, or the time when the block is no longer reserved for a particular service, is the key element in block scheduling. Release times often vary among surgical specialties and institutions.[9] Services performing procedures with some urgency or that have a short lead time, such as cardiac and vascular surgery, will receive shorter release times than services that have a more elective nature of their practice (total joint replacement, hernia repair) (Table 45-3). Once the release time is reached, the remaining hours in the OR would be available to any surgeon on a first-come, first-service basis. The percentage of the ORs blocked is largely dependent on the volume of urgent, emergency, and elective add-on cases. If the hospital has a significant number of these cases, it may be appropriate to have 10% to 15% of the ORs allocated for open scheduling, including leaving an OR unscheduled until the day of surgery.

Block time should be adjusted periodically by assessing surgical service utilization of its allocated block time.[10] Thresholds for adjusting service block time allocation have not been adequately studied, although most institutions would reduce block time allocation for utilization below 70% and increase block time allocation for utilization above 90%.

TIME MANAGEMENT COMPONENTS

On-time starts for the first case of the day, short turn-around times, and a case duration that matches the schedule are desirable time management components in every OR system. Typically, a multidisciplinary team determines targets for OR performance measures; sustaining meaningful improvement in these time components requires participation from anesthesia, nursing, and surgical services.[11] Frequently, anesthesiologists, surgeons, and nursing staff engage in debate regarding causes of OR delays.[12] Each of these disciplines hold perceptual differences regarding

Table 45–3 Service Block Release Times	
Service	**Release Time**
Cardiac	1 day
Vascular	2 days
Surgical oncology	3 days
General	1 week
Orthopedics	1 week
Neurosurgery	1 week
Ear, nose, and throat	1 week
Urology	1 week
Gynecology	1 week
Ophthalmology	1 week
Pediatrics	1 week
Plastic surgery	2 weeks

the cause of delays. Use of a procedural time glossary that incorporates standard terminology for OR events and time periods is helpful in analyzing inefficiencies in the OR.[13] For example, the glossary defines start time as the time that the patient enters the OR. Because induction of anesthesia and preparation depend on the patient's medical condition and type of surgery, the time from patient entry into the OR to surgical preparation and draping will vary.

On-Time Starts for the First Case

Starting the first surgical procedure of the day on time is perceived as an important indicator of OR efficiency. The morning start time often sets the pace for the OR for the rest of the day. Specific strategies have been suggested to facilitate on-time starts (Table 45-4).

PATIENT AND PREOPERATIVE HOLDING AREA RESPONSIBILITIES

Ideally, preoperative evaluation of the patient's medical condition should take place 1 or more days before surgery, with the results of laboratory testing being available before patient arrival in the preoperative holding area. Likewise, all necessary paperwork, including the history, physical examination, and surgical consent, should be completed before patient arrival in the preoperative area. Anesthesiologists should review these data the day before the planned surgery. The preoperative area should be organized and sufficiently staffed to facilitate efficient patient check-in and make patients available to the anesthesiologist and surgeon.

ANESTHESIA TEAM RESPONSIBILITIES

The anesthesia machine and other equipment should be checked, drugs prepared, special needs assessed, intravenous line inserted, and preanesthesia evaluation completed with ample time before the scheduled start time.

SURGICAL TEAM RESPONSIBILITIES

The surgeon is responsible for completion of the patient's history, physical examination, and consent. In addition, the surgeon must be available to answer patient questions, address special needs for the planned procedure, and perform operative site marking when applicable.

NURSING SERVICE RESPONSIBILITIES

The ORs should be set up overnight with adequate supplies and equipment to perform the procedures. The circulating and scrub nurses should confirm the general readiness of OR supplies and equipment on their arrival in the morning. The circulating room nurse would complete the final patient check-in. Anesthesiologists, nurses, and surgeons working in parallel and not in series can save time. For example, induction of anesthesia can proceed while final room setup is being completed.

VI

Table 45–4 Keys to Improving On-Time Starts

Administrative/System Organization

Accurate scheduling system

Personnel availability

Equipment, instrument, implant readiness

Ensure that the operating room environment is functional

Patient Issues

Clarify all questions at the preoperative visit

Completion of prescribed preoperative testing

Follow preoperative instructions

On-time arrival

Arrange postoperative transportation

Anesthesia

Complete and timely operating room preparation

Equipment maintenance

Adequate supplies

Thorough preoperative evaluation before the day of surgery

Review patient information in advance

Nursing

Adequate staffing

Well-maintained supplies, equipment, and instruments

Service-specific organization

Timely patient check-in

Surgeon

Accurate booking

Ensure on-time personal availability

Resolve consent issues at the preoperative visit

Complete documentation in advance of the day of surgery

Timely patient site marking

MONITORING ON-TIME STARTS

Although most hospitals would agree on a goal of an 80% on-time start for the first case of the day, most institutions fail to achieve this goal.[11,14] Many institutions permit a 10-minute window before categorizing it as a late start. Common causes of surgical delay include surgeon unavailability, no history and physical examination on the patient's record, informed consent not completed, operative site marking absent, and incorrect booking of the case. Anesthesia delays include difficult technical procedures, such as placement of an intravenous catheter or epidural placement in the preoperative holding area rather than in the OR. Patient-related delays are mostly due to late arrival or failure to follow preoperative NPO instructions. Nursing service delays include late arrival of personnel and issues related to equipment, supplies, and instruments, as well as systems issues such as delays related to transport (Fig. 45-2).

Turnover Time

Turnover time between procedures is often a focal point for discussion at OR committee meetings as a means for improving OR efficiency. Surgeons consider any time when they are unable to operate as "downtime." Thus, they often consider turnover time to be the time from the end of the surgical procedure on one patient to the start of the surgical procedure on the next patient. A clear definition of turnover time should be adopted and is the time interval between the previous patient's exit from the OR to the succeeding patient's entry in the OR.[13] Because this definition attempts to include the time spent cleaning and preparing the OR for the next procedure, it should be calculated only if a subsequent case is scheduled to immediately follow.

Strategies to facilitate rapid turnover times are similar to those for ensuring on-time starts for the first case of the day. Preparation for the next patient should occur before the first case is completed. Ideally, the holding room nurse would start an intravenous catheter. The circulating room nurse would call the next patient's case cart and have an organized turnover team ready to clean and prepare the OR for the next case. The anesthesiologist prepares drugs and any special equipment for the next case. In some circumstances, if an epidural is planned for the next case, placement in the holding area might save time. The surgeon must remain available between cases and confirm that the workup is complete and the operative site is marked, if appropriate, for the next patient.

Turnover times are dependent on the type of surgical procedure and the setting in which it is being performed. It is often suggested that turnover times be 30 minutes for inpatient ORs and 15 to 20 minutes for ambulatory centers.[15] Although it is acceptable to have a goal of 30 minutes for turnover times for inpatients, in reality, complex cardiac or orthopedic procedures take longer and often average 40 or more minutes.[11,16] Reductions in turnover times might save 10 to 15 minutes per case, but these times do not usually permit additional procedure to be scheduled unless there is a large number of turnovers, as might occur with short cases in the ambulatory setting.[17] Nevertheless, given an improvement of 10 to 15 minutes per case and three turnovers per room, 30 to 45 minutes could be saved each day. In the inpatient setting, such time saving is important because it may result in reduced

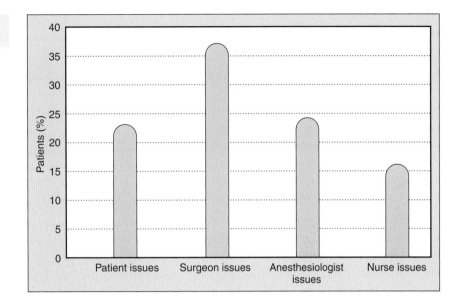

Figure 45-2 Causes of first-case delays by category.

overtime expenses. It is estimated that at academic medical centers, 10- to 19-minute reductions in turnover time would result in a 2.5% to 4% reduction in staffing costs.[2] Perhaps equally as important, reducing turnover time produces an atmosphere of cooperation and enhanced satisfaction among all members of the operative team.

Case Length

For most facilities, turnover time represents only 10% to 20% of the total case time, and therefore improvements in OR time management should also address case length. Case length may be defined as the time from patient entry into the OR until patient departure from the OR. This time frame includes anesthesia induction and procedures, surgical positioning and preparation, operative time, dressing placement, and emergence from anesthesia and transfer to the postanesthesia care unit (PACU). Although these actions occur in series, whenever possible, minimizing the time between these sequences will dramatically decrease case length. For example, surgical positioning and preparation should begin as soon as possible after induction of anesthesia. Operative time can be decreased by the attending surgeon's presence throughout the procedure. Anesthesia emergence can be improved by using shorter-acting anesthetics when indicated.

MANAGEMENT OF THE SCHEDULE ON THE DAY OF SURGERY

Although great effort is expended in creating a long-term schedule, proper management of the schedule on the day of surgery is equally important. Many events occur that produce changes in the planned schedule. To deal efficiently with changes in the schedule, a single person (often an anesthesiologist) is partnered with an OR nursing leader to make decisions regarding running the daily schedule. Running an efficient schedule on the day of surgery begins by reviewing the schedule the evening before and then again on the morning of surgery. The review would determine potential problems related to patient flow, as well as opportunities for add-ons.

Add-On Cases

A carefully structured daily OR list can easily be disrupted by add-ons, emergencies, and cancellations.[18] Ideally, the elective surgery schedule should be protected from these interruptions. If the elective schedule is often interrupted by emergency or urgent cases, it is sensible to maintain an unoccupied OR with available staff during the day to minimize disruption of the electively scheduled cases.

A clear policy and algorithm should exist regarding scheduling and proceeding with the add-on cases. A common approach is to proceed with cases in the order of their booking. However, this sequence of proceeding with add-on cases can be interrupted on the basis of medical need (emergency, urgent, and elective cases). Emergency cases are those that must come to the OR immediately because of threat to life, limb, or organ. Urgent cases encompass the large majority of add-on surgeries that need to be performed within a 12- to 24-hour period to prevent morbidity. Many of these cases should in fact proceed within a 4- to 6-hour period. Examples include appendectomy, ectopic pregnancy, open fractures, and kidney transplantation. Depending on the urgency, if no OR is available, the case would bump the surgeon's elec-

VI

tive scheduled case or bump a procedure within the same surgical service. If there were no cases scheduled in the same surgical service, the urgent case would proceed to the OR with the shortest surgical list. Elective add-on cases should follow elective cases in the first available OR.

ECONOMIC ANALYSIS OF THE OPERATING ROOM

The OR is the driving engine for revenue and expense in any hospital. It is estimated to be responsible for as much as 70% of hospital revenue while incurring as much as 40% of the cost.[1] Understanding the basic concepts of economic analysis in the OR is important to be able to participate effectively in the decision-making process regarding OR management. Two fundamental concepts of health care economics are cost and benefits. Three types of economic analysis that are often studied include cost identification, cost-effectiveness, and cost-benefit ratio.[19]

Costs

Costs are divided into fixed and variable, and within these two broad categories the cost can be apportioned into direct and indirect components. Direct costs are identified specifically with patient care, whereas indirect costs are incurred to support the clinical service. Fixed costs constitute a major portion of the cost of providing health care in the hospital and in the ORs.[20] These costs include buildings, depreciation of the surgical suite, capital equipment, salaries of the full-time equivalent personnel, and administrative overhead.

Fixed costs can be modified up or down by opening or closing ORs. Variable costs are incurred when supplies, pharmaceuticals, medical devices, and implants are consumed and increase or decrease with surgical volume. Variable costs for labor become a consideration when the number of OR cases extends past the normal workday and overtime pay is needed for staff members. For example, the fixed cost of performing additional surgeries remains constant up to the point at which it is necessary to provide overtime pay. At that point what was a fixed cost now becomes a semivariable cost and increases in direct proportion to the increased workload.

COST-TO-CHARGE RATIO
Although the amount of money that a patient is charged by a hospital represents a cost for the patient, it is not a true indicator of the actual cost incurred by the provider to deliver the service to the patient. The cost-to-charge ratio is defined as the total cost of providing the service divided by the amount charged.[21] In practice, the institution determines how much it costs to provide a service, builds in a markup to generate a profit, and then relates the cost to the charge as a ratio. Cost-to-charge ratios

vary widely for different services throughout a hospital. For example, the cost-to-charge ratio may range from 0.92 in the surgical admission unit, to 0.5 in the laboratory, to a low of 0.29 for anesthesia services.[21] These varying ratios reflect attempts to achieve reasonable profit margins and to use collections from a revenue-producing department to support non–revenue-producing hospital functions.

Profit

Profit represents revenue minus fixed and variable costs.[22] There are a variety of mechanisms for enhancing profitability. Short-term strategies are designed to lower variable costs, with much effort centered on decreasing the cost of consumables. Profitability can also be enhanced even when the ORs are functioning at less than full capacity. In this circumstance, fixed costs have been incurred and covered by all the preceding cases. Thus, if performing an additional case or cases produces a marginal profit (revenue minus variable costs), the contribution margin is positive and will be beneficial to the overall enterprise.[23]

Analysis of Operating Room Costs

The basic cost of the OR, exclusive of procedure-specific needs, has been estimated as $13.54 per minute.[24] Of this amount, 62% of the costs are fixed and 38% are variable and amenable to changing physician practice. Cost attributed to the ORs accounts for 33% of the hospital bill.[21] Anesthesia costs represent 6% of the total hospitalization bill, with about half of that being classified as direct or variable costs. Thus, 3% of the total hospital bill was influenced by the anesthesiologist's clinical decision-making and is potentially available for cost savings. The PACU accounts for approximately 3.7% of the total hospital bill, with a majority of the cost (67%) being fixed.

The influence of anesthesiologists on perioperative costs extends beyond the operative period.[25] For example, enhanced pain management (epidural infusions) initiated as part of the anesthetic care results in fewer (less costly) complications and shorter length of stay in the hospital. Typically, these increased costs of analgesic therapy, but not the benefits of earlier discharge, have been assigned to anesthesia services. A wider perspective considering the entire surgical experience should be used to identify the cost and benefits of anesthetic interventions.

DATA MANAGEMENT-INFORMATION SYSTEMS

There is an old adage that states, you cannot manage what you cannot measure. For ORs to perform efficiently, detailed information about the surgical procedures must be easily retrieved from an OR information system (Table 45-5).[26] Commercially available systems may be used to gather this information. Data are automatically fed to a central-

Table 45–5 Desired Information regarding Surgical Procedures Performed in the Operating Room

Type of cases
Cost
Length
Downtime between cases
Steps to improve efficiency

ized mechanism of data recording. There must be some mechanism to compile, extract, and present the information in a format that is useful. Data collection, data storage, and data presentation are the three essential components of an OR information system.

Recording the standard information of patient, procedure, surgeon, anesthesiologist, nurses, and multiple time points for each case is the minimum standard that will create a large database. These data can be used to (1) analyze patterns in flow of patients through the ORs and correct this flow to make the ORs more efficient, (2) determine the accuracy of the allotted times for cases on the schedule, and (3) create strategies for effective matching of staff shifts to the actual OR occupancy at different times on different days of the week. Data analysis can be automated to process these data in the same way for each successive month. Information (actual room entry time, actual incision time, actual surgical time, actual turnover time, reasons for any delays) will ultimately improve OR efficiency only if the participants use the information and change behavior.

CONTINUOUS QUALITY IMPROVEMENT AND IMPLEMENTATION OF CLINICAL GUIDELINES

The medical director is in a leadership position with influence and authority to implement positive change in improving the quality of medical care for surgical patients. It is widely believed that meaningful reductions in complications depend on surgeons, anesthesiologists, perioperative nurses, pharmacists, infection control specialists, and hospital executives working together to improve surgical care. The frequency of on-time starts, turnover times, and patient satisfaction should be routinely monitored.

Surgical Care Improvement Project

The Surgical Care Improvement Project (SCIP) is a national partnership of organizations (Center for Medicare and Medicaid Services [CMS], Centers for Disease Control and Prevention, Leapfrog, ASA) committed to improving the safety of surgical care through reduction of post-

operative complications.[27] Launched in 2005, the SCIP endorses a multiyear national campaign to substantially reduce surgical morbidity and mortality through the use of evidence-based care processes and designing of systems of care with redundant safeguards. Quality improvement efforts focus on reducing postoperative complications in four broad areas in which the incidence and cost of complications are high (Table 45-6).

To evaluate and report on performances in specific clinical areas, the SCIP will collect data on measures that intimately involve anesthesia care. For example, in the area of surgical site infections, preoperative antibiotics are often administered by the anesthesiologist in the OR at the request of the surgeon. Thus, selecting the appropriate antibiotic and administering it within 1 hour of surgery will frequently become the responsibility of the anesthesiologist.[28] In the area of reducing the frequency of perioperative myocardial infarctions, the anesthesiologist often initiates and informs the surgeon to maintain perioperative β-blockade in high-risk surgical patients.[29]

REGULATORY OVERSIGHT

A large number of agencies and regulations govern the function of ORs today. These regulatory bodies are both internal to the organization (OR committee, patient safety committee, bylaws of the medical staff) and external (JCAHO, CMS). The medical director must be familiar with the rules and regulations ensuring compliance within the OR not only to satisfy requirements for hospital accreditation but also to enhance patient and employee safety. Areas of concern include infection control, fire and laser safety, and proper tracking of controlled medications and other medical devices and implants.

Sentinel Event Policy

Since 1995, JCAHO has promulgated a sentinel event policy as part of the accreditation process. Recently, the policy has been refined with the addition of national patient safety goals and sentinel event alerts. In 2004, JCAHO launched seven national safety patient goals, several of which had a major impact in OR function.[30] Perhaps the most important one for the OR was the universal protocol

Table 45–6 Areas to Reduce Postoperative Complications and Associated Costs

Surgical site infections
Perioperative myocardial infarctions
Venous thromboembolism
Postoperative pneumonia

VI

for preventing wrong-site, wrong-procedure, and wrong-person surgery. From 1995 to 2004, 370 events of wrong-site surgery were reported to JCAHO. The universal protocol is separated into three components.[31]

PREOPERATIVE VERIFICATION PROCESS

The health care team ensures that all relevant documents and studies are available before the start of the procedure and that they are consistent with each other and with the patient's expectations and understanding of the intended procedure.

MARKING THE OPERATIVE SITE

In procedures in which laterality, multiple levels (spinal procedures), or multiple structures (fingers and toes) are applicable, the surgeon performing the procedure will confirm and mark the surgical site or sites with the marker's initials using a skin marker. Surgical site marking should occur in the preoperative area with involvement of the patient. The site mark should be visible after the patient is prepared and draped.

TIMEOUT

Immediately, before starting the procedure, the operative team (circulating nurse, surgeon, and anesthesiologist) will take a "timeout" together and verbally verify the patient, the procedure, the surgical site, the position, and the availability of correct implants and special equipment. The timeout policy may also be extended to include whether indicated preoperative antibiotics have been administered.

Review and Evaluation

JCAHO's sentinel event policy requires that all serious complications undergo careful review.[32] The policy also encourages self-reporting of these adverse events to JCAHO so that the relative frequencies and underlying causes of sentinel events are reviewed and lessons learned can be shared with other health care organizations to reduce the risk for future sentinel events in other organizations.

A sentinel event is defined as an unexpected occurrence (not related to the natural course of the patient's illness or underlying condition) involving death or serious physical or psychological injury. Surgery on the wrong patient or wrong body part would be categorized as a sentinel event. Such events are called "sentinel" because they signal the need for immediate investigation and response.

ROOT CAUSE ANALYSIS

Typically, the process starts with an executive group meeting within 24 hours of knowledge of the event, and it is decided whether the case meets sentinel event criteria. If a sentinel event is determined to have occurred, a root cause analysis team is assembled. The multidisciplinary team includes participation by hospital leadership and by individuals most closely involved in the process and systems under review. The root cause or causes of the event should be determined and changes made in the organization's systems and processes to reduce the probability of such an event in the future. The analysis focuses primarily on systems and processes, not on individual performance. A report is written in which the root cause or causes of the event are identified, and an action plan is issued and monitored by a specific individual assigned to ensure that the plan is in place. Although these reviews are complex and time consuming, they are informative and provide an avenue for anesthesiologists to have input in developing solutions to problems.

SENTINEL EVENT ALERTS

Information about specific sentinel events and how they can be prevented may be disseminated by JCAHO through its newsletter *Sentinel Event Alert*. Examples of sentinel event alerts that involve anesthesia practice have included (1) Preventing Surgical Fires—2003, (2) Preventing and Managing the Impact of Anesthesia Awareness—2004, and (3) Patient-Controlled Analgesia by Proxy—2005.

REFERENCES

1. Rutter T, Brown A. Contemporary operating room management. Adv Anesth 1994;11:174-214.
2. American Society of Anesthesiologists: Standards, Guidelines and Statements. Available at http://www.asahq.org/index.htm.
3. Joint Commission on Accreditation of Healthcare Organizations: Hospital Accreditation Standards. Oakbrook Terrace, IL, 2004.
4. Dexter F, Abouleish AE, Epstein RH, et al. Use of operating room information system data to predict the impact of reducing turnover times on staffing costs. Anesth Analg 2003;97:1119-1126.
5. Mazzei W. Guidelines for the Role of Clinical Director of Anesthesiology. Available at http://www.aacdhq.org/Members/DirectorRole.asp.
6. Ozkarahan I. Allocation of surgeries to operating rooms by goal programming. J Med Syst 2000;24:339-378.
7. Dexter F, Macario A, Traub R, et al. An operating room scheduling strategy to maximize the use of operating room block time: Computer simulation of patient scheduling and survey of patients' preferences for surgical waiting time. Anesth Analg 1999;89:7-20.
8. Dexter F. How can ORs best manage block time for scheduling surgical cases? OR Manager 2003;19:20-24.
9. Dexter F, Traub R, Macario A. How to release allocated operating room time to increase efficiency: Predicting which surgical service will have the most underutilized operating room time. Anesth Analg 2003;96:507-512.
10. Strum DP, Vargus L, May JH. Surgical subspecialty block utilization and capacity planning: A minimal cost analysis model. Anesthesiology 1999;90:1176-1185.

11. Overdyk FJ, Harvey S, Fishman RL, Shippey F. Successful strategies for improving operating room efficiency at academic institutions. Anesth Analg 1998;86:896-906.

12. Udelsman R: The operating room: War results in casualties. Anesth Analg 2003;97:936-937.

13. Donham RT, Mazzei WM, Jones RL. Glossary of times used for scheduling and monitoring of diagnostic and therapeutic procedures. Am J Anesth 1996;23:4-12.

14. Shelver SR, Winston L. Improving surgical on-time starts through common goals. AORN J 2001;74:506-513.

15. Kaiser shares ambulatory surgery benchmarks. HealthCare Benchmarks 1998;Jan:5-6.

16. Mazzei W. Operating room start times and turnover times in a university hospital. J Clin Anesth 1994;6:405-408.

17. Dexter F, Coffin S, Tinker JH. Decreases in anesthesia-controlled time cannot permit one additional surgical operation to be reliably scheduled during the workday. Anesth Analg 1995;81:1263-1268.

18. Dexter F, Macario A, Traub R. Which algorithm for scheduling add-on elective cases maximizes operating room utilization? Use of bin packing algorithms and fuzzy constraints in operating room management. Anesthesiology 1999;91:1491-1500.

19. Sperry RJ: Principles of economic analysis. Anesthesiology 1997;86:1197-1205.

20. Roberts RR, Frutos PW, Ciavarella GG, et al. Distribution of variable and fixed costs of hospital care. JAMA 1999;281:644-649.

21. Macario A, Vitez TS, Dunn B, McDonald T. Where are the costs in perioperative care? Analysis of hospital costs and charges for inpatient surgical care. Anesthesiology 1995;83:1138-1344.

22. Dexter F, Macario A, Cerone SM. Hospital profitability for a surgeon's common procedures predicts the surgeon's overall profitability for the hospital. J Clin Anesth 1998;10:457-463.

23. Macario A, Dexter F, Traub R. Hospital profitability per hour of operating room time can vary among surgeons. Anesth Analg 2001;93:669-675.

24. Macario A. How do hospitals account for costs in the operating room? Can anesthesiology make a difference? Curr Rev Clin Anesth 1999;19:193-204.

25. Orkin FK. Meaningful cost reduction: Penny wise, pound foolish. Anesthesiology 1995;83:1135-1137.

26. Dexter F, Macario A: Applications of information systems to operating room scheduling. Anesthesiology 1996;85:1232-1234.

27. Surgical Care Improvement Project: A national partnership. Available at http://www.medqic.org/scip/.

28. Bratzler DW, Houck PM, for the Surgical Infection Prevention Guidelines Writers Workgroup. Antimicrobial prophylaxis for surgery: An advisory statement from the National Surgical Infection Prevention Project Clinical Infectious Diseases 2004;38:1706-1715.

29. Mangano DT, Layug EL, Wallace A, Tateo I, for The Multicenter Study of Perioperative Ischemia Research Group: Effect of atenolol on mortality and cardiovascular morbidity after noncardiac surgery. N Engl J Med 1996;335:1713-1721.

30. http://www.jcaho.org/accredited+organizations/patient+safety/04+npsg/index.htm.

31. http://www.jcaho.org/accredited+organizations/patient+safety/universal+protocol/wss_universal+protocol.htm.

32. http://www.jcaho.org/accredited+organizations/sentinel+event/se_index.htm.

VI

APPENDICES

BASIC STANDARDS FOR PREANESTHESIA CARE

(Approved by the House of Delegates on October 14, 1987, and amended October 25, 2005)

These standards apply to all patients who receive anesthesia care. In exceptional circumstances, these standards may be modified. When such is the case, the circumstances shall be documented in the patient's record.

An anesthesiologist shall be responsible for determining the medical status of the patient and developing a plan of anesthesia care.

The anesthesiologist, before the delivery of anesthesia care, is responsible for the following:

1. Reviewing the available medical record
2. Interviewing and performing a focused examination of the patient to
   a. Discuss the medical history, including previous anesthetic experiences and medical therapy
   b. Assess aspects of the patient's physical condition that might affect decisions regarding perioperative risk and management
3. Ordering and reviewing pertinent available tests and consultations as necessary for the delivery of anesthesia care
4. Ordering appropriate preoperative medications
5. Ensuring that consent has been obtained for the anesthesia care
6. Documenting in the chart that the above has been performed

STANDARDS FOR BASIC ANESTHETIC MONITORING

(Approved by the ASA House of Delegates on October 21, 1986, and last amended on October 25, 2005)

These standards apply to all anesthesia care, although in emergency circumstances, appropriate life support measures take precedence. These standards may be exceeded at any time according to the judgment of the responsible anesthesiologist. They are intended to encourage quality patient care, but observing them cannot guarantee any specific patient outcome. The standards are subject to revision from time to time, as warranted by the evolution of technology and practice. They apply to all general anesthesia, regional anesthesia, and monitored anesthesia care. This set of standards addresses only the issue of basic anesthesia monitoring, which is one component of anesthesia care. In certain rare or unusual circumstances, (1) some of these methods of monitoring may be clinically impractical, and (2) appropriate use of the described monitoring methods may fail to detect untoward clinical developments. Brief interruptions in continual[†] monitoring may be unavoidable. In extenuating circumstances, the responsible anesthesiologist may waive the requirements marked with an asterisk (*); it is recommended that when this is done, it should be so stated (including the reasons) in a note in the patient's medical record. These standards are not intended for application to the care of obstetric patients in labor or in the conduct of pain management.

STANDARD I

Qualified anesthesia personnel shall be present in the room throughout the conduct of all general anesthesia, regional anesthesia, and monitored anesthesia care.

OBJECTIVE
Because of rapid changes in patient status during anesthesia, qualified anesthesia personnel shall be continuously

present to monitor the patient and provide anesthesia care. In the event of a direct known hazard (e.g., radiation) to the anesthesia personnel that might require intermittent remote observation of the patient, some provision for monitoring the patient must be made. In the event that an emergency requires temporary absence of the person primarily responsible for the anesthesia, the best judgment of the anesthesiologist will be exercised in comparing the emergency with the anesthetized patient's condition and in selecting the person left responsible for the anesthesia during the temporary absence.

STANDARD II

During all anesthesia, the patient's oxygenation, ventilation, circulation, and temperature shall be continually evaluated.

Oxygenation

OBJECTIVE
To ensure adequate oxygen concentration in the inspired gas and blood during all anesthesia.

METHODS
1. Inspired gas: During every administration of general anesthesia via an anesthesia machine, the concentration of oxygen in the patient breathing system shall be measured by an oxygen analyzer with a low–oxygen concentration limit alarm in use.*
2. Blood oxygenation: During all anesthesia, a quantitative method of assessing oxygenation such as pulse oximetry shall be used.* When a pulse oximeter is used, the variable-pitch pulse tone and the low threshold alarm shall be audible to the anesthesiologist or the anesthesia care team personnel. Adequate illumination and exposure of the patient are necessary to assess color.*

[†]Note that "continual" is defined as "repeated regularly and frequently in steady rapid succession" whereas "continuous" means "prolonged without any interruption at any time."

Ventilation

OBJECTIVE

To ensure adequate ventilation of the patient during all anesthesia.

METHODS

1. Every patient receiving general anesthesia shall have the adequacy of ventilation continually evaluated. Qualitative clinical signs such as chest excursion, observation of the reservoir breathing bag, and auscultation of breath sounds are useful. Continual monitoring for the presence of expired carbon dioxide shall be performed unless invalidated by the nature of the patient, procedure, or equipment. Quantitative monitoring of the volume of expired gas is strongly encouraged.*
2. When an endotracheal tube or laryngeal mask is inserted, correct positioning must be verified by clinical assessment and by identification of carbon dioxide in the expired gas. Continual end-tidal carbon dioxide analysis, in use from the time of endotracheal tube/laryngeal mask placement until extubation/removal or initiation of transfer to a postoperative care location, shall be performed with a quantitative method such as capnography, capnometry, or mass spectroscopy.* When capnography or capnometry is used, the end-tidal CO_2 alarm shall be audible to the anesthesiologist or the anesthesia care team personnel.*
3. When ventilation is controlled by a mechanical ventilator, there shall be in continuous use a device that is capable of detecting disconnection of components of the breathing system. The device must give an audible signal when its alarm threshold is exceeded.
4. During regional anesthesia and monitored anesthesia care, the adequacy of ventilation shall be evaluated by continual observation of qualitative clinical signs and/or monitoring for the presence of exhaled carbon dioxide.

Circulation

OBJECTIVE

To ensure adequacy of the patient's circulatory function during all anesthesia.

METHODS

1. Every patient receiving anesthesia shall have the electrocardiogram continuously displayed from the beginning of anesthesia until preparing to leave the anesthetizing location.*
2. Every patient receiving anesthesia shall have arterial blood pressure and heart rate determined and evaluated at least every 5 minutes.*
3. Every patient receiving general anesthesia shall have, in addition to the above, circulatory function continually evaluated by at least one of the following: palpation of a pulse, auscultation of heart sounds, monitoring of a tracing of intra-arterial pressure, ultrasound peripheral pulse monitoring, or pulse plethysmography or oximetry.

Body Temperature

OBJECTIVE

To aid in maintenance of appropriate body temperature during all anesthesia.

METHODS

Every patient receiving anesthesia shall have temperature monitored when clinically significant changes in body temperature are intended, anticipated, or suspected.

VII

STANDARDS FOR POSTANESTHESIA CARE

(Approved by the House of Delegates on October 12, 1988, and last amended on October 27, 2004)

These standards apply to postanesthesia care in all locations. They may be exceeded according to the judgment of the responsible anesthesiologist. The standards are intended to encourage quality patient care but cannot guarantee any specific patient outcome. They are subject to revision from time to time as warranted by the evolution of technology and practice. In extenuating circumstances, the responsible anesthesiologist may waive the requirements marked with an asterisk (*); it is recommended that when this is done, it should be so stated (including the reasons) in a note in the patient's medical record.

STANDARD I

All patients who have been given general anesthesia, regional anesthesia, or monitored anesthesia care shall receive appropriate postanesthesia management.[†]

1. A postanesthesia care unit (PACU) or an area that provides equivalent postanesthesia care (for example, a surgical intensive care unit) shall be available to receive patients after anesthesia care. All patients who receive anesthesia care shall be admitted to the PACU or its equivalent, except by specific order of the anesthesiologist responsible for the patient's care.
2. The medical aspects of care in the PACU (or equivalent area) shall be governed by policies and procedures that have been reviewed and approved by the department of anesthesiology.
3. The design, equipment, and staffing of the PACU shall meet requirements of the facility's accrediting and licensing bodies.

[†]Refer to Standards of Post Anesthesia Nursing Practice 1992, published by the American Society of Post Anesthesia Nurses (ASPAN), for issues of nursing care.

STANDARD II

A patient transported to the PACU shall be accompanied by a member of the anesthesia care team who is knowledgeable about the patient's condition. The patient shall be continually evaluated and treated during transport, with monitoring and support appropriate to the patient's condition.

STANDARD III

On arrival in the PACU, the patient shall be re-evaluated and a verbal report provided to the responsible PACU nurse by the member of the anesthesia care team who accompanies the patient.

1. The patient's status on arrival in the PACU shall be documented.
2. Information concerning the preoperative condition and the surgical/anesthetic course shall be transmitted to the PACU nurse.
3. The member of the anesthesia care team shall remain in the PACU until the PACU nurse accepts responsibility for nursing care of the patient.

STANDARD IV

The patient's condition shall be evaluated continually in the PACU.

1. The patient shall be observed and monitored by methods appropriate to the patient's medical condition. Particular attention should be given to monitoring oxygenation, ventilation, circulation, level of consciousness, and temperature. During recovery from all anesthetics, a quantitative method of assessing oxygenation such as pulse oximetry shall be used in the initial phase of recovery.* This is not intended for appli-

cation during recovery of an obstetric patient in whom regional anesthesia was used for labor and vaginal delivery.

2. An accurate written report of the PACU period shall be maintained. Use of an appropriate PACU scoring system is encouraged for each patient on admission, at appropriate intervals before discharge, and at the time of discharge.
3. General medical supervision and coordination of patient care in the PACU should be the responsibility of an anesthesiologist.
4. There shall be a policy to ensure the availability in the facility of a physician capable of managing complications and providing cardiopulmonary resuscitation for patients in the PACU.

STANDARD V

A physician is responsible for discharge of the patient from the PACU.

1. When discharge criteria are used, they must be approved by the department of anesthesiology and the medical staff. They may vary, depending on whether the patient is discharged to a hospital room, to the intensive care unit, to a short-stay unit, or home.
2. In the absence of the physician responsible for the discharge, the PACU nurse shall determine that the patient meets the discharge criteria. The name of the physician accepting responsibility for discharge shall be noted on the record.

VII

INDEX

Note: Page numbers followed by f refer to figures; page numbers followed by t refer to tables.